GATEWAYS IN VASCULAR SURGERY: AN OPERATIVE ATLAS

Timur P. Sarac, MD

Professor of Surgery
University of Virginia
Professor of Surgery Emeritus
The Ohio State University

Vikram S. Kashyap, MD

Endowed Chair, Frederik Meijer Heart and Vascular Institute
Vice President, Cardiovascular Health, Corewell Health
Professor of Surgery, Michigan State University College of Human Medicine

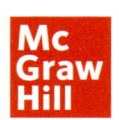

NOTICE

Medicine is an ever-changing science. As new research and clinical experience broaden our knowledge, changes in treatment and drug therapy are required. The authors and the publisher of this work have checked with sources believed to be reliable in their efforts to provide information that is complete and generally in accord with the standards accepted at the time of publication. However, in view of the possibility of human error or changes in medical sciences, neither the authors nor the publisher nor any other party who has been involved in the preparation or publication of this work warrants that the information contained herein is in every respect accurate or complete, and they disclaim all responsibility for any errors or omissions or for the results obtained from use of the information contained in this work. Readers are encouraged to confirm the information contained herein with other sources. For example and in particular, readers are advised to check the product information sheet included in the package of each drug they plan to administer to be certain that the information contained in this work is accurate and that changes have not been made in the recommended dose or in the contraindications for administration. This recommendation is of particular importance in connection with new or infrequently used drugs.

This book was set in Minion Pro by KnowledgeWorks Global Ltd.
The editors were Sydney Keen Vitale and Christina M. Thomas.
The production supervisor was Richard Ruzycka.
Project management was provided by Radhika Jolly, KnowledgeWorks Global Ltd.
The cover designer was W2 Design.

Library of Congress Cataloging-in-Publication Data

Names: Sarac, Timur, editor. | Kashyap, Vikram S., editor.
Title: Gateways in vascular surgery : an operative atlas / [edited by]
    Timur Sarac, Vikram Kashyap.
Description: New York : McGraw Hill, [2025] | Includes bibliographical
    references and index. | Summary: ""Gateways to Vascular Surgery" edited
    by Drs. Sarac and Kashyap is a remarkable atlas of surgical operations.
    It is meant to be a companion to Zollinger's Atlas of Surgical
    Operations. The idea for the atlas was born from a student surgical
    course they developed together where Harvard Medical students would
    rotate through various surgical duties as they performed basic surgical
    procedures and techniques on dogs. The two conceived a text with
    illustrations of common operations for general surgeons in training and
    in practice. From its inception, the authors determined that medical
    illustration would play an important role in the atlas and serve as a
    visual guide to the procedures. The first edition was organized in an
    oversized folio format which allowed paragraphs of text on the left-side
    page and a full page of multiple surgical illustrations on the
    right-side page. This way, text, and the illustrations from the
    surgeon's point of view could be viewed simultaneously"—Provided by
    publisher.
Identifiers: LCCN 2024006464 (print) | LCCN 2024006465 (ebook) | ISBN
    9781260474299 (hardcover) | ISBN 9781260474305 (ebook)
Subjects: MESH: Vascular Surgical Procedures | Atlas
Classification: LCC RD598.5 (print) | LCC RD598.5 (ebook) | NLM WG 17 |
    DDC 617.4/13—dc23/eng/20240528
LC record available at https://lccn.loc.gov/2024006464
LC ebook record available at https://lccn.loc.gov/2024006465

McGraw Hill books are available at special quantity discounts to use as premiums and sales promotions, or for use in corporate training programs. To contact a representative please visit the Contact Us pages at www.mhprofessional.com.

DEDICATION

Our first and foremost dedication goes to our wives, Sangeeta Kashyap, MD and Judy Sarac, whose unparalleled support allowed us to spend the usual nights and weekends to see this through.

We also dedicate this to our children Tejas Kashyap, Anjali Kashyap, MD, Rohit Kashyap, Rebecca Sarac, MD, Nikolas Sarac, MD, and Benjamin Sarac, MD, who inspire us every day.

Finally, we would like to specially acknowledge Thomas Forbes, MD, who contributed early on as we started the project but stepped aside due to other obligations.

CONTENTS

SECTION XIII: LOWER EXTREMITY SFA, TIBIAL OCCLUSIVE DISEASE AND ANEURYSM ENDOVASCULAR

CHAPTER

SECTION XIV: VEINS AND INFERIOR VENA CAVA

CHAPTER

CONTRIBUTORS

Steven Abramowitz, MD
Associate Professor of Surgery
Department of Vascular Surgery
MedStar Heart and Vascular Institute
Georgetown University School of Medicine
Washington, DC

Mark Ajalat, MD
Vascular Surgery Resident
Division of Vascular Surgery
Ronald Reagan Medical CenterUniversity of California
Los Angeles, California

Afsha Aurshina, MD
Post-doctoral Research Fellow
Vascular Institute of New York
Johnson City, New York

Martin R. Back, MD, MS, FACS
Professor of Surgery
Division of Vascular Surgery
University of Florida College of Medicine
Gainesville, Florida

Robert J. Beaulieu, MD, MSE
Assistant Professor of Surgery
Division of Vascular Surgery
University of Michigan
Ann Arbor, Michigan

Asha Behdinan, MD
Resident Physician
Department of Vascular Surgery
University of Toronto
Toronto, Ontario, Canada

Michael Belkin, MD
Professor of Surgery
Department of Surgery
Brigham and Women's Hospital
Boston, Massachusetts

Marton Berczeli, MD
Vascular Surgeon
Budapest, Hungary

James H. Black, III, MD
Professor of Surgery
Division of Vascular Surgery
Johns Hopkins University
Baltimore, Maryland

Thomas Bower, MD
Professor of Surgery
Division of Vascular Surgery
Mayo Clinic
Rochester, Minnesota

April J. Boyd, MD, PhD
Professor of Surgery
Division of Vascular Surgery
University of Manitoba
Winnipeg, Manitoba

John Bozinovski, MD, MSc
Professor of Surgery
Division of Cardiac Surgery
The Ohio State University
Columbus, Ohio

Drew J. Braet, MD
Resident in Vascular Surgery
Division of Vascular Surgery
University of Michigan
Ann Arbor, Michigan

Anand Brahmandam, MBBS
Assistant Professor of Surgery
Division of Vascular Surgery and Endovascular Therapy
Northwestern University
Chicago, Illinois

Matthew D. Breite, MD
Vascular Surgeon
Mercy Clinic Vascular Specialists
St. Louis, Missouri

Jonathan A. Cardella, MD
Associate Professor of Surgery
Division of Vascular Surgery and Endovascular Therapy
Yale University School of Medicine
New Haven, Connecticut

Cassius Iyad Ochoa Chaar, MD, MS
Associate Professor of Surgery
Division of Vascular Surgery and Endovascular Therapy
Yale University School of Medicine
New Haven, Connecticut

Elliot L. Chaikof, MD, PhD
Professor of Surgery
Division of Vascular and Endovascular Surgery
Beth Israel Deaconess Medical Center
Boston, Massachusetts

Jesse Chait, DO
Resident Physician
Division of Vascular and Endovascular Surgery
Mayo Clinic
Rochester, Minnesota

Venita Chandra, MD
Clinical Professor of Surgery
Division of Vascular and Endovascular Surgery
Stanford University
Stanford, California

Michael J. Cheng, MD
Vascular Surgeon
Kaiser Permanente
Woodland Hills, California

Jae S. Cho, MD
Professor of Surgery Department of Surgery
Division of Vascular Surgery and Endovascular Therapy
Case Western Reserve School of MedicineUniversity Hospitals
Cleveland, Ohio

Elizabeth Chou, MD
Assistant Professor of Vascular Surgery
Division of Vascular Surgery
Cedars, Sinai Medical Center
Los Angeles, California

C. Yvonne Chung, MD
Assistant Professor of Surgery
Division of Vascular surgery
University of Maryland Medical Center
Baltimore, Maryland

Daniel Clair, MD
Professor of Surgery
Department of Vascular Surgery
Vanderbilt University
Nashville, Tennessee

W. Darrin Clouse, MD
Professor of Surgery
Division of Vascular and Endovascular Surgery
University of Virginia
Charlottesville, Virginia

Jill Colglazier, MD
Assistant Professor of Surgery
Division of Vascular Surgery
Mayo Clinic
Rochester, Minnesota

Dawn M. Coleman, MD
Professor of Surgery
Division of Vascular Surgery
Duke University Medical Center
Durham, North Carolina

Michael S. Conte, MD
Professor of Surgery
Division of Vascular Surgery
University of California, San Francisco
San Francisco, California

R. Clement Darling III, MD
Professor of Surgery
Division of Vascular Surgery
Albany Medical College/Albany Medical Center Hospital
Albany, New York

Alan Dietzek, MD
Professor of Vascular Surgery
Division of Vascular Surgery
Western Connecticut Health Network
Danbury, Connecticut

Luc Dubois, MD, MSc
Associate Professor of Surgery
Western University
Division of Vascular Surgery and Department of Epidemiology and
   Biostatistics
Schulich School of Medicine
London, Ontario, Canada

Julie M. Duke, MD
Assistant Professor of Surgery
Division of Vascular Surgery
University of Minnesota
Minneapolis, Minnesota

Audra A. Duncan, MD
Professor of Surgery
Western University
Division of Vascular Surgery and Department of Epidemiology and
   Biostatistics
Schulich School of Medicine
London, Ontario, Canada

Mark K. Eskandari, MD
Professor of Vascular Surgery
Division of Vascular Surgery
Northwestern University Feinberg School of Medicine
Chicago, Illinois

Armin Farazdaghi, MD
Resident in Vascular Surgery
Mayo Clinic College of Medicine
Division of Vascular and Endovascular Surgery
Rochester, Minnesota

Javairiah Fatima, MD, RPVI, FACS, DFSVS
Associate Professor of Surgery
MedStar Heart and Vascular Institute
Georgetown University School of Medicine
Washington, DC

Amanda C. Filiberto, MD
Fellow in Vascular Surgery
Division of Vascular Surgery
University of Alabama Birmingham
Birmingham, Alabama

Amanda G. Fobare, MD
Vascular Surgeon
Kaiser Permanente Medical Center
Clackamas, Oregon

Thomas L. Forbes, MD
Professor of Vascular Surgery
Division of Vascular Surgery
University of Toronto
Toronto, Ontario, Canada

Julie A. Frieschlag, MD
Professor of Surgery
Wake Forest Baptist Health, Wake Forest School of Medicine
Winston-Salem, North Carolina

Asvin M. Ganapathi, MD
Assistant Professor Surgery
Division of Cardiac Surgery
The Ohio State University
Columbus, Ohio

Hugh Gelabert, MD
Professor of Surgery
Division of Vascular Surgery
Ronald Reagan Medical Center University of California
Los Angeles, California

Patrick Geraghty, MD
Professor of Surgery
Division of Vascular Surgery
Washington University
St. Louis, Missouri

Angela Giese, MD
Assistant Professor of Surgery
Division of Vascular Surgery
University of California Davis
Sacramento, California

Alexandra Gobble, MD
Resident in Vascular Surgery
Division of Vascular Surgery
The Ohio State University
Columbus, Ohio

Clara Gomez-Sanchez, MD
Assistant Professor of Surgery
Division of Vascular Surgery
University of California, San Francisco
San Francisco, California

Brian Grant, MD
Vascular Surgeon
Med Center Health
Bowling Green, Kentucky

Randolph Guzman, MD, FRCSC
Professor of Surgery
Section of Vascular Surgery
Rady Faculty of Health Sciences Max Rady College of Medicine
University of Manitoba
Winnipeg, Manitoba, Canada

Joseph Hart, MD
Associate Professor of Surgery
Division of Vascular Surgery
Medical College of Wisconsin
Milwaukee, Wisconsin

Karem Harth, MD
Associate Professor of Surgery
Division of Vascular Surgery
University Hospitals Case Western Reserve University
Cleveland, Ohio

Rebecca B. Hasley, MD, MPH
Assistant Professor of Surgery
Department of Surgery
Boston University Medical Center
Boston, Massachusetts

Mounir J. Haurani, MD, MPH
Professor of Surgery
Division of Vascular Surgery
Eastern Carolina University
Greenville, Norh Carolina

Matthew C. Henn, MD
Assistant Professor of Surgery
Division of Cardiac Surgery
The Ohio State University
Columbus, Ohio

Kara Hessel, DO
Assistant Professor of Surgery
Division of Vascular Surgery
University of Kansas
Kansas City, Missouri

Anil Hingorani, MD
Professor of Surgery
Division of Vascular Surgery
NYU Lagone University
New York, New York

Kathryn L. Howe, MD, PhD
Associate Professor of Surgery
Department of Surgery
University of Toronto
Toronto, Ontario, Canada

Thomas S. Huber, MD, PhD
Professor of Surgery
Division of Vascular Surgery and Endovascular Therapy
University of Florida College of Medicine
Gainesville, Florida

Misty D. Humphries, MD, MAS, FACS
Professor of Surgery
Division of Vascular Surgery
The University of California Davis
Sacramento, California

Mohamad A. Hussain, MD, PhD
Associate Professor of Surgery
Division of Vascular and Endovascular Surgery
Brigham and Women's Hospital
Boston, Massachusetts

Momodou L. Jammeh, MD
Assistant Professor of Surgery
Division of Vascular Surgery
Medical College of Wisconsin
Milwaukee, Wisconsin

William Jordan Jr, MD
Professor of Surgery
Department of Surgery
Medical College of Georgia
Augusta, Georgia

Manju Kalra, MBBS
Professor of Surgery
Division of Vascular and Endovascular Surgery
Mayo Clinic
Rochester, Minnesota

Vikram S. Kashyap, MD, FACS
Endowed Chair, Frederik Meijer Heart and Vascular Institute
Vice President, Cardiovascular Health, Corewell Health
Professor of Surgery, Michigan State University College of Human Medicine
Grand Rapids, Michigan

Sean A. Kennedy, MD, FRCPC
Resident in Radiology
Division of Vascular and Interventional Radiology
University of Toronto
Toronto, Ontario, Canada

Vipul Khetarpaul, MD
Associate Professor of Surgery
Division of Vascular Surgery
Washington University
St. Louis, Missouri

Amanda Kistler, MD
Assistant Professor of Surgery
Division of Vascular Surgery
University of Nebraska
Omaha, Nebraska

Ezra Y. Koh, MD
Fellow in Vascular Surgery
Division of Vascular Surgery
Houston Methodist Hospital
Houston, Texas

Emilia Krol, MD
Vascular Surgeon
OSF HealthCare Cardiovascular Institute
Rockford, Illinois

Nathan Kugler, MD
Assistant Professor of Surgery
Medical College of Wisconsin
Milwaukee, Wisconsin

Norman H. Kumis, MD
Professor of Surgery
Division of Vascular Surgery and Endovascular Therapy
University Hospitals
Case Western Reserve University, School of Medicine
Cleveland, Ohio

John Landau, MD, MSc
Assistant Professor of Surgery
Division of Vascular Surgery and Department of Critical Care Medicine
Schulich School of Medicine
London, Ontario, Canada

Patric Liang, MD
Assistant Professor of Surgery
Division of Vascular and Endovascular Surgery
Beth Israel Deaconess Medical Center
Boston, Massachusetts

Joseph V. Lombardi, MD
Professor of Surgery
Division of Vascular Surgery
Cooper University
Camden, New Jersey

Allan Lumsden, MD
Professor of Vascular Surgery
Department of Cardiovascular Surgery
Houston Methodist Hospital
Houston, Texas

Sebastian Mafeld, MBBS
Assistant Professor
Division of Vascular and Interventional Radiology
Department of Medical Imaging
University of Toronto
Toronto, Ontario, Canada

Randall R. De Martino, MD, MS
Professor of Surgery
Division of Vascular and Endovascular Surgery
Mayo Clinic
Rochester, Minnesota

Daniel Mason, DO
Radiologist
Tripler Army Medical Center
Honolulu, Hawaii

Katherine K. McMackin, MD
Assistant Professor of Surgery
Division of Vascular Surgery
Cooper University
Camden, New Jersey

Christopher McQuinn, MD
Vascular Surgeon
Wakemed Medical Center
Raleigh, North Carolina

Ross Milner, MD, FACS
Professor of Surgery
Section of Vascular Surgery and Endovascular Therapy
The University of Chicago Medicine & Biological Sciences
Chicago, Illinois

Gregory Modrall, MD
Professor of Surgery
Division of Vascular Surgery
University of Texas Southwestern
Dallas, Texas

Gregory Moneta, MD
Professor of Surgery
Division of Vascular and Endovascular Surgery
Oregon Health and Science University
Portland, Oregon

Samuel R. Money, MD, MBA
Professor of Surgery
Division of Vascular Surgery
Ochsner Health
New Orleans, Louisiana

Wesley S. Moore, MD
Professor of Surgery
Division of Vascular Surgery
University of California
Los Angeles, California

Sudhir K. Nagpal, MD
Professor of Surgery
Division of Vascular and Endovascular Surgery
University of Ottawa
Ottawa, Ontario, Canada

Gustavo S. Oderich, MD
Professor of Surgery
Department of Cardiothoracic and Vascular Surgery
The University of Texas Health Science Center at Houston
Houston, Texas

Mohammed al-Omran, MD, MSC
Professor of Surgery
Division of Vascular Surgery, St. Michael's Hospital
University of Toronto
Toronto, Ontario, Canada

Kristine Orion, MD, RPVI
Associate Professor of Surgery
Division of Vascular Surgery
The Ohio State University Wexner Medical Center
Columbus, Ohio

Michael Paisley, MD
Vascular Surgeon
Santa Barbara Vascular Specialists
Santa Barbara, California

Jean M. Panneton, MD
Professor of Surgery
Division of Vascular Surgery
Eastern Virginia Medical School
Norfolk, Virginia

Giuseppe Papia, MD, MSc
Professor of Surgery
Department of Vascular Surgery
University of Toronto
Toronto, Ontario, Canada

Eric K. Peden, MD
Professor of Vascular Surgery
Department of Cardiovascular Surgery
Houston Methodist Hospital
Houston, Texas

Amani Politano, MD, MS
Associate Professor of Surgery
Division of Vascular and Endovascular Surgery
Oregon Health and Science University
Portland, Oregon

Bala Ramanan, MD
Associate Professor of Surgery
Division of Vascular Surgery
University of Texas Southwestern
Dallas, Texas

Todd E. Rasmussen, MD
Professor of Surgery
Division of Vascular Surgery
Mayo Clinic
Rochester, Minnesota

Derek J. Roberts, MD, PhD
Assistant Professor of Surgery
Division of Vascular and Endovascular Surgery
University of Ottawa
Ottawa, Ontario, Canada

Graham Roche-Nagle, MD
Associate Professor of Surgery
Division of Vascular Surgery
University of Toronto
Toronto, Ontario, Canada

Rae S. Rokosh, MD
NYC Health and Hospitals-Bellevue
New York, New York

Russell H. Samson, MD
Vascular Surgeon
Sarasota Vascular Specialists
Sarasota, Florida

Timur P. Sarac, MD
Professor of Surgery
Division of Vascular Surgery
University of Virginia
Charlottesville, Virginia
Professor of Surgery Emeritus
The Ohio State University
Columbus, Ohio

Hosam El Sayed, MD
Associate Professor of Surgery
Division of Vascular Surgery
Eastern Virginia Medical School
Norfolk, Virginia

Salvatore T. Scali, MD
Professor of Surgery
Division of Vascular Surgery and Endovascular Therapy
University of Florida College of Medicine
Gainesville, Florida

Andres Schanzer, MD
Professor of Surgery
Division of Vascular and Endovascular Surgery
University of Massachusetts Medical School
Worcester, Massachusetts

Marc L. Schermerhorn, MD
Professor of Surgery
Division of Vascular Surgery
Beth Israel Deaconess Medical Center
Boston, Massachusetts

Peter Schneider, MD
Professor of Surgery
Division of Vascular and Endovascular Surgery
University of California, San Francisco
San Francisco, California

Sherry D. Scovell, MD
Assistant Professor of Surgery
Division of Vascular Surgery
Massachusetts General Hospital
Boston, Massachusetts

Rebecca Scully, MD, MPH
Assistant Professor of Surgery
Division of Vascular and Endovascular Surgery
Dartmouth-Hitchcock Medical Center
Lebanon, New Hampshire

Ocean Setia, MBBS
Vascular Surgery Resident
Division of Vascular Surgery and Endovascular Therapy
Yale University School of Medicine
New Haven, Connecticut

Murray Shames, MD
Professor of Surgery
Department of Surgery
University of South Florida Health Morsani School of Medicine
Tampa, Florida

Jessica P. Simons, MD, MPH
Associate Professor of Surgery
Division of Vascular Surgery
University of Massachusetts Medical School
Worcester, Massachusetts

Jeffrey J. Siracuse, MD
Professor of Surgery
Division of Vascular Surgery
Boston University School of Medicine
Boston, Massachusetts

Matthew R. Smeds, MD
Professor of Surgery
Division of Vascular and Endovascular Surgery
Saint Louis University
St. Louis, Missouri

Kristine L. So, MD
Assistant Professor of Surgery
Division of Vascular Surgery
Penn State University
Hershey, Pennsylvania

Ina Y. Soh, MD, MS
Assistant Professor of Surgery
Division of Vascular and Endovascular Surgery
Mayo Clinic
Rochester, Minnesota

Sunita D. Srivastava, MD
Professor of Surgery
Division of Vascular and Endovascular Surgery
Massachusetts General Hospital
Boston, Massachusetts

Lars Stangenberg, MD
Assistant Professor of Surgery
Division of Vascular Surgery
Beth Israel Deaconess Medical Center
Boston, Massachusetts

Benjamin Starnes, MD
Professor of Surgery
Division of Vascular and Endovascular Surgery
University of Washington School of Medicine
Seattle, Washington

Julianne Stoughton, MD
Assistant Professor of Surgery
Division of Vascular and Endovascular Surgery
Massachusetts General Hospital
Boston, Massachusetts

David Szalay, MD
Associate Professor of Surgery
Division of Vascular Surgery
University of Toronto
Toronto, Ontario, Canada

Emanuel R. Tenorio, MD, PhD
Vascular Surgery Resident
Department of Cardiothoracic and Vascular Surgery
The University of Texas Health Science Center at Houston
Houston, Texas

Angelyn Thayer, MD
Vascular Surgery Integrated Resident
Division of Vascular Surgery
University of South Florida Health Morsani School of Medicine
Tampa, Florida

Robert W. Thompson, MD
Professor of Surgery
Division of Vascular Surgery
Washington University
St. Louis, Missouri

Tadaki M. Tomita, MD
Assistant Professor of Surgery
Division of Vascular Surgery
Northwestern University Feinberg School of Medicine
Chicago, Illinois

Gilbert R. Upchurch Jr.
Professor of Surgery
Department of Surgery
University of Florida College of Medicine
Gainesville, Florida

Patrick Vaccaro, MD
Professor of Surgery Emeritus
Division of Vascular Surgery
The Ohio State University
Columbus, Ohio

R. James Valentine, MD
Professor of Surgery
Division of Vascular Surgery
University of Minnesota
Minneapolis, Minnesota

Harold Davis Waller, MD
Vascular Surgeon
St. Mary's Healthcare System
Athens, Georgia

Courtney J. Warner, MD
Associate Professor of Surgery
Division of Vascular Surgery
Albany Medical College/Albany Medical Center Hospital
Albany, New York

Blair E. Warren, MD
Division of Vascular and Interventional Radiology
Department of Medical Imaging
University of Toronto
Toronto, Ontario, Canada

Aric A. Wogsland, MD
Vascular Surgeon
Centracare Heart and Vascular Center
St. Clous, Minnesota

Virginia L. Wong, MD
Assistant Professor of Surgery
Division of Vascular Surgery
Case Western Reserve University
Cleveland, Ohio

Edward Woo, MD
President, MedStar Medical Group
MedStar Heart and Vascular Institute
Professor of Surgery
Georgetown University School of Medicine
Washington, DC

Mathew Wooster, MD, MBA
Associate Professor of Surgery
Division of Vascular Surgery
Medical University of South Carolina
Charleston, South Carolina

Bian Wu, MD
Vascular Surgeon
Kaiser Permanente San Francisco Medical Center
San Francisco, California

FOREWORD

Gateways to Vascular Surgery, edited by Drs. Sarac and Kashyap, is a remarkable atlas of surgical operations. It is meant to be a companion to *Zollinger's Atlas of Surgical Operations*. The first edition of the atlas was conceived and developed by two giants in the world of surgery, Elliot Carr Cutler, MD, Mosely Professor of Surgery at Harvard Medical School and Surgeon-in-Chief at Peter Bent Brigham Hospital (PBBH), and Ohio State's Robert M. Zollinger, Sr., MD. Zollinger received his BA and MD at Ohio State before joining Cutler first at University Hospitals, Cleveland, and then the PBBH. Zollinger served as chief resident and then as Chief of Surgery for the PBBH Harvard 5th General Hospital in World War II. Following the premature death of Cutler in 1947, Zollinger returned to Ohio to serve as chair of the Department of Surgery at The Ohio State University College of Medicine from 1947 to 1974.

The idea for the atlas was born from a student surgical course that Cutler and Zollinger developed together, in which Harvard medical students would rotate through various surgical duties as they performed basic surgical procedures and techniques on dogs. The two conceived a text with illustrations of common operations for general surgeons in training and in practice. From its inception, the authors determined that medical illustration would play an important role in the atlas and serve as a visual guide to the procedures. The first edition was organized in an oversized folio format which allowed paragraphs of text on the left-side page and a full page of multiple surgical illustrations on the right-side page. This way, text and the illustrations from the surgeon's point of view could be viewed simultaneously.

Over the years, the table of contents grew to include many surgical procedures as they became refined and accepted. The first vascular operations were introduced in the 1967 third edition Volume 2, with Resection of Abdominal Aortic Aneurysm. This text introduced advanced surgical procedures which today form the basis of many surgical specialties. Since then, new vascular procedures, when proven and established, were added. The 11th edition included 161 chapters, including 19 chapters covering essential information concerning vascular surgery. In discussion with Dr. Sarac, it was clear that there was much more material to include than would fit into the *Zollinger Atlas*. Hence, a specialized vascular atlas was developed using the trademark organization and underpinnings that have made the *Zollinger's Atlas of Surgical Operations* the go-to guide for surgical procedures.

Drs. Sarac and Kashyap have assembled an exceptional group of vascular surgeons as contributors to this essential atlas of vascular surgery. Included are 77 chapters divided into 14 sections. This atlas is appropriate for the trainee as well as the practicing vascular surgeon. For trainees, introduction to surgical dissection of arteries and the appropriate use of vascular clamps as well as how to perform an endarterectomy and vascular anastomoses are provided. A description of the basic concepts in endovascular surgery is essential. In addition, excellent descriptions of exposure are provided. For the practicing vascular surgeon, the content is comprehensive, providing clear and well-illustrated descriptions of open and endovascular techniques. We think that this is an outstanding companion to *Zollinger's Atlas of Surgical Operations*.

E. Christopher Ellison, MD
Robert M. Zollinger Professor Emeritus
Department of Surgery
The Ohio State University College of Medicine

Robert M. Zollinger, Jr., MD
Professor Emeritus
Case Western Reserve University School
Clinical Professor
University Arizona College of Medicine

PREFACE

The rapid evolution of vascular surgery over the past 25 years has been spectacular. New devices, iterative improvements of old devices, and hybrid techniques have transformed patient care and vascular training. These changes have forced us to adapt educating our colleagues, partners, and trainees through mini-fellowships, going from 1 to 2 clinical years of vascular fellowship to allow time for extra training on new techniques, and finally adding vascular surgery residency directly from medical school. In addition, new clinical trial results have brought an increasing number of innovations to the bedside.

As new surgical and endovascular therapies advance and mature, we felt a new comprehensive atlas of vascular surgery accounting for all procedures was needed. We were honored to have McGraw Hill and Dr. Christopher Ellison approach us with the idea of coalescing *Gateways in Vascular Surgery: An Operative Atlas*, a contemporary and concise atlas of vascular surgery, as a sister atlas to *Zollinger's Atlas of Surgery*. This marquee atlas format is ideal for learning, providing both text and illustrations in an easy-to-use format for all residents, fellows, and practicing vascular surgeons. We chose the title *Gateways in Vascular Surgery*, as frequently a case has a few steps for which, when the "gateway" is opened, the case proceeds more expeditiously.

When compiling a list of contributing authors, we chose expert clinical vascular surgeons who are also expert educators and are currently leaders in the field. Most of the authors are surgeons we have directly or indirectly worked with and are respected on all levels.

The *Atlas* has truly been a labor of love that took 4 years to complete from start to finish. We are incredibly grateful to McGraw Hill for helping us stay the course and see this through, as the *Atlas* survived a pandemic with the accompanying world and workplace changes. For us, this included three separate McGraw Hill senior editors and three separate illustrators help us see this through. We hope you are as delighted as we are with the product, *Gateways in Vascular Surgery*.

Timur P. Sarac, MD
Vikram S. Kashyap, MD

ACKNOWLEDGMENTS

Special acknowledgment goes to our mentors who helped us develop our visions in this field. Thank you Ken Ouriel, MD, Wesley Moore, MD, Richard Cambria, MD, Frank Veith, MD, Enrico Ascher, MD, Thomas Huber, MD, and James Seegar, MD (in memory).

Section I
BASIC CONCEPTS: OPEN SURGICAL TECHNIQUES

Surgical Exposure of Arteries

Vikram S. Kashyap, MD • Kristine L. So, MD

INTRODUCTION One of the greatest skills of a vascular surgeon is the ability to reach and isolate the human body's major blood vessels. This requires extensive knowledge of anatomy, the course of arteries and veins, and substantial technical skill and experience. To provide the panorama of surgical procedures outlined in this book, the vascular surgeon must master the ability to expose and control the aorta and yet be able to delicately dissect free tibial vessels. In this chapter, we discuss the key components of arterial dissection.

PREPARATION A few principles apply to almost all vascular operations.

1. Study any preoperative imaging prior to making an incision. Invariably, patients will have ultrasound, computed tomography (CT), magnetic resonance (MR), and/or angiographic images that provide a roadmap of the vasculature.
2. The liberal use of bedside duplex ultrasound after anesthesia induction and positioning, but prior to prepping, allows the surgeon to finalize the trajectory of peripheral arteries and the incision.
3. As in all surgery, proper visualization of the operative field is a key component to accurate dissection, arterial control, and repair. Loupe magnification of 2.5× to 3.5× is a commonly used adjunct, especially in the setting of smaller blood vessels. The positioning of surgical lights is key to illuminating the operative field. However, in cases where the wound is deep or the aperture is small, overhead surgical lighting may be insufficient. The use of fiberoptic headlamps worn by the surgeon or assistant will further enhance visualization of the field in cases of deep or angled exposures.

EXPOSURE Adequate exposure to the operative field begins in the preoperative phase. Planning the optimal incision for the target vessel(s) allows the surgeon to utilize the incision made to most efficiently and successfully expose the operative field with proper placement of retractor clamps. Each of the ensuing chapters in this book will discuss the optimal incision for its associated procedure. Most commonly, a longitudinal incision over a blood vessel is used for exposure, thus allowing for the ability to extend the incision should further exposure be necessary. An incision approximately 2 cm longer than the desired visual field is made so as to prevent overtraumatizing of the skin once retractor clamps are placed. The placement and length of the incision is a key first step. The surgeon needs enough space for proximal and distal control, and often an anastomosis between. If excessive bleeding, thick muscle tissue, or other major obstructions are encountered, the surgeon should reassess the approach. The type of retractor clamp used depends on the depth of the operative field and may vary as the dissection progresses down to the target vessel. For example, one may begin with a Weitlaner retractor at skin level and progress to the cerebellar retractor for a femoral artery exposure. In the abdomen, a hand-held abdominal wall retractor may suffice initially but is often replaced by a fixed retraction system to allow adequate exposure of the retroperitoneum. Once an initial incision is made, the principle of traction and countertraction is utilized to carefully traverse subcutaneous tissue. Understanding the vascular anatomy is essential to arterial dissection, as a pulse may not be present as a guide for arterial exposure.

As the target vessel is visualized, atraumatic (non-toothed) instruments should always be used. Electrocautery that may have been previously used to traverse more superficial tissues will be exchanged for sharp dissection. With the use of the traction–countertraction technique, sharp dissection is carried out along the top of the artery with the correct plane exposing the overlying adventitial layer (**FIGURE 1-1**).

This adventitial layer is a soft, gray/pink color that can be utilized to atraumatically lift the target vessel and dissect it free from the perivascular investing tissues. It is essential to be able to differentiate this layer from the surrounding tissues, as circumferential dissection of the artery allows for further arterial manipulation, such as clamp or vessel loop placement for proximal and distal control. It is also important to differentiate this layer because over-dissection can denude an artery of its adventitia, which may cause unnecessary bleeding in an operative field and will also remove a potential strength layer for future anastomoses.

During arterial isolation, the anterior and lateral surfaces of the artery are dissected free. Fine, atraumatic forceps and sharp dissection with scissors can be used. Scissors can be used to gently spread in a perpendicular manner to the artery, cut the periarterial tissue, and identify branches (**FIGURE 1-2**).

Blunt-angled clamps can be passed posterior to the artery and away from the adjacent venous structures to allow for placement of silastic vessel loops of different widths, or cotton umbilical tapes. Also, manual palpation of the artery with an angled clamp behind it will identify a less diseased site for eventual arterial clamping (**FIGURE 1-3**). This is especially important to assess for intravascular calcification and avoiding clamp-associated damage.

A vessel loop placed around the artery can serve as a simple way to achieve gentle countertraction (usually by the assistant) without the use of forceps for further dissection in either a cranial or caudal direction (**FIGURE 1-4**).

Dissection and exposure of larger vessels including the aorta can be accomplished in a similar manner, except for the more frequent use of manual retraction. Spread fingers over a moist sponge can allow for gentle and broad displacement of the aorta more effectively than forceps, which can cause focal injury.

Vascular exposure in the reoperative field poses a unique challenge to the vascular surgeon. The famed "re-do groin," for example, is composed of dense scar formation and destruction of normal anatomic vascular planes. Often, the surgeon may forego the usual fine, atraumatic forceps and utilize more sturdy toothed forceps such as a rat tooth forceps or Bonney forceps in order to better grasp the underlying scar tissue to employ an effective countertraction technique. Sharp dissection with a scalpel blade may prove to be more successful than use of scissors.

With experience, exposure and dissection of most arteries can be done expeditiously. Even though arterial exposure can become routine, this still remains the important first step for a successful vascular operation. ■

SUGGESTED READINGS

Chaikof E, Cambria R. *Atlas of Vascular Surgery and Endovascular Therapy: Anatomy and Technique.* Philadelphia, PA: Saunders, Elsevier; 2014.

Greenhalgh R. *Vascular Surgical Techniques.* London: Butterworth; 1984.

Hans SS, Shepard A, Weaver M, Bove P, Long G. *Endovascular and Open Vascular Reconstruction.* Boca Raton, FL: CRC Press; 2018.

Sidawy AN, Perler BA. *Rutherford's Vascular Surgery and Endovascular Therapy.* 9th Ed. Philadelphia, PA: Elsevier; 2019.

Stanley J, Veith F, Wakefield T. *Current Therapy in Vascular and Endovascular Surgery.* Philadelphia, PA: Saunders, Elsevier; 2014.

Walberg E, Olofsson P, Goldstone J. *Emergency Vascular Surgery.* Berlin: Springer; 2007.

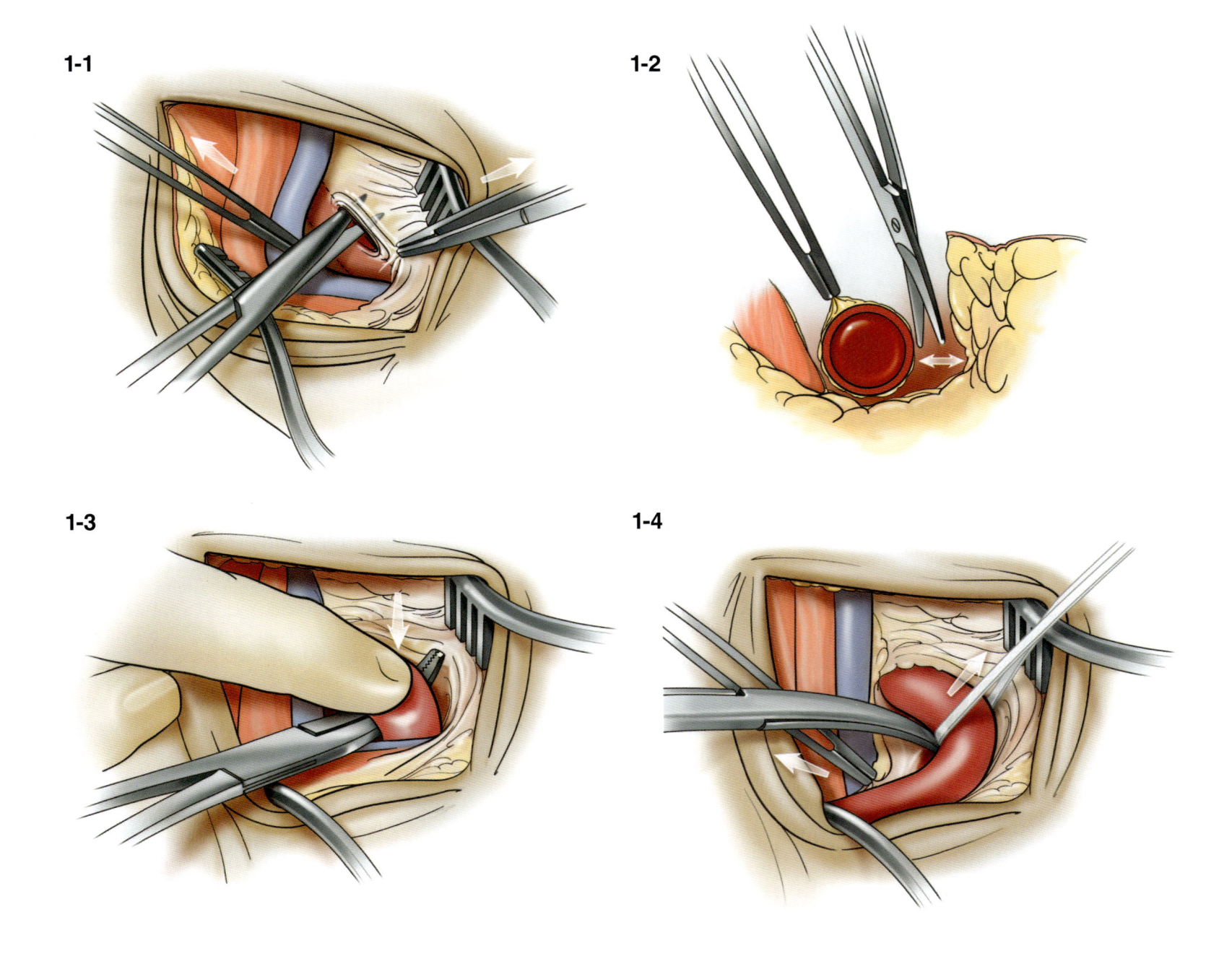

1-1

1-2

1-3

1-4

Use of Clamps, Loops, and Other Devices to Interrupt Blood Flow

Jae S. Cho, MD

INTRODUCTION Operating on blood vessels requires the ability to obtain control of the vessel to minimize blood loss, optimize visualization of the surgical field, and facilitate safe and efficient vascular reconstruction; all of this directly impacts the conduct of the surgery and the eventual outcome. It may be achieved by a variety of instruments and techniques. It is certainly beyond the scope of this chapter to discuss every available instrument, as there are multiple derivatives and permutations of any given instrument, each with its own distinct features and advantages. It is neither practical nor possible to familiarize oneself with all the different instruments and tools. The intent of this chapter is to provide an understanding and guiding principles of various ways to achieve hemostasis effectively and efficiently.

CHOICE OF TECHNIQUE The method for interruption of blood flow is dictated by the need for complete or partial control and the vessel size. While complete control can be obtained with any of the available instruments and techniques, partial control can only be achieved with the use of clamps. In general, large vessels are best controlled with clamps, medium-size vessels with either clamps or vessel loops, and small vessels with other devices (occluders, clips, or pneumatic tourniquets).

CLAMPS Many different types of clamps can be found on an operating room instrument table, some of which are vascular and some not. It is necessary to understand the parts and features of a clamp, as they determine the different functionality of each clamp.

ANATOMY AND FEATURES OF A CLAMP

1. Jaws (blades): The working end of a clamp.
2. Teeth: The prongs at the top of an instrument allowing firm grasp. Vascular clamps (or forceps) do not have teeth.
3. Serration: The grooves that allow for firm holding of tissue. The serrations are delicate compared to nonvascular clamps so as to avoid trauma to the vessel.
4. Box-lock: The hinge point.
5. Shank: The run from the joint to the finger ring.
6. Ratchet: The interlocking parts between finger rings that allow the instrument to be closed.

It is important to differentiate an atraumatic vascular clamp from a nonvascular clamp so as to avoid crush injuries that may arise from application of a nonvascular clamp. One simple way to test a clamp is to apply it to one's little finger; if it does not cause discomfort, it can be safely applied to a blood vessel.

Although considered atraumatic, malfunctioning or inappropriately applied clamps may cause significant vessel injury. This can particularly be the case in the presence of a heavily calcified plaque or fragile vessel, as seen in patients with connective tissue disorders. Ideally, vascular clamps should be applied to a disease-free segment of the artery. Palpating the artery against a right-angle clamp can help determine the presence and extent of an atherosclerotic plaque, which is often in the posterior aspect and not appreciated by only palpating the anterior aspect of the artery (see Chapter 1, Figure 1-3). In the presence of significant plaque, the artery should be dissected further proximally and distally to identify a site suitable for clamping. If clamping is necessary across an area of a diseased artery, the clamp should be applied in a manner that apposes the soft part of the artery against the plaque without causing plaque fracture or vessel tear.

Fine interdigitating serrations allow clamping of the vessel without slippage or significant crush injury. It is noteworthy, however, that these serrations may also tear adjacent veins as the clamp is being applied. Thus, due caution should be taken when a clamp is being applied to the vessel. In addition, in patients with a high risk for vessel injury or those undergoing an operation for an acute aortic dissection, serrations may injure the vessels. Thus, in such cases, Fogarty-Hydragrip clamps (FIGURE 2-1) should be used. Another situation in which Fogarty-Hydragrip clamps are invaluable is when controlling an aortic endograft with an endoskeleton, such as

Endologix endoprosthesis. The endoskeleton precludes appropriate apposition of the fabric resulting in persistent and marked blood loss. The rubber inserts provide blood-tight graft occlusion around the endoskeleton.

The majority of blood vessel control is attained by clamps. A full spectrum of sizes and shapes has been developed and refined to accommodate different anatomic and clinical circumstances, such as the quality of the vessel/graft and the need for complete or partial occlusion.

CLAMPS FOR COMPLETE OCCLUSION: Complete occlusion is required when the blood vessel needs to be disconnected or resected with an end-to-end anastomotic reconstruction. It is achieved by cross-clamping a blood vessel. A clamp is chosen based on the size and depth of the vessel and the angle of approach.

For control of the aorta, the most versatile clamp is the Cherry clamp (FIGURE 2-2). It has a sufficient posterior angle at the shank such that it stays out of the way of the surgical field. The distance from the box-lock to the tip of the jaws is sufficiently long even for morbidly obese patients. It can be applied to supraceliac as well as infrarenal aorta in most cases. In rare cases where a longer clamp is needed, either a C-shaped DeBakey aortic clamp (FIGURE 2-3) will provide additional depth. Another use of a C-shaped Sklar DeBakey aortic clamp is for preparation of a retroperitoneal tunnel during aortobifemoral bypass grafting and a suprapubic tunnel during cross-femoral bypass grafting. The curvature of the C-shaped clamp allows the leverage to direct the jaw of the instrument anteriorly at the level of aortic bifurcation. The posteriorly bent shank of the S-shaped clamp renders such a maneuver difficult because the shank comes in immediate contact with the patient's thigh.

When working in an area with a tighter bending radius with limited space, Cosgrove flex clamps with rubber inserts are ideal (FIGURE 2-4). They are available in different lengths and jaw shapes. This clamp is useful not only for calcified aorta but also for reaching deep into the proximal thoracic aorta such as in thoracoabdominal aortic repair.

Other clamps useful for aortic occlusion or control of renovisceral and iliac vessels are Wiley hypogastric (FIGURE 2-5) and Zanger clamps (FIGURE 2-6). They have a very similar appearance, except that Zanger clamps have a longer shank, which allows a deeper reach. These clamps can also be used to control the limbs of an aortic prosthetic graft after completion of proximal anastomosis.

For smaller, superficial vessels (femoral or iliac arteries in thin patients), an angled DeBakey clamp or its variants, such as a Leland-Jones clamp, are widely used. Another clamp that is most useful for occlusion of the proximal common femoral/distal external iliac artery is the Derra clamp (FIGURE 2-7), allowing anterior-posterior occlusion of the vessel, which is necessary more often than not. It is also very useful to obtain control of a vessel in deep and tight spaces such as the proximal axillary artery and the proximal subclavian artery (during subclavian-carotid transposition).

Some special clamps designed for specific arteries are also available. For example, the Gregory profunda clamps (FIGURE 2-8) are designed for control of the profunda femoris artery with a gently curved and sufficiently long jaw. Another example is the Kitzmiller carotid clamp. It is an elegant, delicate clamp that allows control of the distal internal carotid arteries. They come in left- and right-angled configurations.

Bulldog clamps of various sizes and shapes are effective in providing hemostasis of small vessels and branch vessels.

CLAMPS FOR PARTIAL OCCLUSION: Partial occlusion is utilized when there is no need to resect the vessel segment or when continuous flow to the distal organ is desired. It is used for ascending aorta-, descending thoracic aorta-, supraceliac aorta-, or infrarenal aorta-based inflow construction in an end-to-side fashion. This is an important technique as it allows distal perfusion and mitigates complications of end-organ ischemia, particularly paraplegia. It also minimizes blood loss from back-bleeding through the intercostals and lumbars that may be encountered with cross-clamping of the aorta. **CONTINUES** ▶

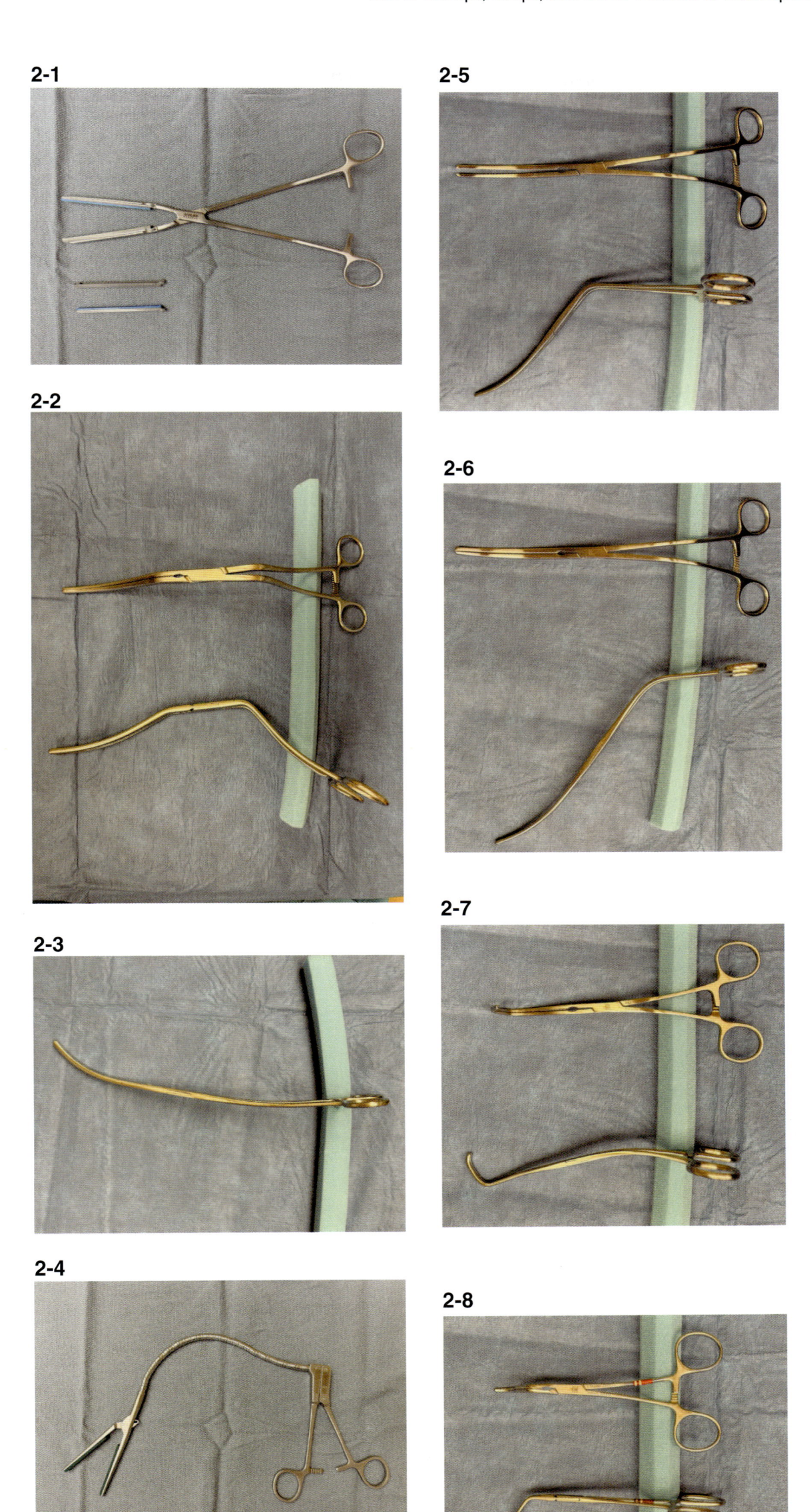

CLAMPS `CONTINUED` The most well-known side-biting clamp of its kind is the Satinsky clamp. A variant is the Lemole-Strong clamp (FIGURE 2-9), characterized by heart-shaped jaws that allow better access to deep tissue while displacing adjacent tissue out of the field of anastomosis. This clamp also provides an excellent grasp that assures hemostasis without slippage. Side-biting clamps with a rubber insert are also available. However, due precaution should be taken as these partial clamps with inserts are somewhat prone to slipping and loss of hemostasis.

The aforementioned Derra clamp can be useful for a medium-sized vessel (i.e., common femoral artery or vein).

For the rarely performed innominate endarterectomy, Wylie J clamp is utilized. The deep curve provides exposure of the origin of the innominate artery well into the ascending aorta, allowing adequate removal of plaque spilling into the orifice and beyond. Unfortunately, this operation is becoming a lost art with the advances in endovascular solutions and preference for ascending aorta-based direct reconstructions.

SHUNT CLAMPS: The need to place a shunt may be encountered during carotid reconstruction and in traumatic settings. While a shunt may be secured in place by a variety of mechanisms, a Javid shunt clamp, available in different sizes, provides an effective means of secure hemostasis.

VESSEL LOOPS AND TAPES Vessel loops are widely used to occlude medium- and small-size vessels (i.e., common femoral, common carotid, popliteal, and internal carotid arteries or equivalents thereof). Although a variety of materials may be used (silastic, umbilical tape, plasma tubing), the most common is the silastic type. They are available in different colors, which is helpful for denoting different vessels in the operative field.

While less traumatic than clamps, vessel loops and tapes are not without shortcomings. First, when used with excessive tension, vessel loops can cause vessel injuries. Furthermore, excessive tension applied from both proximal and distal ends closes off the arteriotomy and hampers repair or anastomosis. Application of a vessel loop on the proximal end and a Yasargil clip on the distal end remedies such a condition. Second, when applied over calcified vessels, hemostasis cannot be assured, requiring adjunct measures such as clamps or intraluminal occlusion with a Fogarty balloon. Third, loops may clutter the field and get caught in the prongs of a self-retaining retractor. Fourth, vessel loops invariably require more dissection, albeit not extensive, because when the loops are pulled up, the vessel is crimped/constricted above and below the loop. This limits visualization of the inside of the vessel and may require more dissection of the vessel.

With that said, the advantages of vessel loops include avoidance of clamp-induced injury and the ability to bring up the vessel out of deep space (such as the below-the-knee popliteal artery) so as to allow easier execution of anastomoses.

The most common way to control the blood vessel using loops is a double loop technique (Potts technique) (FIGURE 2-10). Another method is the Rummel technique, in which an umbilical tape is passed around a vessel and both ends are brought through a short red rubber catheter (or its equivalent), which is then cinched against the vessel (FIGURE 2-11). This technique is often used to secure an intraluminal shunt solely or in conjunction with a shunt clamp. Another area where it effectively provides hemostasis is in the setting of persistent bleeding around a sheath or cannula. While an effective technique, it may cause arterial wall damage in the presence of significant plaque and should not be used without an intraluminal device because the tape will fracture the vessel. Due precaution should be taken to avoid such a mishap.

PNEUMATIC TOURNIQUET An orthopedic tourniquet provides an effective means of hemostasis in the setting of exsanguinating traumatic injuries, major amputations, and distal bypass grafting during which direct clamping or looping is best avoided to prevent intimal injury or spasm. It allows for minimal dissection limited to the anterior surface of the vessel, which mitigates vessel spasm as well as the risk of vessel injury. A tourniquet can be placed around the distal thigh or below the knee. After a soft roll is applied at the site of tourniquet placement, the limb is elevated and wrapped with an Esmarch bandage to drain the venous blood. The tourniquet is then inflated to 300 mm Hg and the Esmarch is released.

This technique may not be effective in the setting of calcified vessels. When persistent bleeding is encountered, hemostasis can be achieved by increasing the pressure in the tourniquet or by application of a clamp on the profunda femoris artery.

Tourniquets are also used effectively in the setting of exsanguinating traumatic injuries as well as in elective major amputations.

INTRALUMINAL VESSEL OCCLUDER When bleeding persists despite the aforementioned maneuvers after an arteriotomy is made in the distal target vessel, an intraluminal artery occluder (FloRester; http:www.Lamed.de) can be utilized to provide hemostasis. Oversizing should be avoided to prevent intimal damage during insertion.

BALLOON OCCLUSION Balloon occlusion may be employed in a wide range of clinical situations. Resuscitative endovascular balloon occlusion of aorta (REBOA) in the setting of a ruptured aorta or other exsanguinating emergency situations can be a life-saving maneuver. Several compliant occlusion balloons can be used to occlude the aorta, including the Gore Molding and Occlusion Balloon (W.L. Gore, Flagstaff, AZ), the Reliant balloon (Medtronic, Minneapolis, MN), the Coda balloon (Cook, Bloomington, IN), and the Equalizer balloon (Boston Scientific, Natick, MA). It is important to have a 12 or 14 French sheath to support the balloon so as to help withstand the hemodynamic forces and prevent distal migration of the balloon.

One common situation where balloon occlusion is used is during femoral endarterectomy. The plaque in the common femoral artery often extends proximally and requires exposure and control of the mid to distal external iliac artery so as to enable endarterectomy of the latter vessel. In such a setting, balloon occlusion of the external iliac artery essential. A #4 or #5 Fogarty balloon embolectomy catheter will provide hemostasis. Alternatively, an angioplasty balloon may be used. It also provides rapid and effective hemostasis in the setting of iatrogenic injury to the iliac vessels during endovascular interventions while definitive repair modalities are being prepared.

Other uses of balloon occlusion include control of the iliac arteries during open aortic surgery to prevent back-bleeding, inflow control during repair of a femoral pseudoaneurysm, and control of renovisceral vessels during a thoracoabdominal aortic aneurysm repair. Although not exactly a balloon, Foley catheters have been used to stop common iliac artery back-bleeding during aortic surgery.

SUMMARY Principles for attaining control of blood vessels have been outlined in this chapter. Proficiency with various means of achieving hemostasis shall draw the surgeon one step closer to mastery of the art. ■

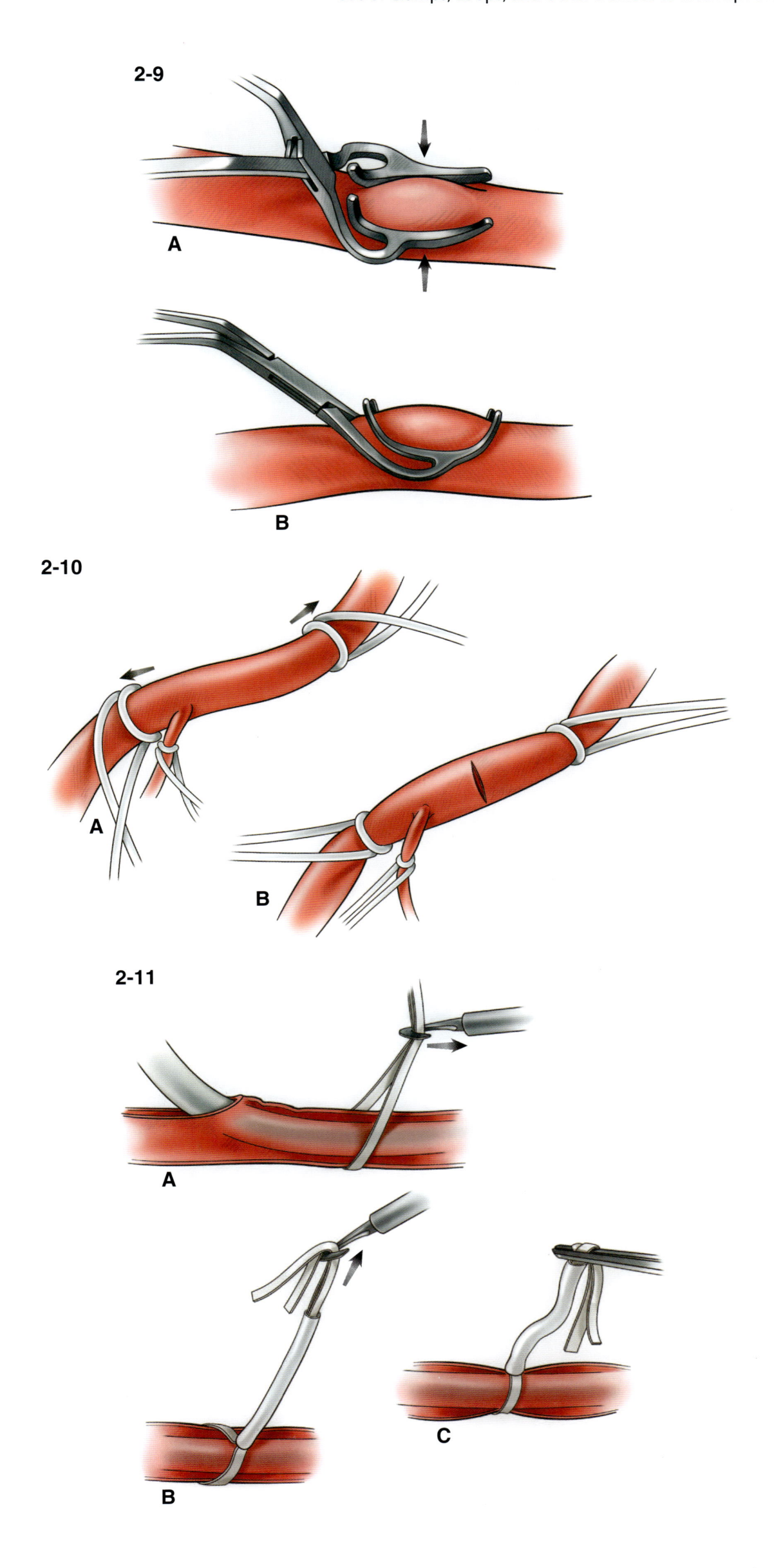

2-9

A

B

2-10

A

B

2-11

A

B

C

Rebecca Scully, MD, MPH • Michael Belkin, MD

INDICATIONS Knowledge of the various approaches to vascular anastomoses is a critical component of the vascular surgeon's toolkit. Anastomoses are core to open vascular surgery and an essential component of the open replacement or bypass of both arterial and venous disease, particularly occlusive, aneurysmal, or traumatic injuries. While the general technique of a vascular anastomosis remains similar across arterial beds, specific considerations apply when approaching anastomoses in large (aortic), medium (femoropopliteal), and small (tibial, pedal, distal upper extremity, mesenteric) vessels.

EXPOSURE Maximizing exposure and setup prior to initiating an anastomosis is one of the more important steps in ensuring success. Regardless of location, when setting up for an anastomosis it is critical to place retractors and clamps in such a fashion that exposure allows for appropriate visualization for both operator and assistant while completing the anastomosis. This becomes particularly important while operating in more constrained spaces such as in the pelvis or tibial vessels. Extensive exposure simplifies the performance and improves the odds of technical success.

DETAILS OF PROCEDURE

LARGE VESSEL (AORTIC) ANASTOMOSES: As with any anastomosis, we begin an aortic anastomosis by ensuring adequate exposure for proximal and distal control. When at all possible, candidate clamp points should be identified based on preoperative imaging to allow for expeditious dissection. Circumferential dissection of the aorta is generally unnecessary and is avoided given the risk of avulsion of lumbar vessels which can be difficult to control. If lumbar vessels are readily apparent and there is concern for disruption of these vessels with proximal or distal clamping, they can be divided prior to making an aortotomy. It is vital to ensure the aorta is cleared of perivascular tissue down to the spine posterior to the aorta and that this plane is completely clear prior to clamping or the proximal aortic clamp may be incomplete or become dislodged. A large part of this dissection is often completed with blunt finger dissection along the lateral aspects of the aorta.

Clamping A reverse-curved DeBakey or straight atraumatic aortic clamps can offer good inflow control while also falling out of the operator's way. An umbilical tape can be looped around the handle of the clamp and tagged with a Kelly clamp to hold the clamp out of the way and stable. It is vital to make certain the clamp is placed such that it is completely down to the spine without additional tissue, to ensure it does not become dislodged. Often a self-retaining retractor is utilized in these cases, and if a retractor blade is present at the apex, it should be positioned to facilitate optimal clamp positioning. Distal clamp sites depend on the nature of the disease being treated. When constructing an end-to-side anastomosis we prefer not to use side-biting clamps (e.g., a Satinsky clamp) as it does not give optimal exposure for removal of atherosclerotic debris or completion of the anastomosis. Clamps with atraumatic inserts of various sizes can often be used for distal aortic control or for control of common iliac arteries.

Vessel Preparation In the case of aneurysmal disease we typically score the anterior surface of the aorta and then enter the aneurysm wall using cautery followed by opening of the aneurysm with Metzenbaum or Mayo scissors. Scoring the aneurysm can help improve hemostasis and oozing from the aneurysm wall. In the case of aneurysmal disease, when making

the aortotomy it is important to preserve the proximal and distal "sewing ring" of normal aorta and to not carry the aortotomy too far proximally. We prefer to leave the back wall of the aorta intact as originally described by Creech rather than completely transecting it, and as such the aortotomy is taken transversely to the left and right to create a "T" shape (FIGURE 3-1A). This should extend across the anterior wall of the aorta from approximately the 9 o'clock to 3 o'clock positions. When doing this it is important to bring the superior horizonal incision toward the feet and the inferior toward the head to prevent shortening of the usable aortic neck. This will preserve the back wall of the aorta and the sewing ring described above. In the case of aortic occlusive disease, when an end-to-end anastomosis is planned the aorta is completely divided between clamps and/or using a TA stapler for the distal aorta. In an aorta with a juxtarenal occlusion, the aorta can be divided and any atherothrombotic plug removed prior to reclamping more distally, allowing for a potentially infrarenal clamp site. There is often a calcific plaque component in the aortic neck, and a focal endarterectomy should be performed to allow for improved needle passage. Care must be taken to not overly endarterectomize the aorta as the wall can become thinned out, compromising the integrity of the suture line.

Graft An appropriately sized tube or bifurcated graft should be selected. Graft sizers can be used to help in this decision. Typically 18- or 20-mm grafts are adequate for aortic aneurysm repairs. For end-to-end anastomoses the graft typically does not need to be beveled, but in the case of bifurcated grafts can be shortened proximally to improve the lie of the bifurcation.

Anastomosis The anastomosis is typically completed with 3.0 polypropylene sutures. We prefer a double-armed 3.0 polypropylene on an SH needle for the proximal anastomosis, though 2.0 polypropylene (Prolene) on an MH needle can also be helpful in some situations. We begin our proximal anastomosis with a horizontal mattress stitch [or suture] at the direct posterior or 6 o'clock position (FIGURE 3-1A). Contrary to arterial anastomoses elsewhere in the body, we routinely sew outside-to-in into the aorta to allow the operating surgeon (standing on the patient's right side) to take large, deep forehand bites across the posterior wall of the aorta. Conversely, the surgeon standing on the patient's left side will sew in-to-out in a forehand fashion on the posterior wall. Using each arm of the suture, we begin with a horizontal mattress at the 6 o'clock position then tie the sutures outside of the graft in an anchor technique. The suture passes are carried out in a radial fashion as in a clock face around the aorta, with care to advance a similar distance on the graft compared to the aorta (FIGURE 3-1B). As stated above, preparation of the aortic wall with removal of calcified plaque is essential no matter the direction of sewing. Particularly in the case of a suprarenal or supraceliac clamp it is important to remain cognizant of the renal and visceral vessels to avoid inadvertent injury or occlusion to these vessels while completing the anastomosis. We advocate tying the sutures at the 12 o'clock position rather than offset and doing so over a pledget. It is important to back-flush the anastomosis with heparinized saline to help identify any large leaks, particularly posteriorly, prior to unclamping. These are often best repaired using pledgeted sutures. As with other anastomoses, the graft is then antegrade flushed and the clamp may be repositioned onto the proximal graft. The suture line should again be policed for hemostasis.

CONTINUES ▶

3-1

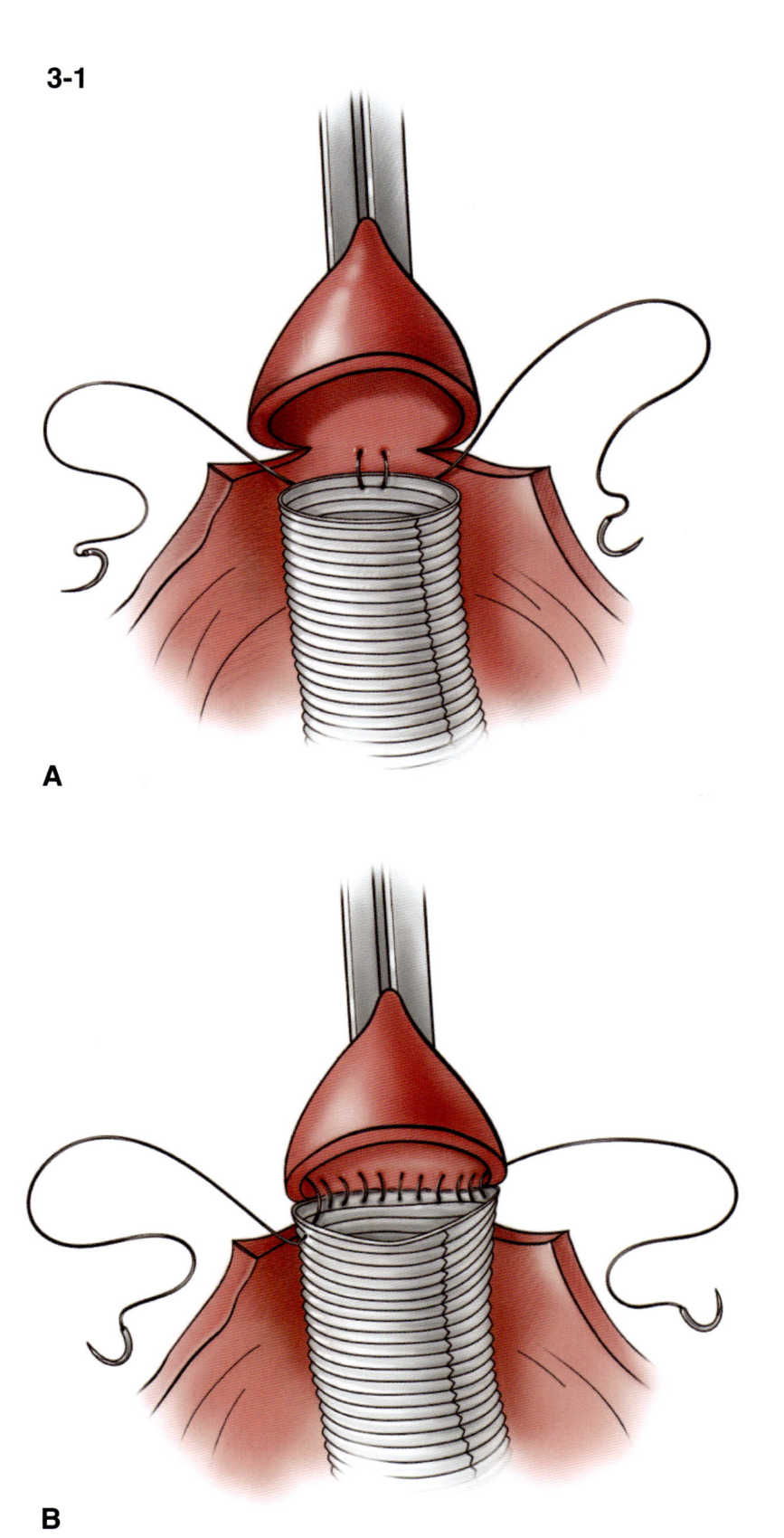

A

B

LARGE VESSEL (AORTIC) ANASTOMOSES: End-to-Side Aortic Anastomoses CONTINUED Similar to the end-to-end anastomoses in the aorta, when completing an end-to-side anastomosis we advocate for the use of straight rather than side-biting clamps when at all possible. The aortotomy should be of sufficient length to accommodate the graft material in question. As with elsewhere, this is typically performed using an 11-blade and Potts or Metzenbaum scissors. Contrary to end-to-end aortic anastomoses, we typically sew in-to-out on the aorta (again in a forehand fashion) when performing end-to-side anastomoses. As with above, double-armed 3.0 polypropylene sutures are used. The graft should be beveled at least 45 degrees to allow the graft to lie parallel to the native aorta (**FIGURE 3-2**). The anastomosis is begun with an anchor stitch at the heel at the 6 o'clock position and then each arm of the suture is carried radially to the 3 o'clock and 9 o'clock position and a second suture is then started with an anchor stitch at the toe at the 12 o'clock position.

Role of the Assistant The assistant plays a vital role in the completion of any anastomosis, but particularly in the case of aortic anastomoses given the need to complete them in an expeditious fashion and the importance of adequate visualization and maintaining constant tension on the suture so that it does not loosen. The assistant plays a dynamic role, maintaining appropriate tension on the suture while manipulating the graft to optimize visualization of the suture site for the operator.

MEDIUM VESSEL (FEMOROPOPLITEAL) ANASTOMOSES: Anastomoses to medium-sized vessels have many of the same considerations as those of larger vessels; however, there are some specific techniques that can be employed to improve outcomes.

Clamping Clamps should be selected based on the caliber of vessel in question and should be placed in such a manner as to optimize visualization and access of the operating surgeon. Clamps may also be placed so as to improve exposure and lift the vessel in question up and into the field in a manner that is advantageous to creation of the anastomosis in question. For vessels with posterior plaque, a clamp can be placed in an AP orientation to flatten the vessel against the plaque without disrupting it. Damp laparotomy pads or towels draped over retractors after clamping and prior to beginning an anastomosis can be useful in holding retractors out of the way and can protect the suture from snagging on clamps and retractors. In the groin we typically employ atraumatic insert clamps or Satinsky clamps (for AP clamping) proximally and straight or angled PV or peripheral DeBakey clamps distally. Small profunda clamps can also be quite helpful, as can Kitzmiller clamps.

Vessel Preparation For bypasses that are coming in medial or lateral to a vessel, it is important to keep in mind the orientation of the bypass to the inflow and outflow vessels. For example, in a femoral-femoral bypass, creating an arteriotomy on a slight angle will help avoid kinking. The arteriotomy is typically started with an 11-blade and then carried to size using Potts scissors. Endarterectomy may be required and should be carried out

to acceptable proximal and distal endpoints. We prefer to extend the arteriotomy several millimeters past the endarterectomy endpoint to ensure adequate visualization and combat stenosis. Handling of the vessels should be done with care, and the unendarterectomized segment of the vessel should be manipulated gently to avoid disruption of the intima and creation of a flap. We avoid tacking sutures unless necessary. In the case of an extended endarterectomy we will typically patch the vessel using bovine pericardium or vein prior to creating a new arteriotomy in the patch to which the anastomosis is performed.

Graft The conduit should be cut to length to mirror the arteriotomy (**FIGURE 3-3A**). A small size discrepancy can been adjusted for; however, a good size match can improve technical outcomes. For prosthetic conduits (Dacron, PTFE) we typically will use a tonsil clamp to create a template to follow for creating a bevel. It can be placed at an angle across the conduit to create a gentle curve. An 11-blade is then run across the top of the clamp's jaws to divide the conduit. It is easier to do this from the heel to the toe rather than the opposite direction.

Anastomosis Similar to end-to-side anastomoses in the aorta, we typically employ an anchor technique beginning at the heel or 6 o'clock position (**FIGURE 3-3A**). At the femoropopliteal position we typically employ 5.0 or 6.0 polypropylene (Prolene) on a BV-1 or C-1 needle. The operator and their assistant typically stand across the table from each other and take turns completing the side of the anastomosis ipsilateral to themselves. In cases where visualization may be difficult, it can be beneficial to complete the more difficult side of the anastomosis first, as this will improve visualization. As with end-to-side anastomoses in the aorta, the one suture is run from the heel to the 3 o'clock and 9 o'clock positions, the arteriotomy and the hood are checked to ensure a size match, and a second suture is then started in an anchor fashion at the toe and run to the midpoint of the anastomosis on each side where it is tied (**FIGURE 3-3B**). Prior to completing the final quadrant of the anastomosis it is important to retrograde and antegrade flush the vessel to clear any potential embolic material and to ensure that inflow or outflow have not been compromised with the suture.

SMALL VESSEL (TIBIAL, PEDAL, DISTAL UPPER EXTREMITY, MESENTERIC) ANASTOMOSES: Small vessel anastomoses can be challenging. Technical precision and gentle handling of the artery and conduit are paramount to success.

Clamping Adequate exposure is of paramount importance prior to clamping tibial vessels to afford adequate hemostasis and access for the arteriotomy and anastomosis. Generally a soft bulldog clamp applied to a soft segment of the vessel is optimal (See Chapter 2, Figure 2-4). In certain cases (e.g., deep vessels or reoperative cases) a tourniquet placed around the distal thigh may offer better control, minimizing the need for distal exposure and avoiding any clamps in the surgical field. In cases of severe arterial calcification, intraluminal control with appropriately sized Fogarty embolectomy balloons can also be used. CONTINUES

3-2

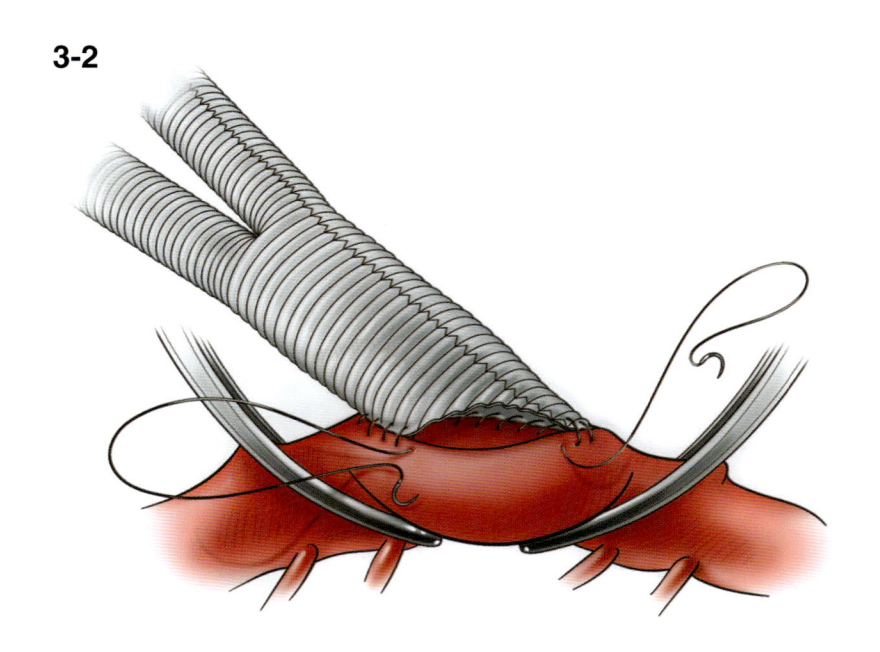

3-3

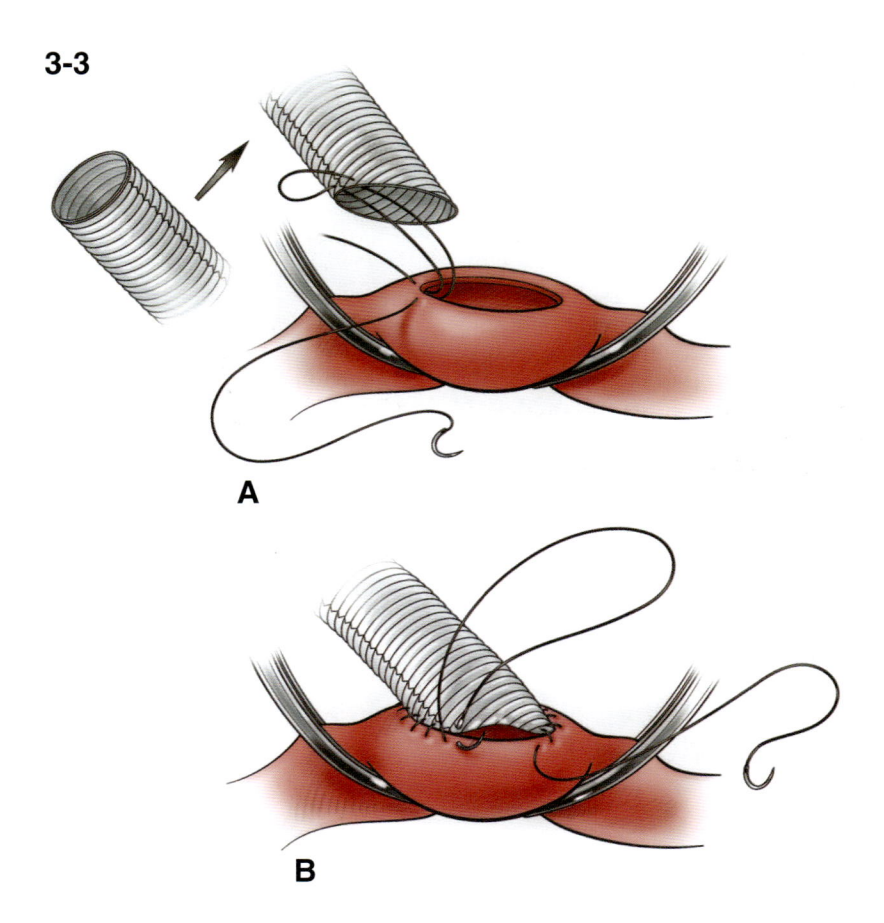

A

B

SMALL VESSEL (TIBIAL, PEDAL, DISTAL UPPER EXTREMITY, MESENTERIC) ANASTOMOSES: Vessel Preparation CONTINUED When making the arteriotomy it is important to remember in small vessels particularly to approach the vessel at a shallow angle so as to not disrupt the backwall of the vessel with the blade. A Beaver blade can also be useful in small calcified vessels. The arteriotomy is then extended, typically using Potts scissors. In calcified vessels a focal removal of calcified shards from the vessel wall at the edge of the arteriotomy is sometimes necessary. Similarly, a focal endarterectomy can be performed if necessary, although this is best avoided by selection of the optimal site for the arteriotomy. The most critical factor for success is continuing the arteriotomy for a distal anastomosis to a widely patent vessel at the anastomotic endpoint or toe.

Conduit Autogenous vein is the preferred conduit in the vast majority of cases. To avoid kinking of the distal anastomosis we perform the proximal anastomosis first. The graft is then pressurized via inflow and both tunneled and measured for length with the conduit fully distended. This helps to prevent twisting of the conduit as well as reduces the risk of cutting the conduit to be either too short, which can place tension on the anastomosis, or too long, which can lead to kinking. The fully pressurized graft is then brought down to the arteriotomy site and a DeBakey forceps is used to grasp the conduit at a 45-degree angle immediately adjunct to the endpoint of the arteriotomy (FIGURE 3-4A). The graft is then cut using an 11-blade or scissors to allow precise orientation of length and angle of the vein graft. The graft is then incised further to match the length of the arteriotomy (FIGURE 3-4B). This creates an optimal "cobra-head" shape to the end of the vein graft (FIGURE 3-4C).

Parachute Parachuting, or beginning the anastomosis without an anchor suture, can be a helpful technique in distal targets when anchoring a bypass graft may compromise exposure to complete the anastomosis. This is particularly helpful in the case of deep or small tibial vessels. A double-armed 6.0 or 7.0 polypropylene suture with a small, typically BV-1, needle is used. The anastomosis is begun offset from the heel of the arteriotomy contralateral to the operator with sufficient distance to allow for two stitches to be placed proximal to the heel (FIGURE 3-5). The anastomosis is started outside-to-in on the conduit and then inside-to-out on the artery, and then protected using a shodded clamp. The suture is then run toward the operating surgeon without bringing the conduit to the artery. The suture is then run around the heel with two bites prior to the heel, one at the heel, and two bites to the side of the operator, for a total of five around the heel. The sutures are then moistened with saline and the conduit is brought down to the artery by pulling gentle tension on the sutures in a see-saw technique. It is important to put equal tension on both arms of the suture to avoid foreshortening one arm of the suture compared to the other. Once this has been completed the anastomosis can be carried out as one would any end-to-side anastomosis; however, it should be noted that a stitch must be taken back out-to-in on the graft to reverse its direction and allow for in-to-out sewing through the artery. Particularly in distal anastomoses it is important to take small but full-thickness bites of the artery with particular attention to the suture at the toe of the anastomosis as a stenosis. We do not advocate for the creation of anastomotic toe using interrupted sutures.

Venous Anastomoses Venous anastomoses can be completed in a similar fashion to arterial anastomoses; however, there are some specific considerations. It is particularly important to be vigilant against inadvertent narrowing of venous anastomoses. One technique to attempt to avoid this is to deliberately introduce redundancy into the suture when creating the anastomosis by way of creating an "air knot" to leave a loop when tying down the suture. An alternative technique is to release the vessel clamps to expand the vessels prior to tying the suture down to allow the suture to be tied down under pressure to avoid stenosing the anastomosis.

PITFALLS Completion examination with physical exam, Doppler, duplex ultrasound, and/or angiography is essential following anastomosis creation to evaluate for intimal flap or stenosis. Early complications of arterial anastomoses include bleeding, dissection, and thrombosis, which should all be identified prior to skin closure based on exam and/or imaging. Stenosis or flap can sometimes be corrected locally; however, revision may be required if the anastomosis appears compromised. Revision can be carried out by taking down and redoing the anastomosis, by patching the anastomosis, or by patching the arteriotomy and completing the anastomosis at a different location, though this may require extension of the conduit. ■

SUGGESTED READINGS

Ailawadi G. Chapter 36. Operative management of aortoiliac occlusive disease. In: Minter RM, Doherty GM, eds. *Current Procedures: Surgery.* McGraw-Hill; Accessed May 17, 2021. https://accesssurgery-mhmedical-com.ezp-prod1.hul.harvard.edu/content.aspx?bookid=429&sectionid=40112050

Aortofemoral bypass. In: Ellison C, Zollinger RM, eds. *Zollinger's Atlas of Surgical Operations.* McGraw Hill, 2016;522–525.

Arnaoutakis DJ, Belkin M. Surgical management of aortoiliac occlusive disease. In: Moore WS, Lawrence PF, Oderich GS, eds. *Vascular and Endovascular Surgery: A Comprehensive Review.* Elsevier, 2019;358–369.

Femoropopliteal reconstruction. In: Ellison C, Zollinger RM, eds. *Zollinger's Atlas of Surgical Operations.* McGraw Hill, 2016;530–539.

Kabbani LS, Henke PK. Chapter 37. Surgical revascularization of infrainguinal arterial occlusive disease. In: Minter RM, Doherty GM, eds. *Current Procedures: Surgery.* McGraw-Hill; Accessed May 17, 2021. https://accesssurgery-mhmedical-com.ezp-prod1.hul.harvard.edu/content.aspx?bookid=429&sectionid=40112051

Sidawy AN, Neville RF. Technique: Open surgical. In: Sidway AN, Perler BA, eds. *Rutherford's Vascular Surgery and Endovascular Therapy.* Elsevier, 2019;727–746.

3-4

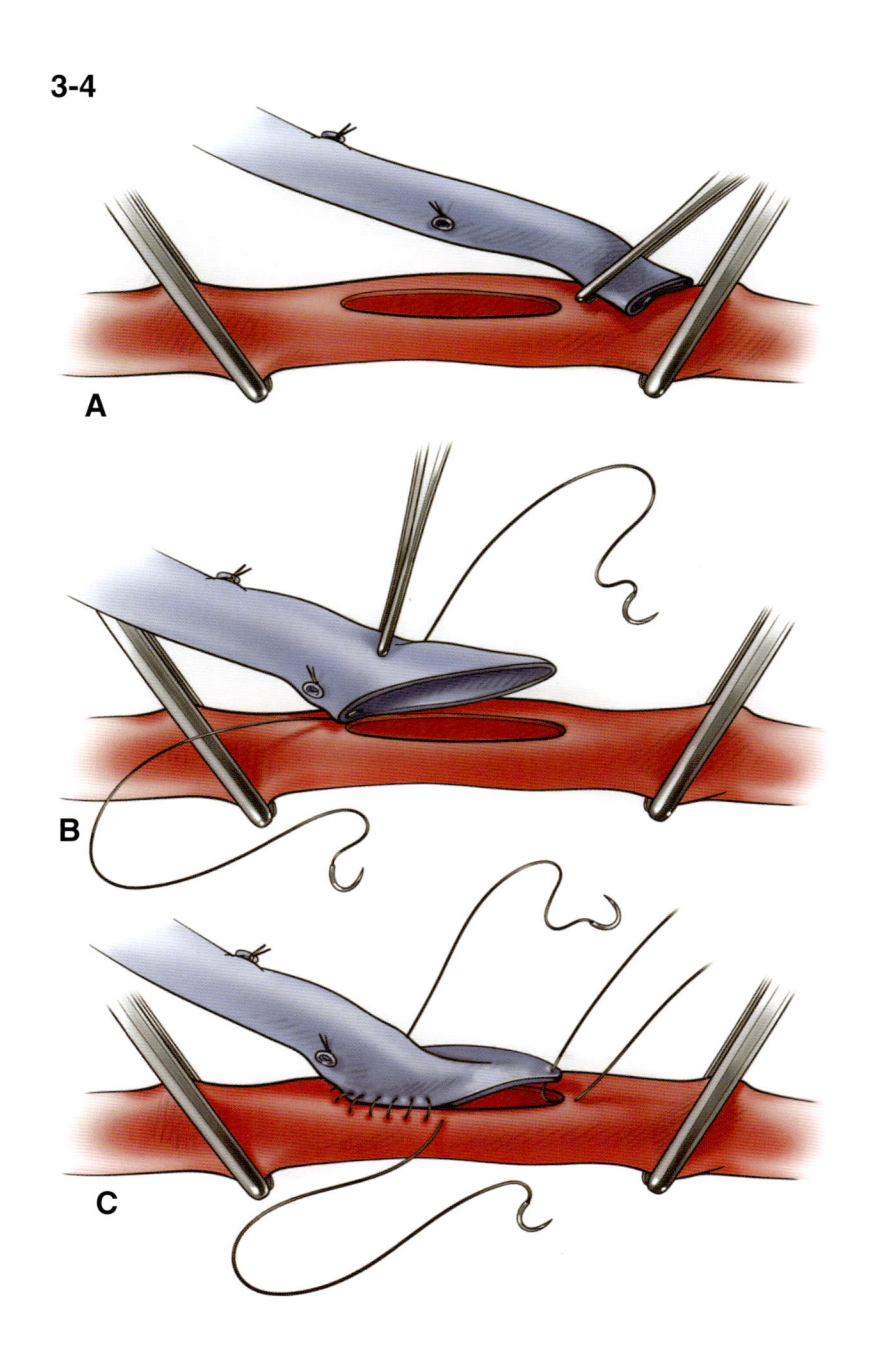

A

B

C

3-5

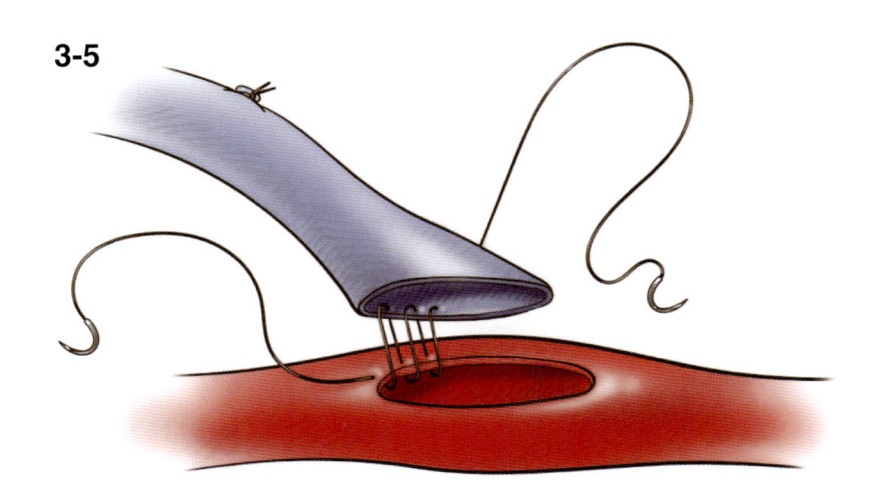

Harvesting and Preparing Vein Conduit

Bala Ramanan, MBBS • Greg Modrall, MD

HARVESTING GREAT SAPHENOUS VEIN

PREOPERATIVE PREPARATION

Duplex Ultrasound Bilateral venous duplex ultrasonography assessing the size and conduit suitability is essential prior to vascular reconstruction using great saphenous vein (GSV). Typically GSVs <3 mm or with evidence of inflammation, occlusion, or calcification are not utilized as conduits for bypass surgeries.

DETAILS OF PROCEDURE

Open Vein Harvest The course of the vein should be marked using preoperative ultrasound to identify its location and to avoid creating flaps during harvest. The whole leg is prepped and gently angled to expose the complete GSV (FIGURE 4-1). An initial 3- to 5-cm incision is made at the saphenofemoral junction, which is usually located 2.5 to 4 cm inferior and lateral to the pubic tubercle. The vein is located and carefully dissected with closed fine scissors to identify its course under the skin. The subcutaneous tissue is divided with electrocautery or scissors. Care should be taken to open the fascia above the GSV to fully expose the vessel (FIGURE 4-2A).

Skip incisions have been shown to decrease wound complications and should be used if feasible (FIGURE 4-2B). The required length of the GSV is exposed. Once the vein is exposed throughout its course, a vessel loop is passed around the vein to facilitate circumferential dissection using "no-touch" technique. Injury to the adjacent saphenous nerve must be avoided to prevent postoperative neuralgias. The vein side branches are carefully dissected with fine scissors and ligated with silk sutures (FIGURE 4-3). Side branch ligatures should be placed at an appropriate distance from the vein wall to allow complete distension of the vein and to prevent local narrowing of the vein lumen that may be difficult to correct later (FIGURE 4-4). Side branch stumps that are too long may be snagged during tunneling and result in damage to the conduit. Side branches that are missed and inadvertently transected flush with the vein are repaired with fine (7-0) polypropylene suture when the vein is distended. After the dissection is complete, the vein is left in situ until the arterial exposure is complete. Once arterial exposure is complete, the length of vein exposed is confirmed to be adequate prior to dividing it. The GSV is harvested by dividing it at the saphenofemoral junction, which is oversewn with a two-layer vascular closure consisting of 5-0 or 6-0 polypropylene sutures. **CONTINUES ▶**

4-1

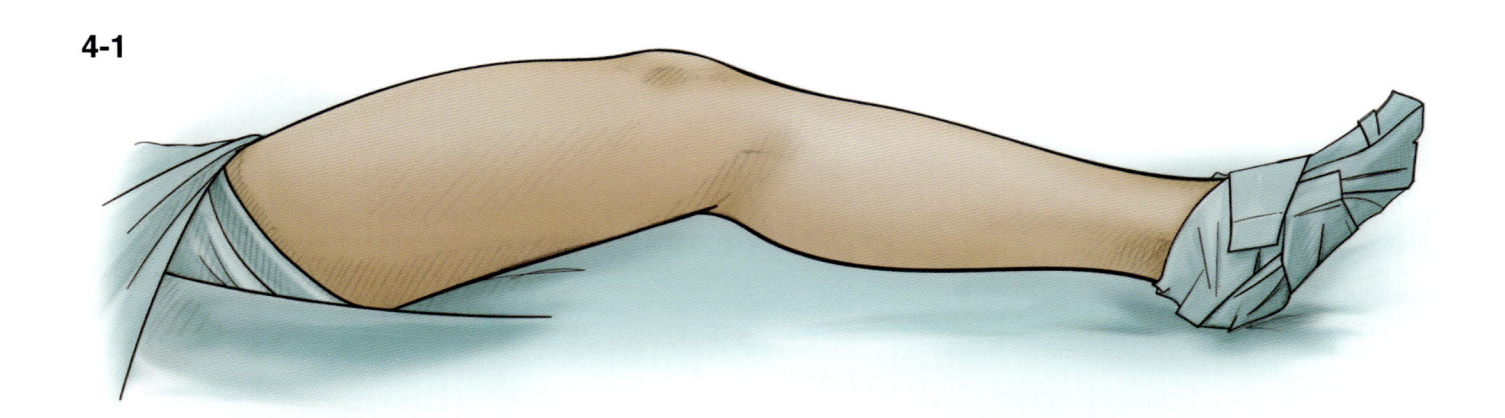

4-2

Saphenous vein

A

Saphenous vein

B

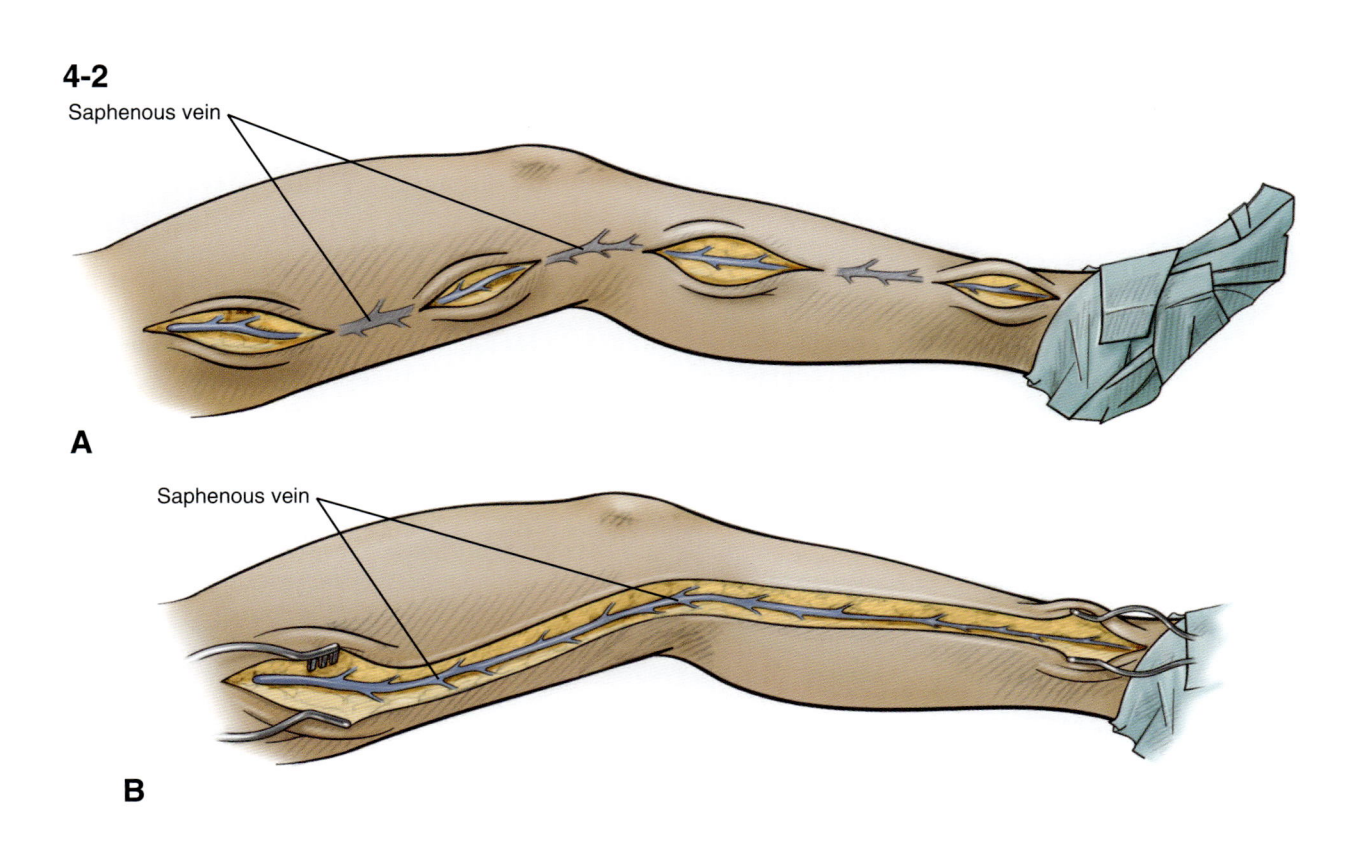

4-3

4-4

Avoid constriction

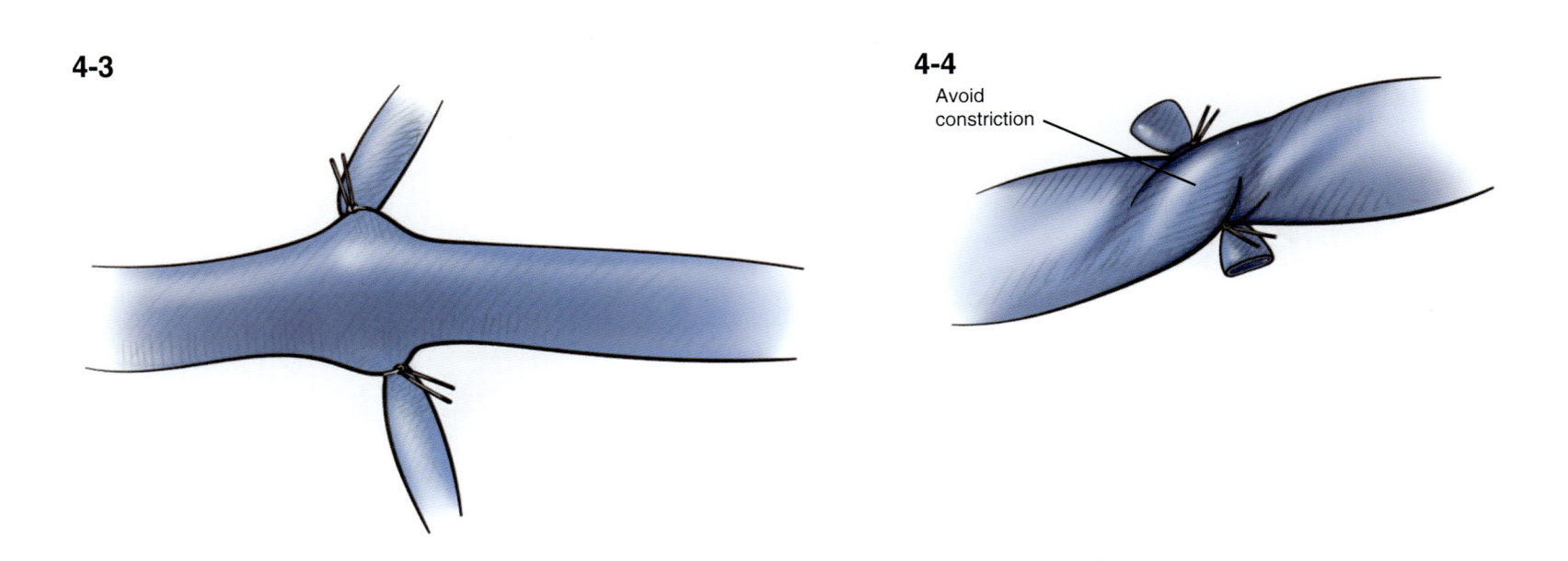

DETAILS OF PROCEDURE: *Ex Vivo Preparation of the Vein* **CONTINUED** The caudal end of the vein is canulated with a fine plastic or metal canula. Gentle dilation of the orifice with a fine mosquito clamp may facilitate cannulation (FIGURE 4-5). Some operators fix the canula in place with a tie. The GSV is then flushed with a physiologic solution to identify leaks or damage to the vein wall (FIGURE 4-6). Overdistension of the vein should be avoided to prevent endothelial damage, which may affect graft patency. If a branch stump is visible at the site of the leak this can be repaired with a ligature. All holes or tears in the vein wall need to be repaired with 7-0 polypropylene sutures. The vein is then kept in the physiologic solution until implantation.

After ensuring hemostasis, the incisions are closed in layers with absorbable sutures for the subcutaneous and deep dermal tissues. The skin is closed with either a running subcuticular suture with absorbable monofilament or skin staples.

POSTOPERATIVE CARE: Open vein harvest techniques are associated with a higher risk of surgical site infections (SSIs), with reported incidences ranging from 2 to 25, so postoperative close follow-up is necessary. Use of a continuous incision to harvest the GSV has been associated with a higher risk of SSIs in some studies. Endoscopic vein harvest was developed as a minimally invasive alternative to the traditional open harvest. Endoscopic harvesting is associated with improved wound healing and cosmesis, but the coronary artery bypass literature suggests that long-term graft patency may be inferior.

DEEP VEIN HARVEST

INDICATIONS: Femoropopliteal vein (FPV) graft, or "deep vein," is most commonly used for in situ reconstruction of the aortoiliac segment after removal of infected aortic grafts. However, this graft can be used for multiple major vascular reconstructions due to its large caliber, durability, infection resistance, compliance, kink resistance, and ability to accommodate tortuous anatomy.

PREOPERATIVE PREPARATION: Bilateral venous duplex ultrasonography is essential when planning vascular reconstruction using FPV. Duplex ultrasound allows assessment of the diameter and suitability of the conduit. FPVs <6 mm or evidence of prior DVT preclude use of the FPV. Depending on the body habitus, the vein has a usable length of 40 to 50 cm. Duplications are found in 25% of patients and are not contraindications for vein harvest. In 7%, congenital abnormalities such as diminutive or absent FPVs are found. If the FPV is absent or incomplete, there is often a profunda femoris vein that is located posteriorly in the thigh and connects with the popliteal vein, which can used as a conduit. However, an enlarged profunda femoris vein may be indicative of prior FPV thrombosis. The GSV is also mapped, in the event that a lower extremity bypass is required. Whenever possible, concurrent FPV and GSV harvest in the same leg should be avoided due to the increased risk of acute compartment syndrome in this scenario.

DETAILS OF PROCEDURE

Exposure The patient is positioned supine with the donor leg or legs bent at the knee and externally rotated in "frog-leg" position. Sterile iodine-impregnated drapes are applied to limit contamination of the thigh incisions. A two-team approach may be used to optimize operative time if bilateral vein harvest is necessary. The incision is placed over the lateral border of the sartorius muscle from the anterior superior iliac spine to the medial condyle of the tibia (FIGURE 4-7A). If a short segment of the vein is needed, a smaller incision can be used. The sartorius muscle is reflected medially to preserve its blood supply. The subsartorial canal is entered and the fascia overlying the femoral vessels is incised (FIGURE 4-7B). To expose the popliteal vein, the adductor magnus tendon is divided and the adductor canal is entered. Care is taken to preserve the great saphenous vein in the event that it needed for a concomitant or future bypass. Injury to the saphenous nerve either directly or by traction should be avoided to prevent postoperative neuralgia. Arterial collaterals, especially those near the adductor hiatus, should be preserved to prevent unexpected limb ischemia in patients with preexisting occlusive disease in the femoropopliteal arterial segments.

Harvest The FPV is always harvested from the confluence with the profunda femoris vein extending distally. It is important to avoid a creating a stump where the FPV is detached from the common femoral vein (FIGURE 4-8). A stump at this location may become a nidus for thrombus formation that can cause a pulmonary embolism. The FPV has multiple large and small side branches. Small side branches are doubly ligated in close apposition to the vein wall with 3-0 silk suture and are divided at least 2 mm distal to the ligature. This technique contrasts with the technique for ligating saphenous vein branches in which side branches are ligated away from the vein wall to prevent narrowing of the lumen. Due to the large size of the FPV, the closely applied ligature does not compromise the lumen. Furthermore, the vein wall is thin at branch points and the suture helps gather the thin wall of the vein into the ligature. Branches larger than 3 mm are suture-ligated with 5-0 polypropylene suture. These measures are taken to prevent exsanguinating hemorrhage from rupture of a thinned-out vein wall or from a dislodged, or "popped," tie, which carries a 36% mortality risk.

Ex Vivo Preparation The vein can be left in situ until needed for arterial reconstruction. Although Clagett and colleagues described the FPV harvesting, infected graft excision, use of the FPV for aortoiliac reconstruction in one setting, Ali and colleagues described a modification of this approach in which the veins are fully exposed and all branches divided with the vein left connected proximally and distally one day prior to the graft excision. This approach breaks the operation into two smaller components, avoiding an arduous, lengthy operation at one setting. After the FPV is harvested, the graft is completely everted and the valves are excised under direct vision with fine scissors (FIGURE 4-9). This technique was developed because FPV valves are large and often incompletely lysed by valvulotomies, which can lead to vein graft stenosis and early graft failure. The graft is then inverted back prior to implantation. Usually two closed drains are left in the harvest bed before closing the incisions in multiple layers.

POSTOPERATIVE CARE: Drains are removed once the output is serous and less than 30 mL for 24 hours. As many as 15–20% of patients require fasciotomy due to acute compartment syndrome after deep vein harvest. Risk factors for acute compartment syndrome after FPV harvest include low preoperative ankle-brachial index (ABI) and concurrent ipsilateral GSV harvest. Leg edema is almost universal in the early postoperative period. However, duplex of the lower extremity veins is not necessary. Many will have a thrombus in the ligated popliteal vein stump, but the significance of this is unknown and patients are not anticoagulated based on this finding. In the long term, clinical evidence of chronic venous morbidity (C3–C6) is found in only 15% of harvested limbs and the majority (85%) have no significant chronic venous insufficiency. Patients with FPV graft reconstructions are followed postoperatively with ABIs, toe pressure, and duplex scan of the graft every 6 months. ■

SUGGESTED READINGS

Chung J, Clagett GP. Neoaortoiliac System (NAIS) procedure for the treatment of the infected aortic graft. *Semin Vasc Surg.* 2011;24(4):220-226.

Domingos SR Souza, Arbeus M, Pinheiro BB, Filbey D. The no-touch technique of harvesting the saphenous vein for coronary artery bypass grafting surgery. *Multimed Man Cardiothorac Surg.* 2009 Jan 1;2009(731):mmcts.2008.003524.

Smith ST, Clagett GP. Femoral vein harvest for vascular reconstructions: pitfalls and tips for success. *Semin Vasc Surg.* 2008;21(1):35-40.

Zingaro C, Cefarelli M, Berretta P, Matteucci S, Pierri M, Di Eusanio M. Endoscopic vein-graft harvesting in coronary artery bypass surgery: Tips and tricks. *Multimed Man Cardiothorac Surg.* 2019 Jul 9:2019. doi: 10/1510/mmcts.2019.019.

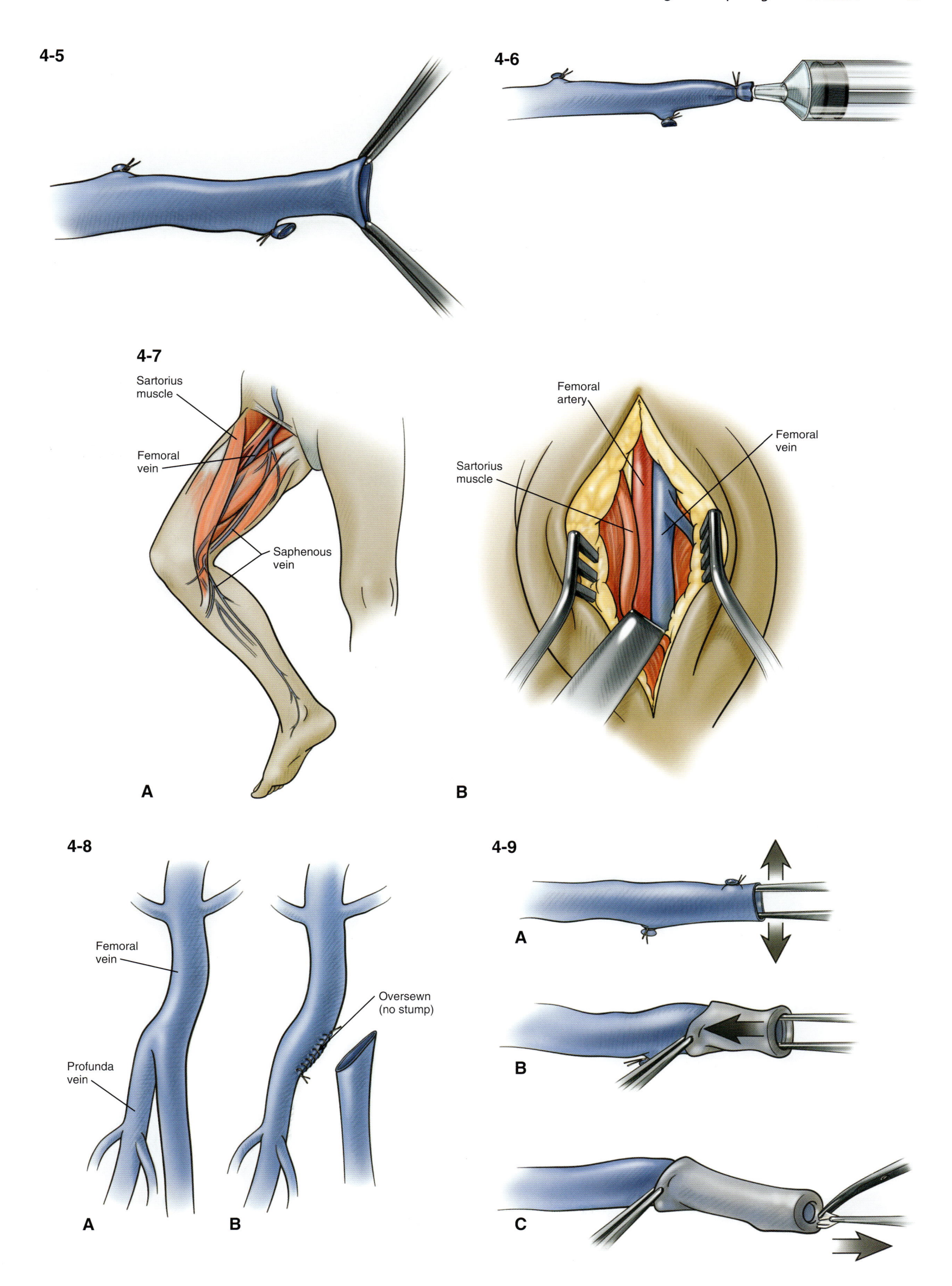

4-5

4-6

4-7

Sartorius
muscle

Femoral
vein

Saphenous
vein

Femoral
artery

Sartorius
muscle

Femoral
vein

A

B

4-8

Femoral
vein

Profunda
vein

Oversewn
(no stump)

A   **B**

4-9

A

B

C

BASIC CONCEPTS: ENDOVASCULAR TECHNIQUES

Vascular Access, Sheaths, and Guiding Catheters

Ocean Setia, MBBS • Jonathan A. Cardella, MD, FRCS, FACS

INDICATIONS Endovascular techniques have become a quintessential skill for vascular surgeons. The core principles of endovascular surgery are comprised of establishing safe access, appropriate selection of devices (sheaths, wires, catheters, and treatment devices), and a secure closure. Endovascular therapy has gained massive popularity for many different vascular pathologies as it enables treatment to be performed in a minimally invasive fashion, while allowing for expedited patient recovery. Endovascular procedures are performed for a number of indications including, but not limited to, atherosclerotic occlusive disease, aneurysmal disease, arteriovenous malformations (AVM), cerebrovascular disease, deep venous thrombosis (DVT), traumatic vascular injuries, iatrogenic injuries, dialysis access, and central venous access.

ACCESS SITE SELECTION Determination of an appropriate access site is a key first step in endovascular surgery, with several factors considered. An optimal access site is easily accessible, has the ability to achieve hemostasis with manual pressure, and allows safe and quick conversion to open. The site of entry should always be tailored to the type intervention being performed, as it should allow a straightforward approach to the vascular bed of interest. The access vessel should be able to accommodate the size of endovascular devices being used during the procedure, and thus a careful assessment should be made of the vessel diameter and size of intended devices. In addition, review of preoperative imaging can help identify vessel calcification, stenosis, occlusion, and tortuosity, which could be limiting factors in obtaining access or traversing devices to the vascular bed of interest.

The most common site for endovascular access is the common femoral artery (CFA). It allows access to a number of vascular beds in the body, such as the lower extremities, aorta and arch vessels, visceral vessels, and cerebral vasculature. It is easily palpable in the groin region, can be compressed against the femoral head for hemostasis, and has adequate caliber to accommodate most commonly used endovascular devices, making it an ideal access vessel for most endovascular procedures. The CFA is accessed in a retrograde or antegrade fashion, depending on the vascular bed requiring treatment. Review of imaging to determine vessel tortuosity, calcification, and distance of the vascular bed of interest from the access site will help guide a retrograde or antegrade approach.

The second most common access site is the brachial artery. Similar to the CFA, it satisfies the criteria of an optimal access and has ease of access to various areas of body, including upper extremities, aorta and visceral vessels, and cerebral vessels; however, it is of smaller diameter, and this needs to be considered when choosing devices. Some of the other less commonly used access sites include popliteal artery, tibial arteries, carotid artery, radial artery, and axillary artery, any of which can be utilized depending on the type of planned procedure. For most venous interventions, femoral or popliteal veins are the most common site of access. The use of other options for venous access sites, such as greater saphenous vein, internal jugular vein, upper extremity veins, and so on, varies with location of the pertinent lesion and procedure type. Occasionally, an open cutdown should be considered, particularly if large-bore devices are being planned or if the point of access is not over a bony, prominence.

POSITIONING AND ANESTHESIA For most endovascular procedures, patients are laid supine on the operating table. The arms are secured to the sides to allow for efficient maneuvering of the imaging unit around the operative table. Our usual practice is to sterilely prepare both groins when using CFA access, and instituting a wide area of sterile preparation in case of conversion to open. If brachial access is used, the arm should be extended, supinated, and appropriately secured on an arm board. A circumferential extremity sterile preparation is employed for brachial access.

Prone positioning is usually required if popliteal access is being planned, with wide sterile preparation of the lower extremity circumferentially. A vascular exam is performed and the pulses and/or Doppler signals are marked preoperatively.

Choice of anesthesia for endovascular procedures should be tailored to the patient and procedure. Most procedures can be performed under moderate sedation with monitored anesthesia care and local anesthesia, but more complex cases with longer operative times require general anesthesia. Patient factors such as high-risk comorbidities, increased aspiration risk, anxiety, and inability to maintain immobility during the procedure should also be considered when selecting the right type of anesthesia.

DETAILS OF PROCEDURE Although several access techniques such as manual palpation, double wall puncture, and ultrasound (US)-guided access have been described in various texts, our preference is to use the micropuncture technique with dual image guidance. Fluoroscopy helps identify the appropriate puncture location in relation to the anatomical landmarks, while US allows for direct visualization of the needle passing through the tissue into the vessel. This technique enables a safe and precise access with minimal vessel trauma, reducing postoperative access–related complications.

MICROPUNCTURE ACCESS TECHNIQUE: For CFA access, the femoral pulse is palpated in the groin between the bony landmarks of the anterior superior iliac spine and the pubic symphysis. We place a hemostatic clamp on the skin and use fluoroscopy to confirm location of the instrument tip over the mid-femoral head (**FIGURE 5-1**). This area is then marked with a skin marker. US is then used to identify the CFA, femoral bifurcation, superficial femoral artery (SFA), and profunda artery (**FIGURE 5-2**). The additional benefit of ultrasonography is real-time assessment of the access vessel for calcification, size, patency, and/or tortuosity. Any heavily calcified areas should be avoided.

Once the site of entry is determined, local anesthetic is injected into the skin and subcutaneous tissue. The US probe is stabilized, with one hand keeping the access vessel in the middle of the image field. Using the other hand, a 21-gauge micropuncture needle is advanced. The entry point of the needle on the skin is 1 to 2 cm away from the US probe at a 45- to 60-degree angle (**FIGURE 5-3**). The CFA is punctured under direct visualization. Brisk arterial flow indicates presence of the needle tip in the vessel lumen. A short 0.018-inch guidewire is then passed into the vessel and visualized in the lumen with the US. Fluoroscopy is used to confirm the location of the needle tip and guidewire (**FIGURE 5-4**). Once satisfactory positioning of the tip over the mid-femoral head is confirmed, a small skin incision is made at the site of needle entry and a hemostatic clamp is used to dilate the track in the subcutaneous tissue. The micropuncture needle is removed and the introducer sheath is placed. Next, the inner dilator and the short 0.018-inch guidewire is removed, and a 0.035-inch wire with a soft, atraumatic tip is advanced under fluoroscopic guidance. The introducer sheath is then exchanged over the wire for the desired sheath for the procedure, and placement is confirmed with fluoroscopy. A number of wires, catheters, and specialized devices can be introduced via the sheath to carry out the procedure.

Vascular access at other sites, including the brachial artery, is obtained with a similar micropuncture technique. During venous access, brisk flow is usually not encountered on puncture due to the low-pressure venous system. A syringe attached to the micropuncture needle can be used for aspiration during the puncture. A flash of blood indicates needle entry into the vessel lumen.

5-1

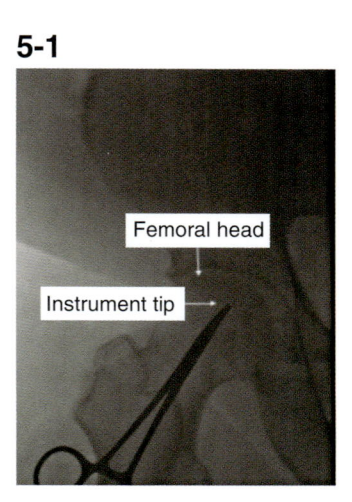

Figure 5-1 Fluoroscopic image showing use of hemostatic clamp to locate the mid femoral head.

5-2

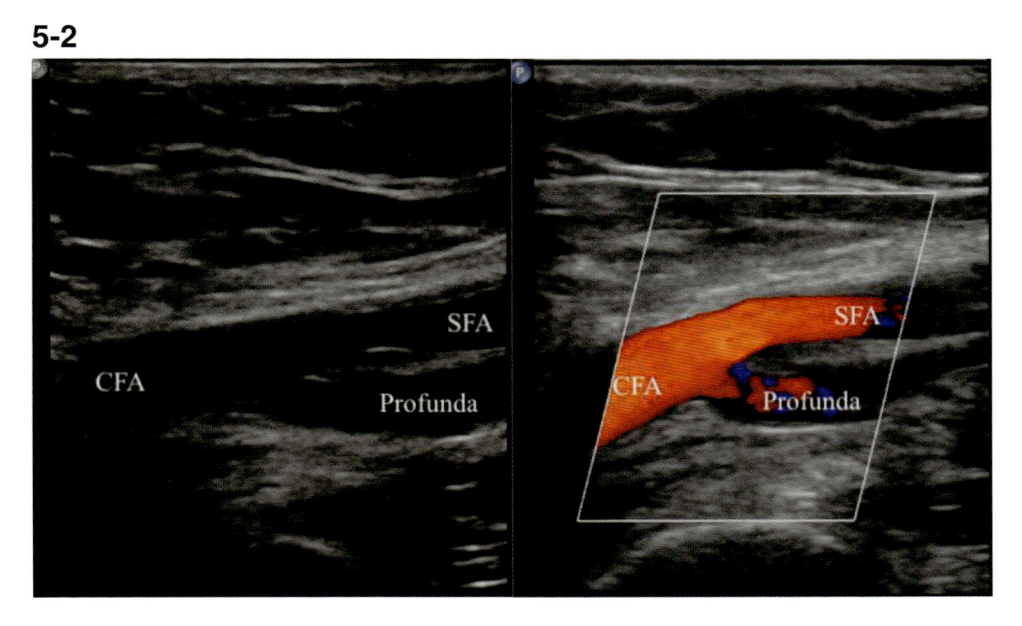

Figure 5-2 Ultrasound image showing common femoral artery (CFA), femoral bifurcation, superficial femoral artery (SFA), and profunda artery.

5-3

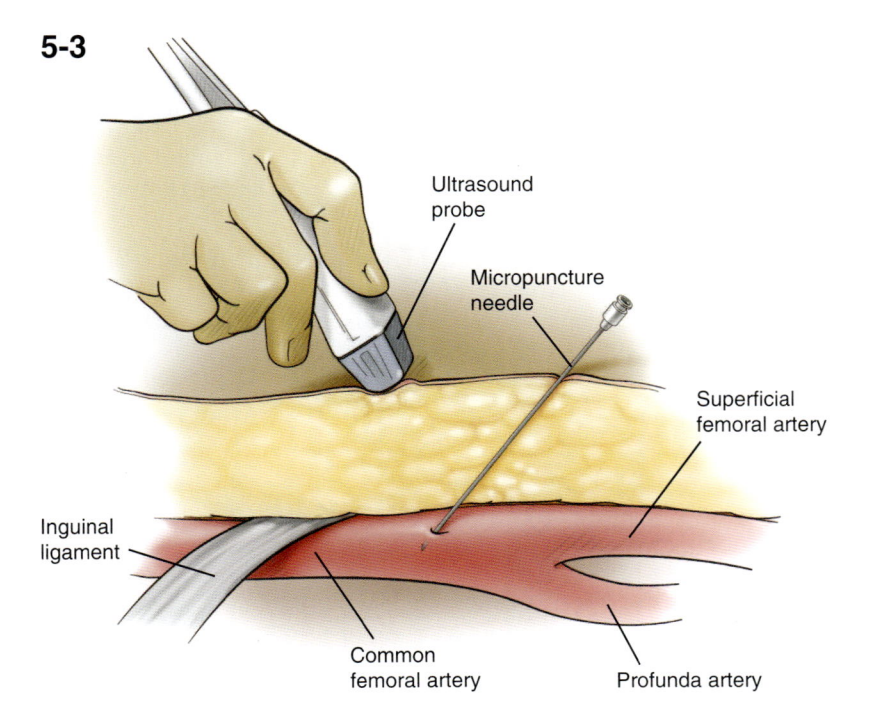

Figure 5-3 Image depicting positioning of needle in relation to ultrasound probe and correct angulation at the entry point.

5-4

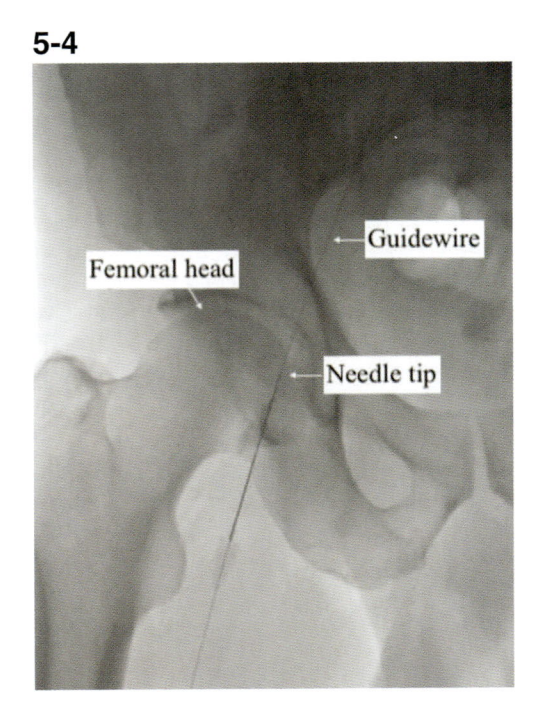

Figure 5-4 Fluoroscopy image showing micropuncture needle tip and guidewire location in relation to the femoral head.

SHEATHS Sheaths are placed to maintain access to the vessel throughout the duration of an endovascular procedure and serve as a conduit for insertion of a variety of devices into the vascular system. Sheaths have a tapered tip inner dilator which prevents injury to the vessel during insertion. The inner dilator is removed once the sheath is placed. Some sheaths have radiopaque markers at the tip for easy identification during fluoroscopy. Sheaths have a hemostatic valve which prevents back-bleeding whether or not there is an indwelling wire or device in the vessel lumen. All sheaths have a side port which allows contrast injection or administration of fluids and medications (FIGURE 5-5).

Sizing of a sheath is based on the inner diameter and is measured in French size (1 French [F] = 1/3 mm). Commonly used sheath sizes range from 4F to 11F (sizes ranging to 24F) and have universal color-coded hubs for quick and easy identification. There is also a wide range of sheath lengths. Generally, a longer sheath should be used to hold position near the vascular bed to be treated, to ease in device exchange. Stiff sheaths can be used if the access vessel has heavy calcification or if there is extensive scar tissue at the site of insertion, or flexible hydrophilic sheaths can be used to negotiate tortuous anatomy. Thus, the sheath size, length, and type should be personalized for each case based on lesion location, device compatibility, vessel characteristics, and access site of choice.

Some noteworthy specialty sheaths that we use in our practice are mentioned below:

- TourGuide steerable sheath (Medtronic): The tip of this sheath can be deflected up to 180 degrees and has the advantage of retaining the tip curve at the desired deflection angle. It is an excellent tool that facilitates efficient navigation through difficult anatomy and engaging angulated vessel takeoff (e.g., visceral vessels) while maintaining a stable platform for insertion and exchange of various catheters and devices through the sheath lumen. It is available in three working lengths— 45, 55, and 90 cm.
- GORE DrySeal Flex Introducer Sheath (W.L. Gore & Associates, Inc.): This large-bore sheath can house multiple devices simultaneously, thus minimizing the need for multiple exchanges. This sheath has a special GORE DrySeal valve which can be pressurized by injecting saline into it to create a seal that maintains excellent hemostasis, even when multiple devices are accommodated in the lumen. This sheath is especially useful in complex aortic interventions where multiple devices are needed through a single access point.

GUIDING CATHETERS Guiding catheters are delivery devices that provide a sturdy, supportive platform for working catheters, wires, and other specialized devices such as microcatheters to reach the anatomical destination from a remote access site during an endovascular procedure.

Guiding catheters have certain distinctive characteristics that differentiate them from diagnostic catheters. These catheters are hydrophilic, have stiffer shafts, and are have reinforced two- to three-layer construction. The internal lumen diameter is larger due to thinner walls, and the diameter remains constant throughout the catheter length, allowing easy advancement and exchange of working devices. Guiding catheters are rather similar in function to guiding sheaths, but unlike sheaths, they lack hemostatic valves and inner dilators. They have short and more angulated tips, and are available in numerous tip configurations, sizes, and lengths. Guiding catheters facilitate the selective cannulation of vessels and aid in keeping the ostium engaged while working catheters, wires, and devices are maneuvered through. In addition, they can be used for contrast injections at the target vascular bed, thus acting as diagnostic catheters if needed.

Although not as widely used in the scope of vascular surgery practice except in procedures involving renal, visceral, or aortic arch vessels, they are popular in cardiovascular and neurovascular interventions.

CLOSURE Direct manual pressure is held over the access site with two or three fingers to compress the access vessel against the underlying bony structures (e.g., femoral head for CFA access). Manual pressure can be held for 15 to 30 minutes depending on sheath size, anticoagulation status, and vessel calcification. For venous access, shorter duration of manual pressure (5–10 minutes) is usually adequate to achieve hemostasis.

Assisted compression devices, such as FemoStop Gold Femoral Compression System (Abbott), SafeGuard Pressure Assisted Device (Merit Medical), and TR BAND Radial Compression Device (Terumo Medical), can provide external compression at the access site. These can be used if a prolonged period of direct external pressure is required; however, they are likely not as effective as manual compression, and if left unattended for extended periods can be dangerous.

There are several commercially available vascular closure devices that can be used to close the arteriotomy, thus allowing immediate hemostasis and enabling expedited postoperative ambulation. Some examples of widely used closure devices are:

- Perclose ProGlide (Abbott): utilizes suture-mediated closure of the arterial puncture site (FIGURE 5-6A and B).
- StarClose SE Vascular Closure System (Abbott): employs use of a nitinol clip to close the arteriotomy.
- ANGIO-SEAL VIP Vascular Closure Device (Terumo Medical): uses a bioabsorbable copolymer anchor and a collagen plug to create a mechanical seal at the arteriotomy site.
- MYNXGRIP Vascular Closure Device (Cordis, Cardinal Health): utilizes a polyethylene glycol (PEG) sealant at the arteriotomy site and tissue tract to achieve hemostasis. ∎

SUGGESTED READINGS

Balceniuk MD, Sebastian A, Schroeder AC, et al. Regional variation in usage of ultrasound-guided femoral access in the vascular quality initiative. *Ann Vasc Surg.* 2021 Apr; Epub 2020/09/20. doi: 10.1016/j.avsg.2020.08.156.

Bazan HA, Le L, Donovan M, et al. Retrograde pedal access for patients with critical limb ischemia. *J Vasc Surg.* 2014 Aug; 60(2), 375-382. doi:10.1016/j.jvs.2014.02.038.

Christopher W. McQuinn and Kristine C. Orion. Endovascular diagnostic technique. In: Sidaway A, Perler B, eds. *Rutherford's Surgery and Endovascular Therapy.* 10th ed. Philadelphia, PA: Elsevier. pp 790-802.

Lumsden AB. Ultrasound Guided Femoral Access [Video]. Debakey Institute for Cardiovascular Education & Training: Houston Methodist Debakey Heart & Vascular Center. https://mdvideos.houstonmethodist.org/videos/ultrasound-guided-femoral-access

Maeda K, Ohki T. Endovascular therapeutic technique. In: Sidawy A, Perler B, eds. *Rutherford's Vascular Surgery and Endovascular Therapy.* 9th ed. Philadelphia, PA: Elsevier.

Perry M, Callas PW, Alef MJ, Bertges DJ. Outcomes of peripheral vascular interventions via retrograde pedal access for chronic limb-threatening ischemia in a multicenter registry. *J Endovasc Ther.* 2020 Apr; 27(2), 205-210. doi:10.1177/1526602820908056.

Ramirez JL, Zarkowsky DS, Sorrentino TA, et al. Antegrade common femoral artery closure device use is associated with decreased complications. *J Vasc Surg.* 2020 Nov; 72(5), 1610-1617. doi: 10.1016/j.jvs.2020.01.052.

5-5

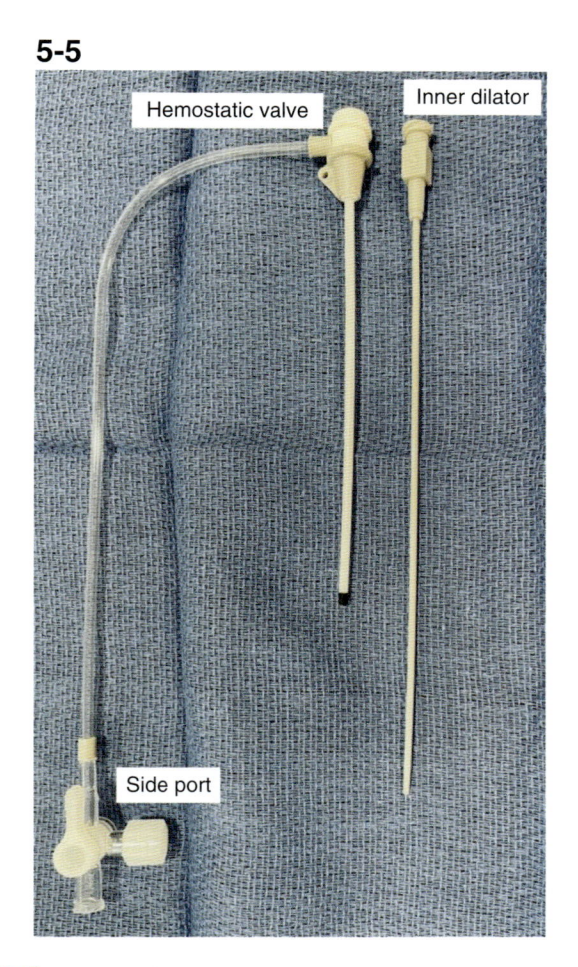

Figure 5-5 Image of a sheath depicting hemostatic valve, side port, and inner dilator.

5-6

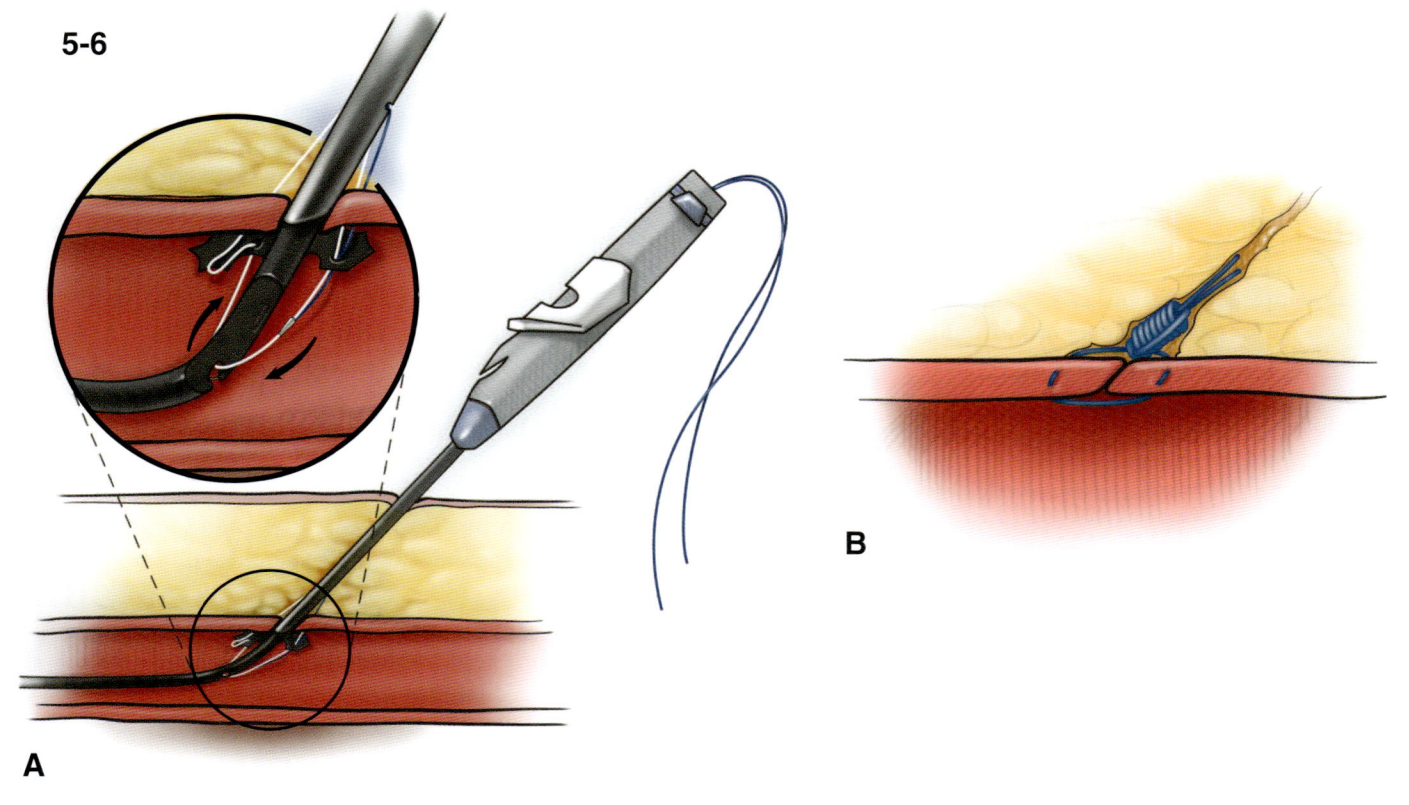

Figure 5-6 ProGlide closure technique.

WIRES AND CATHETERS

Karem Harth, MD

INDICATIONS Successful application of endovascular therapies involves knowing and understanding which wires and catheters will allow the interventionalist to maximize success of the proposed therapy. Like most vascular surgery, it is important to have a good understanding of the available tools to assure optimal outcome as one maneuvers through challenging anatomy and pathologies. Modern-day endovascular therapies are approached in many different ways, and how one chooses to approach the lesion will also define the selection of wires and catheters. Some key examples that highlight the growing diversity of approaches include radial artery-based interventions, antegrade femoral access, and retrograde pedal access. Mastery of the available endoluminal wires and catheters prepares the operator for success.

WIRES Wires are crucial throughout the procedure, as they help us navigate within the vessels to a desired destination, and once we get to that point, they provide the necessary support to carry out endovascular therapies. A single wire is often not sufficient to provide a therapy. Factors that determine selection of a wire include how far away from the access point the lesion is located, how much support is necessary, the size of the vessel being treated, the underlying pathology being treated, the challenges associated with that lesion, and the therapy being delivered.

Wires come in standard sizes measured in inches and commonly include an 0.014-, 0.018-, 0.035- and 0.038-inch wires. Strength and support increase with increasing wire diameter. The diameter chosen for intervention is related to the size of the target vascular bed, and one will often downsize or alternate wires during the navigation of complex anatomy. (Aortoiliac requires 0.035 while tibial, renal, and carotid usually require 0.018- and 0.014-diameter to ultimately deliver therapy.) The lengths vary, and commonly include 180, 260, and 300 cm. Slight variations in available lengths do exist, and choice of length should be dictated by distance from access point to the final destination and should include additional length to ensure support beyond the point of intended therapy. Required length of wire is often less when using a monorail versus an over-the-wire device.

Wires are engineered to have a core, body, and variable tips and coatings (FIGURE 6-1). This ultimately leads to variety of wires of diverse composition, with characteristics that affect steering, tracking, support, pushability, and flexibility [1–3]. The core runs along the length of the wire from tip to end of the shaft. It affects flexibility, support, and tracking ability. The core is generally made of a composite of stainless steel and nitinol. Stainless steel is stiffer, retains its shape better, and is important in supportive wires. Nitinol is malleable and flexible, allowing for better tracking in tortuous vessels and less kinking. For initial access, a less stiff wire with a soft tip is desired but once the lesion has been crossed and the device is ready to be delivered, then a stiffer wire with better support is required.

When the core goes all the way to the tip of the wire, it is called a "core to tip design." These tips allow for better steerability, durability, and tactile feedback, necessary for challenging lesions. In comparison, a "shaping ribbon design" is more delicate and soft, as the core does not go all the way to the tip. In the latter design, the core is interrupted and replaced by areas of constant core diameter or grinds. These tips are easier to shapeand less likely to injure a vessel.

A short, tapered core is flexible but does not track very far into a branch vessel before the stiffer portion encounters the angle and may cause the tip to prolapse out of the desired branch/target vessel. A long taper has a tip that is less supportive but can advance further into a branch vessel before encountering the stiffer portion of the wire.

Wire polymer coatings can be hydrophilic or hydrophobic. Hydrophilic coatings provide increased lubricity to aid in better tracking but at the expense of reducing tactile feedback. Wires will track and steer better in tortuous vessels and allow for lesion crossing. In comparison, hydrophobic coatings provide less tracking due to increased friction but provide better tactile feedback to the user.

The relative characteristics of a guidewire relate to how steerable they are, how they track along a vessel, how much support they provide, and their relative pushability and flexibility (FIGURE 6-2; guidewires from left to right: Spartacore 0.014″, Glidewire 0.035″, Rosen 0.035, Lunderquist 0.035″). Nonsteerable wires are often floppy-tipped, and the core provides the support needed to exchange catheters and sheaths. The tip is often straight or J-shaped (e.g., Bentson and J-wire, respectively). Steerable wires are often hydrophilic and provide the ability to navigate angles and challenging anatomy (e.g., Glidewire; Roadrunner). The most supportive wires are the larger diameter wires and ones that have a core-to-tip design. This is important at the time of endovascular therapy delivery.

Pushability relates to the ability to manipulate the direction and advancement of the wire from outside the body—done manually and often with the help of a torque device.

Flexibility helps maneuver through challenging anatomy and angles, and from an engineering standpoint is balanced out with pushability characteristics, such as the stiffness of the wire, to achieve the desired effect.

CATHETERS Catheters help direct wires and devices to locations distal to the access site. Catheters are made in various sizes (measured in Fr by the outer diameter; 3Fr = 1 mm), lengths (65–150 cm), shapes, materials (polyurethane, polyethylene, Teflon, or nylon), and number and locations of openings. Their basic components include the hub, shaft, and tip. They may have radio-opaque markers at their end spaced out toward the shaft in predetermined lengths. In peripheral interventions, their size ranges from 4Fr to 6Fr, allowing for a 0.035- or 0.038-inch wire to traverse.

Flush catheters allow for contrast pump injection and will have maximum flow rates (mL/sec) and injection pressures or pounds per square inch (PSI), and this information is generally found on the packaging. Longer catheters that are meant for more distal locations often require longer sheaths and/or guiding catheters ("guides") to provide support on the back end. This support is important as it also helps with catheter manipulation and the proper translation of movement of the preshaped tip in a desired direction.

Catheters are generally grouped into nonselective and selective functions. Non selective catheters are best used for diagnostic imaging and in larger vessels (i.e., aorta or IVC) [4]. Nonselective flush catheters have an end-hole and multiple smaller side-holes toward the shaft in order to deliver a rapid homogenous bolus of contrast (FIGURE 6-3). They come in curved and straight configurations. A pigtail marker and Omni catheter are examples of curved configurations. Removal of pigtail or curved catheters should be done over a wire so that they straighten out and vessel trauma can be avoided. When a vessel is too narrow to accommodate the curve, a straight marker catheter with multiple-side holes can be used. Selective catheters generally only have an end-hole and come with a wide variety of tips to facilitate vessel cannulation. These can also be used for angiography and work best in smaller caliber vessels, and should be injected at slower rates through power injector or via handheld injections. **CONTINUES ▶**

6-1

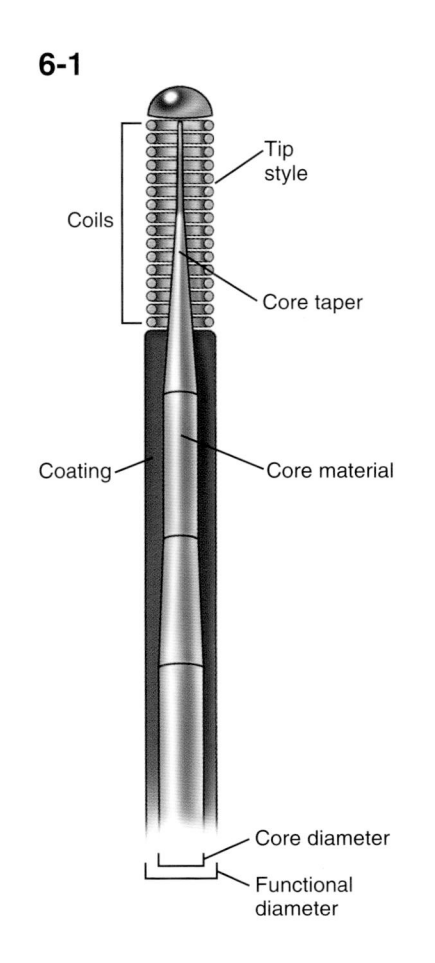

Tip style
Coils
Core taper
Coating
Core material
Core diameter
Functional diameter

6-2

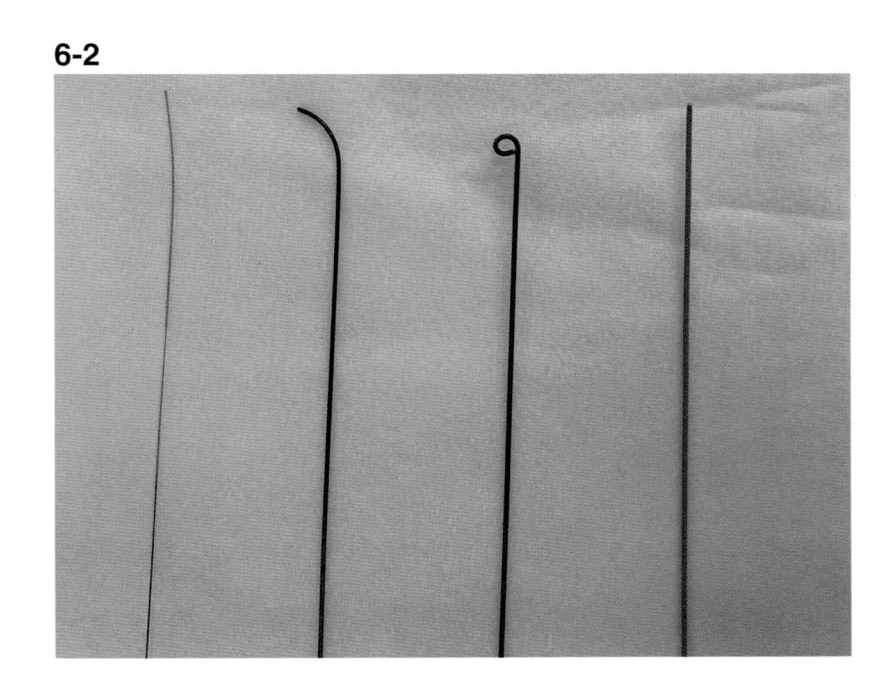

6-3

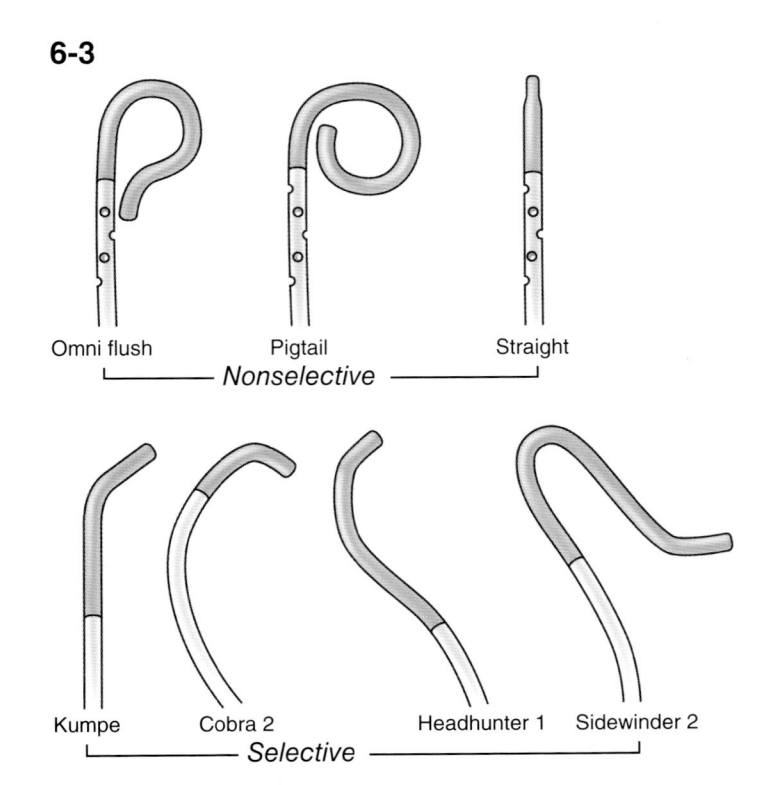

Omni flush   Pigtail   Straight
Nonselective

Kumpe   Cobra 2   Headhunter 1   Sidewinder 2
Selective

CATHETERS ◀CONTINUED▶ The tip has the greatest diversity, can be variably coated, and is designed with the anatomy of the various vascular beds in mind. Tips increase from complexity from straight, single-curved (Kumpe, FIGURE 6-4A), double-curved (C2, FIGURE 6-4B) to reverse-curved (SOS, FIGURE 6-4C). These shapes ultimately determine how a catheter will move within a vessel and how it will engage the orifice of the vessel of interest when externally manipulated [5]. The shape will also be variably affected depending on if the catheter is passed over a stiff, floppy, or no wire. The latter allows for reshaping as long as the vessel size allows. The direction of steering achieved by the tip of the catheter is affected by use of either a straight or angle wire.

For example, cannulation of the renal artery can be performed with multiple types of catheters. Using a reverse-curved catheter (i.e., Simmons) is common in down-sloping renal arteries. The reverse-curved catheter is shaped in the aorta (FIGURE 6-5A) above the target renal artery. A floppy-tipped guidewire is advanced carefully into the renal artery, and the catheter is slowly pulled downward (FIGURE 6-5B). With continued downward traction, the catheter extends into the renal artery over the tip of the wire until the apex of the catheter approximates the renal orifice (FIGURE 6-5C). To deselect the vessel, the catheter is pushed cephalad. Cannulation of a vessel does not imply that that same catheter will then track well once the wire is advanced. This will often require changing over to a simpler catheter (i.e., a crossing catheter) with better trackability to then advance over the wire to the target vessel.

Catheters can have additional components to their anatomy that influence handling and success in crossing challenging lesions. Braiding catheters with wire reinforcement increase torque and stiffness of the catheter. They can have various coatings, which if hydrophilic makes them more steerable and trackable. Additional coatings, such as barium coating or placing of a platinum band, can improve visibility of the catheter tip and can often be used as distance reference. One example is the Terumo, Navicross catheter, which has a double-woven stainless steel wire and a hydrophilic coating to allow pushability, steerability, and durability during the crossing of complex and challenging lesions.

For supraselective catheterization, microcatheters are available in smaller 2- or 3Fr sizes, of long lengths and meant for 0.018- and 0.014-inch wires. They are often used in a coaxial technique with an additional supporting catheter behind it. When there is a smaller wire in a larger catheter, there are a couple of things to consider. On the front end, the tip of the catheter will not be flush with the wire and may cause vessel injury upon advancement, particularly at an ostial level. A tapered tip on the catheter will decrease this somewhat, but appropriately sized wires and catheters help mitigate this issue. On the back end, the hub of the catheter will have a slow continuous bleed and can be made hemostatic with use of a Tuohy-Borst adapter. ■

REFERENCES

1. George JC, Trayer T, Kovach R. Wired for success. Guidewire escalation and techniques for successful crossing of chronic total occlusions. *Endovasc Today* (Suppl) March 2014;16-19.

2. Northcutt BG, Shah AA, Sheu YR, Carmi L. Wires, Catheters, and More: A Primer for Residents and Fellows Entering Interventional Radiology. September-October 2015. https://pubs.rsna.org/doi/pdf/10.1148/rg.2015130155

3. Walker C. Guidewire selection for peripheral vascular interventions. *Endovasc Today*. May 2013;80-83.

4. Beck AW, Lee WA. General principles of endovascular therapy: Guidewire and catheter manipulation. Chapter 4. *Atlas of Vascular Surgery and Endovascular Therapy*. Elsevier 2014;41-49.

5. Kaufman JA. Fundamentals of angiography. Chapter 2. *Vascular and Interventional Radiology: The Requisites*. Elsevier 2013;25-55.

6. Saw J. Carotid Artery Stenting: The Basics. pp 171-192|. Humana: Secaucus, NJ.

6-4

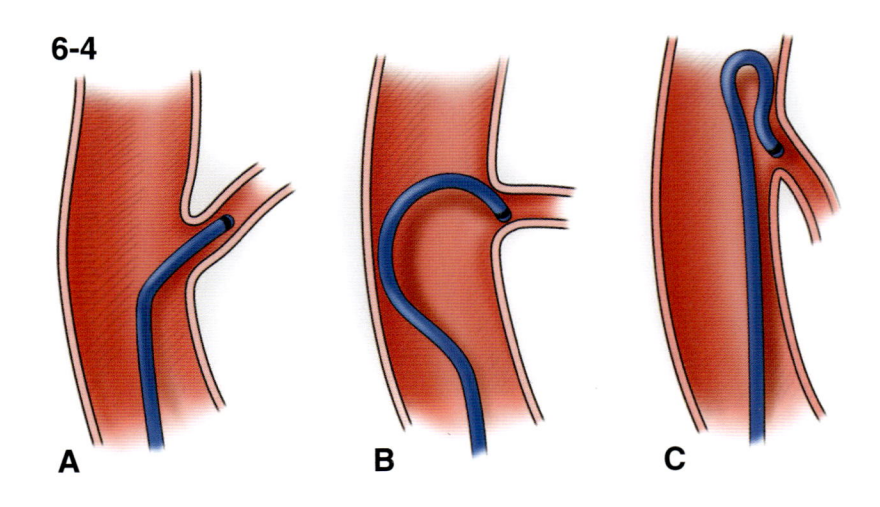

A   B   C

6-5

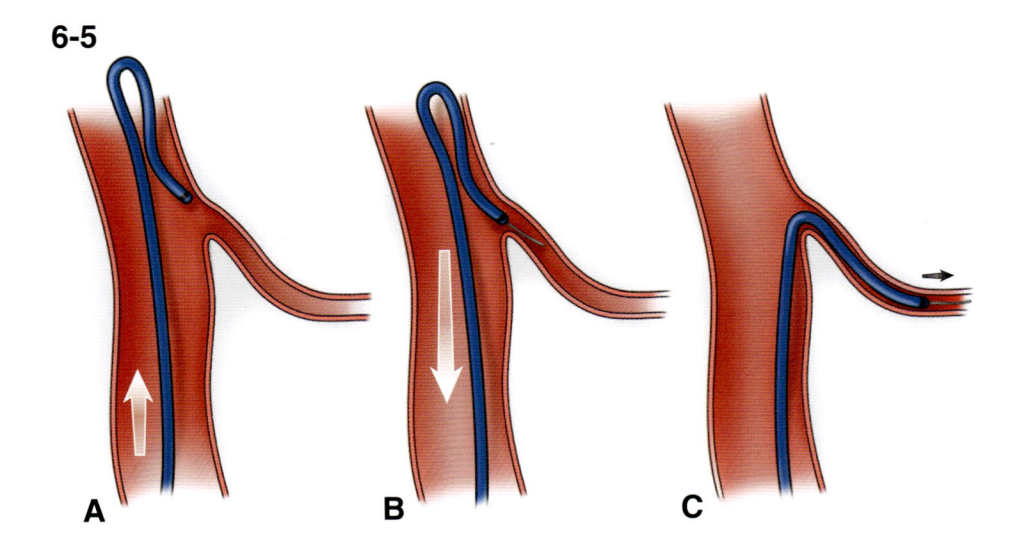

A   B   C

RECANALIZATION AND RE-ENTRY TECHNIQUES

Vipul Khetarpaul, MD • Patrick Geraghty, MD

INDICATIONS Chronic limb-threating ischemia (CLTI) patients often have multilevel disease with chronic total occlusions (CTOs). Ability to cross these lesions is the rate-limiting step in endovascular revascularization. Multiple factors—plaque morphology, location, length, collateral and cap morphology, and arterial access site—affect CTO crossing success.

PREOPERATIVE PREPARATION Preoperative exam is important for identifying access sites and coming up with a strategy to access and cross. Body habitus and previous scars and surgeries impact arterial access. Doppler and duplex studies localize lesions and provide information about potential access sites. In cases of poor inflow with diminished or absent common femoral pulses, CT angiography or MR angiography of the aorta and runoff aids in procedural planning. A careful pulse exam and chest CT angiography are useful when upper extremity access is contemplated. Key things to note are quality of access sites, steepness of aortic bifurcation, presence of inflow lesions and stents, location and nature of CTOs, and quality of runoff vessels (for possible retrograde approach).

ANESTHESIA Conscious sedation with local anesthesia is adequate in most cases. General anesthesia can be used judicially for patient comfort in complex endovascular cases and hybrid cases, and for airway protection in high-risk cases. Ultrasound-guided injection of local anesthetic next to calcified SFA/popliteal lesions can reduce discomfort during intervention under sedation.

POSITION Position the patient in the supine position with arms tucked and both groins prepped to preserve the option of utilizing both contralateral femoral and antegrade femoral approaches. Prepping the target limb/foot facilitates access to popliteal and tibial arteries when the crossing strategy requires escalation.

DETAILS OF PROCEDURE The ideal goal of CTO recanalization is to cross the lesion within the true lumen to preserve collaterals, reduce the chances of perforation, and keep all the interventional options open, including atherectomy/plaque modification. Frequently, though, part or all of the crossing may occur in the subintimal plane, especially when a looped wire technique is used.

Considering all possibilities, being patient, and staying flexible during the intervention are key to successfully crossing and treating difficult CTO lesions. In one's early experience, it is important not be deterred by failure. Staged repeat intervention using a different access and/or crossing technique is often successful.

ACCESS Choice of access is very important in CTO crossing. Lesion morphology (location/length/complexity), patient body habitus, and availability of alternate access sites figure into the selection of the initial access site.

Tortuous iliacs, acute aortic bifurcation angle, and heavy calcification can make it difficult to achieve up-and-over access to the contralateral side while maintaining adequate pushability for crossing difficult infrainguinal CTOs. In these instances, an antegrade common femoral artery approach may be better if the lesion is not flush at the SFA origin and body habitus is suitable. Complex popliteal and tibial CTOs—especially in tall patients—are best managed from an antegrade approach, which improves pushability across calcified CTOs and ensures adequate platform length to deliver therapy. Antegrade access also facilitates advanced techniques like transcollateral recanalization and pedal loop interventions.

Every CTO has a proximal and distal cap. If crossing from above is not feasible, considering alternate sites of access during the intervention can expedite safe crossing of CTOs in a retrograde fashion. Micro channels in the distal cap are generally wider and numerous, which makes retrograde crossing easier in most cases.

Sometimes, direct retrograde access into the CTO lesion itself can help get a wire across the proximal cap and make it feasible to cross the cap in an antegrade fashion and work on the distal cap. This technique can be used for flush proximal SFA CTOs, distal tibial occlusions, or in-stent occlusions where an occluded SFA stent is directly accessed with a long spinal needle under fluoroscopy and a wire is advanced across the proximal cap to create a channel.

For common iliac CTO, if the retrograde ipsilateral approach fails, consider antegrade crossing using a reverse curve catheter from contralateral common femoral access or the inline pushability afforded by brachial/radial access.

Pedal access belongs in every vascular surgeon's toolbox. In most cases, ultrasound-guided pedal access is sheathless, using the inner cannula of a micropuncture set. Subsequently, bareback 0.018″ profile crossing catheter and a hydrophilic tip wire are used to cross the CTO, and the wire is externalized through the antegrade access. Intervention is then undertaken in antegrade fashion. If retrograde intervention is needed, thin-walled 4 to 6Fr sheaths are introduced into the pedal vessels. To prevent spasm and access complications, intraarterial vasodilators and heparin are infused immediately after access. Some centers have published feasibility of proximal tibial artery access under ultrasound and fluoroscopic guidance with low complication rates. The concern for compartment syndrome would presumably be higher at these sites, but that trend was not detected in these small studies. External blood pressure cuffs were used for compression in these cases with confirmation of hemostasis by angiogram from antegrade access. Similarly, distal SFA and popliteal access sites can be controlled by external pressure along with internal balloon inflation.

CATHETER- AND WIRE-BASED STRATEGIES Initial lesion crossing usually involves the use of hydrophilic, braided support catheters paired with specialty hydrophilic wires. Thick fibrotic caps, heavy calcifications, or presence of large collaterals can pose a challenge. Using directional catheters and pointing the wires toward the lesion can help with penetration of the cap. Gradual escalation of CTO wires is often needed to penetrate these difficult caps, starting with a standard CTO 4- to 6-gmf wire and gradually escalating to a penetrating tip/heavier gram tip wire for fibrotic/calcified lesions. It is important to utilize adequate catheter support, keep the wire tip straight, and use a rotational "drilling" technique to achieve wire penetration into the CTO caps.

Building a triaxial system is useful in select cases to improve pushability. If support catheters are bending excessively, inflating a short balloon (1:1 sizing) just proximal to the cap aids CTO wire passage through calcified CTOs. Specialized CTO catheters like Corsair Armet (Asahi) or Viance (Medtronic) are used over 4- to 6-gmf CTO wires and use rotational force to cross difficult lesions. Branch points should be avoided using this technique and care should be taken to avoid engaging collaterals.

Subintimal tracking and re-entry (STAR) technique (**FIGURE 7-1**) is another basic strategy for CTO crossing. A hydrophilic guidewire is formed into a loop within the subintimal space (**FIGURE 7-1A**), then advanced until the plaque feathers out and the wire reenters the distal true lumen (**FIGURE 7-1B**). Care should be taken to keep the loop narrow (less than the native vessel diameter) to avoid perforation. The primary limitation of this technique is that re-entry is not guaranteed. Furthermore, if a capacious dissection flap is formed, alternate re-entry techniques may not work as well. There are variations of this technique where a smaller caliber wire is used to maintain options for re-entry and limit the subintimal dissection. Mini-STAR technique (or limited antegrade subintimal tracking [LAST]) involves crossing the proximal cap using a loop wire technique as described above to create a channel and then using an angled low-profile support catheter along with a higher tip load CTO wire to penetrate the subintimal flap in order to reenter the true lumen distally. It is important to take orthogonal views during this re-entry to ensure that catheter and wire tips are directed toward the true lumen at the planned re-entry site.

When using 0.014″ or 0.018″ microcatheters and wires, the parallel wire technique can assist in CTO crossing. The first wire that has lodged in CTO subintimal plane (**FIGURE 7-2A**) is left in place to keep the false entry site closed. A second wire and catheter are then introduced parallel to the first wire (**FIGURE 7-2B**), improving chances of successful CTO traversal and distal true lumen re-entry (**FIGURE 7-2C**). **CONTINUES ▶**

7-1

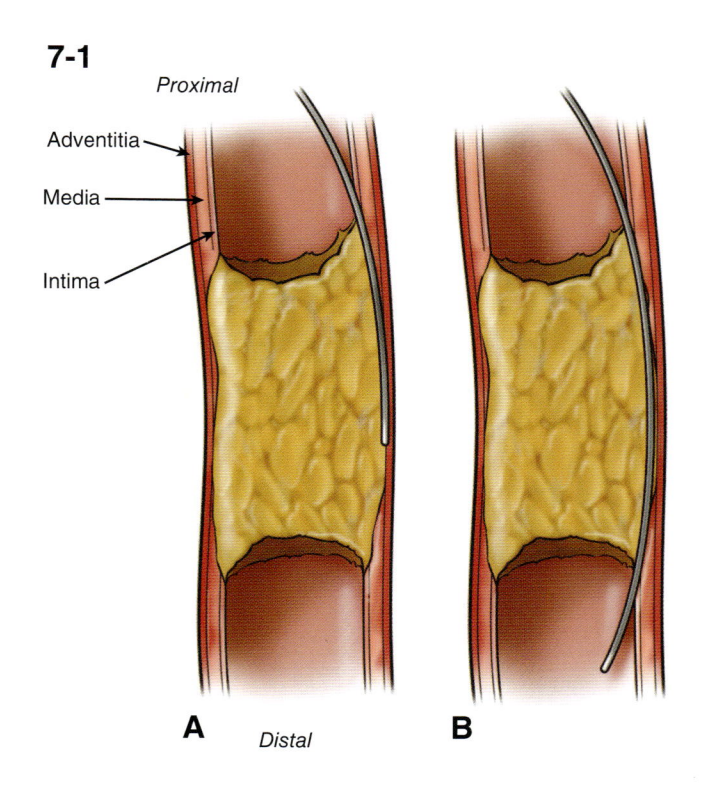

Proximal

Adventitia

Media

Intima

A   *Distal*   **B**

7-2

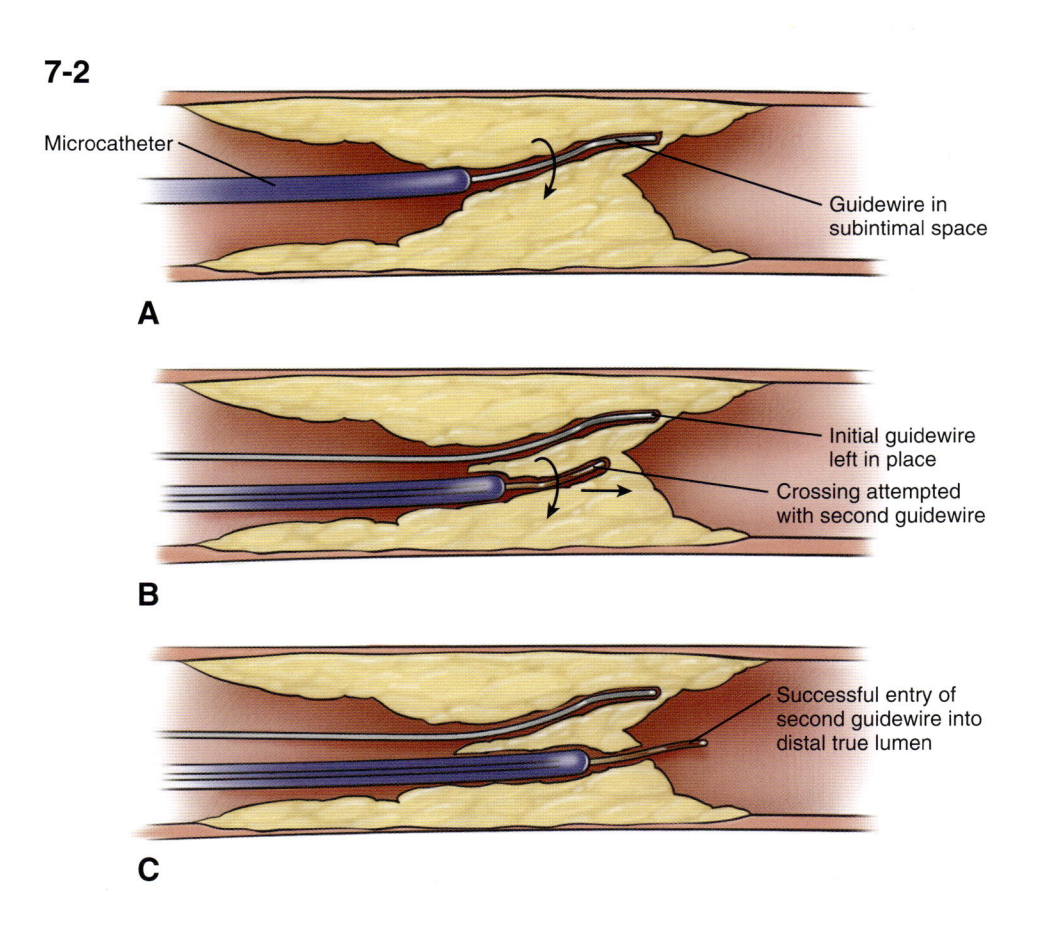

Microcatheter

Guidewire in subintimal space

A

Initial guidewire left in place

Crossing attempted with second guidewire

B

Successful entry of second guidewire into distal true lumen

C

CATHETER- AND WIRE-BASED STRATEGIES CONTINUED When antegrade crossing is not feasible, retrograde access sites are used to cross CTOs, which results in true lumen crossing fairly often. The wire can be snared from above to have true lumen access across the lesion. In the majority of cases, distal access with only a 0.018″ catheter or inner cannula of a micropuncture sheath along with a 0.018″ CTO wire is adequate for crossing the lesion. In cases where both antegrade and retrograde wires are in different subintimal planes, additional maneuvers are required to get through the lesion in the same plane. Since the retrograde access is mostly sheathless, the next best step is to use a reverse controlled antegrade and retrograde subintimal tracking (CART) technique (FIGURE 7-3). Wires are advanced from true lumen access from both antegrade and retrograde access sites across the CTO (FIGURE 7-3A). Orthogonal views are taken to ensure that they are in different planes, and once standard ways of redirecting wires in the same plane fail, balloon inflation (1:1 vessel size) from antegrade access is used to disrupt the subintimal plane (FIGURE 7-3A). Wires can now be directed into the same plane (FIGURE 7-3B) and snared to establish access across the lesion (FIGURE 7-3C). If this technique fails, CART can be used (FIGURE 7-4), which involves advancing a balloon from retrograde access (FIGURE 7-4A) and inflating it to disrupt the flap (FIGURE 7-4B) and facilitate crossing from the antegrade access (FIGURE 7-4C). CART and reverse CART can be used in different segments of the CTO to disrupt the subintimal planes, because it is difficult to predict where the flap is thin. If these techniques fail, confluent balloon technique is used to disrupt the subintimal flaps. This involves simultaneous inflation of balloons (1:1 to vessel size) from both antegrade and retrograde approaches. It is important to make sure that the tips of the balloons are touching each other but not overlapping.

DEVICE-BASED STRATEGIES Numerous devices are marketed for CTO crossing and re-entry. While these devices have not displaced thoughtful catheter/wire-based technique, they can be used in select circumstances to cross CTOs. An optical coherence tomography (OCT)-guided CTO crossing system (Avinger) was recently approved for use. It uses distal tip OCT technology to image and utilizes fast rotational speeds to penetrate tough lesions. Other devices like Crosser (Bard) use high-frequency mechanical vibration to cross CTO lesions.

For re-entry, self-centering flat balloons like Enteer (Medtronic) can be inflated in the subintimal plane and the re-entry wire can be used to penetrate the subintimal flap to re-enter in true lumen. Sharp re-entry can be performed using catheters like GoBack (Upstream Medical) and Outback Elite catheter (Cordis). The GoBack catheter is available in 4Fr, which opens up possibilities of use from a retrograde approach. Both these devices depend on fluoroscopy to direct the needle toward true lumen. The Pioneer intravascular ultrasound (IVUS)-guided re-entry catheter (Phillips) uses IVUS to help orient the needle throw into true lumen. The depth of the needle throw is adjustable in these devices. IVUS-guided re-entry is very successful and safe in common iliac CTOs as well. In steep aortic bifurcations, upsizing to a 7Fr sheath and pre-dilating long calcified CTO subintimal plane with a 2.5- to 3-mm balloon can help with tracking of the Pioneer catheter and prevent damage to the catheter tip for optimal imaging.

IVUS-guided re-entry can also be used to perforate two different subintimal planes when using CART/reverse CART techniques. Re-entry in P2/P3 segment of popliteal artery can be very challenging, and early escalation to an alternate access site should be considered. In some cases, it is possible to inflate a balloon in true lumen of native vessel from retrograde approach and using a needle-based re-entry catheter from antegrade approach to intentionally perforate the balloon and advance wire into true lumen distally.

CLOSURE Manual compression for femoral access along with use of closure devices are standard of care for common femoral access sites. For alternate access sites like pedal access, radial bands can be used selectively but external compression works well in most circumstances. For pedal/tibial/SFA access, balloon inflation across the site while holding external pressure also is commonly employed. For proximal tibial access, an external blood pressure cuff inflated above systolic pressure for several minutes has been utilized. Alternate access site hemostasis is confirmed with angiography whenever possible.

POSTOPERATIVE CARE Bed rest with sterile dressing at access site. Close monitoring of vital signs, access sites, and pedal pulses/Doppler signals in the postoperative period. ■

SUGGESTED READINGS

Saab F, Jaff MR, Diaz-Sandoval LJ, Engen GD, McGoff TN, Adams G, et al. Chronic total occlusion crossing approach based on plaque cap morphology: the CTOP classification. *J Endovasc Ther*. 2018 Jun;25(3):284-291. doi: 10.1177/1526602818759333. Epub 2018 Feb 27. PMID: 29484959.

Schwindt AG, Bennett JG Jr, Crowder WH, Dohad S, Janzer SF, George JC, et al. Lower extremity revascularization using optical coherence tomography-guided directional atherectomy: final results of the EValuatIon of the PantheriS OptIcal COherence Tomography ImagiNg Atherectomy System for Use in the Peripheral Vasculature (VISION) Study. *J Endovasc Ther*. 2017 Jun;24(3):355-366. doi: 10.1177/1526602817701720. Epub 2017 Apr 10. PMID: 28393673.

Walker CM, Mustapha J, Zeller T, Schmidt A, Montero-Baker M, Nanjundappa A, et al. Tibiopedal access for crossing of infrainguinal artery occlusions: a prospective multicenter observational study. *J Endovasc Ther*. 2016 Dec;23(6):839-846. doi: 10.1177/1526602816664768. Epub 2016 Aug 24. PMID: 27558463; PMCID: PMC5315197.

Zhuang KD, Patel A, Tan BS, Irani FG, Gogna A, Chan SX, et al. Outcome and distal access patency in subintimal arterial flossing with antegrade-retrograde intervention for chronic total occlusions in lower extremity critical limb ischemia. *J Vasc Interv Radiol*. 2020 Apr;31(4):601-606. doi: 10.1016/j.jvir.2019.12.006. Epub 2020 Feb 29. PMID: 32127314.

7-3

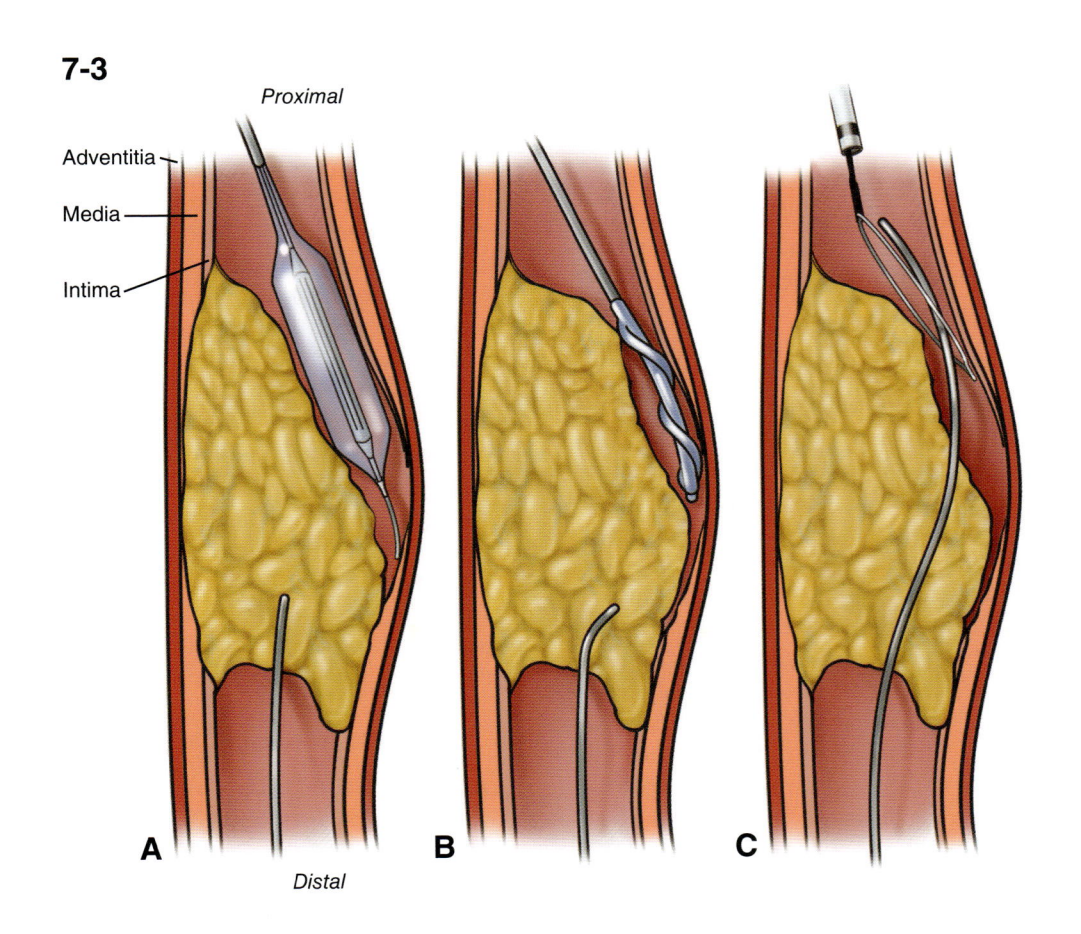

7-4

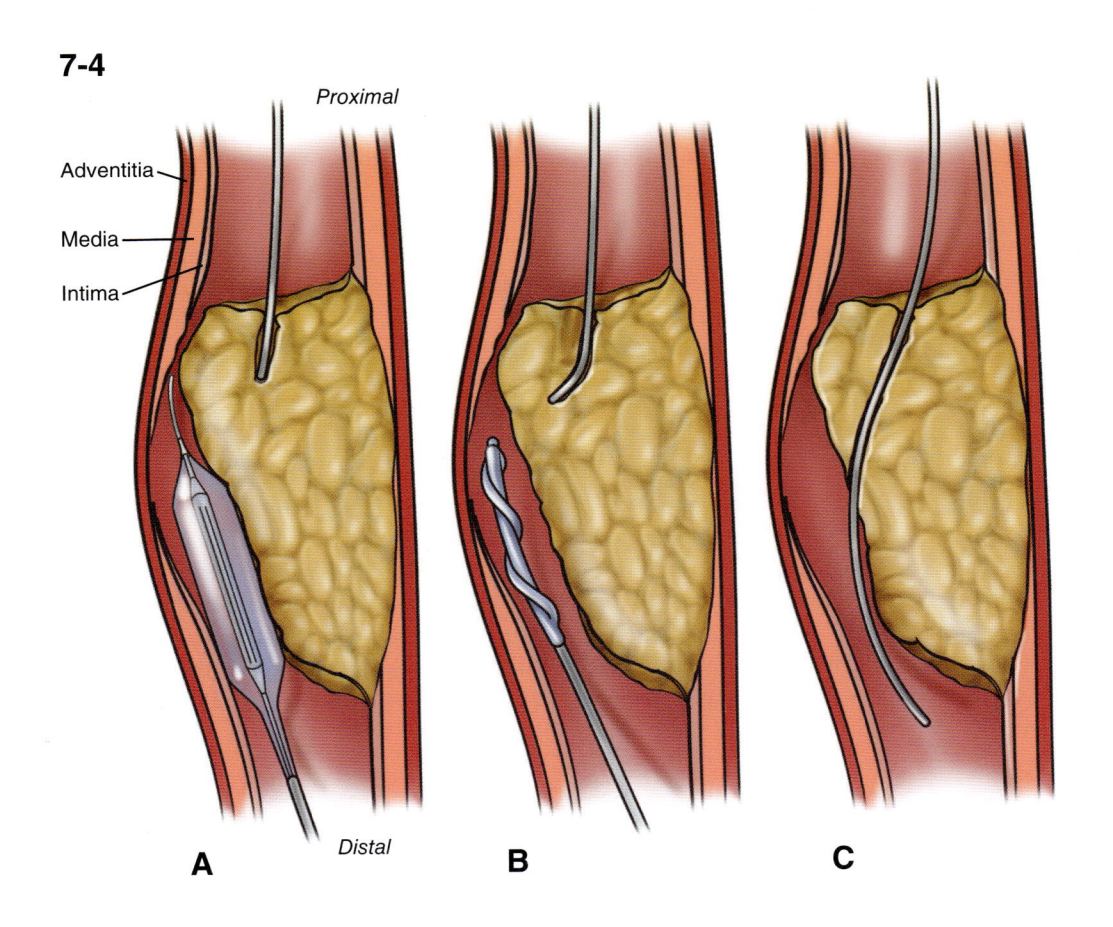

CHAPTER 8

ANGIOPLASTY BALLOONS AND TECHNIQUE

Norman H. Kumins, MD

INTRODUCTION Transluminal balloon angioplasty is a catheter-based procedure that increases the diameter of a narrowed or diseased artery or vein thereby improving blood flow. Arterial dilation was first described by Dotter and Judkins in the mid-1960s. They described a technique of passing a series of sequentially larger dilators through a narrowed arterial segment. Arterial dilation using a balloon catheter was first described by Gruntzig and Hopff for the treatment of an atherosclerotic plaque in a coronary artery.

Currently, dilation of vascular structures is performed using a catheter with a balloon mounted on the end of the shaft. The balloon is inflated inside the vessel within the narrowed region. Often balloon dilation of arterial lesions is referred to as "angioplasty" and of venous lesions is referred to as "venoplasty." The term "angioplasty" will be used in this chapter to describe treatment of all vascular structures.

ANGIOPLASTY-MECHANISM OF ACTION Angioplasty is the most basic catheter-based interventional procedure which uses a simple removable balloon to dilate vascular pathology. When performed in an atherosclerotic arterial plaque (FIGURE 8-1A), angioplasty causes a longitudinal fracture of the plaque-lined intima, separating it from the media and adventitia (FIGURE 8-1B). Arterial lumen size is increased by the flattening of the plaque and stretching of the vessel wall media and adventitia. This results in a controlled dissection, which initiates a positive remodeling process (FIGURE 8-1C) ending with re-endothelialization. The intentional arterial injury causes much of the endothelium to be denuded, leading to the deposition of platelets on the treated arterial surface. Platelet-derived growth factor (PDGF) and other cytokines are released, which leads to vessel healing and remodeling. The loss of the endothelium and the recruitment of cytokines and growth factors can also initiate uncontrolled overgrowth of the underlying smooth muscle cells leading to restenosis, a process referred to as neointimal hyperplasia (FIGURE 8-1D).

The goal following balloon angioplasty is arterial lumen expansion. A variety of factors contribute to achieving this goal, including lesion length and lesion composition. Ideal lesions for angioplasty are short, with atherosclerotic plaque that is soft and compliant. On the other hand, long, heavily calcified lesions would not be expected to yield an optimal outcome. Arteries are elastic and instead of dilating may recoil after treatment.

BALLOON DESIGN Angioplasty balloons are manufactured using a variety of materials and come in a wide range of configurations. The device is created by securing a balloon to the distal end of a dual-lumen delivery catheter. One lumen is for the passage of the catheter over a guidewire. The other lumen is connected to the balloon to allow for its inflation. Typically, there are one or more radiopaque markers mounted to the catheter, which can be seen under fluoroscopy. These markers indicate the location of the balloon on the catheter so it can be appropriately positioned. Most balloons use a marker to identify both ends of the balloon. Some short coronary balloons have only a single marker in the center of the balloon, while long peripheral balloons may have markers on each end and another in the middle.

Balloons can be designed to pass over a guidewire in two ways. If the entire length of the balloon catheter passes over the guidewire it is called "over the wire" (FIGURE 8-2A). This is a standard balloon design. Balloons may also be available as "rapid exchange" or "monorail" (FIGURE 8-2B) which means that the wire passes out of the catheter close to the balloon end, allowing the balloon and wire to be controlled by a single operator and the balloon to be more quickly loaded and removed. Common elements include the wire exit port (1) which exits at the rear of the over-the-wire balloon and closer to the balloon end of the monorail catheter. Other elements are the balloon inflation port (2), the balloon itself (3, inflated state), radiopaque markers indicating the treatment zone (4), and wire entrance (5).

BALLOON SIZE: Balloons are available in multiple size configurations corresponding to the balloon diameter, balloon length, length of the balloon catheter, and diameter of the balloon catheter. Balloon diameters start as small as 1.0 mm and can go beyond 45 mm for some specialty balloons. Balloons typically increase in diameter by 0.5-mm increments until they reach a diameter of 6 mm. Diameters then increase by 1 mm until they reach 10 mm and then increase by 2 mm up to about 24 mm. Specialty balloons for use in aortic dilation can reach diameters in excess of 45 mm. Balloon length describes the length of the balloon segment on the shaft, and ranges from 6 to 300 mm.

The catheter itself that delivers the balloon can be as short as 40 cm or as long as 200 cm. Selection of the catheter length depends on both the vascular access site and the location of the lesion to be treated. If they are in close proximity, access a short shaft is adequate. A longer device is needed if the access site and lesion are far apart, as in the case of femoral access with the lesion distal in the contralateral limb.

The balloon catheter is delivered to the target lesion over a guidewire. The catheter diameter correlates to the wire diameter over which it will pass. Balloon catheters typically are sized by passing over standard wire sizes of 0.014-, 0.018-, and 0.035-inch. Thus, when using a balloon that passes over a smaller wire, the balloon shaft and mounted balloon will be smaller, resulting in a diminished crossing profile.

BALLOON STRUCTURE: Available angioplasty balloons have multiple structural parameters. A key feature of each balloon is its compliance, which is defined by the level of elasticity or deformability at a given applied force. Balloons can be created from a variety of materials, each of which responds differently to pressure. Balloons can be compliant, allowing them to deform in direct relation to the pressure applied, or be noncompliant, where the balloon stays the same size irrespective of the pressure applied. Most peripheral balloons are semi-compliant. Each balloon is packaged with a chart that lists the expected size of the balloon at a given pressure. The nominal pressure describes the pressure at which the balloon reaches its indicated size. The rated burst pressure describes the maximum pressure for the balloon. A noncompliant balloon allows adequate force to be applied to a specific lesion without significant overdistension. On the other hand, compliant balloons increase size in direct proportion to the pressure delivered. These should be used cautiously, since the balloon can be expanded beyond the vessel diameter and lead to vessel rupture.

ANGIOPLASTY TECHNIQUE The operator selects an appropriate balloon, taking into account wire size, balloon diameter, balloon length, shaft length, and balloon compliance. Estimation of vessel diameter can be made by measuring the vessel immediately proximal or distal to the stenosis. The vessel and the lesion of interest must be mapped to allow correct balloon placement under fluoroscopy. There are a number of ways this can be accomplished, including the use of bony landmarks, road-mapping, or contrast angiography next to a radio-opaque marking ruler. The balloon is inflated (FIGURE 8-3A) with a mixture of contrast and saline. This allows visualization of the balloon under fluoroscopy. The balloon is left inflated (FIGURE 8-3B) for a period of time, then deflated and removed. A post-angioplasty angiographic image is then obtained. **CONTINUES ▶**

8-1

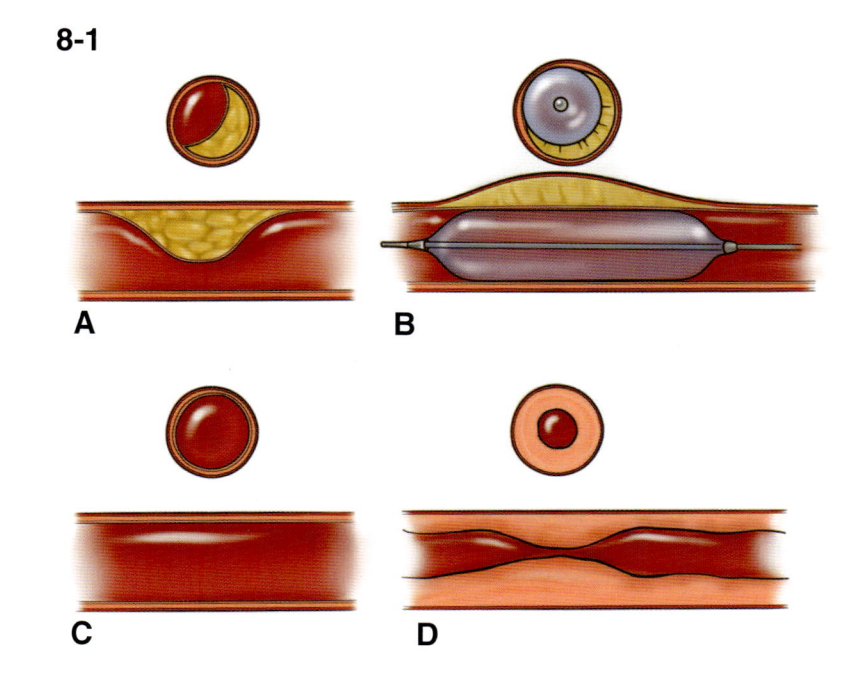

8-2

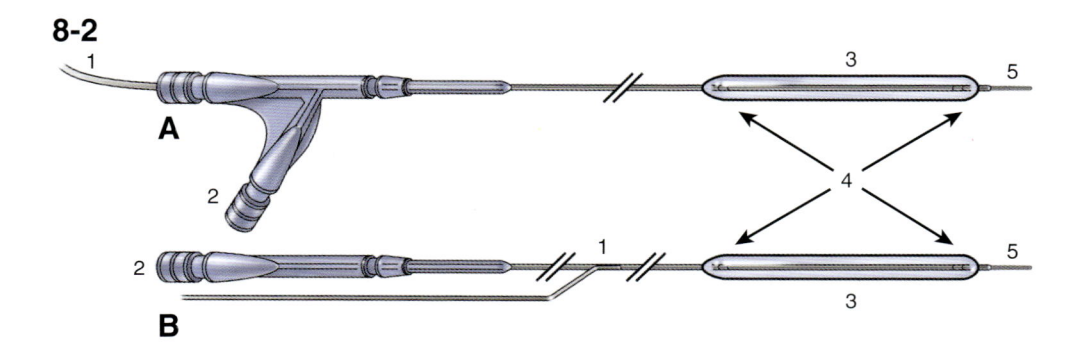

8-3

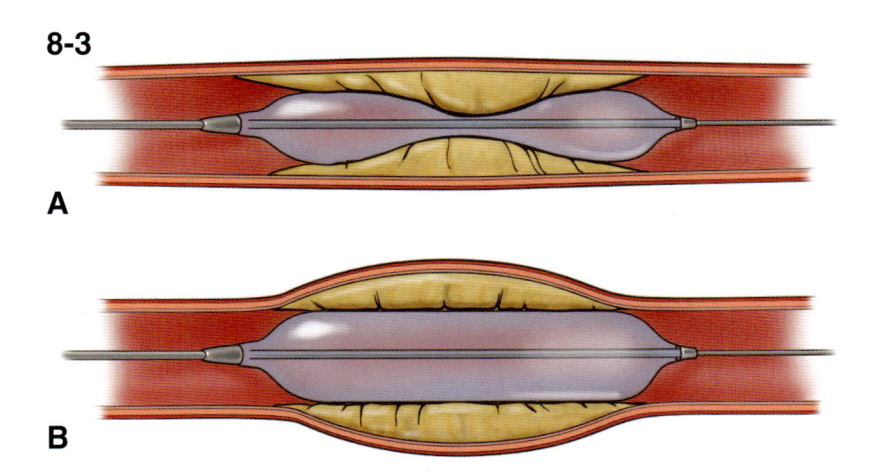

ANGIOPLASTY TECHNIQUE `CONTINUED` Usually, the balloon is inflated using an insufflator, a device which has a chamber that contains the diluted contrast medium connected to a threaded plunger (**FIGURE 8-4**). This allows the gradual delivery of the contrast mixture to fill the balloon. The insufflator has a gauge that measures the pressure applied to the balloon. This chamber is connected to the inflation port on the balloon with a Luer lock.

When treating arterial stenosis, sequential dilation of the lesion is often desirable. This gradual dilation is helpful to decrease arterial dissection and perforation. A balloon with a diameter smaller than the target vessel is inflated within the lesion prior to a nominally sized balloon.

SUBINTIMAL ANGIOPLASTY: There are two pathways the wire and balloon may take in crossing an artery. If the artery is not occluded, the wire can pass through the stenosis or stenoses and remain in the true lumen (**FIGURE 8-3**). On the other hand, the artery may be totally occluded by atherosclerotic plaque and chronic thrombus, a condition termed chronic total occlusion (CTO). When crossing a CTO the wire may stay in the true lumen or may intentionally or unintentionally enter the vessel wall under the diseased intima and cross in a subintimal plane (**FIGURE 8-5A**). After wire re-entry into the true lumen, angioplasty is performed (**FIGURE 8-5B**).

Results/Complications The ideal lesion for angioplasty is a short focal stenosis. The longer the lesion length, the more of the vessel is at risk for restenosis. Controlled arterial dissection is an intended consequence of angioplasty; it is how the balloon dilates the vessel. This dissection, however, can be uncontrolled and severe enough to be flow limiting. Untreated, flow-limiting dissections can cause arterial thrombosis. Additionally, angioplasty-treated lesions may recoil or fail to dilate, especially if they are heavily calcified. Balloon angioplasty, therefore, is often not adequate stand-alone therapy. It may be combined with other modalities such as atherectomy or stent placement. If the lesion is especially dense, calcified or bulky angioplasty can lead to arterial perforation. The operator must keep the possibility of perforation in mind, and techniques to treat this complication should be considered before intervention takes place.

SPECIALTY BALLOONS

Cutting or Scoring Balloons Some balloons are designed to cut or score the lesion. Cutting balloons have small, longitudinally mounted blades protruding from the balloon which score or cut into the lesion when the balloon is inflated. This technique is useful to treat stiff or calcified plaque, allowing for improved vessel expansion. Scoring balloons are similarly designed but have wires mounted to the outside of the balloon instead of blades. They work in a similar fashion but make a less aggressive cut on the lesion. The end result of treatment with these strategies is to appropriately expand the target lesion without dissection or vessel recoil.

Drug-Coated Balloons One of the most exciting advances in balloon angioplasty has been the development of drug-coated peripheral balloons (DCBs). These balloons are coated with paclitaxel and have been used to treat stenoses in femoropopliteal arteries, tibial arteries, and within arteriovenous fistulas used for hemodialysis access. The Achilles heel of any vascular intervention is neo-intimal hyperplasia, which is the development of smooth muscle overgrowth incited by the denudation of the vessel endothelium. This overgrowth can be arrested by paclitaxel, which is an antimitotic drug used to treat cancer. Paclitaxel-coated peripheral balloons have been shown to be especially beneficial in treating femoropopliteal arterial atherosclerotic disease and have shown promise in treating venous stenoses in arteriovenous fistulas and grafts. Current studies using DCB in tibial arteries are ongoing.

Lithotripsy Balloons Balloons have been developed that use sonic pressure waves to disrupt calcium-containing plaque in the arterial wall. This technology uses the same principles as shock wave lithotripsy for the dissolution of kidney stones. The lithotripsy balloon contains a miniaturized array of emitters that generate sonic waves to break up calcium. The balloon is gently inflated at low pressures inside of a calcified lesion. When the lithotripsy emitters are activated, the calcium in the arterial wall is fractured into small pieces which remain in situ. This calcium disruption allows the vessel to expand with minimal pressure. These balloons are currently approved for use in coronary and peripheral arteries.

Cryoplasty Balloons This specialty device uses liquid nitrous oxide instead of dilute contrast to insufflate the balloon. This has the effect of freezing a thin layer of vessel wall exposed to the balloon surface, the goal of which is to induce cellular apoptosis and limit neointimal hyperplasia. ■

8-4

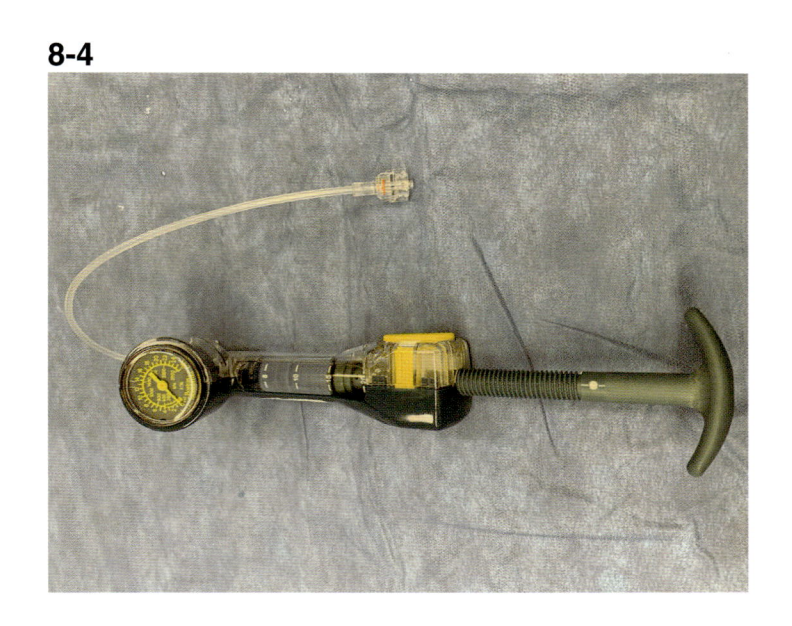

8-5

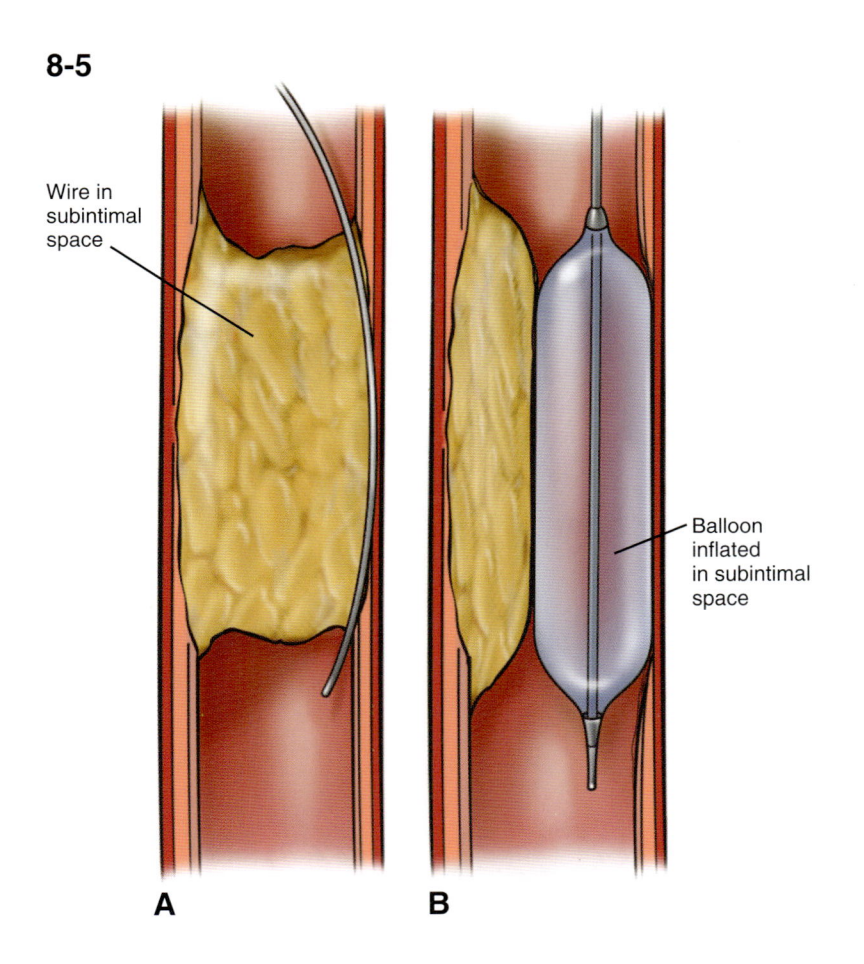

Wire in subintimal space

Balloon inflated in subintimal space

A

B

Stents and Stent-Grafts

Matthew D. Breite, MD • **Todd E. Rasmussen, MD**

OVERVIEW Endovascular stents, or those placed within a blood vessel, rely on an interwoven metal wire framework to expand or maintain a target vessel lumen diameter. They are categorized primarily by manner of deployment as either balloon-expandable or self-expanding. Both stent types can have either bare metal or covered designs, the latter often referred to as "stentgrafts." Selection of stent type should involve consideration of the anatomic location and characteristics of the lesion undergoing treatment, as each stent has specific physical properties that influence its technical placement, effectiveness, and durability.

The decision to place an endovascular stent can be considered as a selective or primary scenario. In selective stenting (i.e., in some but not all cases), a stent is placed following balloon angioplasty and/or atherectomy, after which a radiographic or flow-limiting abnormality persists (e.g., a pressure gradient or residual luminal stenosis). In these scenarios, the stent is placed to optimize the initial endovascular treatment that failed to completely treat the target lesion. In contrast, primary stenting refers to treatments in which stent delivery serves as the planned or initial treatment method.

BALLOON-EXPANDABLE STENTS Balloon-expandable stents combine a high radial force and a rigid structure, also referred to as "hoop strength," to provide precise deployment at a target lesion. These most commonly employ a stainless-steel framework. Due to their relatively low flexibility, these stents have difficulty traversing tortuous vessels and can suffer permanent deformation if placed in a mobile target vessel or compressed during a future intervention. When sizing, these stents should be matched one-to-one with the target vessel.

For deployment of a balloon-expandable stent, the lesion should first be crossed with a delivery catheter or sheath to prevent detachment of the exposed stent as it traverses the stenosis. The guiding catheter or sheath can then be withdrawn proximally, exposing the stent and allowing for its deployment. An embolic protection wire or device may be considered to reduce the likelihood of distal embolization when treating high-risk target lesions. The balloon-expandable stent will detach once the nominal pressure of the balloon has been reached. Inflation results in simultaneous balloon expansion at the proximal and distal ends to minimize movement of the stent from its desired location (**FIGURE 9-1A**). The stent will then maintain the size to which the balloon was expanded (**FIGURE 9-1B**), although a larger diameter can be reached with post-dilation using a 1- to 2-mm larger angioplasty balloon to improve vessel apposition. Over-dilation of the stent does carry a risk of stent foreshortening and structural weakening.

Common sites of deployment include the origin of the celiac, superior mesenteric, renal, and subclavian arteries. Balloon-expandable stents are also used for bilateral simultaneous deployment in the common iliac arteries, as well as in short-treatment segments of the common and external iliac

system where a caliber change is not traversed. A relative contraindication exists for deployment in the venous system due to increased risk of perforation with the high radial force (i.e., hoop strength) of these stents.

SELF-EXPANDING STENTS Self-expanding stents have low radial force, with a flexible structure. These are most commonly composed of the nickel and titanium alloy nitinol. The flexible nature of the metal framework allows the stent delivery system to navigate tortuous vessels without risk of permanent stent deformation. The device can also then be deployed at sites that undergo frequent movement or involve a change in vessel caliber. Recommended sizing should be 10 to 15% greater than target vessel diameter.

Deployment occurs when the outer sheath of the delivery system is proximally retracted by the delivery mechanism (**FIGURE 9-2A**). No additional protective catheter or sheath is needed to cross the target lesion. The stent deploys in a distal to proximal fashion until it is completely unsheathed (**FIGURE 9-2B**), requiring careful attention under live fluoroscopy to prevent the stent from jumping forward or being pulled proximally by the operator. Post-stent deployment angioplasty can still be performed if there is significant narrowing. However, if further expansion is needed to obtain vessel wall apposition because the original stent size was too small, post-dilation is not an option due to the inherent stent flexibility. Instead, a larger diameter second stent must be deployed within the first, typically requiring a balloon-expandable design to utilize its greater radial force.

Typical target vessels include the carotid bifurcation, distal aspects of the superior mesenteric artery, long segments of the iliac system to account for caliber change and external iliac tortuosity, and the left common iliac vein in the setting of May-Thurner syndrome. The flexibility and resistance to permanent deformation of these stents also makes them the preferred design for infra-inguinal arterial use.

STENT-GRAFTS (COVERED STENTS) For areas requiring complete vessel wall coverage at the site of deployment, fabric-coated stents exist which can have either balloon-expandable or self-expandable deployment mechanisms. Polytetrafluoroethylene (PTFE) or polyester are the most used fabrics for these devices (**FIGURE 9-3**). The deployment mechanism for balloon-expandable designs remains similar to their bare metal counterparts. However, self-expanding covered stents exist in both distal-to-proximal and proximal-to-distal deployment designs.

Covered stents are of greatest utility when excluding vessel wall defects such as aneurysm, perforation, or plaque or thrombus deemed prone to embolization. The fabric can also be used to exclude a site of arteriovenous fistula or pseudoaneurysm. However, the operator must be aware that these stents will also cover all branch and collateral vessels originating along the treatment length. ■

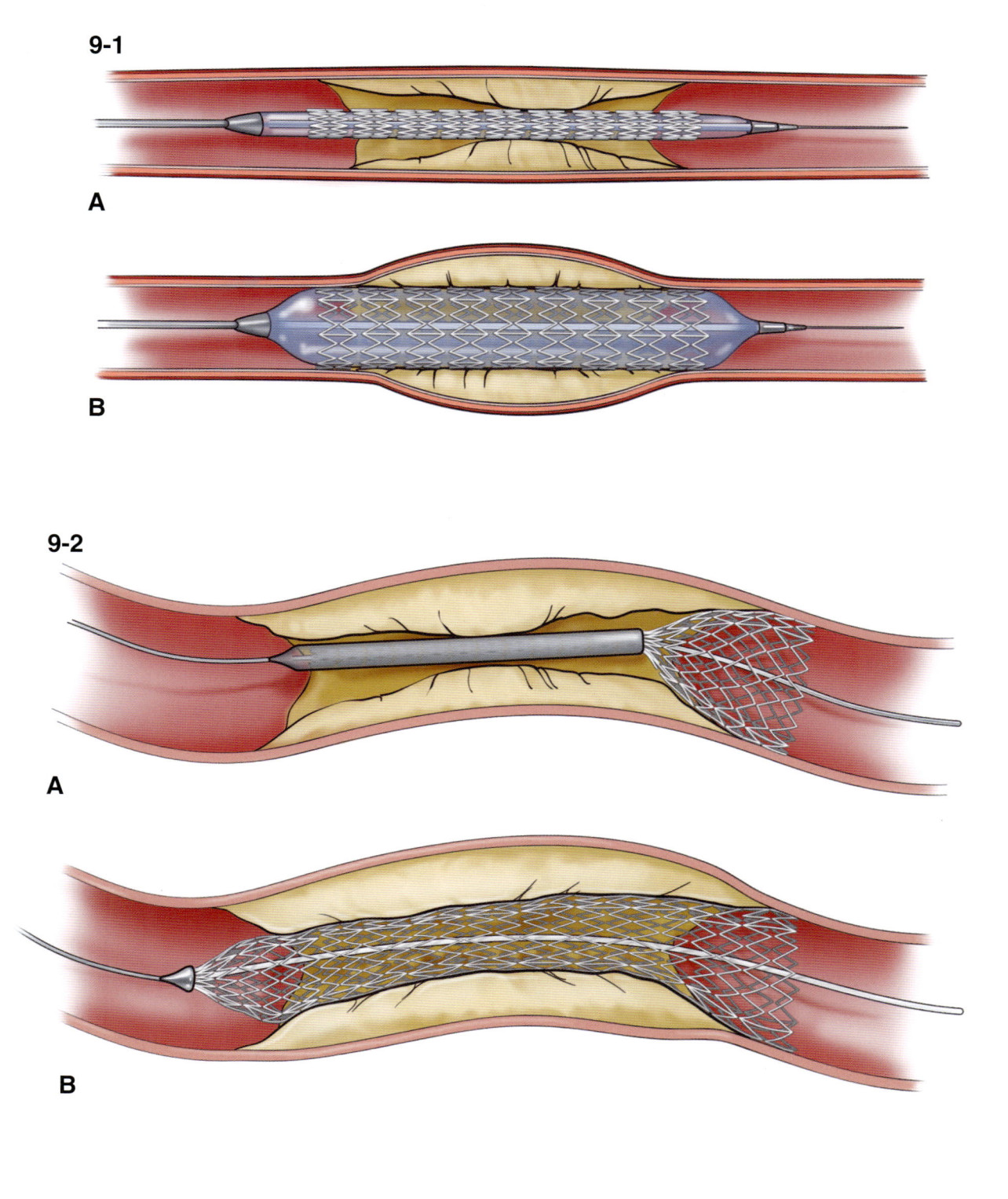

9-1

A

B

9-2

A

B

9-3

Section III
CEREBROVASCULAR

Longitudinal Arteriotomy and Patch Closure

Wesley S. Moore, MD

PREOPERATIVE PREPARATION Patient comorbidities should be optimized prior to surgical intervention. Hypertension should be well controlled, ideally with a systolic blood pressure around 130 mmHg. All patients with atherosclerosis should be on a statin with their LDL level maintained at 70 mg/dL or less. If they are intolerant or resistant to statin medication, then use of a PCSK-9 inhibitor is advised. If the patient is diabetic, then their HbA1c level should be around 5.5%. Since one of the major causes of postoperative morbidity and mortality is myocardial infarction, patients should be evaluated for covert coronary artery disease with a preoperative cardiac evaluation and stress testing.

ANESTHESIA AND PATIENT POSITIONING Carotid endarterectomy can be performed using cervical block or general anesthesia. My preference is general anesthesia for several reasons, which include patient comfort, maintenance of a quiet operative field, and my ability to concentrate on the operation without my attention being diverted by patient discomfort.

The patient should be asked to void before coming into the operating room. A urinary catheter can be avoided if the anesthesiologist restricts intravenous fluids to a minimum.

The patient is positioned supine on the operating table with a small roll under the shoulders to provide mild neck extension, with the head turned away from the side of operation. Extensive hyperextension and cervical rotation should be avoided to prevent cervical spine and nerve injury.

PLACEMENT OF SKIN INCISION Once the patient is appropriately positioned, we identify the carotid bifurcation with the aid of a portable duplex ultrasound unit. Once the bifurcation is identified, it can be marked with an indelible marker on the skin.

The skin is then surgically prepared and the patient is appropriately draped. It is my practice to use an iodinated adhesive applied to the surgical field, which should allow access from the clavicle to the mastoid process.

A short (usually 3-inch) skin incision is marked and centered over the carotid bifurcation, as previously marked with an indelible arrow based upon duplex ultrasound insonation. I prefer an incision that runs along the anterior border of the sternomastoid muscle (**FIGURE 10-1**), although some surgeons may choose to use a modified oblique incision, placed in a skin crease, for cosmetic considerations.

EXPOSURE OF THE CAROTID BIFURCATON Following skin incision, the platysma muscle is divided and the anterior edge of the sternomastoid muscle is exposed. An avascular plane is incised between the edge of the muscle and midline structures to reveal the underlying carotid sheath containing the jugular vein, carotid artery, and vagus nerve. The next key step is to identify the common fascial vein as it drains into the jugular vein, as the carotid bifurcation usually resides immediately beneath it. The common fascial vein is circumferentially mobilized, doubly ligated, and divided between suture. In the case of a high carotid bifurcation, the 12th cranial nerve can lie immediately behind the common fascial vein, so care must be taken to ensure that the nerve has not been encircled together with the vein before ligation and division. The jugular vein is then fully mobilized along its medial edge for the entire length of the incision. As the surgeon proceeds cephalad, along the vein, small accessory fascial veins may be encountered. These should be individually ligated and divided to provide optimal exposure.

The common carotid artery is then circumferentially mobilized in the perivascular plane (the plane of LeRiche) and exposure carried toward the bifurcation. Before proceeding further, the location of the vagus nerve should be ascertained. It usually resides posterior and medial to the artery, but can be anywhere within the sheath (**FIGURE 10-2**). When it lies anterior to the artery it can give rise to the nerve to the vocal cord (so called nonrecurrent, recurrent laryngeal nerve). **CONTINUES▶**

10-1

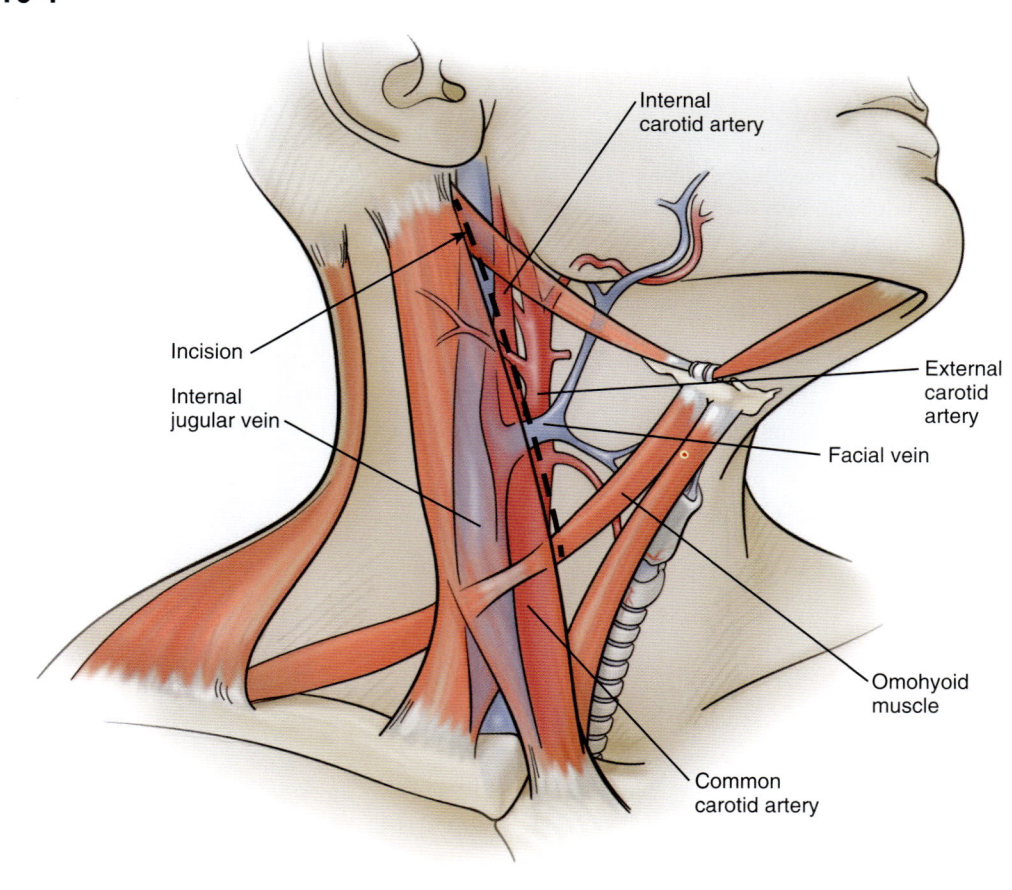

- Internal carotid artery
- Incision
- Internal jugular vein
- External carotid artery
- Facial vein
- Omohyoid muscle
- Common carotid artery

10-2

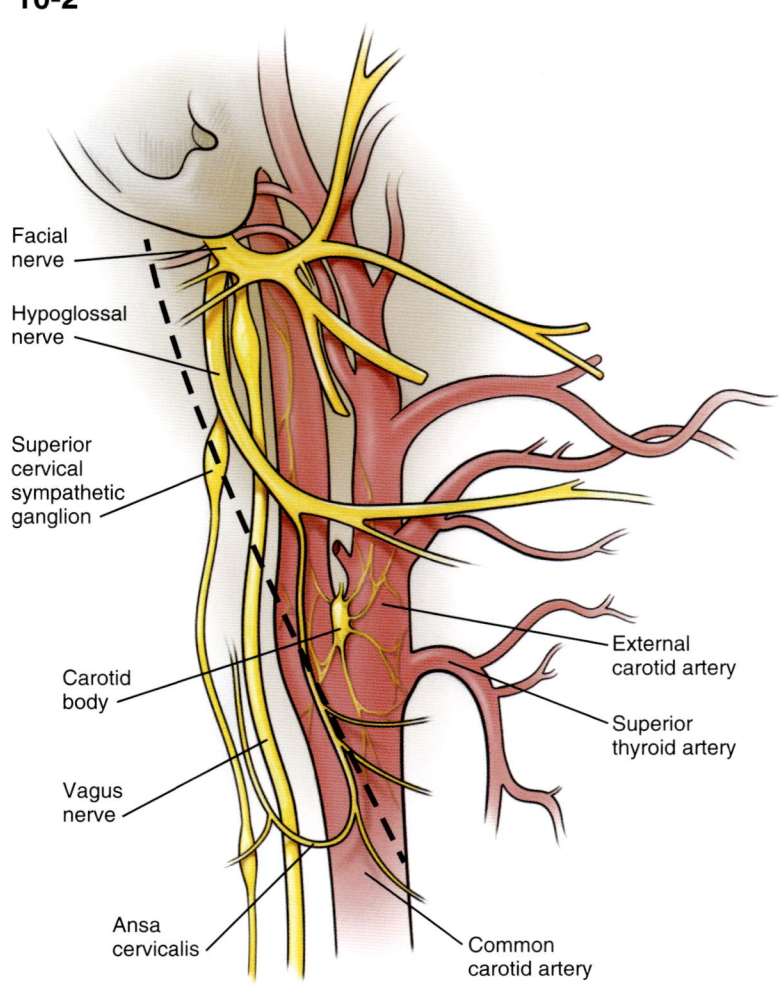

- Facial nerve
- Hypoglossal nerve
- Superior cervical sympathetic ganglion
- Carotid body
- Vagus nerve
- Ansa cervicalis
- External carotid artery
- Superior thyroid artery
- Common carotid artery

EXPOSURE OF THE CAROTID BIFURCATON ◄CONTINUED The carotid bifurcation is then gently mobilized, keeping in mind that it is at this point that any loose atherothrombotic material can be dislodged with the risk of embolization to the brain. The internal and external arteries are separated and the internal carotid artery is mobilized well beyond palpable plaque (FIGURE 10-3). The external carotid artery is circumferentially mobilized. I usually divide the superior thyroid artery to provide additional mobility. The structures between the internal and external carotid arteries include the nerve to the carotid sinus and occasionally the ascending pharyngeal artery. It is prudent at this point to inject 1% lidocaine into the nerve in order to prevent a reflex bradycardia. In the case of a high carotid bifurcation, the nerve to the carotid sinus serves as a suspensory ligament. Dividing the nerve will permit the bifurcation to drop caudally and permit additional exposure for the internal carotid artery (FIGURE 10-4).

EVALUATING NEED FOR SHUNT PLACEMENT At this point, surgeons are divided into three groups: routine shunters, selective shunters, and never shunters. I am a selective shunter. I originally worked out the parameters for measuring internal carotid back pressure as an estimate of hemispheric arterial perfusion pressure. While this proved to be a very accurate method of identifying the approximately 10% of patients who were intolerant to prolonged carotid clamping, it represented only a single measurement in time. We currently employ continuous EEG monitoring as a more convenient method. If the ipsilateral hemisphere EEG shows drop in amplitude or slowing, we use that as an indication for shunt placement. I prefer the use of a long Javid shunt. The distal end of the shunt is first placed in the internal carotid artery and held in place with a Rumel torniquet. The shunt is back-bled and clamped. The proximal end is placed in the common carotid artery and held in place with a Rumel torniquet. The clamp on the shunt is slowly released, watching for air bubbles or atheromatous debris. If seen, the shunt is promptly clamped, the proximal end taken out, back-flushed, and the process repeated. Alternative shunts are displayed (FIGURE 10-5. Photograph of multiple shunt types. Top to bottom: Javid shunt, in-line Bard shunt, and Pruit-Inahara double balloon shunt).

10-3

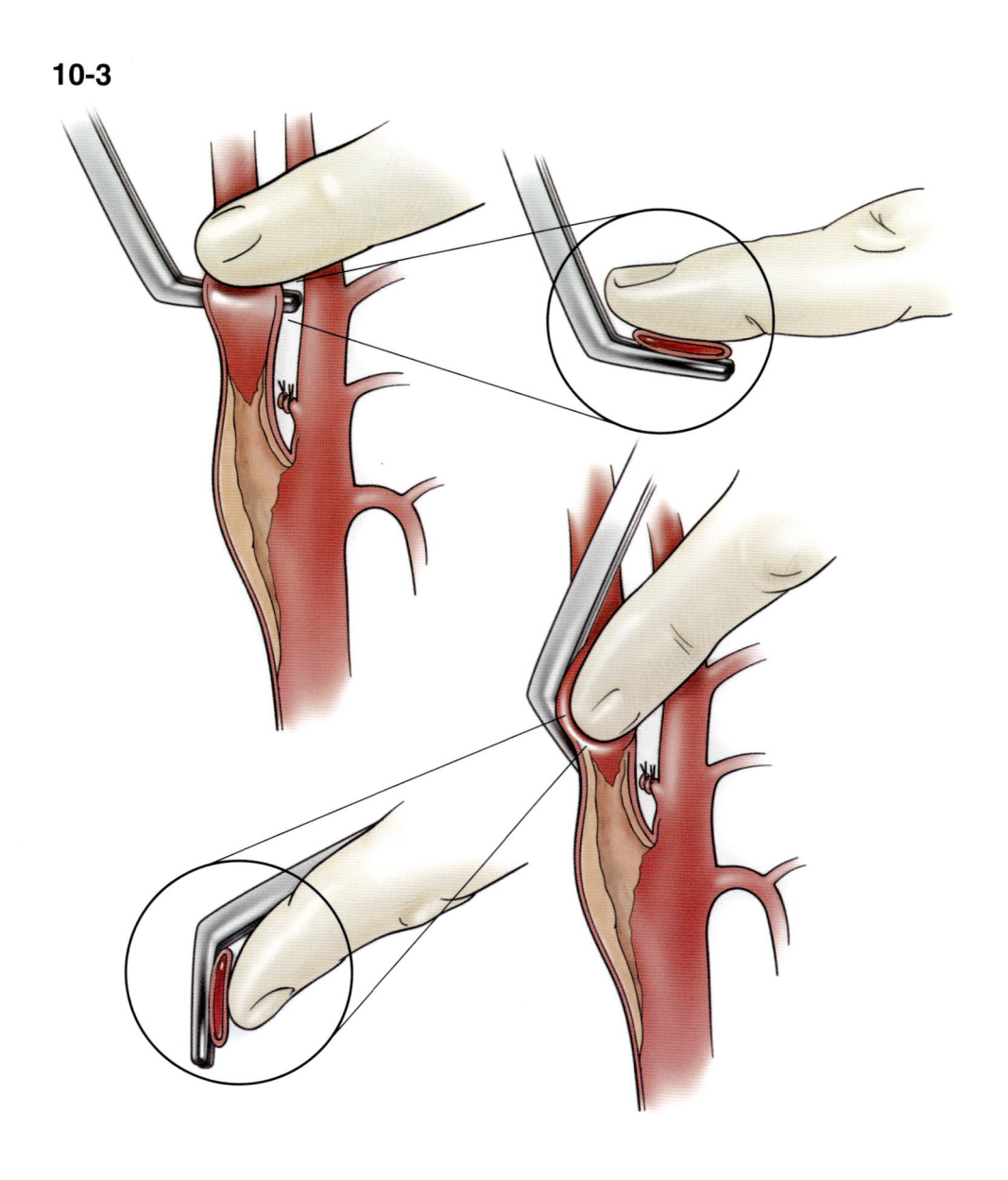

10-4

Ascending pharyngeal artery

Internal carotid artery

Autonomic nerve to carotid body

A   B

10-5

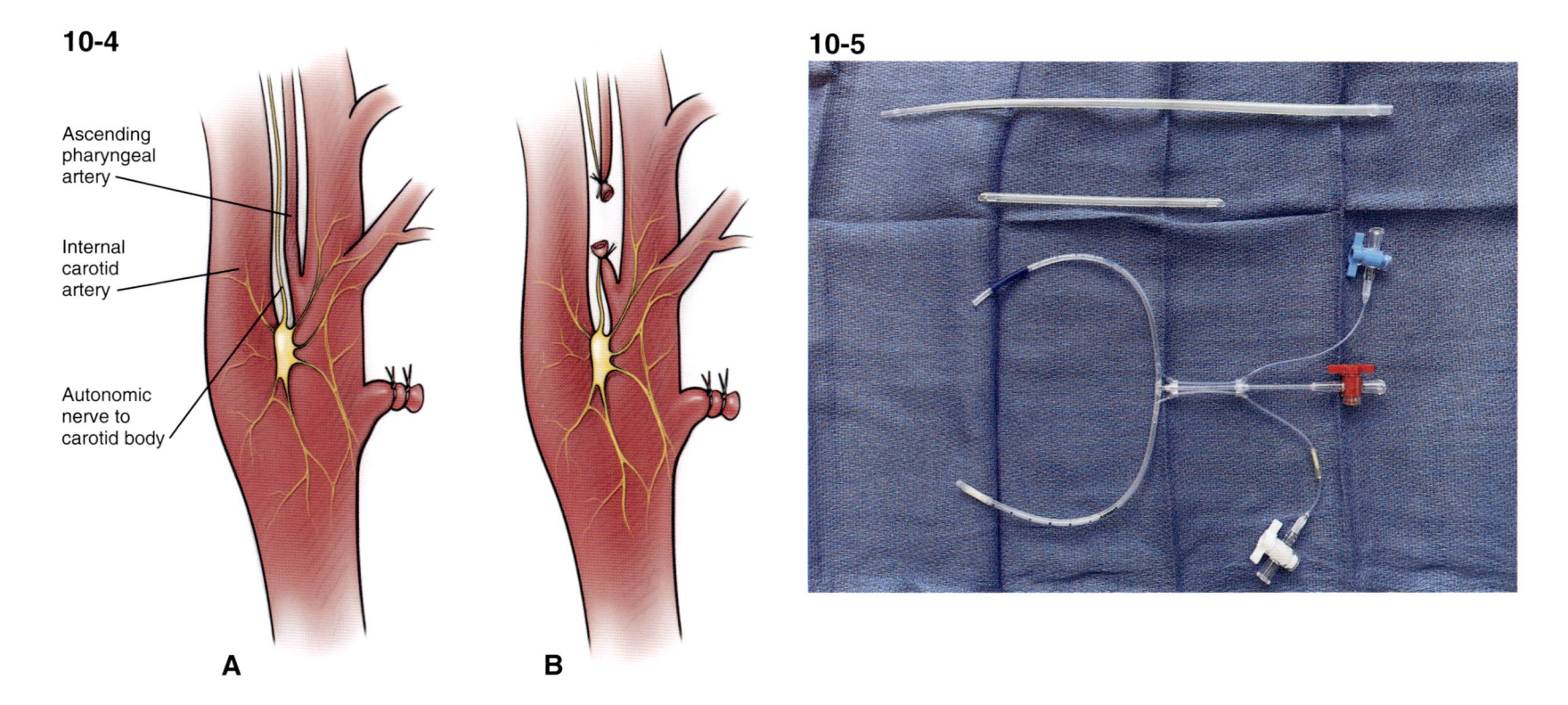

TECHNIQUE OF ENDARTERECTOMY AND PATCH PLACEMENT   Once the carotid bifurcation is fully mobilized, I usually administer about 5000u of heparin prior to clamping, unless the patient has been on dual antiplatelet drugs. In that case, I cut the heparin dose back to about 3500u. I clamp the internal carotid artery first, then the external carotid artery, then I place a clamp on the common carotid artery such that I can rotate the bifurcation placing the carotid bulb and the internal carotid artery in an anterior position. An arteriotomy is made with a #11 blade and extended through the plaque into the internal carotid artery, well beyond the end of the plaque (FIGURE 10-6). If a shunt is required, it is placed at this time (FIGURE 10-7). The endarterectomy is usually done where the major portion of the plaque is present since it is at this point that it is easiest to separate the plaque from the arterial wall (FIGURE 10-8). The plaque separation is continued distally. As the endpoint is approached, care is taken to enter a plane between the plaque and the arterial media. This will provide the best opportunity to achieve a tapered and feathered endpoint. The arteriotomy on the internal carotid artery should be extended as far distally as needed to enable the operator to achieve a clean feathered endpoint under direct vision (FIGURE 10-9). I never use tacking sutures to secure the distal endpoint. The endarterectomy is then continued proximally to clear the external carotid orifice, and when the end of the plaque is reached in the common carotid artery it is sharply transected, leaving normal intima attached to the arterial wall. The intimectomized artery is then irrigated with heparinized saline. Any residual bits of floating media are carefully removed. The artery is now ready for patch placement. I continue to use a collagen-impregnated Dacron patch, with suturing beginning distally and progressing proximally (FIGURE 10-10). The artery is back-bled and flushed prior to completion. Flow is begun first to the external carotid artery, then to the internal carotid artery.

ASSESSMENT OF TECHNICAL RESULT   The objective of carotid endarterectomy is to prevent stroke. One of the major causes of periprocedure stroke is thromboembolism due to technical error. We have one chance to do a technically perfect operation. Therefore it is incumbent upon the surgeon to be assured of technical perfection before leaving the operating room. My preference is to do a completion angiogram using a portable C-arm fluoroscopy unit. An alternative would be to use a duplex scan, paying particular attention to the distal endpoint.

WOUND CLOSURE   Following careful inspection for hemostasis, I close the platysma with a continuous absorbable suture and the skin with a subcuticular suture that does not require removal. I do not use a drain.

POSTOPERATIVE MONITORING AND FOLLOW-UP   Patients should be monitored in the recovery room with careful attention paid to neurologic status and maintenance of optimum blood pressure. If the patient is neurologically intact and blood pressure is well maintained without the use of intravenous medication, they are transferred to a regular hospital room for overnight monitoring. If all is well in the following morning, they are discharged on their regular medication, including aspirin. The first postoperative visit will be in 3 weeks, at which time I will obtain a duplex scan. The next visit will be in 6 months and again at 1 year, then yearly thereafter. ■

SUGGESTED READINGS

Ahn SS, Jordan SE, Nuwer MR, Marcus DR, Moore WS. Computed electroencephalographic topographic brain mapping. A new and accurate monitor of cerebral circulation and function for patients having carotid endarterectomy. *J Vasc Surg.* 1988;8:247–254.

Goldberg JB, Goodney PP, Kumbhani SR, Roth RM, Powell RJ, Likosky DS. Brain injury after carotid revascularization: outcomes, mechanisms, and opportunities for improvement. *Ann Vasc Surg.* 2011;25(2):270–286.

Goldstein LB, Bushell CD, Adams RJ, Appel LJ, Braun LT, Chaturvedi S, et al. Guideline for the primary prevention of stroke: A Guideline for Healthcare Professionals from the American Heart Association/American Stroke Association. *Stroke.* 2011;42(2):517–584.

Moore WS, Barnett HJM, Beebe HG, Bernstein ER, Brener BJ, Brott T, et al. Guidelines for carotid endarterectomy. A multidisciplinary consensus statement from the ad hoc committee, American Heart Association. *Stroke.* 1995;26:188–201.

Moore WS, Yee JM, Hall AD. Collateral cerebral blood pressure. An index of tolerance to temporary carotid occlusion. *Arch Surg.* 1973;106:520–523.

Moore WS, et al. Carotid angiographic characteristics in the CREST trial were major contributors to periprocedural stroke and death differences between carotid artery stenting and carotid endarterectomy. *J Vasc Surg.* 2016;63(4):851–857.

10-6

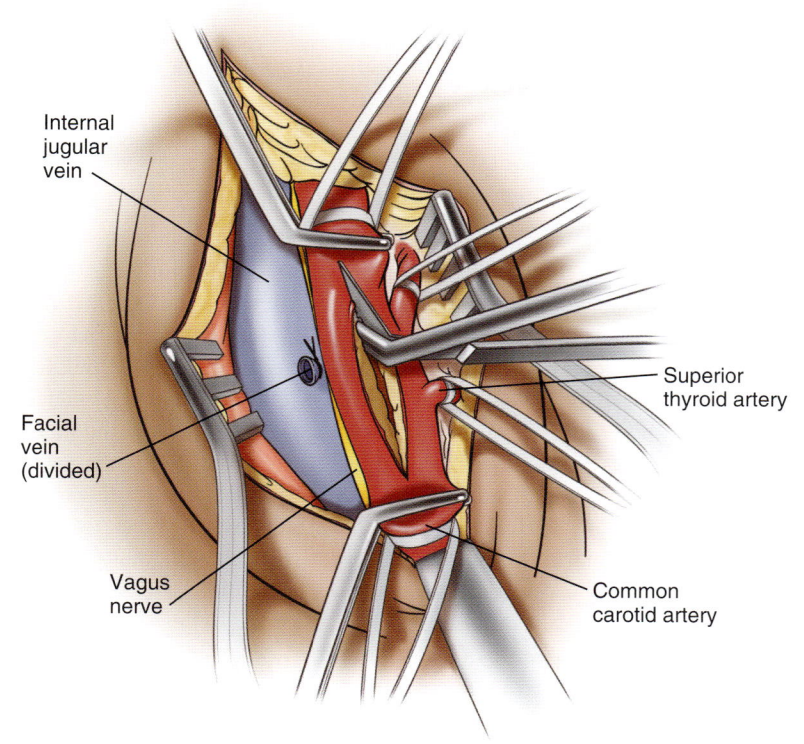

Internal jugular vein

Facial vein (divided)

Vagus nerve

Superior thyroid artery

Common carotid artery

10-9

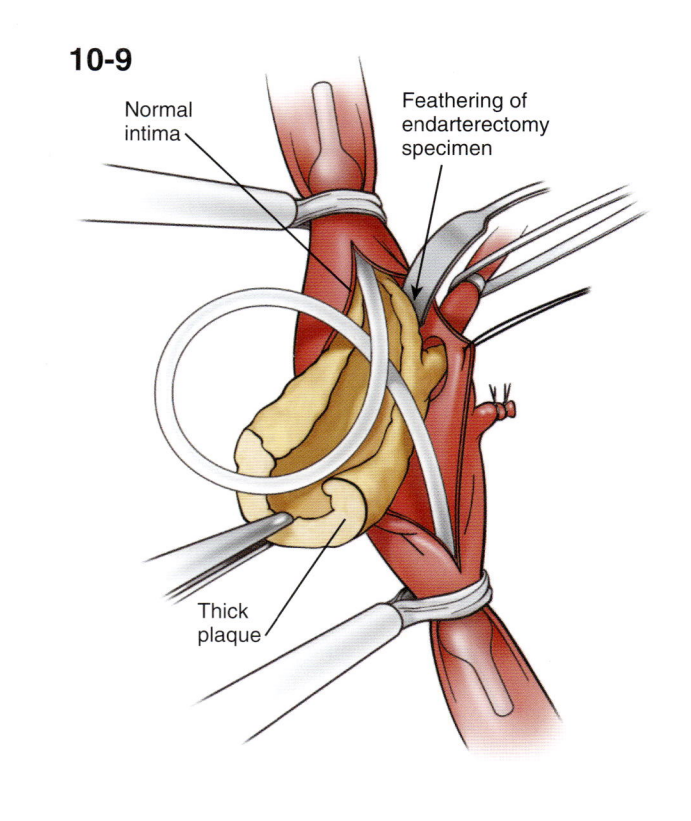

Normal intima

Feathering of endarterectomy specimen

Thick plaque

10-7

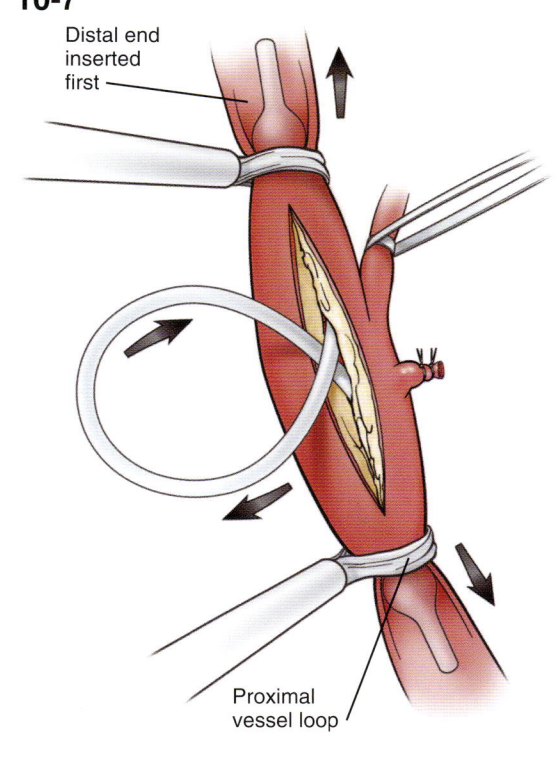

Distal end inserted first

Proximal vessel loop

10-10

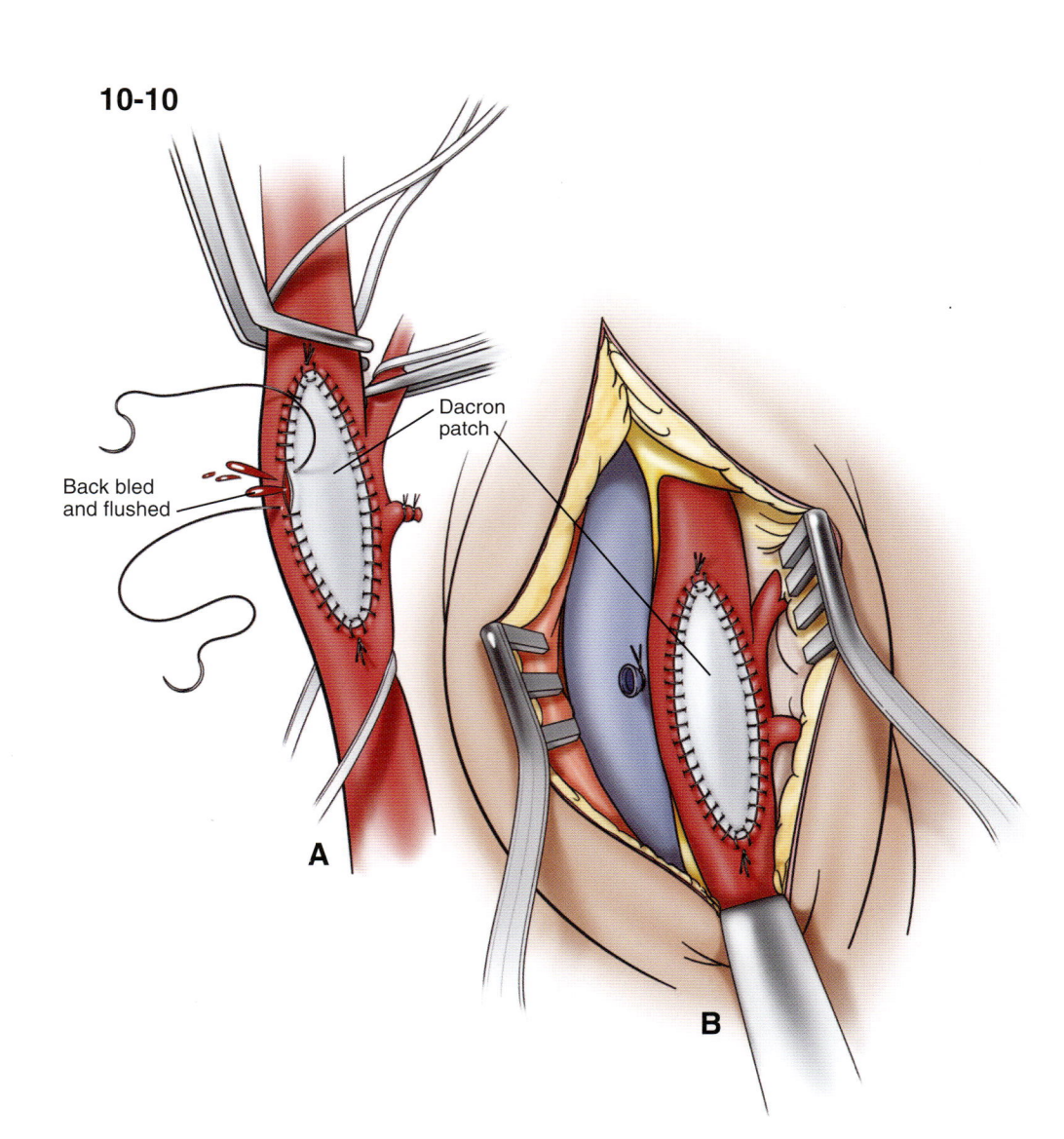

Back bled and flushed

Dacron patch

A

B

10-8

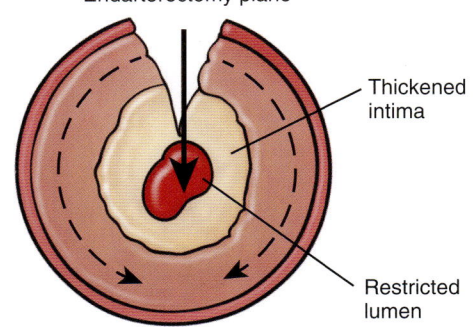

Endarterectomy plane

Thickened intima

Restricted lumen

CEREBROVASCULAR EVERSION ENDARTERECTOMY

Amanda Kistler, MD • Courtney J. Warner, MD • R. Clement Darling III, MD

BACKGROUND There are two well-documented open surgical approaches to treating carotid stenosis: carotid endarterectomy with conventional patch angioplasty and eversion endarterectomy. Eversion endarterectomy was first described by DeBakey in 1959 in an article published in *Postgraduate Medicine* whereby the common carotid artery was transected 1 cm proximal to the carotid bifurcation with eversion of both the internal and external carotid arteries as one unit. This was modified by Kierny et al. with transection and eversion limited to the internal carotid artery. As this technique gained more widespread acceptance, data demonstrated favorable operative, perioperative, and long-term outcomes.

Comparing eversion to traditional patch angioplasty, multiple studies have demonstrated a reduced risk of restenosis due to the longer oblique anastomosis in the mid- and long-term outcomes; however, there is a lack of consensus as to whether this is clinically significant for stroke risk. This is echoed in the EVEREST study. Other advantages of eversion endarterectomy are shorter operating times, decreased clamp time, decreased time spent in the ICU, and decreased length of stay. There is controversy as to whether perioperative stroke risk and death is improved with eversion as compared to traditional patch angioplasty, and studies show no change in rates of peri- and postoperative arrhythmias, transient ischemic events, and cumulative postoperative complications. Two points of controversy regarding the eversion technique are postoperative hypertension and risk of cerebral hyperperfusion syndrome associated with transection of the carotid baroreceptor and perceived difficulties with establishing an endpoint. Nonetheless, literature and case history have established that eversion endarterectomy is a safe and effective technique for extracranial carotid artery stenosis.

PREOPERATIVE EVALUATION In many circumstances, carotid imaging has already been obtained at the time of presentation to a vascular surgeon. A duplex ultrasound should be obtained and any stenosis should be quantified following the NASCET index. Computed tomography angiography may be considered for asymptomatic patients with borderline stenosis, to identify arch or more proximal stenosis, for operative planning, or as confirmation of duplex findings. As patients are awaiting surgery, efforts should be made to improve modifiable risk factors associated with carotid atherosclerosis, namely addressing hypertension, hyperlipidemia, diabetes, and smoking. Patients should be optimized preoperatively by cardiology as well as undergo risk stratification. Consultation with the anesthesia provider may be useful, as many patients undergoing eversion endarterectomy will do so under a regional block. Antiplatelet agents are continued through the perioperative period.

OPERATIVE TECHNIQUE

POSITIONING AND STANDARD PREPARATION: Operative technique for eversion endarterectomy is similar to typical carotid artery exposure with a few modifications. Once in the operating room, the patient is positioned supine on the operating table. Anesthesia will perform a regional block, which is followed by typical surgical positioning with the neck slightly extended and the face turned contralateral to the operative side. The surgical site is prepped and draped to include the angle of the mandible and the inferior portion of the ear lobe superiorly. The prep extends to the sternal notch with the inferior limit of the clavicle and laterally to ensure that the styloid process is within the sterile field.

OPERATIVE EXPOSURE: The incision will be made along the anterior border of the sternocleidomastoid (SCM) muscle extending 7 to 8 cm; however, this may vary based on individual anatomy. If cephalad extension of the incision is needed, it is recommended that the incision be carried posteriorly toward the styloid process, allowing for maneuvers that will facilitate distal exposure. Next, Bovie electrocautery is used to carry the incision through the platysma, followed by sharp dissection with Metzenbaum scissors to deepen the wound through the deep cervical fascia along the anterior border of the SCM. The SCM will be retracted posteriorly, exposing the carotid sheath. Entering the carotid sheath, the internal jugular vein (IJV) is identified and the common facial vein is ligated and divided to facilitate exposure. The IJV is retracted laterally, allowing better visualization of the carotid artery. Exposure of the common, internal, and external carotid arteries follows typical technique while ensuring adequate identification of the vagus and, if necessary, hypoglossal nerves (see **FIGURES 11-1** and **11-2**). The exception to the usual exposure here is that periadventitial tissue will need to be cleared circumferentially from the distal internal carotid artery, beyond the location of atherosclerotic disease, which is seen as the artery takes a bluish hue. This site is where eventual clamping will occur.

EVERSION AND ENDARTERECTOMY TECHNIQUE: After adequate exposure is obtained (**FIGURE 11-1**), intravenous heparin is administered, and the internal carotid artery (ICA) is clamped using Yasargil clips in the aforementioned location. The common carotid artery (CCA) and external carotid artery (ECA) are subsequently clamped again with Yasargil clamps. At this point and moving forward, frequent commands are given by the anesthesiology staff to the patient to demonstrate appropriate neurologic status. Selective shunting will be undertaken if neurologic status declines. The ICA is transected obliquely (**FIGURE 11-2**) angling anteriorly at its origin at the bifurcation using an 11 blade, and any remaining periadventitial tissue is cleared from the CCA and circumferentially from the ICA (**FIGURE 11-3**). An arteriotomy is created on the medial side of the ICA for 1 to 2 cm followed by a similar arteriotomy on the CCA.

Endarterectomy is now undertaken of the ICA using the eversion technique. First, a dissection plane is identified in the proximal ICA (**FIGURE 11-4**). Care is typically taken to handle the endarterectomized artery with fine ring tipped forceps to facilitate removal as a single continuous sheet. **CONTINUES ▶**

11-1

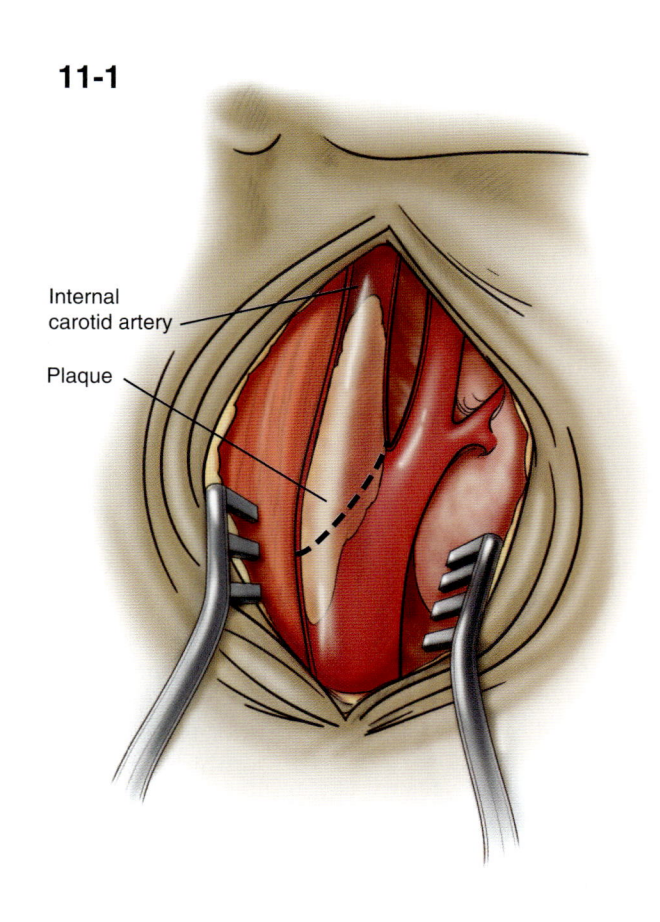

Internal
carotid artery

Plaque

11-2

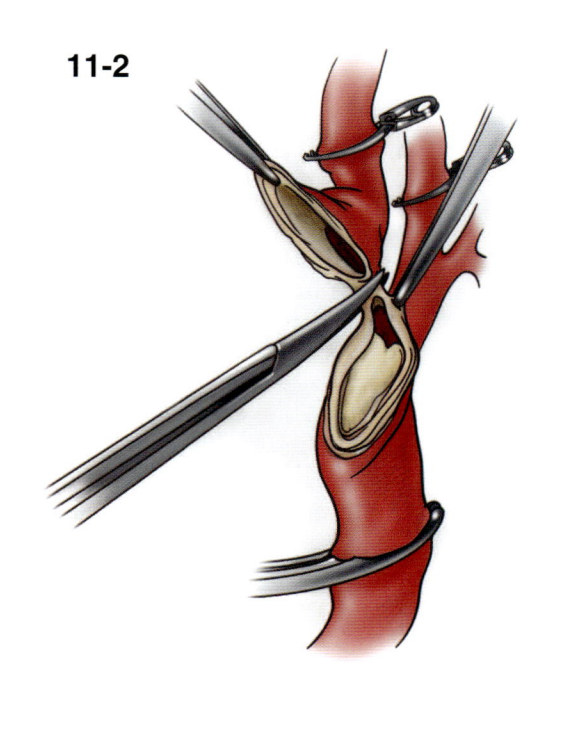

11-3

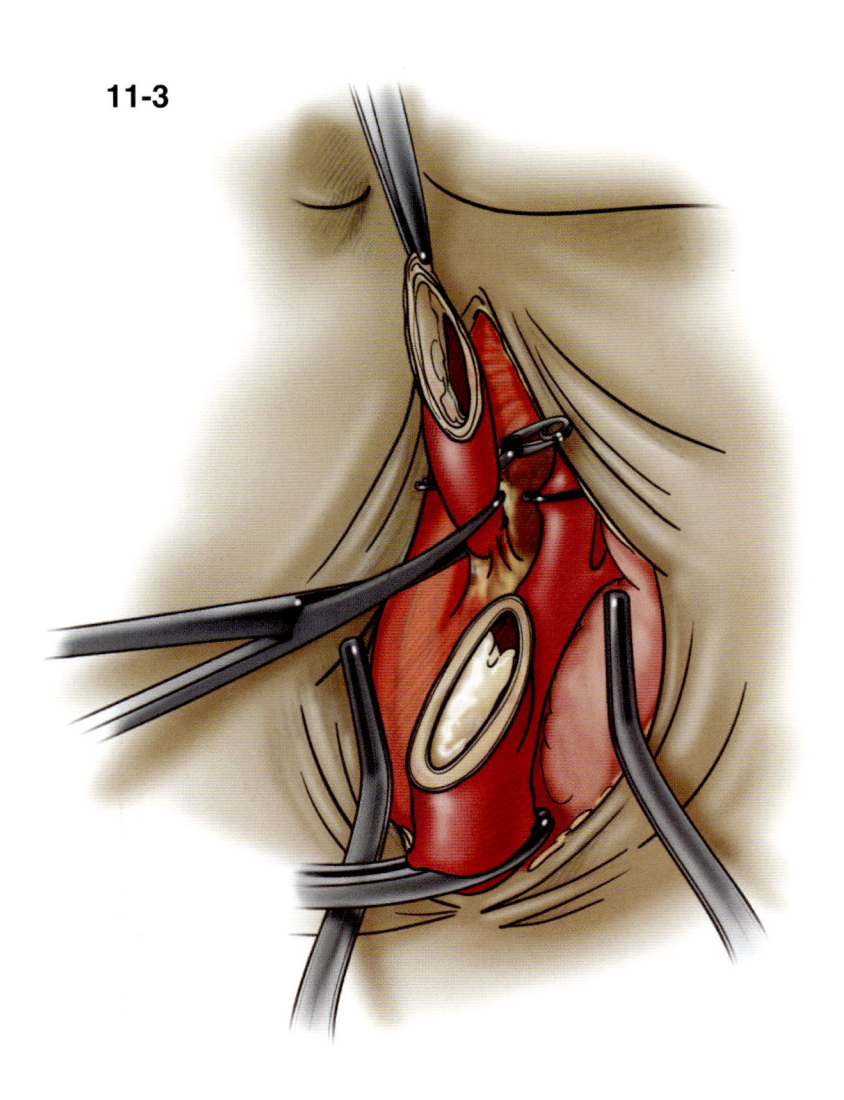

11-4

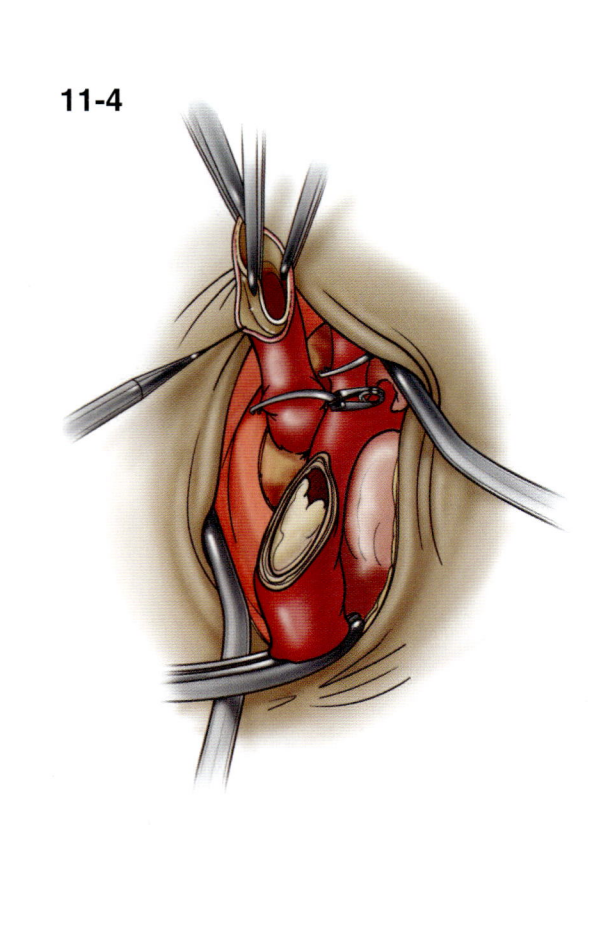

OPERATIVE TECHNIQUE *EVERSION AND ENDARTERECTOMY TECHNIQUE:* ◀ CONTINUED The plaque is separated from the adventitia as the ICA is everted (FIGURE 11-5), resembling the turning out of a sock where the plaque remains stationary (FIGURE 11-6). Once the plaque fully separates from the adventitia, any residual debris is removed in a spiral motion to prevent cephalad dissection. The end point should be clearly visible at this stage (FIGURE 11-7) and if not, the Yasargil clamp should be moved more cephalad on the ICA until this is achieved. Irrigation with heparinized saline is used to identify any residual strands that need removal. Subsequent endarterectomy of the CCA is performed in traditional fashion and is transected proximally with Metzenbaum or Potts scissors. If there is extensive plaque involving the CCA, the arteriotomy may need to be extended proximally to ensure appropriate endarterectomy, necessitating primary closure of such segment with a 6-0 polypropylene to allow for appropriate size match of the eventual ICA-CCA anastomosis (FIGURE 11-8). In some cases, endarterectomy of the proximal ECA is performed in a modified eversion fashion.

Once both arteries are successfully endarterectomized, the ICA is anastomosed to its origin on the CCA with a continuous 6-0 or 7-0 polypropylene suture (FIGURE 11-8). Prior to completion, the ICA clamp is flashed, allowing the artery to back-bleed, and the lumen is irrigated with heparinized saline to remove any stasis thrombus that may have formed. The clamps are then released in the order of ECA, CCA, and finally the ICA. Flow is confirmed by Doppler insonation. Hemostasis is meticulously obtained through the wound bed and the platysma is closed in a running fashion with a 3-0 vicryl followed by stapled closure of the skin.

POSTOPERATIVE CARE Postoperatively, endarterectomy patients are admitted into the vascular surgical floor or neuroprogressive unit where they undergo frequent neurologic checks as well as blood pressure monitoring. Each patient is continued on their home medications as well as an antihypertension protocol with goals of systolic blood pressure less than 180 mmHg. On postoperative day one, if the patient remains medically stable and does not require significant intravenous antihypertensives, the staples are discontinued, quarter inch steristrips are applied, and the patient is discharged with warning signs and symptoms of hyperperfusion syndrome. As advised previously, all patients should undergo risk factor reduction and be discharged on aspirin and statin therapy.

TROUBLESHOOTING As with any other operation, technical issues may be encountered. One perceived limitation to the eversion technique is the inability to establish a distal endpoint. Although this is an exceptionally rare occurrence, it is possible that the distal plaque becomes incorporated in the remaining intima or that upon removal of the plaque the distal intima lifts or dissects. In the former situation, the endarterectomy is stopped in a location that appears relatively free of disease and without significant luminal compromise and is sharply transected. If the intima remains secure, the operation proceeds as previously discussed. However, if there is concern that the remaining intima is unsecure, tacking sutures with 7-0 or 8-0 polypropylene may be used. In the most severe cases, the decision may be made to resect the ICA and perform an interposition bypass with saphenous vein or prosthetic graft.

Another controversial issue not specifically related to eversion endarterectomy is shunting. Substantial data and anecdotal evidence exists to support both obligate and selective shunting. At our institution, we typically employ selective shunting with regional anesthesia. As mentioned previously, as soon as the ICA is clamped, the anesthesiology staff frequently ask the patient to perform tasks, specifically to squeeze a saline bag that is secured to the contralateral hand and connected to an arterial line tracing, at regular intervals. The patient will also intermittently respond to questions. If upon clamping or at any point in the operation the patient is unable to perform these activities, a shunt is inserted if a considerable portion of the surgery remains. It is our practice to use a Javid shunt inserted first into the ICA and then CCA and secured carotid shunt clamps. Care must be taken while inserting the shunt, specifically distally, to not create intimal damage or dissection that would be prone to thrombose in the perioperative period.

Upon completion of the anastomosis and Doppler interrogation, if no flow is detected in the ICA, re-exploration is necessary whether or not the patient is experiencing a neurological deficit, as this implies thrombosis. When investigating the thrombus, etiology will dictate further management. Red thrombus usually indicates a local problem such as the end point. Once opened, retrograde flow through the ICA will often flush out the thrombus but this is not always the case. In circumstances where thrombus remains, a No. 2 or 3 Fogarty embolectomy catheter may be used to remove the thrombus. Still, the anastomosis and end points need to be investigated and revised. If, however, white thrombus is encountered, aberrant platelet aggregation has occurred. If no technical issue is encountered, replacement of the segment with a vein interposition graft may be considered as well as a more potent antiplatelet regimen. Heparin-induced thrombocytopenia should be considered and ruled out.

SPECIAL CIRCUMSTANCES Special considerations when contemplating approach for endarterectomy should include underlying etiology. Eversion endarterectomy is particularly well suited when ICA kinks or coils are present. With coils, the redundancy of the ICA lends itself well to the eversion technique because the artery is mobilized and can be stretched to an appropriate length, excised, and anastomosed in a more anatomic orientation. ICA kinks may be handled in a similar fashion.

CONCLUSION Eversion endarterectomy is a safe and effective management of extracranial carotid artery stenosis as well as circumstances such as carotid artery kinks and coils. As explained, the positioning and vascular exposure remain quite typical and the procedure is therefore adoptable with adequate experience by many vascular surgeons. Eversion endarterectomy incurs shorter operative times, clamp times, and length of stay without significant increases in postoperative neurologic events or incidence of cerebral hyperperfusion syndrome. ■

SUGGESTED READINGS

Brott T. Carotid Revascularization and Medical Management for Asymptomatic Carotid Stenosis Trial (CREST-2) [Internet]. Available from: https://clinicaltrials.gov/ct2/show/NCT02089217

Chaturvedi S, Lalla R, Raghavan P. Trends and controversies in carotid artery stenosis treatment. *F1000Res* 2020;9:1–10.

Cheng SF, van Velzen TJ, Gregson J, Richards T, Jager HR, Simister R, et al. The 2nd European Carotid Surgery trial (ECST-2) [Internet]. Available from: http://s489637516.websitehome.co.uk/ECST2/index2.htm

Davidovic LB, Tomic IZ. Eversion carotid endarterectomy: A short review. *J Korean Neurosurg Soc* 2020;63(3):373–9.

DeBakey M. Regarding "A randomized study on eversion versus standard carotid endarterectomy. Study design and preliminary results: The Everest Trial." *J Vasc Surg* 1998;28:753.

Djedovic M, Mujanovic E, Hadzimehmedagic A, Totic D, Vukas H, Vranic H. Comparison of results classical and eversion carotid endarterectomy. *Med Arch* (Sarajevo, Bosnia Herzegovina). 2017;71(2):89–92.

Hathout GM, Fink JR, El-Saden SM, Grant EG. Sonographic NASCET Index: A New Doppler Parameter for Assessment of Internal Carotid Artery Stenosis. *AJNR Am J Neuroradiol* 2005;(January):68–75.

Kieny R, Hirsch D, Seiller C, Thiranos JC, Petit H. Does carotid eversion endarterectomy and reimplantation reduce the risk of restenosis? *Ann Vasc Surg* 1993;7:407–13.

Marsman MS, Wetterslev J, Vriens PWHE, Bleys RLAW, Jahrome AK, Moll FL, et al. Eversion technique versus conventional endarterectomy with patch angioplasty in carotid surgery: Protocol for a systematic review with meta-analyses and trial sequential analysis of randomised clinical trials. *BMJ Open* 2020;10(4):1–9.

Ricotta JJ, Aburahma A, Ascher E, Eskandari M, Faries P, Lal BK. Updated Society for Vascular Surgery guidelines for management of extracranial carotid disease. *J Vasc Surg* [Internet]. 2011;54(3):e1–31. Available from: http://dx.doi.org/10.1016/j.jvs.2011.07.031

11-5

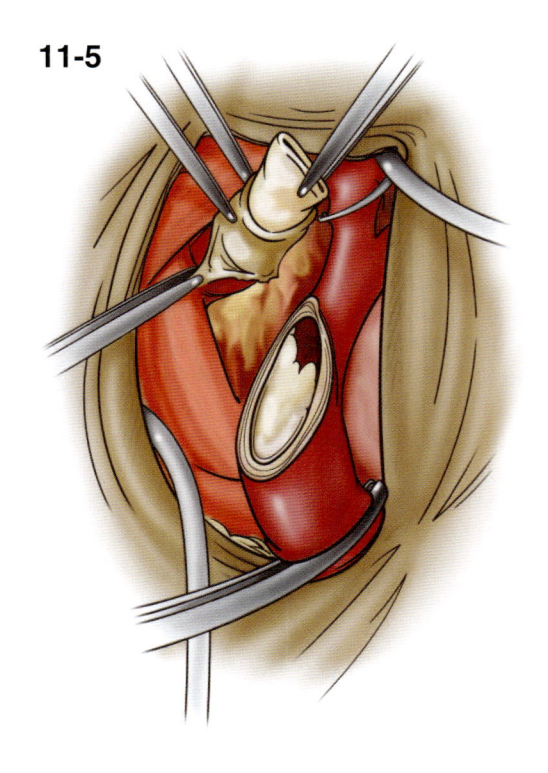

11-6

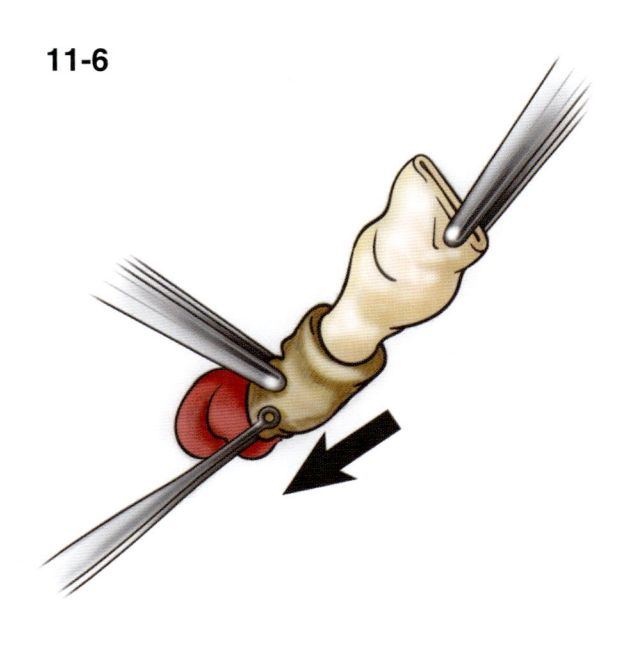

11-7

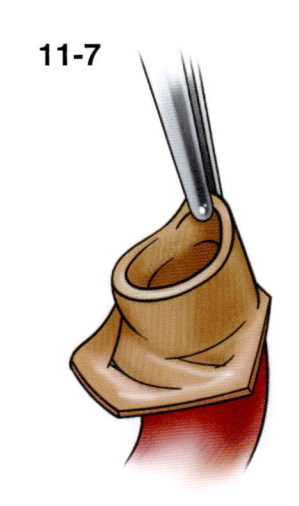

11-8

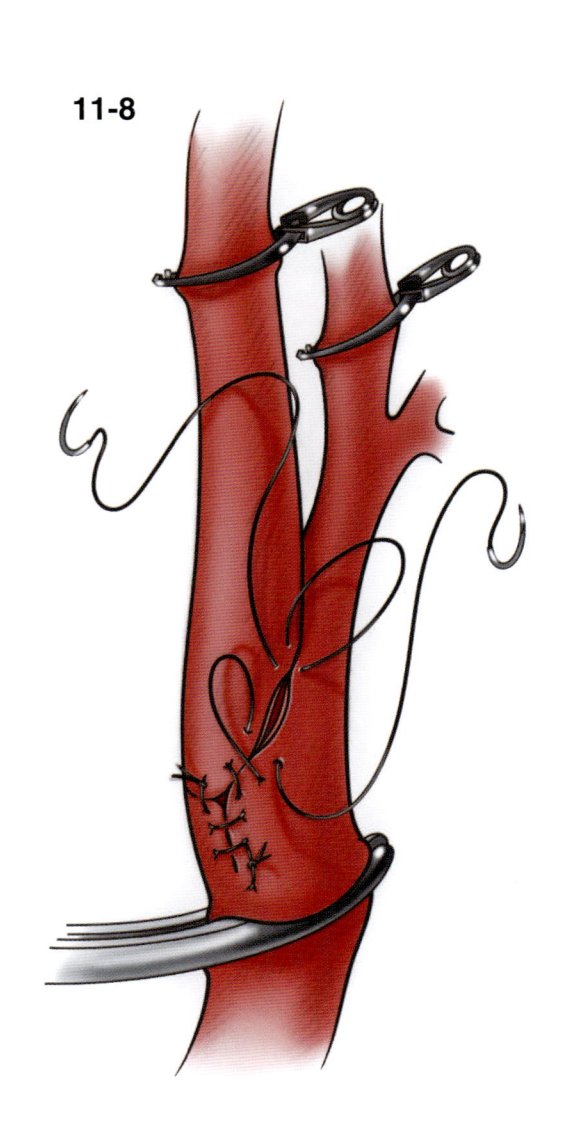

Carotid Subclavian Bypass and Transposition

Tadaki M. Tomita, MD • Mark K. Eskandari, MD

INDICATIONS Historically carotid subclavian bypass or transposition has been performed on patients with atherosclerotic occlusive disease that require revascularization; however, in the endovascular era most subclavian revascularizations are done as an adjunct procedure for endovascular treatment of aortic pathology. Currently, the most frequent indication for subclavian revascularization is in the setting of left subclavian coverage during thoracic endovascular aortic repair (TEVAR). Our preference is to perform carotid subclavian bypass (CSB) over subclavian transposition (ST) since it is technically more straightforward. The drawback is that in cases of TEVAR coverage of the left subclavian artery, coil embolization of the origin of the subclavian is required to prevent a type II endoleak. Subclavian revascularization for atherosclerotic disease should be reserved for patients with symptoms of upper extremity ischemia, subclavian steal syndrome, or any patient with a significant subclavian stenosis proximal to an internal mammary artery coronary artery bypass. CSB is preferred in these coronary bypass patients over ST as well as in patients with a very proximal vertebral artery. The benefit of ST is there is a single anastomosis without a need for a prosthetic implant. Here we describe both methods for subclavian revascularization.

POSITION After being placed under general anesthesia with endotracheal tube taped to the contralateral side, the patient is placed in the supine position with the arms tucked. A small shoulder roll is placed under the scapula transversely. The head is supported and rotated to the contralateral side. For patients undergoing concomitant TEVAR, this procedure can be done on an endovascular table with ease. Patients who are not undergoing a combined procedure are done on a standard bed to allow placement in the beach chair position.

OPERATIVE PREPARATION For both CSB and ST, the patient is prepped from the margin of the mandible to the nipple line. Laterally the neck is prepped to the bed, over the shoulder and medially past 3 cm past the midline. Chlorohexidine prep is preferred with adequate drying time. To drape, scrunched up blue towels are first placed on either side of the neck. Folded up blue towels are then used to towel off the operative field. An adhesive antimicrobial incise drape is then placed on the skin and over the towels. A universal drape is then used to cover the remainder of the patient.

INCISION AND EXPOSURE For CSB, a transverse incision is made 1 cm cephalad to the clavicle, starting 1 cm lateral to the clavicular head of the sternocleomastoid muscle (SCM) and extending 6 to 8 cm laterally (FIGURE 12-1). The incision and exposure for ST differs slightly and is more medial—centered between the two heads of the SCM—than for CSB. This incision is then carried down through the platysma with electrocautery. Subplatysmal flaps are then created to maximize exposure. The lateral border of the clavicular head of the SCM is then mobilized longitudinally and medially. The inferior belly of the omohyoid muscle is divided with electrocautery. Along with a self-retaining retractor, a hand-held retractor is used to retract the lateral aspect of the SCM medially to facilitate exposure of the common carotid artery. Division of the clavicular head of the SCM is rarely required. The carotid sheath is entered sharply and opened longitudinally. The internal jugular vein (IJ) is typically identified first, mobilized along its lateral border and retracted medially. Care must be taken to observe the vagus nerve and preserve it. The common carotid artery is then circumferentially dissected for several centimeters within the field (FIGURE 12-2).

Next, the scalene fat pad is mobilized laterally. Crossing vessels and lymphatics are divided between clips or ties. On the left side, the thoracic duct is ligated when encountered. Care is taken to identify the phrenic nerve, which travels from lateral to medial over the anterior scalene muscle. This muscle is palpated at the base of the incision and acts as the gateway to the subclavian artery. With the phrenic nerve preserved in the field, the anterior scalene muscle is then divided transversely directly over the subclavian artery (FIGURE 12-3). Once the subclavian artery is visualized it can be mobilized as medial in the field as possible. As the artery is dissected the thyrocervical trunk, vertebral and internal mammary can be encountered and each should be circumferentially controlled. The subclavian artery is then controlled at the lateral extent of the incision. **CONTINUES ▶**

12-1

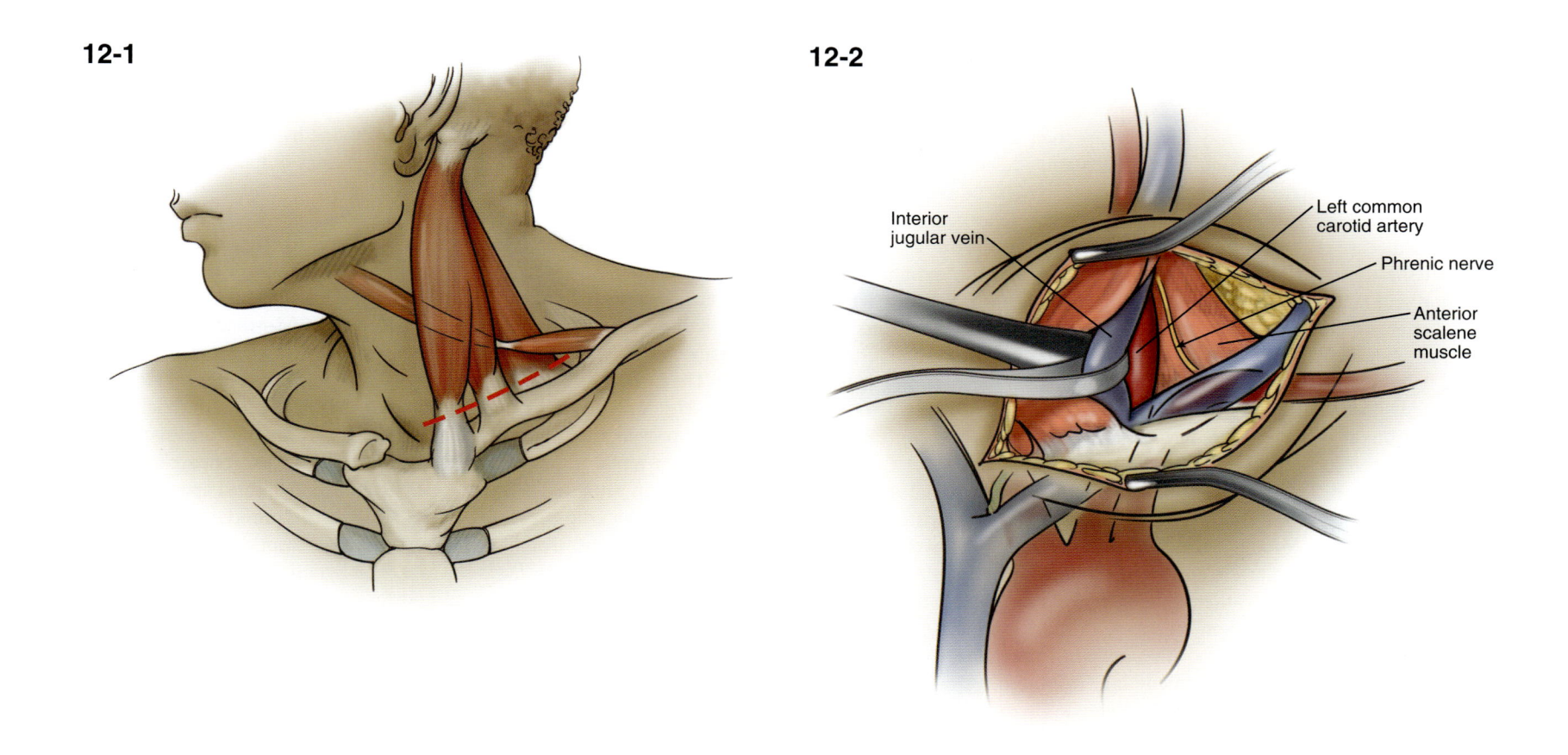

12-2

Interior jugular vein

Left common carotid artery

Phrenic nerve

Anterior scalene muscle

12-3

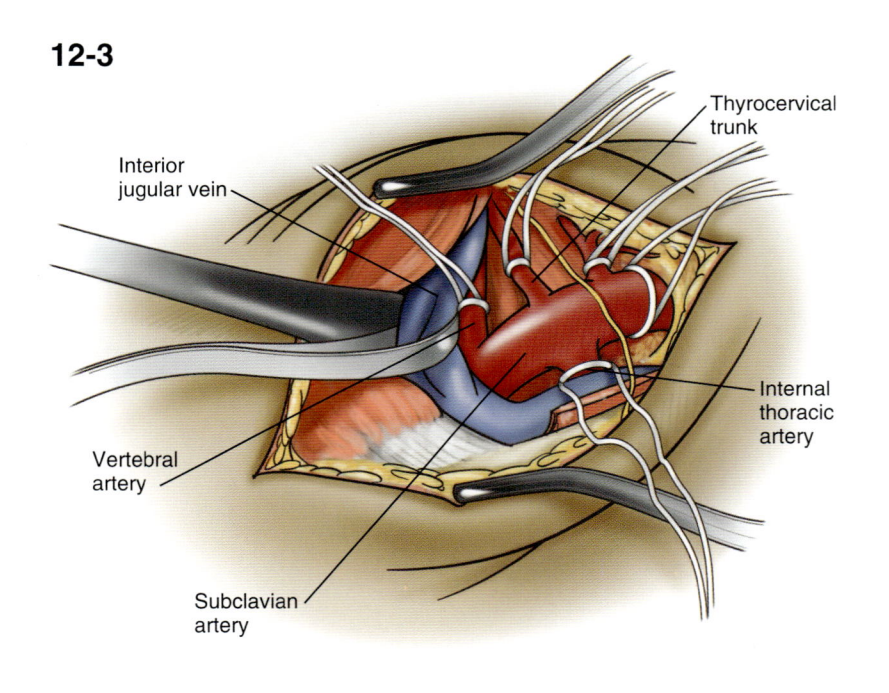

Interior jugular vein

Thyrocervical trunk

Internal thoracic artery

Vertebral artery

Subclavian artery

INCISION AND EXPOSURE `CONTINUED` The incision for a ST is more medial than the incision for CSB and is centered between the heads of the SCM. After dividing the platysma, subplatysmal flaps are raised to aid in the exposure. The two bellies of the SCM are then separated in the avascular plain that runs longitudinally between them, and self-retaining retractors are placed. Deep to this, the omohyoid muscle will be encountered and divided using electrocautery. Next, the internal jugular vein is mobilized, and in this case is retracted laterally. The common carotid artery is then dissected as centrally and cranially as possible to allow for maximal mobilization and facilitate exposure of the subclavian artery. Working between the IJ laterally, and the carotid and vagus nerve medially, the dissection is carried posteriorly (FIGURE 12-4). The thoracic duct on the left side will need to be ligated; however, smaller lymphatics can be present on either side and will also need to be ligated. The gateway to the subclavian artery in this location is the vertebral vein. Ligation of this vein allows for exposure of the proximal subclavian artery and its branches (FIGURE 12-5). Care must be taken when dissecting out the vertebral artery and internal mammary, as the origins of the vessels are fragile and can be located posterior to the subclavian artery. Crossing sympathetic nerves should be avoided in this region of the subclavian artery and travel cephalad with the vertebral artery. The proximal subclavian is then dissected proximally under the clavicle. It is important to stay directly on the artery in this location to prevent entry into the pleural cavity. To get distal control of the subclavian artery, the medial portion of the anterior scalene may need to be retracted out of the way, and typically does not need to be divided. Thyrocervical trunk vessels may be encountered laterally and should be controlled.

DETAILS OF THE PROCEDURE For CSB, the subclavian anastomosis is performed first. After administration of heparin, micro bulldogs are placed on any branches within the field and profunda clamps are placed on the distal and proximal extent of the subclavian artery. In the setting of an internal mammary–based coronary bypass, the proximal subclavian clamp should be distal to this vessel to prevent coronary ischemia. With the vessels clamped, a longitudinal arteriotomy is made in the subclavian artery. An 8-mm polytetrafluoroethylene (PTFE) graft is our preferred graft for this bypass and has superior durability to vein. The graft is spatulated and sewn end-to-side to the subclavian artery. Care should be taken when placing stitches into the subclavian artery as it is typically very thin-walled and prone to dissection or tearing. In cases where the anatomy is challenging, a parachute technique may be required to perform this anastomosis. After completion of the anastomosis, the flow is directed down the bypass prior to restoring flow to the arm. A padded clamp is then placed on the PTFE graft. The anastomosis should be inspected at this point for any technical issues, as it will be easier to fix at this stage. When satisfied, the padded clamp is moved as close as possible to the subclavian anastomosis. Attention is then replaced to the common carotid artery. Profunda clamps are used to clamp proximal and distal on the common carotid artery. Neuromonitoring or stump pressures are typically not required. A longitudinal arteriotomy is then made in the lateral common carotid artery with an 11 blade and extended with Potts scissors. The bypass is positioned anterior to the phrenic and vagus nerves and posterior to the IJ (FIGURE 12-6). The IJ should be retracted medially in the field at this point. The graft is then trimmed to length and sewn end-to-side to the common carotid artery using a running 5-0 polypropylene suture. This anastomosis is typically started at the inferior aspect of the bypass. It is important to sew the posterior wall of the anastomosis first and the anterior portion last. Prior to completion of the anastomosis the clamps are flashed and the arteriotomy is irrigated with heparinized saline. Flow is then directed down the subclavian bypass prior to restoring flow to the brain. `CONTINUES`

12-4

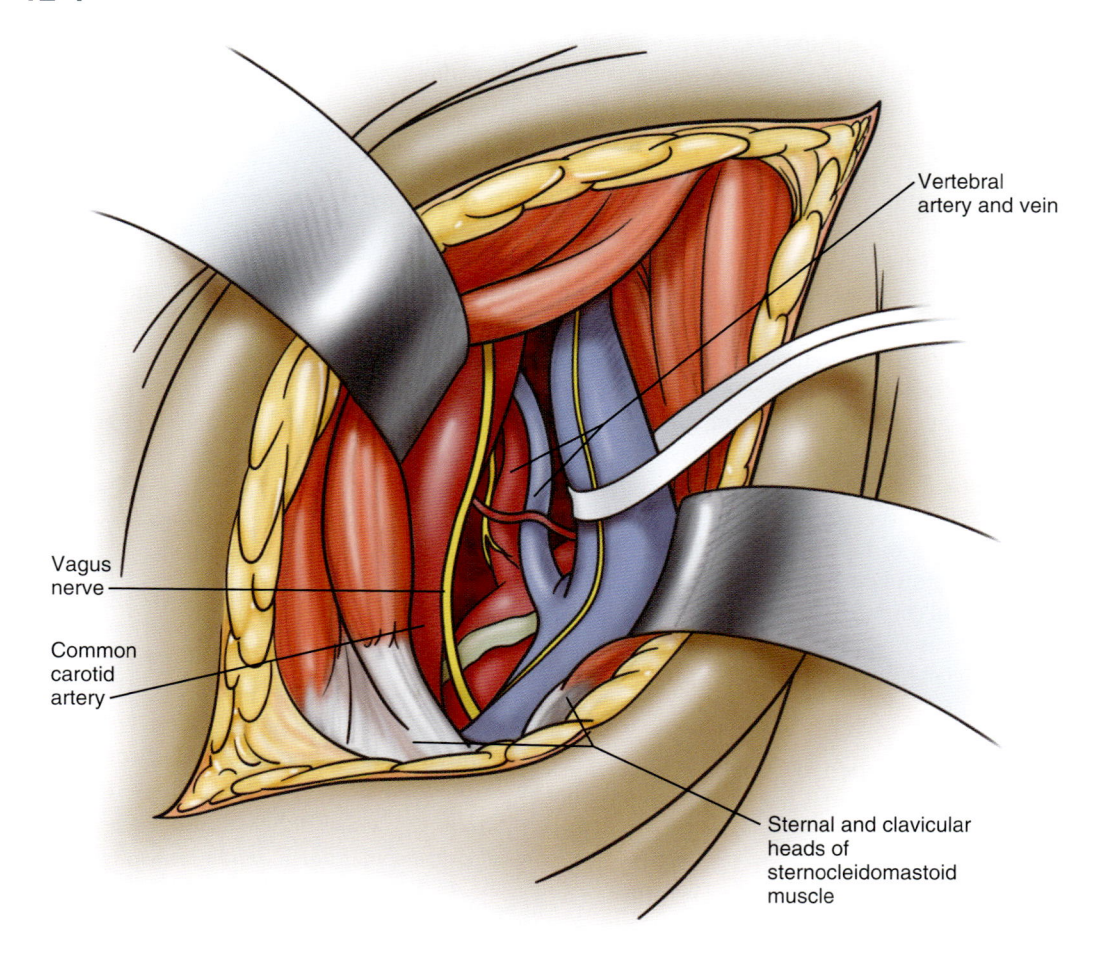

Vertebral artery and vein

Vagus nerve

Common carotid artery

Sternal and clavicular heads of sternocleidomastoid muscle

12-5

12-6

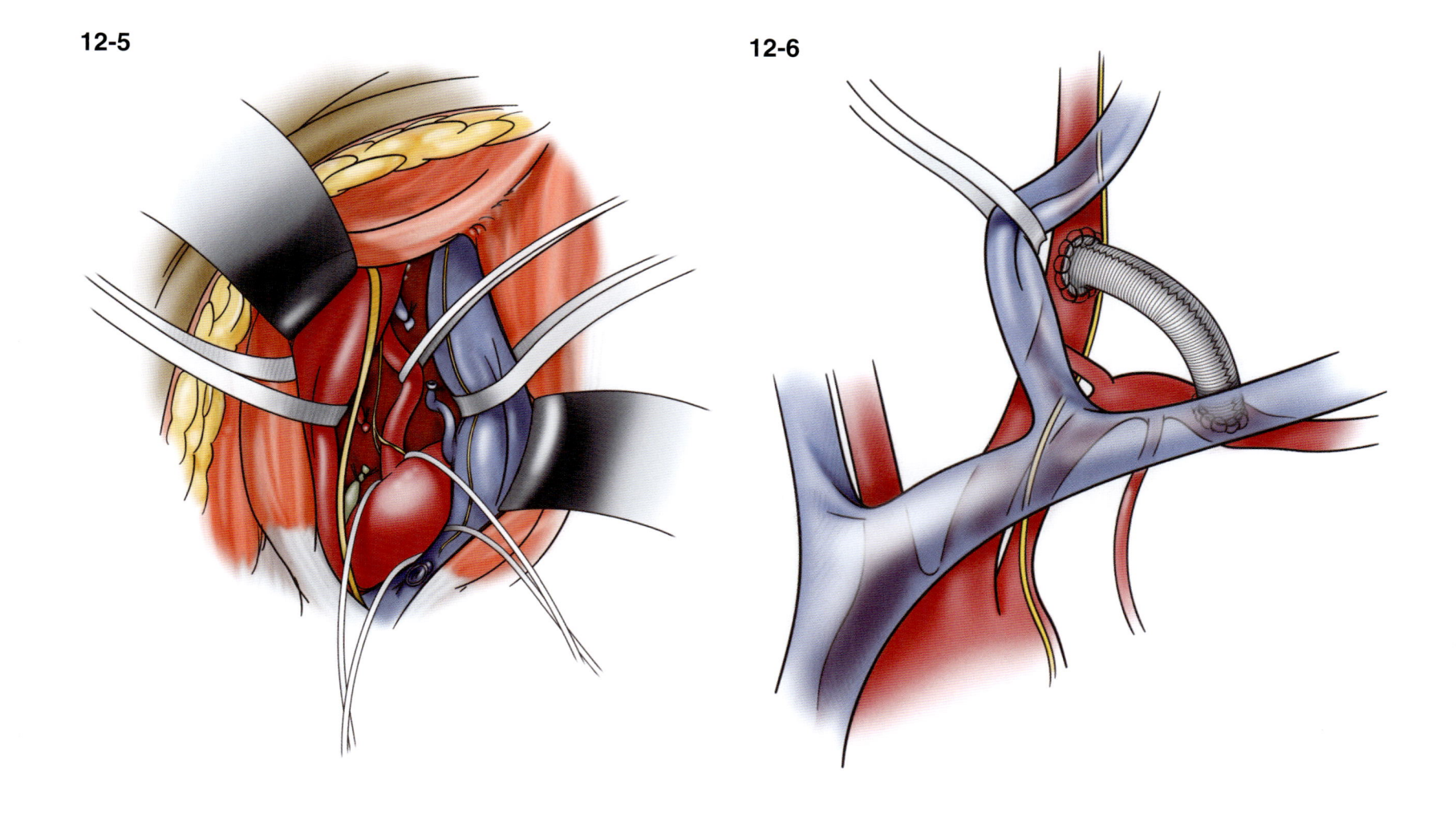

DETAILS OF THE PROCEDURE `CONTINUED` The first step for a ST is division of subclavian artery and ligation of the stump. After administration of heparin, the vertebral artery and other branches are clamped using micro bulldogs. A profunda clamp is placed on the distal subclavian artery and a right-angle clamp is placed on the proximal subclavian artery. A 5-0 polypropylene stay suture is then placed on either side of the proximal subclavian artery just distal to the clamp to prevent retraction of the vessel after transection. The subclavian artery is then transected 1 cm distal to the proximal clamp. The stump is over sewn using a running 5-0 polypropylene suture in two layers; the first is a running horizontal mattress suture followed by a simple running suture (**FIGURE 12-7**). The clamp is removed prior to cutting the sutures to prevent vessel retraction in the setting that hemostasis is not achieved. It is critical to ligate the stump prior to proceeding with the reconstruction, as it is technically easier and loss of control of this vessel while working on the reconstruction could be catastrophic.

Next, the common carotid artery is rotated and clamped with profunda clamps in a way to expose the posterolateral portion of the vessel (**FIGURE 12-8A**). An arteriotomy is made in the segment of the common carotid artery adjacent to the distal edge of the transected subclavian artery. The end of the subclavian artery is then sewn to the side of the common carotid artery starting with the posterior aspect of the anastomosis. If the subclavian is too redundant, it may need to be trimmed to prevent kinking. If there is not enough length, the carotid can typically be further mobilized to allow it to move laterally. Prior to completion of the anastomosis, the clamps are flashed and the arteriotomy is irrigated with heparinized saline. Flow is then directed down the subclavian prior to restoring flow to the brain (**FIGURE 12-8B**).

CLOSURE Prior to closing, protamine is given to reverse the heparin, and hemostasis is ensured. For CSB the scalene fat pad is reapproximated to the lateral margin of the SCM using interrupted absorbable sutures. For both SCB and ST, a drain is placed in the wound bed and brought out through the skin lateral to the incision. The platysma muscle is then closed using a running absorbable suture over the drain. Interrupted deep dermal sutures are then placed to approximate the skin margin and the skin is closed using a monofilament absorbable suture in a subcuticular fashion. Topical skin adhesive is placed as a dressing. A drain sponge is placed over the drain site followed by a clear adhesive dressing.

POSTOPERATIVE CARE The patient is extubated in the operating room, where a neurological exam is performed to evaluate for possible signs of stroke. Distal pulses and a blood pressure are also evaluated to confirm patency of the revascularization. In the recovery area, a chest x-ray is performed to evaluate for possible sign of phrenic nerve palsy with an ipsilateral raised hemidiaphragm or evidence of a pneumothorax. A clear liquid diet is followed the evening after surgery. On postoperative day 1 the diet is advanced to a regular diet and the patient is allowed to ambulate with assistance. The drain is left in place until the patient is tolerating a regular diet and there is less than 30 cc of output per 24-hour period. Most patients are discharged on postoperative day 2 without the drain on full-dose aspirin and a statin. Patients are then seen 1 month postoperatively for noninvasive vascular testing and the aspirin is typically reduced to 81 mg. The long-term patency for both CSV and ST is very good and rarely requires reinterventions. ■

SUGGESTED READINGS

Eskandari MK. Aortic debranching procedures to facilitate endografting. *Perspect Vasc Surg Endovasc Ther.* 2006;18(4):287–292.

Delafontaine JL, Hu B, Tan TW, et al. Outcome comparison of TEVAR with and without left subclavian artery revascularization from analysis of nationwide inpatient sample database. *Ann Vasc Surg.* 2019;58:174–179.

D'Oria M, Kärkkäinen JM, Tenorio ER, et al. Perioperative outcomes of carotid-subclavian bypass or transposition versus endovascular techniques for left subclavian artery revascularization during nontraumatic zone 2 thoracic endovascular aortic repair in the vascular quality initiative. *Ann Vasc Surg.* 2020;69:17–26.

Morasch MD. Technique for subclavian to carotid transposition, tips, and tricks. *J Vasc Surg.* 2009;49(1):251–254.

Zamor KC, Eskandari MK, Rodriguez HE, et al. Outcomes of thoracic endovascular aortic repair and subclavian revascularization techniques. *J Am Coll Surg.* 2015;221(1):93–100.

Ziomek S, Quiñones-Baldrich WJ, Busuttil RW, et al. The superiority of synthetic arterial grafts over autologous veins in carotid-subclavian bypass. *J Vasc Surg.* 1986;3(1):140–145.

12-7

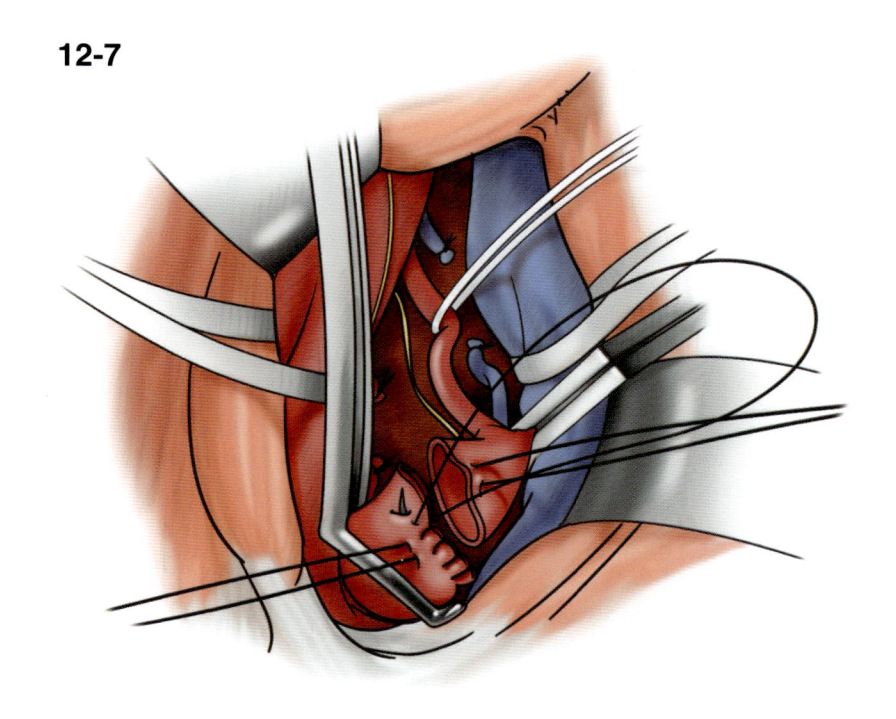

12-8

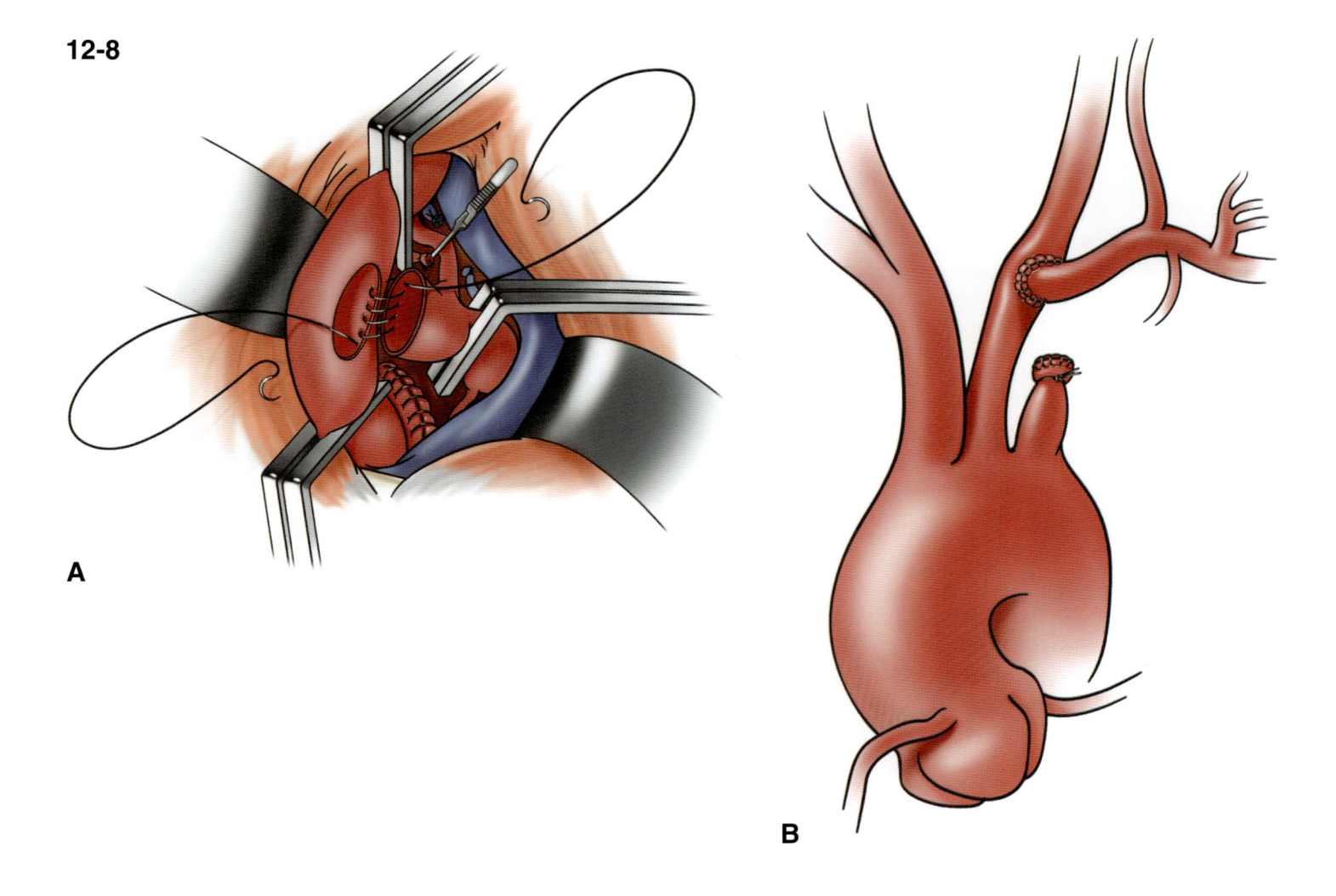

A

B

INNOMINATE ARTERY RECONSTRUCTION (ENDARTERECTOMY AND BYPASS)

Jill Colglazier, MD • Thomas Bower, MD

INDICATIONS The most common indication for innominate artery endarterectomy or bypass in the United States is symptomatic atherosclerotic occlusive disease, with embolism the primary mechanism. Neurologic symptoms can be anterior or posterior circulation-related and include upper or lower extremity weakness or paralysis, amaurosis, facial droop, aphasia, dysarthria, vertigo, or imbalance and nausea. Right upper extremity symptoms are less frequent and include exertional arm pain or fatigue or digital ischemia from distal embolization. The combination of neurologic symptoms and arm ischemia is reported in 18 to 39% of patients.

The second leading cause of innominate artery disease is arteritis, of which Takayasu arteritis (TA) is most common. TA causes long segment tapered stenoses or occlusions of the supra-aortic trunks (SAT), most commonly in women of childbearing age and of Asian descent, though anyone can be affected. TA manifests initially as a systemic illness with fever, malaise, night sweats, weight loss, arthralgias, or fatigue. Symptoms result from low flow states, as opposed to thromboembolism. Upper extremity exertional fatigue, orthostasis, global cerebral ischemia, visual impairment, or vertebrobasilar symptoms are common.

PREOPERATIVE PREPARATION The diagnosis and etiology of innominate artery disease can be determined from the history and physical examination. Imaging confirms the diagnosis and is critical for operative planning. Computed tomographic angiography (CTA) or magnetic resonance angiography (MRA) of the head, neck, and chest defines the severity and extent of disease in the ascending aorta, arch, innominate and other SATs. It is essential that the ascending aorta and arch be free from calcification to provide a safe area for clamping for bypass or endarterectomy. If needed, carotid duplex ultrasonography provides additional anatomic information about the cervical carotid and vertebral arteries.

Choice of direct aortic-origin bypass or endarterectomy is determined by medical risk for surgery and when endovascular therapy is not an option. One-fourth of patients with atherosclerotic disease have coexisting coronary artery disease. Those with TA may have valve disease, pulmonary hypertension, or left ventricular hypertrophy from longstanding hypertension. Therefore, cardiac stress testing and/or coronary angiography and echocardiography are needed prior to operation. Pulmonary risk is evaluated with pulmonary function tests and an arterial blood gas.

ANESTHESIA AND PATIENT POSITIONING General anesthesia is needed. The left radial artery is used for blood pressure monitoring provided there is no left subclavian artery disease. A central venous line is placed into the left internal jugular or left subclavian vein. We use intraoperative electroencephalography for neuro-monitoring in all cerebrovascular revascularizations. Transcranial Doppler or cerebral oximetry can also be used.

The patient is placed supine on the operating room table with arms tucked at the sides. A rolled towel is placed vertically under the spine between the scapulae to open the chest. The head is extended and the neck supported. Both sides of the neck, chest, and upper abdomen are prepared and draped into the sterile field.

INCISION AND EXPOSURE A partial or full median sternotomy is used to expose the ascending aorta and innominate artery. A full sternotomy is done through a vertical incision from the suprasternal notch to below the xiphoid process. The incision can be extended into the right neck as necessary to expose the innominate artery bifurcation or the proximal subclavian and common carotid arteries (**FIGURE 13-1A**). The latter may require division of the sternal muscle attachments. A partial sternotomy is used if the innominate artery disease is focal and the ascending aorta can be accessed. The sternum can be divided horizontally in the third or fourth interspace to facilitate exposure. This approach is avoided in patients with extensive SAT disease or in emergency cases.

DETAILS OF THE PROCEDURE To perform the median sternotomy, the sternal incision is deepened through the subcutaneous tissue to the periosteum. Blunt finger dissection is used behind the sternal notch and beneath the xiphoid to clear the posterior surface of the sternum. A sternal saw or vertical oscillating blade is used to divide the sternum in the midline. Retraction and exposure is gained by opening a sternal retractor a few turns at a time to avoid fractures (**FIGURE 13-1B**).

Thymic and mediastinal fatty tissue is divided and resected if bypass is to be done, to make room for grafts. The left brachiocephalic vein crosses anteriorly over the innominate artery and the aortic arch. It is circumferentially dissected free and preserved to avoid postoperative left upper extremity venous congestion. The innominate artery origin is visualized by retracting the brachiocephalic vein caudally. The origin is not controlled until the distal clamp sites have been isolated and the patient heparinized to avoid atheroembolization. The pericardial sac is incised vertically to expose the ascending aorta, which is often free from atherosclerotic disease and is the preferred location for the proximal graft anastomosis.

Exposure of the distal clamp sites usually involves isolation of the proximal right subclavian and common carotid arteries and requires transection of the right-sided strap muscles. The vagus and recurrent laryngeal nerves are identified and protected. The recurrent laryngeal nerve loops beneath the proximal right subclavian artery (**FIGURE 13-2**). The vagus nerve descends along the lateral or posterolateral edge of the right common carotid artery, crosses on top of the proximal right subclavian artery, and continues into the mediastinum posterior to the right brachiocephalic vein. If further exposure of the right subclavian is required to find a disease-free segment, the incision is carried into the supraclavicular space. This may necessitate the mobilization of the scalene fat pad and requires identification of the phrenic nerve, which lies on the anteromedial surface of the anterior scalene muscle and descends from lateral to medial. The anterior scalene muscle is divided fully or in part with bipolar cautery to visualize the artery. Similarly, if more common carotid artery requires isolation, the sternotomy incision can be extended along the anterior border of the sternocleidomastoid muscle. If both arteries must be isolated in the neck, the sternotomy incision is carried obliquely between the anterior border of the sternocleidomastoid muscle and the clavicle. Once the distal clamp sites are isolated, the patient is given intravenous heparin to achieve a therapeutic activated clotting time. The origin of the innominate artery and the adjacent arch are then dissected free, with minimal manipulation of the artery.

Rarely, if atherosclerotic disease is isolated to the innominate artery, does not involve the aortic arch, and there is no common brachiocephalic trunk, an innominate artery endarterectomy can be performed. The mean arterial pressure is raised to between 90 and 100 mmHg. The distal arteries are clamped first. Then an all-purpose aortic or similar shaped clamp is placed beneath the innominate artery origin on the aortic arch. The innominate artery is opened vertically with the arteriotomy extended onto the arch. An endarterectomy is performed. Proximal and distal tacking sutures for the endpoints may be needed, particularly in the arch, to avoid an intimal flap and dissection. The artery is closed primarily or with a patch using running 4-0 or 5-0 polypropylene suture.

Innominate artery bypass is done with an 8-, 9-, or 10-mm diameter polyester graft. If the right common carotid and subclavian arteries have to be separately reconstructed, our preference is to use a single limb to one artery, with reimplantation or a separate graft to the other. Bifurcated grafts are bulky and can kink or be compressed with sternal closure. The proximal end of the graft is spatulated to prepare for sewing. The systolic blood pressure is lowered to between 90 and 100 mmHg for placement of an all-purpose aortic or Kay Lambert clamp on the anterolateral ascending aorta (**FIGURE 13-3**). The aorta is opened vertically. The proximal anastomosis is performed using running 4-0 polypropylene suture. The suture line is buttressed with a felt strip as needed. The graft is filled with saline to test the anastomosis. Suture line leaks are controlled with interrupted horizontal mattress pledgeted sutures. The partial occlusion clamp is released, the graft flushed, and a coarctation clamp placed on the graft just distal to the anastomosis. Blood is stripped from the graft, it is irrigated and the fluid suctioned to be certain the graft is clean. **CONTINUES ▶**

13-1

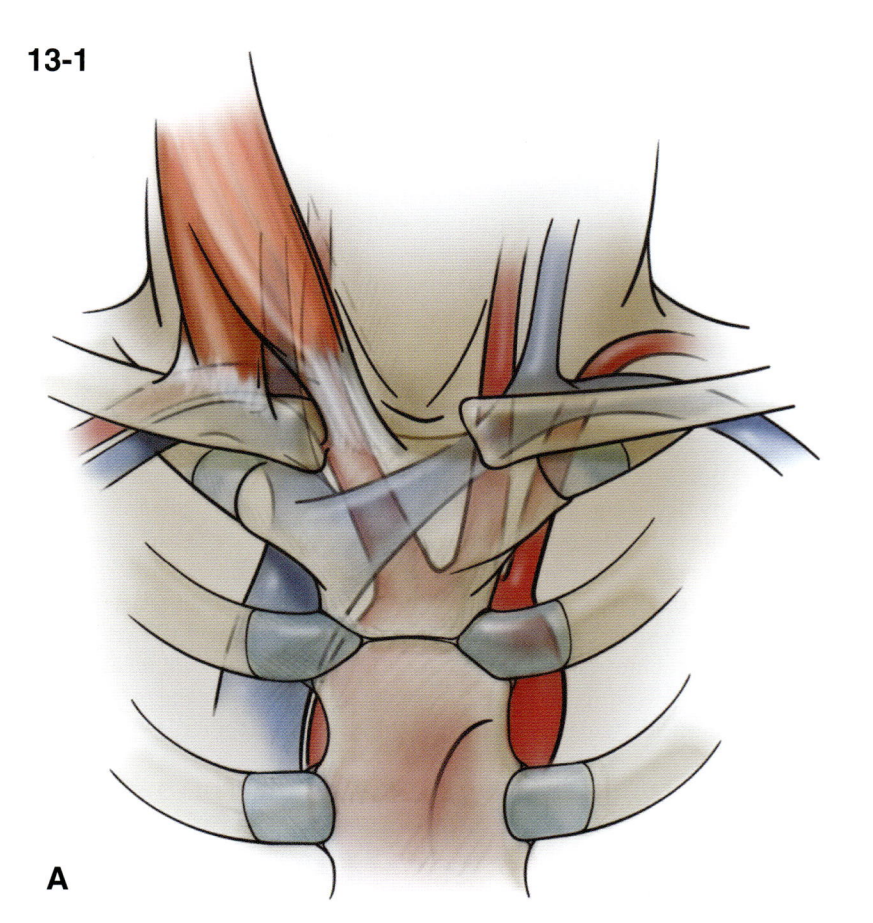

A

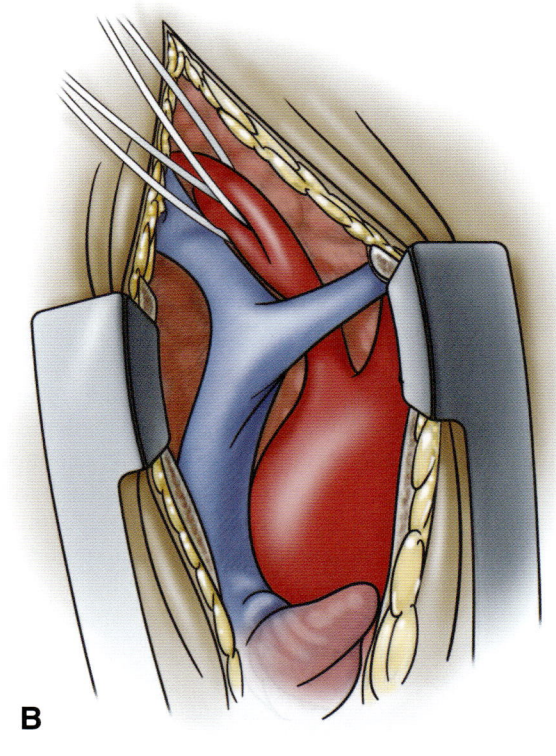

B

13-2

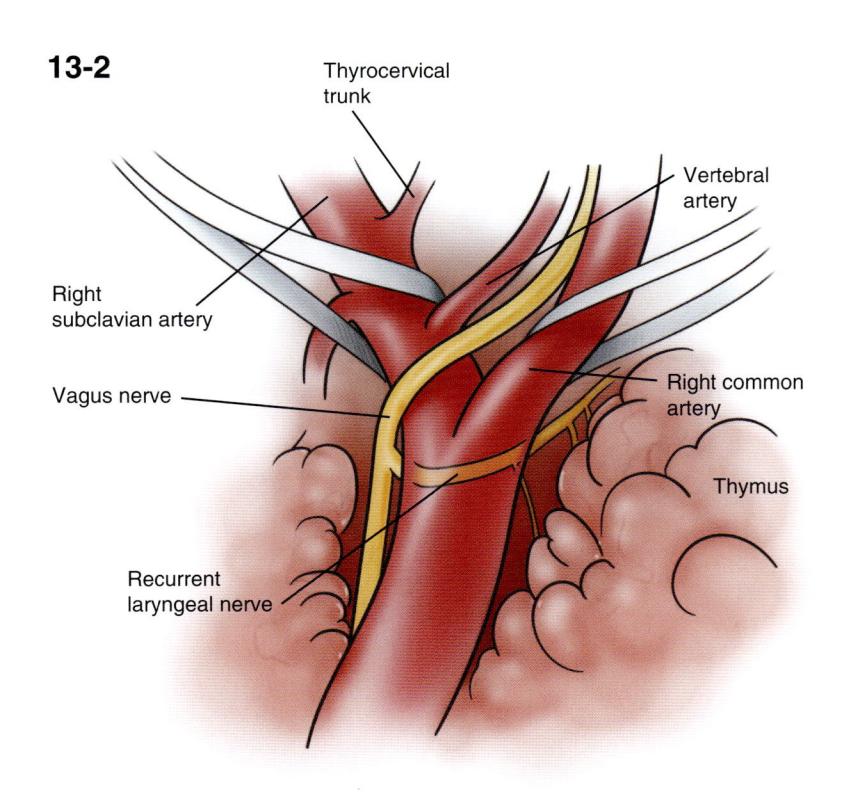

Thyrocervical trunk

Vertebral artery

Right subclavian artery

Vagus nerve

Right common artery

Thymus

Recurrent laryngeal nerve

13-3

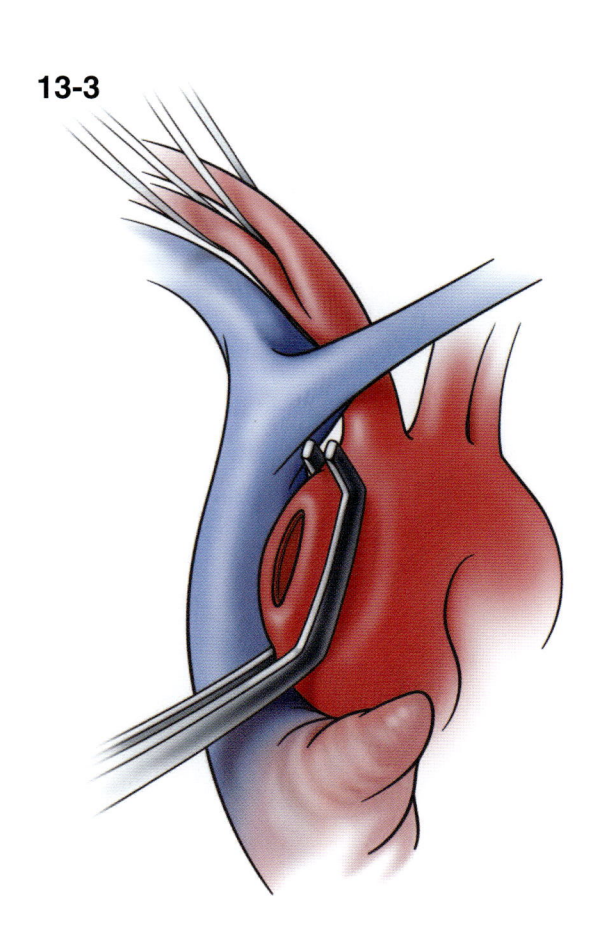

DETAILS OF THE PROCEDURE ◄ CONTINUED The mean arterial blood pressure is raised as for endarterectomy. Distal clamps are placed first. A shunt is rarely needed during innominate artery reconstruction, and only when there is significant disease in the other SATs, at the carotid bifurcations or involving the vertebral arteries. The proximal innominate artery is clamped near its origin and divided. The stump is oversewn with a double layer of running 4-0 polypropylene suture, with one layer a running horizontal mattress stitch and the other an over-and-over stitch. An endarterectomy of the proximal artery may be needed to obtain a secure stump closure. Horizontal mattress 4-0 polypropylene pledgeted sutures buttress the stump closure if there is bleeding from it when the clamp is released.

If the bifurcation of the innominate artery is an adequate distal target, the distal artery is divided and spatulated. A segment of innominate artery can be resected to make room for the graft. The graft is passed beneath the left brachiocephalic vein. If the graft is placed on top of the vein, compression of the vein has to be avoided. The graft is cut to length, spatulated, and sewn end-to-end to the artery with running 4-0 polypropylene suture (FIGURE 13-4). As the anastomosis nears completion, the mean arterial blood pressure is lowered to baseline or approximately 80 mmHg. Back-bleeding and forebleeding are performed and the graft irrigated with heparinized saline prior to completing the anastomosis. The distal clamp on the subclavian artery is released first, the graft is de-aired, and the proximal clamp on the graft removed. Blood flow is allowed into the subclavian artery for 15 to 20 seconds before the clamp on the right common carotid artery is released. The flow in the common carotid and subclavian arteries can be checked with Doppler insonation, but we obtain an intraoperative completion Duplex ultrasound scan of the graft and its anastomoses to assess technical outcome.

When arterial disease extends beyond the innominate artery origin, then the common carotid and subclavian arteries need to be separately reconstructed. This revascularization can take several forms depending on anatomy and surgeon discretion. Most often, a graft from the ascending aorta is sewn end-to-end to the common carotid artery and a side-arm polyester graft is used to reconstruct the subclavian. Usually, the subclavian anastomosis is at or proximal to the vertebral origin, except in some patients with TA where the anastomosis is further distally. If there is enough length of normal subclavian, it can be reimplanted onto the carotid graft. Alternatively, the aortic-based graft can be sewn end-to-end to the subclavian, and the common carotid artery reimplanted or reconstructed with a short interposition graft.

Isolated innominate artery reconstruction is uncommon. Direct aortic-origin reconstructions are often relegated to good risk patients with atherosclerotic or TA involvement of multiple SATs, or for patients with a diseased common brachiocephalic artery trunk. Complex reconstructions are needed in these circumstances and require one (FIGURES 13-5 and 13-6) or two sidearm grafts from the main aortic-based graft. Almost always, the sternotomy incision is carried into the right or left neck to afford adequate exposure of the carotid and/or subclavian arteries. Typically, the main graft from the ascending aorta is sewn to the right common carotid artery, and side-arm grafts are used to reconstruct the right subclavian and left common carotid arteries (FIGURE 13-6). The left subclavian rarely needs reconstruction if the left vertebral artery is patent. The sequence of distal anastomoses depends on how best to maintain cerebral perfusion when each artery is clamped, and on the working room available in the mediastinum and neck. Simultaneous clamping of both common carotid arteries is avoided. The side arms are sewn end-to-side to the main graft with their origins staggered, which allows separate clamping of them when blood flow is restored into the first reconstructed artery. Care must be taken to cut these grafts to appropriate length for the distal anastomoses to avoid tension or kinking.

Once the anastomoses are completed and blood flow restored after the bypass(es) or endarterectomy, and the duplex scan shows the graft anastomoses to all be widely patent, Protamine is given in small incremental doses to partially reverse the heparin effect. Hemostasis is secured and the mediastinum and/or neck incisional sites are irrigated. Mediastinal chest tubes are placed. The sternal closure must be done carefully to avoid compression of the grafts by the manubrium and its underlining muscular and fibrous tissues. Some of the muscle and soft tissue may need excision so the grafts lie freely. The sternum is reapproximated with wires, the fascial and subcutaneous tissues are closed in layers, and the skin closed with a running subcuticular stitch. If a neck incision is done, the platysma is closed. A sterile dressing or incisional wound VAC is applied.

POSTOPERATIVE MONITORING AND FOLLOW-UP The patient should undergo an immediate neurologic and right upper extremity pulse examination upon waking from general anesthesia and before leaving the operating room. The patient is extubated and transferred to a postoperative unit where invasive continuous blood pressure monitoring can be performed and vasoactive medications given to manage blood pressure. Neurologic checks and right upper extremity pulse examinations are done hourly the first night. A chest x-ray is done after surgery and repeated daily until the mediastinal and pleural chest tubes have been removed. Patients return at 4 to 6 months for a recheck and a CTA of the neck and chest. Subsequent follow-up and imaging is based on the etiology of the disease and the results of the first postoperative CTA. ∎

13-4

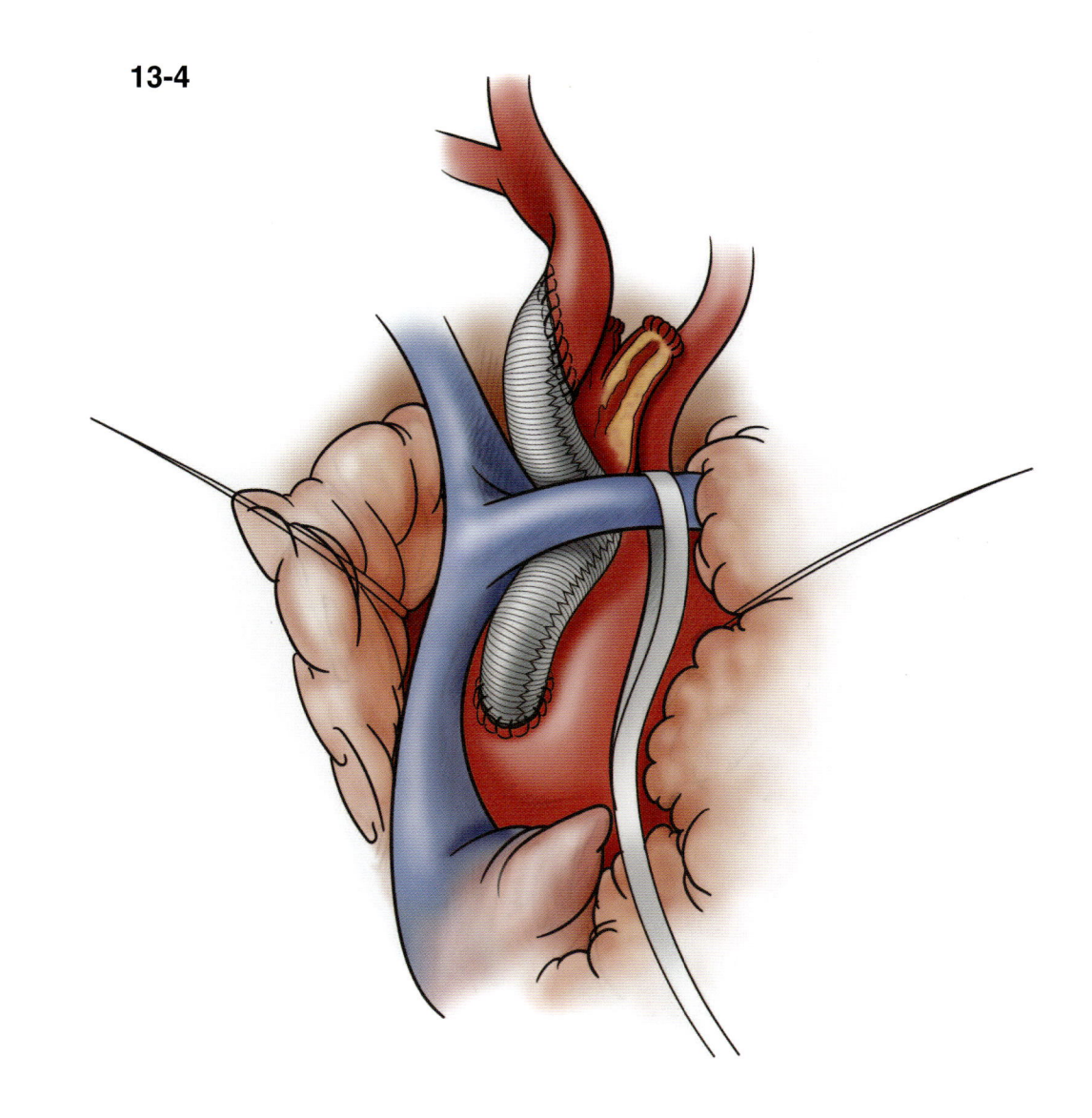

13-5

13-6

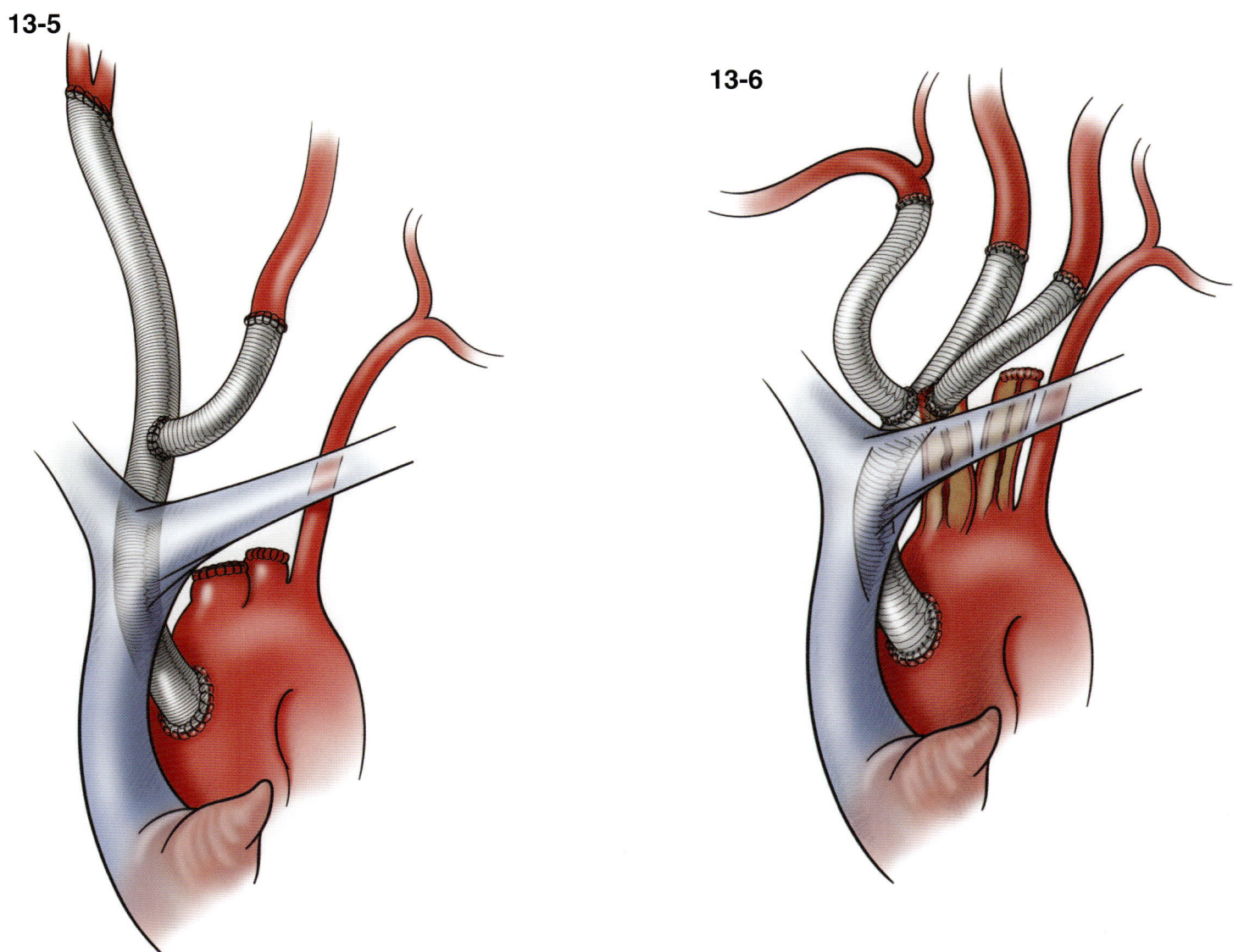

Vertebral Artery Transposition and Bypass

Alexandra Gobble, MD • **Robert J. Beaulieu, MD, MSE**

INDICATIONS The vertebral artery most often arises off the subclavian artery and supplies the posterior circulation of the brain. Symptoms of vertebrobasilar ischemic symptoms can be varied, and include dizziness, vertigo, drop attacks, diplopia, tinnitus, dysphasia, and ataxia. Ostial atherosclerosis resulting in stenosis of the vertebral artery is an important consideration in evaluating vertebrobasilar insufficiency. In patients with posterior circulation occlusive disease, extracranial vertebral artery stenosis is the most common site of occlusion. Symptoms resulting from low flow disease are typically limited in duration and repetitive. Vertebral artery atherosclerotic plaque may also be a source of distal embolization. Though less frequent than ischemia resulting from low-flow states, embolic ischemia is more likely to cause a debilitating or fatal stroke.

The diagnosis of vertebral artery disease is made more difficult by the intraosseous course of the second segment of the artery (V2). Duplex sonography evaluation is typically limited to detecting reversal of flow but can sometimes show tardus parvus, indicating more proximal stenosis. Noninvasive cross-sectional imaging with MRA and CTA are more useful to establish the presence of atherosclerotic disease within the vertebral artery. Diagnostic angiography remains the gold standard imaging modality, especially for preoperative planning. This allows for identification of flow-limiting disease, can help establish dominance, and can incorporate provocative maneuvers in instances when vertebral artery compression (typically in the V3 segment) is suspected.

Surgical access of the vertebral artery is typically limited to the V1 and V3 segments (FIGURE 14-1). Transposition or bypass to the V1 segment is a useful and preferred treatment for ostial narrowing resulting in vertebrobasilar insufficiency. Narrowing or occlusion of the V2 segment or narrowing resulting from external compression of the V3 segment with maneuvers

is treated with bypass or transposition of the V3 segment. Bypass conduit for these segments is most commonly the saphenous vein, though the radial artery has also been used.

PATIENT POSITIONING The patient is positioned supine on the operating room table. A shoulder roll or table that allows for a semi-Fowler ("beach chair") positioning is helpful to extend the neck. The patient's head should be rotated away from the operative side, with care to adhere to the endotracheal tube on the opposite side of the mouth as well.

OPERATIVE PREPARATION Prior to entering the operating room, it is of paramount importance to review the CT scan to specifically determine the relationship of the course of the vertebral to the common carotid artery. This information will be crucial when performing this aspect of the exposure to limit blind dissection in this critical area. The operative field should be prepped to include the angle of the sternum medially, the chin superiorly, the angle of the jaw and ipsilateral ear lobe superiorly, the trapezius posteriorly, and the clavicle inferiorly.

PROXIMAL VERTEBRAL ARTERY (V1)

Incision and Exposure Exposure of the vertebral artery is best assisted with a transverse incision over the clavicle. The incision should start approximately 1 to 2 cm above the clavicle, medially at the sternal notch, and extending laterally out 7 to 8 cm (FIGURE 14-2). The underlying platysma should then be divided to reveal the underlying sternal head of the sternocleidomastoid. It is not necessary to divide both heads of the sternocleidomastoid for exposure. CONTINUES ▶

14-1

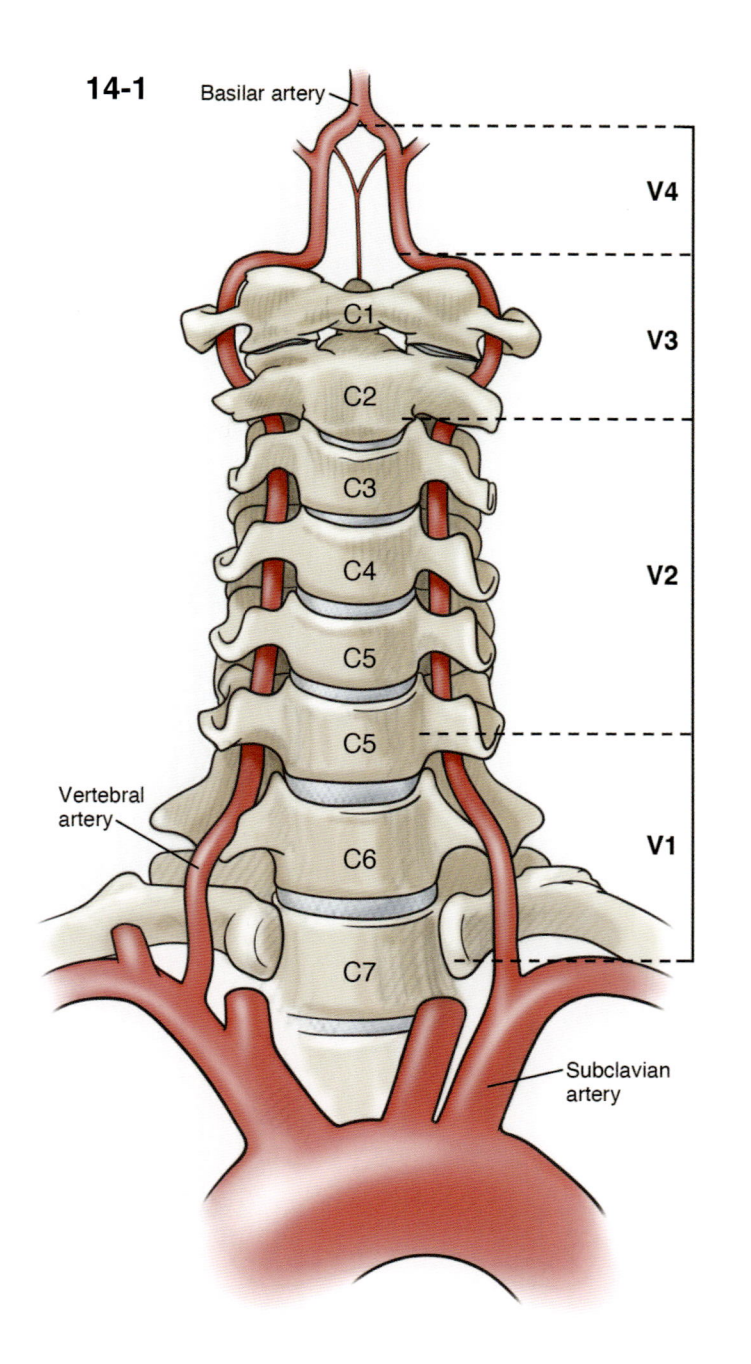

Basilar artery

V4

C1

V3

C2

C3

C4

V2

C5

C5

Vertebral artery

V1

C6

C7

Subclavian artery

14-2

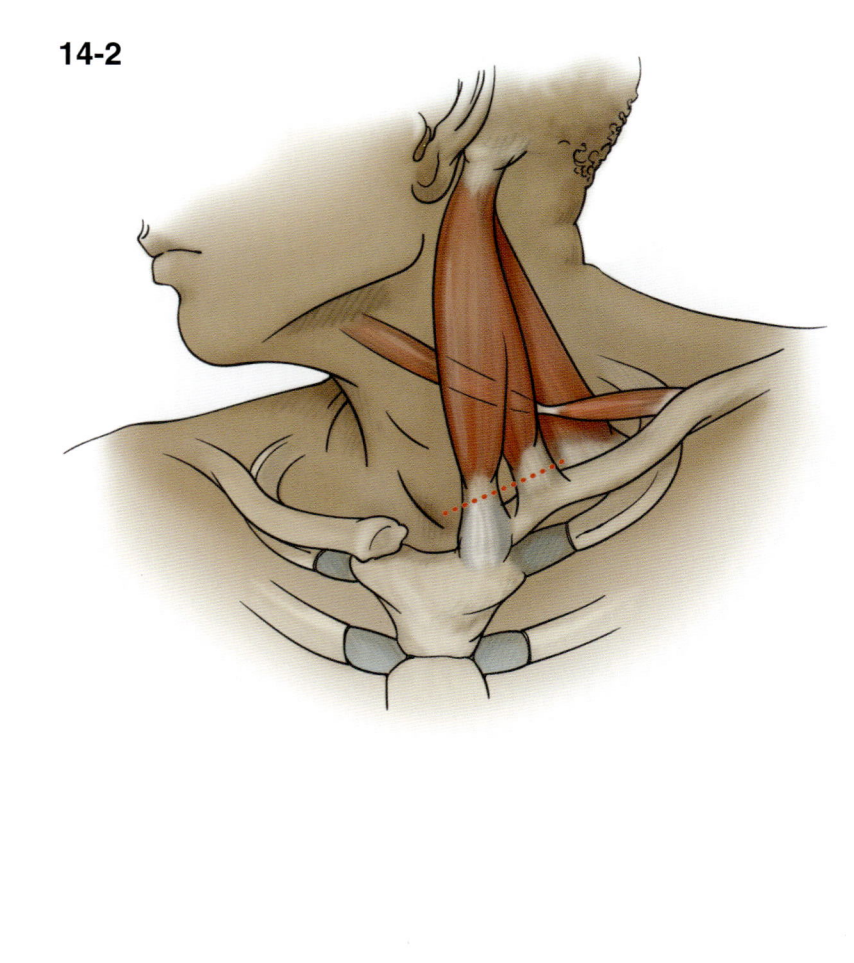

OPERATIVE PREPARATION *PROXIMAL VERTEBRAL ARTERY (V1)*
Incision and Exposure   `CONTINUED` Exposure can often be obtained by
dividing just the sternal head of the sternocleidomastoid. Upon doing so,
the common carotid artery and internal jugular vein will be revealed. The
carotid sheath containing these structures should be incised. At this point
of the operation, the use of electrocautery should be limited. In cases in
which it must be used, the bipolar electrocautery is strongly preferred to
prevent spread and injury of the nearby nerves, including the vagus nerve.
The internal jugular vein and vagus nerve are retracted laterally and the
common carotid artery is retracted medially (**FIGURE 14-3**). The dissection is then carried out medially to the anterior scalene. Visualization of
the anterior scalene should raise concern that the dissection is progressing
too laterally. Dissection in this area is marked by the appearance of several
important structures that require identification to reduce the risk of injury.
On right-sided dissections, the recurrent laryngeal nerve progresses around
the subclavian and can be visualized at the base of the dissection. On the
left side, the thoracic duct should be identified and ligated to prevent leak
in the postoperative period (**FIGURE 14-4**). Deep to this dissection, the deep
cervical fascia is identified and entered to allow for visualization of the fatty
and nerve tissue surrounding the vertebral artery. The expected location
of the vertebral artery can be determined based on the preoperative CT
scan. Preoperative determination of the anatomic relationship between the
vertebral artery and common carotid artery can reduce unnecessary dissection in this area which may increase the risk of injuring the vertebral
veins. The vertebral artery can now be identified. The vertebral does not
have any branches in this segment, a fact which can aid in the identification of the correct vessel, especially to differentiate it from the thyrocervical
trunk, which has multiple branches. The artery should be dissected for a
segment long enough to allow for ligation of the proximal portion, mobilization to the carotid or exposure for the distal anastomosis of a bypass,
and appropriate clamp placement. It is sometimes necessary to divide
the overlying sympathetic fibers, which may increase the risk of Horner
syndrome. `CONTINUES`

14-3

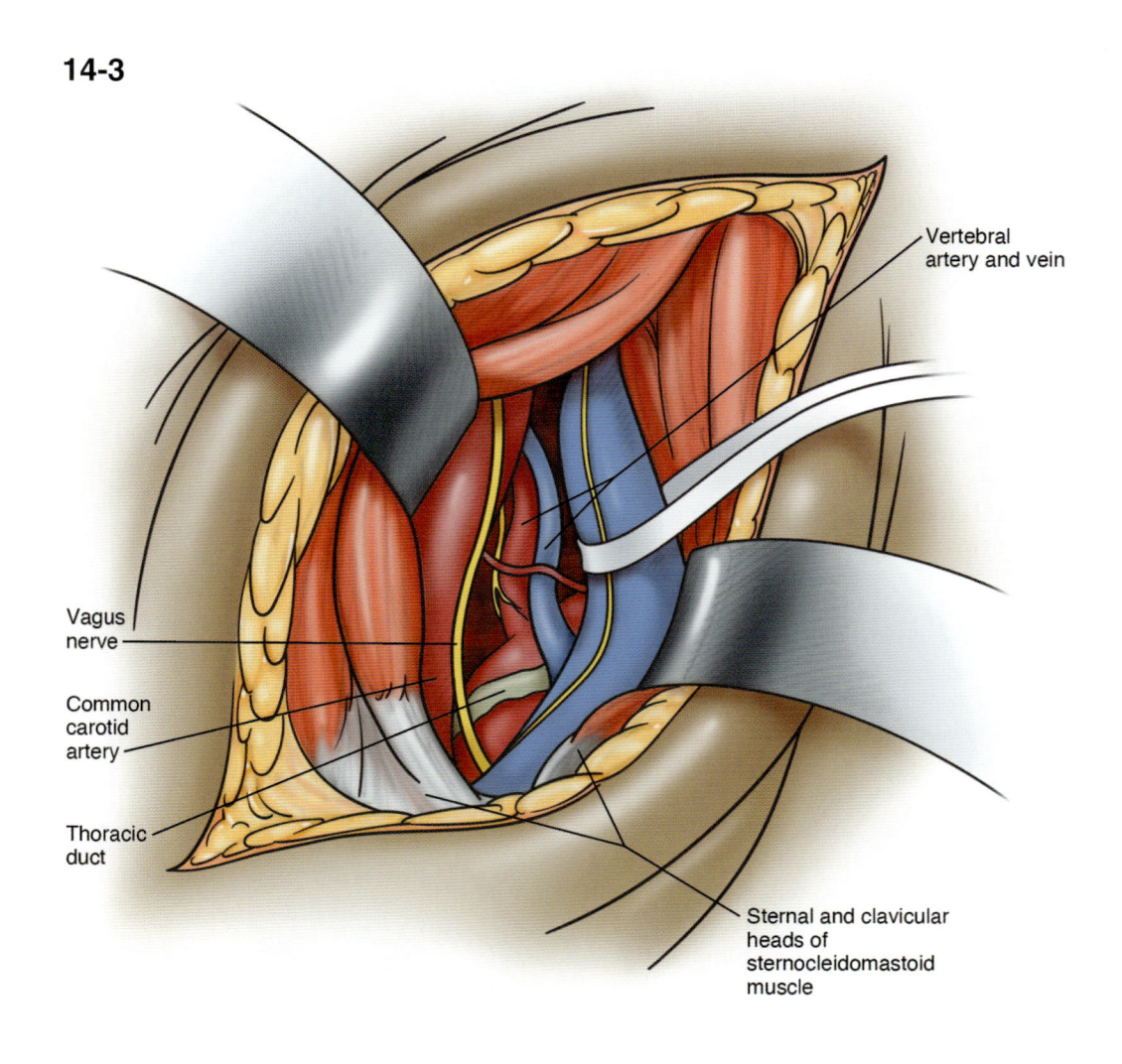

Vertebral artery and vein

Vagus nerve

Common carotid artery

Thoracic duct

Sternal and clavicular heads of sternocleidomastoid muscle

14-4

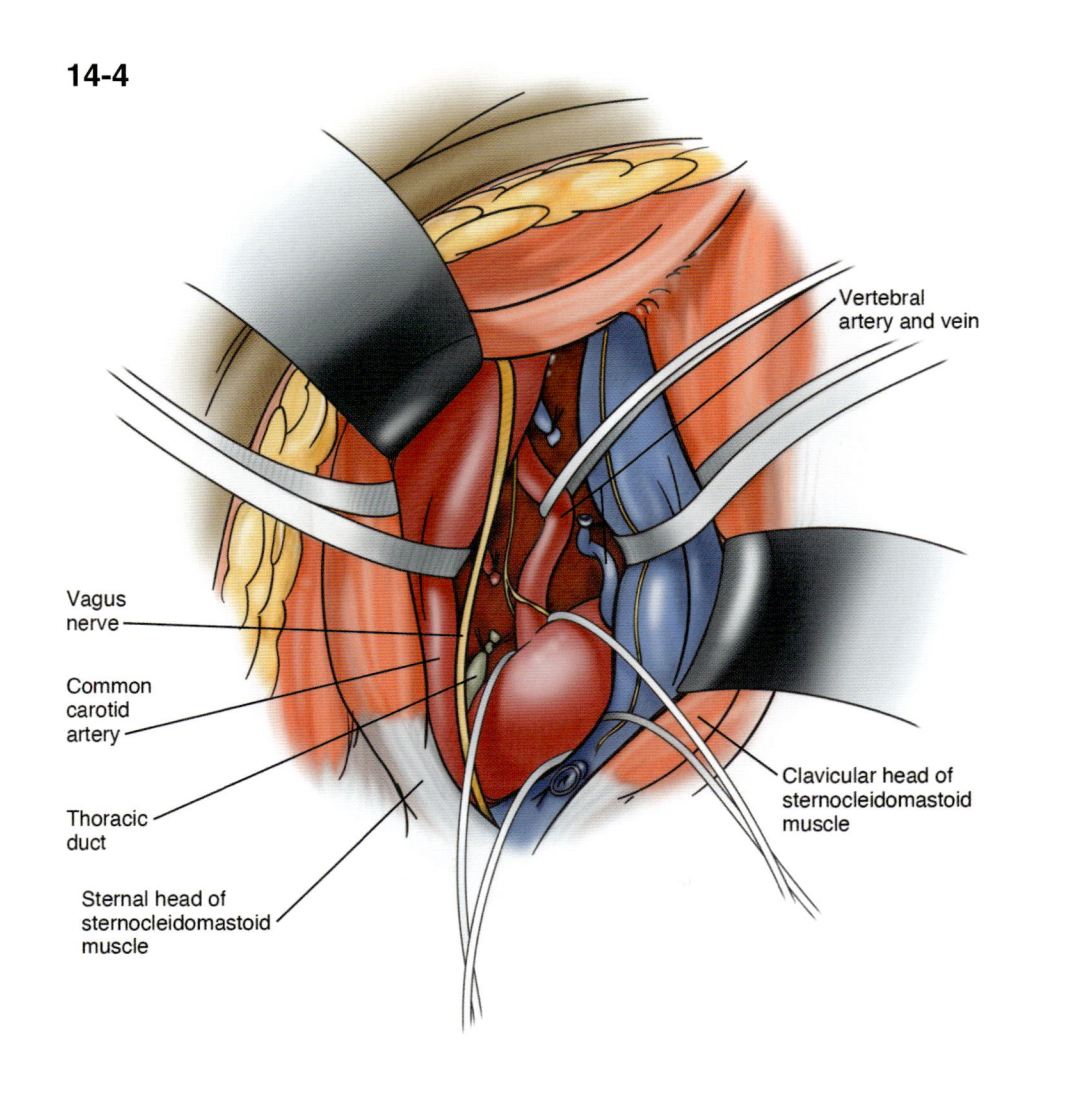

Vertebral artery and vein

Vagus nerve

Common carotid artery

Thoracic duct

Clavicular head of sternocleidomastoid muscle

Sternal head of sternocleidomastoid muscle

OPERATIVE PREPARATION *PROXIMAL VERTEBRAL ARTERY Vertebral Artery Transposition* `CONTINUED` In instances in which the artery has appropriate mobilization, transposition to the common carotid artery can reduce the number of anastomoses and the difficulty of these anastomoses when compared to vertebral bypass. The common carotid artery should already be exposed for anastomosis as a part of the dissection. At this point, the patient should be anticoagulated with intravenous heparin to achieve an activated clotting time (ACT) greater than 250 seconds. The blood pressure should be maintained at systolic pressures greater than 150 mmHg in anticipation of clamping the common carotid for anastomosis. The vertebral artery is dissected to the transverse process of C7, which should be immediately behind the artery. It is carried this high to allow for a better lie on the anastomosis. The proximal vertebral artery is ligated. Our preference is to perform ligation using a 5-0 prolene suture through the artery as a suture ligation. This ligation can be further buttressed with a large clip. The vertebral artery is then divided distal to the ligation. The distal end of the vertebral artery is then rotated up to the common carotid to ensure a lie with no kinking or twisting. The position on the common carotid that will allow for the best lie on the transposition is marked with a marking pen. The common carotid is then clamped with vascular clamps. Optimal exposure of the vertebral artery implantation site can be assisted by rotating the vascular clamps toward the patient's shoulder after clamping. Once the correct site is well visualized, an arteriotomy is made with an 11 blade. Due to the small size of the vertebral artery, we prefer to extend the arteriotomy using a vascular punch, typically a 4 mm punch. The anastomosis is carried out in standard fashion with 6-0 prolene (**FIGURE 14-5**). Once the anastomosis is completed, hemostasis can be assessed by releasing the distal clamp on the vertebral or common carotid. The distal clamp on the vertebral should be replaced prior to releasing common carotid clamps and then can be removed when the common carotid clamps are both off.

In rare cases, the vertebral artery may enter into the foramen at C6 instead of C5, which may preclude transposition. In such cases, saphenous vein bypass may be used. It is necessary to dissect a portion of the subclavian artery to allow for proximal anastomosis. This can be accomplished by following either the vertebral artery or the thyrocervical trunk back to its origin. The common carotid artery can also be used for inflow. Once the proximal anastomosis is performed, the vein graft is brought to length to ensure no buckling. The distal anastomosis can be done as an end-to-side or end-to-end anastomosis. If an end-to-side anastomosis is performed, the artery is occluded between two microvascular clips and a longitudinal arteriotomy is made. Alternatively, if an end-to-end anastomosis is performed, the proximal portion is ligated and the distal is controlled with an endovascular clip. Great care must be taken to ensure the endovascular clip is secure. Loss of control of the vertebral artery in this area may allow for retraction and continued bleeding. The anastomosis is performed with 6-0 or 7-0 prolene in the standard vascular fashion.

DISTAL VERTEBRAL ARTERY (V3)

V3 Exposure While experience with the distal vertebral exposure is becoming less frequent, the tenets of the operation are similar to carotid artery endarterectomy exposure. The skin incision is made similar to a carotid artery exposure with extension to beneath the earlobe. The platysma is divided, typically with cautery, and the dissection then takes place on the anterior border of the sternocleidomastoid down to the jugular vein. The spinal accessory nerve is encountered on the anterior border of the sternocleidomastoid and is followed cranially toward C1. The levator scapulae muscle is then identified. The ramus of C2 is palpated and the levator scapulae is transected. The C2 ramus is then clearly visible overlying the V3 portion of the vertebral artery (**FIGURE 14-6**). It is divided using sharp dissection with either Metzenbaum scissors or a scalpel. The effects of cutting the ramus are limited to posterior scalp numbness, which often resolves without therapy. Care is taken to separate the artery from its venous attachment and encircle the artery with a silastic vessel loop. These venous attachments can be a source of significant bleeding during this exposure and therefore care should be taken to prevent inadvertent injury to these vessels during the exposure.

Distal Vertebral Artery Bypass There are multiple inflow options for bypass to the V3 segment of the vertebral artery. Most commonly, common carotid artery to vertebral artery bypass can be completed by exposing the distal portion of the common carotid. The patient is then systemically anticoagulated with heparin to achieve an ACT greater than 250 seconds. Microvascular clamps are placed on the vertebral artery and a longitudinal arteriotomy is made and extended with Pott's scissors. The distal anastomosis is then completed to the vein or arterial conduit using 7-0 prolene sutures. Once completed, microvascular clamps on the vertebral artery are released and one is placed on the graft. The graft is then passed beneath the jugular down to the identified portion of the common carotid. The common carotid is then clamped proximally and distally. An arteriotomy is made with an 11 blade and extended with Potts scissors. The proximal anastomosis is completed with 6-0 prolene sutures ensuring there is no kinking or twisting of the conduit.

An alternative reconstruction technique is also possible where the external carotid artery can be transposed in an end-to-end fashion to the vertebral (**FIGURE 14-7**). In this instance, the branches of the external carotid must be ligated to allow for mobility.

CLOSURE It is important to obtain meticulous hemostasis when preparing to close to prevent cervical hematoma. In this distribution, we favor using bipolar electrocautery if cautery is necessary. Protamine sulfate is typically used to reverse the coagulopathy induced by heparinization. The wound is closed in two layers, reapproximating the platysma and then the skin.

POSTOPERATIVE CARE Care should be taken to observe for postoperative hematoma that may result from suture line bleeding, improper hemostasis, or postoperative hypertension, often with awakening and coughing. Swelling in the postoperative setting may also be secondary to a lymphocele or chylothorax, especially if the occurrence of the swelling coincides with the patient resuming a diet. Postoperatively, Horner syndrome may be recognized due to nerve injury to the sympathetic chain. Symptom onset may occur as late as 1 week after the operation. Up to 30% of patients will resolve at a variable time period after the operation from 3 months to 3 years.

Patients should be closely monitored for neurologic deficit in the postoperative setting. Stroke rates for proximal reconstruction have been reported as less than 1%, with distal reconstructions having a higher risk at 3%. Kinking and subsequent thrombosis of the vertebral artery may results in a posterior stroke, highlighting the importance of fashioning the conduit or vertebral artery to appropriate length during that portion of the operation. Additionally, postoperative hypotension should be avoided to reduce the risk of low-flow thrombosis in the vertebral artery. ■

SUGGESTED READINGS

Berguer R, Bauer RB. Vertebral artery reconstruction. A successful technique in selected patients. *Ann Surg.* 1981 Apr;193(4):441-447.

Coleman DM, Obi A, Criado E, Arya S, Berguer R. Contemporary outcomes after distal vertebral reconstruction. *J Vasc Surg.* 2013 Jul;58(1):152-157.

Diaz FG, Ausman JI, de los Reyes RA, Pearce J, Shrontz C, Pak H, Turcotte J. Surgical reconstruction of the proximal vertebral artery. *J Neurosurg.* 1984 Nov;61(5): 874-881.

Morasch M. Chapter 97. Vertebral artery dissection and other conditions. Sidawy AN, Perler BA, eds. *Rutherford's Vascular Surgery and Endovascular Therapy, 10th edition.* Elsevier, 2019;1277-1291.

Rangel-Castilla L, Kalani MYS, Cronk K, Zabramski JM, Russin JJ, Setzler RF. Vertebral artery transposition for revascularization of the posterior circulation: a critical assessment of temporary and permanent complications and outcomes. *J Neurosurg.* 2015 Mar;122(3): 671-677.

14-5

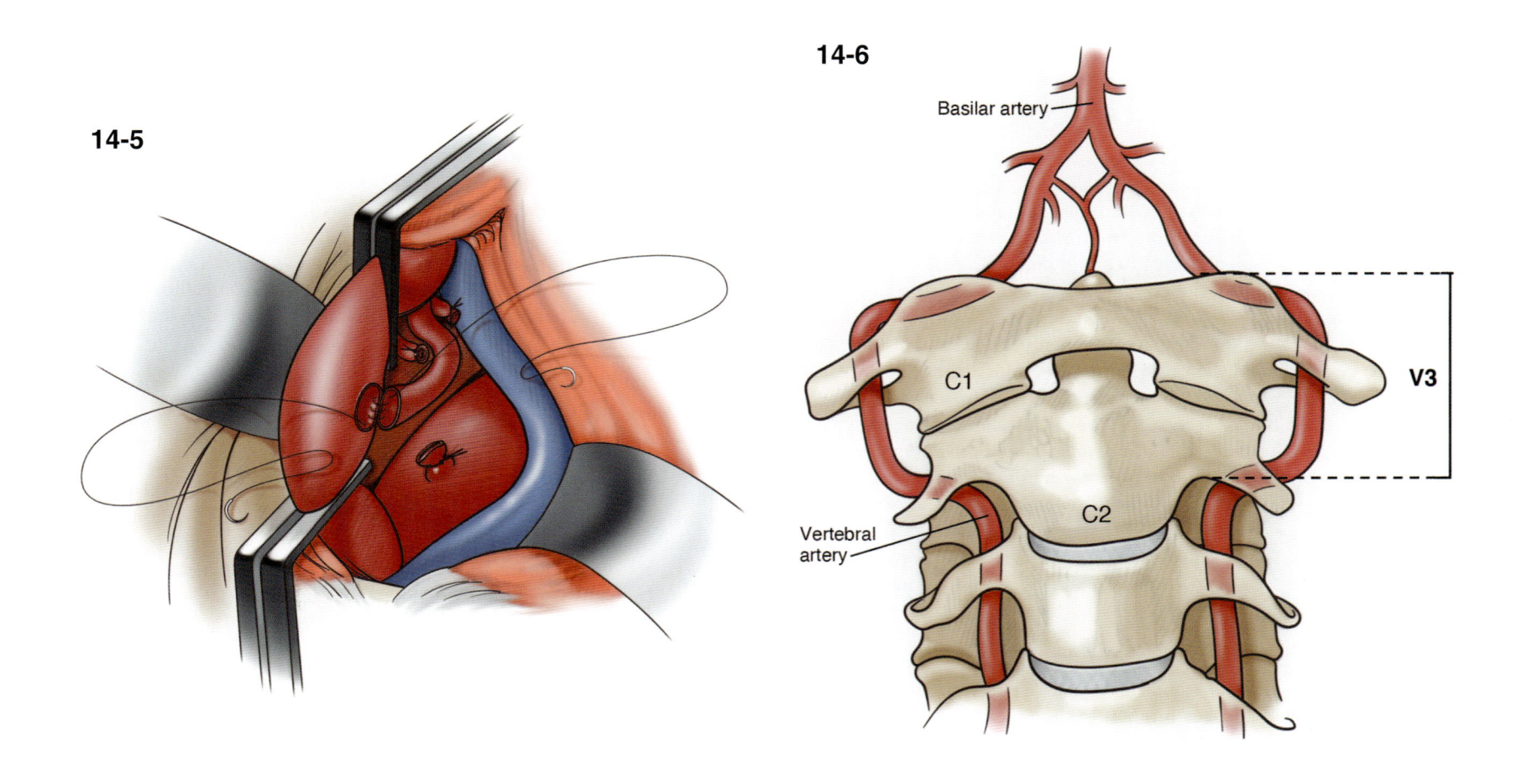

14-6

Basilar artery

C1

C2

Vertebral artery

V3

14-7

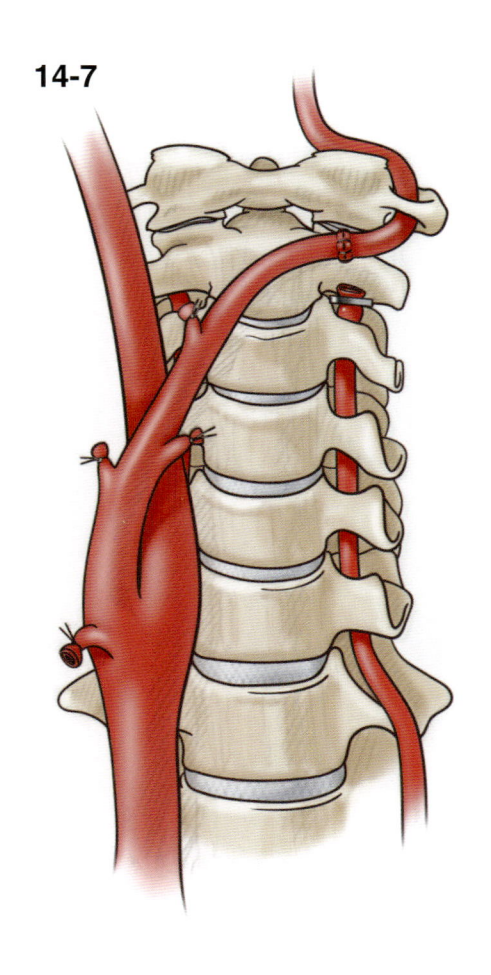

Transcarotid Artery Revascularization

Aric A. Wogsland, MD • Vikram S. Kashyap, MD

INDICATIONS Transcarotid arterial revascularization (TCAR) is a novel minimally invasive hybrid procedure designed to treat atherosclerotic carotid disease and minimize the risk of stroke. TCAR provides a less invasive approach for higher-risk surgical patients and provides neuroprotection by utilizing a cerebral flow reversal device (ENROUTE Transcarotid Neuroprotection System [NPS], Silk Road Medical, Inc.). The reversal of flow (ROF) prevents macro- and microemboli during the intervention. TCAR is a safe alternative for patients with physiological or anatomical conditions that put them at higher risk for adverse events with carotid endarterectomy. TCAR also avoids complications associated with aortic arch and branch artery manipulation seen with transfemoral carotid artery stenting (TFCAS) and provides neuroprotection prior to crossing the lesion. It is important to select patients that fit certain anatomic parameters prior to performing TCAR. Anatomic contraindications are specific to common carotid artery (CCA) access and sheath placement. The sheath must be able to cannulate a CCA of >6 mm that is free of atherosclerotic disease. There must also be adequate distance from the CCA puncture site to the carotid bifurcation. The ENROUTE NPS requires a clavicle-to-carotid bifurcation distance of at least 5 cm on imaging, as the carotid sheath tip extends 2.5 cm into the CCA and the sheath dilator extends an additional 1.5 cm. Increased depth (>4 cm) of the CCA must also be taken into consideration, as it can increase the complexity of the procedure. Other anatomical contraindications to TCAR are similar to TFCAS, including small caliber distal internal carotid artery (ICA) (<4 mm) or string sign, aneurysmal or dilated ICA that exceeds the largest carotid stent size (9 mm), as well as heavy circumferential atherosclerotic plaque.

PREPARATION AND ANESTHESIA Dual antiplatelet therapy (aspirin and clopidogrel), as well as statin therapy, are critical through the perioperative period. The patient is brought to the operating room and placed in supine position on a fluoroscopically capable table. TCAR can be performed with either a local, regional, or general anesthesia. A radial arterial line is routinely placed for continuous monitoring of hemodynamics. Both arms are tucked and the C-arm is positioned cranially. A shoulder bump may be utilized for more adequate exposure of anatomical landmarks with neck extension. Duplex ultrasound insonation is used to identify the CCA at the base of the neck and the location marked. Hair removal, surgical prep, and antibiotic prophylaxis per routine are performed.

DETAILS OF THE PROCEDURE

INCISION AND EXPOSURE: The CCA is exposed with a 2- to 4-cm transverse or longitudinal incision that is 1 cm cephalad to the clavicle and between the heads of the sternocleidomastoid muscle. Prior ultrasound-guided marking of the CCA will help guide the incision. Platysma flaps are developed down to the clavicle and cephalad for approximately 1 cm.

Dissection should remain proximal to the omohyoid muscle in the avascular plane. Identifying the avascular plan between the heads of the sternocleidomastoid muscle is the key step in exposure (**FIGURE 15-1**). The carotid sheath is incised longitudinally and the internal jugular vein is partially dissected and retracted laterally. Care is taken to avoid the vagus nerve that may be located lateral and posterior to the CCA. The proximal CCA is dissected for 3 to 4 cm circumferentially. A cotton umbilical tape without a Rummel tourniquet is placed on the most proximal CCA under direct vision. A 5-0 or 6-0 polypropylene U-stitch is placed on the proximal CCA in anticipation for arterial access closure at the cessation of the procedure. Common femoral venous access is obtained with a micropuncture system under ultrasound guidance per routine. An 8F venous return sheath with a 4-mm radiopaque tip is advanced over a 0.035" wire, both contained in the ENROUTE NPS kit. After removal of the dilator and wire, the side port is aspirated and flushed with heparinized saline and secured to the patient with suture.

COMMON CAROTID ARTERY ACCESS: Prior to arterial access, a baseline activated clotting time (ACT) is obtained and the patient is heparin bolused with 80 to 100 μ/kg, with an ACT goal of 250 to 300 seconds. Confirm ACT goal levels every 30 minutes, as additional heparinization may be needed. The proximal CCA is held under tension with the use of the previously placed cotton umbilical tape. It is critical to avoid lesion manipulation prior to flow reversal to prevent intraoperative thromboemboli. The CCA can be accessed between the previously placed U-stitch with a standard 4Fr micropuncture kit. The 21-G micropuncture needle gains CCA access and a micropuncture supportive 0.018" wire is advanced 3 to 4 cm, followed by needle removal. The micropuncture sheath is then advanced over the wire approximately 2 cm into the CCA. Care must be taken to avoid wire or sheath entry into the carotid bifurcation. Pulsatile bleeding through the microsheath confirms proper placement. A short extension tubing with a three-way stopcock is attached to the 4F microsheath and used for contrast injections. Angiography via the micropuncture sheath confirms the carotid bifurcation and lesion location. If the atherosclerotic disease is confirmed to be confined to the ICA, the external carotid artery (ECA) may be selected with the microwire and sheath for extra wire purchase. A 90-cm extra support 0.035" J-tipped guidewire is inserted into the micropuncture sheath, entering either the ECA or just proximal to the bifurcation (**FIGURE 15-2A AND B**). The micropuncture sheath is removed and the 8F marked ENROUTE Transcarotid Arterial Sheath is positioned 2.5 cm into the CCA with gentle caudad traction of the umbilical tape and visualization of the stiff 0.035" guidewire. A sheath stopper is attached to the arterial sheath that is positioned on the CCA surface and prevents cephalad migration of the sheath. The sheath is then secured in place with suture through grooves and eyelets after proper positioning is confirmed under fluoroscopy. **CONTINUES ▶**

15-1

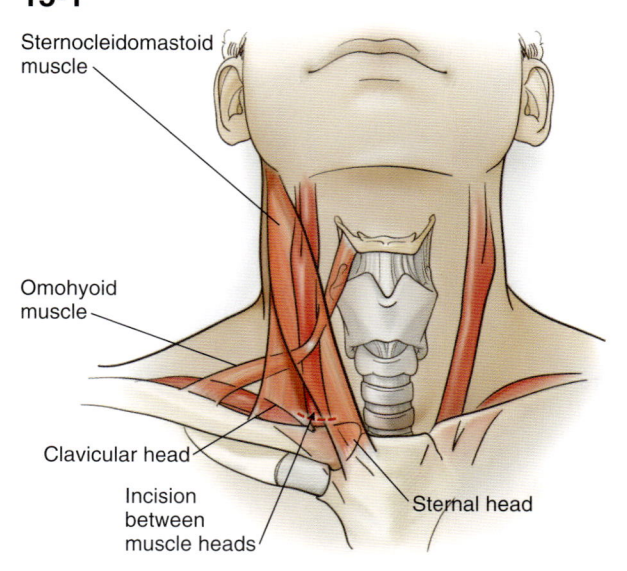

Sternocleidomastoid muscle

Omohyoid muscle

Clavicular head

Incision between muscle heads

Sternal head

15-2

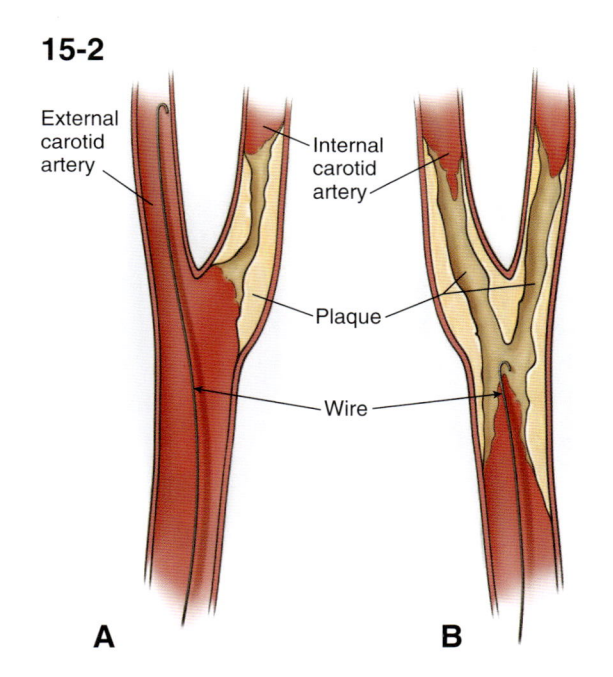

External carotid artery

Internal carotid artery

Plaque

Wire

A   B

DETAILS OF THE PROCEDURE *REVERSAL OF FLOW:* `CONTINUED`
After placement of the sheaths, the ENROUTE NPS flow controller tubing is connected to the arterial sheath and allowed to fill with arterial blood. The NPS flow controller has a High/Low switch and should be set to Low while preparing. The venous end of the tubing is raised vertically while filling to remove bubbles. Once blood has filled the NPS filter and the remainder of the flow controller tubing, it is connected to the venous sheath and de-aired. Prior to the arterial intervention, set the High/Low switch to High. After ensuring adequate anticoagulation, proximal control of the CCA is obtained ideally by using an atraumatic clamp. Cessation of blood flow via traction on the umbilical tape or Rummel tourniquet should be avoided since this can lead to CCA dissection. Flow reversal is now established (FIGURE 15-3). ROF times can be minimized if all interventional devices are prepared ahead of time. Flush the venous sheath with heparinized saline to confirm ROF. Carotid angiography can be performed through the arterial side arm with a 10-cc contrast-filled syringe and holding the Flow Stop button. After contrast is injected, the red Flow Stop button is released to reestablish flow reversal.

CAROTID INTERVENTION: Prior to crossing the atherosclerotic lesion, ensure systolic blood pressure is 140 to 160 mmHg to optimize ROF. Stenting is similar to other carotid artery stenting procedures. The lesion is crossed with a 0.014″ wire. An angled tipped catheter may be utilized to cross difficult lesions. Pre-dilation can be performed using a rapid exchange 3- to 4-mm angioplasty balloon. The ENROUTE Transcarotid Stent System (TCSS) consists of a nitinol self-expanding stent and stent sizes range from a diameter of 5 to 10 mm, with a length of 20 to 40 mm. Due to self-expansion of the nitinol stent, the stents are placed in vessels 1 to 2 mm smaller than the unconstrained diameter. The TCSS has a short 57-cm delivery system platform that is ergonomic and eliminates stored energy, allowing for precise stent deployment. After stent deployment, post dilation can be performed and carotid angiography confirms proper stent placement and an adequate technical result.

SHEATH REMOVAL AND CLOSURE: After all intervention is completed, the guidewire is removed. Reversal of flow may continue for a minute or longer to prevent embolization. The CCA clamp is then removed and antegrade carotid blood flow is restored. Flow through the arterial sheath is stopped by using the attached stopcock. The arterial sheath is removed and the previously placed polypropylene U-stitch is tied down for hemostasis. Heparin is reversed with protamine administration. The platysma

flaps are approximated over the CCA and closed with 3-0 vicryl suture. The skin is closed with a running subcuticular 4-0 monocryl suture. Thrombin-gel foam and other hemostatic agents may be used in the incision prior to closing for adequate hemostasis. The femoral vein sheath is removed and manual pressure applied.

POSTOPERATIVE CARE AND FOLLOW-UP After extubation and ensuring patient is neurologically intact, they are transferred to the post-anesthesia care unit (PACU). We routinely observe patients in a monitored unit for 4 hours after the operation for incisional and groin hematoma as well as neurological and hemodynamic monitoring. Patients are admitted overnight to monitor any immediate postoperative complications. Patients are discharged on postoperative day one after tolerating a regular diet, spontaneously voiding, and with adequate hemodynamics. Dual anti-platelet therapy with aspirin and clopidogrel is continued upon discharge. Follow-up is scheduled for 1 month for incisional wound examination and duplex ultrasound of the carotid stent. Plavix may be discontinued after 90 days with continuation of other medical therapy. Routine follow-up with carotid duplex ultrasound surveillance is scheduled at 6 months postoperatively and yearly thereafter. ∎

SUGGESTED READINGS

Kashyap VS, King AH, Mazin FI, et al. A multi-institutional analysis of transcarotid artery revascularization compared to carotid endarterectomy. *Journal of Vascular Surgery*. 1 July 2019;70(1):123-129.

Kashyap VS, Schneider PA, Foteh M, Motaganahalli R, et al. Early outcomes in the ROADSTER 2 study of transcarotid artery revascularization in patients with significant carotid artery disease. *Stroke*. 19 Aug 2020;51(9):2620-2629.

Kumins NH, Kashyap VK. Learning curve and proficiency of transcarotid artery revascularization compared to transfemoral carotid artery stenting. *Seminars of Vascular Surgery*. Jun-Sep 2020;33(1-2):16-23.

Kwolek CJ, Jaff MR, Leal JI, et al. Results of the ROADSTER multicenter trial of transcarotid stenting with dynamic flow reversal. *Journal of Vascular Surgery*. Nov 2015;62(5):1227-1234.

Malas MB, Leal J, Kashyap VK, et al. Technical aspects of transcarotid artery revascularization using the ENROUTE transcarotid neuroprotection and stent system. *Journal of Vascular Surgery*. Mar 2017;65(3):916-920.

15-3

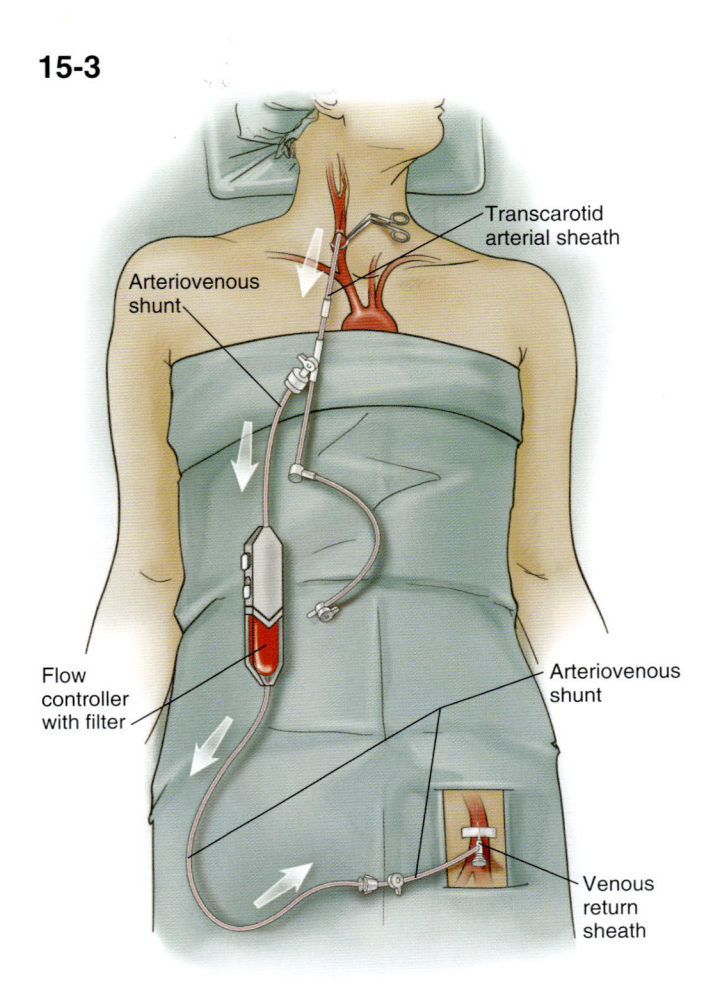

Transcarotid arterial sheath

Arteriovenous shunt

Flow controller with filter

Arteriovenous shunt

Venous return sheath

TRANSFEMORAL CAROTID ARTERY STENTING

Lars Stangenberg, MD • Marc L. Schermerhorn, MD

INDICATIONS Cerebrovascular disease is a leading cause of morbidity and mortality in the United States. There are approximately 800,000 new or recurrent strokes annually, of which about 87% are ischemic in nature. Eighteen percent of all ischemic events are due to large vessel cervical etiology. Stenosis of the carotid artery due atherosclerotic disease is at the core of those ischemic events.

Asymptomatic Carotid Atherosclerosis Study (ACAS) and North American Symptomatic Carotid Endarterectomy Trial (NASCET) clearly proved the benefits of carotid endarterectomy to reduce the risk of stroke. In some instances, carotid endarterectomy (CEA) is not feasible, for anatomic or medical concerns. One alternative is transfemoral carotid artery stenting (tfCAS). Several landmark papers in the 2000s, most notably Carotid revascularization endarterecomy vs stenting trial (CREST), evaluated both techniques in randomized controlled trials, and are the basis for current practice. tfCAS is non-inferior to CEA in a composite endpoint of stroke, myocardial infarction, or death. The trial did show, however, higher stroke risk (4.1% vs. 2.3%, P = 0.01) with the benefit of lower myocardial events (1.1% vs. 2.3%, P = 0.03) in the tfCAS group during the perioperative period.

tfCAS is now considered an excellent alternative to CEA but is not first choice in the treatment algorithm for the majority of patients. Since the advent of transcervical carotid artery revascularization (TCAR), the role of tfCAS has become even more nuanced. Currently, we recommend tfCAS in patients with asymptomatic or symptomatic stenosis of the carotid artery when they are high risk for CEA and TCAR. Surgical risks include presence of a tracheostomy, prior contralateral nerve palsy, high lesions beyond the C2 vertebral body, and scarring or fibrosis of the neck from prior ipsilateral surgery or external beam radiotherapy. Medical risks are severe heart-related comorbidities such as congestive heart failure, low left ventricular ejection fraction <35%, significant coronary artery disease, unstable angina, or recent myocardial infarction, and severe pulmonary disease.

The indication for any endovascular approach has to be made carefully, as 7% of patients have very unfavorable anatomy for any stenting. For tfCAS in particular, the literature documents increased stroke risk for older patients, for intervention immediately post stroke, and for patients with complex arch or adverse carotid anatomy.

PREOPERATIVE PLANNING Key to successful tfCAS is careful planning of the procedure. A high-quality, thin-cut computed tomography angiography (CTA) starting at the aortic valve and covering the entire neck and head is absolutely essential. We pay particular attention to arch type, degree and location of aortic and carotid calcifications, carotid tortuosity proximal and distal to the lesion, and lesion characteristics such as length, calcification, and relation to bifurcation. Ideally, the carotid lesion is around the bifurcation, short, and has only mild to moderate calcium, while the common carotid artery (CCA) and internal carotid artery (ICA) are free of any tortuosity or calcium. It is a matter of experience to gauge which complex lesions are ultimately safe to stent and which ones portend an unacceptably high stroke risk.

The stent and angioplasty balloons are carefully sized. The external carotid artery is evaluated to determine whether it can be cannulated safely. This is important during initial sheath positioning not only to allow for a more distal and stable wire position but also for a flow arrest system (Mo. Ma, Medtronic), if used.

Finally, we highly recommend the use of modern image fusion technology. We showed that it reduces procedural time and radiation exposure. We also believe it to be safer, as it reduces catheter manipulations in the aortic arch.

PREPARATION, POSITION, AND ANESTHESIA In the preoperative area, the operating surgeon confirms that the patient has taken dual antiplatelet therapy (DAPT), usually aspirin 81 mg and clopidogrel 75 mg daily, for at least 7 days prior to the procedure, including the day of surgery. If the patient has asymptomatic disease and has not taken DAPT, the procedure is cancelled and rescheduled ensuring compliance with DAPT. We also confirm use of statins. Should the patient be symptomatic and similarly not have been compliant with DAPT, it is the surgeon's discretion to follow the asymptomatic pathway to reschedule or to proceed with the operation if a

delay is deemed unsafe. In that case, we recommend a 600-mg loading dose of clopidogrel 4 hours before the procedure and performing the procedure under a drip of eptifibatide. Alternatively, the patient can be loaded with 180 mg ticagrelor with a shortened delay to surgery.

The anesthesia provider should ensure sufficient intravenous access. An arterial line is placed to closely monitor blood pressure during the intra- and postoperative period. The patient is brought to the hybrid operating room and placed in supine position. The patient is then connected to the standard monitoring equipment. Care is taken not to obscure crucial anatomic areas with cords or electrodes. Gentle monitored anesthesia care is started to ensure a comfortable and relaxed but responsive patient. This allows for intermittent neuromonitoring during the procedure, for example by squeezing a squeaky toy with the contralateral hand. Patients that are too deeply sedated can enter the excitement stage of anesthesia and can act erratically. Glycopyrrolate or atropine is administered to prevent undue bradycardia or asystole during carotid angioplasty.

OPERATIVE PREPARATION The groins are prepped with chlorhexidine. We usually leave the head uncovered to allow access for anesthesia if necessary. Ancef is given preoperatively. We prepare anticipated sheaths, wires, and catheters on the back table. The previously chosen balloons and stents are prepped with utmost diligence to remove any air in the system. We have copious amounts of syringes with heparinized saline and full-strength contrast at hand. These should never be completely emptied, to avoid air embolism. At this point a standard time-out is performed.

DETAILS OF THE PROCEDURE We evaluate the right common femoral artery (CFA) with duplex ultrasonography. We identify the femoral bifurcation in short-axis view and then stay proximal to that. The view is then changed to long axis to allow for assessment of CFA in its entirety. We pick a safe spot over the femoral head, free from calcium or posterior plaque. Using real-time B-mode ultrasound the vessel is then entered, and access is confirmed with fluoroscopy.

We place a Perclose Proglide (Abbott) device in pre-close technique if Mo.Ma is employed and standard post-close if a 6F sheath is used. The patient is heparinized systemically to an activated clotting time (ACT) >250 seconds before entering the aortic arch with any wire or catheter. We check the ACT every 20 minutes thereafter and re-dose heparin as needed.

ACCESS TO COMMON CAROTID ARTERY: We prefer using CT image fusion roadmapping to help us traverse the aortic arch, delineate the height of the lesion, and reduce contrast dose and radiation exposure. A preoperative, high-quality CTA is co-registered to an on-table cone beam CT using 3D–3D alignment based on small aortic calcifications that serve as fiducials. This allows a live fusion mask of the aortic arch and supra-aortic branches without any aortogram, which carries a small risk of stroke. If fusion technology is not available, we will still avoid an arch aortogram if a preoperative CT of the arch is available. In the rare situation when no noninvasive arch imaging has been performed, an arch angiogram is performed in the appropriate left anterior oblique (LAO) projection, usually around 45 degrees when the catheter in the arch is maximally splayed, to best visualize the common carotid artery origin of interest (FIGURE 16-1A AND B).

Next, the common carotid artery is selected. We would like to re-emphasize the importance of gentle and deliberate catheter and wire manipulations in this stage of the procedure to avoid any cerebral embolism. For left carotid lesions, we usually choose a JB1 catheter to select the CCA. A floppy glidewire is advanced into the ascending aorta followed by the JB1 catheter to just proximal to the left CCA origin. The wire is withdrawn into the catheter. In a gentle counterclockwise motion, the catheter is pulled back and the CCA is selected. Correct location of the catheter is confirmed by contrast injection. At this point, the floppy glidewire is advanced to the distal CCA with a good 2-cm safety distance of the carotid bifurcation followed by the catheter. The wire is exchanged for an Amplatz Super Stiff wire, over which the working sheath is advanced. Usually, selection of the external carotid artery (ECA) is preferable to ensure sufficient stability of the stiff wire to allow for sheath advancement. In such a case, CCA or bifurcation disease must not be present. **CONTINUES** ▶

16-1

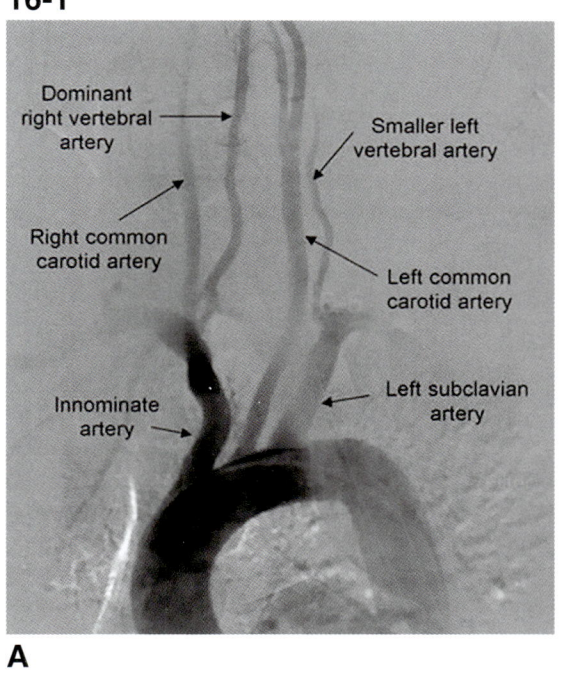

A

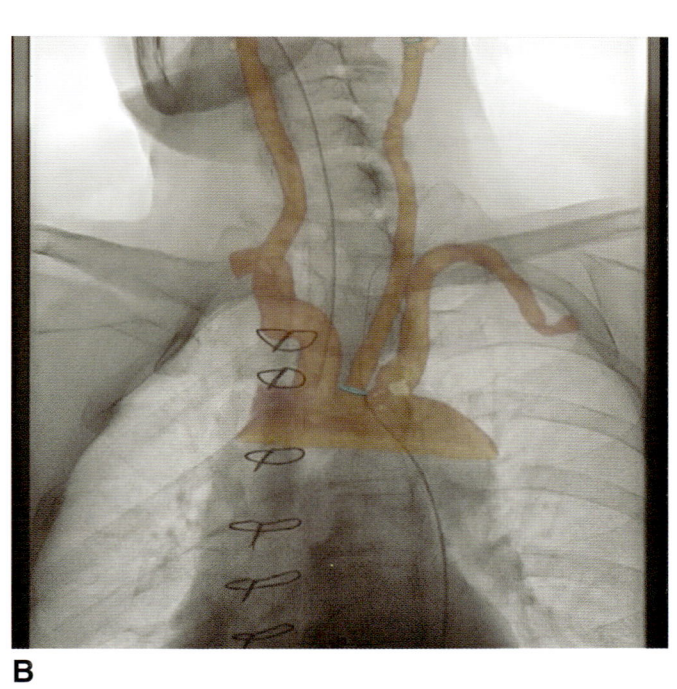

B

DETAILS OF THE PROCEDURE *ACCESS TO COMMON CAROTID ARTERY:* **CONTINUED** For right carotid lesions, selecting the CCA may be more difficult. Often the approach described above using a JB1 catheter is successful. With type II and especially type III arches, reverse-curve catheters such as Simmons 2 or Vitek are needed. These are large catheters that are at times hard to re-form, but several options exist to achieve it. (1) The left subclavian artery is selected. The catheter is advanced to the halfway point of the reverse curve. Then the wire is pulled back enough to be out of the curve. Finally, the catheter is advanced, at which point it should follow the aortic arch contour and be re-formed in the arch (**FIGURE 16-2A**). (2) The floppy glidewire can be advanced to and then coiled over the aortic valve, thus creating a loop. The catheter is advanced sufficiently to regain its original shape (**FIGURE 16-2B**). (3) The contralateral iliac artery is selected with a separate catheter such as an Omni. The Simmons catheter is then advanced and reformed similarly to the Left subclavian artery (L SCA) technique and advanced halfway into the iliac. The wire is again pulled back, and the catheter is advanced into the infrarenal aorta, re-formed, and advanced into the arch, avoiding branch origins along the way (**FIGURE 16-2C**).

Care must be taken to avoid embolization during these maneuvers. Once the catheter is re-formed and in the ascending aorta, it is gently rotated with a counterclockwise motion right at the origin of the innominate artery. This should allow for cannulation of the right CCA with the floppy glidewire. The remainder is similar to left CCA access. It has to be stressed, though, that the wire and catheter manipulations have to be executed carefully to avoid losing access, especially in type II and III arches, due to built-up torque in the system and poor initial stability.

A rare but very difficult situation for cannulation arises from type II or III arch anatomy combined with a bovine variant when the lesion is on the left side. In this case, the innominate is cannulated as described above and the Simmons 2 is advanced to the curve into the right CCA. The catheter is then advanced into the ascending aorta while rotating 180 degrees such that the catheter tip is facing the origin of the left CCA. The catheter tip will drop into the origin of the left CCA, at which time the wire can be gently advanced while simultaneously pulling the catheter back (which will advance the tip into the CCA) and reversing the 180-degree rotation (unwinding the catheter) (**FIGURE 16-3A–D**).

Once the CCA has been cannulated, an injection is performed to confirm the level of the bifurcation. The appropriate obliquity for this injection can be determined from the preoperative CTA but is typically at about 30 degrees ipsilateral oblique or preferably, the neck is rotated away from the side of the lesion and minimal obliquity is needed.

If the ECA is cannulated, a stiff glidewire may be used instead of the combination of a floppy glidewire and Amplatz Super Stiff. However, if the ECA cannot be cannulated, it is preferred to use a braided super stiff wire in the distal CCA as this is less likely to advance across the lesion during delivery of the stiff sheath which straightens (shortens) the path from groin to CCA. ECA cannulation is a requirement for use of the Mo.Ma device per Instructions for Use (IFU).

A telescope technique can facilitate delivery if a standard 6F 90-cm sheath (e.g., Cook shuttle) is employed using 6.5F catheter. In this case, the sheath is advanced to the proximal descending aorta and the catheter and wire are advanced first into the ECA (or CCA) and the sheath is then advanced over the catheter/wire combination. Sheaths with a rotating hemostatic valve are necessary to allow proper de-airing with the introduction of any catheter or device.

Finally, in very rare circumstances, a curved guide catheter may be left in the arch and the angioplasty and stenting may be performed through this. However, this is not recommended when the above methods are possible, as the position of the guide catheter will not be as stable and it is possible that the access across the lesion may be lost during the procedure, with a high likelihood of adverse events. **CONTINUES**

16-2

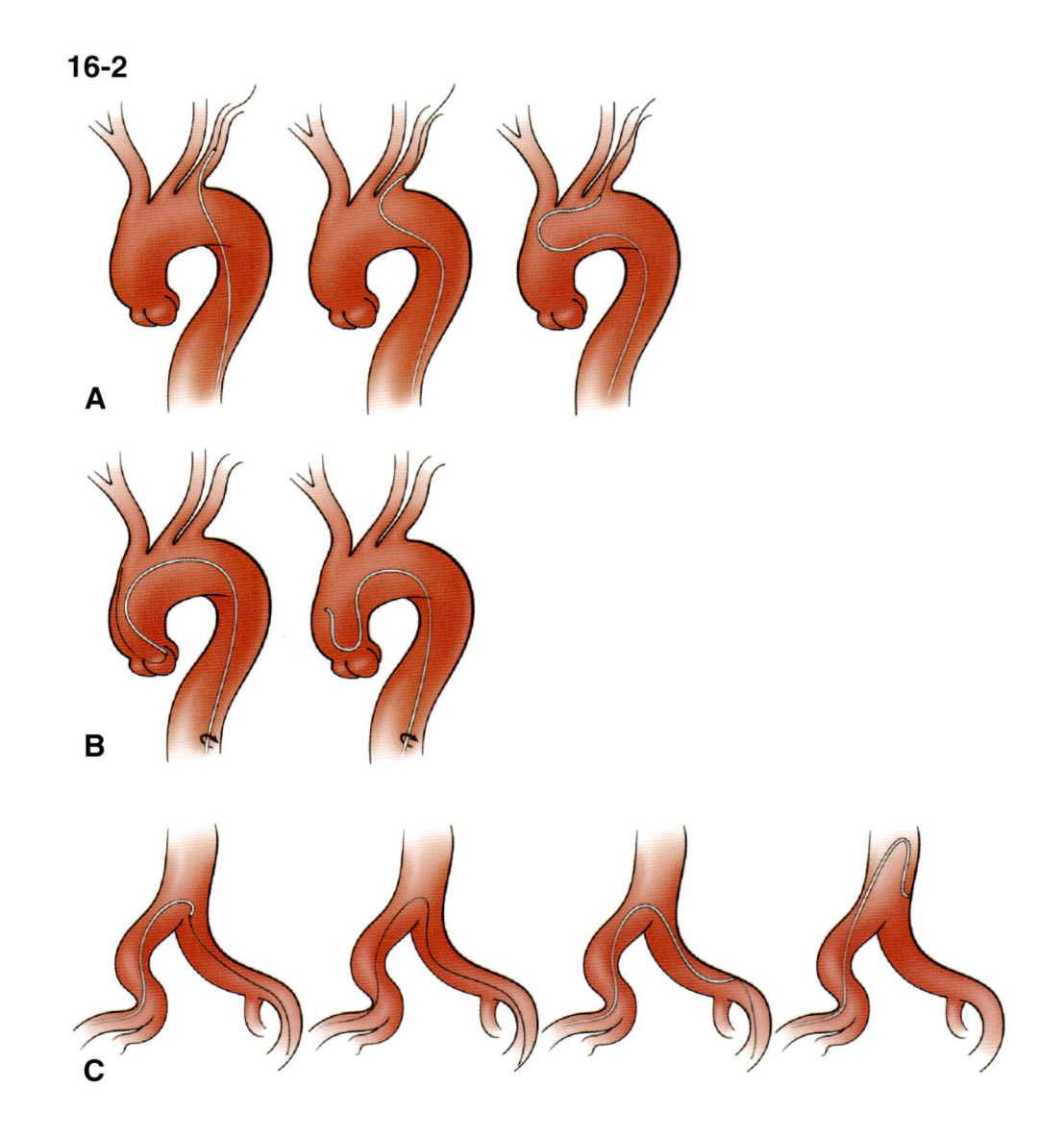

16-3

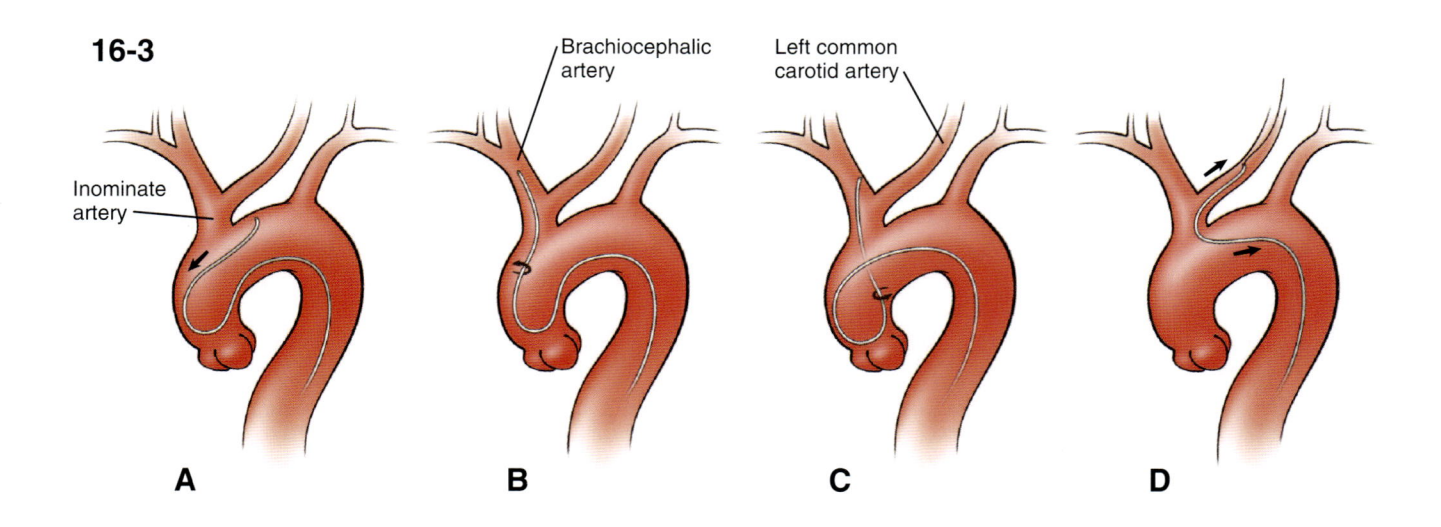

DETAILS OF THE PROCEDURE *CROSSING THE LESION AND CEREBRAL PROTECTION:* `CONTINUED` A simple hand injection is performed to show the carotid bifurcation and location of the lesion. We typically avoid power injections to speed the procedure and limit radiation exposure although occasionally the extra detail is needed, in which case we use low-flow rates, for example 6 mL/sec for 9 mL with a pressure limit of 200 psi. With very careful and deliberate motions, a distal protection system is advanced through the lesion and deployed in healthy, distal ICA. We use the Emboshield Nav6 system (Abbott) as it allows some axial wire motion during loading of angioplasty balloons and stents without motion of the filter (**FIGURE 16-4**).

Should we employ proximal embolic protection, we introduce the Mo.Ma Ultra device. This approach requires the lesion to be in the ICA, as the Mo.Ma system is rather bulky (9Fr outer diameter [OD]) and requires access to the ECA. There is a distal ECA balloon and a proximal CCA balloon. Once both balloons are inflated, there is flow arrest in the ICA preventing distal embolization. Intermitted flow reversal can be achieved via gentle aspiration during periods when there is no obstruction in the center lumen from angioplasty balloon or stent. Once correct position and flow arrest have been confirmed, the lesion is carefully crossed with a 0.014″ wire.

DILATION AND STENTING: We routinely employ a vigorous predilation technique in which the balloon is sized to the healthy ICA just distal to the lesion. We oversize the stent by at least 2 mm and often choose a tapered model. We prefer one-time angioplasty over the dual approach with smaller predilation and larger postdilation balloons, as it shortens the procedure and may be safer. This will avoid pushing the stent into the lesion and with debris from the plaque protruding through the interstices. If a significant residual stenosis is present, repeat angioplasty may be considered with a larger balloon (**FIGURE 16-5**).

We recommend pretreating all patients with anticholinergic agents (glycopyrrolate is preferred over atropine as it causes less dry mouth) and avoiding prolonged inflation to reduce the risk of irritating the carotid baroreceptors. Should, despite pretreatment, hypotension and bradycardia or asystole occur, we deflate the balloon immediately and ask the anesthesiologist to administer additional glycopyrollate, IV fluids, and potentially pressors to reverse the effect. If neurological changes occur with hypotension during a case with the Mo.Ma system, the CCA balloon may be deflated after aspiration of debris and then reinflated when the blood pressure and neurological function are normalized. Next, the chosen stent is brought into the patient and deployed in standard fashion. Angiography of the stent is performed to confirm correct placement and expansion of the stent. A second injection in an opposite oblique projection may be added if there is any question of significant residual stenosis, and intravascular ultrasound (IVUS) may be used for this purpose as well, although this may add undue time and expense. If an issue is identified such as missing coverage of parts of the lesion or insufficient expansion of the stent, a second stent or postdilation balloon angioplasty is performed until a satisfactory result is achieved. In our experience, careful preoperative planning makes this event a rare occurrence. We make no attempt to precisely match stent length with lesion length and prefer extra length to avoid the need for a second stent, which is associated with higher adverse event rates. This also allows faster stent deployment. We make use of gentle syringe aspiration between these steps to reduce the risk for embolization when using flow arrest/reversal. We usually choose a closed-cell design stent (e.g., Xact, Abbott) to prevent embolization. We use an open-cell stent when there is excessive tortuosity.

COMPLETION: We usually do not perform a cerebral angiogram unless there are neurologic changes. The preop CTA serves as a baseline cerebral angiogram for comparison if neurologic changes arise. In that case we recommend performing a Towne's view in posterior-anterior with cranial angulation to the point where the petrous bones line up with the upper margin of the orbits, as well as a lateral view with the floor of the left and right anterior fossa and the auditory canals directly overlapping. If a filling defect is identified in the cerebral vascular beds, we call for immediate assistance from neurointerventional colleagues.

After confirmatory angiography of the stent itself, we carefully remove all hardware from the carotid artery. We make sure to remove the sheath over a stiffer wire. The access is then closed with a Perclose Proglide. We like the device for its ability to maintain wire access if a second closure device is necessary to achieve hemostasis. Protamine is safe to administer without any detrimental effect on the stent if deemed necessary. A small dry sterile dressing is applied over the access site, allowing intermittent groin checks.

POSTOPERATIVE CARE The patient is brought to the recovery area and kept there for 2 to 3 hours. Frequent checks of the neurological function (every 15 minutes for the first hour, then every 30 minutes) are performed. The blood pressure is invasively monitored and kept between 100 and 140 mmHg. If necessary, hypotension is treated by infusion of crystalloid combined as needed with phenylephrine. In the case of hypertension, we start a nicardipine drip. The access is intermittently assessed for hemostasis. From the recovery area the patient is transferred to the intermediary care unit. Frequency of neuromonitoring checks and vital signs is reduced to hourly at this point. Bedrest is lifted 2 hours after access closure and definitive hemostasis. The patient is usually discharged on the first postoperative day. All patients are discharged on dual antiplatelet therapy for at least 1 month. A high-intensity statin is prescribed indefinitely. ■

SUGGESTED READINGS

Chaikof EL, Cambria RP. *Atlas of Vascular Surgery and Endovascular Therapy*, 1st Edition, Elsevier, 2024.

Osborn AG. *Diagnostic Cerebral Angiography*, 2nd Edition, Lippincott, 2023.

Sidawy AN, Perler BA, eds. *Rutherford's Vascular Surgery and Endovascular Therapy*, 10th Edition, Elsevier, 2022.

Stanley JC, Veith F, Wakefield TW. *Current Therapy in Vascular and Endovascular Surgery*, 5th Edition, Elsevier, 2014.

16-4

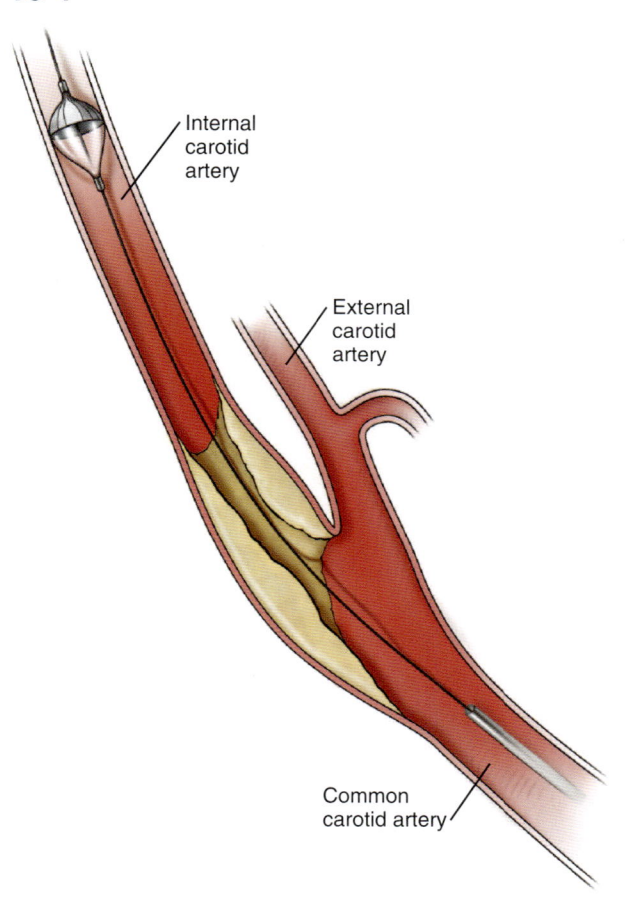

Internal carotid artery

External carotid artery

Common carotid artery

16-5

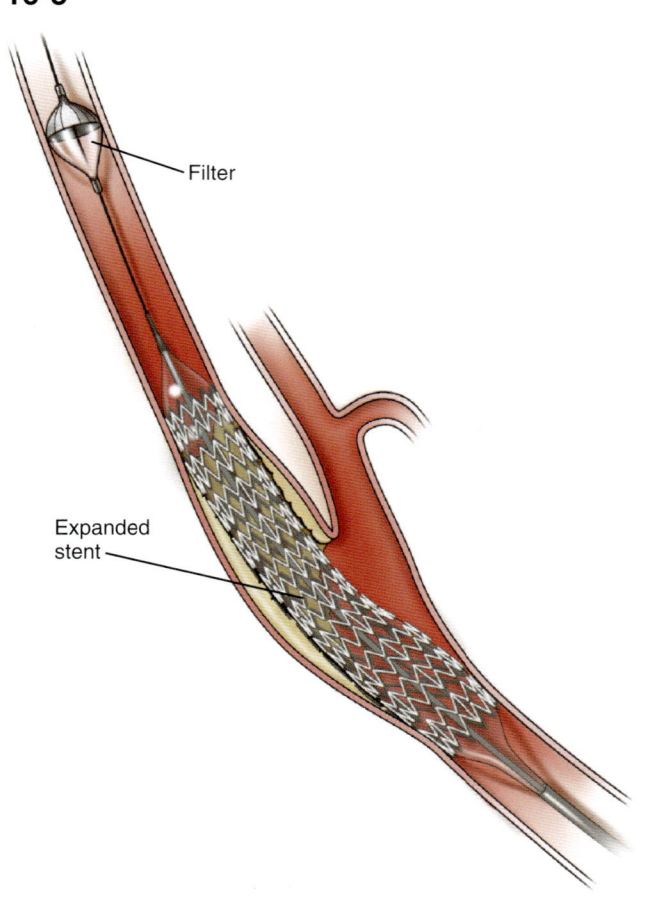

Filter

Expanded stent

BRACHIOCEPHALIC INTERVENTIONS

Bian Wu, MD • Peter Schneider, MD

INTRODUCTION TO ENDOVASCULAR INTERVENTIONS FOR ARCH VESSEL DISEASE

INDICATIONS: Atherosclerosis may involve the aortic arch and its branch vessels: the innominate, right subclavian, right common carotid, left common carotid, and left subclavian arteries. The left subclavian artery is the most frequently involved arch vessel affected by atherosclerosis, followed by the innominate and left carotid arteries. As is the case in other vascular beds, not all stenoses (or occlusions) warrant treatment. Revascularization may be indicated for either occlusive symptoms (i.e., upper extremity pain/fatigue, global cerebrovascular hypoperfusion, vertebrobasilar "steal" syndrome) or atheroembolic disease (i.e., upper extremity digit ischemia or ischemic strokes).

Endovascular interventions for occlusive disease of the arch vessels offer lower perioperative risks, faster recovery times, and acceptable durability when compared with open surgical approaches. Although the risk–benefit profile is generally more favorable than for open procedures, the decision to proceed with an intervention still requires careful consideration. Thoughtful anatomic assessment is also critical for appropriate patient selection and case planning. Less common causes of arch vessel disease include inflammatory arteritis, radiation arteritis, dissection, aneurysm, and trauma. These pathologies may also have endovascular solutions, if clinically indicated and anatomy allows. Potential endoluminal strategies for traumatic and aneurysmal disease of arch vessels are outside of the scope of this chapter.

PREOPERATIVE PLANNING: A detailed understanding of the patient's anatomy is critical to patient selection and case planning for endoluminal interventions of the arch vessels. Anatomic considerations include arch anatomy, plaque morphology, location of branch vessel origins, and tortuosity of the arch branches. CT angiography is most helpful in providing this information and allows for precise measurements for intended treatments. If possible, contrast for the CT scan should be given through the contralateral arm to minimize artifact from the subclavian and innominate veins. MR angiogram may also be used but is often less helpful, as calcified plaques are not readily visualized and surrounding anatomy is more challenging to reconstruct. Duplex ultrasound may be helpful for hemodynamic evaluation (i.e., degree of stenosis, retrograde flow in vertebral artery) and may help to support specific indications for repair but does not provide the anatomic discrimination necessary for preprocedural planning.

Case planning should include the best approach for endovascular access (antegrade, retrograde, bidirectional, and whether a hybrid component is required) and details for the procedure itself (i.e., to be performed in the interventional radiology suite or hybrid operating room, and with that type of anesthesia). As with all endoluminal procedures, it is critical to ensure proper inventory prior to starting an intervention for arch vessel disease. Specific anatomic and technical considerations are discussed in the following sections.

ANATOMIC CONSIDERATIONS

ARCH ANATOMY: The aortic arch typically has three branches: the innominate (brachiocephalic), the left common carotid, and the left subclavian. The most prevalent anatomic variant in the arch is a shared trunk giving rise to both the innominate and left carotid arteries ("bovine arch"), which occurs in up to 20% of individuals. A single common trunk involving the innominate, left common carotid, and left subclavian arteries ("true bovine arch") is very rare in humans and found in <1% of patients. The right subclavian artery has an aberrant origin distal to the left subclavian artery in approximately 1% of the population. This seemingly random anomaly is caused by aberrant vessel involution during embryology and results in the right subclavian artery arising from the distal arch, distal to the origin of the left subclavian artery. The aberrant right subclavian artery (ARSA) then typically courses posterior to the esophagus as it goes on to perfuse the right arm and may be associated with dysphagia, with or without aneurysmal degeneration (Kommerell diverticulum). Another anomaly is the left vertebral artery originating directly from the aortic arch, between the left common carotid and left subclavian arteries. A separate left vertebral artery occurs in approximately 6% of the population.

There is also variability as to whether the arch branches arise from the ascending portion of the arch or the top of the arch. Arch anatomy is relevant in endovascular planning as branches arising from the ascending aorta may be more difficult to canulate from a femoral approach due to additional tortuosity in the arch. In such cases a retrograde approach may be more prudent. Of note, advancing age and chronic hypertension contribute to elongation of the arch, with associated increased tortuosity and higher likelihood of branches arising from the ascending arch.

PLAQUE MORPHOLOGY: Plaque morphology is particularly important to consider during endovascular planning and treatment of the arch vessels. Calcified plaques in the aortic arch and arch vessels are prone to embolization (i.e., stroke) with manipulation, and care should be taken to minimize manipulation with wires and devices. Knowledge of specific plaque morphology helps to avoid entering unwanted subintimal planes while crossing lesions and decreases the risk of vessel rupture, which is especially a concern when there are heavily calcified plaques. Rupture of the arch vessels may lead to life-threatening bleeding for which urgent mediastinal exploration may be required.

LOCATION OF CRITICAL BRANCH VESSELS: The target lesion should be evaluated with respect to its proximity to branch origins and other lesions. The most obvious example of this is the bifurcation of the innominate artery to the right common carotid and subclavian arteries, as endoluminal therapies here need to preserve flow to both outflow vessels. Similarly, preservation of the vertebral arteries is important during endoluminal interventions of the subclavian arteries. Plaque near the vertebral artery may be dislodged by interventions and either occlude or embolize, with associated neurologic consequences. Both the left and the right internal mammary arteries may be used as conduits for coronary bypass, and the presence of an internal mammary bypass should clearly be known before attempting an arch procedure.

TECHNICAL DETAILS, TIPS, AND TRICKS

CASE SEQUENCE FOR ANTEGRADE FEMORAL APPROACH

1. **Access.** When considering access for endoluminal procedures it is important to consider not only the potential access vessel itself, but also (and perhaps more importantly) the target lesion. Stable sheath support is essential for technical success. Your sheath tip should be positioned close to the lesion to facilitate crossing and treatment. Of note, the patient should be systemically heparinized (goal ACT 250–300) before any manipulation of the arch to decrease the risk of periprocedural stroke (please see Chapter 16 for additional detail).

2. **Arteriography.** Procedural planning is guided by preoperative cross-sectional imaging, and thus arteriography is typically used as part of the therapeutic intervention rather than for additional diagnostic information. However, obtaining adequate arteriograms to guide the intervention is essential for success. The complex three-dimensional anatomy of the arch and its vessels potentially makes arteriography challenging. For example, the origin of the arch vessels is typically best seen in a steep left anterior oblique (LAO) projection (FIGURE 17-1) as in this 77-year-old patient presenting with symptoms of global cerebral hypoperfusion. Aortogram in a steep LAO projection allows for best visualization of the origin of the great vessels. Another method to estimate LAO projection is to place the wire in the arch and rotate the image intensifier, and observe the narrow upside-down U shape of the arch become a wider U shape. Calcifications in the arch and arch vessels may also be used to help visualize the anatomy and identify the target lesion. There is a critical stenosis at the origin of the brachiocephalic trunk. The left common carotid artery is occluded a few cm past its origin. The innominate bifurcation is typically best seen in a steep right anterior oblique (RAO) projection (FIGURE 17-2). A steep RAO allows for better visualization of the innominate bifurcation; however, it compromises the view of the great vessel origins. The lesion at the origin of the innominate is not seen in this projection. The innominate and proximal left common carotid artery are also superimposed. Incorporating knowledge gained from preoperative imaging with intraoperative fluoroscopy allows for minimization of both contrast use and radiation exposure. Critical branch vessels must be precisely identified before proceeding with intervention. **CONTINUES** ▶

17-1

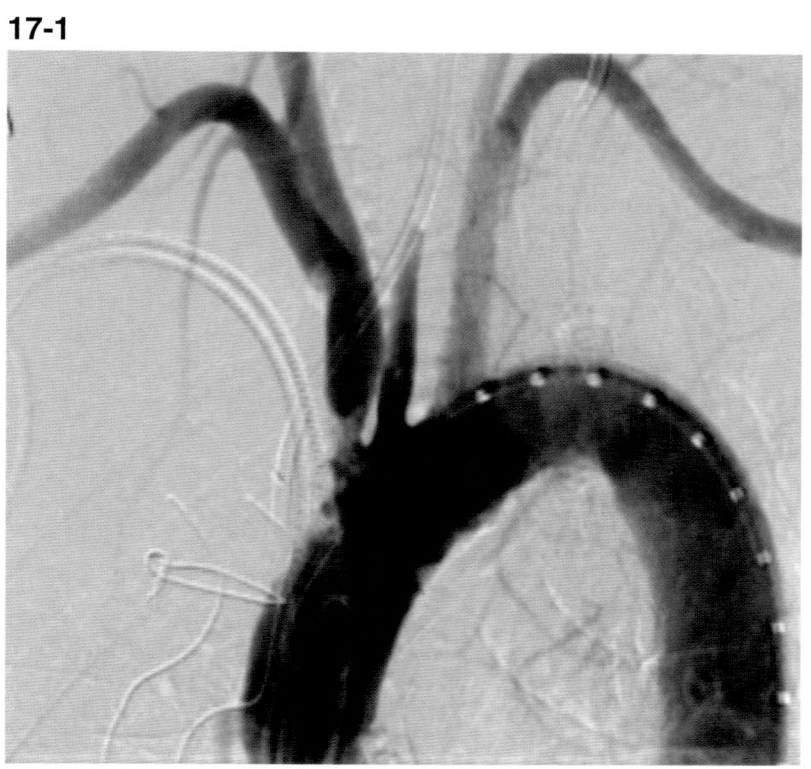

17-2

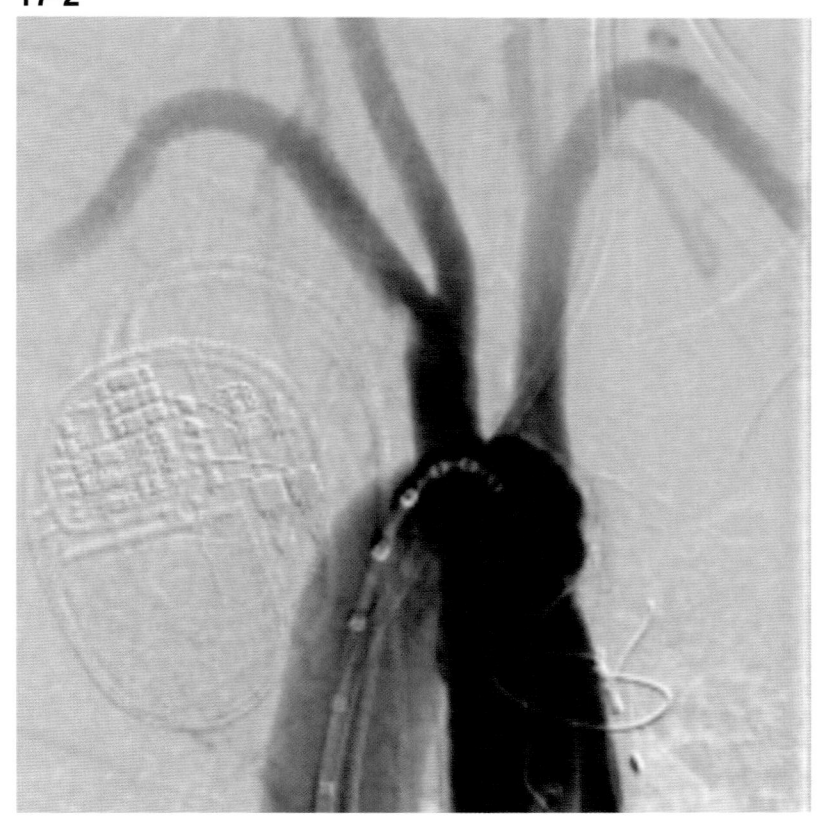

TECHNICAL DETAILS, TIPS, AND TRICKS *CASE SEQUENCE FOR ANTEGRADE FEMORAL APPROACH* ◀ CONTINUED

3. **Crossing the lesion.** As noted above, ensuring stable sheath access near the lesion is critical to maximize chances of technical success when crossing and treating lesions (FIGURE 17-3). For standard transfemoral access, a 70-cm length sheath is typically adequate for the position in the arch. A 90-cm long sheath may be needed for taller patients and/or patients with significant tortuosity. If there is an arch vessel occlusion with a "stump" at its origin (i.e., a non-flush occlusion), the stump may be engaged with a 5F simple curve catheter (FIGURE 17-4). Although this is not a stable position, engaging the stump with the catheter tip may provide just enough support to allow guidewire advancement with a hydrophilic guidewire (potentially even 0.014″ or 0.018″ here). The tip of the wire may be bent to use for "drilling" past the occlusion. Of note, it is important to not permit the wire to buckle. Excessive forward pressure will kick the catheter tip out of the stump. If any progress is made, a catheter may be advanced in short incremental distances. If the wire crosses, the catheter is advanced and intraluminal position is confirmed (FIGURE 17-5). Position of critical branch vessels is again confirmed. As is the case in other vascular beds, occlusions are more difficult to cross than stenoses. CONTINUES ▶

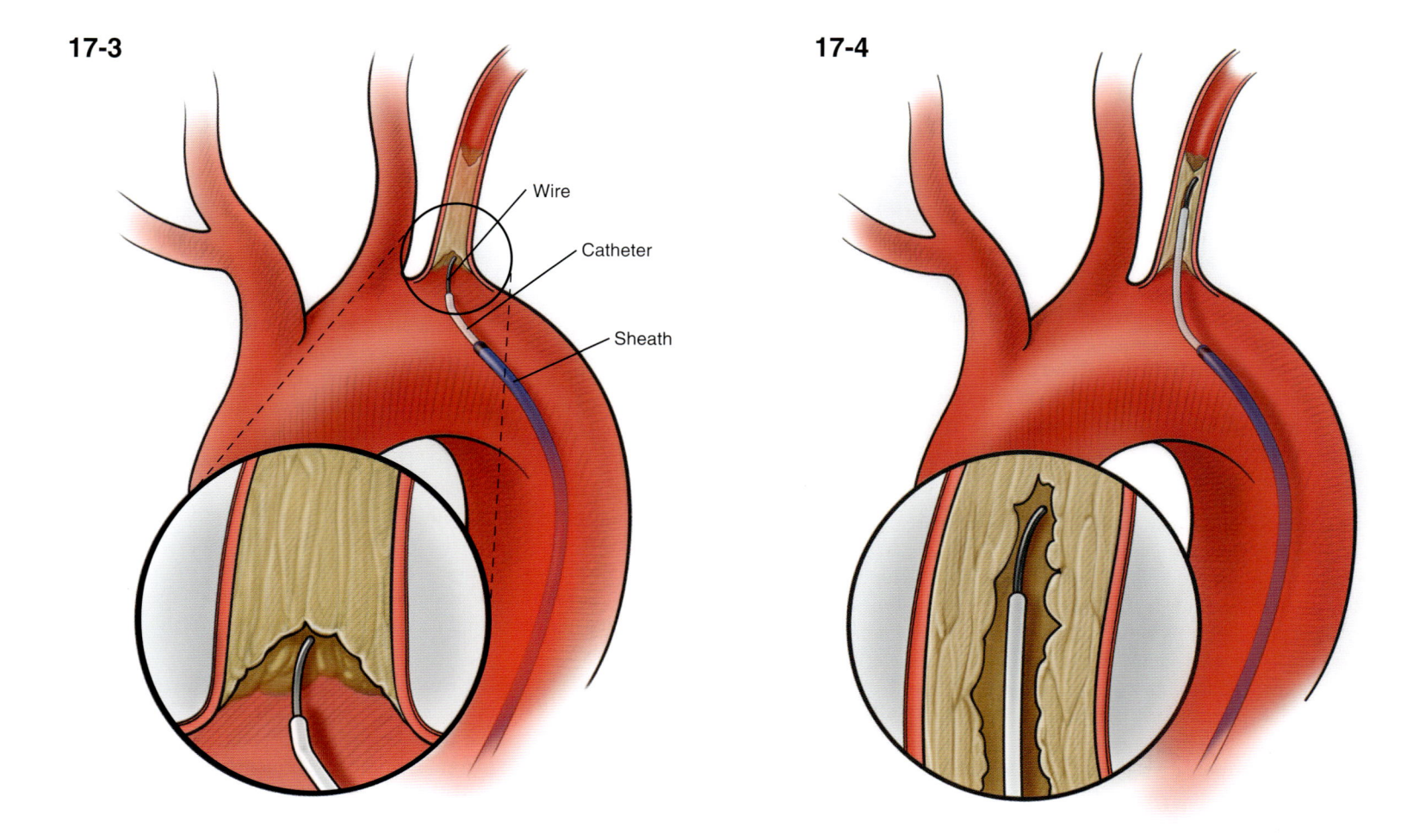

17-3

Wire

Catheter

Sheath

17-4

17-5

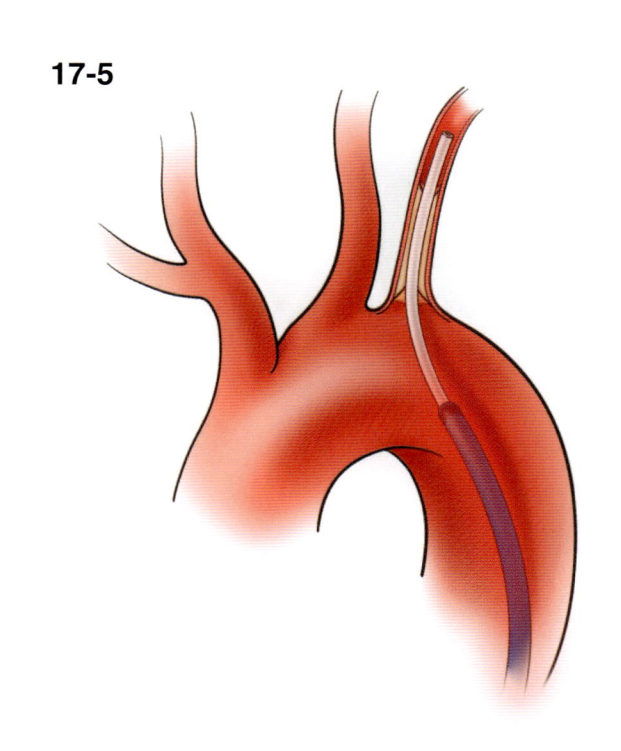

TECHNICAL DETAILS, TIPS, AND TRICKS *CASE SEQUENCE FOR RETROGRADE BRACHIAL APPROACH:* CONTINUED Some lesions may be technically easier and potentially safer to cross retrograde. The above sequence of intervention and additional technical tips and tricks are modified below for a retrograde approach.

1. **Access** can be percutaneous or via a small cut-down in patients with small arm arteries.
2. **Arteriography** should delineate the important branches, especially the vertebral or any prior coronary bypass using a left internal mammary artery (LIMA) graft.
3. **Crossing the lesion.** In some cases it may be prudent to consider retrograde as a primary strategy during preoperative planning (FIGURE 17-6). Retrograde access may also be used to ensure preservation of both the carotid and subclavian arteries while attempting to cross an innominate occlusion. Similarly, retrograde access may be used in cases where occlusive lesions abut the vertebral artery, to avoid reentry distal to (and thus loss of) the vertebral artery. Similar to the antegrade approach, it is important to position the tip of your sheath near the lesion when attempting retrograde recanalization using a drilling technique (FIGURE 17-7). It is important to note that subintimal entry is not necessarily avoided with retrograde access. Entry into a subintimal plane while crossing an arch lesion may result in a dissection that extends to the aorta and potentially along the aorta. The most important angiogram is after crossing and confirming true lumen aortic access (FIGURE 17-8).

Treating the Lesion   Initial endovascular therapy of the arch vessels involved balloon angioplasty alone, which produced reasonable results. Introduction of stents has since improved both the rate of immediate technical success as well as longer-term durability for endovascular treatment of the arch vessels. Most clinicians thus perform primary stenting in this vascular bed. Most clinicians also prefer covered stents over uncovered (bare metal) stents here, although there are no clear data to support this preference. Pre-dilation may be needed to facilitate passage of stents across the lesion. This is typically performed with a 4- to 6-mm plain balloon. It is important that the balloon chosen for pre-dilation is not larger than the vessel distally so as to not induce dissection. Balloon-expandable stents are best suited for interventions of the proximal arch vessels as they provide excellent radial force and hoop strength (FIGURE 17-9). Balloon-expandable stents also afford greater precision for deployment when compared to self-expanding stents, although they should be expected to shorten slightly on both ends as they are expanded.

It is important to extend the stent 1 to 2 mm into the arch to fully cover any "spillover" arch plaque at the vessel origin. Of note, balloon expandable stents may be expanded 1 to 2 mm past their nominal diameters (with associated additional shortening of length on each end). The portion of the stent extending into the arch should be "flared" with a slightly larger balloon to facilitate perfusion and also to accommodate potential future antegrade interventions. Care must be taken not to overexpand, as there is a risk of vessel rupture. Vessel rupture is associated with overdilation of heavily calcified vessels and may be fatal if at the origin of the arch vessels. Self-expanding stents may be preferred for more tortuous lesions distal to the origin of the vessel, especially if the lesion is in a tortuous segment or there is a substantial change in caliber proximal and distal to the lesion. Self-expanding stents will not dilate past their nominal diameters and thus should be oversized 1 to 2 mm to the target vessel diameter. Both pre-dilation and post-dilation are necessary for self-expanding stents. Self-expanding covered stents also afford potential treatment for traumatic and aneurysmal disease of the arch vessels.

ADDITIONAL ADVANCED TECHNIQUES: In some cases a bidirectional approach with a through-and-through wire may be used to both to provide maximal support. After successfully crossing a lesion retrograde, a bidirectional through-and-through wire may be established by snaring the wire from the femoral approach. This allows a larger femoral sheath for delivery of a large stent while maintaining a small sheath access through the brachial artery (FIGURE 17-10). The through-and-through wire also allows for a more stable support. Lastly, in cases where the lesion abuts both the right common carotid and right subclavian arteries, outflow to both vessels may be preserved via a single antegrade access using two 0.014″ wires. The profile of two 0.014″ wires is less than a single 0.035″ wire; thus a 0.035″ device (i.e., stent) may be advanced over the two 0.014″ wires. The device can then be deployed with the smaller wires protecting each branch.

POSTOPERATIVE CARE   Antiplatelet therapy is considered standard of care after angioplasty and stenting; however, the role of dual antiplatelet therapy after endovascular treatment of arch vessels is less clear. Most clinicians treat with at least 1 month of dual antiplatelet therapy after endoluminal therapy in this vascular bed, although there are no definitive data to guide this practice. Surveillance should be continued with either duplex ultrasonography or CT angiography every 6 months for the first 2 years, then annually thereafter. ■

17-6

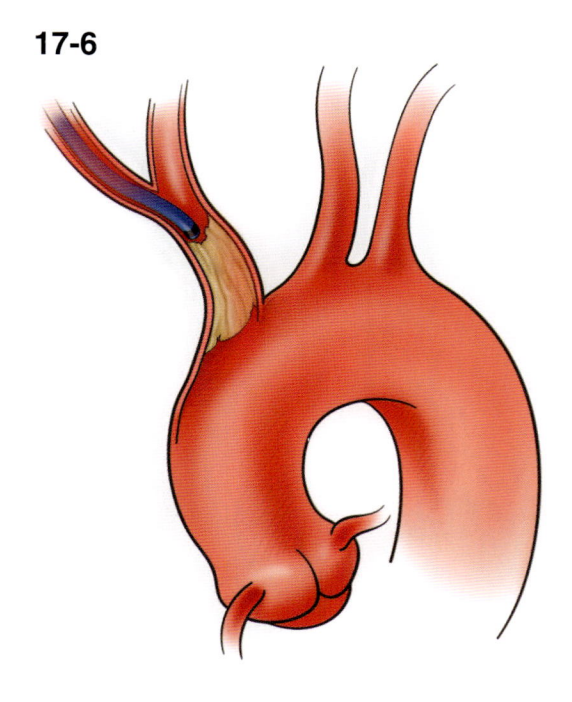

17-7

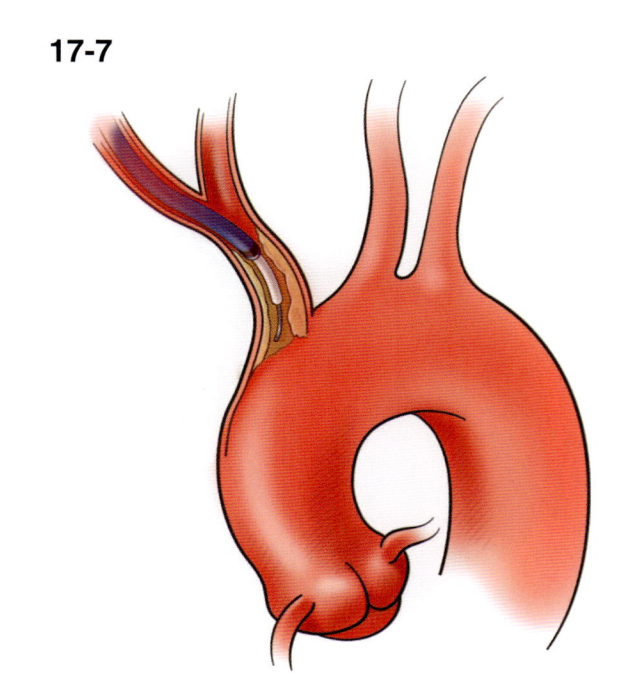

17-8

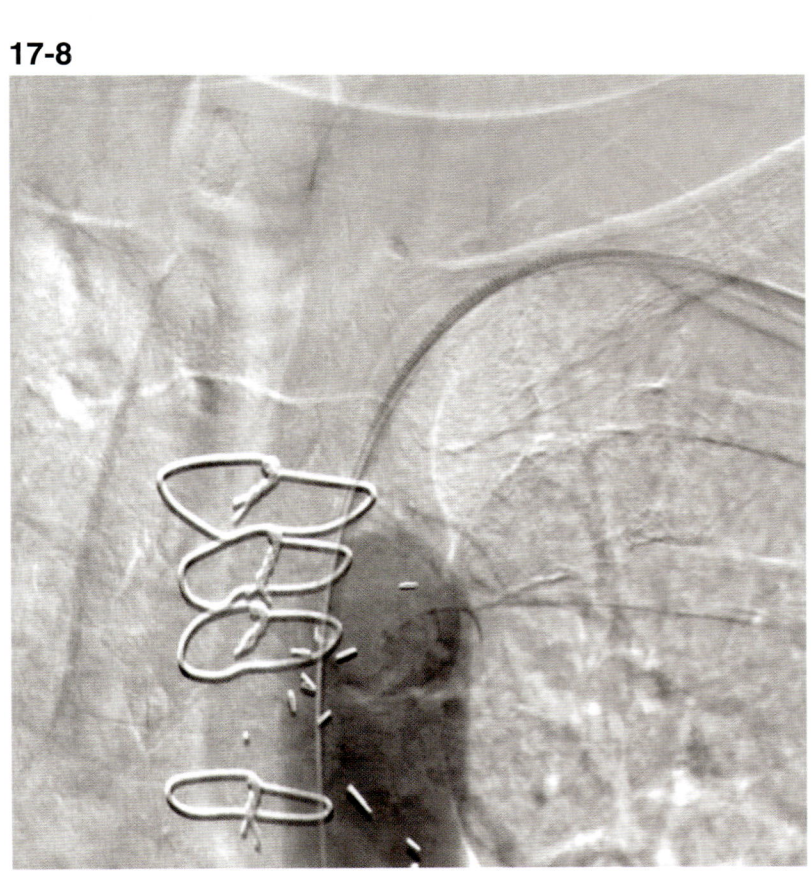

17-9

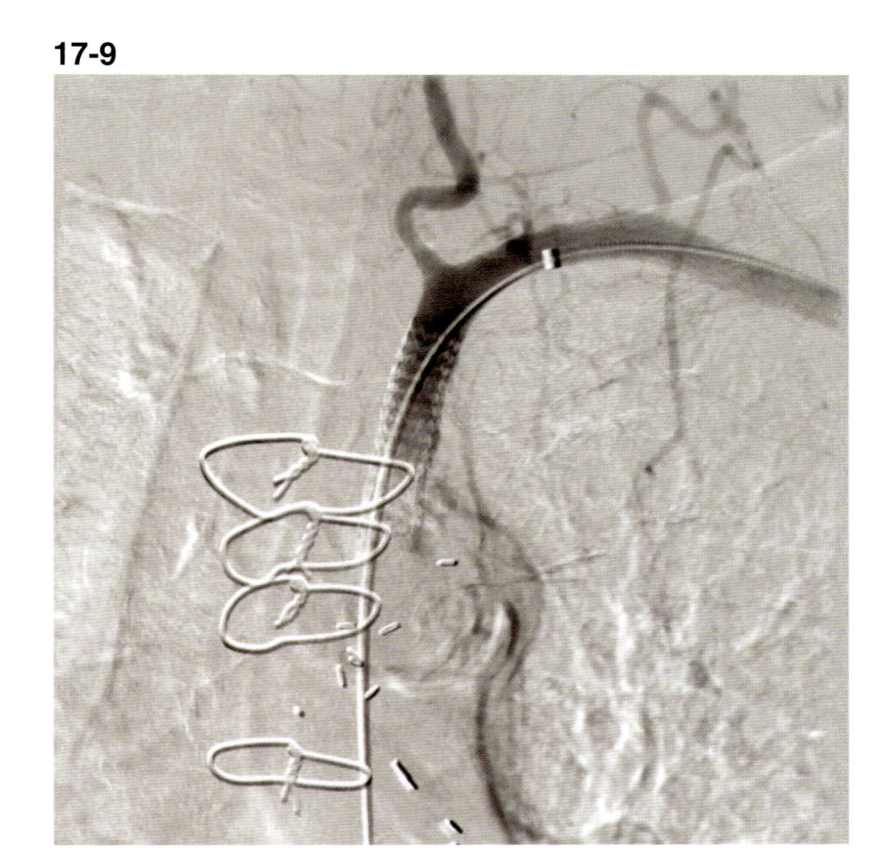

17-10

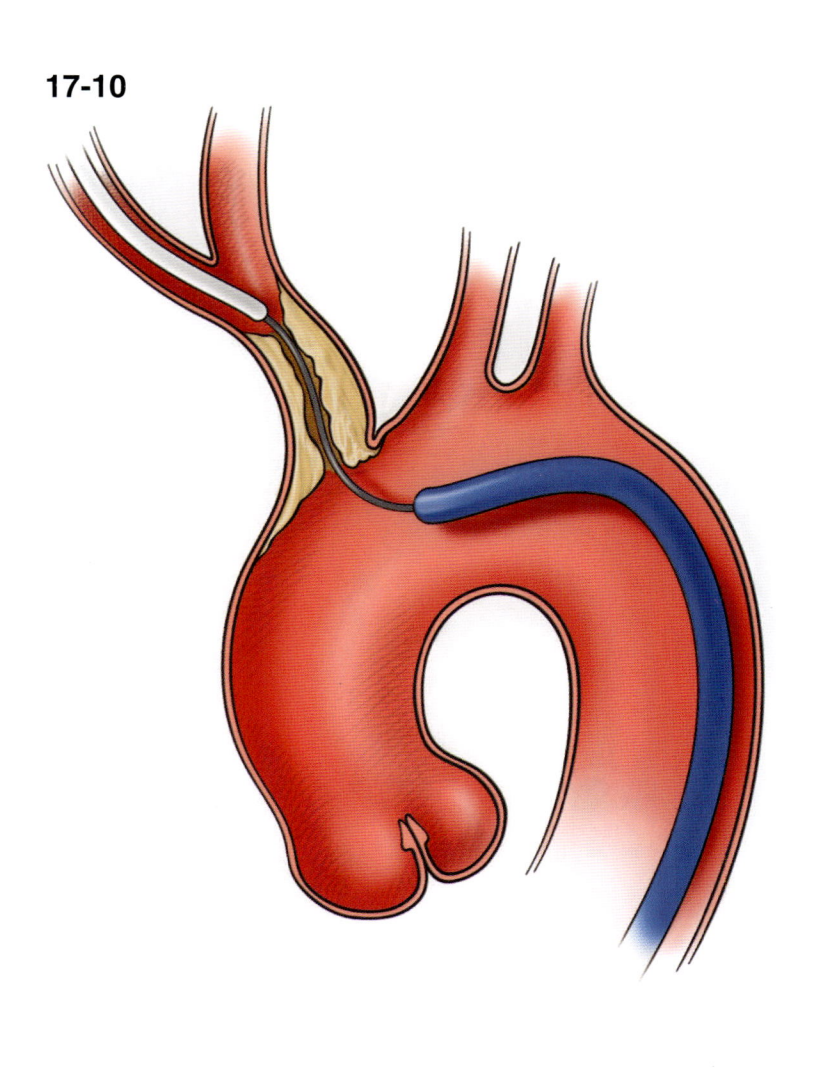

DIALYSIS ACCESS AND UPPER EXTREMITY

ARTERIOVENOUS FISTULA (RADIOCEPHALIC AND BRACHIOCEPHALIC)

Ezra Y. Koh, MD • Eric K. Peden, MD

INDICATIONS Radiocephalic and brachiocephalic arteriovenous (AV) fistulas are created to provide long-term hemodialysis access in patients requiring renal replacement therapy. Indications for the procedure include patients who have end-stage renal diseases as well as those who have stage 5 chronic kidney disease and are expected to progress to end-stage renal disease in the near future. Occasionally, AV access is created for non-dialysis needs, such as for plasmapheresis or exchange transfusions, but these are the minority of cases. AV fistulas have the highest patency rates of dialysis access options and are therefore the preferred initial access option if the patient's anatomy is suitable. However, it is extremely important to avoid a "fistula at all costs" approach and only to create access that has a good chance at maturation, because failure of maturation is very common and leads to dissatisfaction of both patient and provider. Generally, initial access is created as distal in the arm as possible, allowing for future proximal dialysis options to be utilized if necessary. The nondominant arm is preferred for initial fistula creation unless vascular anatomy is far superior in the dominant arm.

PREOPERATIVE EVALUATION Prior to surgery, a comprehensive history and physical is obtained focusing on prior central venous access sites and previous surgery to the upper extremities which could preclude the creation of an AV fistula, along with previous complications of steal or edema from prior access surgeries. Prior history of axillary lymphadenectomy for breast cancer or melanoma and presence of transvenous pacemakers and defibrillators should be noted. Other comorbidities frequently seen in patients with end-stage renal disease, such as poorly controlled diabetes or severe hypertension, should be medically optimized. Examination of obvious visible veins, quality of pulses, and preexisting signs of neuropathy with motor/sensory changes and hand muscle wasting is important, as well as noting signs of central venous obstruction such as chest wall varicosities. To assess the vascular anatomy of the upper extremity, preoperative vessel mapping using duplex ultrasound is obtained. We believe this step is critical, allowing for detailed evaluation of access options to maximize potential for successful fistula creation and avoid complications. The veins are assessed for size, depth, and any flow-limiting lesions such as thrombus or stenosis which could impair outflow and maturation. Threshold cutoffs for vein size adequate for maturation are generally between 2.5 and 3 mm. For a primary transposition fistula, often a bigger vein size is preferred. Arteries are assessed for size, patency, and degree of calcification, as well as anomalies such as a high arterial bifurcation.

Preoperative patient education is very important to discuss rationale for conversion from a catheter to AV access, alternatives such as peritoneal dialysis and renal transplantation, as well as potential complications and need for secondary procedures. Maturation procedures are commonly needed; failures and complications do occur, and patient satisfaction is improved if this is discussed beforehand.

ANESTHESIA Anesthesia options include local anesthetic with or without sedation, regional, or general. Our strong preference for essentially all upper extremity access procedures is regional anesthesia with sedation. The benefits of regional anesthesia are minimizing the cardiopulmonary effects of anesthetics on this frail patient population as well as promoting vasodilation of the vessels in the extremity such that additional AV fistula options may be feasible, particularly for distal wrist fistulas. Our anesthesia team usually performs a suprascapular block with ultrasound and nerve stimulator guidance in the preop area, to help reduce in-room turnover time. One downside to regional anesthesia is that it may delay presentation and recognition of steal or ischemic monomelic neuropathy, emphasizing the need for pre- and postoperative education.

SURGICAL PROCEDURE The entire arm is prepped and draped from centrally beyond the axilla to the fingertips, thereby allowing exposure for various access procedure types. Prior to making the incision, intraoperative ultrasound is crucial for a final evaluation of the veins, decision of fistula type to be created, and deciding where to place the incision for best exposure. If there is one magic tool in access surgery, it is the ultrasound probe in the hands of the surgeon. During ultrasound, location of the arterial bifurcation is noted, arterial size and quality confirmed, and feasibility of various fistula types assessed by vein patency, size, and quality.

RADIOCEPHALIC FISTULAS: For radiocephalic fistulas, the cephalic vein is assessed with ultrasound from the elbow down toward the wrist. When interrogating the vein, particular attention is paid to the size. We commonly find that smaller tributaries join together at the lower third of the forearm along with a significant caliber change, and therefore make the incision at the transition to a larger vein (FIGURE 18-1A). If there is no significant size transition, the incision is made closer to the wrist. The incision is longitudinal and extends approximately 4 to 5 cm. The cephalic vein is mobilized from the surrounding tissues with care taken for gentle tissue handling to avoid damage to the vessel and nearby superficial radial nerve branches (FIGURE 18-1B). Cephalic vein tributaries are ligated as needed for adequate mobilization. Once enough vein is dissected to be transposed to the radial artery without tension, the vein is marked to prevent twisting or kinking. It is subsequently ligated distally and transected. Additional manipulations of the vein with probing or distention with fluids are discouraged.

Next, the radial artery is dissected free from surrounding tissues. Occasionally, the radial artery is hidden under the brachioradialis tendon, in which cases part of the overlying tendon can be excised without significant consequence. For small arteries or those with significant spasm, papaverine can be used topically or with injection into the adventitia. Branches are ligated or controlled to prevent control bleeding during the creation of the anastomosis. The vein must be oriented appropriately without tension or twisting. The vein is spatulated to create an anastomosis 6 to 8 mm in length (FIGURE 18-1C). Generally, systemic heparinization is not required. Proximal and distal arterial control is obtained with delicate clamps or if preferred, a proximal pneumatic tourniquet with arm exsanguination. A longitudinal arteriotomy is then made using a #11 blade scalpel and extended to the desired length using Potts scissors. Stay sutures are placed to help expose the lumen of the artery. The next step is to create the arteriovenous anastomosis. Although options include interrupted sutures and anastomotic devices, we commonly do a continuous anastomosis. An end-to-side anastomosis is created using double-armed 6-0 or 7-0 polypropylene suture, taking care to have small but secure bites of both vessels with tight spacing and avoiding excessive tension on the suture to prevent "purse-stringing." Prior to securing the knot, we flush the anastomotic area with heparinized saline. Once the suture is tied, we generally release the clamps in the following order to detect bleeding and avoid any distal embolization of small clots that may have formed: first the venous clamp, then the distal arterial clamp, and finally the proximal arterial clamp while manually occluding the artery distally. The fistula is palpated to assess for a thrill, and distal pulses are examined.

UPPER ARM CEPHALIC FISTULAS: Options include the standard brachiocephalic AV fistula or a proximal radial artery fistula. Although less common than brachiocephalic AV fistulas, strong consideration should be given to proximal radial artery fistulas over brachiocephalic fistulas to reduce the risk of steal, which is highest with brachiocephalic fistulas. Intraoperative ultrasound determines the feasibility of the proximal radial artery fistula by showing a good-sized perforator vein or proximal forearm median antebrachial vein, because the median cephalic vein frequently will not reach distally to the proximal radial artery for a tension-free anastomosis (FIGURE 18-2).

For the proximal radial artery fistula, either a transverse, or more commonly a longitudinal incision is made and carried down to the target vein, either perforator or proximal median antebrachial vein. The perforator vein frequently has many tributaries at the level of the radial artery that require careful dissection and ligation. The upper forearm median antebrachial vein is more straightforward with few branches. The target vein is dissected free and divided distally and then the fascia is opened to expose the proximal radial artery. Gentle clamps are then applied proximally and distally to the artery, generally without systemic heparin and a 4- to 5-mm arteriotomy created, and an end-to-side tension-free anastomosis done in similar fashion to radiocephalic fistulas with continuous 6-0 polypropylene suture. After clamps are released and patency confirmed, it is important to ligate the perforator branch to the deep system (if not used for the anastomosis) and the cubital branch to the basilic system in order to direct flow up into the cephalic system (FIGURE 18-3). **CONTINUES** ▶

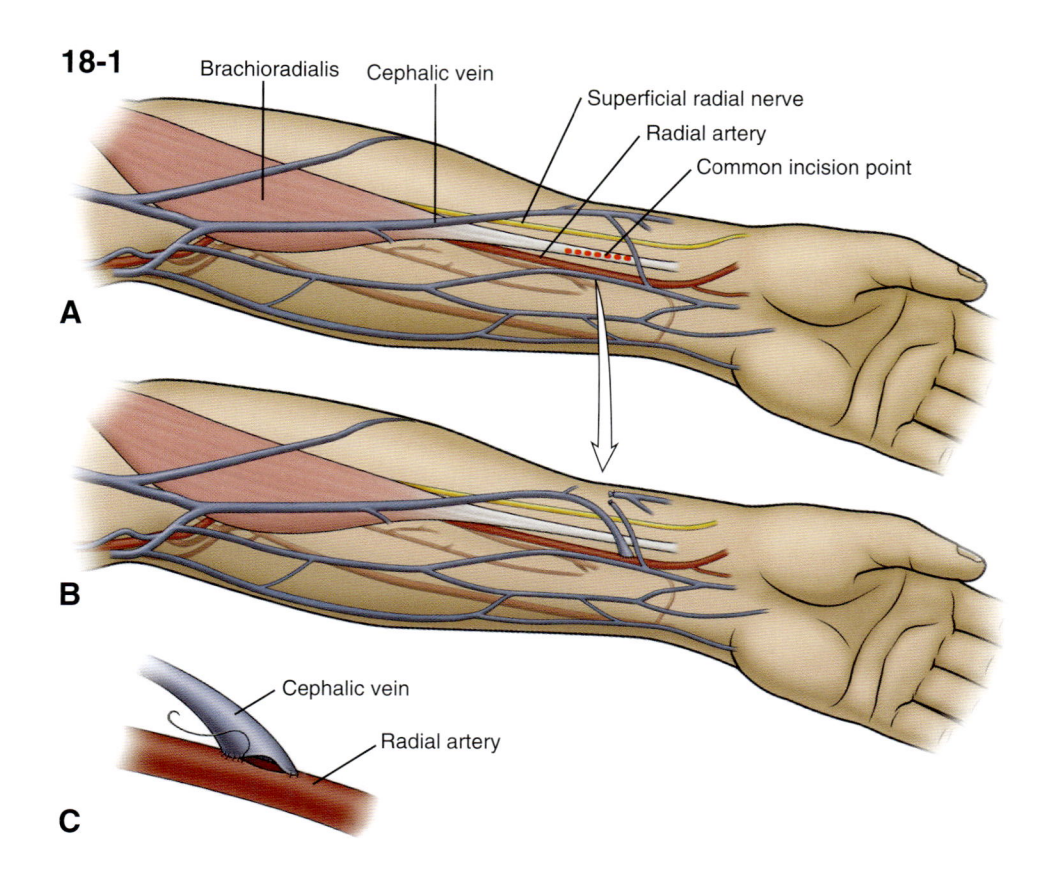

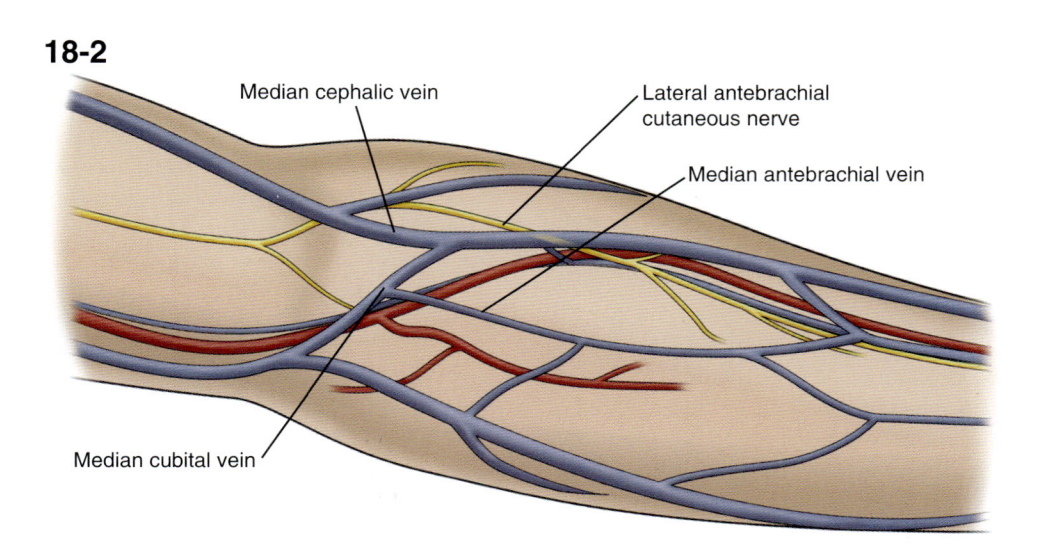

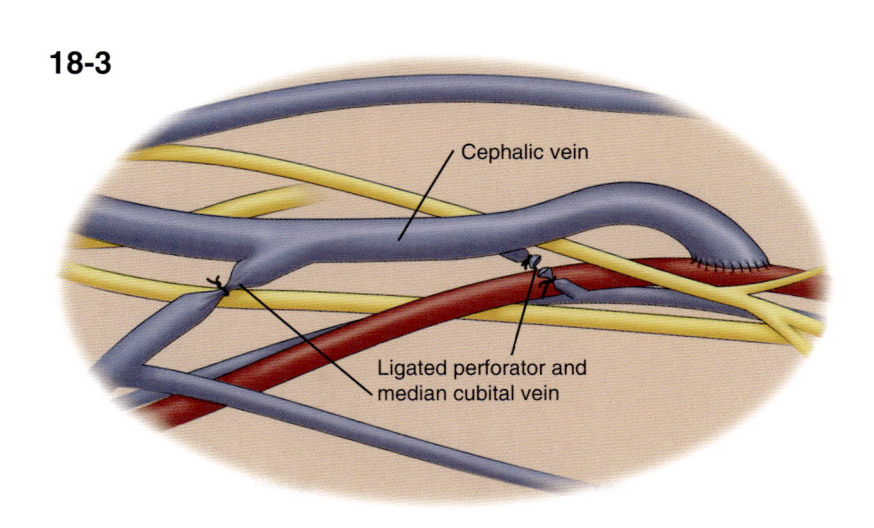

SURGICAL PROCEDURE *UPPER ARM CEPHALIC FISTULAS:* CONTINUED For brachiocephalic fistula creation, the cephalic vein is assessed from the antecubital region up the arm (**FIGURE 18-4A**). It is important to assess the quality of these veins, as they frequently can have previous damage from venous punctures, particularly just at or within the first 2 cm of the antecubital crease. A transverse incision is placed just distal to the elbow crease, approximately 4 to 5 cm in length, although occasionally oblique incisions over the vein are helpful to expose adequate length of vein in cases where the distal vein is sclerotic. Dissection is carried down to the cephalic vein and tributaries are ligated, taking care not to injure the nearby lateral antebrachial cutaneous nerve. Once enough length of vein is dissected free, the vein can be marked to help with orientation. Next, the distal end is ligated and transected.

The brachial artery is then dissected free by dividing the overlying bicipital fascia and mobilizing it from the accompanying veins. The median nerve below the elbow is usually safely tucked away under the pronator muscle group. Proximal and distal control with gentle clamps is obtained and an arteriotomy created with a #11 blade and Potts scissors, generally without systemic heparin. The brachial artery requires gentle tissue handling to avoid injury and separation of vessel wall components during dissection and clamping. The arteriotomy should be kept small to prevent future high flow or steal, commonly around 4 to 5 mm. Stay sutures can be placed to expose the lumen, and an end-to-side anastomosis is created using 6-0 polypropylene suture (**FIGURE 18-4A**). Occasionally, because of sclerotic changes in the vein due to scar tissue from venipunctures, IVs, and so on, the cephalic vein above the elbow will need to be harvested. Attentive intraoperative mapping shows what part of the vein to utilize— commonly the area of tributary confluence 2 to 3 cm above the antecubital crease. This approach also mandates that the brachial artery exposure is higher, frequently just medial to the biceps muscle. The anastomosis in this area is constructed in similar fashion (**FIGURE 18-4B**). After the anastomosis is complete, the vein is assessed for a thrill, and distal pulses are assessed as well.

Important in radiocephalic and upper arm cephalic fistulas is avoidance of nerve injury. The forearm cephalic vein is intimately associated with branches of the superficial radial nerve, and the median cephalic vein is adjacent to the lateral antebrachial nerve. Both nerves have small tributaries that drain into their respected cephalic veins, and injury to those can lead to irritating bleeding. Electrocautery near these nerves should be minimized or avoided, as damage to those nerves can lead to troublesome pain and paresthesias that be quite bothersome to patients.

CLOSURE Prior to wound closure, meticulous hemostasis must be obtained. If heparin has been used, protamine is administered. The anastomosis must be inspected, and if needed additional sutures can be placed or topical hemostatic agents can be used. The wound is closed in layers, commonly with absorbable subcuticular suture for the skin.

POSTOPERATIVE CARE Patients should be given instructions on monitoring for postoperative complications, most importantly to watch for steal symptoms and to report those to the surgeon immediately. We routinely give patients written instructions, a diagram of the procedure, and a follow-up visit appointment prior to discharge. If the fistula is not maturing adequately by 1 month, a duplex is performed and remedial procedures scheduled as needed at that visit. Most commonly, non-maturation at that time point is due to stenosis in the juxta-anastomotic region, and fistulography with angioplasty will frequently suffice to promote maturation. Further delay and observation without intervention rarely leads to spontaneous fistula improvement and maturation.

Ultimately, the goal is to create a fistula that is easy to access with sufficient flow to provide good hemodialysis. In particular in our practice, we find that many fistulas develop but are too deep to access easily. Deep fistulas lead to poor punctures, fistula injury, perhaps aneurysms or loss of the fistula, and dissatisfied patients and dialysis centers. Careful assessment therefore needs to be made of the usability of the fistulas. The KDOQI guidelines of maturation remain relevant with the rule of 6's. The vein should be 6 mm in size, 6 mm or less in depth, and flowing at 600 cc/min. Quick bedside assessment should be able to determine maturation and suitability for accessing. If there is any question, formal duplex study or bedside ultrasound can help the assessment. If the vein is deeper than it is big, consider an elevation procedure. Two elevation procedures—surgical lipectomy or superficialization—are good options, with references listed in the suggested readings. Catheter removal is typically delayed until the AV fistula has been accessed successfully using two needles for 2 weeks consecutively. Clinical surveillance for complications should be available through the dialysis center, and the patient can see the surgical team again as needed. Steal is an uncommon but potentially serious complication. Although beyond the scope of this chapter, we suggest consideration of treatments beyond ligation or distal revascularization with interval ligation, such as proximalization or distalization, as described by some of the suggested readings. ■

SUGGESTED READINGS

Bourquelot P, Tawakol JB, Gaudric J, et al. Lipectomy as a new approach to secondary procedure superficialization of direct autogenous forearm radial-cephalic arteriovenous accesses for hemodialysis. *J Vasc Surg.* 2009 Aug;50(2):369-374, 374.e1.

Inkollu S, Wellen J, Beller Z, et al. Successful use of minimal incision superficialization technique for arteriovenous fistula maturation. *J Vasc Surg.* 2016 Apr;63(4):1018-1025.

Jennings WC, Mallios A, Mushtaq N. Proximal radial artery arteriovenous fistula for hemodialysis vascular access. *J Vasc Surg.* 2018 Jan;67(1):244-253.

Loh TM, Bennett ME, Peden EK. Revision using distal inflow is a safe and effective treatment for ischemic steal syndrome and pathologic high flow after access creation. *J Vasc Surg.* 2016 Feb;63(2):441-444.

Thermann F, Wollert U, Ukkat J, et al. Proximalization of the arterial inflow (PAI) in patients with dialysis access-induced ischemic syndrome: first report on long-term clinical results. *J Vasc Surg.* Apr-Jun 2010;11(2):143-149.

Vein mapping video: https://www.youtube.com/watch?v=EjXcrvJTmYw

18-4

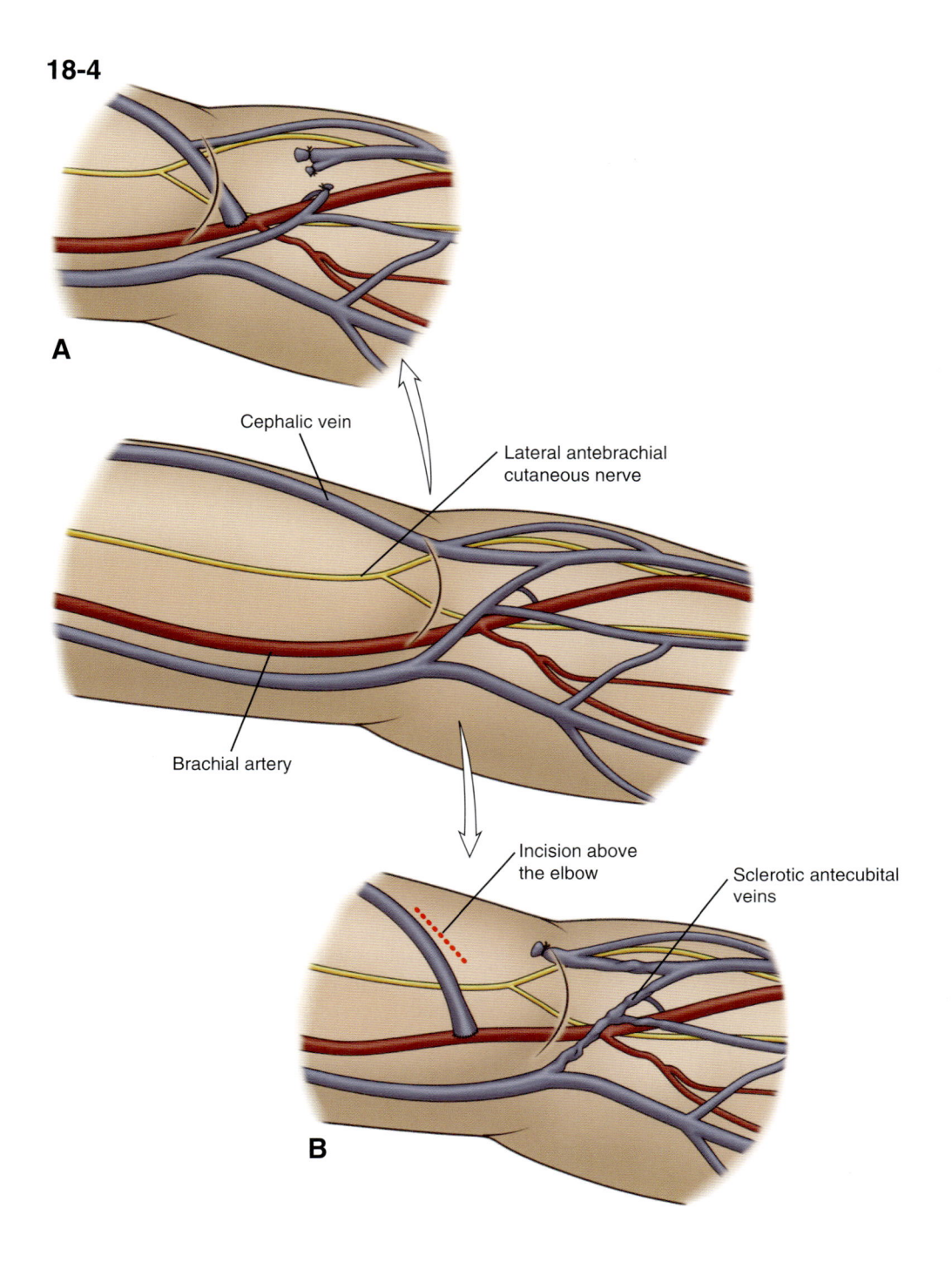

A

Cephalic vein

Lateral antebrachial
cutaneous nerve

Brachial artery

Incision above
the elbow

Sclerotic antecubital
veins

B

BASILIC VEIN TRANSPOSITION

Joseph Hart, MD • Nathan W. Kugler, MD

INDICATION Basilic vein transposition (BVTx) is primarily indicated in those who have no available cephalic vein or in whom this would be inadequate for dialysis access creation. A basilic vein transposition is in line with the goal of "fistula first." Increasingly, basilic vein transposition is accomplished in a staged procedure; the first is a fistula creation only, and the second moves the vein to a usable position after one, it has had a chance to increase in diameter and wall thickness and two, it has proven to remain initially patent. A forearm BVTx is a possible alternative, but is beyond the scope of this chapter.

PREOPERATIVE PREPARATION Avoid vascular access in the intended arm and especially within the basilic vein itself. Many surgeons find formal preoperative vein mapping and marking including the artery as helpful. Certainly at least handheld bedside ultrasound in clinic or on the operating room table will be useful. It is useful to know that there is a solitary brachial artery and that no high radial takeoff is present. Variants of basilic vein anatomy exist. Early termination to the deep system may limit the use of the basilic vein in this setting or relegate it to being part of a combined basilic and brachial outflow; however, this would be a considered a more complex and later stage venous conduit in most algorithms. Optimization of volume, serum glucose, and preoperative electrolytes, especially potassium, is critical in operations on patients with existing or impending renal failure and its attendant comorbidities.

ANESTHESIA Local regional anesthesia with IV sedation is a de facto standard of care in most access surgery. It facilitates outpatient care in most if not all cases. It should be utilized for the vast majority of patients. The first stage of a two-stage facility insurance position should be able to be accomplished under local or regional anesthesia in the vast majority of cases. The second transposition stage, particularly in an obese arm or with other complicating factors, may in some cases be best accomplished under a higher level of anesthesia, such as general. However, with a very skilled regional block and supplemental use of local, the transposition phase of the operation can avoid a full general anesthetic in many cases where patient and operative factors will tolerate this.

POSITION AND OPERATIVE PREPARATION The patient is positioned on the operating table. The upper arm is positioned on an arm table with abduction to approximately 90 degrees, if the shoulder joint will tolerate this. The hand is supinated with the thumb-oriented cephalad in the operator position. This author prefers to prep and drape the arm in its entirety up through the axilla, shoulder, and anterior chest in order to create a boundary of prepared skin beyond a relatively high axillary incision. The primary operator will usually prefer to sit inferior to the arm between the arm and the lower torso. This may vary based on the side of the patient undergoing BVTx, handedness of the surgeon, patient body habitus, and presence/level of training of an operative assistant.

INCISION AND EXPOSURE A transposition is defined as two incisions and a tunnel. If there is a dominant median antecubital tributary that is of the same caliber as the majority of the lower portion of the upper arm basilic vein, this may be useful for the initial anastomosis of a staged series of procedures. In this case it is critical to locate any deep perforator branch at the time of the initial operation. Any small tributary branch should be marked, with a plan to be taken at the initial operation (FIGURE 19-1).

In a single-stage BVTx transposition, the entire basilic vein is exposed and tunneled at the initial operation; in this chapter we will discuss the staged BVTx.

OPERATION At the initial operation, the incision needs to include the target inflow brachial artery and distal basilic vein. The arterial anastomosis

can be optimized by slight angulation of the arteriotomy with the most cephalad or superior portion oriented slightly in the direction of the vein. The apex of the arteriotomy then aligns well with the heel of the spatula to drain for anastomosis; 6-o proline is utilized.

Most surgeons now prefer a staged approach to this procedure. There may be occasional cases with an ideal vein, thin arm, and motivated patient to avoid a second procedure, where single-stage is still appropriate. However, such circumstances are increasingly uncommon. The staged procedure consists of performing an initial anastomosis first, and one month later performing the transposition which may offer some advantages. A tunnel is avoided if for some reason this fistula is destined to not mature, but this is uncommon. The vein is allowed to enlarge and begin to undergo all thickening prior to the more extensive surgery in the two-stage approach. Also, if there is failure to mature, transposition can be avoided and a new access plan developed. Multiple skip incisions maybe useful in some cases (FIGURE 19-2). Ideally, the vein will achieve an 8-mm diameter prior to transposition, though these criteria may vary based on numerous factors and surgeon experience.

Tunneling of the basilic vein is a critical step. A vascular tunneler should be utilized. The goal of tunneling should be for the vein to overlie the apex of the bicep throughout as much of its course as possible and be relatively straight in alignment with the axis of the extremity (FIGURE 19-3). Most operators prefer a venovenous anastomosis at the second operation for a staged transposition, avoiding the need to re-expose the brachial itself. Again, care must be taken not to "pursestring" this anastomosis.

This author prefers a venovenous anastomosis (FIGURE 19-4A) with exposure only of the vein rather than re-exposure of the artery. If necessary due to length considerations, re-anastomosis to the brachial artery more proximally as an alternative. In such a case, the initial anastomosis is managed by formal running proline ligation of a very short segment of vein to serve functionally as a patch at that additional arteriotomy, with a new arteriotomy being created more proximally (FIGURE 19-4B).

Whether being performed in a single or double stage, the most cephalad or central portion of the vein mobilization is critical. There is an encompassing fascia in this location which should be, at a minimum, incised, if not partially removed. Care to avoid excess tension or torsion is critical. This location is a frequent source of venous outflow stenosis which may be quite troublesome in eventual management of an otherwise successful BVTx. Depth of tunneling must be sufficient to provide protective skin without threatening the dermis.

POSTOPERATIVE CARE Careful and meticulous management of skin incisions, especially the one overlying the arterial anastomosis, is critical. Especially on a larger arm, the incision or incisions to expose the basilic vein will generate more pain than typical of other access procedures. Patients may require some additional oral analgesia. It is not infrequent that this more extensive exposure leads to the need to admit the patient, though most guidelines aim to avoid this. Some find an arm sling useful. Any breakdown, dehiscence, or infection should be reviewed by a dialysis access surgeon at its earliest occurrence.

COMPLICATIONS Complications include bleeding, infection, return to the operating room, nerve damage, steal, ischemic monomelic neuropathy, thrombosis, poor maturation, and inability to access, despite a patent fistula and other systemic complications. The large and relatively deep bed of the basilic vein leaves the basilic vein incision or skip incisions more prone to seroma formation than many access procedures.

RE-INTERVENTION Venous outflow obstruction in a basilic vein transposition is often at the so-called "swing portion," or where the vein moves to connect with the deep system. As mentioned above, avoiding torsion, undue tension, and local removal of any fascia may help avoid this complication. ■

19-1

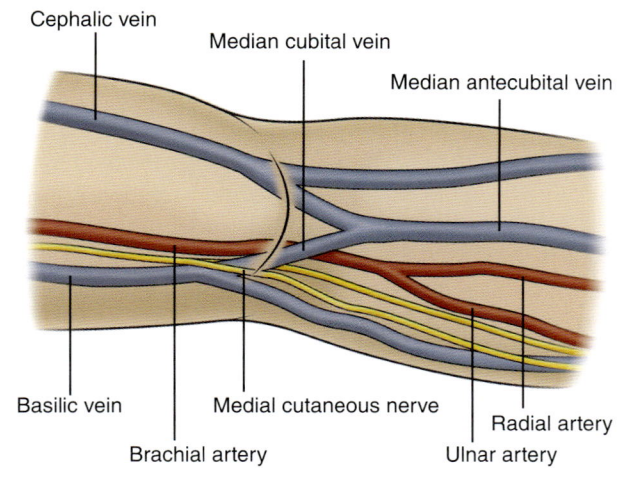

Cephalic vein
Median cubital vein
Median antecubital vein
Basilic vein
Medial cutaneous nerve
Radial artery
Brachial artery
Ulnar artery

19-2

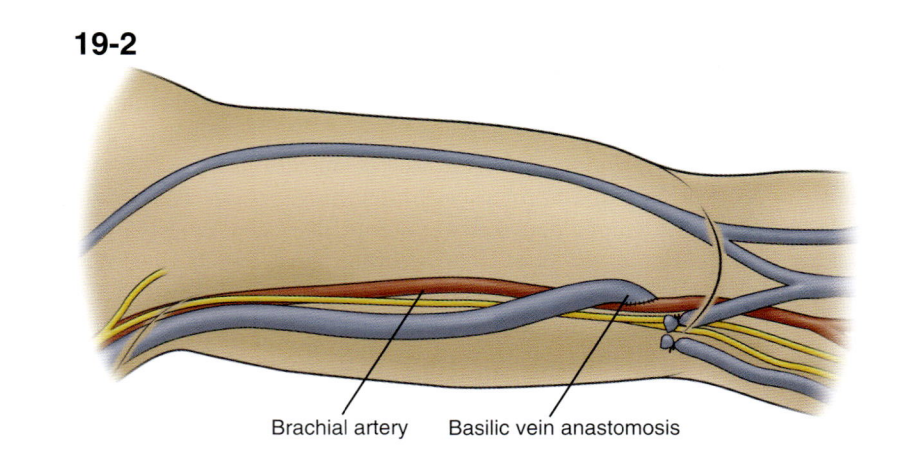

Brachial artery   Basilic vein anastomosis

19-3

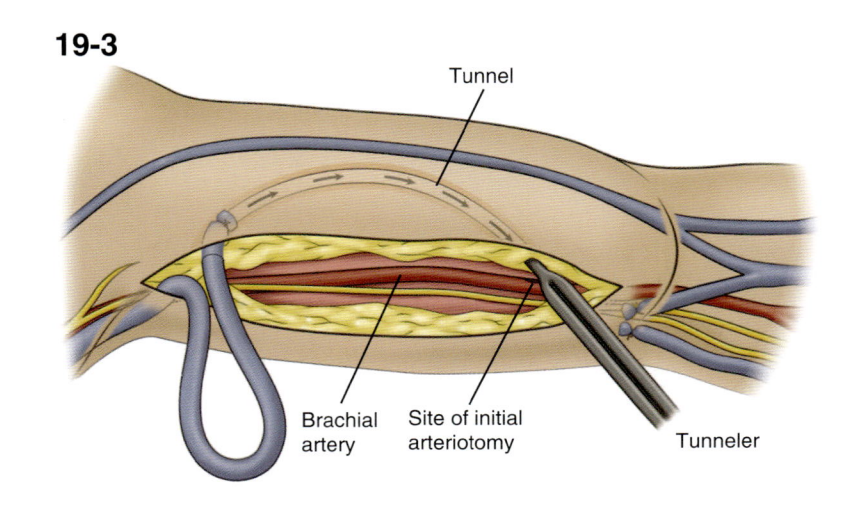

Tunnel
Brachial artery
Site of initial arteriotomy
Tunneler

19-4

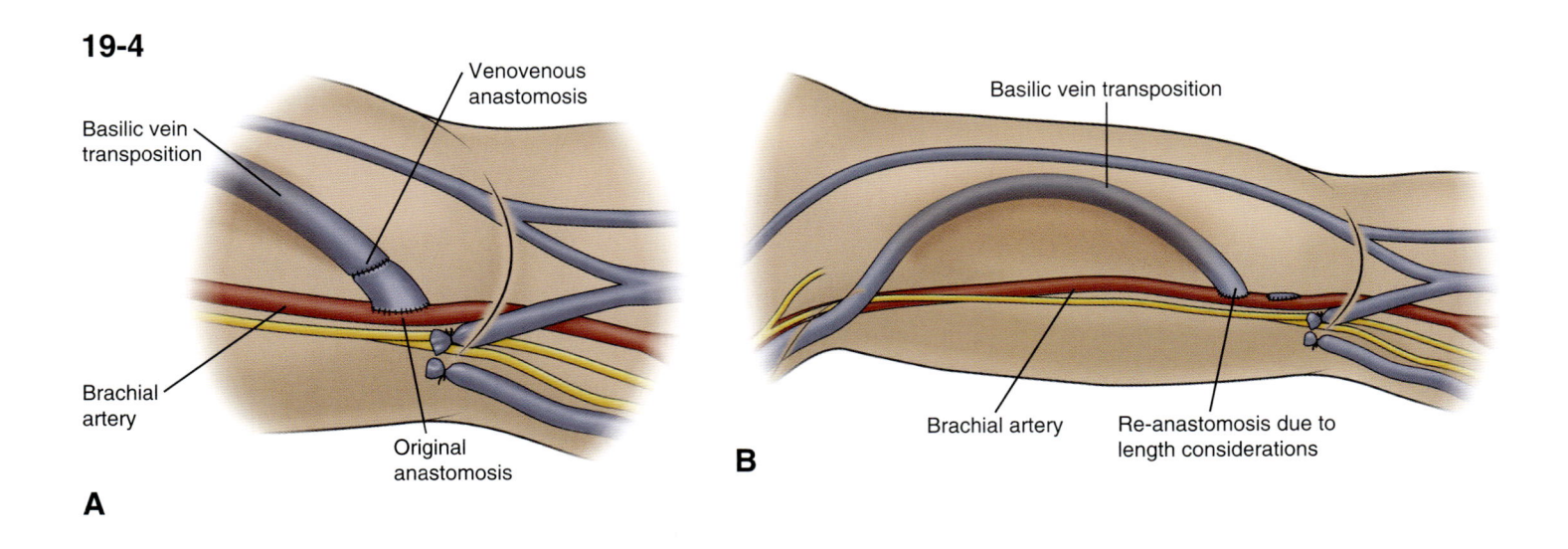

Venovenous anastomosis
Basilic vein transposition
Brachial artery
Original anastomosis

A

Basilic vein transposition
Brachial artery
Re-anastomosis due to length considerations

B

THIGH FISTULA USING FEMORAL POPLITEAL DEEP VEIN

Julie M. Duke, MD • **R. James Valentine, MD**

INDICATIONS The prevalence of end-stage kidney disease continues to increase worldwide. With an aging dialysis population, vascular surgeons face increasing challenges with vascular access options. In patients who have exhausted all options of upper extremity access or who develop severe central venous stenosis, lower extremity dialysis access represents a viable option. Lower extremity dialysis access using greater saphenous vein or prosthetic grafts have been shown to have low patency rates and high complication rates. In this chapter we present another option: thigh fistula using femoral popliteal deep vein transposition.

PREOPERATIVE PREPARATION Adequate preoperative evaluation of both the arterial and venous systems of the lower extremities is crucial prior to this procedure. A venous duplex must be obtained to evaluate for evidence of acute or chronic thrombus, wall thickening, or vein duplication. The diameter of the femoral popliteal vein should be greater than 4 to 5 mm in size. Ipsilateral iliac vein stenosis or occlusion must also be ruled out. For arterial evaluation, ankle-brachial indices (ABIs) are adequate. While controversial, most experts recommend a threshold ABI >0.85 to reduce the risk of developing steal with the operation. Evidence of severe calcific occlusive disease usually represents a contraindication to this procedure. It is important to note that femoral popliteal vein transposition for thigh dialysis access is a more complex operation with longer operative times and larger incisions; therefore, it is important that the patient be medically fit for general anesthesia. Standard deep venous thrombus (DVT) prophylaxis and prophylactic antibiotics are recommended.

ANESTHESIA Most commonly, this procedure is performed under general anesthesia due to the extent of dissection required. If a patient is particularly high risk, this could be done with a spinal block if necessary.

POSITIONING The patient should be positioned supine with the entire lower extremity circumferentially prepped. The leg should be placed in a frog leg position to assist with dissection and visualization.

INCISION AND EXPOSURE The gateway to this procedure is the sartorius muscle. A longitudinal incision is made along the course of the sartorius muscle in a lateral-to-medial direction from the level of the groin to the knee (FIGURE 20-1). The fascia lata is incised to expose the sartorius muscle. The sartorius muscle should be retracted laterally at the level of the groin and medially in the remainder of the thigh to expose the femoral popliteal vein.

DETAILS OF PROCEDURE The adductor canal is exposed by mobilizing the sartorius muscle along its lateral border and rotating it medially. It is important to limit dissection on the medial border of the sartorius muscle to avoid damaging the blood supply to the muscle. The fascia overlying the adductor canal is incised, providing access to the femoral popliteal vein lying medial and deep to the superficial femoral artery (SFA).

The vein is dissected circumferentially along its length from the level of the knee to its confluence with the profunda femoris vein in the groin (FIGURE 20-2; right leg shown). The vein has numerous large branches that should be double-ligated securely with silk ties or suture ligatures to avoid hemorrhage when exposed to arterial pressure. During vein dissection, it is important to protect the saphenous nerve as well as the SFA and its branches. The SFA should be dissected just proximal to the level of the adductor hiatus to prepare for the anastomosis at this level. The popliteal vein at the level of the knee should be transected and oversewn with silk suture. The mobilized femoral popliteal vein should be distended with heparinized saline to ensure that no branches need to be oversewn (FIGURE 20-2, inset). **CONTINUES ▶**

20-1

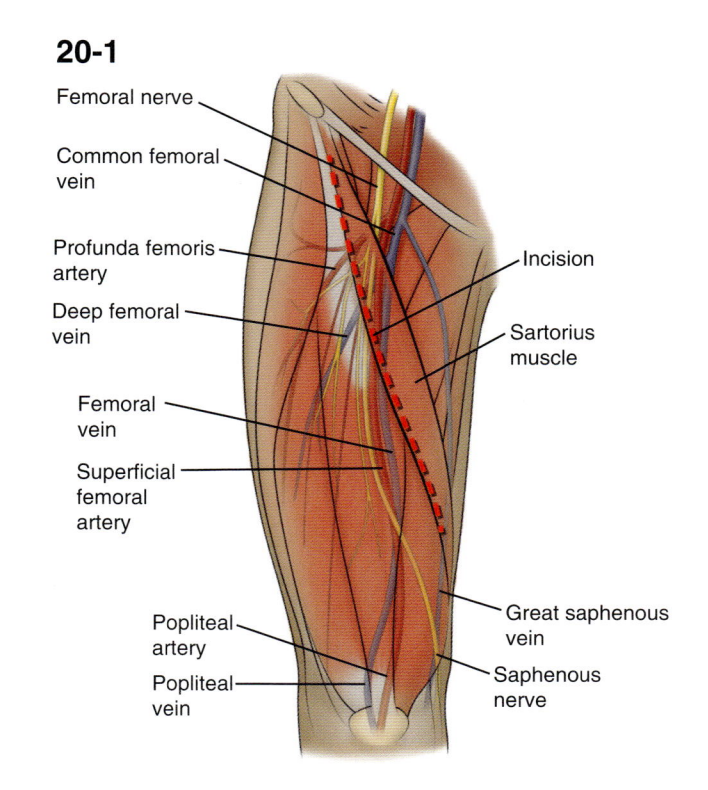

- Femoral nerve
- Common femoral vein
- Profunda femoris artery
- Deep femoral vein
- Femoral vein
- Superficial femoral artery
- Popliteal artery
- Popliteal vein
- Incision
- Sartorius muscle
- Great saphenous vein
- Saphenous nerve

20-2

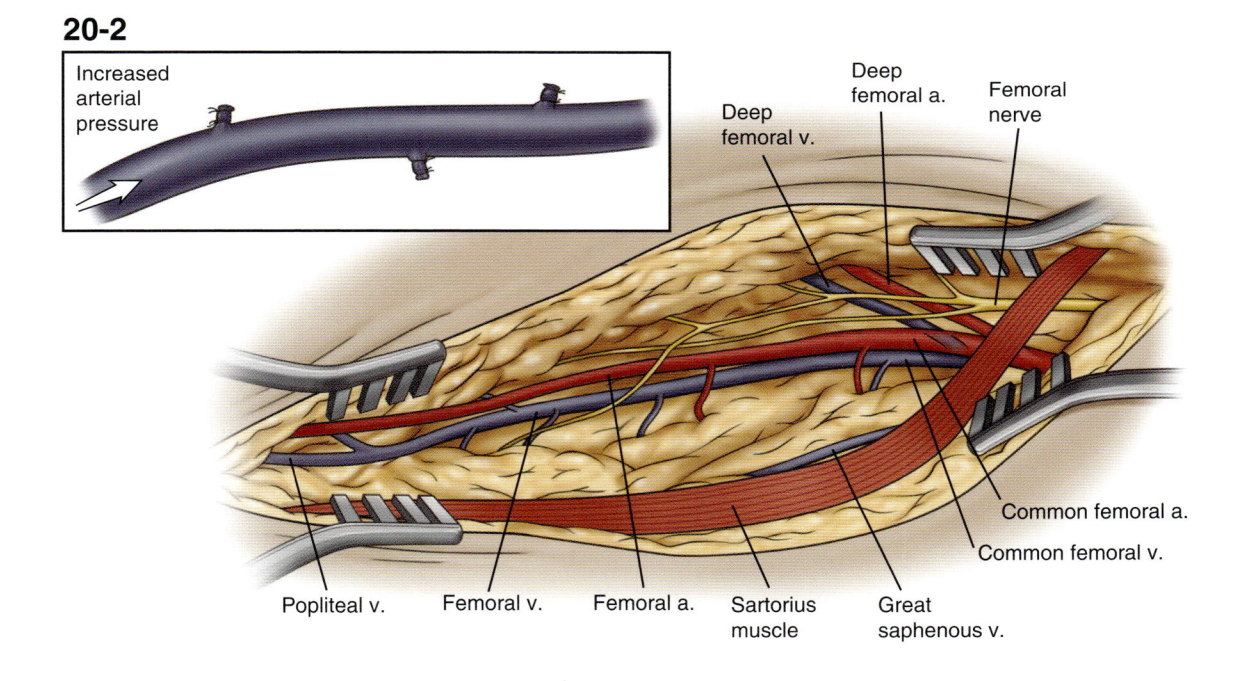

Increased arterial pressure

- Deep femoral v.
- Deep femoral a.
- Femoral nerve
- Common femoral a.
- Common femoral v.
- Popliteal v.
- Femoral v.
- Femoral a.
- Sartorius muscle
- Great saphenous v.

DETAILS OF PROCEDURE `CONTINUED` The subcutaneous tunnel is made in the lateral thigh using two counter incisions. A proximal counter incision should be made 3 to 4 cm lateral to the main incision in the proximal thigh. The vein is then passed beneath the proximal SFA and tunneled over the sartorius muscle to the first counter incision (FIGURE 20-3). A second counter incision is made approximately 15 to 20 cm distal. A superficial tunnel is created between these two incisions (FIGURE 20-4). The vein is then tunneled deep and medial toward the exposed SFA. When tunneling into the adductor canal, liberal incisions should be made in the fascia to avoid compression.

Prior to clamping the artery, the patient should be systemically heparinized. The previously exposed SFA is clamped and an arteriotomy is made on the anterolateral wall of the artery. It remains controversial whether the vein should be tapered prior to the anastomosis to avoid steal syndrome. It is our practice to taper larger veins to a diameter that matches the artery (approximately 4–5 mm) (FIGURE 20-5). An end-to-side anastomosis is performed between the femoral popliteal vein and the distal SFA (FIGURE 20-6). Prior to completion, the artery and vein should be flushed. The clamps are then removed. After the flow is restored, pulses in the foot should be evaluated. If there is concern for steal, the vein can be banded. If there is concern for compartment syndrome, fasciotomies should be performed. `CONTINUES`

20-3

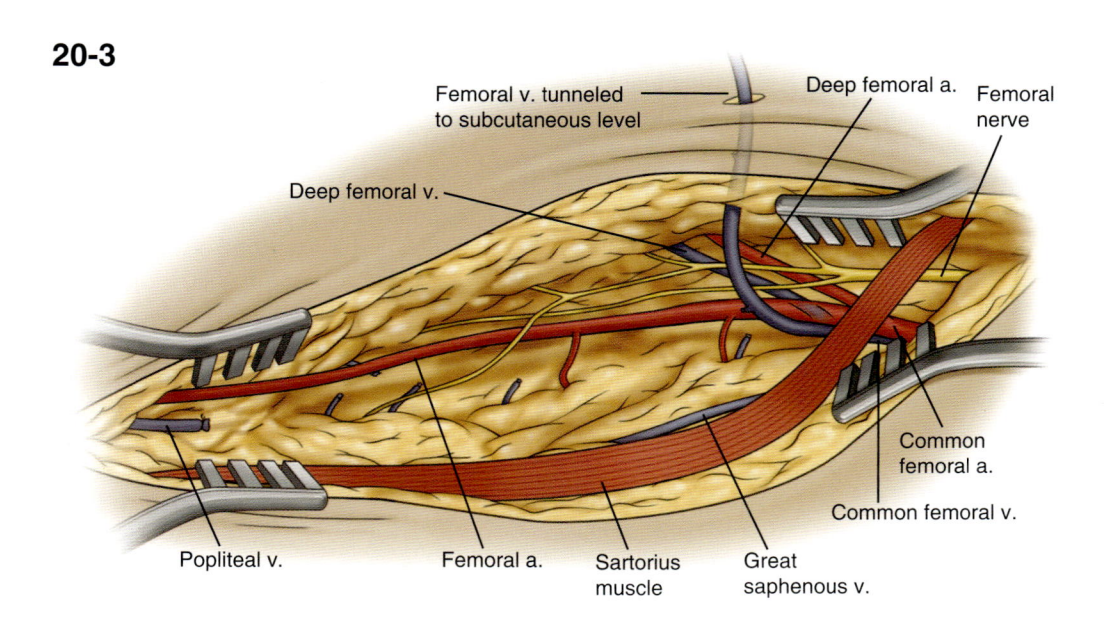

Femoral v. tunneled to subcutaneous level

Deep femoral a.

Femoral nerve

Deep femoral v.

Common femoral a.

Common femoral v.

Popliteal v.

Femoral a.

Sartorius muscle

Great saphenous v.

20-4

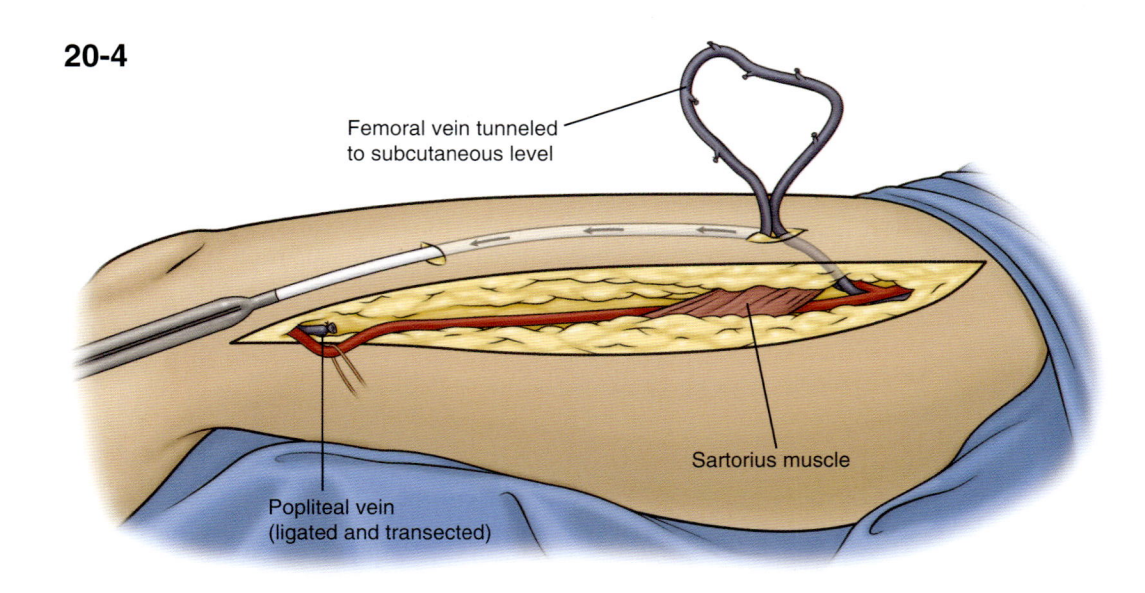

Femoral vein tunneled to subcutaneous level

Sartorius muscle

Popliteal vein (ligated and transected)

20-5

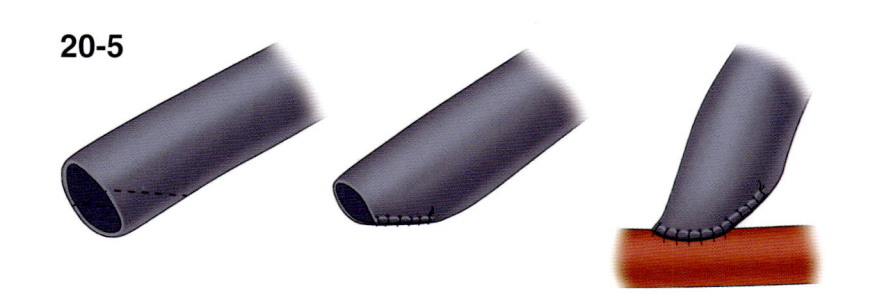

20-6

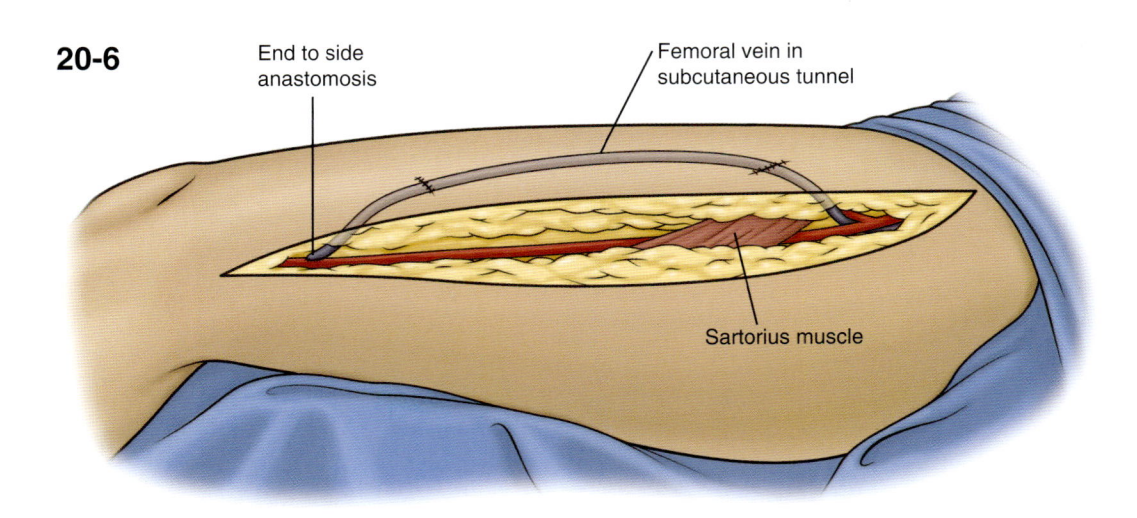

End to side anastomosis

Femoral vein in subcutaneous tunnel

Sartorius muscle

CLOSURE The deep wound should be closed over drains to limit postoperative fluid collections. Two large Jackson-Pratt (JP) drains should be placed within the bed of the vein harvest through distal thigh exit sites. The deep fascia is closed with running vicryl suture. The soft tissue is closed in multiple layers using running vicryl suture. The skin is closed with interrupted nylon sutures or staples that can be left for long periods if necessary (FIGURE 20-7).

POSTOPERATIVE CARE All patients should be admitted to the hospital postoperatively. The patient's leg should be elevated and wrapped with an elastic bandage for compression. DVT prophylaxis should be continued throughout the hospital stay. It is quite common for the drains to have high output, but they should remain in place until the output is less than 30 cc/day.

It is important to monitor the patient for known complications, including steal and compartment syndromes. There is a reported risk of wound complications in up to 30% of patients. To reduce this risk, the incision should be kept dry and drains left in place until there is low output, as noted above.

All patients should be seen at 2 weeks postoperatively for a wound check, and at 6 and 12 weeks to assess for maturation using duplex ultrasound. ∎

SUGGESTED READINGS

Etra JW, Hicks CW, Cooper MA, et al. Feasibility and outcomes of femoral vein harvest for dialysis access and arterial reconstruction. *J Surg Res.* 2019 May;237:50-55. doi: 10.1016/j.jss.2018.11.036. Epub 2019 Jan 24. PMID: 30694791.

Farber A, Cheng TW, Nimmich A, et al. Femoral vein transposition is a durable hemodialysis access for patients who have exhausted upper extremity options. *J Vasc Surg.* 2020 Mar;71(3):929-936. doi: 10.1016/j.jvs.2019.07.062. Epub 2019 Sep 3. PMID: 31492614.

Gradman WS, Cohen W, Haji-Aghaii M. Arteriovenous fistula construction in the thigh with transposed superficial femoral vein: our initial experience. *J Vasc Surg.* 2001 May;33(5):968-975. doi: 10.1067/mva.2001.115000. PMID: 11331836.

Gradman WS, Laub J, Cohen W. Femoral vein transposition for arteriovenous hemodialysis access: improved patient selection and intraoperative measures reduce postoperative ischemia. *J Vasc Surg.* 2005 Feb;41(2):279-284. doi: 10.1016/j.jvs.2004.10.039. PMID: 15768010.

Huber TS, Ozaki CK, Flynn TC, et al. Use of superficial femoral vein for hemodialysis arteriovenous access. *J Vasc Surg.* 2000 May;31(5):1038-1041. doi: 10.1067/mva.2000.104587. PMID: 10805897.

Kim D, Bhola C, Eisenberg N, et al. Long-term results of thigh arteriovenous dialysis grafts. *J Vasc Access.* 2019 Mar;20(2):153-160. doi: 10.1177/1129729818787994. Epub 2018 Jul 25. PMID: 30045660.

Orion KC, Kim TI, Rizzo AN 2nd, et al. Long-term outcomes of transposed femoral vein arteriovenous fistula for abandoned upper extremity dialysis access. *J Vasc Surg.* 2021 Mar 2:S0741-5214(20)32614-8. doi: 10.1016/j.jvs.2020.12.065. Epub ahead of print. PMID: 33348002.

Rueda CA, Nehler MR, Kimball TA, et al. Arteriovenous fistula construction using femoral vein in the thigh and upper extremity: single-center experience. *Ann Vasc Surg.* 2008 Nov;22(6):806-814. doi: 10.1016/j.avsg.2008.08.002. Epub 2008 Sep 21. PMID: 18809277.

Söderman M, Lindholt JS, Clausen LL. The transposed femoral vein arteriovenous fistula for hemodialysis. *J Vasc Access.* 2019 Mar;20(2):169-174. doi: 10.1177/1129729818789315. Epub 2018 Aug 3. PMID: 30073914.

Valentine RJ, Wind GG. *Anatomic Exposures in Vascular Surgery.* 4th ed. Philadelphia, PA: Lippincott Williams & Wilkins; 2020.

20-7

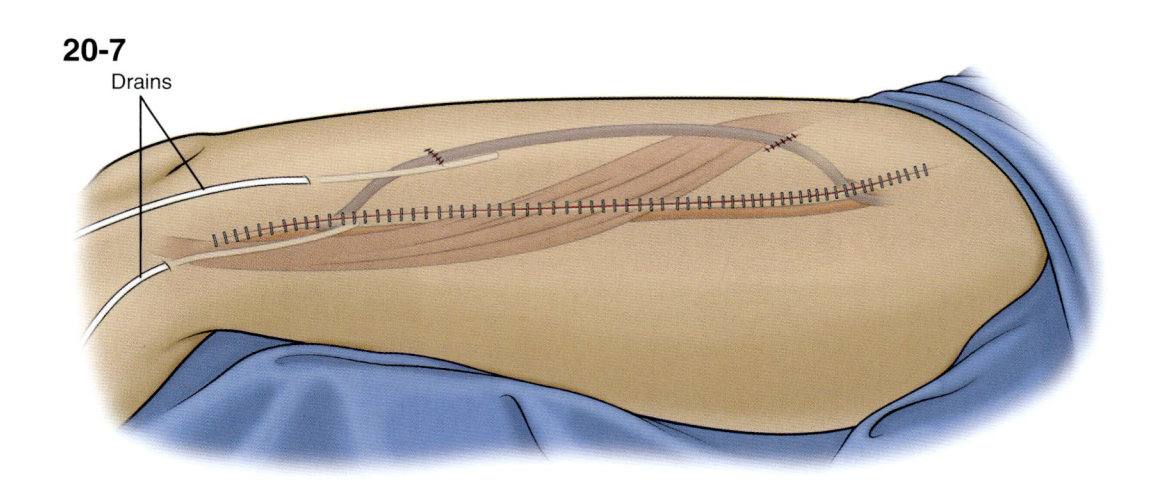

Arteriovenous Grafts for Dialysis: Arm and Forearm

Virginia L. Wong, MD

INDICATIONS An autologous arteriovenous fistula (AVF) is the preferred type of access for patients with end-stage renal disease (ESRD) on hemodialysis (HD). However, a prosthetic arteriovenous graft (AVG) should be considered for those in whom AVF cannot be constructed or established well enough to support HD. AVG may play an important role in avoiding long-term HD catheter use, which has been associated with poor outcomes, including high infection and malfunction rates as well as poor dialysis adequacy, increased hospitalization, and shorter life expectancy on dialysis.

Formal preoperative evaluation by the surgeon should include a thorough history, physical exam, and duplex ultrasound mapping of both upper limb arteries and veins. Finally, contraindications to AVG construction such as bacteremia or other active infection should be ruled out prior to implantation of prosthetic material into the vascular space. Axillary access should be avoided in patients with recurrent infection from *Hidradenitis suppurativa*. Patients at high risk for distal hypoperfusion (steal) due to established arterial insufficiency or who have had this complication previously should be considered carefully for AVG. Finally, patients with severe chronic hypotension or congestive heart failure (CHF) despite medical optimization may not be able to maintain AVG patency or may suffer CHF exacerbation due to increased venous return.

POSITION The patient is positioned supine on the operating table, with the operative limb extended onto an arm table. Ultrasound examination of the limb, performed in the operating room (OR) by the operative surgeon, is recommended. This exam will confirm availability of arterial and venous targets and may alter the operative plan if findings are not exactly as reported on formal preoperative mapping studies. The exact location of prior AVF or AVG anastomoses and venous stents can be identified and incisions planned accordingly.

OPERATIVE PREPARATION Clinical practice guidelines recommend construction of more distal access first when possible. Therefore, forearm looped AVG should be considered before arm grafts. If suitable inflow and outflow vessels cannot be not identified at the antecubital fossa, the arm is used instead. The most common arm option is a brachioaxillary AVG, so named for the origins of its arterial inflow and venous outflow, respectively. However brachio-brachial or looped axillo-axillary AVG may also be constructed, depending on local anatomic or other considerations.

Adequate anesthesia may be achieved by a variety of methods, including local, regional, and general anesthesia, each with benefits and disadvantages that depend on patient medical condition.

Once the exact procedure to be performed has been confirmed, the arm is prepped and draped circumferentially from mid-palm to above the axilla. This allows surgical access to the entire limb and the ability to freely position it in any manner during the case. Additionally, access for monitoring distal perfusion from the surgical field is preserved.

INCISION AND EXPOSURE For a forearm looped AVG, a single transverse or longitudinal incision can be made on the anterior proximal forearm, just below the antecubital crease (FIGURE 21-1A and B; right arm shown). This affords exposure of the terminal brachial artery and the proximal radial artery, both common targets for AVG inflow. For venous outflow, the median cubital, cephalic, and basilic veins, as well as the deep veins, are accessible. The superficial veins lie just beneath the skin and so must be identified from the start and protected from retraction pressure and injury, particularly if they are to be used as an outflow target. Access to the arteries

and the deep veins requires division of the bicipital aponeurosis, which can be fibrous and substantial in some patients. Silastic vessel loop control of the target artery and vein, proximal and distal to the intended anastomosis site, is achieved. Larger side branches may also require loop control, though smaller ones can be temporarily occluded at the time of anastomosis with gently deployed medium Weck clips. The median nerve courses more medially than the vessels at this level. However, more superficially, branches of the medial antebrachial cutaneous nerve may be discovered during the initial dissection and preservation will avoid annoying numbness over the medial aspect of the forearm.

For AVG construction in the arm, incisional placement depends on the planned procedure. Brachioaxillary AVG will require two separate incisions, one for each anastomosis, while an axillo-axillary looped AVG can be accomplished through a single axillary incision used to expose both arterial and venous targets. The distal brachial artery is exposed through a longitudinal skin incision on the anteromedial arm, just above the antecubital crease. The subcutaneous tissue and fascia are opened. The brachial neurovascular bundle is located deep to the medial edge of the biceps muscle, anterior to the course of the more superficial basilic vein. The median nerve is closely associated with the artery at this level and may even lie directly on top of it. More distally, the nerve begins to course medial to the artery. Great care must be taken with the use of cautery in the vicinity of major nervous structures. If necessary, full mobilization of the nerve will allow for gentle vessel loop retraction to expose the underlying artery.

Exposure of the axillary vessels is via a longitudinal incision made on the medial arm at the base of the hair-bearing area or extended up into the axilla along the anterior border of the hair-bearing area, beneath the pectoralis muscle tendon. Below the superficial fascia, the neurovascular bundle can be exposed at the upper aspect of the bicipital groove; the vein is often visible beneath its overlying fascia and is usually encountered before the artery. Superficially, branches of the intercostobrachial sensory nerve may be encountered; division is often necessary in order to gain proper exposure and results in numbness of the axillary skin. Proximally in the deep plane, the medial and lateral cords of the brachial plexus overlie the artery as they join to form the median nerve. The ulnar nerve may be seen as it courses deep to the axillary vein. The basilic vein may enter the deep venous system anywhere along its course; typically this occurs very proximally near the chest wall but sometimes may be identified more distally in the axilla or the arm.

DETAILS OF THE PROCEDURE Following exposure of the target artery and vein, a subdermal tunnel is created through which to pass the prosthetic graft material using a tunneling device (FIGURE 21-2A). Cannulation of the AVG will take place in the tunneled portion of the graft, away from surgical incisions or scar tissue. Sufficient graft length at a suitable depth should be provided to accommodate the required separation for two-needle cannulation and allow for "rope ladder" needle rotation techniques. The intended AVG cannulation zone must lie superficial enough for manual identification, however not so superficially as to risk overlying skin necrosis with repeated needling or graft exposure in the event of dermal breakdown (FIGURE 21-2B). Importantly, tunneling the juxta-anastomotic ends of the graft more deeply within the surgical incision(s), in a "deep to superficial to deep" manner allows for layered closure of subcutaneous tissue over the prosthetic material. This may help prevent graft exposure in the event of postoperative incisional breakdown (FIGURE 21-2C; left arm shown). CONTINUES ▶

21-1

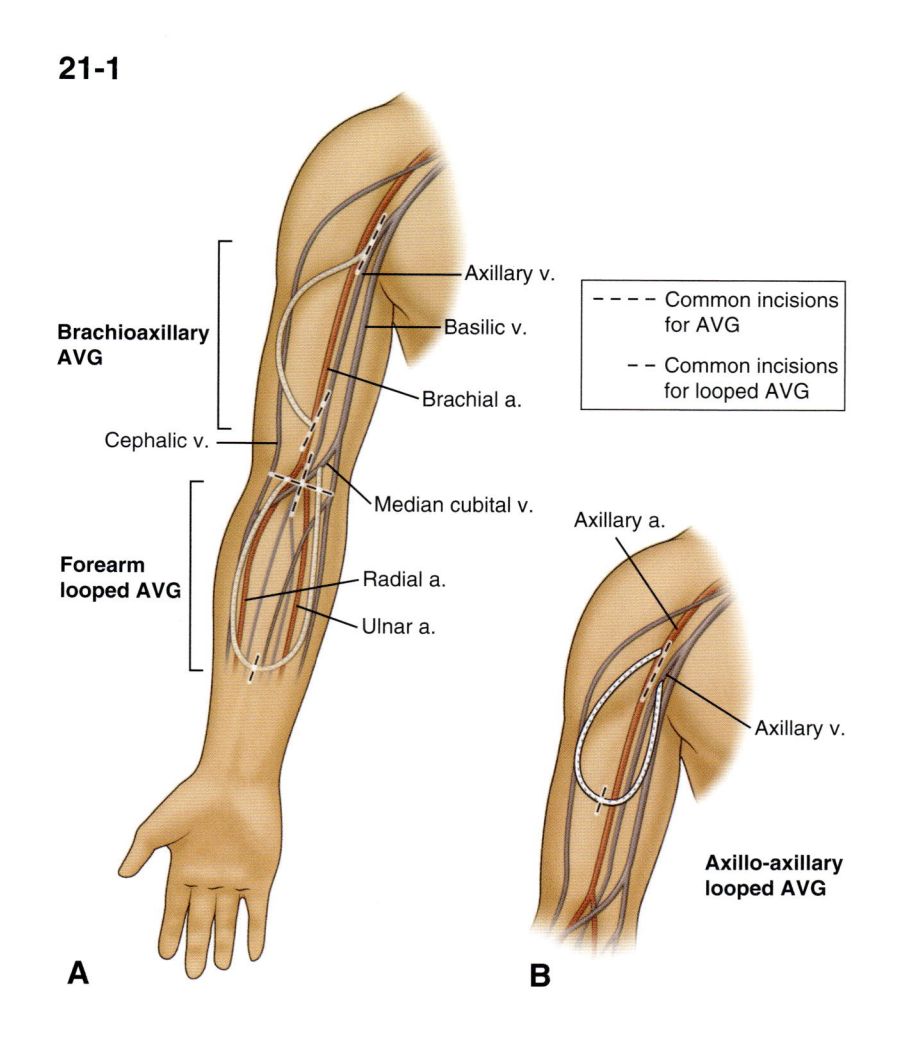

Brachioaxillary AVG

Cephalic v.

Forearm looped AVG

Axillary v.

Basilic v.

Brachial a.

Median cubital v.

Radial a.

Ulnar a.

- - - - Common incisions for AVG
- - Common incisions for looped AVG

Axillary a.

Axillary v.

Axillo-axillary looped AVG

A

B

21-2

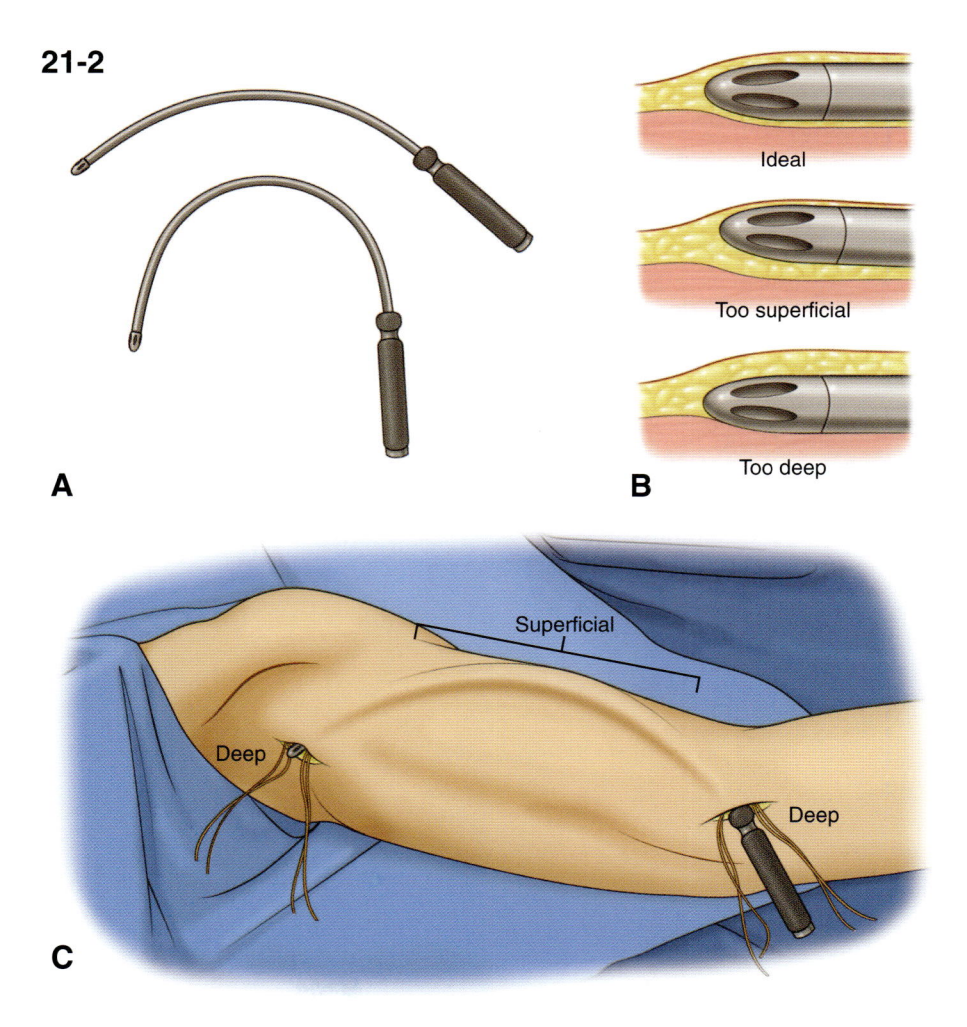

A

Ideal

Too superficial

Too deep

B

Superficial

Deep

Deep

C

DETAILS OF THE PROCEDURE CONTINUED For a brachioaxillary AVG, the prosthetic material is tunneled out laterally in a "C" (right arm), "reversed C" (left arm), or "arch" configuration. For a looped AVG, a small, perpendicular counter-incision placed just to the outside of the loop apex aids bidirectional passage of a tunneling device (FIGURE 21-3A; left arm shown). Additionally, blunt dissection into the subcutaneous plane along the inside edge of the counter-incision will keep the graft from kinking as it changes direction across the curve and prevents the graft from sitting directly beneath the counter-incision. Commonly, the venous (return) limb for a forearm looped AVG is sited laterally on the forearm. If a medial vein is used for outflow, the graft limbs may be crossed over one another proximally (FIGURE 21-3B) within the surgical incision, rather than reversing their subcutaneous positions in the forearm. Maintaining the expected cannulation configuration and following local convention will avoid misidentification or "reversal" of the limbs at dialysis. For axillo-axillary looped AVG, there is no set or common configuration. The orientation of graft limbs may be based on the lie of the inflow artery with respect to the selected outflow vein, or may be influenced by patient body habitus, tunneling to avoid old scar tissue, or other considerations, such as revision of an existing brachioaxillary AVG into an axillo-axillary AVG. Care should be taken to communicate to the patient and to the dialysis unit which limb is which prior to cannulation.

The arterial anastomosis is constructed first, if possible. This allows for pressurization of the prosthetic conduit in its tunnel and, if necessary, adjustments can still be made if the graft cannot be easily palpated in its course. Depending on which venous target is selected for a forearm AVG, and particularly if the graft limbs are to be crossed one over the other, the deeper of the two anastomoses should be constructed first so as maintain access and exposure for the second one. Silastic vessel loops are gently pulled up to occlusive tension on the target artery. A longitudinal arteriotomy is created and 20 mL of heparinized saline (100 units per mL) is flushed distally down the artery. Systemic heparinization is generally not necessary and may result in undesirable bleeding. The arterial end of the prosthetic graft material is trimmed to length and only very slightly spatulated, so as to limit the overall diameter of this anastomosis. Future percutaneous interventions can be simplified by constructing the anastomosis in a way that facilitates retrograde wire access across the anastomosis and into the inflow (proximal) artery. While not an issue for looped AVG configurations, the arterial anastomosis of a brachioaxillary AVG can be slightly retroflexed in a cephalad direction to accomplish this (FIGURE 21-4A, cephalad is left). The anastomosis is constructed in an end-to-side fashion, beginning from the center of the posterior wall and running suture around each side to finish anteriorly (FIGURE 21-4B). Given the small size of this anastomosis, using a "parachute" technique and pulling suture loops taut at the end (with the help of a nerve hook) facilitates full visualization of each bite. Following completion of the anastomosis, the graft material is occluded with a shodded clamp and the arterial vessel loops are released, restoring flow to the distal limb.

The venous anastomosis is then constructed. However, this anastomosis may be larger in diameter and the graft spatulated more severely. The longer anastomosis and narrow angle with respect to the recipient vein allows for easy end-to-side anastomosis using a more typical "heel-first" technique (FIGURE 21-4C). Following completion of the second anastomosis, all vascular occlusion is released and a low-resistance thrill should be palpable through the AVG. Distal limb perfusion should be checked by palpation of wrist pulses and/or the use of continuous-wave Doppler insonation.

CLOSURE Reversal of locally administered heparin is rarely necessary to achieve sufficient postoperative hemostasis. In some patients, particularly those who are predialysis and chronically uremic, persistent intraoperative oozing may be countered with administration of a weight-based intravenous dose of desmopressin (DDAVP) to enhance platelet activity and primary hemostasis.

After final hemostasis is achieved, the incision(s) may be irrigated and closed in standard fashion. Infiltration of additional local anesthetic may be desired. Given the medical comorbidities present in this patient population and the risk of prosthetic graft infection that may occur with incisional dehiscence or breakdown, additional care during closure will help prevent such complications. Take care not to compress the graft or entrap any identified nerve branches with closing sutures. If incisional depth allows, an additional layer of subcutaneous tissue may be closed as well. The choice of skin closure is up to the surgeon, but should aim to provide good dermal apposition and hemostasis. If the skin incision does break down postoperatively, salvage may be possible with local wound care, so long as the deeper protective tissue layer remains intact and all graft material remains covered. The same meticulous closure technique is applied to the apical counter-incision, if one was used to tunnel a looped AVG; exposure of graft material is nearly guaranteed if this incision opens up postoperatively.

POSTOPERATIVE CARE In the post-anesthesia care unit (PACU), patients should be monitored for recovery from anesthesia as well as for immediate complications from surgery. The operative site should be checked for signs of bleeding. Frequent monitoring of AVG patency, distal arterial perfusion, and neuromotor function of the ipsilateral hand is recommended throughout the recovery period. Return to the OR may be required for expanding hematoma or immediate postoperative AVG thrombosis. Profound distal limb ischemia, manifested by hand pallor and pain with absent pulse or Doppler signals, may represent steal by the AVG, but could also result from arterial injury such as dissection or thromboembolism. The immediate onset of significant postoperative ipsilateral hand/finger pain and motor weakness, usually without signs of tissue malperfusion or frank ischemia, is consistent with a diagnosis of severe ischemic monomelic neuropathy (IMN) and mandates immediate return to the OR for AVG ligation to avoid or lessen severe disability.

Most uncomplicated patients can be discharged from the PACU with instructions regarding incisional care, activity restrictions, and resumption of anticoagulant medications. Use of compression, circumferential wraps, and tight sleeves around the AVG should be discouraged. AVG cannulation may be authorized after a few weeks, so long as perigraft edema and bruising have resolved. Thereafter, regular monitoring of AVG function is recommended, with prompt referral for investigation of any concerns before AVG thrombosis occurs. ∎

SUGGESTED READINGS

Davidson I (ed). *On Call In… Vascular Access: Surgical and Radiologic Procedures*, 1st edition. Chapman & Hall; 1996.

Gage S, Lawson J. Forearm versus upper arm grafts for vascular access. *J Vasc Access*. 2017;18(Suppl 1):S77-81.

21-3

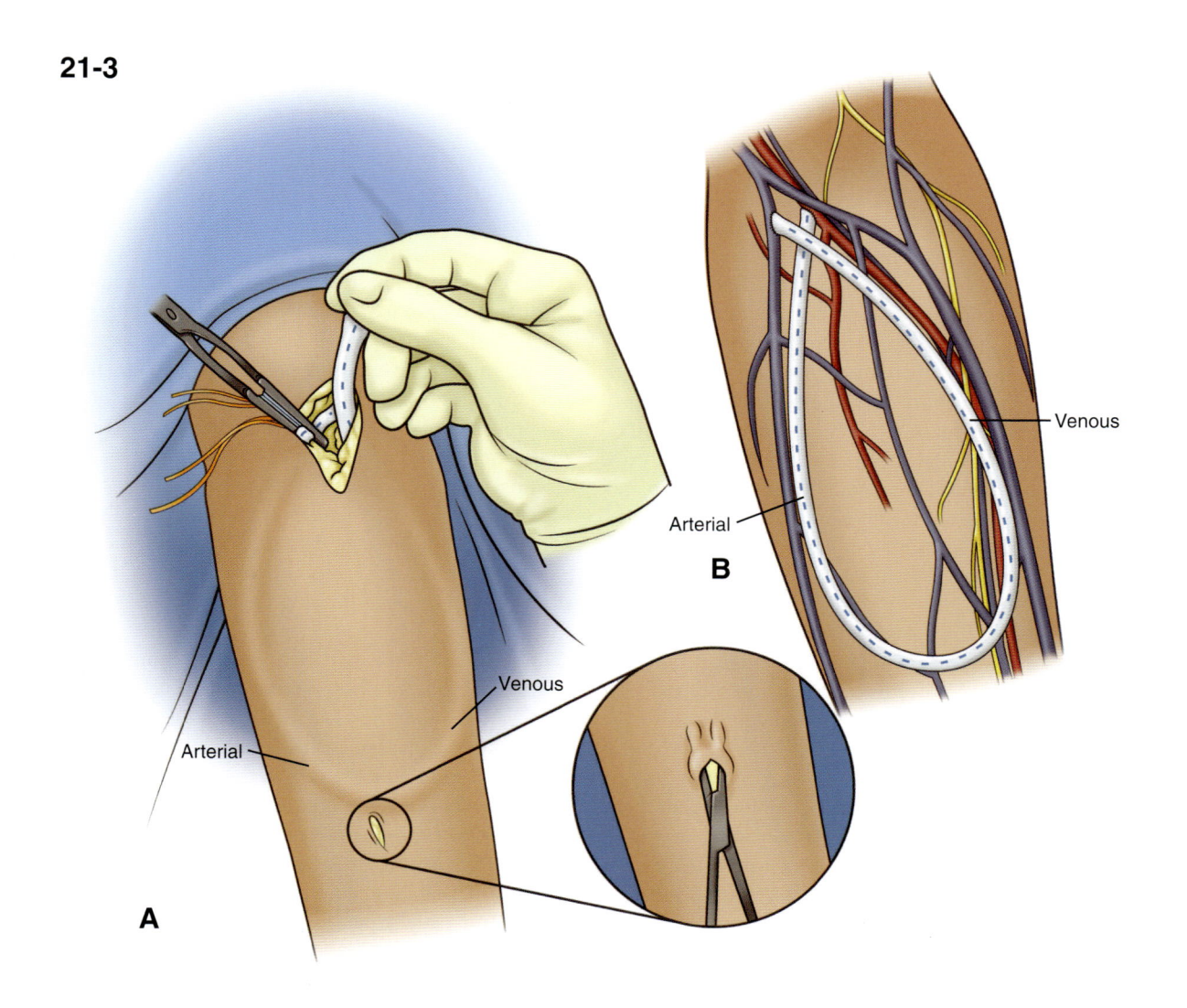

21-4

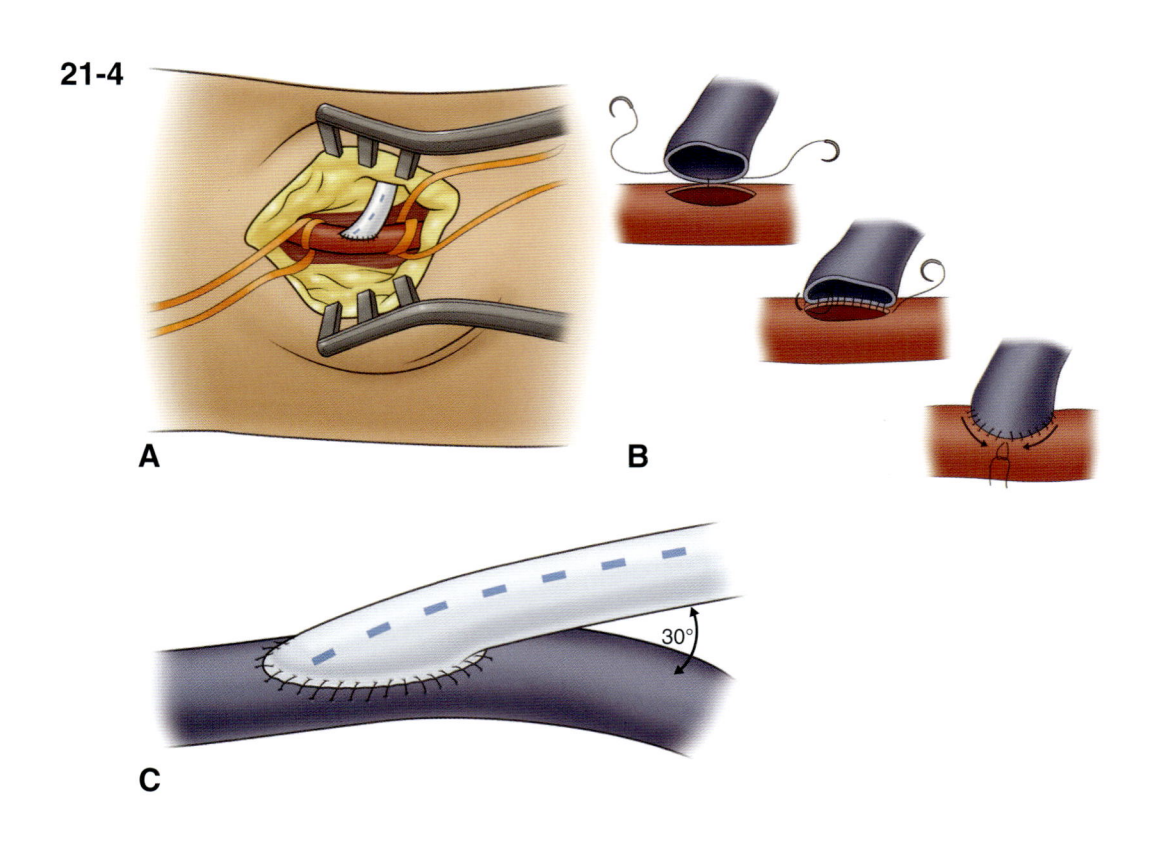

Distal Revascularization and Interval Ligation

Thomas S. Huber, MD, PhD • **Salvatore T. Scali, MD**

INDICATION The construction of an arteriovenous hemodialysis fistula (either an autogenous [AVF] or prosthetic graft [AVG] access) creates a high-flow/low resistance circuit. Indeed, the anastomosis precipitates a "pressure sink" that induces a gradual decrease in the intraluminal pressure from the axillary to the brachial artery for the typical brachial-based access located at the antecubital fossa. The perfusion distal to anastomosis, typically the forearm or hand for an upper extremity access, is reduced and can lead to clinically significant steal. Clinically evident steal syndrome can occur in approximately 20% of all brachial artery-based access procedures, with up to 10% of patients requiring some type of remedial treatment to reverse the ischemic symptoms. The natural history of steal syndrome remains poorly defined, but patients with severe sensory changes, motor changes, and/or tissue loss do not improve without intervention and are at risk for permanent deficits and/or progression of their symptoms.

The treatment goals for patients with severe steal syndrome are to reduce the symptoms, improve the patient's quality of life, and salvage the access. Distal revascularization with interval ligation (DRIL) can accomplish all of these objectives. It is essentially a brachial-brachial artery bypass with the inflow anastomosis sited as proximal on the arterial tree as possible and the distal anastomosis immediately distal to the dialysis-access anastomosis, typically at the antecubital fossa for a brachial artery-based AVF and ligation of the brachial artery between the fistula and distal anastomoses.

OPERATIVE PREPARATION It is important to recognize that the steal syndrome can develop after most access procedures, although it typically occurs after the brachial artery-based procedures at the antecubital fossa. Accordingly, to prevent steal, upper extremity arterial pressures and waveforms should be obtained prior to the index access to identify any arterial inflow or outflow stenosis. It is imperative to exclude a proximal arterial stenosis in patients that *develop* the steal syndrome prior to any remediation, such as the DRIL procedure. A high-quality catheter-based angiogram or CT arteriogram should be performed and any inflow lesion corrected. We have traditionally favored using the saphenous vein, and the target vein should be ≥3 mm and sufficient length for the brachial bypass that comprises the DRIL.

POSITION The procedure is typically performed in a hybrid operating room with a fixed imaging system given the need to interrogate the arterial inflow, although a portable imaging system with an appropriate operative bed is usually sufficient. The patient is positioned supine on the operating bed and the affected upper extremity is abducted 90 degrees and supported with an arm extension or hand table insert. A general endotracheal anesthesia is used given the magnitude of the procedure and the lower extremity vein harvest.

INCISION AND EXPOSURE The proximal brachial artery is exposed over the medial aspect of the upper arm (**FIGURE 22-1**). The artery is usually palpable and located between the groove formed by the biceps and triceps muscles. The exact location of the incision should be dictated by the location of the AVF anastomosis and the length of suitable conduit. We make every attempt to make the DRIL bypass as long as possible, with the proximal DRIL anastomosis at least 7 to 10 cm proximal to the dialysis-access anastomosis. The exposure of the proximal brachial artery requires incising the investing fascial sheath. Care should be exercised during the exposure to prevent damage to adjacent median nerve and the paired brachial veins with their communications. The brachial artery distal to the access anastomosis (**FIGURE 22-2**) is exposed with an incision that incorporates the access incision. This usually involves making a sigmoidal incision incorporating the transverse median antecubital incision. This allows exposure of the brachial artery bifurcation along with the proximal radial and ulnar arteries and requires incising the biceps aponeurosis.

DETAILS OF PROCEDURE The saphenous vein is harvested using standard technique and its proximal and distal ends are suture ligated. The vein can be used in either a reversed or non-reversed configuration. We favor matching the diameter of the proximal and distal arteries with those of the vein and tend to use the vein in the non-reversed fashion with the proximal vein segment (i.e., popliteal end) used for the distal brachial anastomosis. This necessitates lysing the valves, and we usually employ the Mills valvulotome to complete this step. The tunnel for the brachial bypass is created bluntly in a subcutaneous plane using either a Kelly or a small aortic clamp. The clamp usually passes easily between the two incisions, but care should be exercised to not injure or disrupt the arteriovenous anastomosis. The vein can be marked or passed in a distended state to prevent inadvertent kinking or twisting. **CONTINUES**

22-1

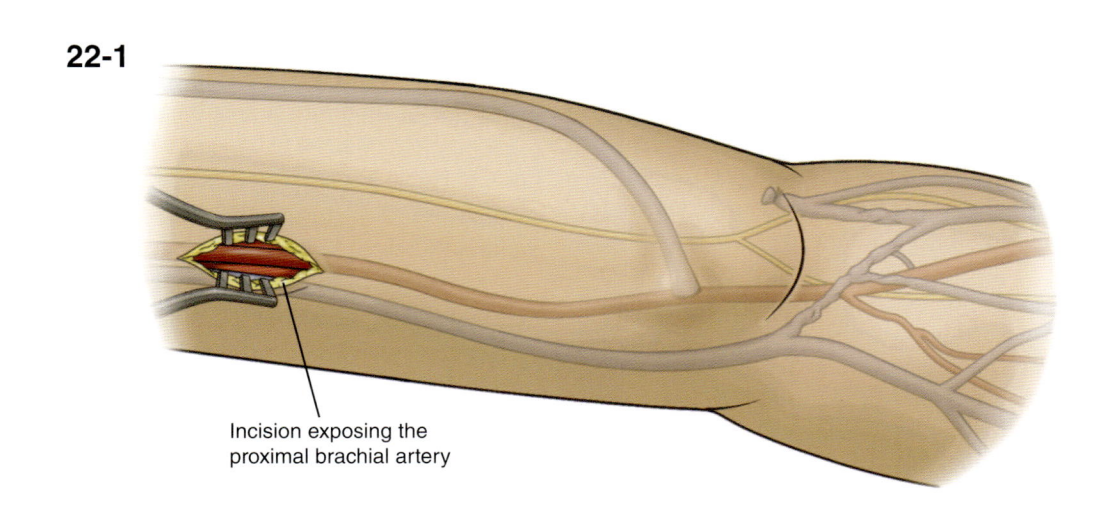

Incision exposing the
proximal brachial artery

22-2

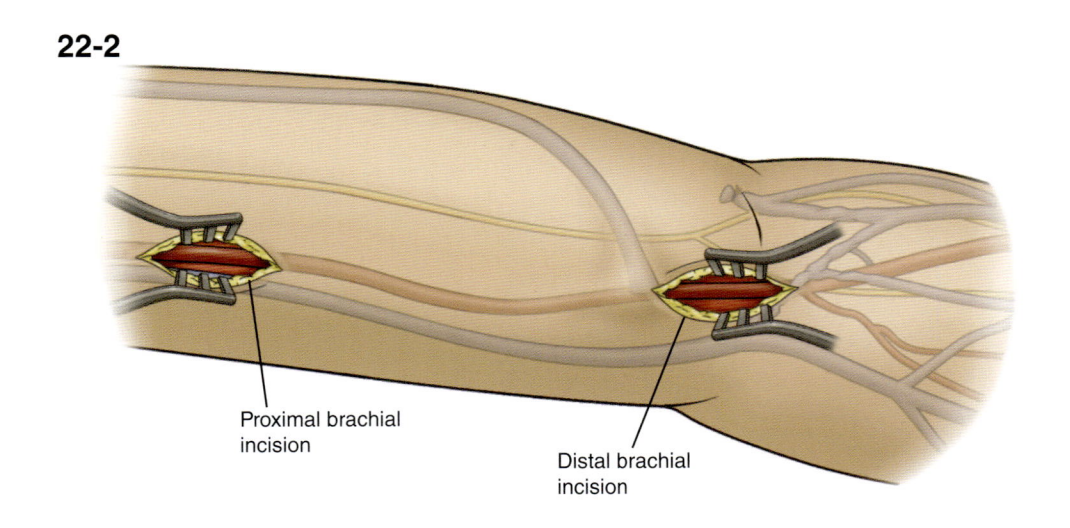

Proximal brachial
incision

Distal brachial
incision

DETAILS OF PROCEDURE `CONTINUED` The anastomoses for the brachial bypass are created using standard technique with a 5-0 or 6-0 monofilament, non-absorbable suture after anticoagulation. We favor using baby profunda or Gregory bulldog clamps to occlude the arteries, with the choice dictated by the size of the vessels and surgeon preference. A suture can be used for proximal control of the distal brachial artery, thereby completing the "ligation" of the DRIL procedure, and we typically use two 2-0 silk sutures for safe measure. This functionally converts the distal brachial end-to-side anastomosis to an end-to-end configuration (FIGURE 22-3). Alternatively, the distal brachial artery can be transected and its proximal end oversewn. The distal anastomosis for the DRIL is usually sited immediately distal to the access anastomosis. Accordingly, care should be exercised to not compromise the access with the axial vessel ligation. The distal anastomosis can be extended onto the radial or ulnar artery after the brachial bifurcation as necessary. We will occasionally perform the distal anastomosis of the brachial bypass first to facilitate performing the proximal anastomosis as proximal as possible on the brachial artery given the length of saphenous vein that was harvested.

The technical adequacy of the completed bypass is assessed using continuous-wave Doppler insonation. The Doppler signals at the wrist are determined with and without compression of the AVF, as well as the new brachial-brachial bypass. Ideally, the wrist signals are not augmented with the compression of the graft but are dependent on the new brachial-brachial bypass. The patient's heparin effect is reversed with protamine. We do not routinely obtain a catheter-based arteriogram as a completion study unless there is a presumed technical problem with the bypass.

CLOSURE The brachial and saphenous incisions are closed using standard technique. We routinely use a 2-0 braided absorbable suture for the deeper subcutaneous/fascial layer(s) and a 3-0 braided absorbable suture for the deep dermal later. The final layer of skin is closed with a running 4-0 monofilament absorbable suture, and a topical skin adhesive is applied. It can be helpful to make transverse marks across the planned sigmoidal antecubital incision at the onset of the DRIL procedure to facilitate reapproximating the skin flaps upon case completion.

POSTOPERATIVE CARE The postoperative care after the DRIL procedure is comparable to any open arterial bypass operation. The patient's preoperative medications and their dialysis schedule are resumed. Patients should have almost immediate relief from any motor compromise noted preoperatively given the significant hemodynamic benefit and augmented blood flow from the DRIL. However, patients may have persistent sensory symptoms, presumed to be secondary to an ischemic neuropathy.

Patients are seen in the outpatient clinic approximately 2 weeks after discharge with upper extremity arterial pressures and a graft scan, similar to our protocol for lower extremity bypass operations, and followed at regular intervals. ∎

SELECTED READINGS

Al-Jaishi AA, Liu AR, Lok CE, Zhang JC, Moist LM. Complications of the arteriovenous fistula: a systematic review. *J Am Soc Nephrol* 2017;28:1839-1850.

Huber TS, Brown MP, Seeger JM, Lee WA. Midterm outcome after the distal revascularization and interval ligation (DRIL) procedure. *J Vasc Surg* 2008;48:926-932.

Illig KA, Surowiec S, Shortell CK, Davies MG, Rhodes JM, Green RM. Hemodynamics of distal revascularization-interval ligation. *Ann Vasc Surg* 2005;19:199-207.

Inston N, Schanzer H, Widmer M, et al. Arteriovenous access ischemic steal (AVAIS) in haemodialysis: a consensus from the Charing Cross Vascular Access Masterclass 2016. *J Vasc Access* 2017;18:3-12.

Kordzadeh A, Parsa AD. A systematic review of distal revascularization and interval ligation for the treatment of vascular access-induced ischemia. *J Vasc Surg* 2019;70:1364-1373.

Lok CE, Huber TS, Lee T, et al. KDOQI Clinical Practice Guideline for Vascular Access: 2019 Update. *Am J Kidney Dis* 2020;75:S1-164.

Rehfuss JP, Berceli SA, Barbey SM, et al. The spectrum of hand dysfunction after hemodialysis fistula placement. *Kidney Int Rep* 2017;2:332-341.

Reifsnyder T, Arnaoutakis GJ. Arterial pressure gradient of upper extremity arteriovenous access steal syndrome: treatment implications. *Vasc Endovascular Surg* 2010;44:650-653.

Scali ST, Chang CK, Raghinaru D, et al. Prediction of graft patency and mortality after distal revascularization and interval ligation for hemodialysis access-related hand ischemia. *J Vasc Surg* 2013:451-458.

Schanzer H, Schwartz M, Harrington E, Haimov M. Treatment of ischemia due to "steal" by arteriovenous fistula with distal artery ligation and revascularization. *J Vasc Surg* 1988;7:770-773.

Wixon CL, Hughes JD, Mills JL. Understanding strategies for the treatment of ischemic steal syndrome after hemodialysis access. *J Am Coll Surg* 2000;191:301-310.

22-3

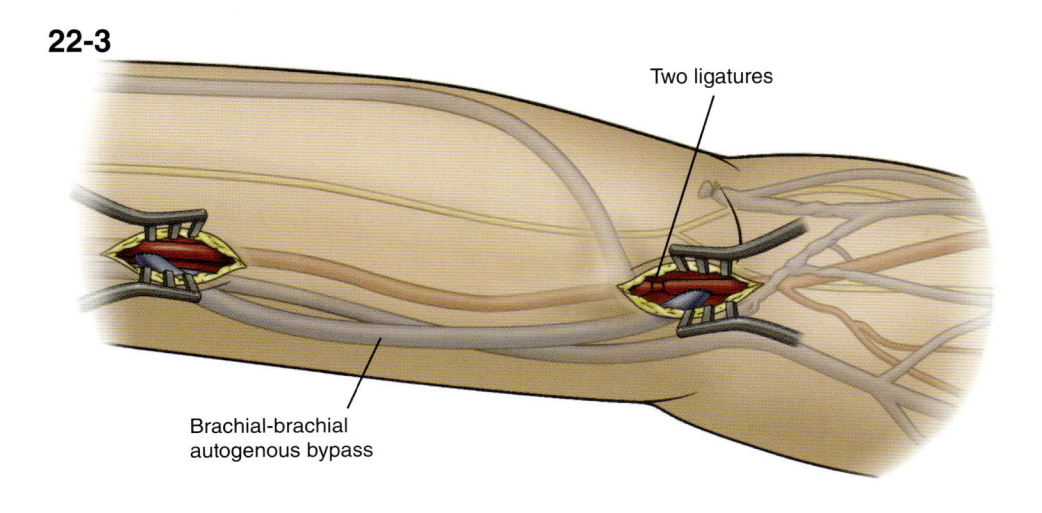

Two ligatures

Brachial-brachial
autogenous bypass

DISTAL ARM BYPASSES

Amani Politano, MS • Gregory Moneta, MD

INTRODUCTION The vast majority of upper extremity arterial diseases are vasospastic or small vessel occlusive problems secondary to cold sensitivity, connective tissue disorders, or vibration injury and are not amenable to surgical correction. However, a myriad of pathologies may result in arterial aneurysms or occlusive diseases throughout the upper extremity arterial tree, and often require surgical intervention. These include atherosclerosis, trauma, Takayasu arteritis, giant cell arteritis, fibromuscular dysplasia, repetitive use injuries, and cervical ribs. Upper extremity aneurysms rarely rupture; rather, their risk is thrombosis and embolization. Thus, the clinical manifestations of either aneurysmal or occlusive pathologies are primarily ischemic, including activity-induced fatigue, ischemic pain, or tissue loss. Surgical correction is based on elimination of the embolic source or occlusive lesion.

INDICATIONS Proximal upper extremity arterial lesions may result from connective tissue disorders (giant cell arteritis), trauma (**FIGURE 23-1**; axillary artery injury secondary to repetitive crutch use), or arterial aneurysmal or atherosclerotic occlusive disease. Lesions may manifest clinically as upper extremity activity–induced ischemia or from microemboli (Raynaud syndrome, ulcerations, or gangrene). In proximal disease, it may be feasible to utilize a proximal great vessel for inflow, which is described in earlier chapters. We will focus on distal arm bypass.

Bypass or interposition grafting of the distal forearm arteries may be indicated in patients with iatrogenic injury from endovascular procedures or invasive monitoring, or from out-of-hospital blunt or penetrating arterial injuries. Such procedures utilize standard vascular surgical techniques, including autogenous venous conduits and spatulated proximal and distal anastomoses.

Procedures with conduits extending distal to the wrist are less common, and in vascular surgical practice are primarily for treatment of ulnar artery "aneurysms," often presenting with distal embolization, as seen in hypothenar hammer syndrome (HHS) (**FIGURE 23-2**, arrow). These lesions most frequently occur in the distal ulnar artery as it passes through the Guyon canal where it overlies the hook of the hamate bone, against which the artery is compressed when the heel of the hand is substituted for a hammer. It should be noted that these processes are distinct from hand-arm vibration syndrome seen with prolonged power tool use that results in primary thickening of digital arterial walls, leading to Raynaud syndrome and eventual arterial occlusion for which treatment is nonoperative (education, behavior modification, and antiplatelet agents).

In many cases, the afflicted artery in HHS or thenar hammer syndrome (THS) is not truly aneurysmal, but contains intraluminal septal lesions more consistent with fibromuscular dysplasia than aneurysmal degeneration. Intervention is performed for patients with severe ischemic symptoms and/or tissue loss, and is concurrent with medical management, including activity modification, smoking cessation, calcium channel or beta blockade, antiplatelet medications, and possibly anticoagulation.

Interposition graft placement is usually necessary. In general, a resection of greater than 2 cm will require an interposition graft. Bypass without resection, especially of an aneurysmal segment, restores perfusion without mitigating the risk of continued emboli; therefore, an interposition graft is preferred.

ANESTHESIA We prefer general anesthesia given the multiple operative sites. Regional blocks in conjunction with general anesthesia may provide potentially favorable vasodilatory effects when smaller diameter, low-flow conduits to high-resistance beds are used. **CONTINUES ▶**

23-1

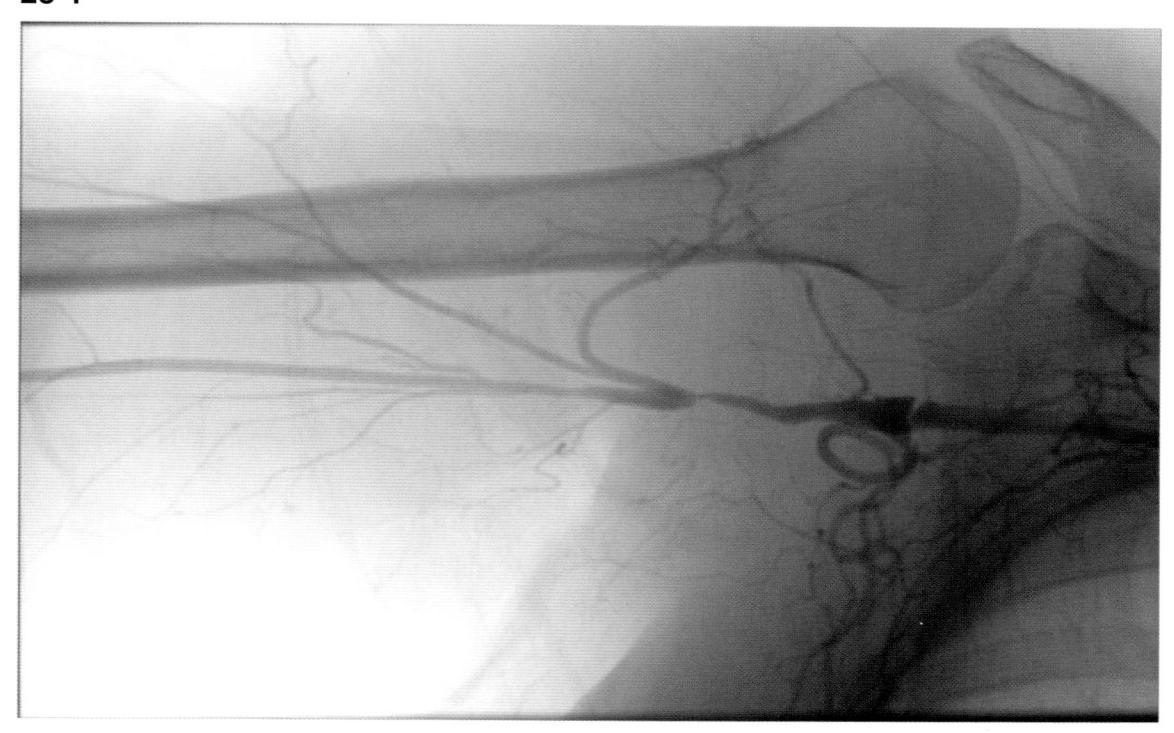

23-2

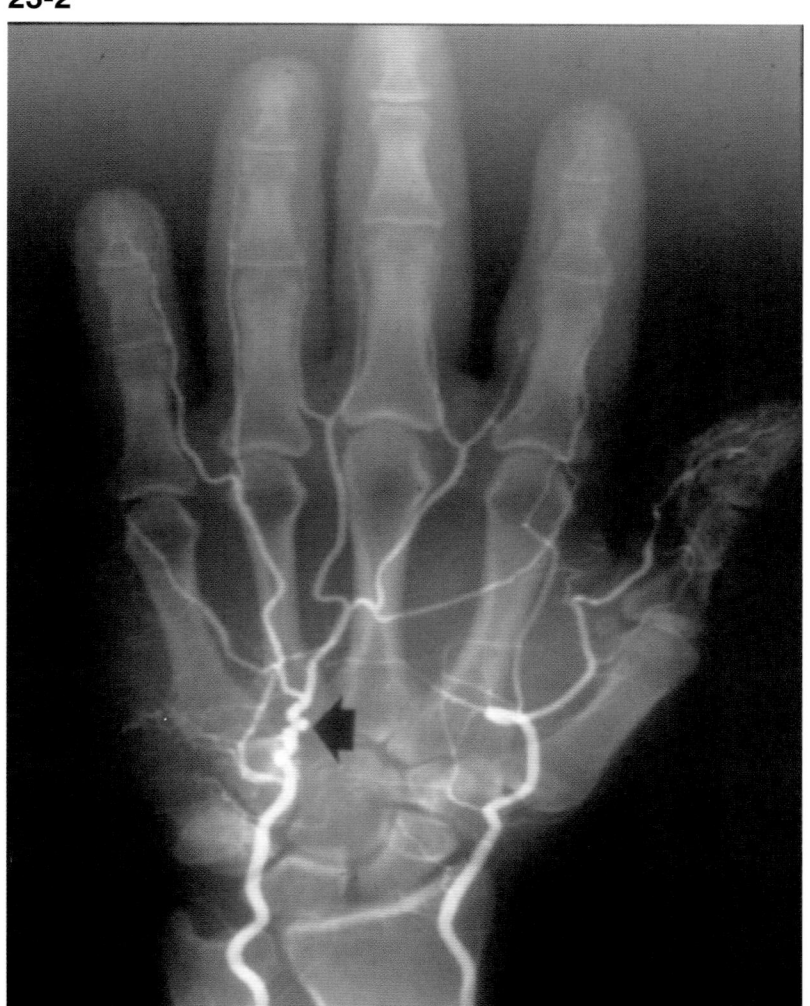

POSITION AND OPERATIVE PREPARATION For a distal upper extremity bypass, the operating table may be rotated 90° relative to the anesthesiologists, with the arm supported on an operative arm board. Care is taken to pad bony prominences and prevent hyperextension. The surgeon and assistant can then be positioned on either side of the arm board, either seated or standing, based on their preference and optimal ergonomics. If conduit from the lower extremity is to be used, positioning of the bed should also consider the optimal lighting and access to all surgical sites.

The operating room should be kept warm to reduce vasospasm. Various hand retractor systems are available to stabilize the hand, extend the fingers, and facilitate exposure (FIGURE 23-3). Operative microscopes are utilized by some surgeons, but most distal ulnar and radial artery procedures can be performed with standard 2.5× or 3.5× loupe magnification.

INCISION AND EXPOSURE Target artery exposure: The precise course of the ulnar artery, if not palpable, should be mapped with continuous wave or duplex ultrasound. Exposure is via a longitudinal incision overlying the hypothenar eminence directly over the artery (FIGURE 23-3). If ulnar artery exposure is needed more proximal to the wrist, a "lazy S" incision can be made, with the horizontal component at the wrist crease. In the hand, the ulnar artery is minimally covered by the tendon of the flexor carpi ulnaris, the palmaris brevis muscle, subcutaneous fat, and skin. Stripping the periadventitial tissue during exposure theoretically results in concurrent sympathectomy, distal vasodilatation, and perhaps aids in perioperative patency.

DETAILS OF THE PROCEDURE Once the ulnar artery is exposed and the venous conduit prepared, systemic heparin is administered. The artery is clamped and the aneurysmal or thrombosed segment excised and sent for pathologic examination. Atraumatic clamps, such as Heifetz clamps, should be used to avoid arterial injury. Alternatively, a tourniquet can be inflated on the upper arm to provide control, though this does not allow assessment of back bleeding to aid in gauging the quality of the outflow. The remaining arterial ends should be inspected for normal appearance of the intima, absence of arterial wall septation, and presence of distal emboli. Fogarty thrombectomy may be performed if loose emboli are noted, though this should be done with care in small vessels. We have on occasion infused lytic agents distally but have found this to be of uncertain benefit.

The distal anastomosis is best performed first to allow optimal manipulation of the conduit while sutures are placed, and to minimize tension on the suture line and the risk of the initial sutures pulling through. If the abnormal artery ends above the branches, a straightforward end-to-end anastomosis with interrupted 7-0 Prolene sutures is appropriate (FIGURE 23-4, completed ulnar artery bypass with vein). If one or two distal branches arise from a mild to moderately abnormal artery, they may be incorporated into a beveled or spatulated end-to-end anastomosis after trimming the diseased artery wall. Reimplantation of digital arteries or side branches is best performed with an operative microscope by a microvascular surgeon.

Inflow should be as distal as possible to decrease the length of the conduit and the incision (FIGURE 23-5A). Exposure of the ulnar artery in the mid and proximal forearm is tedious and difficult, so if the distal forearm ulnar artery is also diseased, proximal inflow can be obtained from the brachial artery in the antecubital fossa. In this scenario, a subcutaneous tunnel between the two incisions should be created, the conduit is marked to ensure orientation and prevent twisting, and any fascia should be relaxed to prevent impingement on the graft (FIGURE 23-5B). Patency of longer bypass grafts is clearly less than that of shorter segments.

CLOSURE Heparin is not reversed. After hemostasis is obtained, closure of the incision is with interrupted deep absorbable sutures, avoiding compression or tension over the bypass graft. Skin closure is with interrupted or running nylon sutures. A volar wrist splint is placed postoperatively to stabilize the joint.

POSTOPERATIVE CARE Following reconstruction, patients are often maintained on single-agent antiplatelet therapy with aspirin. The wrist is kept in the splint for 2 weeks, after which dedicated hand therapy (occupational therapy) may be of benefit.

FOLLOW-UP Surveillance for bypass graft patency may be performed with duplex ultrasound, computed tomography, or magnetic resonance arteriography.

Residual symptoms do not necessarily correlate with bypass graft patency, and may be resultant from the initial ischemic injury, perioperative ulnar nerve palsy, an underlying disease state, or residual digital artery occlusions. Early graft failure or recurrent tissue loss may be indications for thrombectomy or bypass revision. Cold sensitivity and Raynaud syndrome often persist to some degree and may not resolve even with a patent bypass, and in themselves should not prompt reintervention. ■

SUGGESTED READINGS

Cherry KJ Jr, McCullough JL, Hallett JW Jr, Pairolero PC, Gloviczki P. Technical principles of direct innominate artery revascularization: a comparison of endarterectomy and bypass grafts. *J Vasc Surg.* 1989 May;9(5):718-23.

Dalman RL. Upper extremity arterial bypass distal to the wrist. *Ann Vasc Surg.* 1997 Sep;11(5):550-557.

Dethmers RS, Houpt P. Surgical management of hypothenar and thenar hammer syndromes: a retrospective study of 31 instances in 28 patients. *J Hand Surg Br.* 2005 Aug;30(4):419-423.

Ferris BL, Taylor LM Jr, Oyama K, et al. Hypothenar hammer syndrome: proposed etiology. *J Vasc Surg.* 2000 Jan;31(1 Pt 1):104-113.

Hui-Chou HG, McClinton MA. Current options for treatment of hypothenar hammer syndrome. *Hand Clin.* 2015 Feb;31(1):53-56.

Kitzinger HB, van Schoonhoven J, Schmitt R, Hacker S, Karle B. Hypothenar hammer syndrome: long-term results after vascular reconstruction. *Ann Plast Surg.* 2016 Jan;76(1):40-45.

McCarthy WJ, Flinn WR, Yao JST, Williams LR, Bergan JJ. Result of bypass grafting for upper limb ischemia. *J Vasc Surg.* 1986;3:741-746.

McClinton MA. Reconstruction for ulnar artery aneurysm at the wrist. *J Hand Surg Am.* 2011 Feb;36(2):328-332.

Politano AD, Cherry KJ: Chapter 11. Direct surgical repair of aortic arch vessels. In: Chaikof EL, Cambria RP, eds. *Atlas of Vascular Surgery and Endovascular Therapy: Anatomy and Technique.* Elsevier. March 2014; 126-138.

Ravari H, Johari HG, Rajabnejad A. Hypothenar hammer syndrome: surgical approach in patients presenting with ulnar artery aneurysm. *Ann Vasc Surg.* 2018 Jul;50:284-287.

Roddy SP, Darling RC 3rd, Chang BB, et al. Brachial artery reconstruction for occlusive disease: a 12-year experience. *J Vasc Surg.* 2001 Apr;33(4):802-805.

23-3

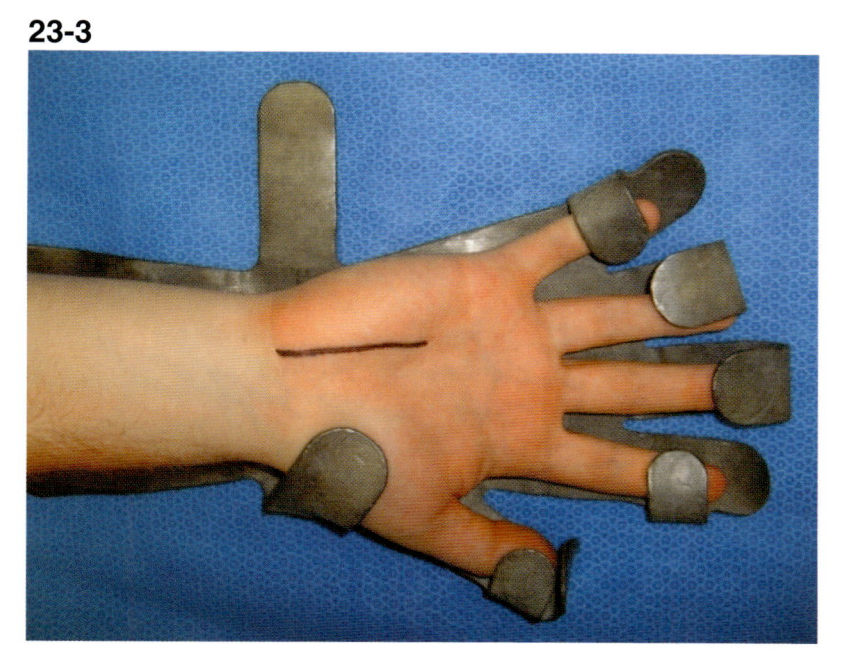

23-4

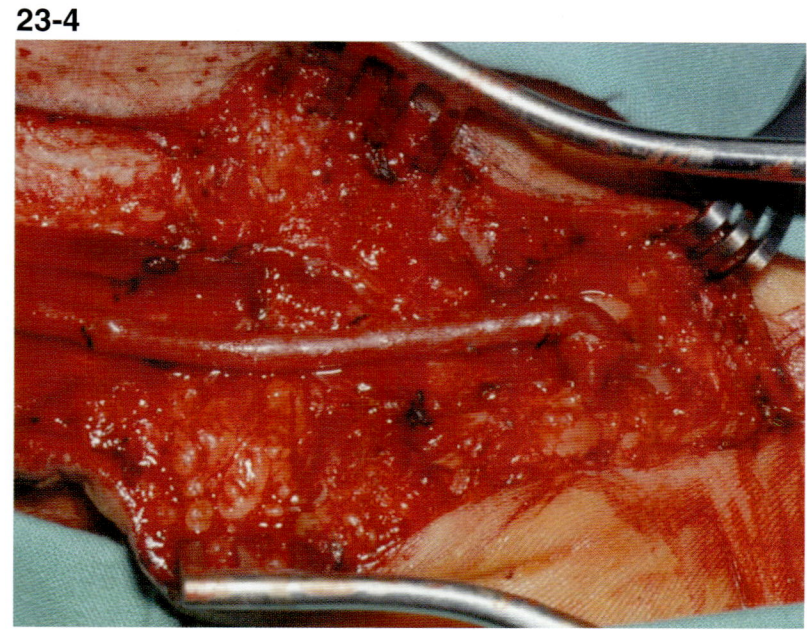

23-5

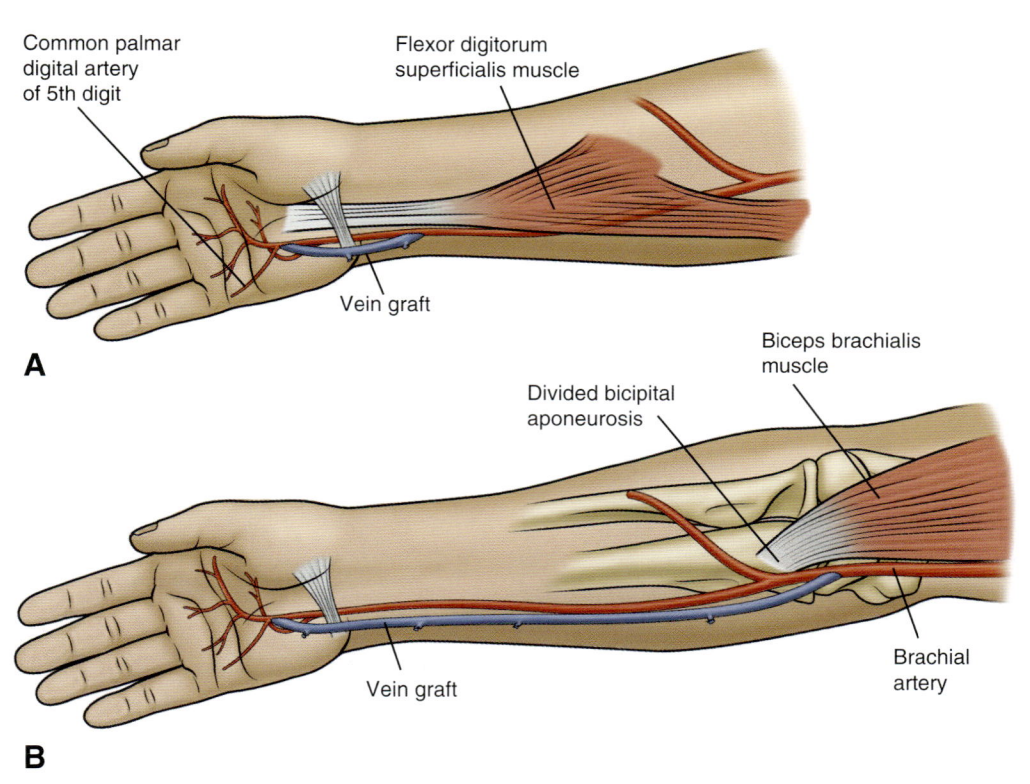

Common palmar digital artery of 5th digit

Flexor digitorum superficialis muscle

Vein graft

A

Divided bicipital aponeurosis

Biceps brachialis muscle

Vein graft

Brachial artery

B

SECTION V
THORACIC OUTLET SYNDROME

SUPRACLAVICULAR THORACIC OUTLET SYNDROME

Mohamad A. Hussain, MD, PhD • Mohammed Al-Omran, MD, MSc

INDICATIONS Thoracic outlet syndrome (TOS) occurs due to compression of the subclavian artery, subclavian vein, brachial plexus, or a combination of these neurovascular structures in the thoracic outlet space. The clinical presentation of patients with TOS is dependent on which structures are compressed. Patients with subclavian artery compression (arterial TOS) can present with arm or hand pain that increases with activity, acute arm or hand ischemia due to arterial thrombosis or embolism, or subclavian aneurysm. Venous TOS (due to subclavian vein compression) symptoms commonly occur due to subclavian vein thrombosis; these include arm edema, bluish discoloration, and presence of collateral veins in the arm, shoulder, and chest. Neurogenic TOS occurs due to compression of the brachial plexus. Symptoms of neurogenic TOS include arm or hand pain, paresthesia, weakness, discoloration, and exacerbation of symptoms with overhead or repetitive activities.

The supraclavicular approach to TOS decompression can be used for the treatment of all three subtypes of TOS, as it allows for complete decompression of the thoracic outlet via anterior scalenectomy, middle scalenectomy, first rib resection, and resection of cervical ribs if present. In addition, this approach can be used to perform brachial plexus neurolysis in patients with neurogenic symptoms, and for arterial reconstruction in those with arterial TOS requiring arterial reconstruction. The supraclavicular incision can be combined with a distal infraclavicular incision to perform arterial bypass in those requiring arterial reconstruction for long-segment subclavian artery occlusion or large aneurysms in order to explore the axillary artery.

Indications for supraclavicular thoracic outlet decompression surgery include signs and symptoms of TOS and/or radiological evidence of vascular compression with provocative maneuvers. Arterial and venous compression can be seen with provocative maneuvers on duplex ultrasound, catheter-based angiography, contrast-enhanced computed tomography (CT), and magnetic resonance imaging (MRI). CT and MRI have the additional benefits of identifying arterial pathology (such as intimal injury, post-stenotic dilatation, or aneurysms), and bony abnormalities (cervical rib, anomalous first rib, elongated C7 transverse process, etc.) that may be contributing to thoracic outlet compression. In cases of isolated neurogenic TOS, decompression can be considered in patients with signs and symptoms of TOS that fail a trial of nonsurgical treatment with physiotherapy.

POSITION AND PREPARATION After general anesthesia is induced and endotracheal intubation is established, the patient is placed in a semi-Fowler 45-degree position with the neck extended and turned toward the contralateral side. The skin is prepared in the standard fashion. The patient is draped to expose the upper neck superiorly, the sternal notch medially, the upper chest inferiorly, and the shoulder laterally. The electrocautery is set to 20/20 monopolar and 15 bipolar. The anesthesia team is instructed to not give any more neuromuscular blocking agents for the duration of the operation after induction to preserve nerve function during dissection, which helps to minimize the risk of nerve injury.

INCISION AND EXPOSURE A supraclavicular incision is made one fingerbreadth above and parallel to the clavicle starting from the clavicular head of the sternocleidomastoid muscle and extending 6 to 7 cm laterally (FIGURE 24-1; right neck shown). The platysma is entered. Wide subplatysmal flaps are created to the level of the cricoid cartilage superiorly, the sternal notch medially, 1 to 2 cm laterally, and the clavicle inferiorly. Self-retaining retractors are then positioned.

The dissection is carried along the lateral border of the sternocleidomastoid muscle and extended superiorly and inferiorly. The omohyoid muscle is identified, isolated, and resected (FIGURE 24-2). Next, the scalene fat pad is mobilized along its superior border, being careful to protect cutaneous nerves; then along its medial border; and finally, the inferior border. Small vessels in the fat pad are ligated using silk ties. Lymphatic channels may also be encountered here that will need to be addressed using hemoclips, electrocautery, or silk ties. The fat pad is then reflected laterally exposing the phrenic nerve and the anterior scalene muscle (FIGURE 24-3). The self-retaining retractors are repositioned after mobilization of the fat pad, which is the gateway to the structures in the thoracic outlet space. **CONTINUES ▶**

24-1

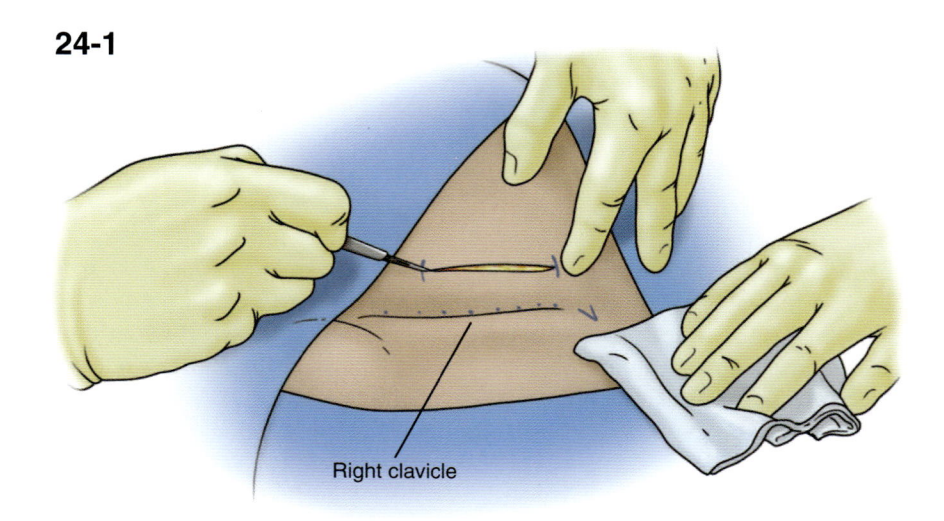

Right clavicle

24-2

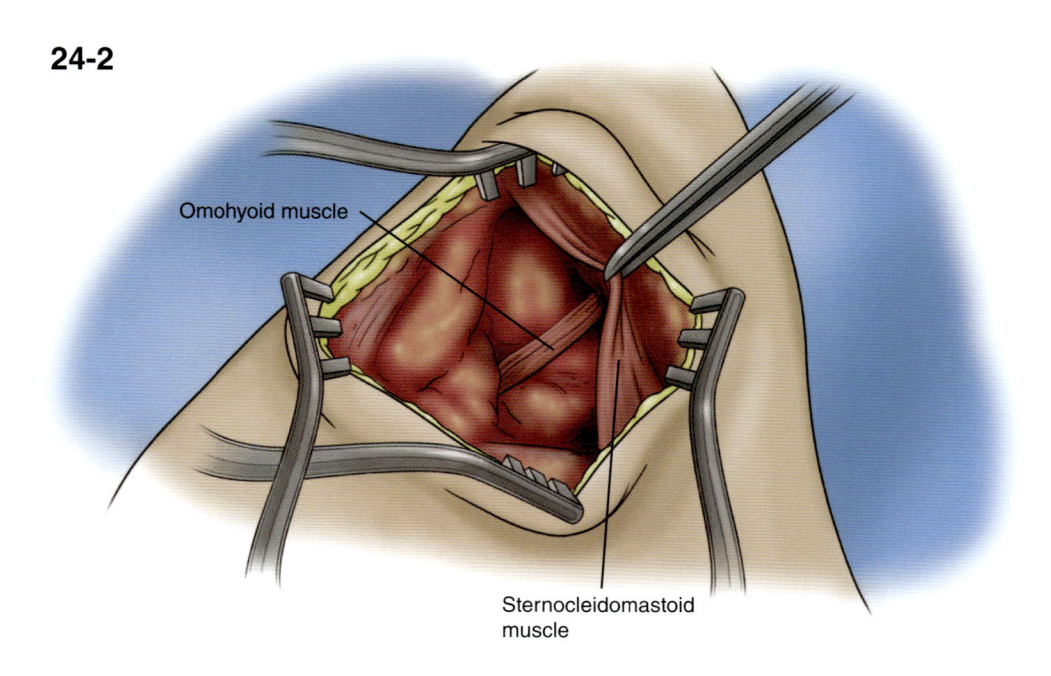

Omohyoid muscle

Sternocleidomastoid muscle

24-3

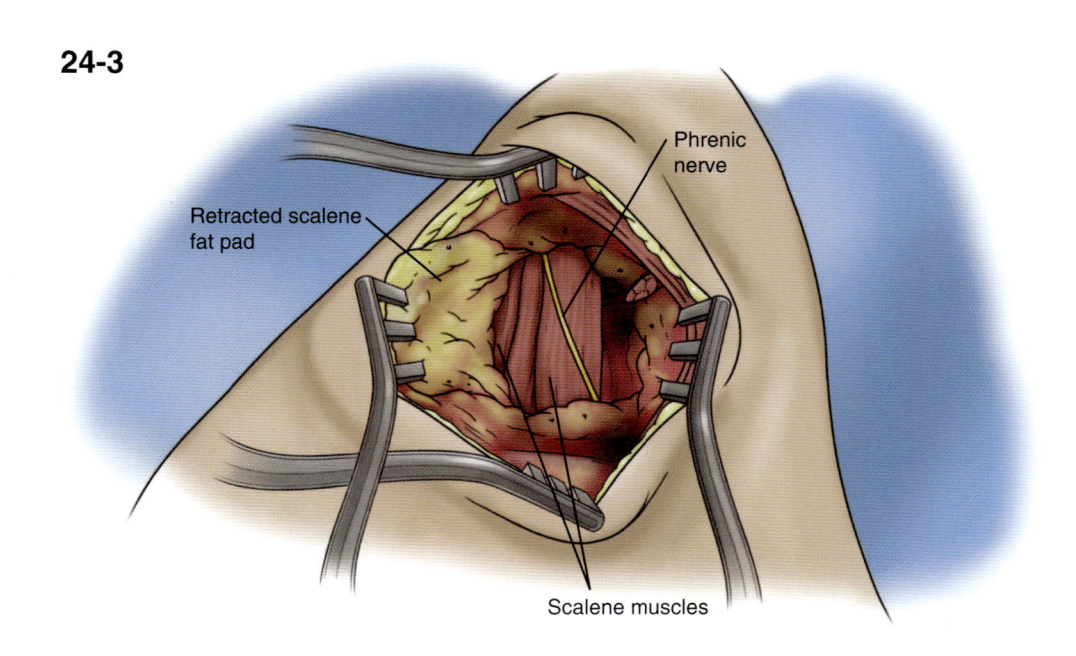

Phrenic nerve

Retracted scalene fat pad

Scalene muscles

ANTERIOR SCALENECTOMY Monopolar electrocautery is switched for bipolar electrocautery at this point to minimize the risk of nerve injury. The medial border of the anterior scalene is first mobilized. The phrenic nerve is then carefully dissected free from surrounding fascia under direct vision using bipolar electrocautery. Aggressive manipulation or injury to the phrenic nerve can lead to postoperative diaphragmatic dysfunction. Next, the lateral border of the anterior scalene is mobilized including any interdigitation with the brachial plexus. The subclavian artery is identified in the inferior portion of the wound behind the anterior scalene and is freed from any adhesions. The anterior scalene muscle is then isolated using umbilical tape (FIGURE 24-4). The subclavian vein is protected using an angled hand-held retractor, and the anterior scalene muscle is divided at its insertion of the first rib a few millimeters at a time under direct vision using bipolar electrocautery. To complete the scalenectomy, the muscle is then divided at its origin of the transverse process a few millimeters at a time (FIGURE 24-5) while being aware of the phrenic nerve location at all times. At this point of the operation, the brachial plexus, phrenic nerve, subclavian artery, and the subclavian vein are all clearly visible.

BRACHIAL PLEXUS NEUROLOYSIS Brachial plexus neurolysis is carried out next. The upper trunk is isolated revealing the C5 and C6 nerve roots. One must be very careful to avoid traction injury to nerves, including the brachial plexus, during this process. Perineural tissues are lysed using bipolar electrocautery to perform the neurolysis. The middle trunk consisting of C7 is isolated and neurolysed next, followed by the lower trunk consisting of C8 and T1. It is critical to identify and isolate all three nerve roots of the brachial plexus to achieve complete neurolysis of the brachial plexus and prevent nerve injury during middle scalenectomy and first rib resection. Retractors are then repositioned for middle scalenectomy.

MIDDLE SCALENECTOMY AND RESECTION OF CERVICAL RIB The middle scalene muscle is identified lateral to the brachial plexus. The dissection is first carried out at the lateral border of the middle scalene muscle. Fibers of the long thoracic nerve on the anterior surface of the middle scalene are identified and protected. Further dissection along the medial border of the middle scalene is carried out, which is followed by isolating the muscle (FIGURE 24-6) with an umbilical tape. The middle scalene is then divided at its origin under direct vision a few millimeters at a time using bipolar electrocautery while protecting the long thoracic nerve. If the patient has a cervical rib, it is identified posterior to the middle scalene muscle at this point and is freed of any adhesions. A Kerrison rongeur is used to resect the cervical rib. The middle scalene muscle is then divided sharply or with bipolar electrocautery at its insertion to the first rib while protecting the long thoracic nerve to complete the middle scalenectomy and remove the specimen. **CONTINUES**

24-4

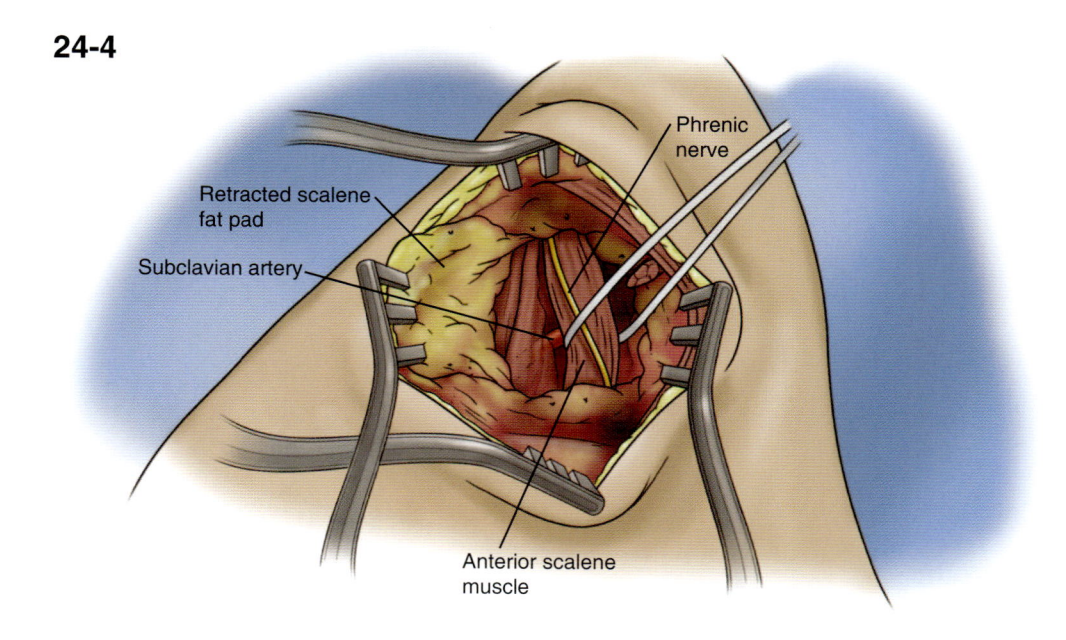

24-5

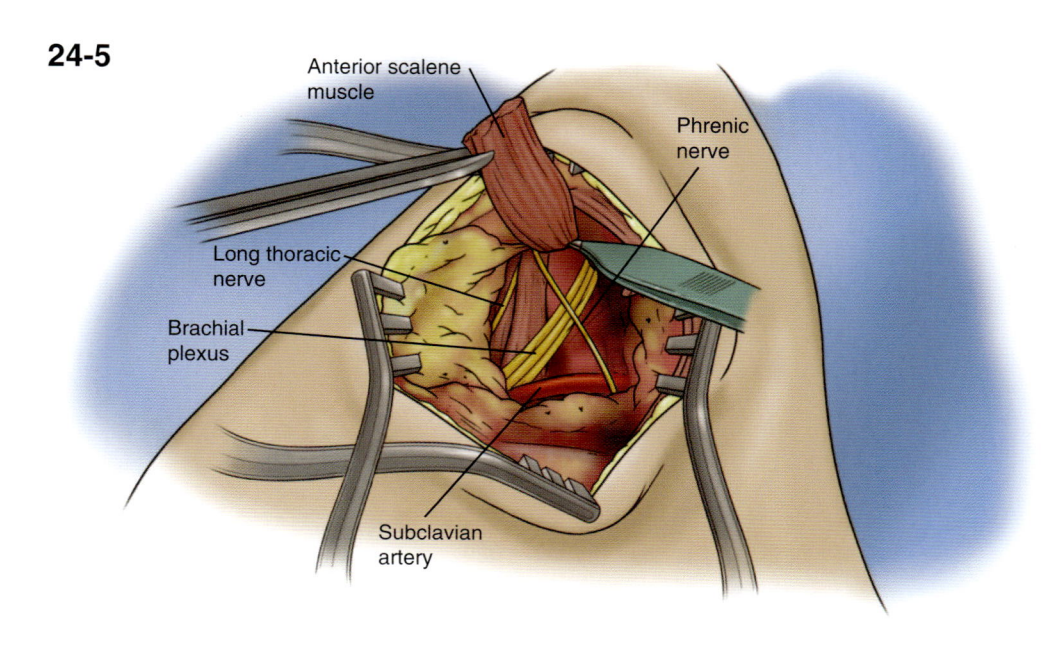

24-6

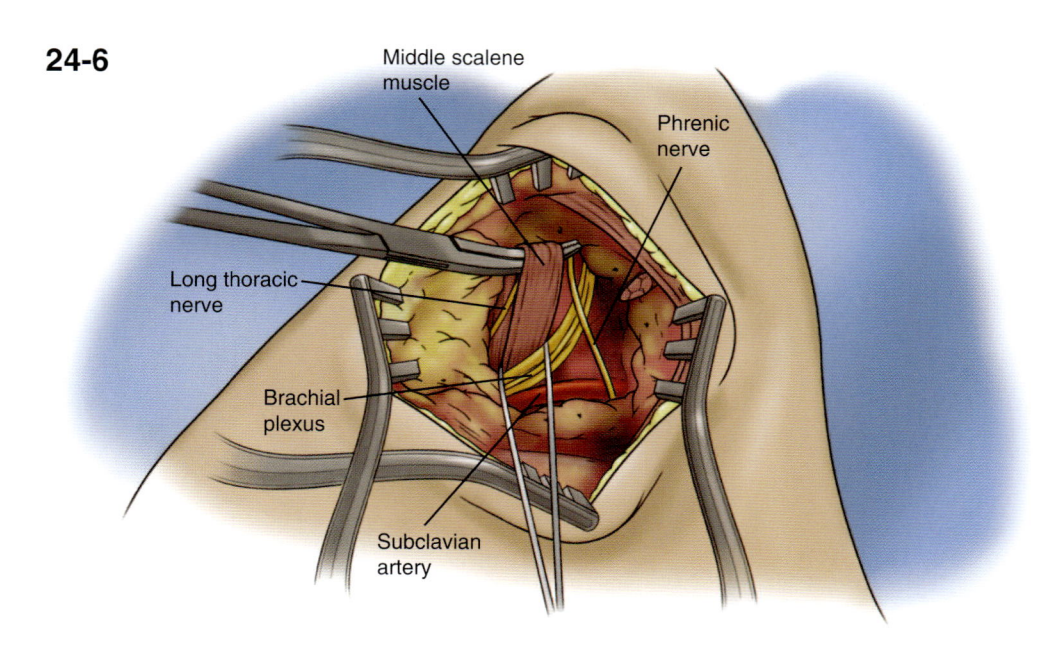

FIRST RIB RESECTION Valve scissors are used to sharply divide any remaining attachments of the intercostal muscles and serratus anterior on the first rib posteriorly. To divide the first rib anteriorly, the subclavian vein is protected with an angled hand-held retractor; the subclavian artery is retracted with a vessel loop; the scalene tubercle on the first rib is identified; and a Kerrison rongeur is used to divide the first rib piecemeal at the scalene tubercle. A bone file is used to smoothen the edges of the remaining bone to prevent any soft tissue injury. Prior to dividing the rib posteriorly, positioning of the T1 nerve root mut be confirmed for protection (FIGURE 24-7). The first rib is then resected with a Kerrison rongeur piecemeal as posteriorly as possible and ideally within 1 cm of the transverse process. The rib is then grasped, pulled, and removed in one piece (FIGURE 24-8). CONTINUES ▶

24-7

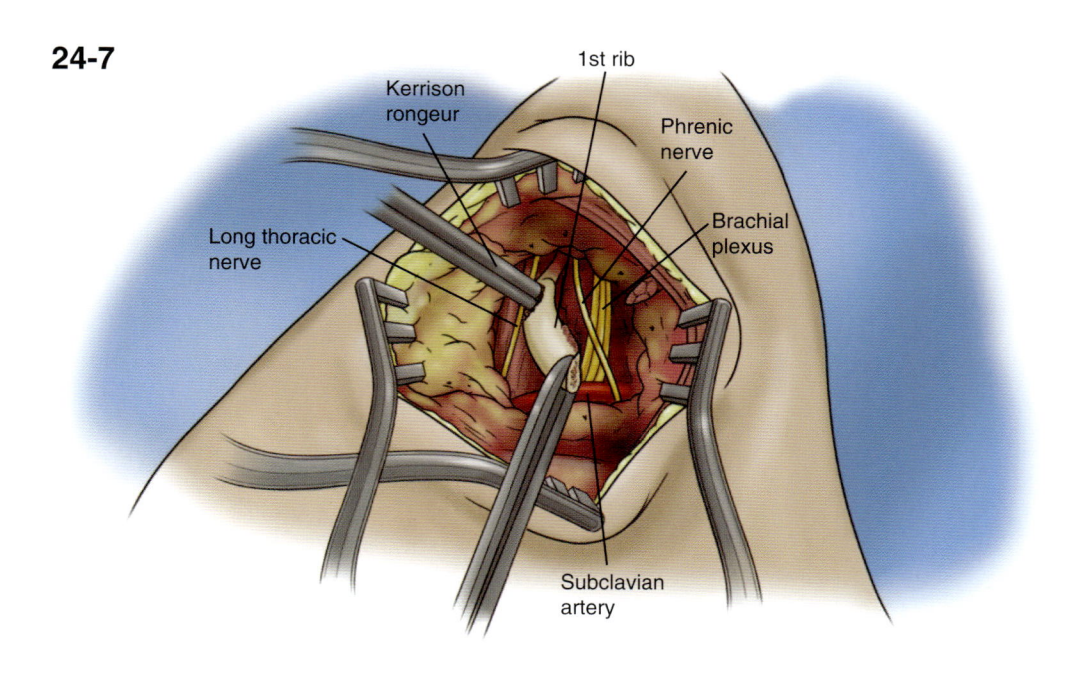

24-8

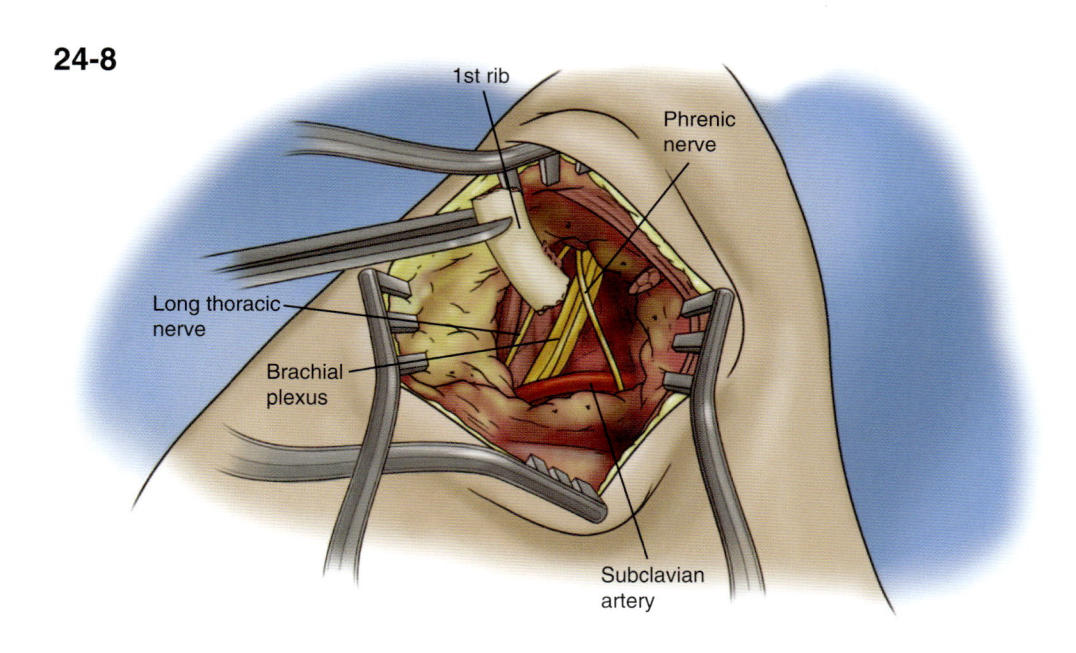

CLOSURE The lung pleura is inspected for any potential defects in the parietal pleura caused during the dissection. These can be repaired primarily using 2-0 Vicryl sutures. Valsalva is done up to 40 mm Hg with saline in the wound for 5 to 10 seconds to rule out bleeding and pneumothorax. The final result should show freed subclavian artery and vein post adhenolysis, intact phrenic nerve, long thoracic nerve, brachial plexus trunks (upper trunk C5–C6, middle trunk C7, and lower trunk C8–T1), and intact lung pleura (**FIGURE 24-9**). The scalene fat pad is closed using interrupted 2-0 Vicryl sutures. A medium-sized suction drain such as Hemovac or Jackson Pratt drain is inserted inferior to the incision; it is placed on the fat pad with 2 cm of its terminal end deep to the fat pad. The purpose of the drain is to collect fluid, but it can also be placed to under water drainage system postoperatively if there is evidence of air on chest x-ray to indicate a pneumothorax. The wound is inspected for lymph leaks, particularly on the left side, before closure. The platysma is closed in a running fashion using 3-0 Vicryl followed by 4-0 Monocryl for skin in subcuticular fashion (**FIGURE 24-10**). Usual dressings are applied to the incision and the drain site.

POSTOPERATIVE CARE The patient should receive a chest x-ray in the recovery room immediately postoperatively to rule out a pneumothorax, pleural effusion, or significant diaphragm elevation due to phrenic nerve neuropraxia.

Neurological assessment in the postoperative period should consist of assessing for neuropraxia of the long thoracic nerve (winged scapula), sympathetic chain (Horner syndrome), and brachial plexus. Pain is generally treated with patient-controlled analgesia, and physiotherapy (chest and shoulder) is immediately initiated.

Drain output should be monitored for both volume and type of fluid. Generally, the drain is removed within 2 to 3 days postoperatively once draining <30 cc/24 hour of pleural fluid. In ~5% of cases, the patient will require a thoracostomy tube to drain a significant pleural effusion. In rare cases, a chyle leak may develop, particularly if the decompression was done on the left side. Our approach is to treat mild chyle leaks with a medium fatty acid chain diet. More severe or persistent chyle leaks may require NPO status, thoracostomy tube, total parental nutrition, octreotide, and/or referral to thoracic surgery for video-assisted thorascopic surgery ligation of the thoracic duct.

Most patients who have an uncomplicated postoperative course are discharged home within postoperative day 2 to 3 after the procedure. If the patient has an indication for postoperative anticoagulation (such as subclavian vein deep venous thrombosis within 3 months prior to decompression), anticoagulation can be initiated on postoperative day 2 to 3 once hemostasis is confirmed. Clinic follow-up is arranged in 2 to 3 weeks for wound check and assessment of symptoms and range of movements. ∎

24-9

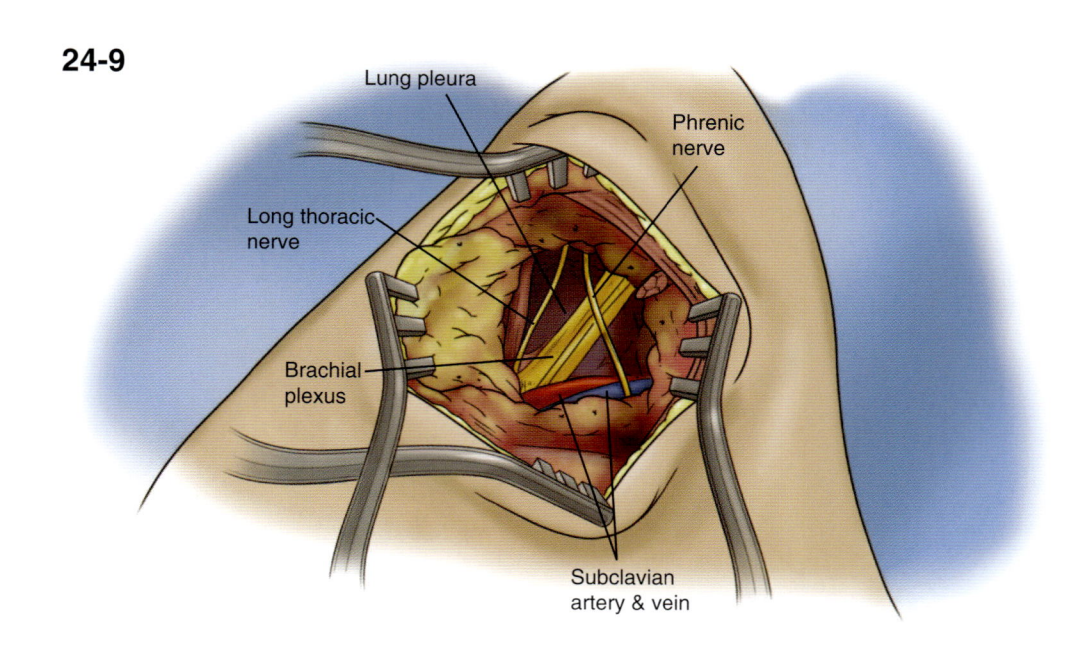

24-10

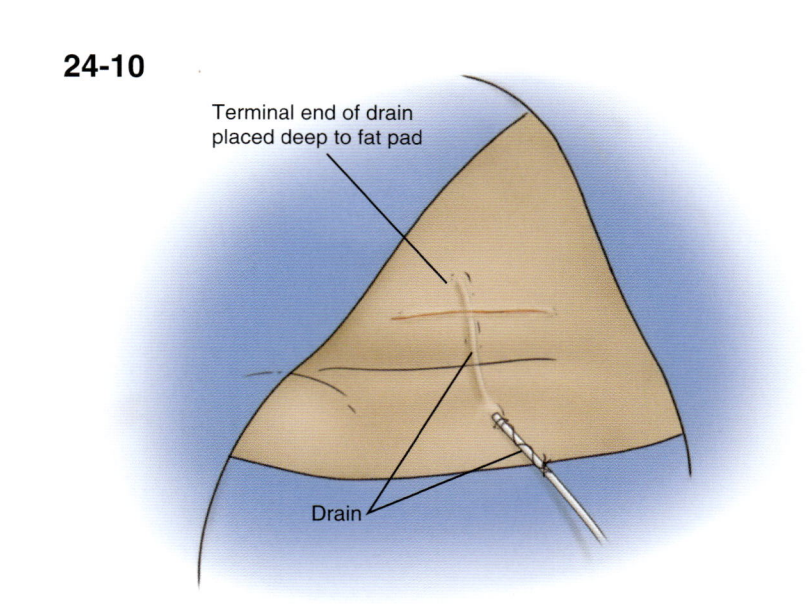

TRANSAXILLARY FIRST RIB RESECTION

Misty D. Humphries, MD, MAS, FACS • Julie A. Frieschlag, MD

INDICATION Treatment of thoracic outlet syndrome (TOS) with first rib resection and scalenectomy to decompress the thoracic outlet (FIGURE 25-1) is highly effective, with excellent long-term outcomes.[1] Roos first described transaxillary first rib resection.[2] The approach can be used in all three types of TOS (neurogenic, venous, and arterial). Because there is no absolute indication for first rib resection and decompression, understanding the contraindications to the transaxillary approach is essential. Vascular reconstruction is the main contraindication to using the transaxillary approach. The approach does not offer the ability to control and treat the subclavian vein with patch angioplasty for open repair. Finally, in patients undergoing first rib resection to maintain dialysis access, the transaxillary approach should be cautiously approached.[3] The arm extension needed to access the rib may compress a functioning fistula and result in thrombosis.

PREOPERATIVE PREPARATION The type of TOS will dictate what preoperative preparation is needed. For patients with venous TOS (vTOS) who are on anticoagulation, this should be held for surgery. Patients who have received recent lytic therapy should have fibrinogen levels checked to ensure they are not at increased bleeding risk during surgery. A chest x-ray with apical views or cervical spine x-ray, including the first thoracic rib, should be performed in patients with cervical ribs. This is imperative to determine if the cervical rib is complete or incomplete and can be entirely removed through the transaxillary approach. There are no differences in outcomes from alternative approaches when resecting cervical ribs.[4] Finally, all patients with cervical ribs should have imaging of the subclavian artery. This can be done by duplex ultrasound or cross-sectional imaging, but a subclavian aneurysm should be ruled out.

ANESTHESIA Transaxillary first rib resection is performed under general anesthesia. A Foley catheter is unnecessary, given the short nature of the case. A peripheral intravenous (IV) catheter should be placed in the nonoperative arm. Because the entire affected arm and hand are prepped into the field, a second IV can be placed in the contralateral arm or lower extremity. An arterial line is not needed. Finally, neuromuscular blocking agents should be limited during anesthesia induction since the operation is performed around the nerves of the brachial plexus.

POSITION AND OPERATIVE PREPARATION The patient is positioned in the lateral decubitus position with the affected arm up. A bean bag can be used to hold the patient, and an axillary roll should be placed under the down arm. The patient is padded appropriately to protect bony prominences. The axillary hair is clipped, and the entire arm is prepped into the field. The Machleder retractor is set up, and the tray is padded with white terrycloth towels (FIGURE 25-2). **CONTINUES**▶

25-1

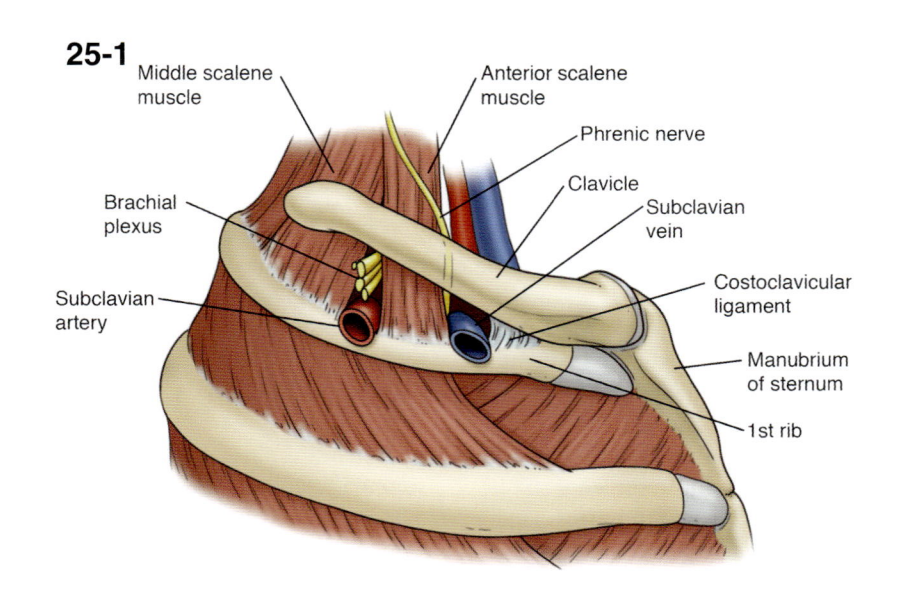

Middle scalene muscle

Anterior scalene muscle

Phrenic nerve

Brachial plexus

Clavicle

Subclavian vein

Subclavian artery

Costoclavicular ligament

Manubrium of sternum

1st rib

25-2

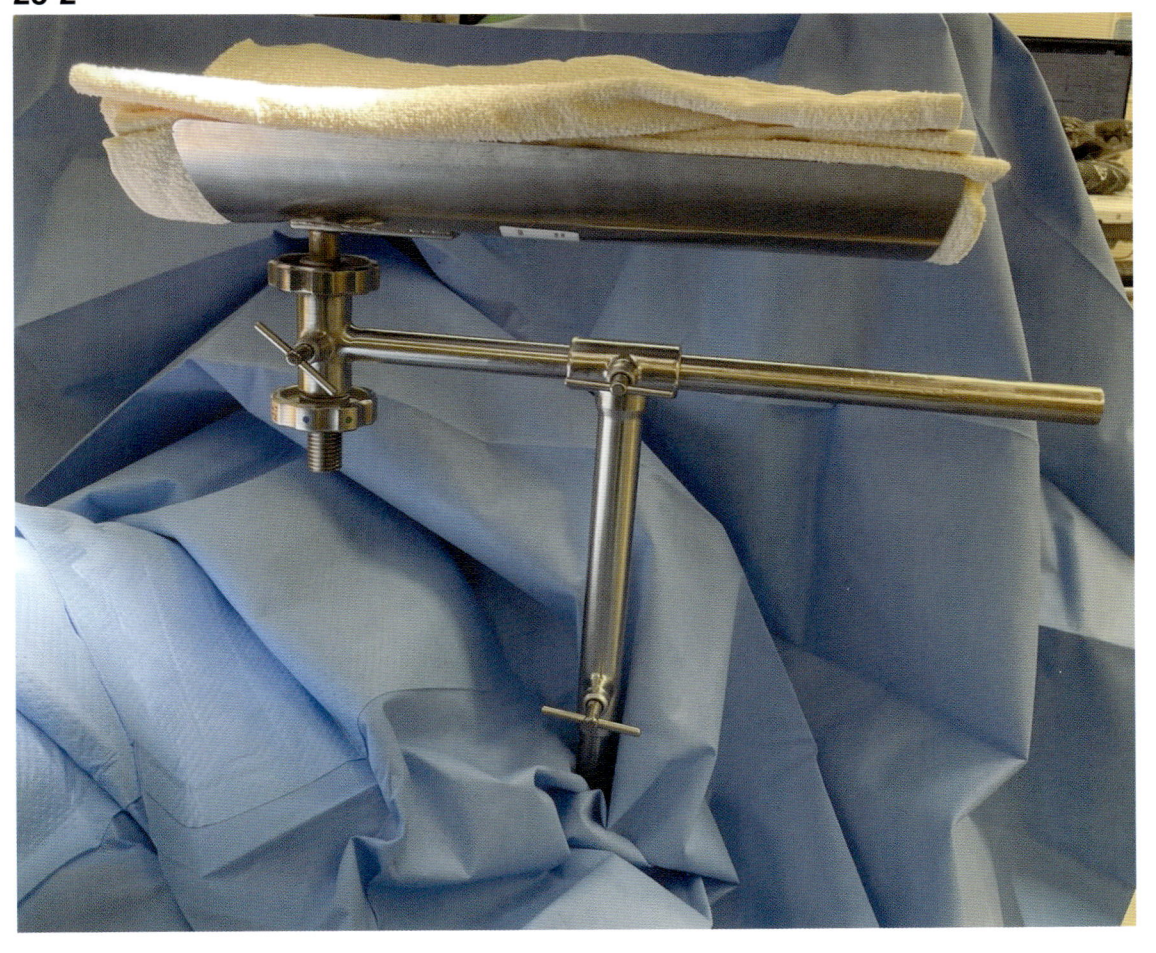

POSITION AND OPERATIVE PREPARATION `CONTINUED` The arm is placed in a stockinette to just above the elbow and wrapped with Kerlix for additional padding. The arm is held in the retractor with Coban (**FIGURE 25-3**). If the retractor is not available, an assistant can hold the arm, but this is not ideal. Manual elevation can allow the person holding the arm to fatigue over time and decrease adequate exposure.

INCISION AND EXPOSURE The external landmarks are marked on the skin once the arm is in the retractor (**FIGURE 25-3**). This includes the latissimus dorsi muscle and the pectoralis major muscle. A transverse incision is made at the base of the hairline. The subcutaneous tissues are dissected down to the chest wall. Once the chest wall is encountered, the arm is lifted in the retractor system. The connective tissue over the thoracic outlet is bluntly dissected following the subclavian vein to the first rib. The arm is raised with the retractor at 10- to 15-minute intervals. Releasing the arm down intermittently prevents any stretch on the brachial plexus. A lighted retractor is used to provide better visibility within the deep space of the thoracic outlet. A second retractor can be used on the opposite side of the incision to hold the tissue back and provide better exposure.

DETAILS OF THE PROCEDURE As the dissection is extended down the subclavian vein to the first rib, small branches can be taken down with clips. The subclavian vein is dissected first, and the dissection is carried from anterior to posterior. Blunt dissection of the vein is carried past the first rib, and care is ensured to separate it from the subclavius muscle (**FIGURE 25-4**). Once the vein is dissected thoroughly, the anterior scalene muscle is cleared of surrounding connective tissue anteriorly and posteriorly. The subclavius muscle and tendon are cut anteriorly. A right-angle clamp is passed posteriorly to the anterior scalene muscle, and the muscle is divided sharply (**FIGURE 25-5**). The phrenic nerve typically separates from the anterior scalene muscle. It enters the chest above where the anterior scalene muscle inserts on the first rib, so it is rarely encountered through the transaxillary approach. The entire anterior scalene muscle does not need to be divided at once. Dividing the muscle slowly allows the surgeon to ensure that no surrounding structures are injured.

Once the subclavius and anterior scalene muscles are cut, a periosteal elevator is used to free up the intercostal muscle fibers along the lateral aspect of the first rib. The muscle fibers of the middle scalene muscle fibers are elevated from the first rib as well. Care is taken to ensure the long thoracic nerve is not injured. This is the reason not to cut those muscle fibers. A smaller periosteal elevator is used to separate the pleura from the inferior aspect of the rib. A pleural tear is common in vTOS, where there may be significant inflammation. If a cervical rib is present, the periosteal elevator is also used to remove any muscle fibers from it. A right-angle clamp is passed under the first rib to separate all medial muscle fibers and attachments to the first rib. At that point, the anterior aspect of the first rib is transected with a Bethune rib cutter. Once the anterior portion is cut, the first rib will lift, and the pleura can be further separated posteriorly. The elevator is then used to clear the muscle fibers from the posterior aspect of the rib. The posterior part of the rib is then cut. It is crucial that the rib is removed to the spine but that the nerve is not injured during the cutting of the rib (**FIGURE 25-6**). This may require the rib to be cut more than once, or cutting the rib and then removing the rest of the residual rib with a first rib rongeur. The cervical rib can be removed with the rongeur as well.

CLOSURE Once the rib is removed, the wound is checked for hemostasis. Any small vessels should be taken down during the dissection with clips to prevent hemithorax. Next, saline is instilled in the field, and a Valsalva maneuver is performed to ensure there is no pleura tear. Small air bubbles may be seen during the Valsalva if there is a tear in the pleura. Another clue that there is a tear is the disappearance of the fluid when the Valsalva is completed as the fluid falls into the chest. If there is a tear in the pleura, a 19 French Blake drain is placed into the chest through the tear. This can be connected to a pleura vac overnight.

Once the wound is irrigated and hemostasis is confirmed, the wound is closed with three layers of an absorbable suture. The deep layer is approximated with a 2-0 absorbable suture in an interrupted fashion. A superficial layer is closed with 3-0 absorbable suture, and the skin is completed with a single layer of absorbable monofilament suture. Dermal glue can be placed as well.

POSTOPERATIVE CARE Postoperative pain control is the main issue in most cases. Multimodal therapy for pain control should be used, including anti-inflammatories, lidocaine patches, and heat/ice. Opioid narcotics can be used but should be tapered appropriately, and patients may need to be sent home on a short course. Patients with long-standing pain on chronic opioids may need to go home on a higher dose with instructions to taper over 6 weeks.

When a drain is placed in the chest for a pleural tear, it can be transitioned from suction to water seal overnight. If a repeat chest x-ray on postoperative day 1 shows no evidence of a pneumothorax, the drain can be removed.

All patients should be started in TOS-specific physical therapy within 7 to 10 days after surgery. This includes soft tissue work to prevent scarring around the brachial plexus and mobilization work to ensure patients have a full range. Physical therapy should continue for 4 to 6 weeks to ensure the patient returns to optimal function and to limit long-term recurrent symptoms. ■

REFERENCES

1. Orlando MS, Likes KC, Mirza S, et al. A decade of excellent outcomes after surgical intervention in 538 patients with thoracic outlet syndrome. *J Am Coll Surg*. 2015;220(5):934-939. doi:10.1016/j.jamcollsurg.2014.12.046

2. Roos DB. Transaxillary approach for first rib resection to relieve thoracic outlet syndrome. *Ann Surg*. 1966;163(3):354-358.

3. Glass C, Dugan M, Gillespie D, Doyle A, Illig K. Costoclavicular venous decompression in patients with threatened arteriovenous hemodialysis access. *Ann Vasc Surg*. 2011;25(5):640-645. doi:10.1016/j.avsg.2010.12.020

4. Jayaraj A, Duncan AA, Kalra M, Bower TC, Gloviczki P. Outcomes of transaxillary approach to cervical and first-rib resection for neurogenic thoracic outlet syndrome. *Ann Vasc Surg*. 2018;51:147-149. doi:10.1016/j.avsg.2018.02.029

5. Urschel HC, Patel AN. Surgery remains the most effective treatment for Paget-Schroetter syndrome: 50 years' experience. *Ann Thorac Surg*. 2008;86(1):254-260; discussion 260. doi:10.1016/j.athoracsur.2008.03.021

6. Kim TI, Orion KC. Advanced Surgical techniques in venous thoracic outlet syndrome. In: Illig KA, Thompson RW, Freischlag JA, et al., eds. *Thoracic Outlet Syndrome*. Springer International Publishing; 2021: 627-634. doi:10.1007/978-3-030-55073-8_69

25-3

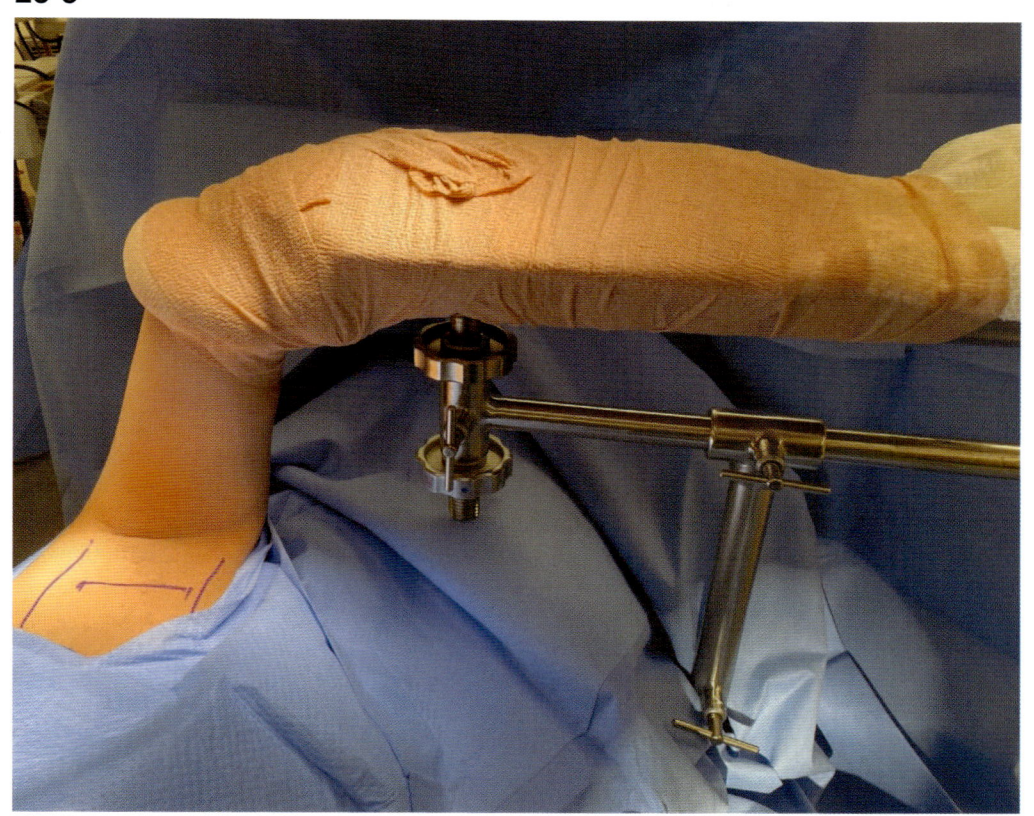

25-4

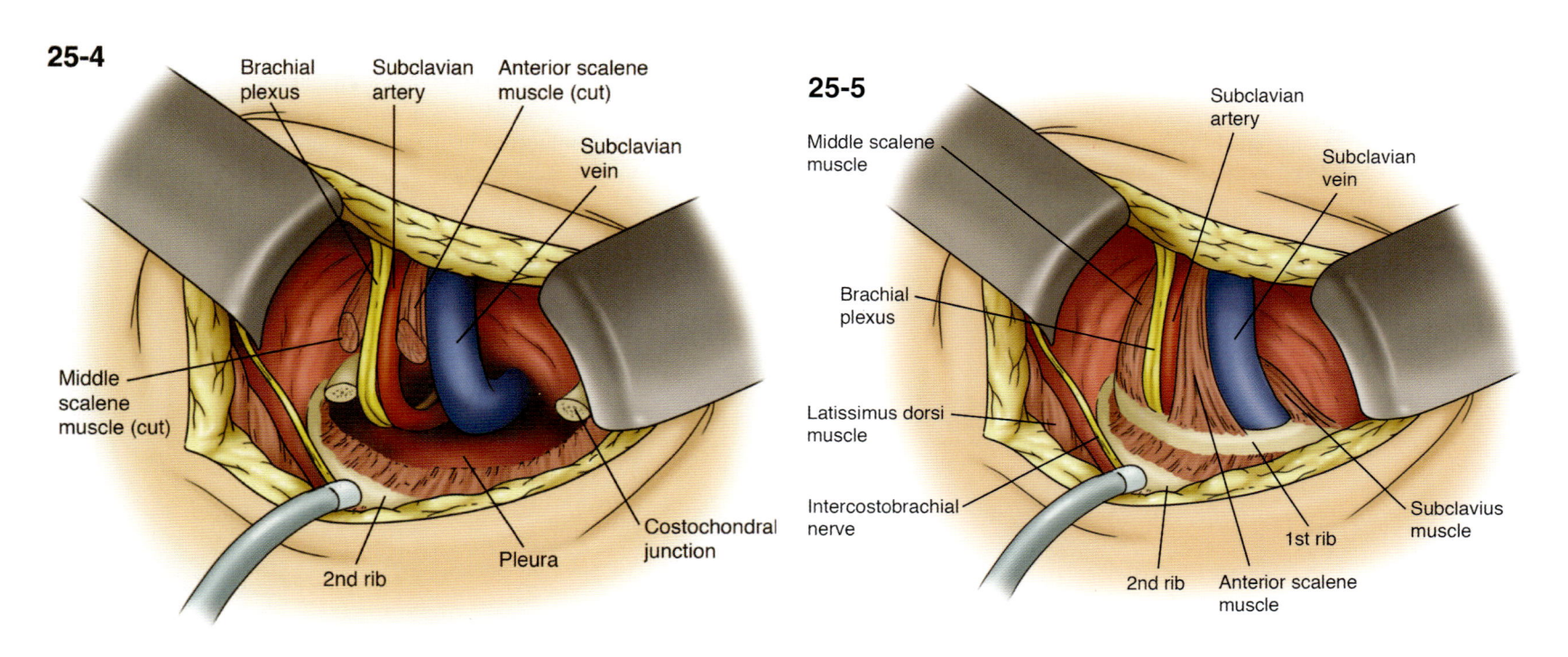

25-5

25-6

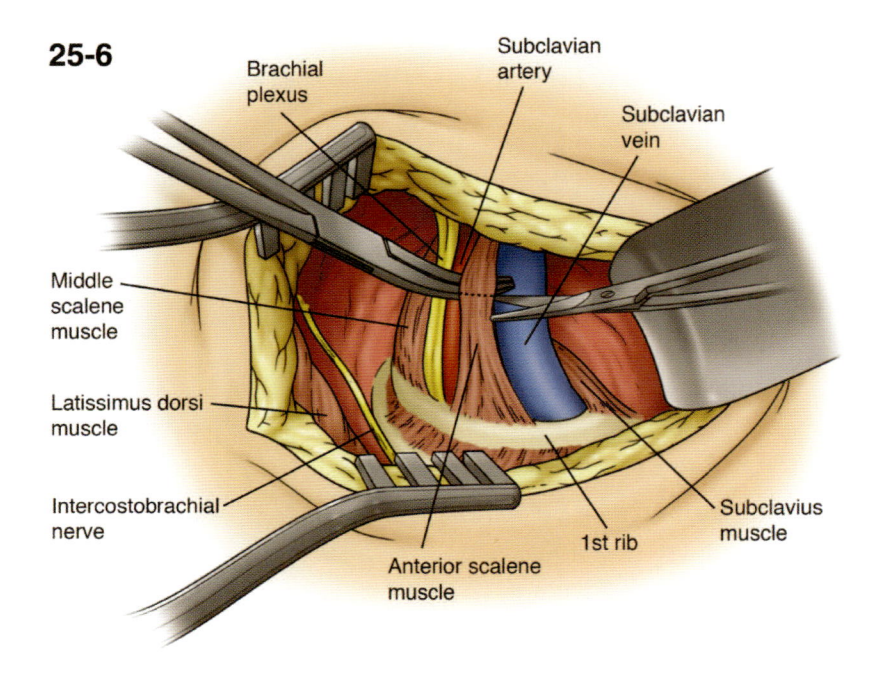

PARACLAVICULAR APPROACHES FOR VENOUS AND ARTERIAL THORACIC OUTLET SYNDROME

Momodou L. Jammeh, MD • Robert W. Thompson, MD

INTRODUCTION Thoracic outlet syndrome (TOS) is an umbrella term that encompasses three distinct conditions: (1) *neurogenic TOS*, caused by compression of the brachial plexus nerve roots within the scalene triangle and/or subcoracoid space; (2) *venous TOS*, caused by compression of the central subclavian vein that can result in the axillary-subclavian vein effort thrombosis syndrome; and (3) *arterial TOS*, caused by chronic compression of the subclavian artery in association with a bony abnormality, leading to post-stenotic arterial dilatation, aneurysm formation, and potential thromboembolism.

Surgical treatment for each form of TOS can be accomplished by anterior or transaxillary approaches, depending on the scope and goals of the operation and the training, experience, and preferences of the individual surgeon. Successful surgical treatment of TOS depends on the sound understanding of the relationships between the musculoskeletal and neurovascular structures in this region, as well as the many anatomical variations likely to be encountered. This chapter is focused on operations that involve "paraclavicular" approaches, with incisions above and below the clavicle, in the treatment of TOS. One of the principal advantages of these approaches is the excellent exposure of the relevant anatomy, allowing more complete decompression and operative management compared to alternative approaches.

PARACLAVICULAR DECOMPRESSION FOR TOS

INDICATIONS: Patients that require both a supraclavicular and infraclavicular incision for TOS will have a venous or arterial TOS pathology. Venous TOS usually presents with axillary-subclavian vein "effort thrombosis," for which upper extremity contrast venography is performed with thrombolysis to reveal focal subclavian vein stenosis or occlusion at the level of the first rib. Surgical decompression with first rib resection is recommended for patients who remain symptomatic despite anticoagulation and restricted activity, as well as those in whom long-term anticoagulation and restrictions on upper extremity activity are undesirable. The paraclavicular approach to venous TOS combines the supraclavicular approach (similar to that for neurogenic TOS) with an infraclavicular exposure, to ensure complete resection of the entire first rib and to facilitate potential axillary-subclavian vein reconstruction when needed.

Arterial TOS is characterized by compressive pathology of the subclavian artery, typically with formation of a post-stenotic subclavian artery aneurysm, and almost always occurs in association with a cervical rib or anomalous first rib. Subclavian artery aneurysms usually arise within several centimeters of the scalene triangle where the subclavian artery crosses over the cervical and first ribs and underneath the clavicle. These lesions are frequently complicated by intimal ulceration, mural thrombus, and distal thromboembolism regardless of size or any potential for rupture. In patients suspected to have arterial TOS, the presence or absence of a subclavian artery aneurysm and the presence of bony abnormality is readily assessed by contrast-enhanced computed tomography or magnetic resonance imaging (**FIGURE 26-1**). Similar imaging studies can be performed in patients who have presented with upper extremity arterial thromboembolism to detect a proximal source of embolism in the subclavian artery. In extensive arterial degeneration, a paraclavicular approach can be utilized.

ANESTHESIA AND POSITION: Anticoagulation is discontinued 24 hours prior to operation and a local anesthesia regional block (erector spinae plane and cervical plexus) is performed in the preoperative holding area. The operation is conducted under general endotracheal anesthesia with the patient in a supine position on a fluoroscopy-compatible table. The neck, upper chest, and affected upper extremity are prepped and draped into the field. To facilitate intraoperative venography in venous TOS, the basilic vein is accessed under ultrasound guidance and a 4-French vascular access sheath is placed just above the elbow. An initial venogram is performed with contrast injection, fluoroscopic imaging, and digital subtraction technique, to help anticipate the need for subclavian vein reconstruction. **CONTINUES** ▶

26-1

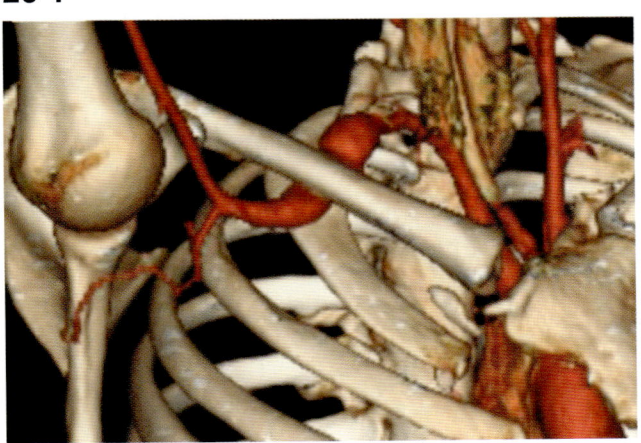

PARACLAVICULAR DECOMPRESSION FOR TOS *INCISION AND EXPOSURE:* CONTINUED A transverse supraclavicular neck incision is made parallel to the clavicle, from the lateral border of the sternocleidomastoid muscle to the anterior border of the trapezius muscle. Subplatysmal flaps are created, the scalene fat pad is mobilized, and the omohyoid muscle is divided. For resection of first rib near the manubrium a separate medial infraclavicular incision is made (**FIGURE 26-2A**). In arterial reconstruction requiring an infraclavicular incision, this incision is more lateral.

DETAILS OF PROCEDURE

PARACLAVICULAR VENOUS DECOMPRESSION: Supraclavicular decompression is initially performed as described in Chapter 25, up to the point when the posterior first rib has been divided. Instead of dividing the anterior first rib from the supraclavicular exposure, a second transverse skin incision is made one fingerbreadth below the medial clavicle. The upper and middle portions of the pectoralis major muscle are spread to expose the anteromedial portion of the first rib. By applying downward fingertip pressure to the divided end of the posterior first rib from the supraclavicular incision, the attachments between the medial first rib and clavicle are placed under tension and the superior edge of the first rib is dissected from its soft tissue attachments through the infraclavicular incision (**FIGURE 26-2B**). After dividing the subclavius muscle tendon, the costoclavicular ligament, and the muscles of the first intercostal space under direct vision (protecting the subclavian vein) (**FIGURE 26-2C**), the first rib can be divided at its sternal edge using a duck-billed rongeur. The entire first rib is then removed from the operative field as a single specimen.

Once the axillary vein is identified through the infraclavicular exposure underneath the clavicle, it is carefully separated from the subclavius muscle and the subclavius muscle is resected along the underside of the clavicle (**FIGURE 26-2D**). The axillary vein is then traced laterally to ensure exposure of a soft compressible segment of vein. If there is chronic occlusion of the subclavicular axillary vein, the infraclavicular exposure can be extended to allow division of the pectoralis minor muscle, in order to further decompress the distal axillary vein and provide exposure for possible vein reconstruction.

Attention is returned to the supraclavicular exposure for further exposure of the subclavian vein, gradually tracing the vein medially toward its junction with the internal jugular and innominate veins. There are typically one or two collateral veins arising from the subclavian vein underneath the medial clavicle, which must be ligated and divided to permit the subclavian vein to fall away from the clavicle. The internal jugular vein is fully exposed above its junction with the subclavian vein, and the innominate vein is exposed into the upper mediastinum. The course of the phrenic nerve is identified as it passes underneath the subclavian vein into the upper mediastinum, and the nerve is protected.

External Venolysis and Intraoperative Venography Once the complete path of the axillary-subclavian vein has been exposed, circumferential external venolysis is completed by excising any residual scar tissue surrounding the vein. When the underlying vein is soft to palpation and easily compressible, with evidence of rapid filling and emptying during respiratory variation, it is likely that no further venous reconstruction is necessary. Using the previously-placed vascular access, an intraoperative contrast venogram is performed to verify that the axillary-subclavian vein is patent with rapid flow to the innominate vein and no filling of collateral pathways. In this event, the operation is completed and the wounds are closed.

Subclavian Vein Reconstruction Additional subclavian vein reconstruction is indicated when external venolysis alone does not alleviate subclavian vein obstruction or when intraoperative venography demonstrates a high-grade residual stenosis despite external venolysis. Systemic anticoagulation is achieved with intravenous heparin, and the distal subclavian (or axillary) vein and the internal jugular vein are controlled with angled DeBakey clamps. The innominate vein is controlled by placement of pediatric Satinsky or spoon clamp through the infraclavicular exposure (**FIGURE 26-2E**), which is then placed around the upper portion of the innominate vein as visualized through the supraclavicular exposure, thereby keeping the clamp handle out of the way. A longitudinal venotomy is created along the superior aspect of the subclavian vein, extending from the normal distal vein, through the stenotic area, and into the normal subclavian-jugular-innominate vein junction. When the luminal surface is relatively smooth and thrombus-free, a simple vein patch angioplasty is performed with either bovine pericardium or a segment of cryopreserved femoral vein allograft. It is important that the patch angioplasty be constructed along the entire length of the affected vessel, proximal and distal to the stenotic segment, usually with extension into the anteromedial aspect of the jugular-innominate vein junction

When the subclavian vein is chronically occluded, when the subclavian vein wall is densely fibrotic despite external venolysis, or when there is extensive surface ulceration and mural thrombus upon inspecting the lumen, the affected segment of the subclavian vein is excised and replaced by an interposition bypass. Our preference has been to use a cryopreserved femoral vein allograft (10–12 mm diameter).

THE GATEWAYS FOR THIS PROCEDURE ARE:

1. Secure a vascular sheath in the basilic/brachial vein for intraoperative venography.
2. From the supraclavicular incision, reflect the scalene fat pad laterally to visualize the operative field exposing the internal jugular vein, anterior scalene muscle, phrenic nerve, brachial plexus, subclavian artery, middle scalene muscle, and long thoracic nerve.
3. Complete supraclavicular decompression as for neurogenic TOS, stopping after division of the posterior first rib.
4. Use transverse infraclavicular incision to split the pectoralis major muscle, expose the anterior first rib to the sternum, and divide the insertion of the subclavius muscle tendon while pressing down upon the divided end of the posterior first rib from the supraclavicular incision.
5. Divide the medial first rib at the edge of the sternum with a duck-billed rongeur, then complete detachment of intercostal muscles and remove the entire first rib.
6. Expose the axillary vein under the clavicle and resect the subclavius muscle.
7. Return to the supraclavicular exposure to complete external venolysis to the junction of the subclavian, jugular, and innominate veins.
8. For subclavian vein reconstruction, place the innominate vein clamp from the infraclavicular incision and open the subclavian vein to the jugular-innominate vein junction.
9. For subclavian vein patch angioplasty, ensure a smooth intimal surface and attach a wide segment of bovine pericardium to the vein wall margins.
10. For subclavian vein bypass, open a wide oval at the innominate junction and perform the central anastomosis first, then pass the bypass graft underneath the clavicle to the axillary vein for an end-to-side distal anastomosis. If needed for distal exposure and control of the axillary vein, extend the infraclavicular incision and perform pectoralis minor tenotomy. CONTINUES

26-2

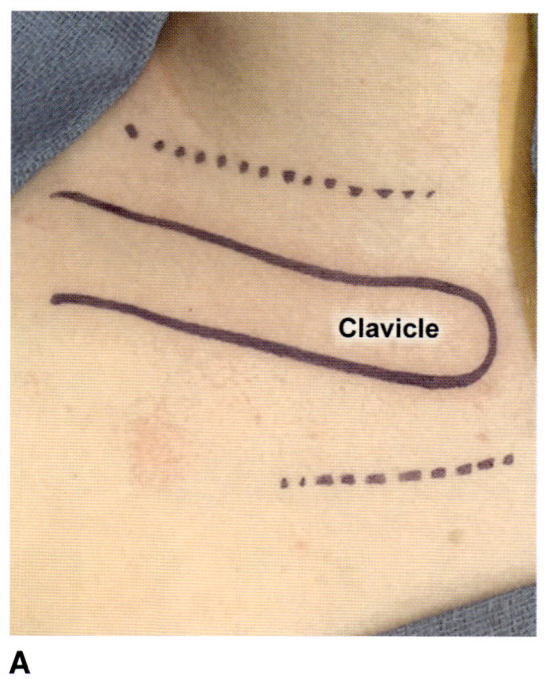

A

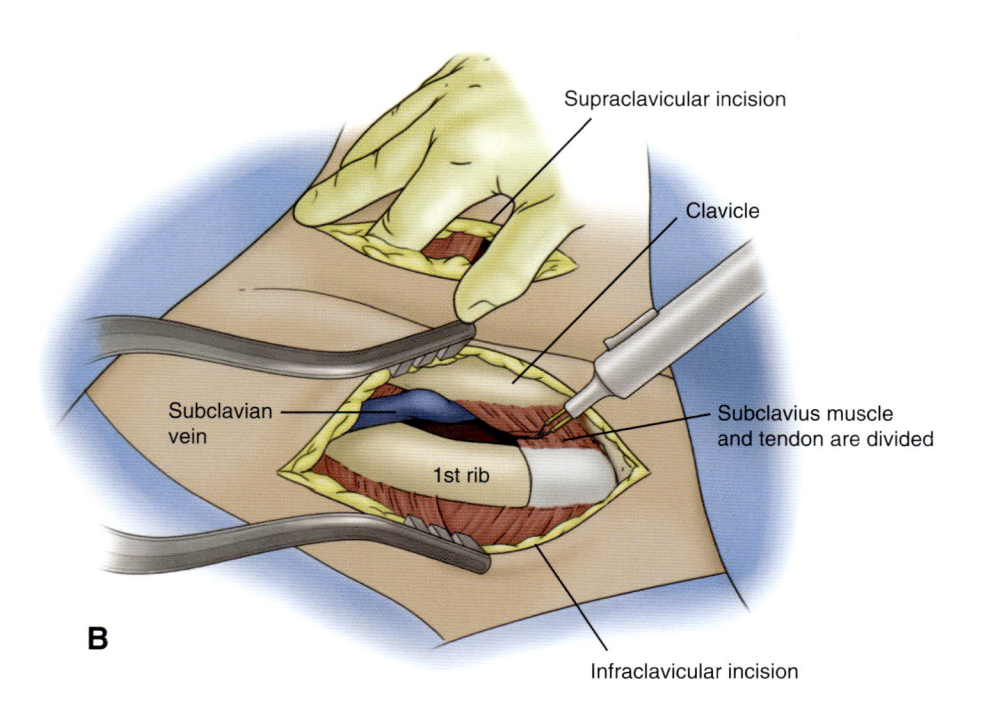

Supraclavicular incision

Clavicle

Subclavian vein

1st rib

Subclavius muscle and tendon are divided

B

Infraclavicular incision

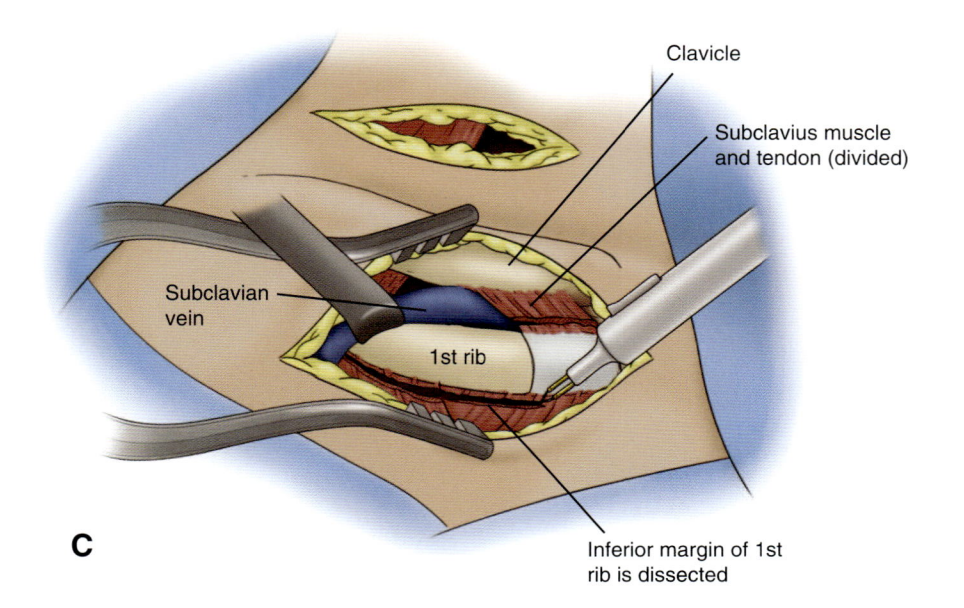

Clavicle

Subclavius muscle and tendon (divided)

Subclavian vein

1st rib

C

Inferior margin of 1st rib is dissected

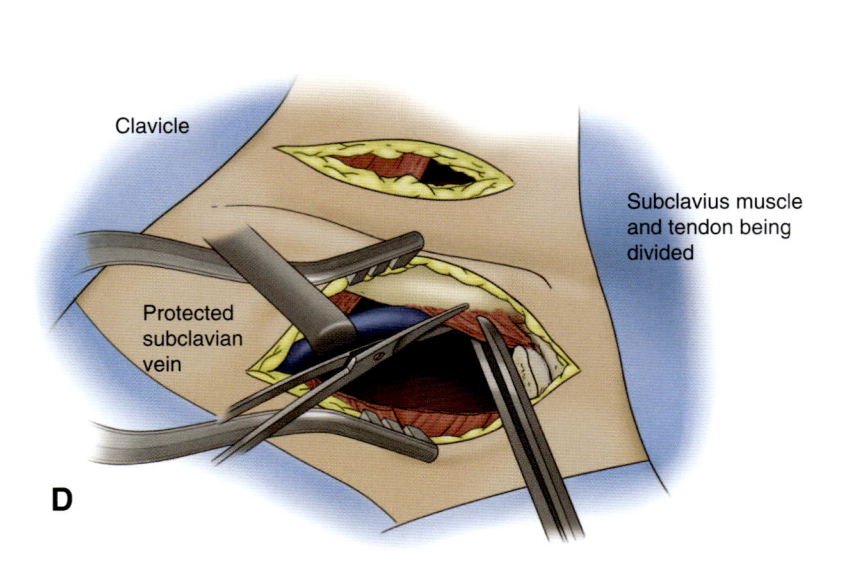

Clavicle

Protected subclavian vein

Subclavius muscle and tendon being divided

D

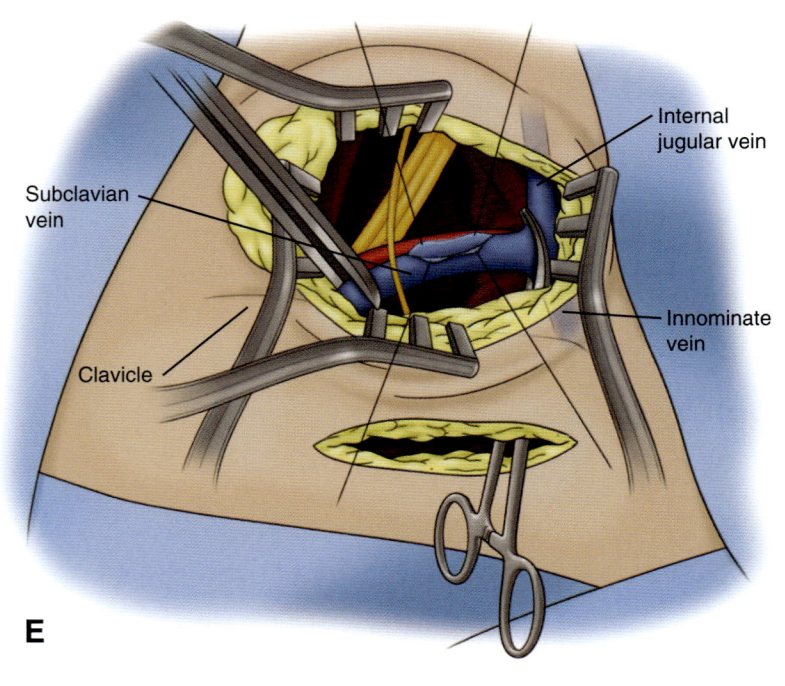

Subclavian vein

Clavicle

Internal jugular vein

Innominate vein

E

PARACLAVICULAR ARTERIAL DECOMPRESSION Decompression is performed as described above. Once the scalene fat pad has been mobilized, the dilatation in the subclavian artery is typically evident immediately lateral to the anterior scalene muscle (**FIGURE 26-3**. Neck is to the left. ASM, anterior scalene muscle; SCA, subclavian artery; BPN, brachial plexus). The scalene muscles are removed, followed by resection of the cervical and first ribs (**FIGURE 26-4**. CR, cervical rib; FR, first rib). The subclavian artery is mobilized and assessed by measuring the diameter of any post-stenotic dilatation, with an aneurysm defined as a diameter at least twice greater than the adjacent normal subclavian artery. If the artery does not meet criteria for aneurysmal dilatation and there is no mural thrombus, ulceration, or previous emboli, the operation is completed without arterial repair.

When arterial repair is indicated, the artery is mobilized in preparation for interposition graft repair of the aneurysmal segment. Distal control of the subclavian artery can often be obtained by elevating the subclavicular portion of the vessel into the supraclavicular exposure to allow clamp control within the same operative field and avoiding a paraclavicular approach. In the event that satisfactory distal control of the normal subclavian artery cannot be obtained from the supraclavicular exposure alone, a second transverse infraclavicular incision is made, encompassing the "paraclavicular" nature of the procedure. This is carried through the fascia between the clavicle and pectoralis major muscle to the axillary space, usually with division of the pectoralis minor muscle tendon (**FIGURE 26-5**), and the axillary artery is isolated for distal vascular control. **CONTINUES ▶**

26-3

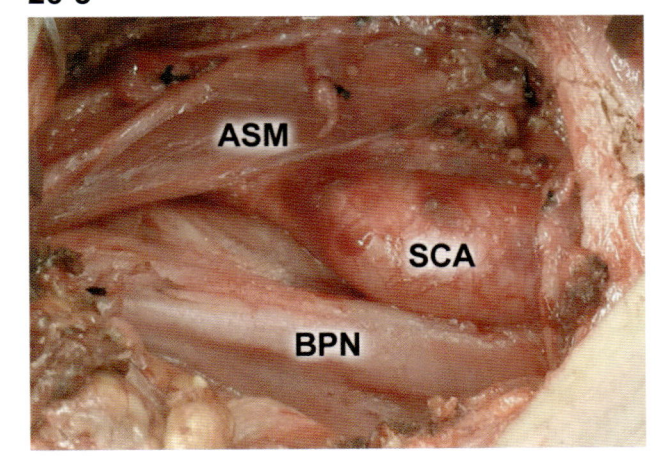

26-4

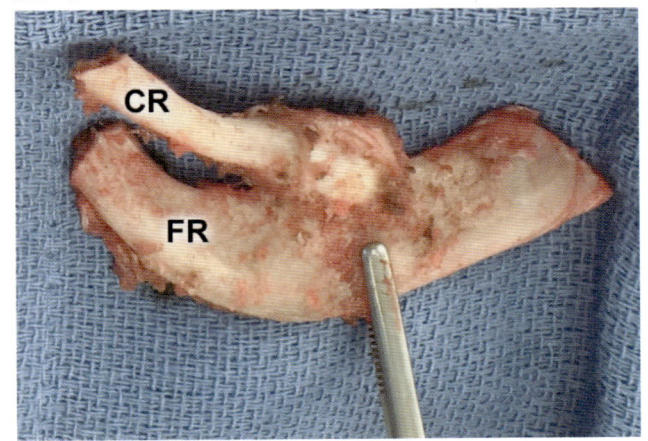

26-5

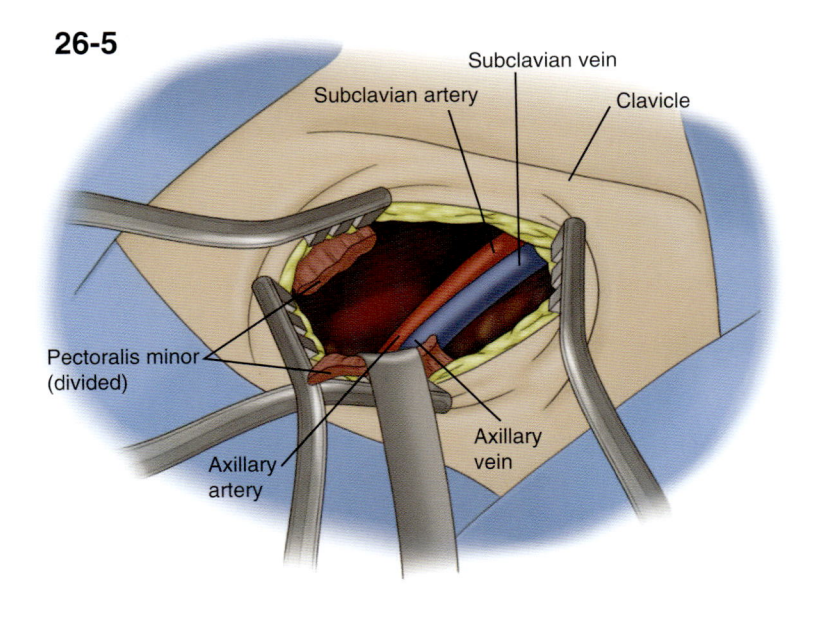

PARACLAVICULAR ARTERIAL DECOMPRESSION `CONTINUED` After systemic anticoagulation with intravenous heparin, an angled DeBakey clamp is placed on the proximal subclavian artery immediately distal to the vertebral artery and the distal subclavian artery is clamped immediately beyond the aneurysm. After excision of the intervening segment of aneurysmal subclavian artery, the opened aneurysm often reveals a focal area of ulceration, with or without mural thrombus (FIGURE 26-6). An interposition bypass graft is created for direct reconstruction of the subclavian artery using beveled end-to-end anastomoses (FIGURE 26-7). BPG, bypass graft; BPN, brachial plexus). Such reconstructions may be performed using reversed autologous saphenous vein grafts, but these conduits are often too small in caliber for subclavian artery replacement. Other conduits that may be more suitable for this type of reconstruction include polyester or polytetrafluoroethylene prosthetic grafts, cryopreserved femoral artery allografts, or autologous grafts (e.g., superficial femoral vein or iliac artery). Following arterial reconstruction, a completion arteriogram may be performed to evaluate the subclavian artery bypass graft, with the arm placed in different positions, and to reassess the distal circulation.

THE GATEWAYS FOR ARTERIAL PARACLAVICULAR APPROACH ARE:

1. From a supraclavicular incision, reflect the scalene fat pad laterally to visualize the operative field exposing the internal jugular vein, anterior scalene muscle, phrenic nerve, brachial plexus, subclavian artery, middle scalene muscle, and long thoracic nerve.
2. Complete anterior and middle scalenectomy as for neurogenic TOS.
3. Divide the posterior portion of the cervical rib and then the posterior portion of the first rib.
4. Divide the anterior portion of the first rib proximal to the junction between the cervical and first ribs, and remove the combined bony specimen intact.
5. Mobilize the subclavian artery to lift the distal artery from under the clavicle, into the supraclavicular operative field, to allow clamp control of the distal artery immediately beyond the aneurysm and the normal artery immediately past the vertebral artery origin.
6. If necessary, make a second infraclavicular incision and perform pectoralis minor tenotomy to expose and clamp the axillary artery beyond the subclavian artery aneurysm.
7. Excise the subclavian artery aneurysm and inspect the opened specimen lumen for ulceration and mural thrombus.
8. Perform interposition bypass graft repair, with the distal end-to-end anastomosis created first, then allowing the distal subclavian artery to retract under the clavicle once the anastomosis is hemostatic and replace the clamp on the bypass graft.
9. Complete the proximal end-to-end anastomosis, remove clamps, and restore arterial flow.
10. Assess the distal circulation of the arm and hand and perform intraoperative arteriography if necessary.

CLOSURE A closed-suction drain is placed through a separate stab wound in the neck and placed into the supraclavicular field extending into the upper posterior pleural space. A second infraclavicular drain is placed after a pectoralis minor tenotomy has been performed for axillary-subclavian vein reconstruction. The scalene fat pad is then reapproximated to the edge of the sternocleidomastoid muscle and periclavicular fascia. The edges of the platysma muscle are reapproximated with interrupted sutures, and the skin is closed with a subcuticular stitch. After reapproximating the pectoralis major muscle fascia with interrupted sutures, the infraclavicular incision is closed in a similar manner.

POSTOPERATIVE CARE/FOLLOW-UP An upright chest x-ray is obtained in the recovery room and each morning after surgery. The closed suction drain is monitored and removed when daily serous fluid output is less than 100 mL. Following surgery for venous TOS, patients are maintained on continuous intravenous Dextran for 48 hours and then switched to intravenous heparin to achieve therapeutic levels of anticoagulation by postoperative day 3. Arterial TOS patients require antiplatelet therapy.

Physical therapy is resumed the day after surgery and continued with home exercises upon hospital discharge. Patients with venous TOS are prescribed an oral anticoagulant at hospital discharge, which will be continued up to 12 weeks after operation, after which anticoagulation is discontinued with resumption of unrestricted normal activities.

SUGGESTED READINGS

Akhmerov A, Thompson RW, Azizzadeh A. Clinical presentation and patient evaluation in arterial thoracic outlet syndrome. In: Illig KA, Thompson RW, Freischlag JA, Donahue DM, Jordan SE, Lum, YW, Gelabert HA, eds. *Thoracic Outlet Syndrome (TOS)*. 2nd ed. Switzerland: Springer Nature; 2021:743-749.

Brownie ER, Abuirqeba AA, Ohman JW, Rubin BG, Thompson RW. False-negative upper extremity ultrasound in the initial evaluation of patients with suspected subclavian vein thrombosis due to thoracic outlet syndrome (Paget-Schroetter syndrome). *J Vasc Surg Venous Lymphat Disord*. 2020;8:118-126.

Caputo FJ, Wittenberg AM, Vemuri C, Driskill MR, Earley JA, Rastogi R, et al. Supraclavicular decompression for neurogenic thoracic outlet syndrome in adolescent and adult populations. *J Vasc Surg*. 2013;57(1):149-157.

Cook JR, Thompson RW. Evaluation and management of venous thoracic outlet syndrome. *Thorac Surg Clin*. 2021;33(1):27-44.

Dadashzadeh ER, Ohman JW, Kavali PK, Henderson KM, Goestenkors DM, Thompson RW. Venographic classification and treatment outcomes for axillary-subclavian vein thrombosis due to venous thoracic outlet syndrome. *J Vasc Surg*. 2023;77(3):879-889.

Goeteyn J, Pesser N, van Sambeek MRHM, Thompson RW, van Neunen BFL, Teijink JAW. Duplex ultrasound studies are neither necessary or sufficient for the diagnosis of neurogenic thoracic outlet syndrome. *Ann Vasc Surg*. 2022;81:232-239.

Illig KA, Donahue D, Duncan A, Freischlag J, Gelabert H, Johansen K, Jordan S, Sanders R, Thompson RW. Reporting standards of the Society for Vascular Surgery for thoracic outlet syndrome. *J Vasc Surg*. 2016;64:e23-e35.

Sheng GG, Duwayri YM, Emery VB, Wittenberg AM, Moriarty CT, Thompson RW. Costochondral calcification, osteophytic degeneration, and occult first rib fractures in patients with venous thoracic outlet syndrome. *J Vasc Surg*. 2012;55(5):1363-1369.

Thompson RW. Complications of surgery for thoracic outlet syndrome. In: Hans SS, Conrad M, eds. *Vascular and Endovascular Complications: A Practical Approach*. Abingdon, CRC Press, Taylor & Francis Group; 2021:233-245.

Thompson RW. Comprehensive management of subclavian vein effort thrombosis. *Semin Intervent Radiol*. 2012;29(1):44-51.

Thompson RW: Management of digital emboli, vasospasm, and ischemia. In: Illig KA, Thompson RW, Freischlag JA, Donahue DM, Jordan SE, Lum, YW, Gelabert HA, eds. *Thoracic Outlet Syndrome (TOS)*. 2nd ed. Switzerland: Springer Nature; 2021:817-826.

Thompson RW, Ohman JW: Surgical techniques: operative decompression using the supraclavicular approach for neurogenic thoracic outlet syndrome. In: Illig KA, Thompson RW, Freischlag JA, Donahue DM, Jordan SE, Lum, YW, Gelabert HA, eds. *Thoracic Outlet Syndrome (TOS)*. 2nd ed. Switzerland: Springer Nature; 2021:265-285.

Thompson RW, Ohman JW: Surgical techniques: operative decompression using the paraclavicular approach for venous thoracic outlet syndrome. In: Illig KA, Thompson RW, Freischlag JA, Donahue DM, Jordan SE, Lum, YW, Gelabert HA, eds. *Thoracic Outlet Syndrome (TOS)*. 2nd ed. Switzerland: Springer Nature; 2021:591-616.

Vemuri C, McLaughlin LN, Abuirqeba AA, Thompson RW. Clinical presentation and management of arterial thoracic outlet syndrome. *J Vasc Surg*. 2017;65:1429-1439.

Vemuri C, Salehi P, Benarroch-Gampel J, McLaughlin LN, Thompson RW. Diagnosis and treatment of effort-induced thrombosis of the axillary subclavian vein due to venous thoracic outlet syndrome. *J Vasc Surg Venous Lymphat Disord*. 2016;4(4):485-500.

26-6

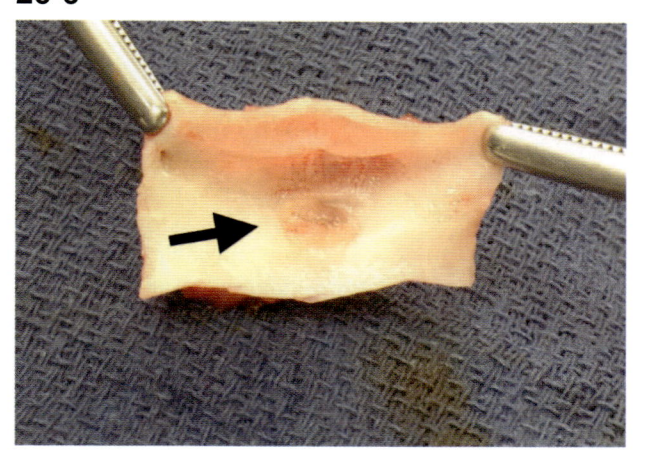

26-7

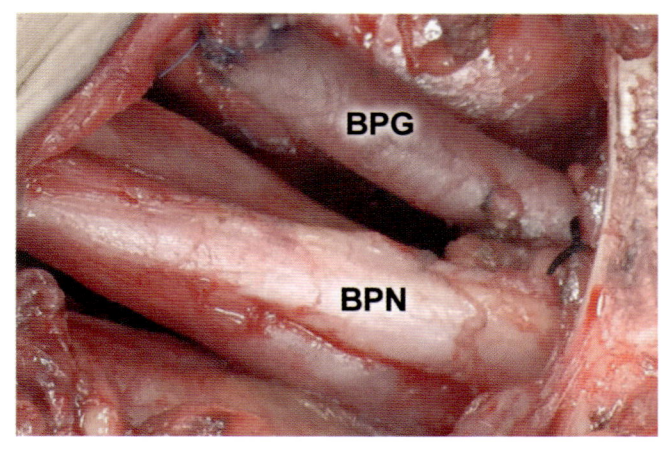

Endovascular Management of Paget-Schroetter Syndrome: Endo, Thrombolysis

Mark Ajalat, MD • Karl Illig, MD • Hugh Gelabert, MD

INTRODUCTION

BACKGROUND: Paget-Schroetter syndrome (PSS) refers to spontaneous thrombosis of the subclavian vein (SCV). The syndrome was named in 1946 by ESR Hughes after combining 300 cases of spontaneous SCV DVT. He named the syndrome after the two physicians who independently first described such cases—Sir James Paget (1886) and Leopold von Schroetter (1889). PSS was recognized as the venous presentation of thoracic outlet syndrome (TOS) in 1956 when the term TOS was coined by Peet.

PATHOPHYSIOLOGY AND ANATOMY: The pathophysiology of PSS involves extrinsic compression of the SCV as it crosses the thoracic outlet where it is bounded by the clavicle and the first rib (FIGURE 27-1). The fist rib is elevated against the clavicle by both the anterior scalene muscle and the subclavius muscle which bracket the SCV. Hypertrophy of these muscles results in reduction of the venous channel through which the SCV courses, impinging on its lumen leading to compression.

The motion of the clavicle and first rib, which is associated with use of the arm, results in periodic compression. This repeated compression causes trauma to the SCV, resulting in fibrosis of the vein wall. Due to this fibrosis, it is common for a partial SCV stenosis to remain in the vein even after surgical decompression. This is the reason that post-decompression venography and angioplasty are necessary.

DIAGNOSIS

The diagnosis of PSS is most often accomplished based on history, exam, and noninvasive testing. The typical history is of acute swelling, pain, and discoloration of the entire affected limb. Often this occurs in the context of an active individual engaged in athletic or physical activity. Physical exam findings include bluish discoloration, swelling of the limb, venous congestion with distension of veins, and prominent venous collaterals across the shoulder and chest. Coexistence of neurological findings is noted in about 15% of cases.

Ultrasound examination is commonly performed to assess possible SCV thrombosis. In such instances where symptoms suggest SCV occlusion and the ultrasound fails to confirm the diagnosis, a CT venogram, MR venogram, or catheter venogram are recommended.

Endovascular techniques (EVT) play a significant role in diagnosis and treatment of PSS. Catheter venography is the gold standard for diagnosis of PSS. Venography coupled with intravenous ultrasound (IVUS) provides the most definitive assessment of the SCV.

Findings that confirm acute PSS include occlusion of the SCV with absence of contrast flowing across the thoracic outlet. Ample collateral veins may be noted coursing around the occluded segment, returning flow to the central veins, most often via the jugular vein. Venography in the setting of chronic PSS may demonstrate post-phlebitic changes with irregular vein wall contours, severe narrowing, ample collateralization, or segmental occlusions (FIGURE 27-2). Positional venography with the arm in neutral and abducted positions may identify compression of the SCV at the thoracic outlet. A benefit of catheter venography is that it allows direct transition to endovascular treatment of the acute thrombus.

INDICATIONS

The presence of thombus in SCV the acute setting (within 14 days of symptom onset) is an established indication for catheter directed threapy. Thrombolysis performed within 14 days of presentation is very effective, while thrombolysis for subacute and chronic thrombosis is not very effective.

PREOPERATIVE PREPARATION

Patients who present with acute PSS and subclavian vein thrombosis should be started on therapeutic anticoagulation. Lytic therapy is contraindicated in the setting of active internal bleeding, cerebral infarction, neurologic/ophthalmologic procedures within 3 months, recent surgery, or known intracranial tumor.

ANESTHESIA

Anesthesia provided for thrombolysis or venography depends on the patient's ability to cooperate during the procedure. If able to follow commands and remain still for the procedure, it is preferred to perform thrombolysis under local anesthesia or monitored anesthesia care (MAC).

POSITION AND OPERATIVE PREPARATION

Patients are placed in the supine position with the ipsilateral arm prepped in its entirety up to the chest wall. Additionally, bilateral groins should be prepped in the event that the occlusion cannot be crossed from the ipsilateral arm. Intravascular ultrasound should be available to assess the quality and structure of the vein.

DETAILS OF PROCEDURE

THROMBOLYSIS AND PHARMACOMECHANICAL THROMBECTOMY IN ACUTE PSS: The preferred access site for venography is the ipsilateral basilic vein just above the antecubital fossa performed under ultrasound guidance. If the basilic vien is inaccessible, access to the brachial vein above the antecubital fossa is another option. A micropuncture 21-gauge needle followed by an 0.018 micro wire is used, confirming wire entry into the vein with the ultrasound. A micro sheath is exchanged and diagnostic venogram of the access site is performed to confirm proper entry into the vein. This is exchanged over a 0.035″ bentson wire for a 5 French short sheath. Diagnostic venography of the upper extremity should include views of the arm (brachial vein, axillary vein), the thoracic outlet (subclavian vein), and the chest (superior vena cava).

Combination of a KMP catheter and floppy glide wire is used to cross the area of occlusion and advance into the superior vena cava. Inability to do so may indicate an instance of acute on chronic thrombus. Caution should be taken with a stiff glide wire as this has a propensity to cause perforation in upper extremity venous structures. Long sheaths for added support and femoral access (snaring a wire from retrograde access) may be of assistance when crossing difficult lesions. On-table lysis may be performed with 2 to 4 mg tPA administered through the extent of the thrombus.

The lysis catheter should be placed across the area of the thrombus, extending into the thoracic outlet. We prefer to use a Cragg-McNamara valved infusion catheter, with size and infusion length depending on the length and site of occlusion.

In addition to thrombolysis, percutaneous pharmacomechanical thrombectomy may be performed to accelerate the dissolution of thrombus in the SCV. AngioJet is one peripheral thrombectomy system that has the ability to perform active aspiration and power pulse delivery using physician-modified solution including lytic agents. The Penumbra Indigo System is another commonly used mechanical thrombectomy device that employs solely aspiration techniques.

Our lysis protocol includes the following: 400 to 500 units/hr heparin infusion through the sheath and 0.5 to 1 mg/hr tPA through the infusion catheter. Patients should be admitted to the ICU postoperatively for serial neurovascular exams as well as serial CBC and fibrinogen q 6 hours. Should the fibrinogen drop by half the initial value or have an absolute value less than 150, the tPA rate is cut by half. Should the patient develop any bleeding episodes or if fibrinogen <100, tPA should be discontinued and cryoprecipitate should be administered. Serial monitoring of the PTT is not necessary, as the dose is subtherapeutic and is used for purposes of sheath patency. The patient should return to the angio suite within 24 hours for repeat venogram. CONTINUES ▶

27-1

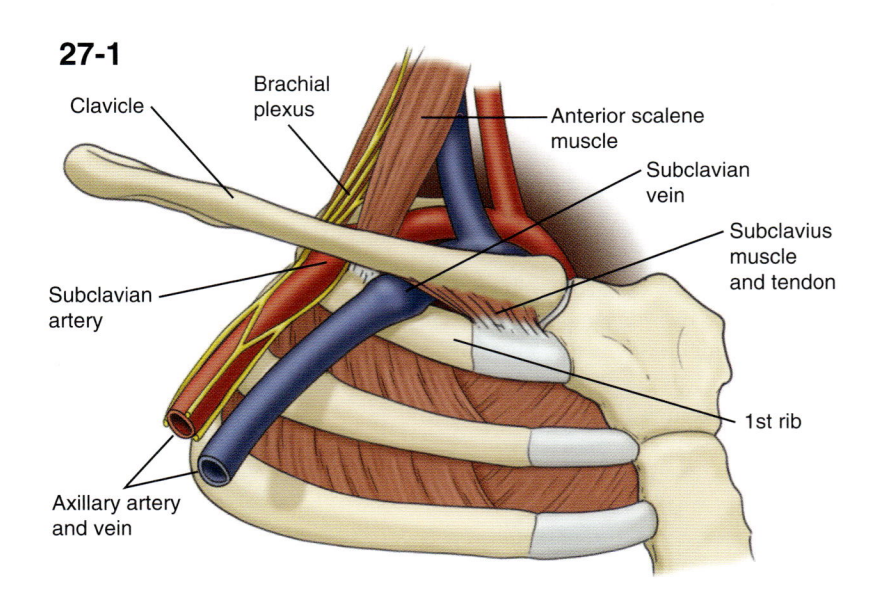

Clavicle

Brachial plexus

Anterior scalene muscle

Subclavian vein

Subclavius muscle and tendon

Subclavian artery

1st rib

Axillary artery and vein

27-2

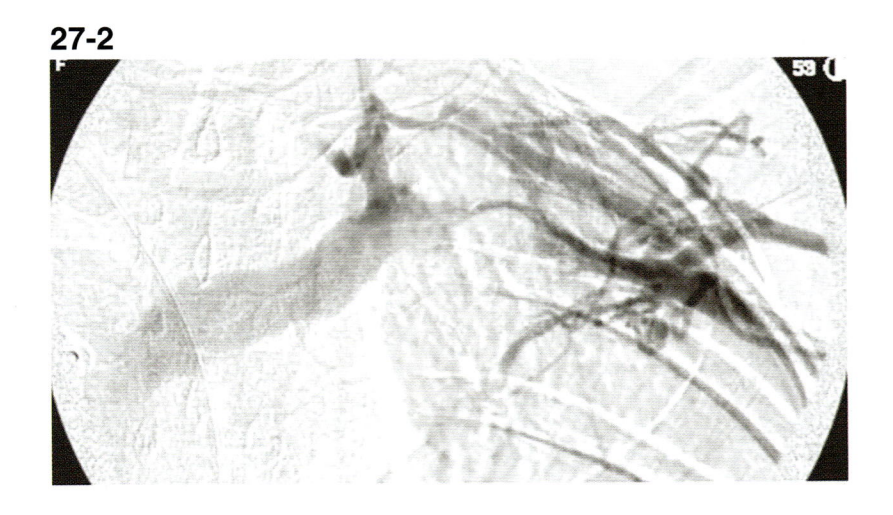

DETAILS OF PROCEDURE *POST-LYSIS VENOGRAPHY:* CONTINUED
Repeat venogram should be performed within 24 hours of initial lysis procedure. If there is residual thrombus, the above-mentioned pharmacomechanical thrombectomy may be performed to lessen the thrombus burden. Once the vein's patency is restored, positional venography may be used to identify compression of the vein at the thoracic outlet (FIGURE 27-3). Should a significant stenosis (>80%) remain after restoration of venous patency, prompt first rib resection may be warranted.

The role of balloon angioplasty in the setting of acute thrombosis is controversial. It may be used to allow more rapid transit of blood across the thoracic outlet. Balloon angioplasty may be used to dilate the vein from 8 to 14 mm depending on the size of the normal adjacent vein. However, there is concern with possible disruption of the vein wall in the setting of thrombolysis. The benefit of angioplasty beyond a momentary enlargement of the venous lumen is unlikely, as the mechanical forces that result from extrinsic compression at the thoracic outlet will persist.

Stenting of the SCV in the course of thrombolysis is contraindicated. Numerous publications have noted that the mechanical forces on the thoracic outlet are far greater than the radial force of the stent, which inevitably results in stent collapse and deformity.

POST-DECOMPRESSIVE VENOGRAPHY AND INTERVENTION
Following first rib resection for TOS decompression, the endovascular approach to reconstruction of the SCV involves post-decompression venography and angioplasty. This may be done at the time of decompression or at a later date. The stenotic subclavian veins are balloon-angioplastied to normal diameter (FIGURE 27-4). Technical considerations include using support catheters such as 6 French 40 cm sheath, and glide wires for recanalization. Balloon angioplasty with low profile balloons (0.014 or 0.018 systems) is used for creating a pathway, then larger balloons to reach 10 to 14 mm (depending on patient size) for the subclavian vein. Success rates have been reported in the vicinity of 90%. The role of stenting in the post-decompression phase is not settled. Those who use stenting sparingly do so with the expectation that the vein will remodel and in most instances return to near-normal dimension and function.

POSTOPERATIVE CARE/FOLLOW-UP Patients who present with acute PSS and undergo thrombolysis should remain on anticoagulation until a thoracic outlet decompression surgery is performed. Anticoagulation is also continued after rib resection until venography and intervention is performed. Duration of anticoagulation is usually determined by the appearance of the vein on IVUS after angioplasty is performed. Additionally, patients may be followed with serial venograms should there be evidence of significant post-phlebitic changes in the SCV. ■

SUGGESTED READINGS

Beygui RE, Olcott C 4th, Dalman RL. Subclavian vein thrombosis: outcome analysis based on etiology and modality of treatment. *Ann Vasc Surg.* 1997;11(3):247-255.

Brownie ER, Abuirqeba AA, Ohman JW, Rubin BG, Thompson RW. False-negative upper extremity ultrasound in the initial evaluation of patients with suspected subclavian vein thrombosis due to thoracic outlet syndrome (Paget-Schroetter syndrome). *J Vasc Surg Venous Lymphat Disord.* 2020 Jan;8(1):118-126. doi: 10.1016/j.jvsv.2019.08.011. Epub 2019 Nov 13.

Chun TT, O'Connell JB, Rigberg DA, et al. Preoperative thrombolysis affords significant benefit in patency and outcome after first rib resection in acute Paget-Schroetter syndrome. *J Vasc Surg.* 2020;72(3):330-331.

de León RA, Chang DC, Hassoun HT, et al. Multiple treatment algorithms for successful outcomes in venous thoracic outlet syndrome. *Surgery.* 2009 May;145(5):500-507. doi: 10.1016/j.surg.2008.09.017. Epub 2009 Mar 21.

Guzzo JL, Chang K, Demos J, Black JH, Freischlag JA. Preoperative thrombolysis and venoplasty affords no benefit in patency following first rib resection and scalenectomy for subacute and chronic subclavian vein thrombosis. *J Vasc Surg.* 2010 Sep;52(3):658-662; discussion 662-663. doi: 10.1016/j.jvs.2010.04.050.

Illig KA, Doyle AJ. A comprehensive review of Paget-Schroetter syndrome. *J Vasc Surg.* 2010 Jun;51(6):1538-1547. doi: 10.1016/j.jvs.2009.12.022. Epub 2010 Mar 20.

Lee MC, Grassi MC, Belkin M, Mannick JA, Whittemore AD, Donaldson MC. Early operative intervention after thrombolytic therapy for primary subclavian vein thrombosis: an effective treatment approach. *J Vasc Surg.* 1998;27:1101-1107.

27-3

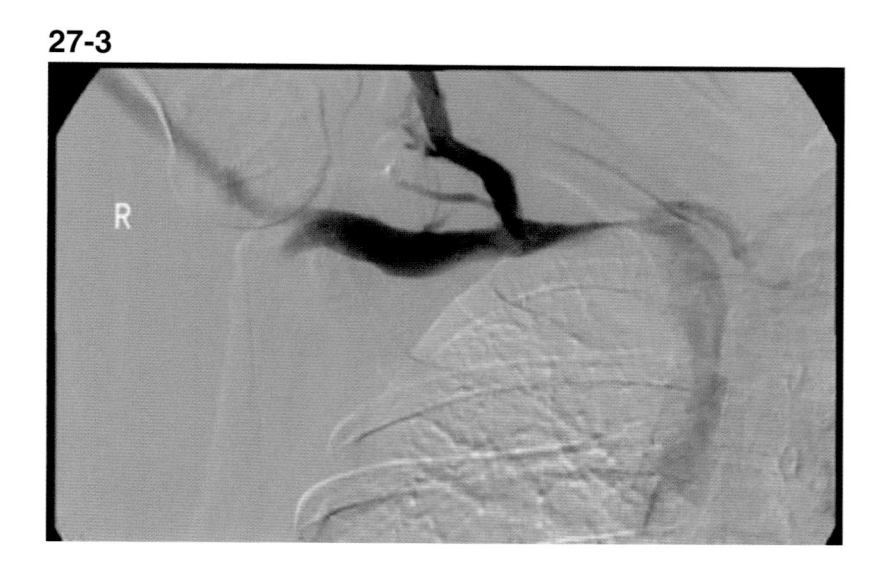

27-4

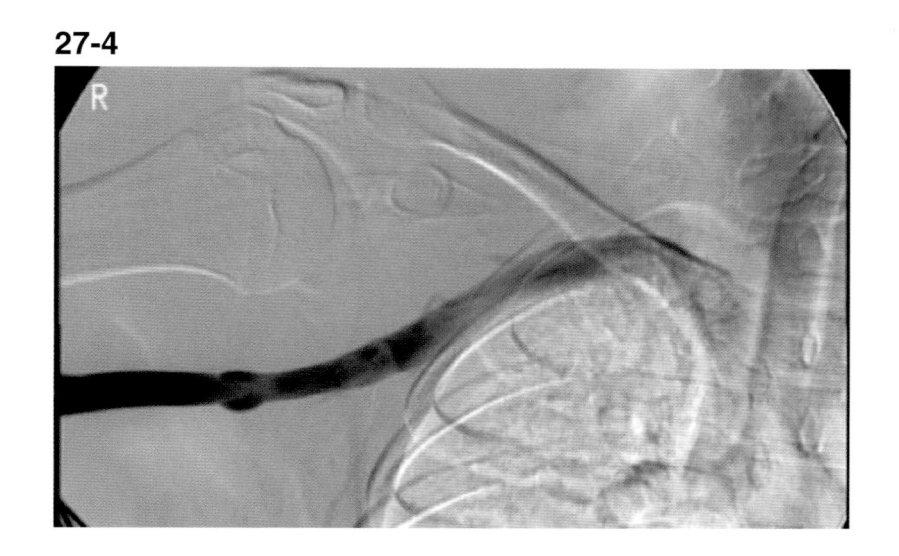

SECTION VI
ABDOMINAL AORTA AND BRANCHES OPEN

Transabdominal Approach to Infrarenal, Juxtarenal, and Iliac Aneurysms

Ina Y. Soh, MD, MS • Samuel R. Money, MD, MBA

INDICATIONS The decision to perform a transabdominal operation for an aortic aneurysm is based on many factors, the most important of which are the patient's overall state of health and aneurysm size. Current guidelines recommend repair of aortic aneurysms with maximum diameters greater than 5.5 cm in males, 5.0 cm in females, or evidence of impending rupture. Over the past 25 years, endovascular aneurysm repair has become the leading treatment modality for aortic aneurysms with favorable neck anatomy. Thus, in the context of adverse neck anatomy, the decision to do an open transabdominal versus complex endovascular operation hinges on patient age, life expectancy, and comorbidity status.

PREOPERATIVE PREPARATION Although ultrasound is the preferred imaging modality for aneurysm screening and surveillance, computed tomography (CT) angiography of the lower chest, abdomen, and pelvis is the recommended study for defining maximum aortic diameter as well as proximal and distal extent of disease. The presence of aberrant anatomy (e.g., posterior left renal vein, renal vein collar, horseshoe kidney, accessory renal arteries) and visceral or iliac occlusive disease is also noted on preoperative CT imaging. If renal function is prohibitive to contrast administration, we obtain an ultrasound and a non-contrast CT scan.

Ischemic heart disease is a common cause of significant morbidity and mortality following open aortic aneurysm repair. For this reason, most patients undergoing elective abdominal aortic aneurysm repair undergo a thorough cardiac evaluation which includes noninvasive stress testing. For patients with a history of symptomatic chronic obstructive pulmonary disease (COPD), long-standing tobacco use, or the inability to climb a flight of stairs, a preoperative pulmonary function test is warranted. Preoperative blood work should include a basic metabolic panel to evaluate renal function, and a complete blood count, which may prompt further hematologic assessment if hemoglobin or platelet counts are abnormally low. Preoperative hydration before aneurysm repair is recommended for non-dialysis–dependent patients with renal insufficiency.

Preoperative discussion with patients undergoing transabdominal aortic or iliac aneurysm repair should include risks of cardiac, pulmonary, renal, wound, and venous thromboembolic complications. There should also be discussion about potential risks of sexual dysfunction, ureteral injury, colon ischemia, limb ischemia, and graft infection.

ANESTHESIA The operation is routinely performed under general anesthesia with endotracheal intubation. The anesthesia team places appropriate monitoring lines, which include an arterial line for continuous blood pressure monitoring, serial blood gas sampling, and intermittent activating clotting time (ACT) checks. Several large bore intravenous catheters or a central venous line are required. Once the patient is intubated, a nasogastric tube is inserted, and a Foley catheter is placed which allows for hourly urine output measurements. Cell salvage or an ultrafiltration device is made available when large blood loss is anticipated. A first-generation cephalosporin or, in the event of penicillin allergy, vancomycin, is administered intravenously within 60 minutes of incision and then continued for 24 hours.

We consider placement of an epidural catheter preoperatively or a transversus abdominis plane (TAP) block postoperatively as adjuncts to pain control.

INCISION AND EXPOSURE The patient is prepped from nipples to mid-thigh, then draped so that access is maintained to both common femoral arteries and to the chest should these exposures become necessary. The standard incision is made in the midline extending from xiphoid to pubic symphysis, although some prefer a modified chevron incision (**FIGURE 28-1**). If more incision is needed or body habitus is demanding, a 1- to 2-cm incision along the lateral border of the xiphoid yields better proximal exposure. The peritoneal cavity is entered through the linea alba, and the peritoneal contents are evaluated for any occult malignancy or other pathology that would preclude proceeding with aortic reconstruction. If additional surgical assistants are unavailable for retraction, a table-mounted retractor system can be set up to facilitate intraabdominal exposure.

Once the abdomen has been fully explored, aortic exposure is begun. The transverse colon and greater omentum are lifted onto the superior abdominal wall. The small bowel is wrapped in a moistened laparotomy towel (**FIGURE 28-2**), reflected to the patient's right, then tucked and contained under a retractor. The third and fourth portions of the duodenum, tethered across the infrarenal aorta, are mobilized carefully toward the patient's right after dividing the ligament of Treitz (**FIGURE 28-3**). It is often helpful to isolate the inferior mesenteric vein and trace it proximally. Ligating this and dividing it helps facilitate this exposure. Be sure to palpate for a meandering mesenteric artery, which may lie next to this. The retroperitoneum is entered, and a thin layer of fibrous preaortic tissue is incised before encountering the anterior surface of the aorta. Lymphatic tissue is ligated. Following the anterior surface of the aorta, the retroperitoneum is opened in the cranial direction in search of the left renal vein, as it usually traverses anterior to the juxtarenal aorta before emptying into the inferior vena cava. In most cases, the renal arteries are found just beneath the cephalad border of the left renal vein. Note the importance of identifying retroaortic left renal veins and circumaortic left renal veins on preoperative CT imaging to avoid inadvertent injury during aortic exposure. In aneurysms with a sufficiently long infrarenal aortic neck, mobilization of the left renal vein is often unnecessary. However, with short infrarenal necks, the left renal vein is frequently mobilized using gentle blunt and sharp dissection, then encircled with a Penrose drain or umbilical tape, which facilitate vein retraction. In the process of mobilizing the left renal vein, it is helpful to ligate the adrenal vein superiorly, and the gonadal and lumbar vein inferiorly. If the aneurysm extends into the juxtarenal aorta, dissection should continue up to the suprarenal aorta for proximal clamp placement so the aortic neck can be sewn to. In these cases, the left renal vein can be safely divided close to its confluence with the inferior vena cava, preserving outflow through the gonadal, adrenal, and lumbar venous tributaries. This maneuver exposes the pararenal aorta. Note that circumferential aortic dissection is not necessary, and injury to posterior lumbar arterial branches should be avoided.

CONTINUES▶

28-1

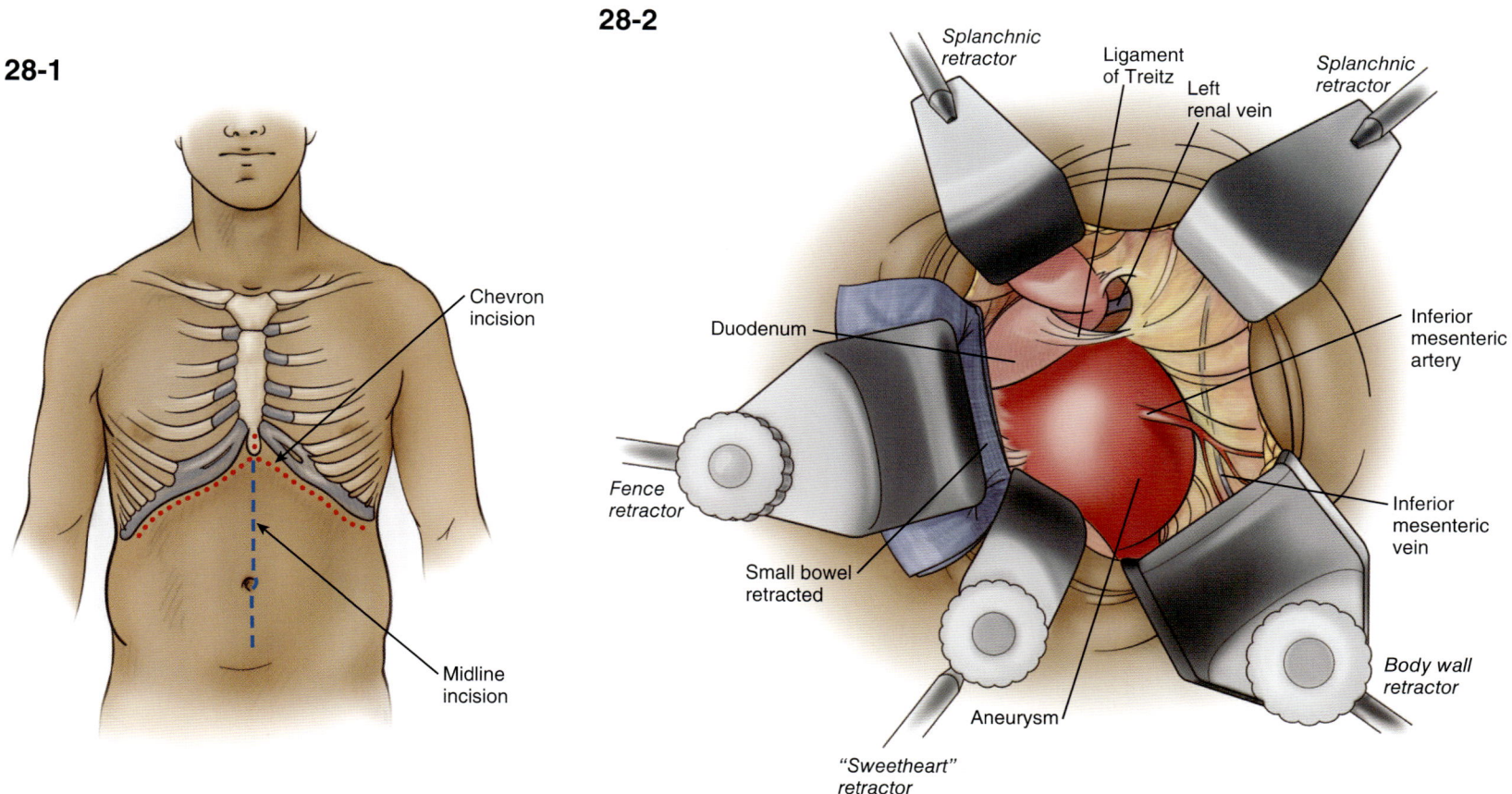

Figure 28-1 Standard and chevron incision.

Figure 28-2 Abdominal contents retracted, and transverse colon elevated.

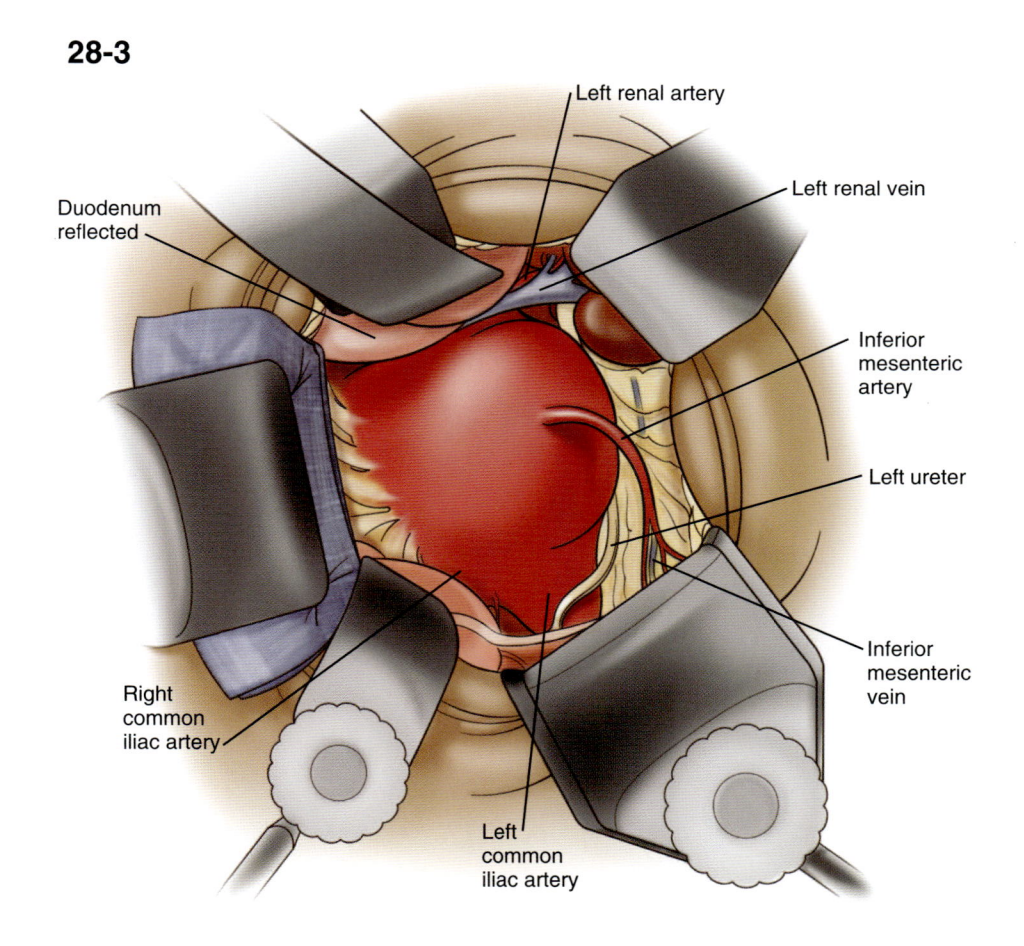

Figure 28-3 Ligament of Treitz, inferior mesenteric vein (IMV), lymphatic tissue, renal and adrenal veins, gonadal veins.

INCISION AND EXPOSURE `CONTINUED` On occasion, it will not be safe to clamp the infrarenal or suprarenal aorta. This may be due to excessive calcification, poor tissue, or proximity to the superior mesenteric artery. In these circumstances, if retroperitoneal exposure is not an option, then plans should be made to clamp the surpaceliac aorta. The technical aspects of this start with mobilization of the left lobe of the liver by taking down the coronary ligament and triangular ligament (FIGURE 28-4A). Next, the gastrohepatic ligament is incised (FIGURE 28-4B). Pay close attention to look for an accessory left hepatic artery in the gastrohepatic ligament. If this is encountered, it usually can be spared by dissecting the vessel for several centimeters throughout its course. The next step involves taking the crus down of the diaphragm. `CONTINUES`

28-4

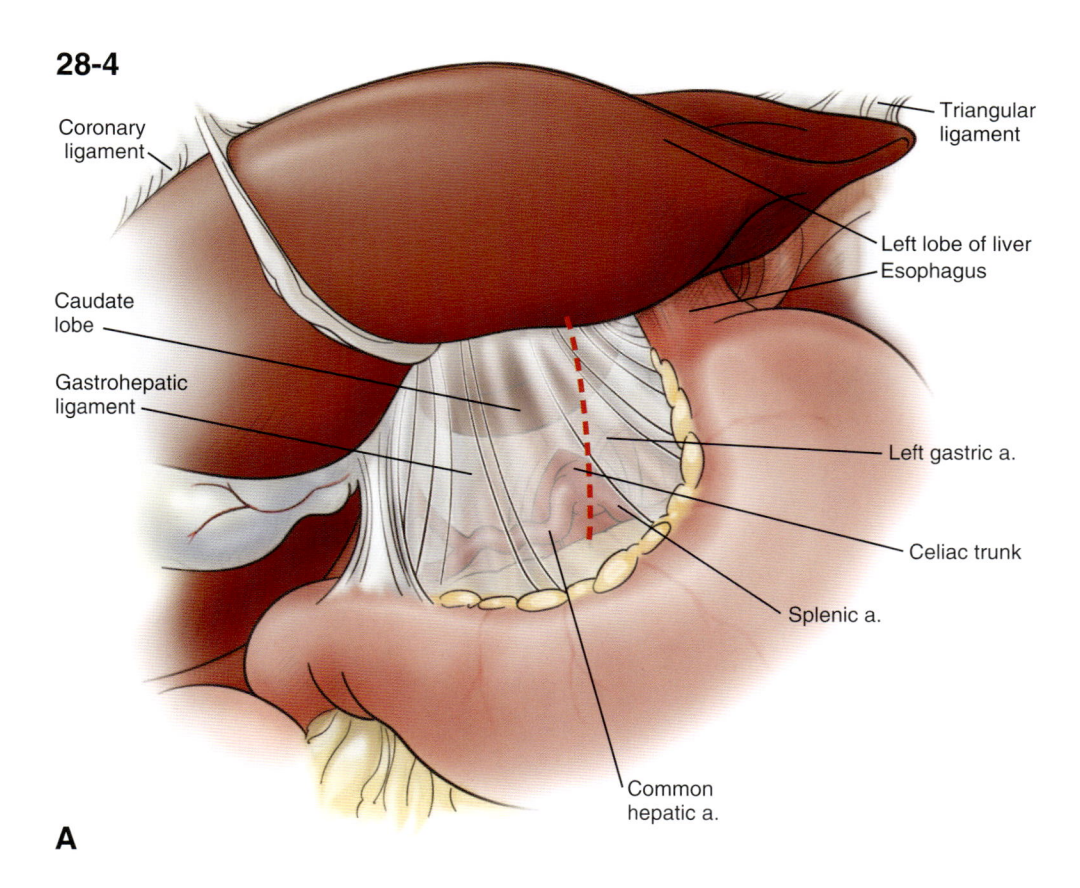

A

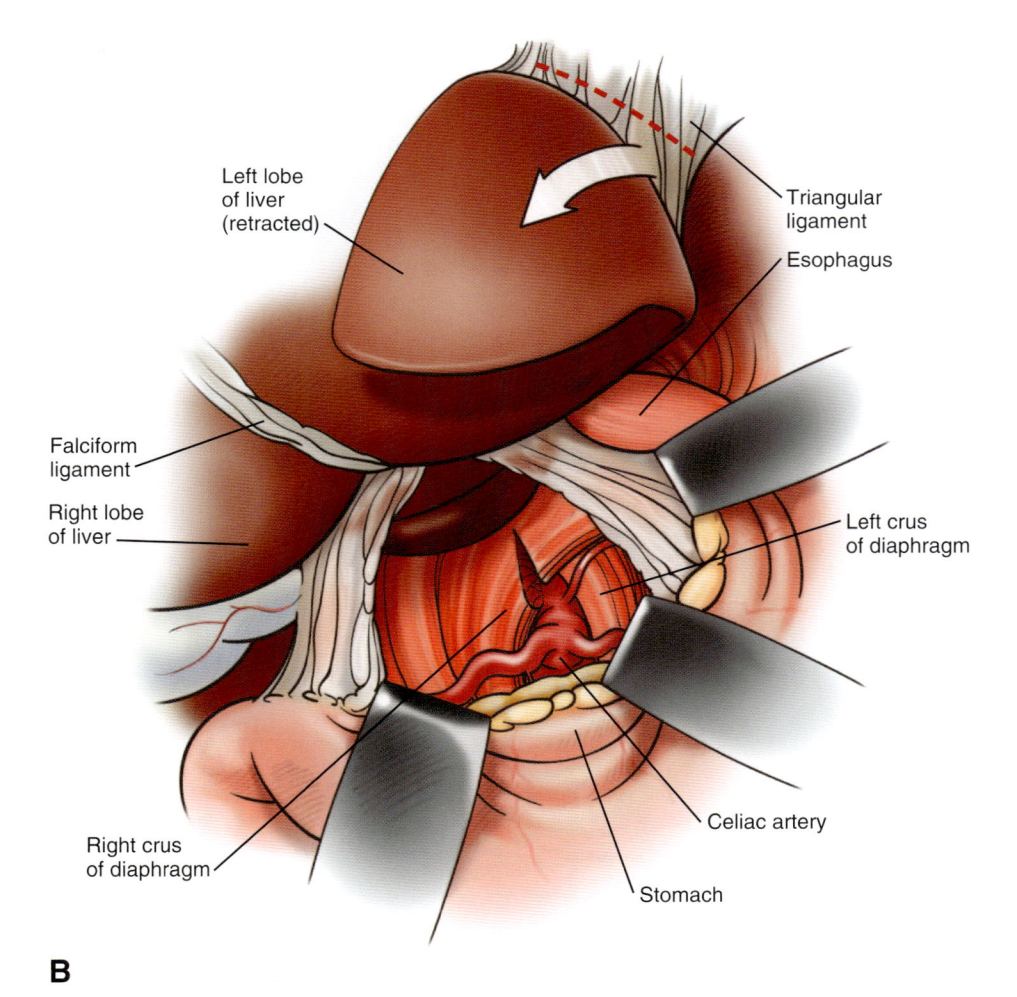

B

Figure 28-4 A and B: Supraceliac exposure.

INCISION AND EXPOSURE CONTINUED Proper retraction is important here (FIGURE 28-5). The left lobe of the liver is retracted with a splanchnic retractor. Too much tension can avulse the caudate lobe from the inferior vena cava. The esophagus is retracted to the left with a long renal vein retractor. This is easily palpated by feeling for the nasogastric tube. Next, the right crus of the diaphragm is carefully transected with bovie cautery, and then part of the left may need be divided to facilitate a clamp. Once complete, dissect along each side of the aorta to feel the spine. It is too dangerous to dissect circumferentially on this area. Aortic clamping is then done after heparinization.

Once the aortic neck is clearly delineated and dissected out, control of the iliac arteries must be obtained. The incised posterior peritoneum and preaortic fibrous tissue is further opened in the caudal direction toward the aortic bifurcation, veering to the right of aortic midline to avoid injuring the inferior mesenteric artery injury and the autonomic nerve plexus, which runs along the anterior surface of the aorta and over the left common iliac artery (FIGURE 28-6). Control of the distal aorta is best obtained at the level of the common iliac arteries. If the aortic aneurysm involves the common iliac arteries, dissection is carried further distally onto the iliac bifurcations. Blood flow through at least one hypogastric artery should be preserved. Care is taken to avoid injuring the ureters and iliac veins. As with proximal aortic control, the iliac arteries do not need to be encircled but rather slotted, leaving the posterior wall untouched and protecting the iliac vein just posterior to the artery. The left common iliac artery may need to be mobilized in the left lower quadrant retroperitoneum for distal control. CONTINUES

28-5

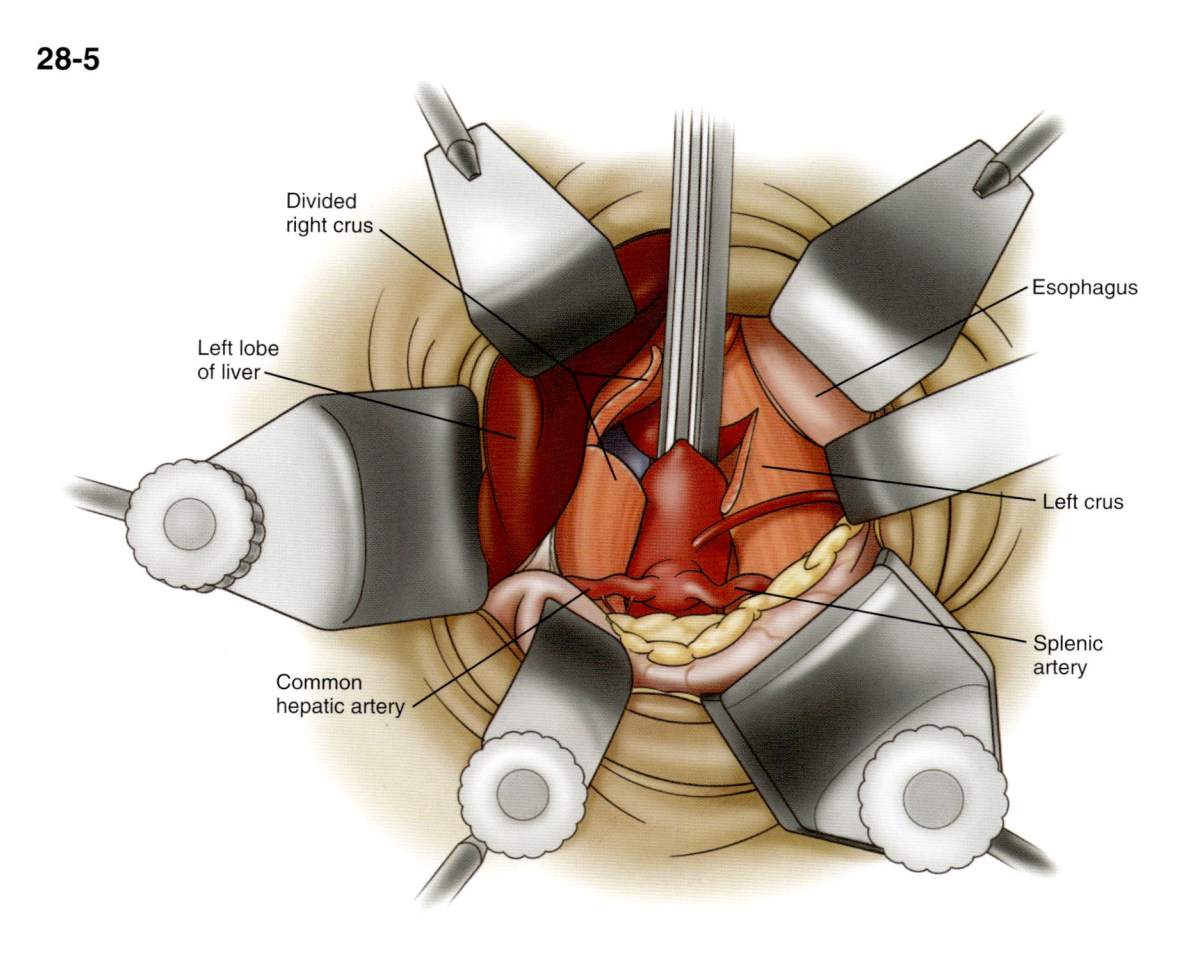

Figure 28-5 Retractors and crus divided.

28-6

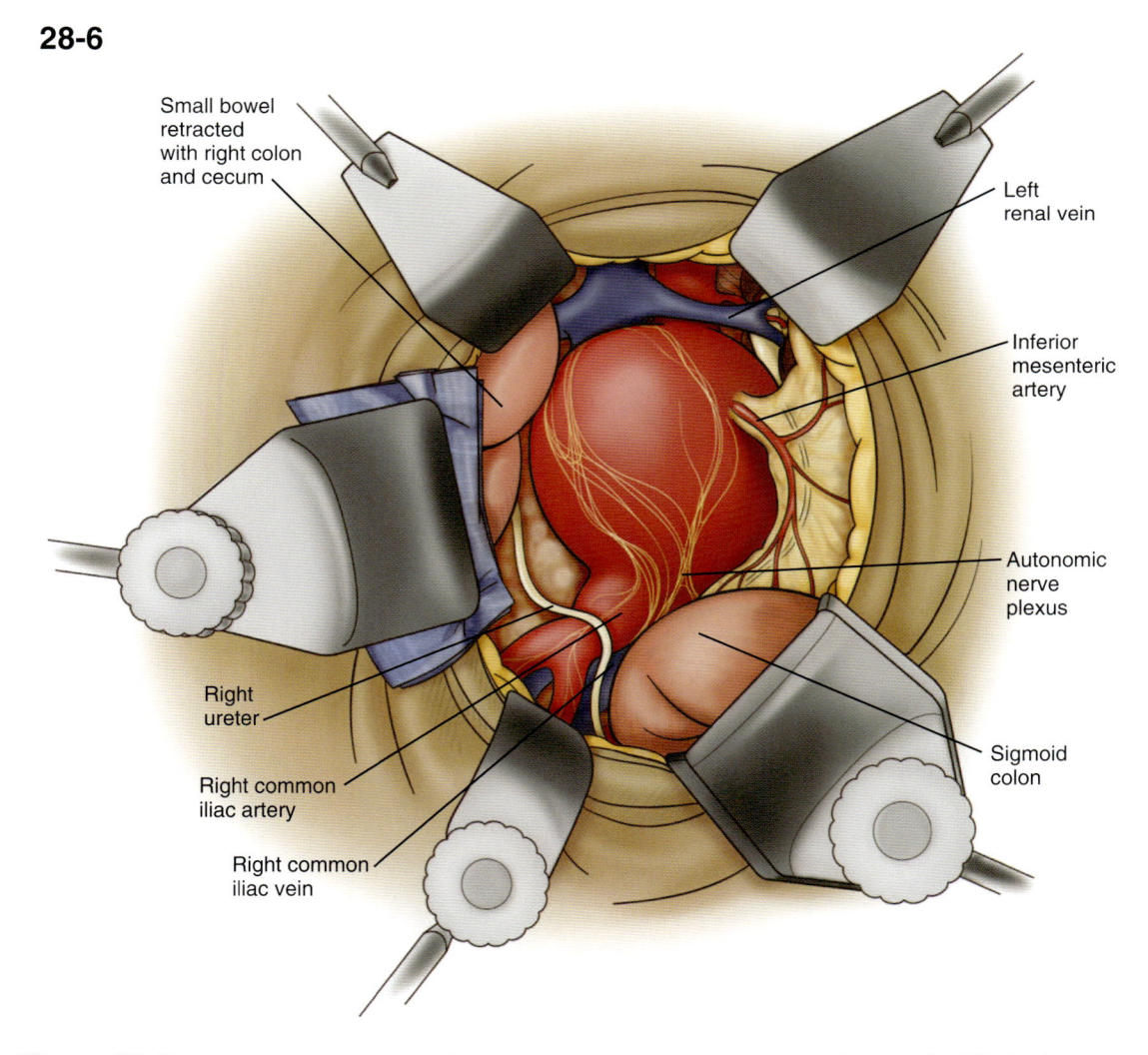

Figure 28-6 Iliac dissection, avoid inferior mesenteric artery (IMA). Avoid ureter, highlight iliac vein.

INCISION AND EXPOSURE CONTINUED This is done by mobilizing the sigmoid colon along the left line of Toldt and paying careful attention to not injure the left ureter as it crosses the left common iliac artery (FIGURE 28-7). Here the left limb of a bifurcated graft is tunneled posterior to the sigmoid mesocolon and ureter.

DETAILS OF PROCEDURE Once proximal and distal control has been established, the patient is systemically heparinized to protect against distal thrombosis during aortic occlusion. During heparin circulation time, an aortic graft that is appropriately sized to the aorta and iliacs is selected and vascular clamps are chosen. After heparin has circulated for 3 minutes or longer, distal clamps are placed prior to the proximal aortic clamp to protect against distal embolization of aortic mural thrombus (FIGURE 28-8). The aneurysm sac is opened through a linear aortotomy, again veering toward the right of aortic midline to avoid injuring the inferior mesenteric artery. With the sac opened, sac contents are extricated and back bleeding from lumbar arteries is controlled with figure-of-eight silk suture ligature. Pulsatile back bleeding from the inferior mesenteric artery is similarly controlled with suture ligature. If back bleeding from the inferior mesenteric artery is meager, reimplantation of this vessel onto the aortic graft may be necessary to minimize the risk of colonic ischemia. In this case, the inferior mesenteric artery is controlled separately with a vascular clamp across its orifice and readdressed following completion of the aortic graft reconstruction.

CONTINUES

28-7

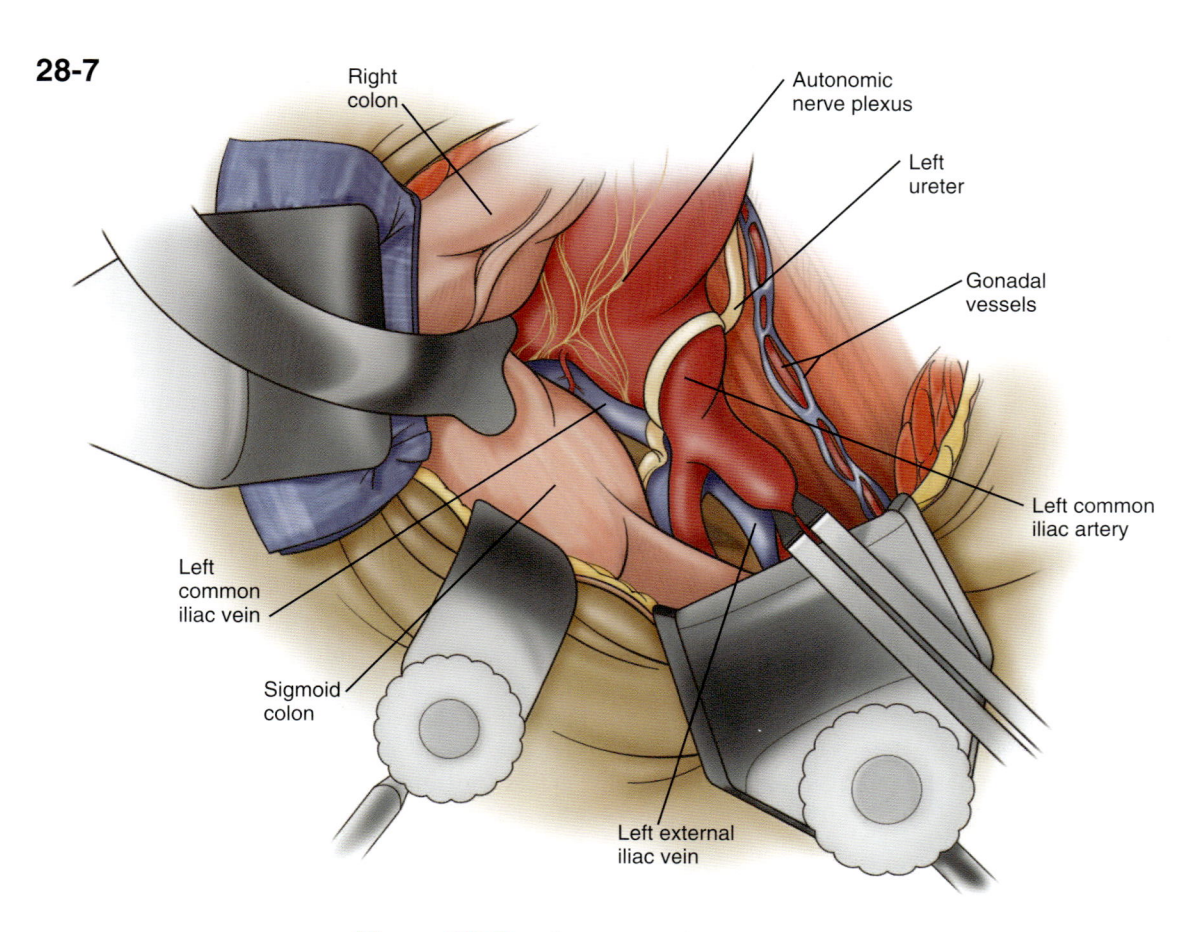

Figure 28-7 Left common iliac exposure.

28-8

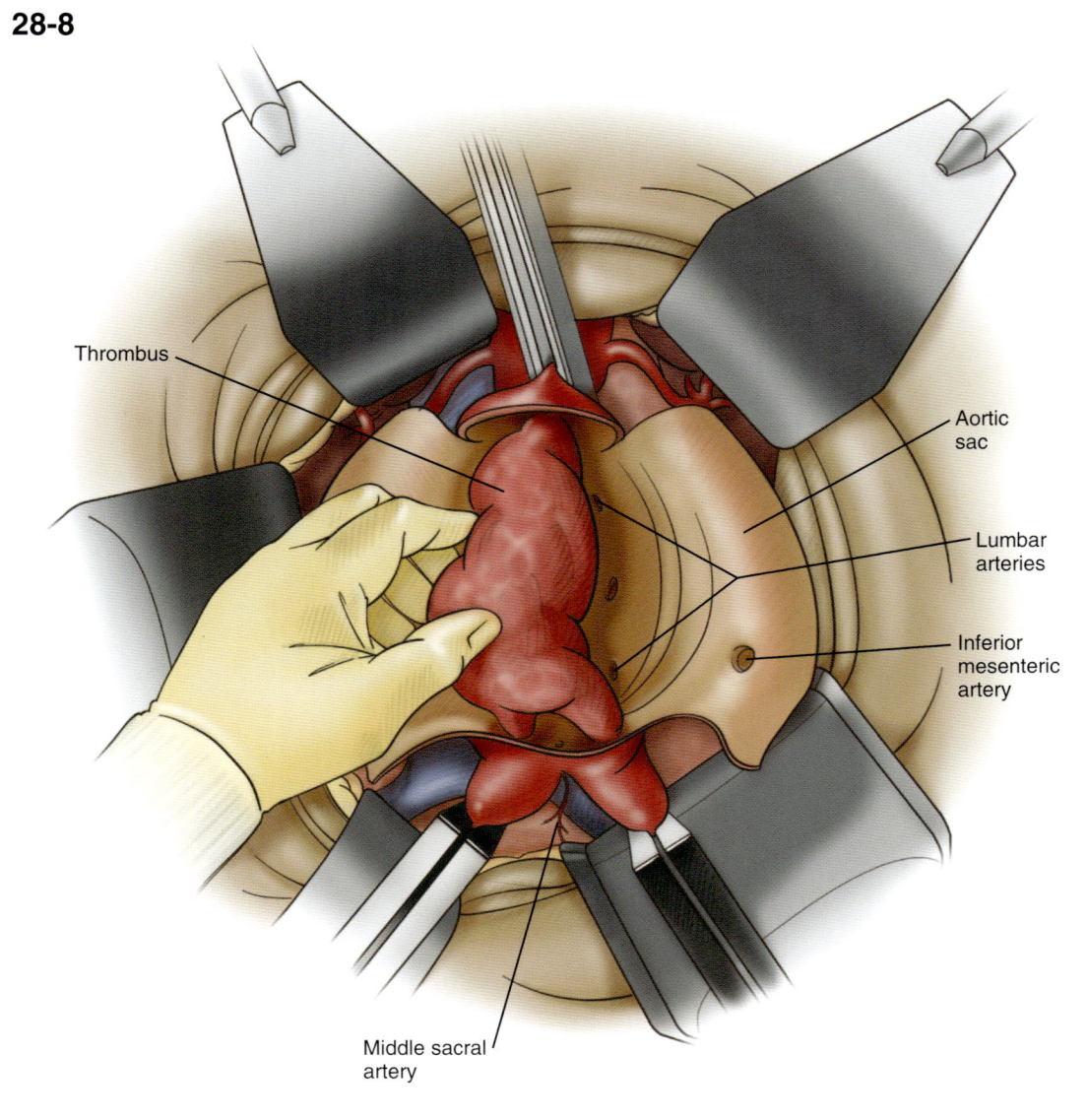

Figure 28-8 Clamps and sac opened, ligate lumbars; ureter retracted.

DETAILS OF PROCEDURE `CONTINUED` Next, we prepare the graft to sew to the proximal aortic neck. The aortic wall is teed off, leaving the posterior wall intact and not 100% transected. The aortic graft is sewn end-to-end to the proximal aortic neck using 3-0 double-armed polypropylene suture (FIGURE 28-9). The aortic back wall is incorporated into the graft suture line starting just a bit left of midline. The double-armed suture is brought up each side of the graft to meet on the anterior surface of the graft. Once the graft is sewn in, the suture line is tested for hemostasis. A clamp is applied to the aortic graft, and the proximal clamp on native aorta is gently released. If there is suture line bleeding, the proximal aortic clamp is reapplied, and the suture line is reinforced with pledgeted polypropylene mattress sutures. Once suture line hemostasis is achieved, the aortic graft is clamped and the proximal clamp on native aorta is released.

If a tube graft is selected, the distal graft is trimmed to appropriate length and sewn end-to-end to the terminal aorta. If aneurysmal disease involves the iliac arteries, a bifurcated aortic graft is chosen with each limb sewn end-to-end to non-aneurysmal iliac artery. Usually, we begin with the right iliac anastomosis first, owing to its easier exposure. Mirroring the proximal aortic anastomosis, the right common iliac artery is teed off, leaving the posterior wall intact and not 100% transected. The graft limb is trimmed to appropriate length and sewn in using 3-0 double-armed polypropylene suture. Prior to completing the suture line, the graft is forward-flushed, and the native iliac artery is back bled, and the graft is pieced with a 20 G de-airing needle. Some surgeons irrigate the graft with heparin–saline solution. The suture line is completed and tested for hemostasis by releasing the distal clamp first. Pledgeted mattress sutures are used if suture line bleeding persists.

Once suture line hemostasis is satisfactory, we hold manual pressure on the ipsilateral femoral artery, then relocate the aortic graft clamp onto the contralateral graft limb. We slowly release manual pressure on the femoral artery allowing controlled reperfusion of the lower extremity. Attention is turned to the contralateral iliac anastomosis and the above steps are repeated.

Once both iliac anastomoses are complete, if inferior mesenteric artery reimplantation is indicated, a Carrel patch including the origin of the inferior mesenteric artery is sewn onto the aortic graft or one of the iliac limbs using 6-0 polypropylene suture (FIGURE 28-10). A side-biting aortic clamp can be used to control the aortic graft during this anastomosis.

We routinely close the aortic sac over the graft reconstruction using running 3-0 Vicryl suture. We also reapproximate the retroperitoneum as an additional barrier between aorta and overlying viscera to protect against future aortoenteric fistula formation (FIGURE 28-11). The abdomen is evaluated again, with special attention to the sigmoid colon. Both lower extremities are evaluated for adequate perfusion by checking Doppler flow and capillary refill. If there is no evidence of ischemic bowel, ischemic extremity, and overall hemostasis is satisfactory, then heparin reversal is achieved by administering protamine sulfate. The abdomen is closed in standard fashion.

POSTOPERATIVE CARE All patients should be admitted to the intensive care unit, and immediate extubation is reserved for those patients with no comorbidities and short clamp times. Postoperative ST-segment monitoring is indicated for all patients following open aortic surgery, in addition to routine EKG. Frequent laboratory studies, volume status management, and lower extremity perfusion assessments are routine components of postoperative care. In the absence of ongoing blood loss, our threshold for blood transfusion after open aneurysm repair is a hemoglobin concentration of <7 to 8 g/dL. Nasogastric decompression is continued after a minimum of 24 to 48 hours, as retracting the duodenum commonly leads to gastric ileus after surgery, and the patient is kept nil per os while awaiting return of bowel function. Following convalescence, our postoperative surveillance includes a non-ontrast CT scan of the entire aorta at 5-year intervals. ∎

28-9

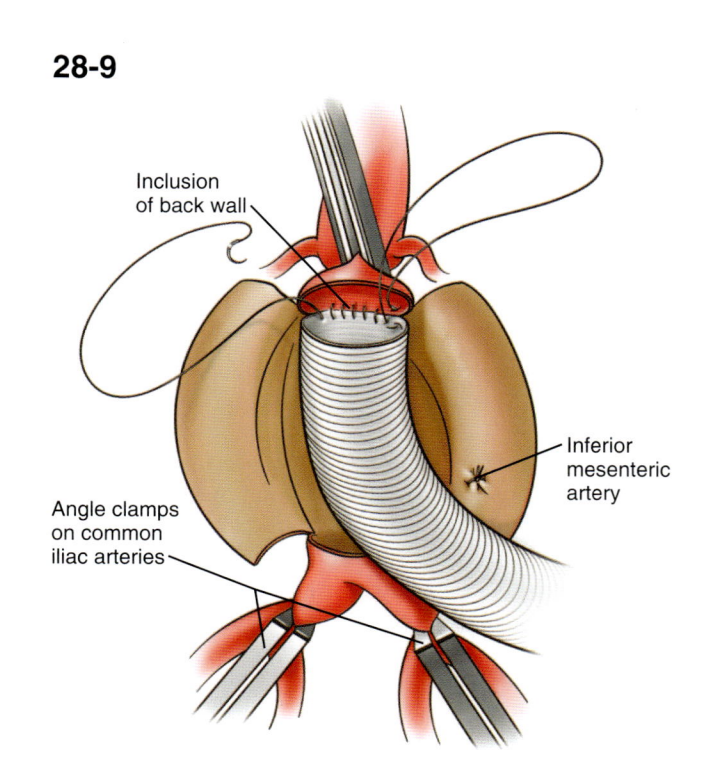

Figure 28-9 Graft sewn, incorporate back wall, left limb or graft tunneled underneath sigmoid and ureter.

28-10

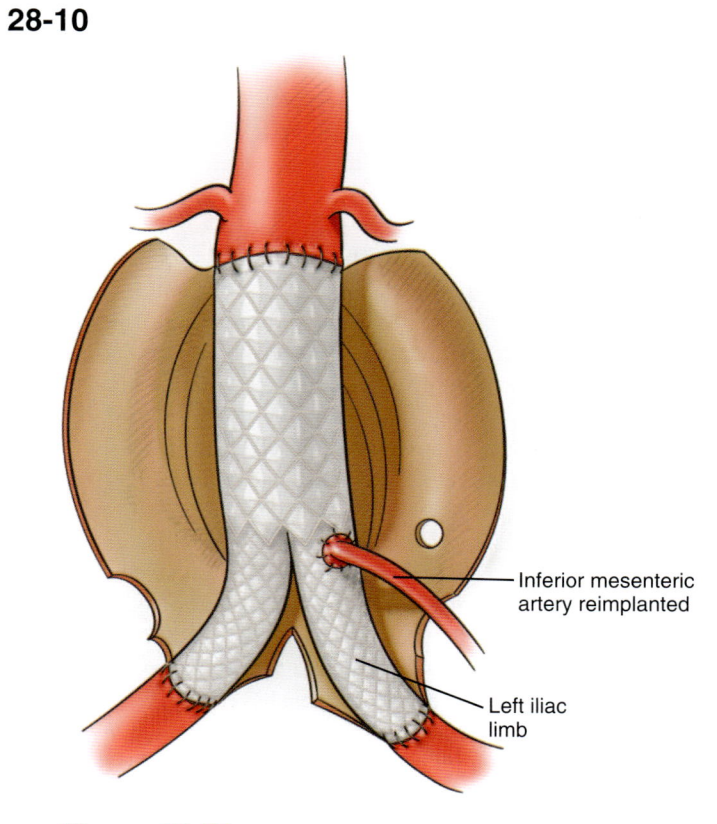

Figure 28-10 IMA reimplanted into left iliac limb.

28-11

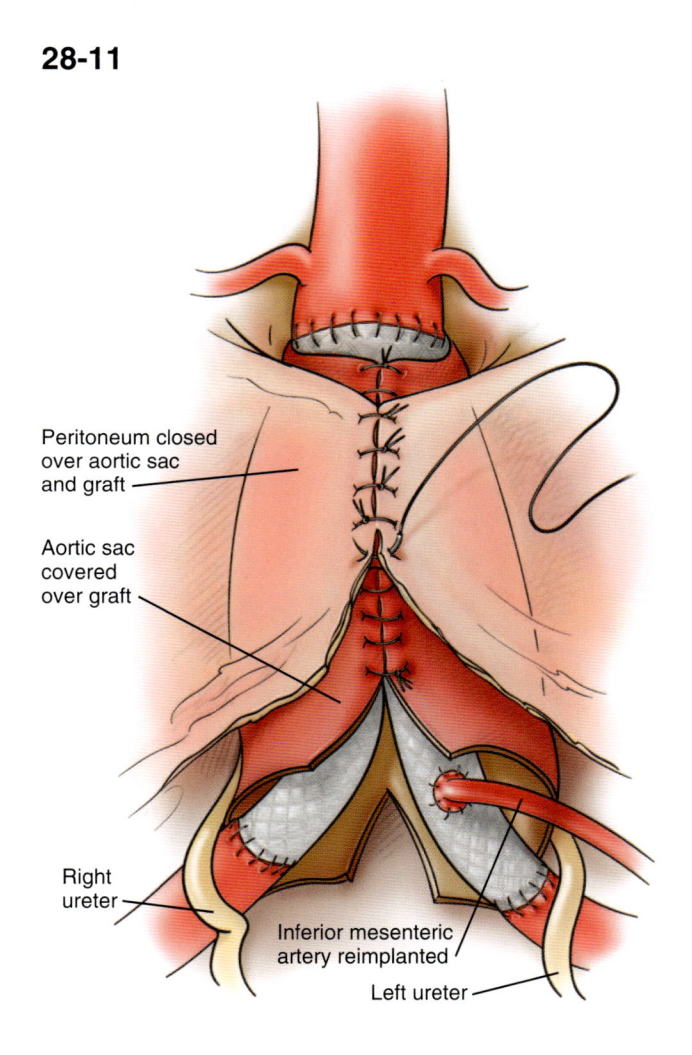

Figure 28-11 Graft covered with sac and retroperitoneum.

Retroperitoneal Approach for Infrarenal, Juxtarenal, and Iliac Artery Aneurysms

Mounir J. Haurani, MD, MPH • Timur P. Sarac, MD

INDICATIONS The retroperitoneal approach is the original described approach for the first successful bypass for aortoiliac occlusive disease and abdominal aortic aneurysm repair.[1,2] Despite this, it is not widely used in current practice. The transabdominal approach is more familiar for many general and vascular surgeons and can be successfully used for most aortic reconstructions. However, there are specific advantages to the retroperitoneal approach that make familiarity with it advantageous. Patients with a prior transabdominal approach for their aortic or other abdominal pathology may be more easily approached in the retroperitoneal plane.[2] There is some suggestion that physiologically the retroperitoneal approach may be less stressful and produces less postoperative ileus, fewer pulmonary complications, and lower overall morbidity than the transabdominal approach.[2-9] However, a metanalysis of five randomized trials showed no clear evidence of a difference between the approaches in terms of mortality.[10] There was some evidence of shorter intensive care unit and overall hospital stays with the retroperitoneal approach.[10]

The retroperitoneal approach can be used for infrarenal, juxtarenal, pararenal, and suprarenal aneurysms. It also allows for aortic reconstructions with revascularization of the left renal or with horseshoe kidneys. It is also particularly useful in cases where mesenteric reconstruction is needed. In morbidly obese patients or those with a hostile abdomen, it also affords more direct access to the aorta and its branches.

While the retroperitoneal approach is versatile for multiple aortic pathologies, it has some limitations. While right iliac and right renal artery reconstruction is feasible from this approach, if extensive or distal intervention is needed, a transabdominal approach may be more appropriate. Additionally, if there is mesenteric reconstruction performed or the inferior mesenteric artery (IMA) is ligated, this approach does not allow for inspection of the intestine. Lastly, care must be taken when retracting the spleen because its intraperitoneal location may mask bleeding or rupture.

POSITIONING The patient is placed in the right decubitus position with the left thorax elevated to about 45 degrees (**FIGURE 29-1**). If a longer incision is anticipated, the angle can be increased some to extend the incision posteriorly; however, the hips should remain somewhat flat. In juxtarenal repair, this angle should be closer to 60 to 70 degrees. The point midway between the thorax and the anterior superior iliac crest should be positioned at the flexion point of the operative table. A vacuum bean bag should be used to help maintain this position. The bean bag should be positioned to avoid covering the rails on the bed and deflated after flexing the bed. The table is flexed to improve exposure to the retroperitoneum by increasing the distance from the thorax to the pelvis. The right arm and brachial plexus should be protected with an axillary roll. The left arm is positioned on a supportive arm board, ensuring the elbow is neutral. Additionally, the arm board should be positioned to avoid interfering with the self-retaining retractor.

PROCEDURE A transverse incision is made extending medially from the lateral edge of the rectus abdominis at the point midway from the umbilicus to the pubic symphysis. The incision is carried laterally toward the 11th intercostal space (**FIGURE 29-2**). The abdominal wall muscles are divided along the length of the incision. After the external and internal obliques are divided, care should be taken as the transverses abdominis muscle and the transversalis fascia are divided, to avoid inadvertently entering the peritoneum. This is more easily accomplished by beginning the division laterally and using a blunt dissection instrument such as a Kittner or Peanut cottonoid sponge on the end of a Schnidt tonsil clamp. Once this plane has been entered, it is bluntly extended by sweeping the peritoneum off the iliac fossa inferiorly and continuing to bluntly dissect it from the remaining abdominal wall. As the dissection continues medially toward the rectus sheath and inferiorly toward the linea semilunaris, the peritoneum thins out considerably and care should be taken to avoid inadvertent tearing of the peritoneum. This medial rotation of the peritoneum and its contents continues until the psoas muscle is identified and the diaphragm is exposed to the aortic hiatus. The spleen may need to be taken down from the diaphragm, and this is done by both blunt and sharp dissection (**FIGURE 29-3**).

CONTINUES ▶

29-1

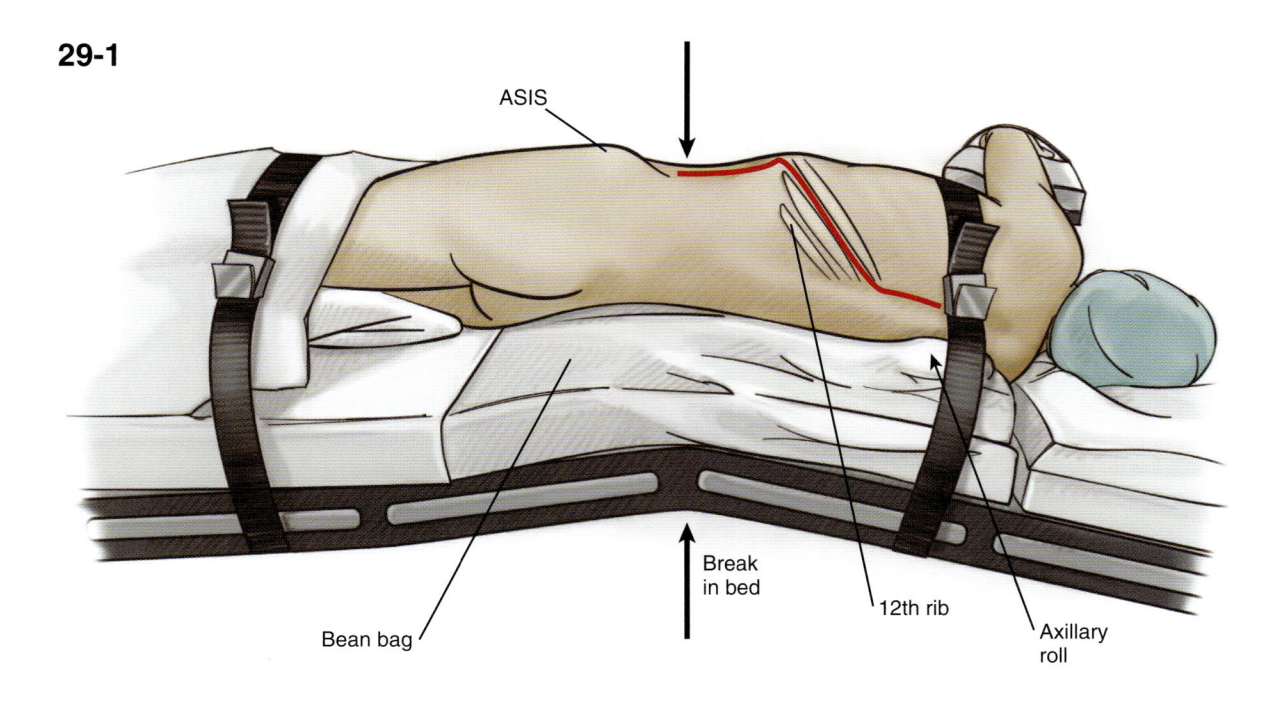

ASIS

Break in bed

Bean bag

12th rib

Axillary roll

29-2

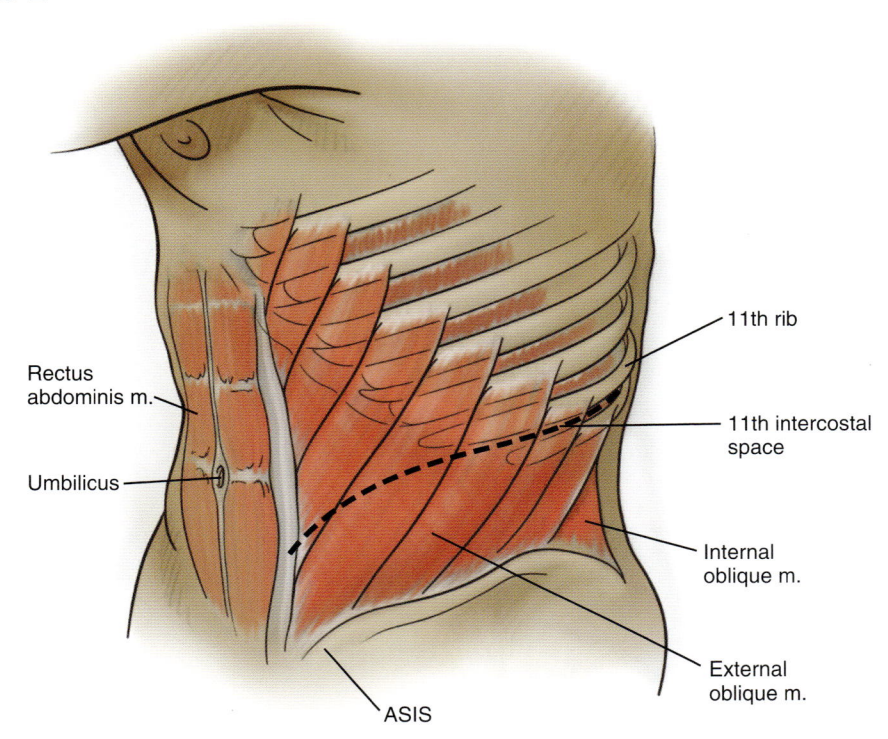

Rectus abdominis m.

Umbilicus

ASIS

11th rib

11th intercostal space

Internal oblique m.

External oblique m.

29-3

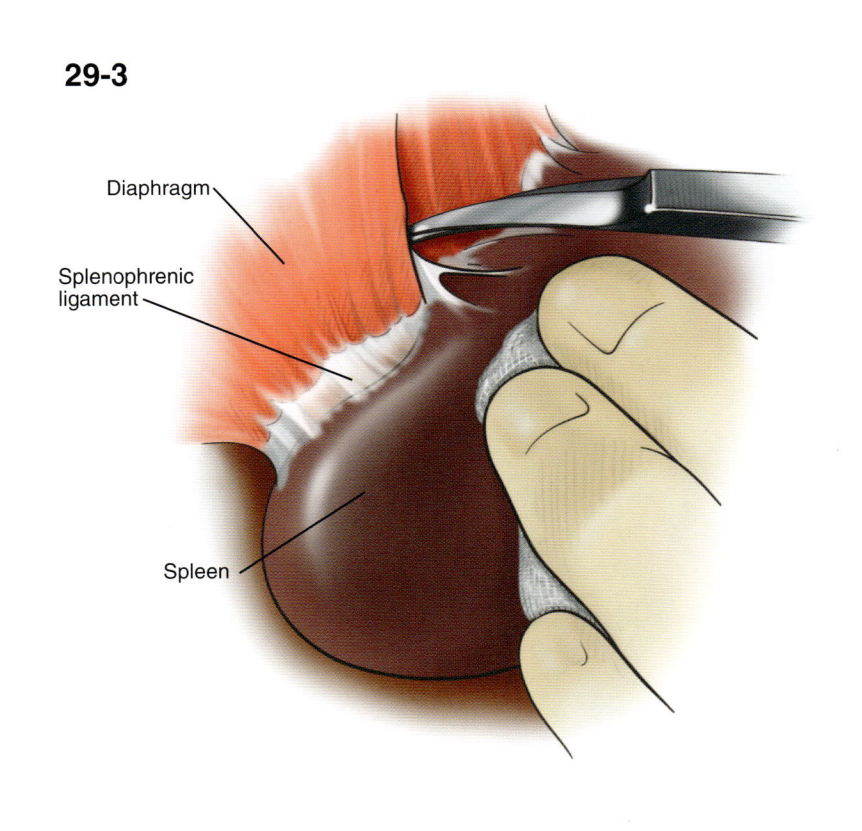

Diaphragm

Splenophrenic ligament

Spleen

PROCEDURE <CONTINUED> The kidney may be left down for further exposure of the visceral vessels or if there is a retroaortic left renal vein (FIGURE 29-4). At this point, a plane posterior to the left kidney and ureter is created along the lumbodorsal fascia. Before placing self-retaining retractors, it is helpful at this point to identify the left renal artery, which commonly is obscured by a lumbar vein branch (renal lumbar vein) which will need to be divided to fully expose the renal artery (FIGURE 29-5). The left renal artery is typically just cephalad to this vein branch. Any retractor system that the surgeon is familiar with is suitable; however, the Omnitract or Thompson retractor allows for less interference posteriorly and slightly more flexibility than ringed retractors.

Once the left renal artery has been located, it provides a convenient reference point to continue the aortic dissection. The retroperitoneum overlying the aorta can then be divided cephalad until a suitable clamp site is identified. The distal dissection continues along the aorta taking care to identify the IMA. If distal exposure to the iliac arteries is needed, the IMA may need to be divided close to its origin and then reevaluated for reimplantation. If the IMA is greater than 3 mm with minimal backflow, consideration should be made to reimplant following completion of the other anastomoses. If needed, the iliac vessels are now dissected. The iliac confluence and left iliac vein course parallel and posterior medially to the arteries (FIGURE 29-6). Careful attention is made to retract the left ureter. While exposure to the right common iliac artery can be cumbersome and difficult, it can be facilitated by extending the incision across the midline and retraction with a long renal vein retractor. Care should be taken to avoid left iliac vein injury and only dissect enough artery necessary to safely clamp and allow adequate anastomotic site. If control of the right iliac artery beyond the proximal vessel is needed, the retroperitoneal approach may prove to be prohibitive; however, it is possible to use balloon occlusion of the distal right iliac artery from inside the aorta once the vessel has been opened. <CONTINUES>

29-4

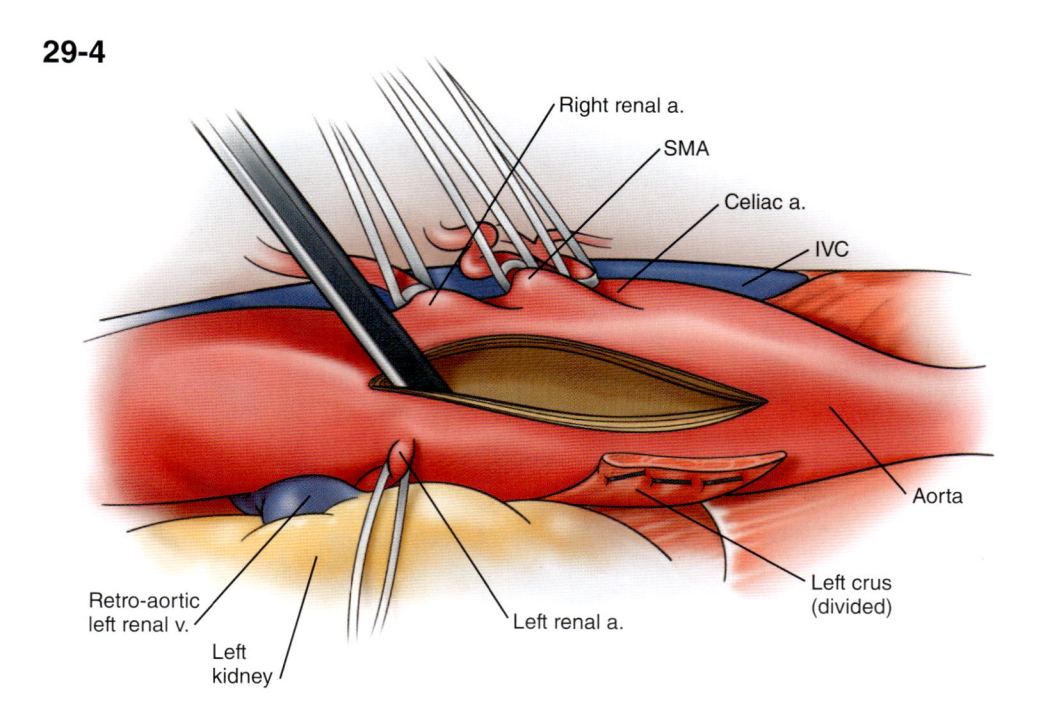

Right renal a.
SMA
Celiac a.
IVC
Aorta
Left crus (divided)
Left renal a.
Left kidney
Retro-aortic left renal v.

29-5

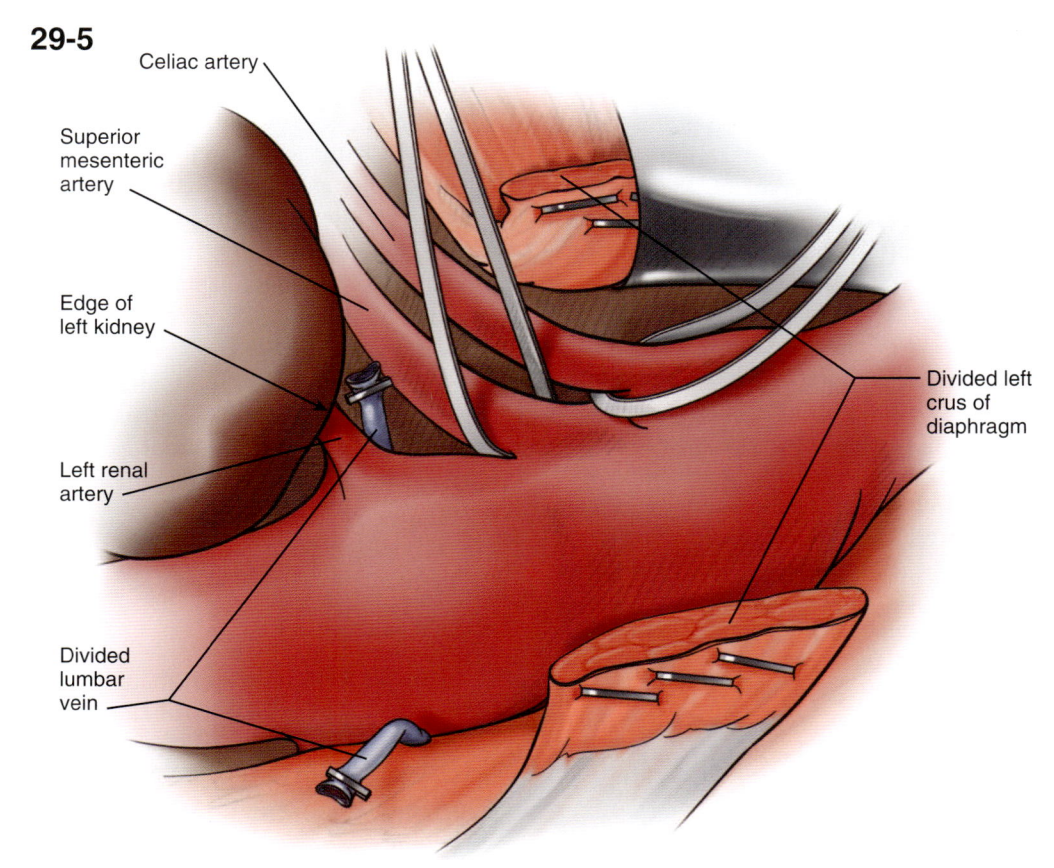

Celiac artery
Superior mesenteric artery
Edge of left kidney
Left renal artery
Divided lumbar vein
Divided left crus of diaphragm

29-6

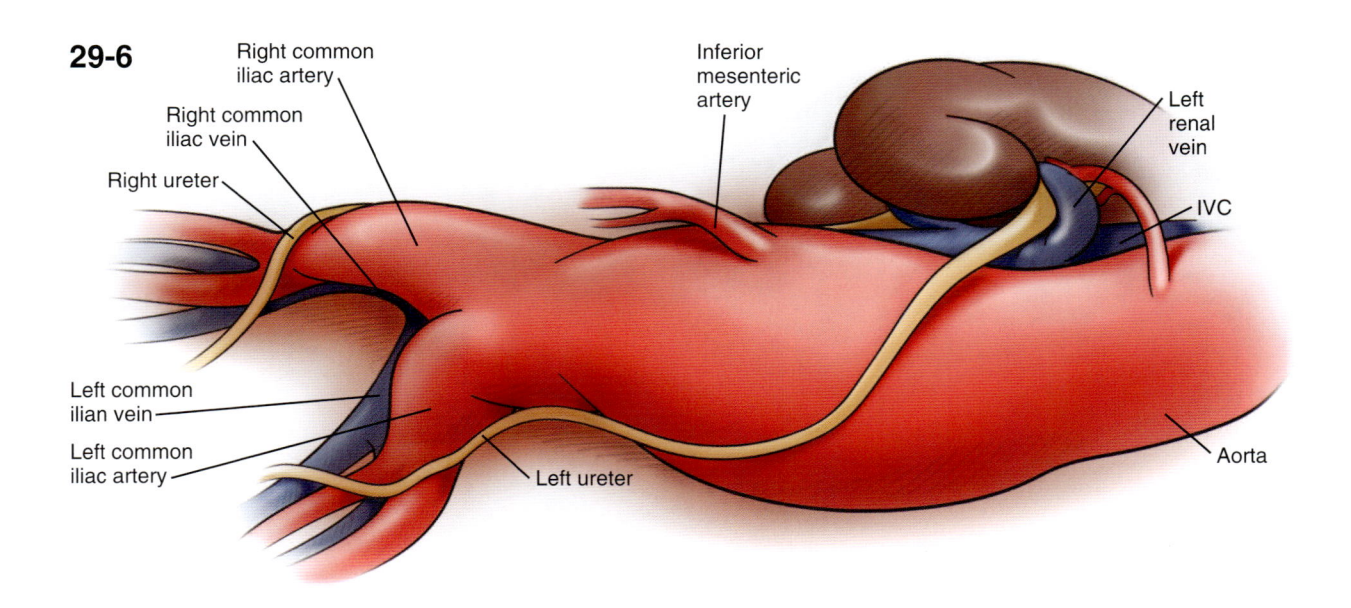

Right common iliac artery
Right common iliac vein
Right ureter
Inferior mesenteric artery
Left renal vein
IVC
Left common ilian vein
Left common iliac artery
Left ureter
Aorta

PROCEDURE <CONTINUED> If the vessels are too inflamed, or it is not safe, back bleeding for both iliac arteries can be controlled by balloon catheter occlusion (4F to 6F balloon catheters) (FIGURE 29-7).

Proximal control will depend on where the aneurysm ends. In general, one will need at least 2 to 3 cm below the left renal artery to clamp and have normal tissue to sew the proximal anastomosis. If more proximal control is needed, the diaphragmatic crus can be divided to expose the suprarenal and supraceliac aorta (FIGURE 29-8). This more proximal clamp site may be desirable in cases where there is significant calcium, inflammation such as an inflammatory aneurysm, or the aneurysm extends up to the renal arteries. The next decision will then need to be made as to whether there is room above the renal arteries to safely place a clamp, or the clamp may need to be placed higher between the renal arteries and superior mesenteric artery (SMA), between the SMA and celiac artery, or above the celiac artery. Dissection in this area can be dangerous, and supraceliac control should always initially be obtained as a bailout. In addition, careful attention should be made to identify posterior lumbar arteries.

Once the clamp sites have been identified and the aorta is opened, back bleeding from the renal ostia and mesenterics can be controlled with external clamps or with occlusion balloons internally. Lumbar arteries are oversewn with nonabsorbable sutures. Pruit occlusion balloon catheters (LeMaitre, Burlington, MA) give the advantage that the vessels can be flushed using the same catheters. This is particularly useful for administering cold renal perfusate or to help protect the vessel origin so that it can be reimplanted or bypassed during reconstruction. Typically, if the repair is not anticipated to take more than 20 to 30 minutes, cold perfusate can be avoided. If the repair is thought to be more complex and reimplantation of renal arteries or bypass is needed, 200 to 300 mL of "kidney cocktail" should be infused into each kidney. This solution consists of 25 grams of mannitol and 1 gram of methylprednisolone in 1 L lactated Ringers cooled to 4°C.

If the aneurysm is infrarenal and there is an adequate length of normal aorta infrarenal, the clamp should still be positioned as close to the lowest renal artery as is safe in order to minimize the length of the residual aorta.

For juxtarenal aortic aneurysms it may be possible to preserve the origin of the right renal artery, but often the left renal will require bypass (FIGURE 29-9). The right renal can be reimplanted with a separate Carell patch if needed. If there is sufficient normal aorta between the right renal and superior mesenteric artery, the origin can be included in a spatulated anastomosis. It is recommended that the left renal bypass is sewn distal on the graft before clamping the renal or aorta. By sewing the sidearm on in a retrograde fashion, distal on the graft, it can be trimmed to the appropriate length just before creating the end-to-end anastomosis with the left renal artery. A ringed ePTFE 6- or 8-mm graft is best used here to prevent kinking. Sewing the bypass to the left renal in this way also allows for it to rotate back into its anatomic location without twisting or kinking the graft.

Once the repair is complete, the aneurysm sac is approximated over the graft. If the crus was divided, the hiatus of the diaphragm is reapproximated with nonabsorbable sutures. The abdominal wall is closed in a single layer with running or interrupted nonabsorbable sutures.

POSTOPERATIVE CARE Extubation should be deferred until the patient is normothermic, coagulation is corrected, and lactate corrected with resuscitation. Since most of these cases do not necessitate entering the left chest, it can be considered early postoperative if parameters are met. Serial hemoglobin levels and hemodynamic monitoring are helpful to ensure hemostasis and stability. Resumption of diet and oral medications is dependent on the usual parameters used to indicate the resolution of ileus. Postoperative mortality after juxtarenal aortic aneurysm repair is 1 to 3%.[11] It is quite common to note deterioration of renal function and thia can be seen in 10 to 20% of patients with a suprarenal clamp site, but dialysis is rarely needed.[12] ■

REFERENCES

1. Oudot J. [Vascular grafting in thromboses of the aortic bifurcation.] *Presse Med.* 1951;59(12):234-236. https://www.ncbi.nlm.nih.gov/pubmed/14816331.

2. Shepard AD, Tollefson DF, Reddy DJ, et al. Left flank retroperitoneal exposure: A technical aid to complex aortic reconstruction. *J Vasc Surg.* 1991;14(3):283-291. doi: 0741-5214(91)90078-9 [pii].

3. Cambria RP, Brewster DC, Abbott WM, et al. Transperitoneal versus retroperitoneal approach for aortic reconstruction: A randomized prospective study. *J Vasc Surg.* 1990;11(2):314-325. doi: 10.1067/mva.1990.17353.

4. Darling C 3rd, Shah DM, Chang BB, Paty PS, Leather RP. Current status of the use of retroperitoneal approach for reconstructions of the aorta and its branches. *Ann Surg.* 1996;224(4):501-508. doi: 10.1097/00000658-199610000-00008 [doi].

5. Jamieson C. Comparison between the transabdominal and retroperitoneal approach for reconstruction of the infrarenal abdominal aorta. *J Vasc Surg.* 1988;8(1):91-92. doi: 0741-5214(88)90254-6 [pii].

6. Kirby LB, Rosenthal D, Atkins CP, et al. Comparison between the transabdominal and retroperitoneal approaches for aortic reconstruction in patients at high risk. *J Vasc Surg.* 1999;30(3):400-405. doi: S0741521499002736 [pii].

7. Nevelsteen A, Smet G, Weymans M, Depre H, Suy R. Transabdominal or retroperitoneal approach to the aorto-iliac tract: A pulmonary function study. *Eur J Vasc Surg.* 1988;2(4):229-232. doi: 10.1016/s0950-821x(88)80031-8 [doi].

8. Sicard GA, Freeman MB, VanderWoude JC, Anderson CB. Comparison between the transabdominal and retroperitoneal approach for reconstruction of the infrarenal abdominal aorta. *J Vasc Surg.* 1987;5(1):19-27. doi: 0741-5214(87)90190-X [pii].

9. Sicard GA, Reilly JM, Rubin BG, et al. Transabdominal versus retroperitoneal incision for abdominal aortic surgery: Report of a prospective randomized trial. *J Vasc Surg.* 1995;21(2):174-3. doi: S0741-5214(95)70260-1 [pii].

10. Ma B, Mei F, Hu K, et al. Retroperitoneal versus transperitoneal approach for elective open abdominal aortic aneurysm repair. *Cochrane Database Sys Rev.* 2021;2021(6):CD010373. https://www.cochranelibrary.com/cdsr/doi/10.1002/14651858.CD010373.pub3. doi: 10.1002/14651858.CD010373.pub3.

11. Knott AW, Kalra M, Duncan AA, et al. Open repair of juxtarenal aortic aneurysms (JAA) remains a safe option in the era of fenestrated endografts. *J Vasc Surg.* 2008;47(4):695-701. https://www.clinicalkey.es/playcontent/1-s2.0-S0741521407020204. doi: 10.1016/j.jvs.2007.12.007.

12. Chong T, Nguyen L, Owens CD, Conte MS, Belkin M. Suprarenal aortic cross-clamp position: A reappraisal of its effects on outcomes for open abdominal aortic aneurysm repair. *J Vasc Surg.* 2009;49(4):873-880. https://www.clinicalkey.es/playcontent/1-s2.0-S0741521408018569. doi: 10.1016/j.jvs.2008.10.057.

29-7

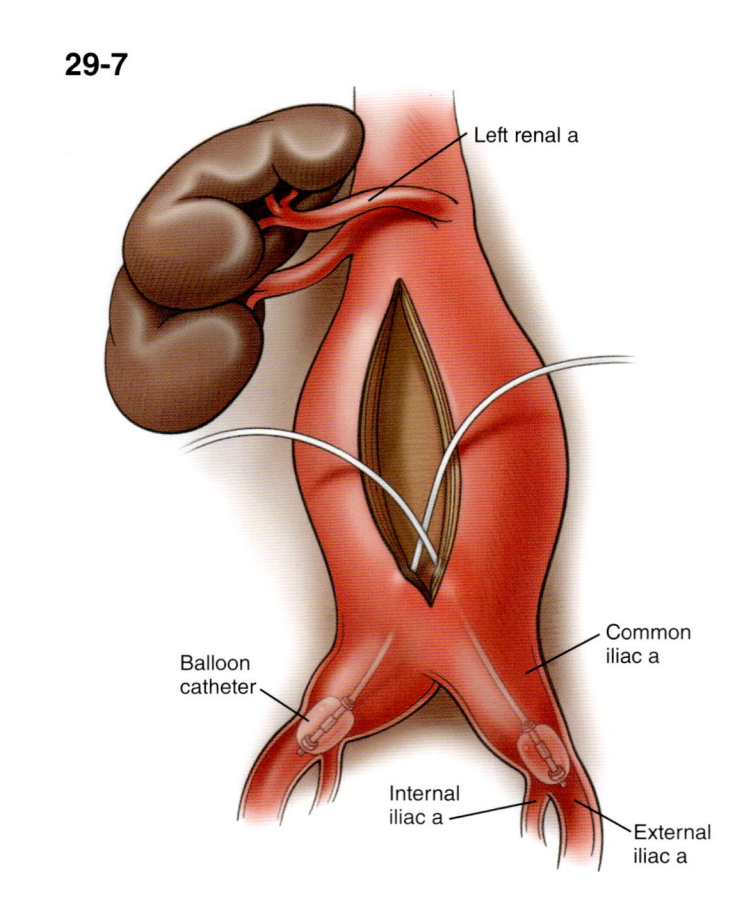

29-8

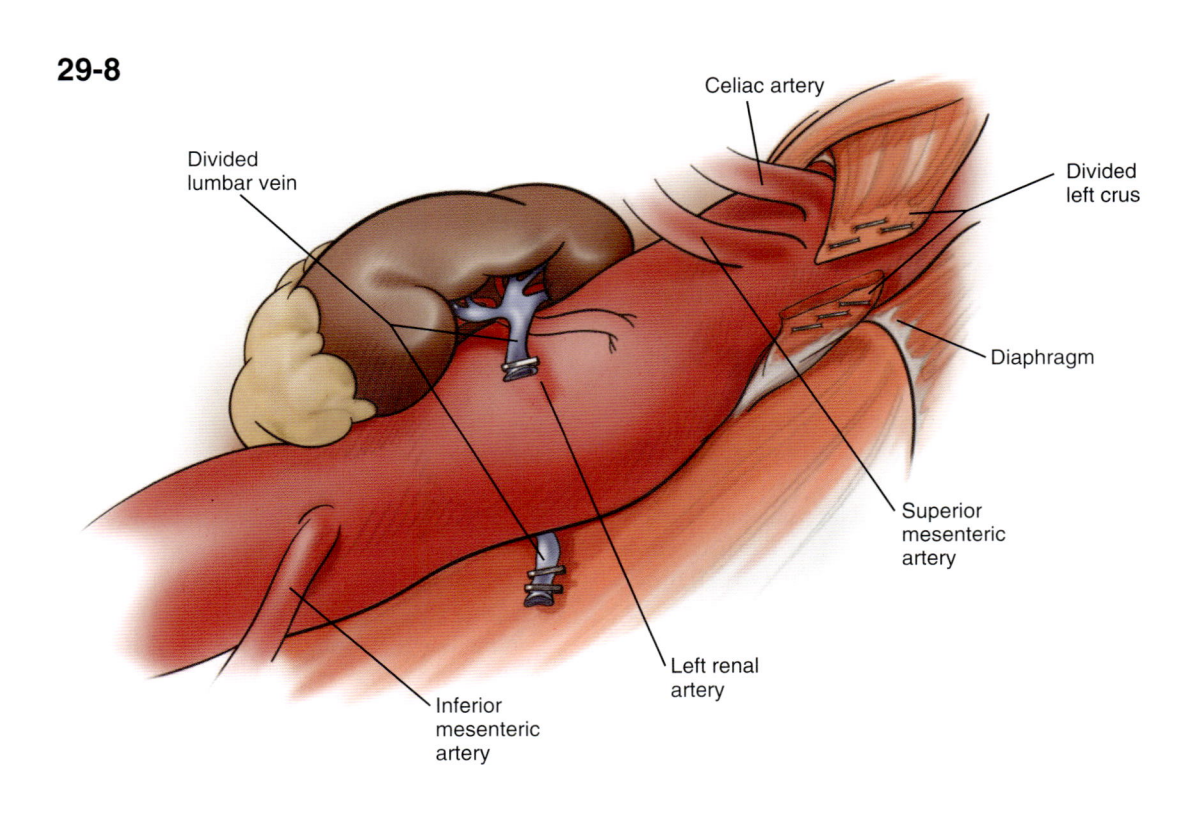

29-9

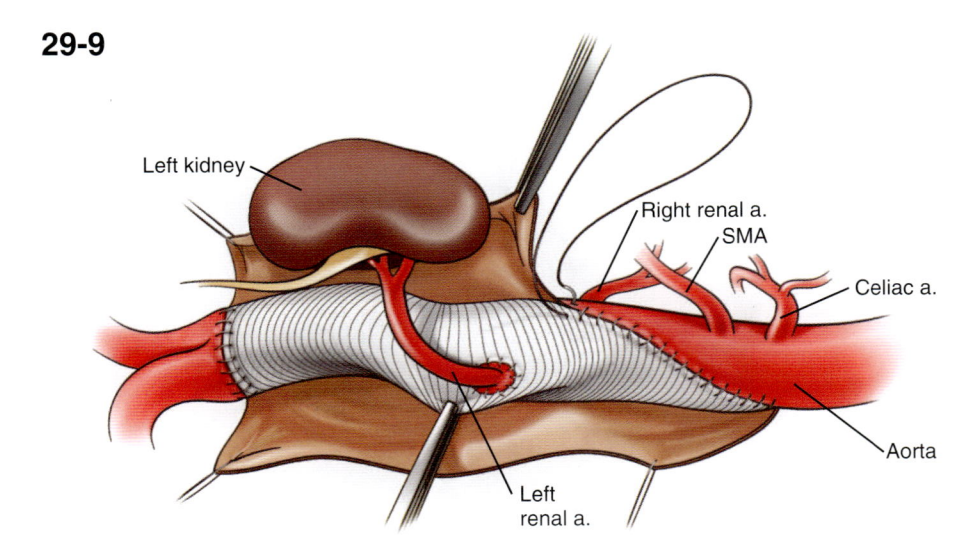

Common and Internal Iliac Artery Aneurysms

Amanda G. Fobare, MD • William Jordan Jr, MD

PEARLS

1. Avoid circumferential dissection of common iliac arteries. The vein is often adherent
2. If vein injury occurs, consider transecting artery to improve exposure of vein
3. If hypogastric perfusion needed and common iliac anastomotic site is not suitable, perform hypogastric anastomosis first, then external iliac anastomosis second.

INDICATIONS When asymptomatic, common and internal iliac artery aneurysms are most commonly discovered incidentally, on cross-sectional imaging. Many of these aneurysms are found in conjunction with aortic ectasia or aneurysmal disease. Consensus statements favor repair of isolated iliac artery aneurysms that measure ≥3.5 cm in otherwise healthy patients. If aortic repair is indicated or there is a concomitant aortic aneurysm of any size, then the iliac repair is done during the same procedure. Symptomatic common and internal iliac artery aneurysms may present with vague abdominal, pelvic, or back pain. Some may demonstrate ureteral obstruction due to compression. Others may complain of tenesmus or constipation. Sudden onset abdominal, flank, or groin pain may indicate rupture.

A full history and physical examination should be obtained from the patient, taking care to elucidate any prior abdominal surgical history that may influence the operative approach. The history should also identify any family members with aneurysmal disease or connective tissue disorders. Smoking cessation is advised in all active tobacco users. Maximal medical therapy is advised to manage all comorbid conditions prior to operative planning. Furthermore, cardiac risk stratification and pulmonary function tests (PFTs) are suggested for all patients with significant risk factors for cardiopulmonary disease.

When considering open repair for common iliac artery (CIA) aneurysms or internal iliac artery (IIA) aneurysms, it is important to obtain contrast CT imaging of the abdomen and pelvis. This imaging will aid in evaluating for any aortic ectasia or aneurysmal disease that would alter operative strategy, with particular attention toward open versus endovascular repair. Furthermore, it is important to clarify the patency of the hypogastric arteries and mesenteric arteries so that an operative approach may be selected that would minimize the risk of pelvic or intestinal ischemia.

Isolated CIA aneurysms may be reconstructed using a Dacron or PTFE interposition graft. Provided there is a cuff of healthy CIA tissue proximally, a short-segment interposition graft may be sewn to nonaneurysmal distal CIA tissue, or the common orifice of the external and internal iliac arteries. Bilateral common iliac artery aneurysms may necessitate reconstruction with an aortobiiliac graft. It is imperative to sew to nonaneurysmal infrarenal aortic or iliac tissue proximally, and nonaneurysmal iliac arteries or common orifice of the distal common iliac to incorporate both the external and internal iliac arteries distally (**FIGURE 30-1A** and **B**).

Isolated internal iliac artery aneurysms pose a greater challenge given their posterior position in the pelvis. It is important to evaluate the pelvic collaterals in the preoperative planning phase. If the contralateral hypogastric artery is patent, sacrificing the aneurysmal IIA is an acceptable option. This is typically done from within the vessel, as circumferential dissection of the aneurysmal IIA is fraught with pitfalls of venous injury and difficult to control bleeding from these friable veins. If injury occurs to the iliac veins, IVC, or the pelvic veins, then one should consider complete division

of the arterial anatomy (**FIGURE 30-2**) with more dissection of the artery from the vein before repair is undertaken for the venous structure. If the venous tissue becomes too friable, then direct venous ligation may be required to control massive hemorrhage. Occlusion balloon catheters may be used for hemostatic control to avoid gaining circumferential control of the vessel, particularly in patients with heavy calcification.

POSITION

1. Transperitoneal approach: The patient is placed supine, arms extended.
2. Retroperitoneal approach: The patient is placed on a bean bag, supine. Following intubation, the patient is placed in a modified lateral decubitus, with the hip positioned at the flex of the bed. The shoulders are at a 45-degree angle, with the arm placed on a sling or arm board anteriorly and superiorly. The pelvis is positioned flat, and the bed is flexed to open the space between the inferior border of the ribs and the anterior superior iliac spine (**FIGURE 30-3**).

OPERATIVE PREPARATION

1. Transperitoneal approach: After routine skin preparation, the operative field is draped to include the xiphoid process, the abdomen, and the groins to the level of the mid-thighs bilaterally. (See Chapter 28 for details of transabdominal exposure.)
2. Retroperitoneal approach: After routine skin preparation, the operative field is draped to include the thoraco-abdomen to the level of the xiphoid process superiorly, the flank laterally, and the mid-thigh (including the groin) inferiorly. (See Chapter 29 for details of the retroperitoneal exposure.)
3. Ureteral stenting: For patients who present with compressive symptoms and evidence of hydronephrosis, preoperative ureteral stenting should be considered for decompression of the kidney and easier intraoperative identification.

INCISION AND EXPOSURE

1. Transperitoneal approach: The incision is made in the midline, with proximal extension based upon the need for aortic exposure and reconstruction. Extension to the pubic bone is important to allow for deep pelvic exposure when the internal iliac repair is planned to a distal target. This incision is deepened through the skin and subcutaneous tissue, until the rectus abdominus facia is reached. The linea alba is incised and the fascia is elevated, taking care not to injure the underlying intestine. The preperitoneal fat is mobilized or divided. The transverse colon and omentum are elevated and retracted superiorly, followed by retraction of the small intestine to the right upper quadrant of the abdomen (**FIGURE 30-4**). If the infrarenal aorta is ectatic or aneurysmal and repair will include replacement of the distal aorta, the duodenum is mobilized off the retroperitoneum to the right upper quadrant. The retroperitoneal tissue overlying the aorta is incised, taking care to err to the patient's right side, to avoid injury to the IMA. The aorta is mobilized below the level of the renal arteries to develop an adequate area for proximal clamping. The peritoneum over the common iliac arteries is incised to expose the vessel wall. Great care must be taken during mobilization and exposure of the iliac arteries, as the iliac veins may be adherent. Circumferential exposure is often not required, to limit injury of the iliac veins and IVC confluence which are adjacent and posterior. **CONTINUES ▶**

30-1

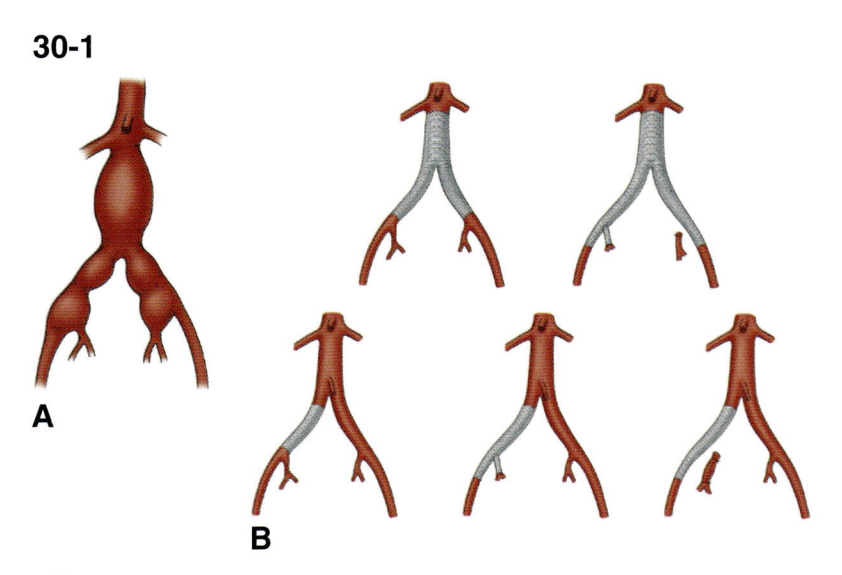

Figure 30-1 A and B. Bilateral common iliac aneurysms before and after.

30-2

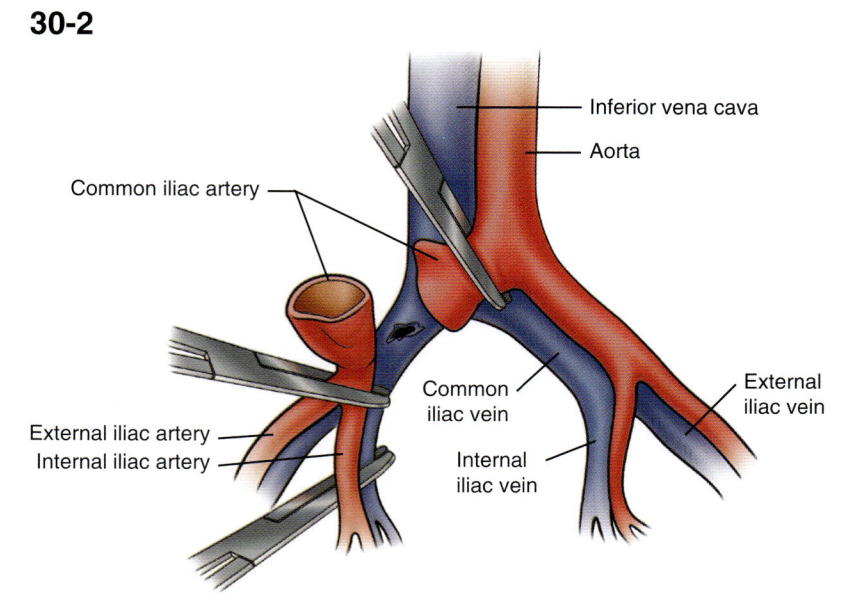

Figure 30-2 Division of iliac artery to expose injured vein.

30-3

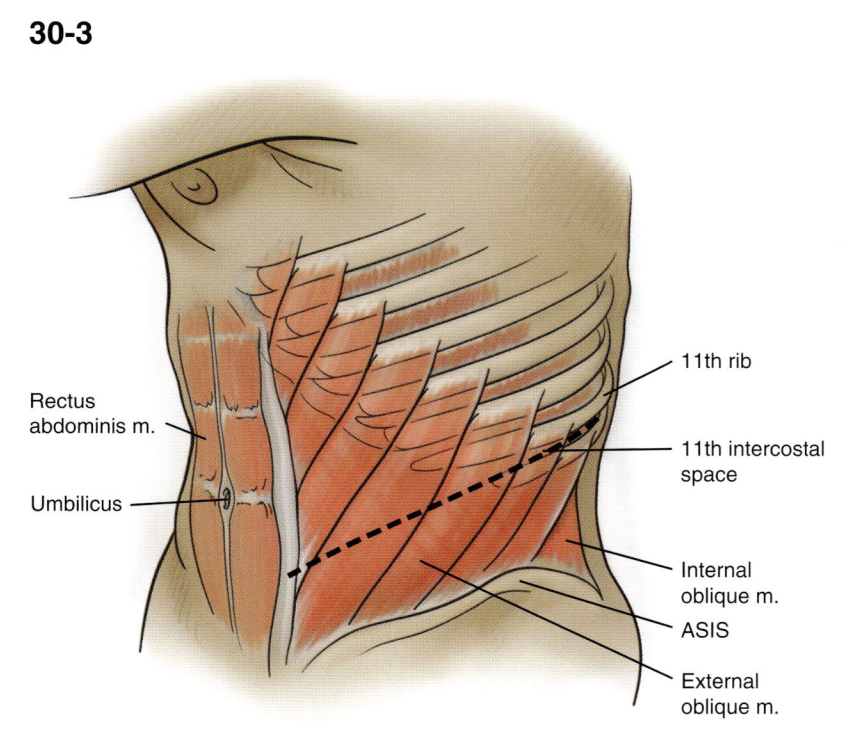

Figure 30-3 Retroperitoneal approach.

30-4

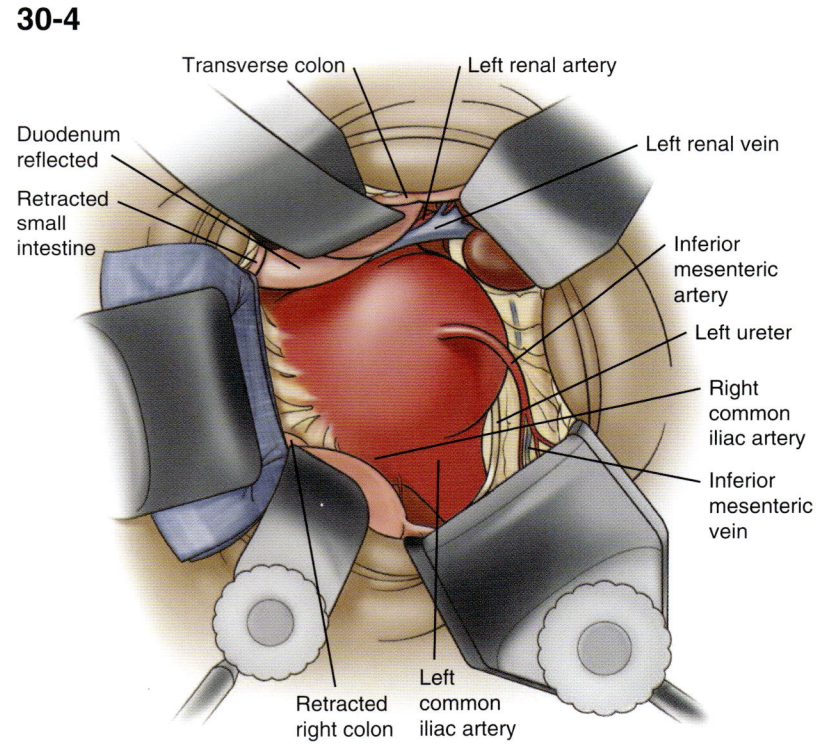

Figure 30-4 Transabdominal. Transverse colon and small bowel reflected.

INCISION AND EXPOSURE CONTINUED

2. Retroperitoneal approach: An incision is made from the edge of the 12TH rib and carried down to just superior to the inguinal ligament on the left side. Electrocautery is used to deepen the incision through the subcutaneous tissues. The external and internal oblique muscles are divided, followed by splitting of the transversus abdominus. Great care is taken to avoid entering the peritoneum, which lies just below the transversus (FIGURE 30-5A). The peritoneum is gently mobilized with a moistened gauze or sponge stick so that the peritoneal contents may be retracted. Care must be taken to identify the ureter, ilioinguinal, or genitofemoral nerves, which lie on the anterior surface of the psoas muscle. If the peritoneum is entered it can usually be closed with a few simple stitches to maintain the advantage of the peritoneal sac containment of the visceral contents

DETAILS OF PROCEDURE The aorta is mobilized as described in Chapter 28. To expose the right common iliac artery and its bifurcation, the right colon and ureter are retracted, and the aortic bifurcation is identified; if possible, the autonomic nerve plexus should be preserved. The retroperitoneal tissue and fat overlying the anterior surface of the artery are carefully divided, paying close attention to identify and gently retract the right ureter (FIGURE 30-5B). In most circumstances, the common iliac aneurysm does not need to be dissected circumferentially, as this is usually densely adherent to left and right common iliac veins. The left common iliac bifurcation is exposed by initially reflecting the sigmoid colon after mobilization through the line of Toldt. Careful attention is also made to gently retract the left ureter (FIGURE 30-5C). A tunnel is then created underneath the sigmoid mesocolon, staying on the anterior surface of the artery.

Following adequate exposure of the target vessels, it is important to gain proximal and distal control. In cases of heavily calcified iliac arteries, where clamping is a concern, occlusion balloon catheters may be utilized in the place of clamps. Furthermore, in the case of internal iliac artery aneurysms, great care must be taken during dissection, as the pelvic veins lie on the posterior wall of the artery and may be densely adherent.

Prior to clamping, the patient is given a therapeutic dose of systemic heparin. The distal clamps are applied, followed by the proximal clamp. In the setting requiring the use occlusive balloons distally, we advocate for proximal clamping first, followed by opening of the aneurysm sac, back bleeding, and then placement of balloon occlusion catheters (FIGURE 30-6). In cases where the proximal anastomosis is the distal aorta, evacuation of thrombus followed by ligation of lumbar and sacral vessels from within the aneurysm sac is completed with 2-0 silk suture. CONTINUES

30-5

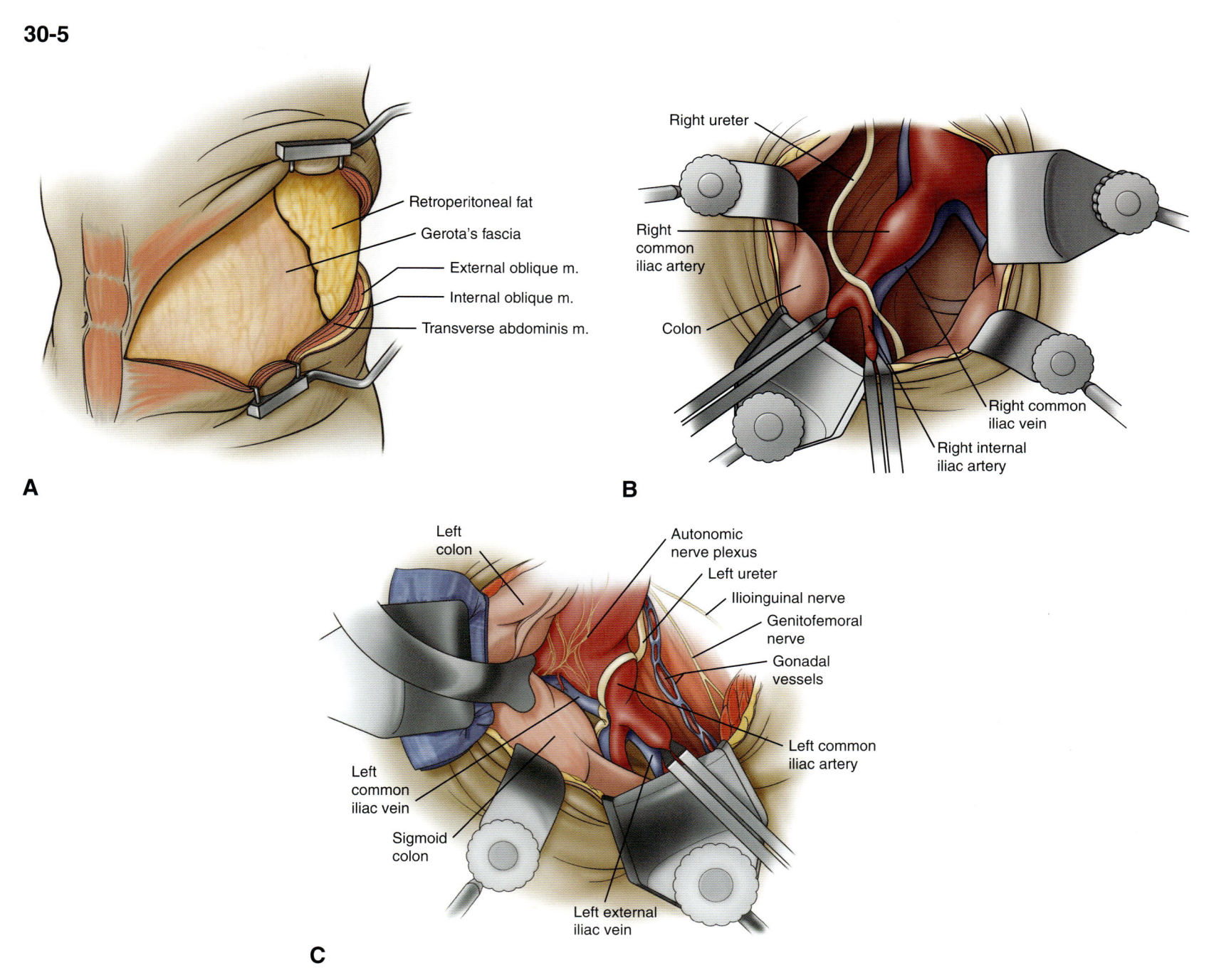

Figure 30-5 A. Retroperitoneal exposure left common iliac. B. Right common iliac artery exposure. C. Left common iliac artery exposure.

30-6

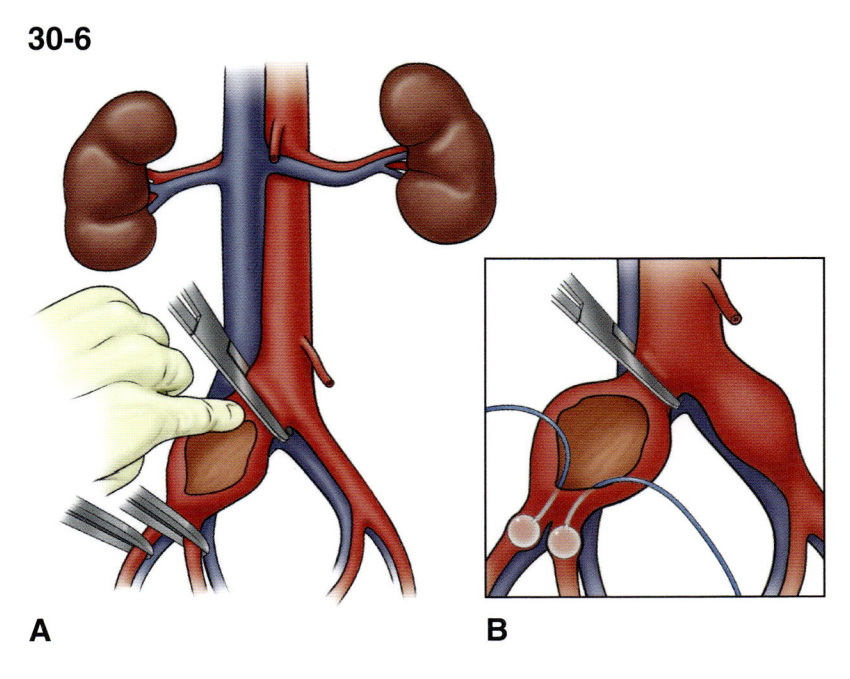

Figure 30-6 A, B. Clamps and balloon occlusion.

DETAILS OF PROCEDURE `CONTINUED` The proximal anastomosis is completed with a 3-0 Prolene for aortic anastomoses, or a 3-0 or 4-0 Prolene if the common iliac artery is the proximal anastomosis site. Distal anastomoses are completed with 3-0 or 4-0 Prolene suture to the appropriate target. If the hypogastric artery is planned for revascularization and the iliac bifurcation is too large for the appropriately sized graft, then a bifurcated anastomosis is prepared. Typically, we construct the anastomosis to the hypogastric artery first and then attach a separate limb of the same graft from the Dacron graft to an appropriate external iliac site (FIGURE 30-7A). Occasionally, the configuration sits better sewing directly to the external iliac artery, and then a jump graft can be taken off the external iliac anastomosis to the internal iliac. If this configuration is selected, it is helpful for visualization to do the distal anastomosis first (FIGURE 30-7B). The left external iliac sometimes can be reimplanted directly on to the graft (FIGURE 30-7C). In the standard fashion, we recommend back bleeding prior to completion of the anastomosis. Repair stitches are placed as needed, taking care not to injure the iliac veins or the vena cava. Felt pledgets may be used to reinforce anastomoses if required.

CLOSURE

1. Transperitoneal approach: If the aneurysm sac was divided, the aneurysm wall is closed loosely over the reconstruction, with interrupted silk suture. The peritoneum overlying the aorta (if divided) is closed with a running 2-0 Vicryl suture. The viscera are returned to the anatomic position, the SMA pulse is confirmed as excessive traction can create an injury, and the omentum is draped over the intestine (FIGURE 30-8). The fascia is closed with two 0-looped PDS suture. The subcutaneous tissue may be approximated with interrupted or running 3-0 suture. Staples are used to reapproximate the skin.

2. Retroperitoneal approach: The transversalis fascia and muscle are reapproximated as a deep layer using a looped 0 PDS suture. The internal and external oblique fascia are reapproximated using a looped 0 PDS suture. Following this, the subcutaneous tissues may be reapproximated with interrupted or running 3-0 Vicryl suture. The skin is reapproximated using staples.

POSTOPERATIVE CARE Patients may be extubated in the operating room if they have been adequately resuscitated without concern for pulmonary compromise. Patients are monitored in the intensive care unit (ICU) following their operation for frequent vascular and neurologic checks. If both internal iliac arteries were ligated or are occluded, special care must be taken to monitor for pelvic and even spinal cord ischemia.

Patients should be monitored with frequent laboratory studies, coagulopathy should be corrected, and resuscitation should continue while monitoring for lactic acid levels and urine output.

A nasogastric tube is typically placed in the operating room and remains for a few postoperative days. Timing varies with surgeon preference, but attention to GI function is important as an ileus can impact the convalescence and extend the hospitalization. Given the extensive mobilization of the intestine and the extent of surgery, postoperative ileus is possible. The diet is advanced slowly back to the preoperative diet so long as the patient continues to have bowel function. If both internal iliac arteries are ligated or occluded, patients must be monitored closely for colonic ischemia.

Early mobilization of patients up and out of bed is a cornerstone of postoperative care. Involvement of physical and occupational therapy is recommended for these often-infirmed patient and can facilitate the recovery period. ■

30-7

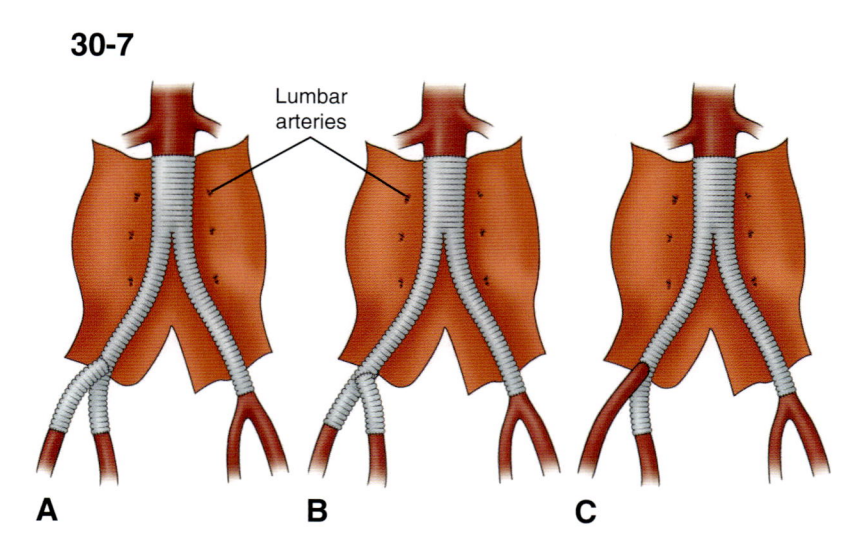

Lumbar arteries

A   B   C

Figure 30-7 A. Aortic limb to internal with jump graft to external. B. Aortic limb to external iliac and jump graft to internal iliac. C. Aorta to internal iliac, reimplant external iliac.

30-8

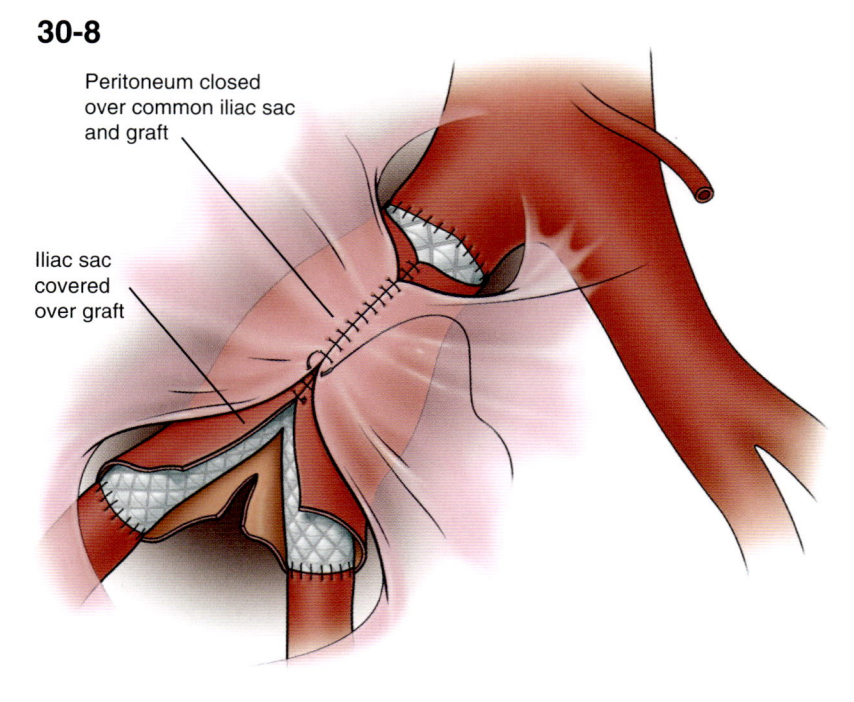

Peritoneum closed over common iliac sac and graft

Iliac sac covered over graft

Figure 30-8 Reperitonealize.

DEBRANCHING: ILIAC, VISCERAL, AORTO-RENAL

Marton Berczeli, MD • **Alan B. Lumsden, MD**

INDICATIONS Patients with thoracoabdominal aortic aneurysm (TAA) or complex abdominal aneurysm that involve the visceral and renal branches of the aorta may benefit from a hybrid approach, which is considered less invasive than conventional open repair. The advantage of this procedure is the reduced renal, visceral, and lower extremity ischemic time, and the absence of aortic cross-clamping and single-lung ventilation or thoracotomy. During the procedure the visceral branches are connected to the common iliac artery/arteries, infrarenal aorta, or a previous graft with retrograde extra-anatomic bypasses followed by an endovascular aneurysm repair (EVAR + TEVAR) (FIGURES 31-1 and 31-2).

The indications for abdominal debranching vary, but when conventional open reconstruction is limited based on significant comorbidities, a hybrid option can be a feasible alternative. Patients with chronic obstructive pulmonary disease (COPD) and concomitant TAA with otherwise acceptable cardiac and renal function benefit most from this approach. Candidates for abdominal debranching are unsuitable for open surgical TAA repair based on their comorbidities, and typically pulmonary status precludes thoracotomy. Hence thorough evaluation of pulmonary, cardiac, and renal functions and existing diseases (diabetes, hypertension, etc.) is fundamental prior to surgery.

Chest, abdomen, and pelvis computed tomography angiography (CTA) or magnetic resonance angiography (MRA) is mandatory to visualize the anatomy of the whole aorta and iliofemoral arteries for operative planning. To obtain good outcomes, the optimal source of inflow and outflow vessels must be present: a calcified, stenotic distal aorta or common iliac arteries are relative contraindications. The potential inflow vessels for debranching include common iliac arteries, external iliac arteries, infrarenal aorta, common hepatic artery, splenic artery, and ascending and descending aorta.

When assessing the outflow, an appropriate caliber vessel should be chosen after careful review for any anatomical variants (accessory renal artery, aberrant visceral take-off, retroaortic renal vein, etc.). Adequate sealing of the endograft must be present in the descending thoracic aorta to complete the hybrid reconstruction: a 2-cm noncalcified wall segment is required. The completion can be done either in a single-staged or a two-staged fashion. The advantage of choosing a single-stage approach is the absence of risk of aneurysm rupture between procedures, but it prolongs surgical time and results in higher morbidity and mortality. Therefore, relative risk of rupture (aneurysm size), patient's general condition, age, and potential operative difficulties during debranching should be encountered that may prolong surgical time. If a single common iliac artery is used as source of inflow, the contralateral side should be used as access for EVAR.

POSITION In general, the patient is placed in a supine position, although on occasion a retroperitoneal approach is applicable if not all vessels need debranching.

OPERATIVE PREPARATION A nasogastric (NG) tube is required along with large bore central venous access. After routine skin preparation, the patient is prepped and draped from nipples to knees.

INCISION AND EXPOSURE A vertical midline incision is made from the xyphoid process to the pubis below the umbilicus, although some prefer a chevron incision. Then the incision is deepened through the subcutaneous tissue and linea alba, and the peritoneum is incised under direct vision. After entering and exploring the peritoneal cavity, the divided abdominal walls are retracted laterally using a self-retracting system.

CELIAC TRUNK EXPOSURE FOR DEBRANCHING: To expose the celiac trunk or outflow branch such as the hepatic artery, the first step involves dividing the triangular ligament of the liver to mobilize the left lobe of the liver to the patient's right. Upon dividing the ligament, the liver is pulled down gently and one's finger can be placed behind the ligament not to injure the left hepatic vein or inferior phrenic vein (FIGURE 31-3). Slightly elevating and mobilizing the left lobe of the liver facilitates exposure of the right the gastrohepatic ligament. The previously placed NG tube can help in identifying the esophagus and the expected location of the celiac trunk. The lesser sac should be opened via a longitudinal incision close to the gastroesophageal junction to the pylorus. Before the procedure, the left hepatic artery should be checked on preoperative imaging, as in approximately 10% of the cases it arises from the left gastric and runs across the incision made on the parietal peritoneum to expose the celiac trunk. After gently retracting the stomach and esophagus to the left and caudally (FIGURE 31-4), the incision of the posterior parietal peritoneum is required. **CONTINUES ▶**

31-1

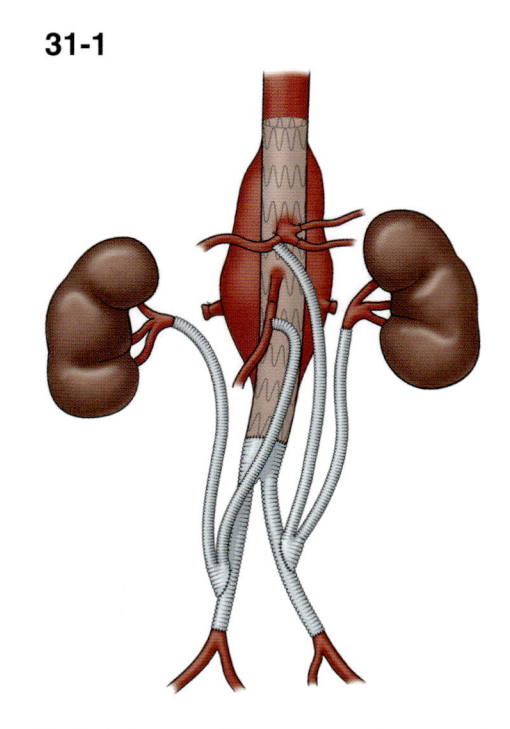

Figure 31-1 Schematic illustrations of a visceral and renal debranching using bilateral preexisting bifurcated Dacron graft as inflow.

31-2

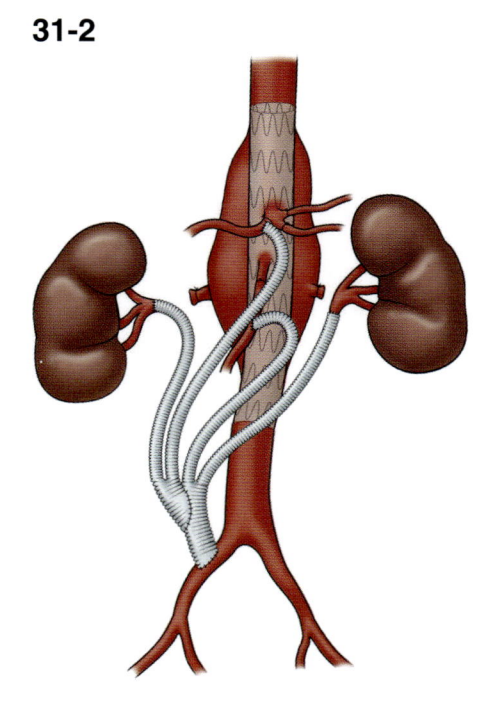

Figure 31-2 Schematic illustrations of a visceral and renal debranching using unilateral preexisting bifurcated Dacron graft as inflow.

31-3

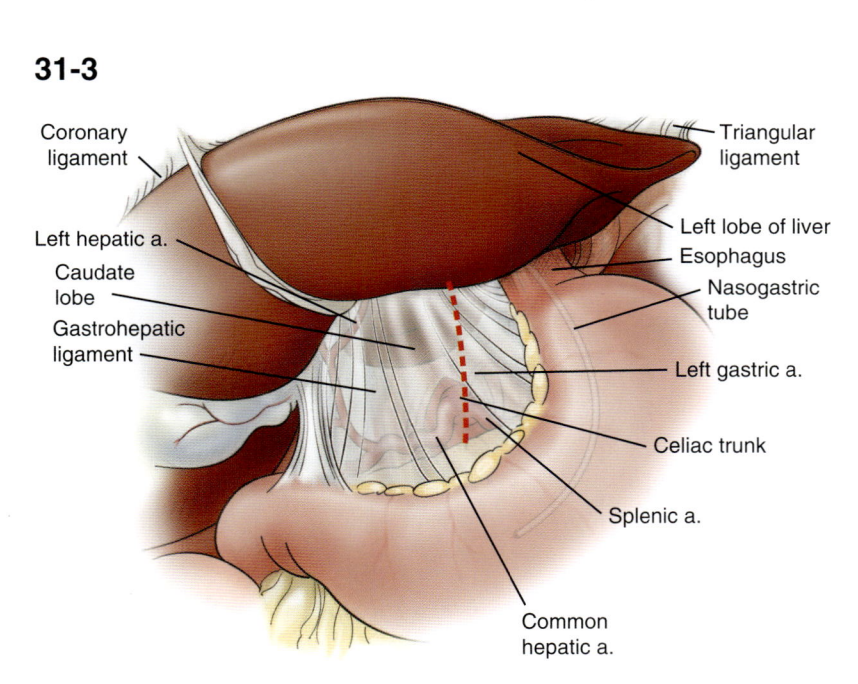

Figure 31-3 Control of the triangular ligament before dividing it to mobilize the liver.

31-4

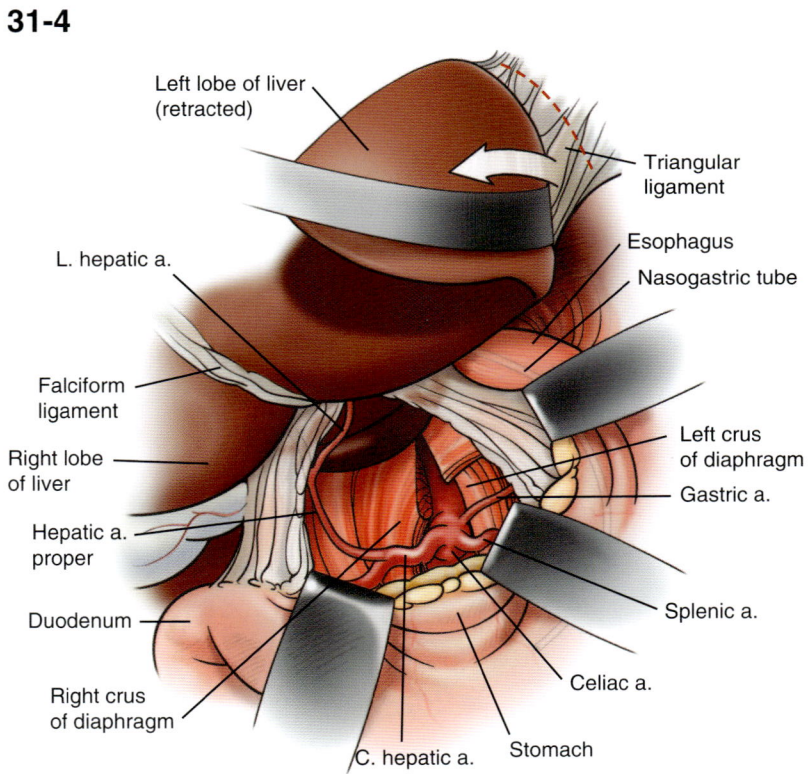

Figure 31-4 Gastrohepatic ligament with the stomach slightly retracted inferiorly.

INCISION AND EXPOSURE *CELIAC TRUNK EXPOSURE FOR DEBRANCHING:* `CONTINUED` To appropriately expose the celiac trunk (FIGURE 31-5), the overlying celiac ganglion must be divided. The common hepatic artery should be exposed by further dissection superior to the pancreas in the porta hepatis to include the proper hepatic artery and the gastroduodenal artery (FIGURE 31-6).

SUPERIOR MESENTERIC ARTERY EXPOSURE FOR DEBRANCHING: For abdominal debranching, inframesocolic or supramesocolic exposure are preferred inferior to the pancreas. For inframesocolic exposure, the transverse colon and the greater omentum are lifted anterior and superior using self-retractors, and the small bowel is packed inferiorly and to the right. The third and fourth segment of the duodenum are identified and the ligamentum of Treitz divided with other attachments of the duodenum to mobilize it to the right. Then the root of the mesentery is incised to the left of to the duodenum; palpation of the superior mesenteric artery (SMA) can help in identification and placing the longitudinal incision on the mesentery (FIGURE 31-7). `CONTINUES`

31-5

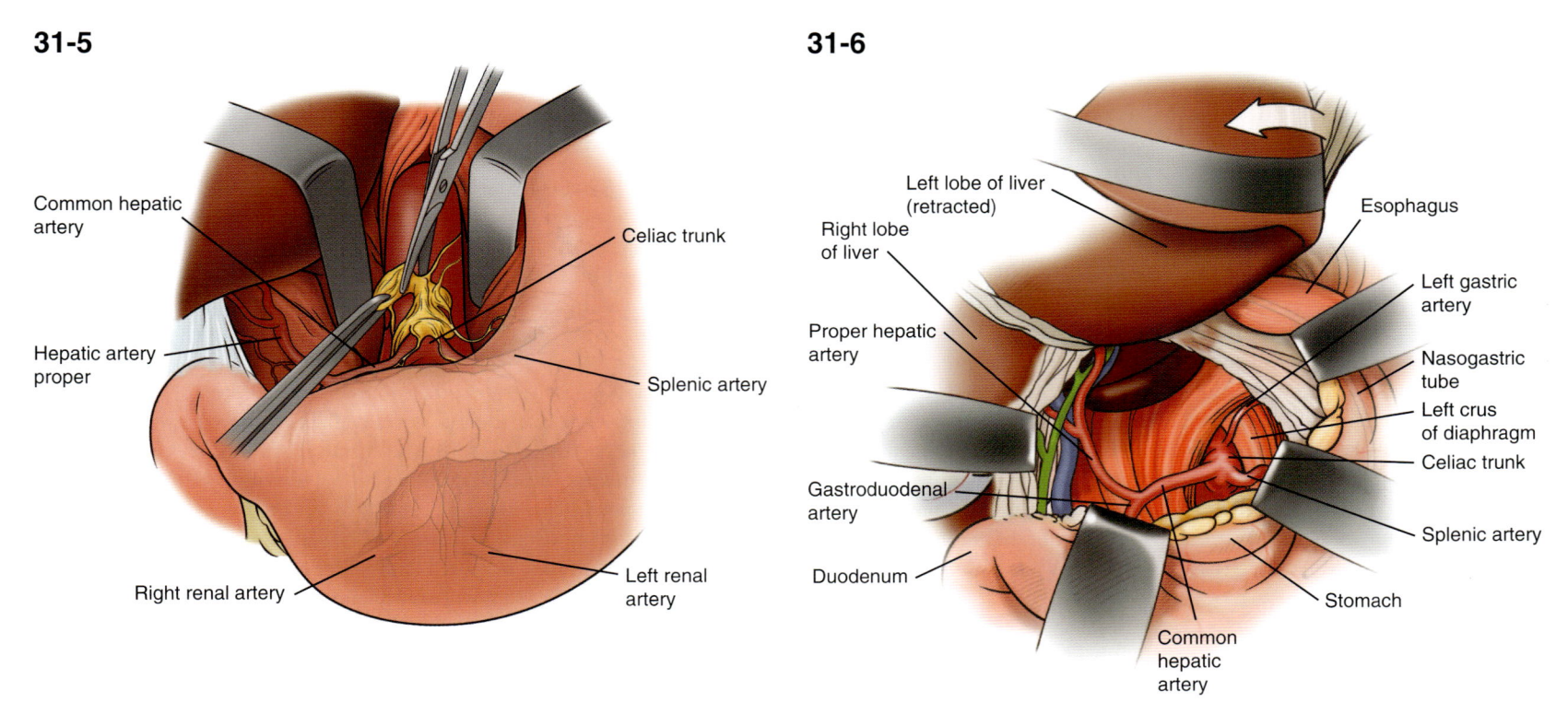

Figure 31-5 Celiac ganglion divided to expose the celiac artery.

31-6

Figure 31-6 Common hepatic artery.

31-7

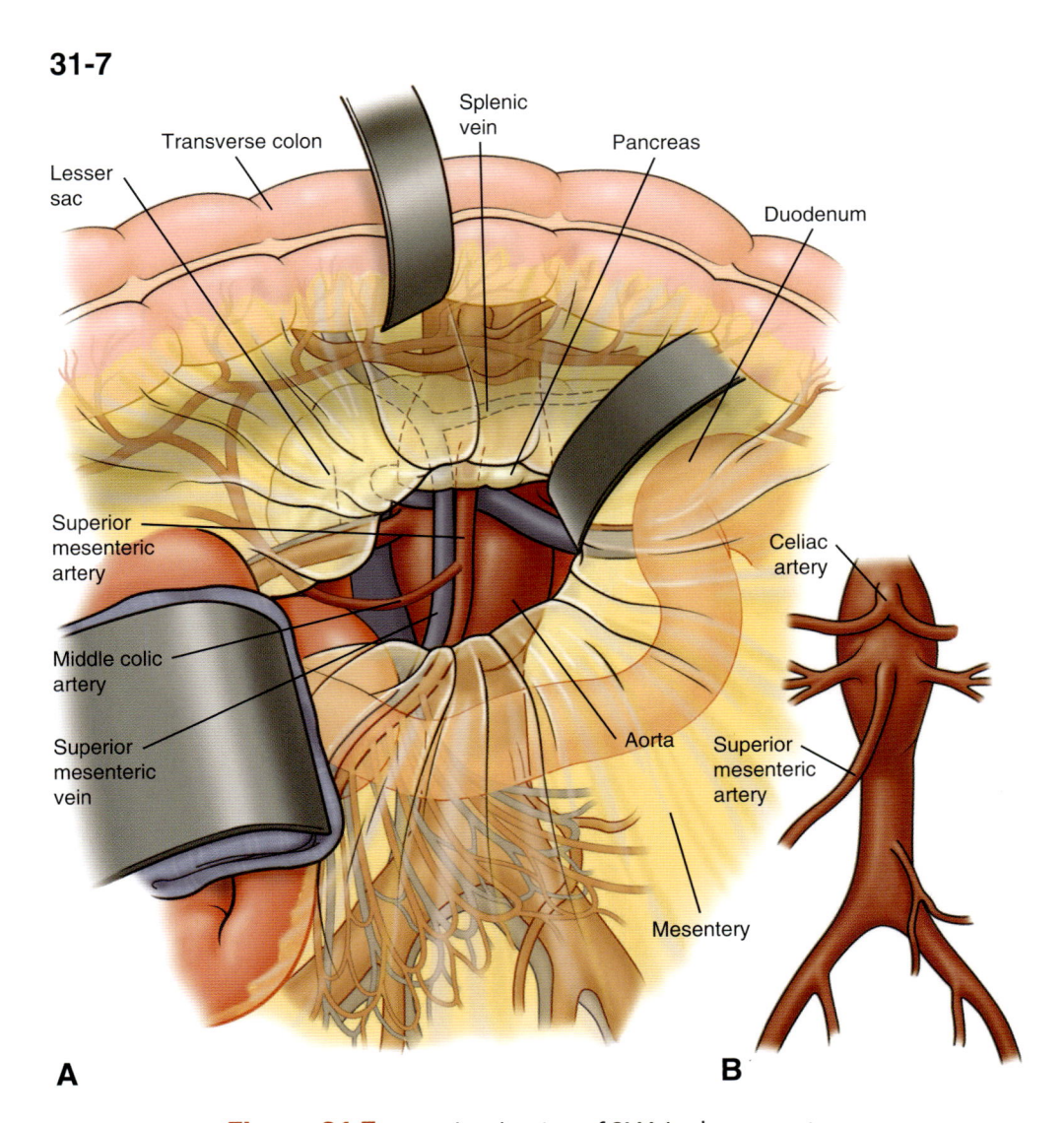

A

B

Figure 31-7 Partial: palpation of SMA in the mesentery.

INCISION AND EXPOSURE *SUPERIOR MESENTERIC ARTERY EXPOSURE FOR DEBRANCHING:* `CONTINUED` Electrocautery with a bipolar cautery is preferred to encounter the small venous bleeding and chyle leak from small lymphatic vessels of the mesentery. A small Weitlaner retractor can be used for better exposure. Multiple branches arise from the side of the SMA, some from the posterior, but none from the anterior surface. These branches should be circled with vessel loops. To create an adequate route for the retrograde bypass, the distal portion of the SMA is preferred to proximal to avoid kinking of the graft. An alternative method is traditional exposure of the SMA caudal to the pancreas through the lesser sac, where the size of the SMA is greater. The artery is on the left side of the superior mesenteric vein. Using this route may avoid having to C-loop the graft (FIGURE 31-8).

RENAL ARTERY EXPOSURE FOR DEBRANCHING: After retracting the midline fascia edges, the transverse colon and the greater momentum are positioned superiorly under moist laparotomy pads, followed by retracting the small bowel to the right. For the left renal artery, the parietal peritoneum is incised to expose the infrarenal aorta, then the ligamentum of Treitz divided with additional attachments of the duodenum to further mobilize the small bowel to the right and facilitate more cephalad exposure. The inferior mesenteric vein should be identified and ligated to further facilitate exposure. The left renal vein (LRV) is the next important structure in the exposure (FIGURE 31-9). This could be either preserved and lifted with an umbilical tape (before elevating the vein additional ligation of lumbar, gonadal, or adrenal branches is highly recommended). Alternately, the LRV can be suture-ligated and divided close to the inferior vena cava (IVC) and divided, making sure to preserve the adrenal and lumbar vein if this is done. After the ligation or mobilization of the left renal vein, the left renal artery can be identified. Further exposure of the artery is gained by horizontally extending the exposure (previous inferior mesenteric vein ligation is mandatory).

Exposing the origin of the right renal artery requires the isolation and retraction of the IVC laterally. The right renal artery is usually localized just posterior to the angle of the IVC and LRV. Lumbar veins encountered are ligated prior retraction of the IVC. The right renal artery will be accessible after gentle retraction of the IVC.

INFRARENAL AORTA AND ILIAC ARTERY EXPOSURES: The exposure for the infrarenal aorta and iliac arteries is through standard approached as previously described.

DETAILS OF PROCEDURE Debranching of the visceral and renal arteries of the aorta is one surgical procedure divided into four individual procedures. Each bypass has its own unique pitfalls, hence anatomical understanding and technical considerations are key to achieve optimal outcome.

CELIAC BYPASS: Once the exposure is completed, a tunnel is created for the bypass in a retrogastric fashion: After gentle elevation of the stomach, a channel must be created underneath the stomach and superficial to the pancreas using blunt finger dissection and electrocautery. Then the transverse colon must be elevated, and the tunnel must be continued through the mesocolon using electrocautery without injuring the mesocolic vessels (FIGURE 31-10).

A bifurcated Dacron graft is the most often used prosthetic graft type. In some countries, a hybrid graft is an available option as well, with preloaded covered stents to perform the distal anastomosis. After systemic heparin administration, the common iliac artery/limb bifurcated bypass is first performed. The proximal anastomosis is beveled and inferiorly angled, as this is important to achieve a "lazy" C-loop for the bypass. The end-to-side anastomosis is created with 3/0 or 4/0 polypropylene suture in a running fashion. After removal of the clamps, the anastomosis is checked for bleeding and the main body of the graft is clamped. Then one limb of the bifurcated graft is brought through the previously created tunnel. The limb is clamped at the level of the proximal anastomosis and cut to length. The graft should have a slight curve before anastomosis to avoid kinking. Then the common hepatic artery is clamped and a longitudinal arteriotomy is made with 11-blade and extended with a Potts scissor. For the end-to-side anastomosis, a 6/0 polypropylene suture is used in a running fashion (FIGURE 31-11). After completion of the anastomosis, intraoperative Doppler should be used to check the outflow vessels. The proximal vessel (distal to the anastomosis) should be ligated if possible, or embolized in the future to avoid a type 2 endoleak. If the hepatic artery bypass is chosen, one needs to ligate either the celiac or all three branches separately.

`CONTINUES`

31-8

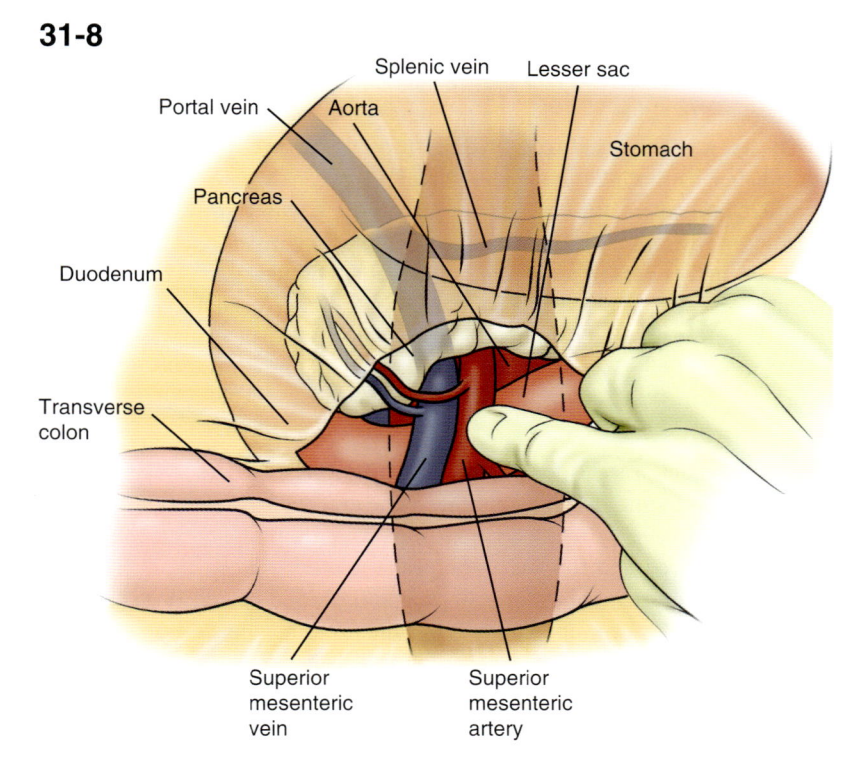

Figure 31-8 Exposed superior mesenteric artery.

31-9

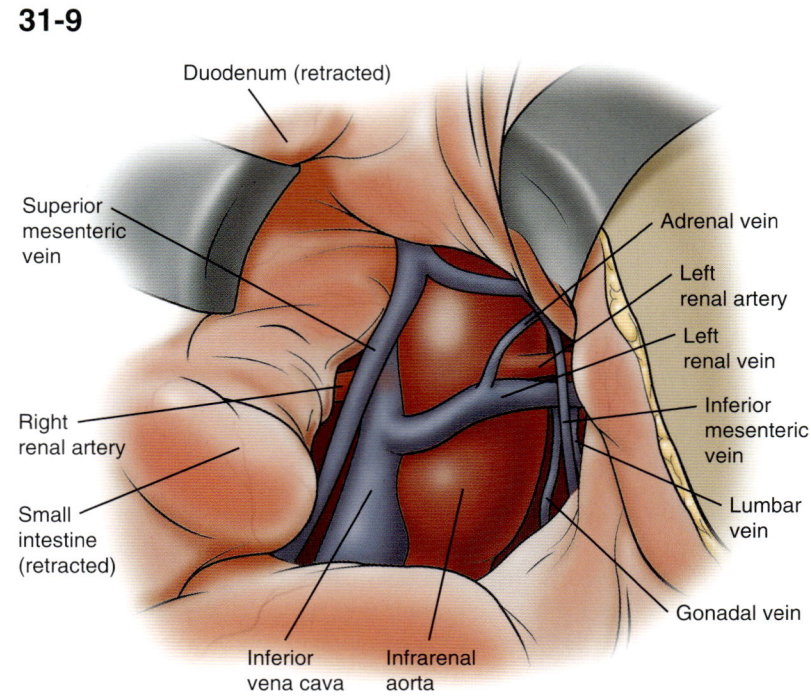

Figure 31-9 Left renal vein exposure.

31-10

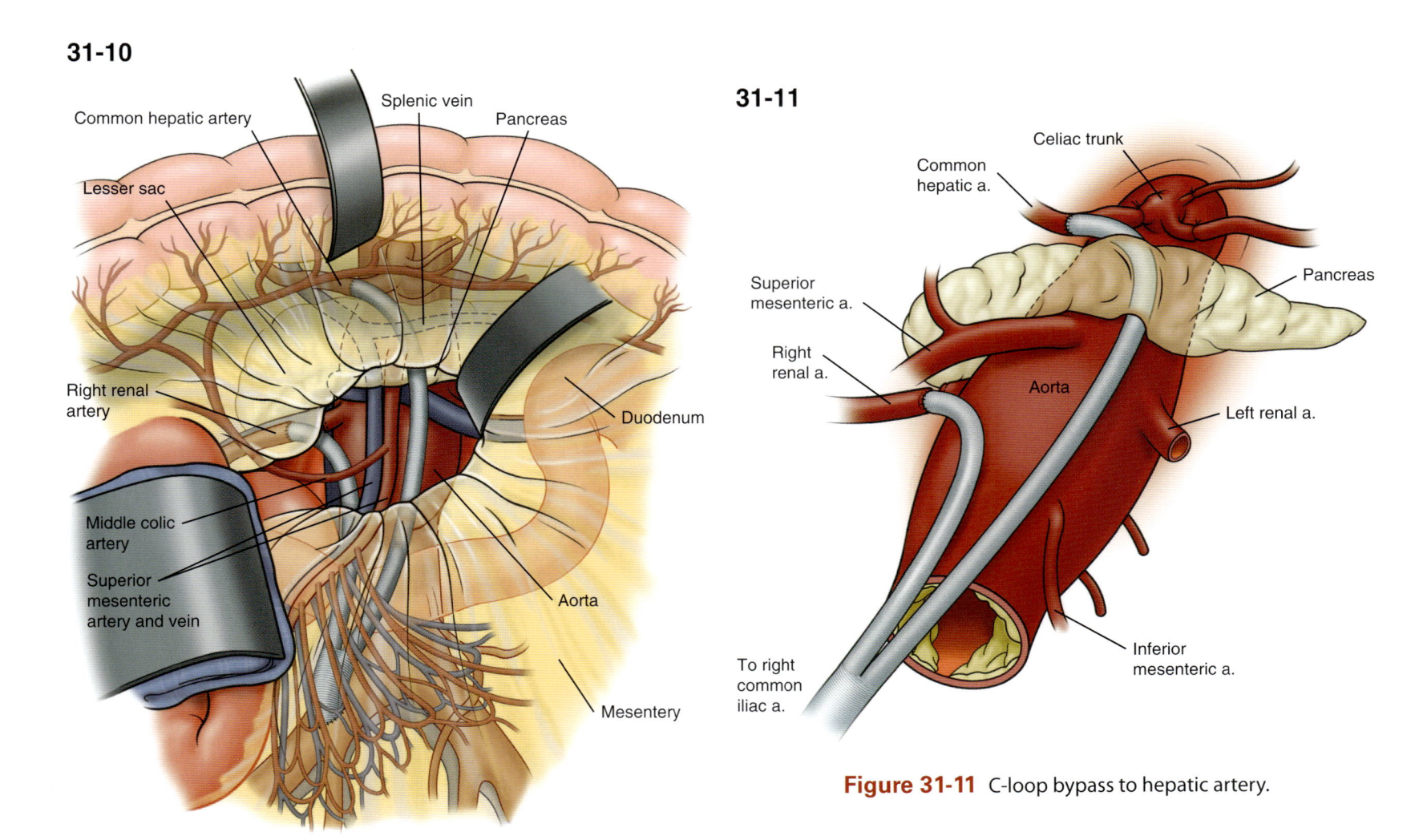

Figure 31-10

31-11

Figure 31-11 C-loop bypass to hepatic artery.

DETAILS OF PROCEDURE *SUPERIOR MESENTERIC BYPASS:* `CONTINUED` After exposure of the inflow vessel and administration of systemic heparin, the vessel is clamped. The proximal bifurcated Dacron graft is done as described to the left common iliac artery. The graft should be routed anterior to the aorta, then in the left paracolic gutter toward the left shoulder in the retroperitoneum, arched over the duodenum, and then it should come down to the anterior surface of the SMA, creating a C-shape for the graft (**FIGURE 31-12**). As indicated, an alternative approach is to tunnel the graft through the transverse mesocolon and perform the anastomosis with a retrograde appearance; however, if performed straight, flow will be bidirectional. It is important to emphasize that the proximal portion of the SMA should not be used for the anastomosis to avoid kinking of the graft after removal of the retractors. The mid-SMA is preferred as a target for the end-to-side anastomosis. During the anastomosis, the SMA is clamped, side-branches are occluded with the vessel loops, and a longitudinal arteriotomy is made using an 11-blade. This is then further extended using Potts scissors. An end-to-side anastomosis is then done using 6/0 polypropylene sutures in a running fashion. After the clamp is removed, the retractors are removed, and the transverse colon is moved back to its original position, the graft is checked to ensure no kinking is present. The outflow is assessed using intraoperative Doppler.

RENAL BYPASSES: Preoperative imaging is paramount in order to identify accessory renal arteries or venous anomalies (circumferential aortic venous collar, retro-aortic left renal vein). If the celiac artery and SMA are not debranched, the most common sites for extra-anatomic bypasses include the common iliac arteries, the common hepatic artery or gastroduodenal artery for the right renal artery, and the splenic artery as the source of inflow for left renal artery bypass.

Transperitoneal exposure is described above. To gain adequate exposure of the renal arteries, it is fundamental to manage the surrounding venous structures. If one chooses the abdominal aorta as the inflow source, the inferior mesenteric vein is usually ligated to gain more exposure for both arteries. For right renal artery revascularization, the next structure to manage is the left renal vein—it is mobilized cephalad superiorly and inferiorly. Subsequently, the left gonadal, lumbar, or adrenal veins are ligated to gain more mobility. If the left renal vein is on top of the right and left renal arteries, it may be suture-ligated with a transfixing 4/0 polypropene and divided. In this case, the left adrenal vein should be preserved. The medial wall of the IVC should be mobilized and slightly retracted from the aorta to better visualize the orifice of the right renal artery if the proximal renal artery is revascularized. Sometimes the aneurysm sac is too bulky, and if additional length is needed to expose the right renal artery, lumbar veins should be ligated to facilitate the mobility of the IVC. However, it is also common to tunnel the limb underneath the IVC (**FIGURE 31-13**). If the common iliac artery is chosen as the inflow, it can be tunneled anteriorly or retroperitoneally by mobilizing the right colon and performing a Kocher maneuver. The grafts are then routed on top of the aorta or previous infrarenal graft. If a concomitant infrarenal aortic repair is done, the proximal anastomosis of the renal bypass can be fashioned as a limb off the side of the aortic graft prior to sewing the aortic graft. The right renal artery is exposed as medial to the IVC as possible. It is also doubly clipped or suture-ligated at its origin, transected, and an end-to-end anastomosis is performed. Cold perfusion of the kidney is usually not necessary.

The left renal artery is exposed directly off the aorta or through the retroperitoneum by mobilizing the left colon and spleen. The left renal artery is clamped, and an end-to-end anastomosis is done with a 5/0 polypropylene suture in a running fashion (**FIGURE 31-14**). It is clamped and transected a few centimeters beyond its origin and doubly clipped or suture-ligated to minimize ischemia. The distal artery may be cold perfused, but usually this is not required for a quick anastomosis. After removal of the clamp, the anastomoses is checked for bleeding and with a Doppler to confirm distal flow.

CLOSURE Each anastomosis is meticulously rechecked to avoid a postoperative hematoma that may compress the graft or be a source for subsequent infection. Heparin is reversed using protamine sulfate. Self-retractors are then removed and the lay of the grafts is rechecked to avoid kinking. The retroperitoneal is reperitonealized, and if needed an additional greater omentum flap can be mobilized to cover the proximal anastomosis and the graft to prevent future fistula. The abdominal wall is closed in multiple layers; for the rectus sheath a 3/0 q suture is used, and a 2/0 synthetic absorbable monofilament suture should be used for subcutaneous tissue.

POSTOPERATIVE CARE Early postoperative care is done in the intensive care unit. Since this patient population is unsuitable for open TAA reconstruction, comorbidities, such as COPD, diabetes, and hypertension are monitored. Every anastomosis is a potential source of bleeding, especially when anticoagulation is needed postoperatively. Graft occlusion can occur but should be rare; however, a decrease in urine output, or elevated serum lactate level are early signs for graft occlusion. Liver and pancreatic enzymes and renal function are all monitored as well. If there is a concern for graft occlusion, additional imaging such as a CTA or duplex ultrasound is valuable before taking the patient back for re-exploration. The patient should remain under physiologic monitoring, and bowel movements and urine output monitored. Approximately 6 weeks after discharge, the second-stage endovascular repair should be undertaken, but a CT scan of the repair is performed prior to deployment. ■

31-12

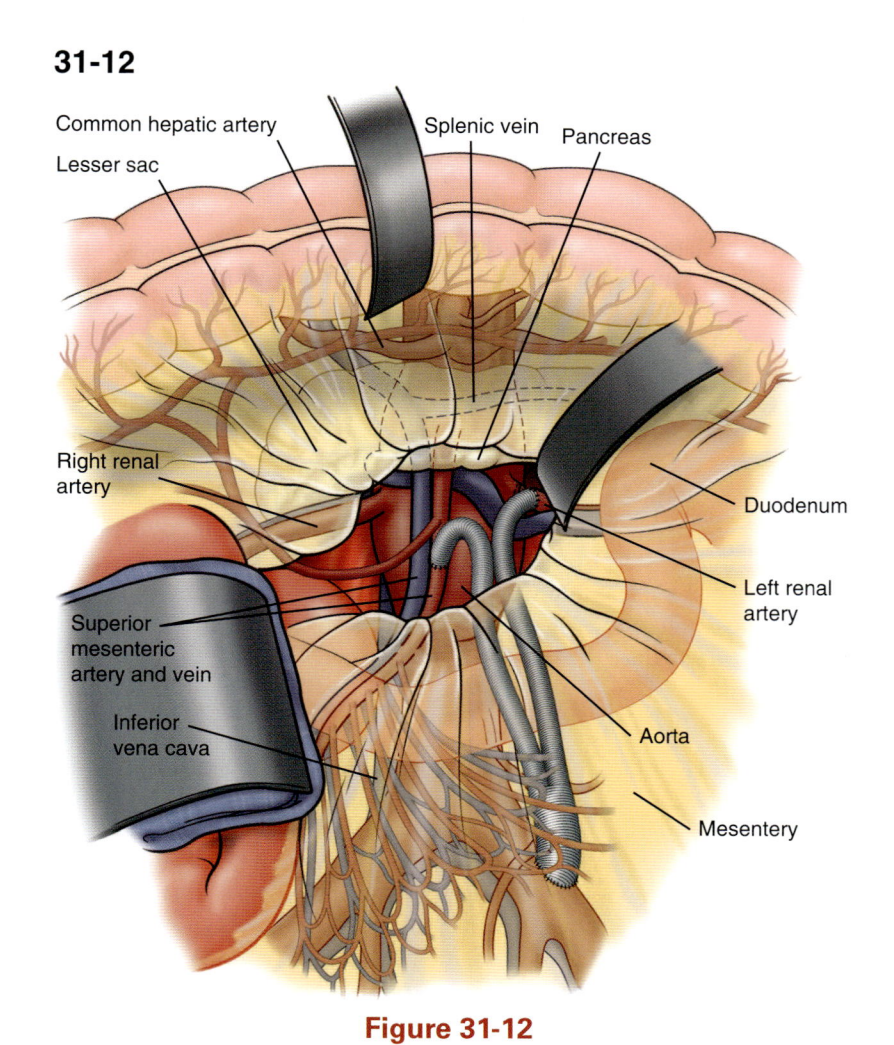

Common hepatic artery
Lesser sac
Splenic vein
Pancreas
Right renal artery
Superior mesenteric artery and vein
Inferior vena cava
Duodenum
Left renal artery
Aorta
Mesentery

Figure 31-12

31-13

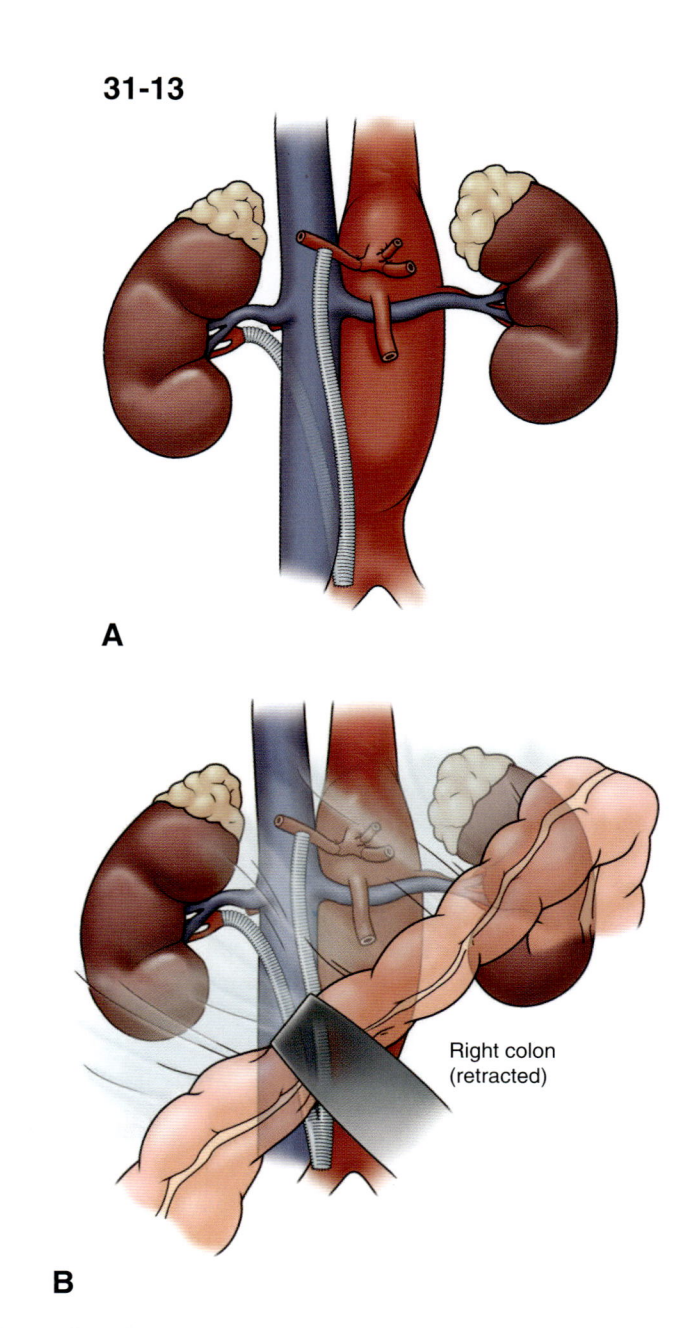

A

B

Figure 31-13 (A) A right renal artery under aorta or tunneled under IVC from aorta, or (B) a right renal artery retrograde from right iliac retroperitoneal.

Right colon (retracted)

31-14

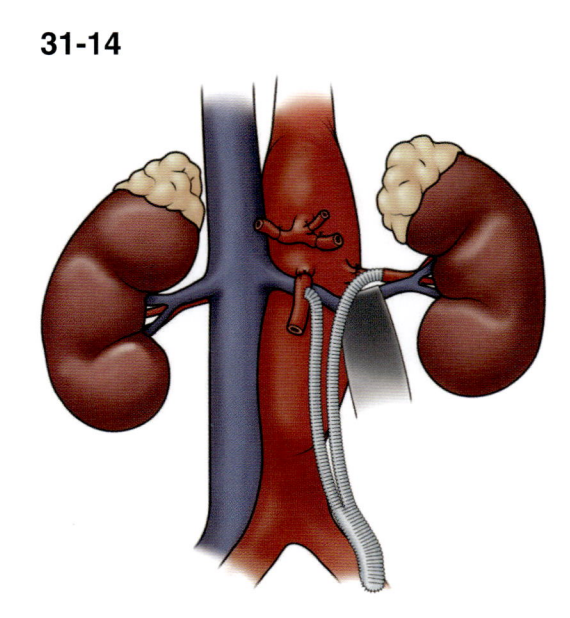

Figure 31-14 Left renal artery exposure; left renal artery anastomoses.

Graft Infections: Neo-Aortoiliac System

Audra A. Duncan, MD

INDICATIONS Replacement of a primarily infected aorta or infected aortic prostheses is one of the most challenging undertakings, even for an experienced vascular surgeon. It can be accomplished by many techniques, including one-stage and two-stage reconstructions. Many consider the neo-aortoiliac system (NAIS) to be the gold standard of reconstruction, due to its durability and low risk of reinfection. First described by Patrick Claggett, MD, NAIS (sometimes called the "Claggett procedure") is an aortic graft constructed of bilateral superficial femoral and popliteal veins which are resected between the geniculate tributaries and the profunda femoris veins to maintain as much collateral venous drainage as possible. The femoral veins are then refashioned to create a tube or bifurcated graft that is used as the conduit in an in-situ one-stage reconstruction. NAIS is typically considered for younger patients and/or those with virulent organisms, and at centers familiar with NAIS that can provide two surgical teams to be efficient in the operating room.

OPERATIVE PREPARATION Aortic graft infection, aorto-enteric erosions, or primary aortic infection are typically diagnosed by history and physical exam including fever, chills, septic emboli, back pain, abscess or draining incisional sinus tracts, elevated inflammatory markers, and possible positive blood cultures. Suspected aortic infections are confirmed by computed tomography angiography with the presence of perigraft fluid, air, abscess, as well as soft tissue thickening or stranding. In severe prolonged infection, destruction of surrounding tissues and bone can occur. MRI or duplex scanning may also be used to differentiate between perigraft infection and hematoma. Tagged WBC or PET scans can support the diagnosis by confirming the presence of infection and may also guide decision-making by assessing the extent of infection. For example, infection of only one limb of an aorto-bifemoral graft based on WBC scan may indicate that partial graft excision could be successful. In general, nuclear scans are best interpreted in late infections, because there is a high false-positive rate in early postoperative patients. When in doubt, the most definitive way to make the diagnosis is open exploration.

Once the extent of infection is identified, preoperative assessment of bilateral superficial femoral veins should be done with duplex imaging. Assessment for patency, wall thickening, or duplicate femoral veins should be included, as well as identification of large suprapopliteal geniculate veins. If there is a concern about the length of conduit required to replace the infected aorta, estimated length measurement of deep vein can be made to complete surgical decision-making. If femoral vein is inadequate, great saphenous vein may be reconfigured as an aortic conduit, but this is not optimal due to its thin wall and smaller size. Finally, a second operative team to simultaneously harvest vein while aortic exposure is performed can be mobilized in order to minimize operative time and improve patient outcomes.

POSITION The patient should be supine on the table. If not already imaged, the deep veins may be visualized on-table with ultrasound. The prep should extend from nipples to include both lower limbs circumferentially, with each foot protected in plastic bags or with towels. Alternatively, the legs can be "frog-legged" and prepped if the patient's body habitus allows for adequate exposure of the entire medial thigh. If the groin sites are involved, groin hair should be clipped and cultures taken of fluid from draining sinuses, if present.

INCISION AND EXPOSURE In order to harvest the femoral veins, a medial thigh incision is made along the border of the sartorius muscle from the groin to above the knee (**FIGURE 32-1**). If an infected graft involves a limb anastomosed to the femoral artery, the vein harvest incision should be separated by a skin bridge to keep the vein harvest sites clean. The incision is initially made on the lateral birder of the sartorius which is reflected medially, and distally may need to be reflected in the opposite direction (**FIGURE 32-2**); the superficial femoral artery (SFA) is identified adjacent to the superficial femoral vein in the subsartorial space. The profunda femoral vein and substantial above-knee tributaries must be left intact to prevent post-procedure venous complications, as this collateral network is critical in lower limb drainage after the femoral vein is removed. Care is taken to preserve branches of the SFA and popliteal arteries to avoid potential limb ischemia, and to leave the saphenous nerve intact to avoid postoperative neuralgia.

A midline abdominal incision and femoral artery exposure is made to resect the infected aortic graft. Although the laparotomy can occur simultaneously during vein harvest, exposure of grossly infected material may be delayed if possible until the femoral incisions are closed and covered to prevent cross-infection. The use of separate "clean" and "dirty" instruments and teams may reduce the risk of cross-infection.

DETAILS OF PROCEDURE

SUPERFICIAL FEMORAL/POPLITEAL VEIN HARVEST: The exposure and dissection of the femoral veins requires meticulous dissection, as the venous tributaries can be friable or short and may easily tear during mobilization. Although the tributaries may be securely ligated or suture ligated, suture ligation may result in tearing of the fragile vessel wall. Any bleeding points can be repaired with 6-0 or 7-0 polypropylene suture. Once adequate exposure is accomplished, the veins are left in-situ until the exact length required for replacement is determined. The patient is fully heparinized before vein harvest. Once completed dissected out, the superficial femoral vein is divided flush with the profunda vein (**FIGURE 32-3**) and sutured at both ends with 5-0 polypropylene suture to avoid the creation of a venous stump, which can harbor thrombus. The vein is prepared by distending it under pressure and ligating any leaking points with 6-0 or 7-0 polypropylene suture and removing adventitial constricting bands. Valves may be removed in order to place the vein conduit in a non-reversed fashion. However, traditional valvulotomies may injure the fragile vein or incompletely lyse the valves, and therefore complete vein eversion and open resection of the valve leaflets is preferred. The vein is stored in heparinized saline until time for creation of the aortic replacement. **CONTINUES ▶**

32-1

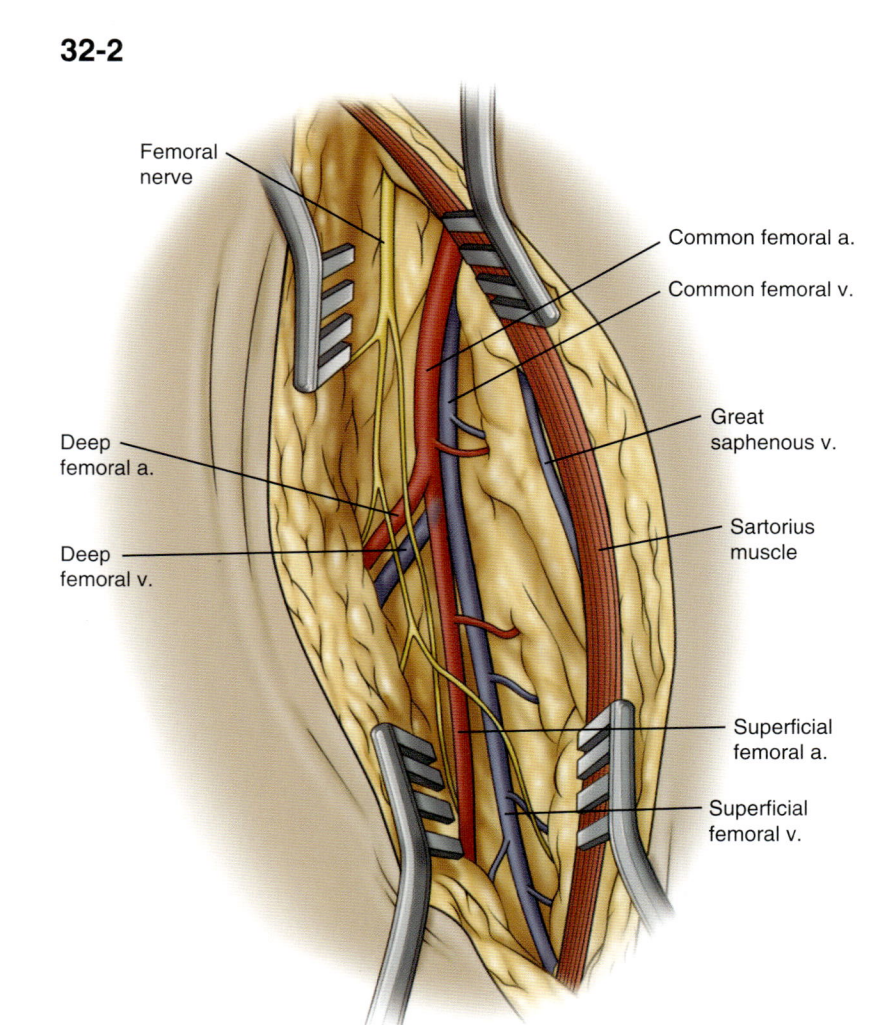

Figure 32-1 Harvest of superficial femoral vein 1.

32-2

Figure 32-2 Harvest of superficial femoral vein 2.

32-3

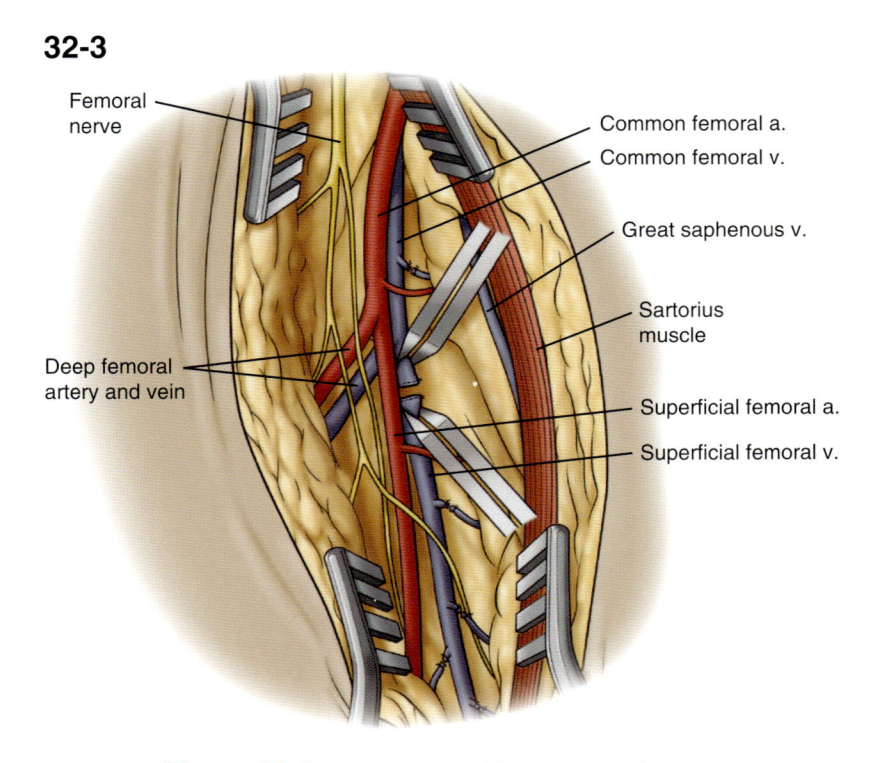

Figure 32-3 Completion of femoral vein harvest.

DETAILS OF PROCEDURE *AORTIC GRAFT RESECTION:* `CONTINUED` When excising an aortic graft, it is necessary to get proper proximal control of the aorta, which can either be surpaceliac or suprarenal (**FIGURE 32-4A** and **32-4B**), and distal control if the graft is only in the abdomen. Dissecting out the limbs of a bifurcated graft can be treacherous; therefore, having ureteral stents placed preoperatively will help avoid ureteral injury. It is not unusual to have a calcified rind around the limbs, and once this is identified, careful incision will expose the infected graft (**FIGURE 32-5**). Additionally, the iliac veins and inferior vena cava are in proximity, and careful attention should be paid in dissecting in these areas, as the inflammatory reaction will obscure tissue planes. Prior to clamping, the patient is systemically heparinized, and ACT maintained greater than 220 secs. The proximal aorta site is chosen for clamping and the infected graft is excised. After the aorta or aortic graft is resected completely and sent for cultures, necrotic tissue is carefully removed. Too aggressive debridement can result in injury to the inferior vena cava and iliac veins. Next, clean instruments are used, and new gowns and gloves are donned. The deep veins can then be assessed for length and optimal configuration for aortic reconstruction determined. The femoral vein is often smaller than the native aorta, and for an end-to-end anastomosis the size mismatch can be managed by beveling the vein (**FIGURE 32-6A**), resecting a wedge of native aorta (**FIGURE 32-6B**), or oversewing the aortic stump and coming off anteriorly as an end-to-side anastomosis (**FIGURE 32-6C**). The latter will result in the loss of significant length. Additionally, when oversewing the aorta, one should sew the lumen closed in an anterior-to-posterior direction to minimize the length of the posterior wall. The proximal anastomosis is completed with 3-0 or 4-0 polypropylene suture. `CONTINUES`

32-4

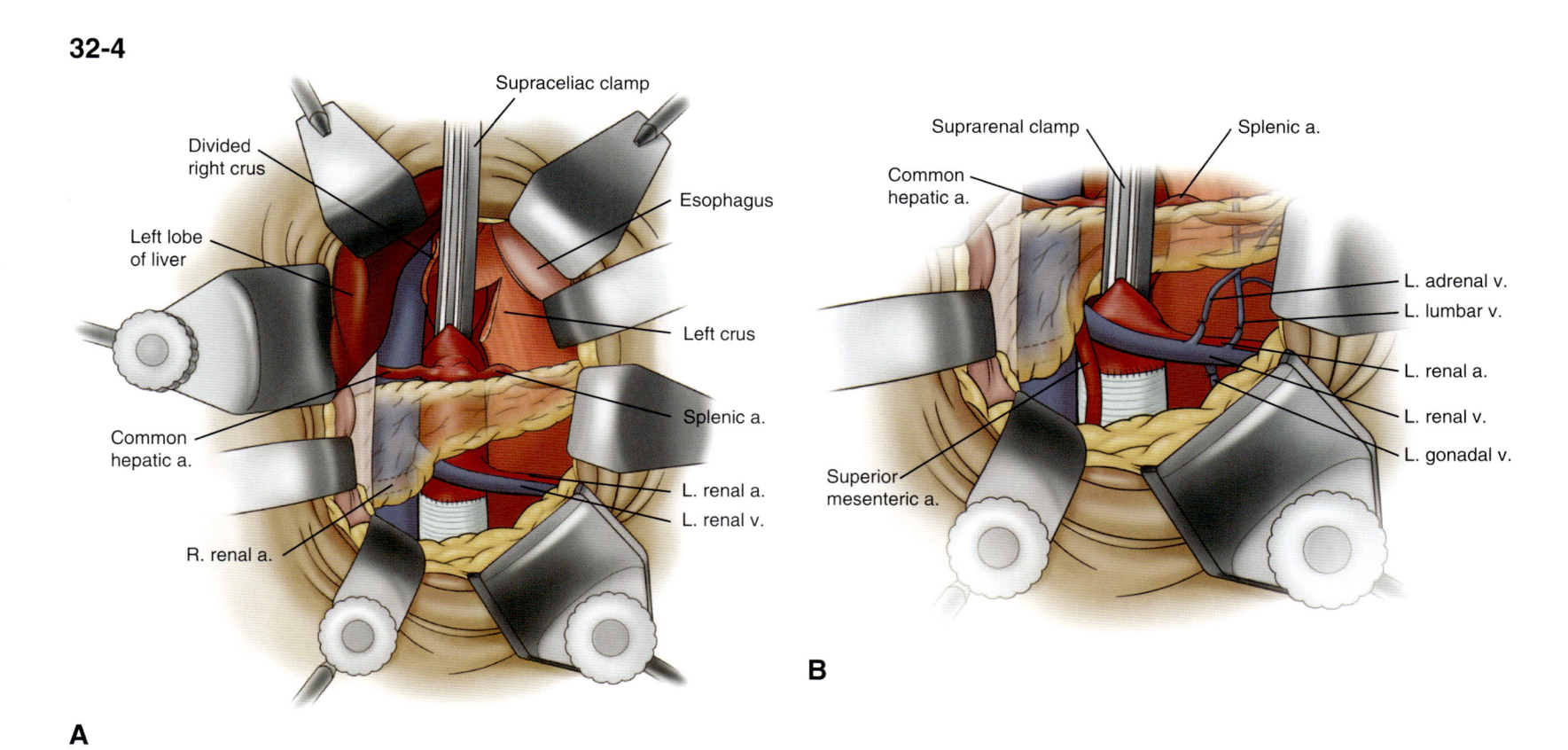

Figure 32-4 Suprarenal and supraceliac control.

32-5

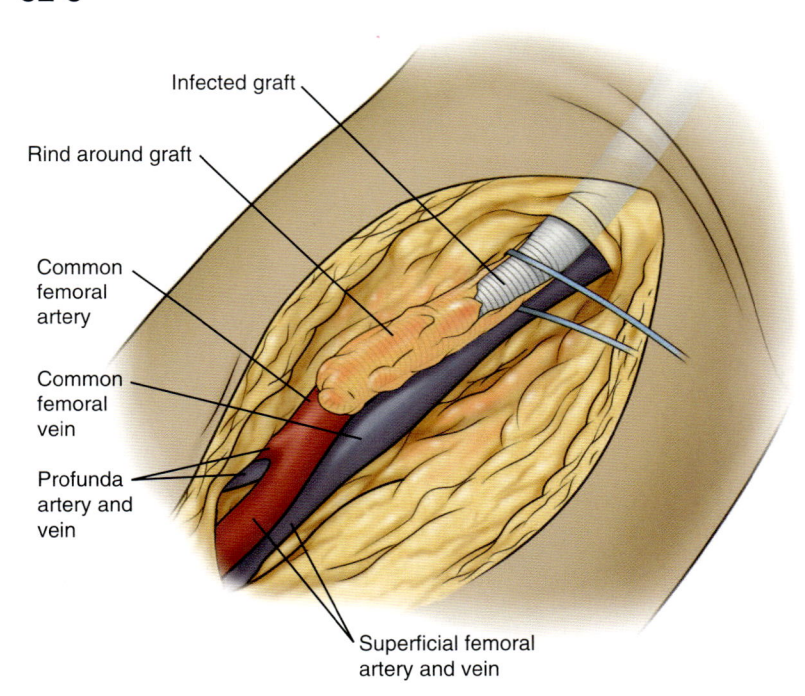

Figure 32-5 Infected limb and rind, iliac veins, and IVC.

32-6

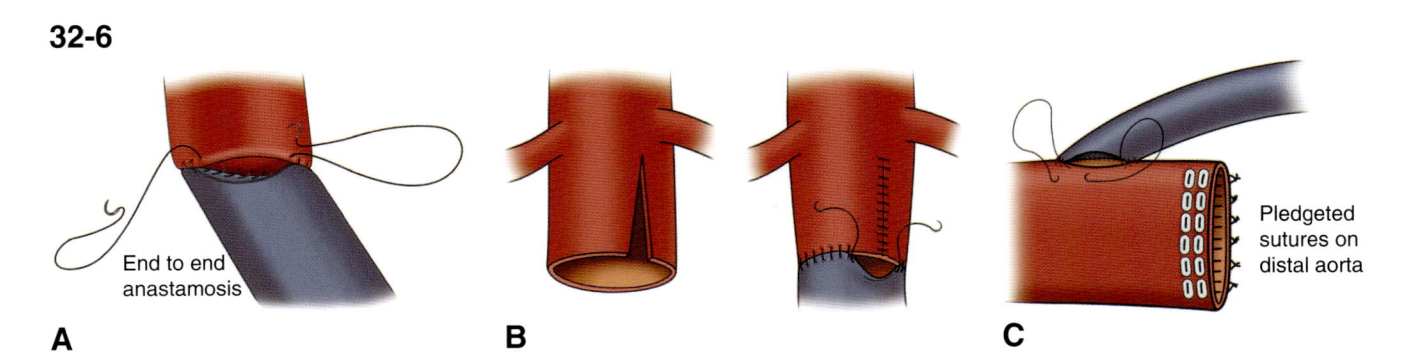

Figure 32-6 Proximal anastomosis configuration options.

DETAILS OF PROCEDURE *AORTIC GRAFT RESECTION:* **CONTINUED** When constructing the combined veins, a veno-venous anastomoses in the optimal configuration for the patient's anatomy is performed by using at least two 4-0 polypropylene sutures to avoid purse-stringing of the anastomosis with concomitant constriction (**FIGURE 32-7**). The femoral or iliac anastomoses are done with 5-0 polypropylene suture, possibly including long, beveled anastomoses if required. If length is an issue, creating a distal external iliac and common femoral endarterectomy with bovine patch can buy you several centimeters. In rare cases if the femoral veins are not adequate to use for aortic reconstruction, the great saphenous veins can be conjoined to create a bifurcated graft (**FIGURE 32-8**). The lower limbs are assessed for perfusion using a Doppler probe. The bowel is inspected for viability, and 15 to 30 mg of protamine may be administered. If a bowel fistula or erosion was present, it is now repaired in layers. Prior to closure, an omental flap is mobilized and wrapped 360° around the NAIS conduit (**FIGURE 32-9**).

CLOSURE The abdomen is closed along the fascia with adsorbable monofilament suture, and the skin left open and packed if gross contamination was evident. Similarly, the femoral vein harvest incisions are closed in layers to reduce the risk of seromas or hematomas. Closed-suction drains may be used in these incisions to reduce the risk of fluid collections.

POSTOPERATIVE CARE Venous morbidity is a significant concern with this operation, therefore intermittent pneumatic compression, subcutaneous heparin, and early mobilization are critical. Despite these maneuvers, there is a 30% risk of developing edema. There is also a significant risk of compartment syndrome, and the patient should be monitored closely; some surgeons opt to perform prophylactic fasciotomies. Long-term anticoagulation is not indicated. Well-fitted 30- to 40-mmHg graduated compression stockings should be ordered for outpatient wear. Intravenous antibiotics are continued in the perioperative period and adjusted based on intraoperative cultures, with an overall course of 4 weeks, or longer in the case of Candida (6 weeks) or in those with extensive polymicrobial infections or immuno-compromise patients (4–6 weeks). ■

SUGGESTED READINGS

Ali AT, Modrall JG, Hocking J, Valentine RJ, Spencer H, Eidt JF, Clagett GP. Long-term results of the treatment of aortic graft infection by in situ replacement with femoral popliteal vein grafts. *J Vasc Surg.* 2009;1:30-39.

Chung J, Clagett GP. Neoaortoiliac system (NAIS) procedure for the treatment of infected aortic graft. *Semin Vasc Surg.* 2011;4:220-226.

Clagett GP, Valentine RJ, Hagino RT. Autogenous aortoiliac/femoral reconstruction from superficial femoral-popliteal veins: feasibility and durability. *Vasc Surg.* 1997 Feb;25(2):255-66; discussion 267-270.

Smeds MR, Duncan AA, Harlander-Locke MP, Lawrence PF, Lyden S, Fatima J, Eskandari MK; Vascular Low-Frequency Disease Consortium. Treatment and outcomes of aortic endograft infection. *J Vasc Surg.* 2016 Feb;63(2):332-340.

Valentine RJ, Clagett GP. Aortic graft infections: replacement with autogenous vein. *Cardiovasc Surg.* 2001 Oct;9(5):419-425.

32-7

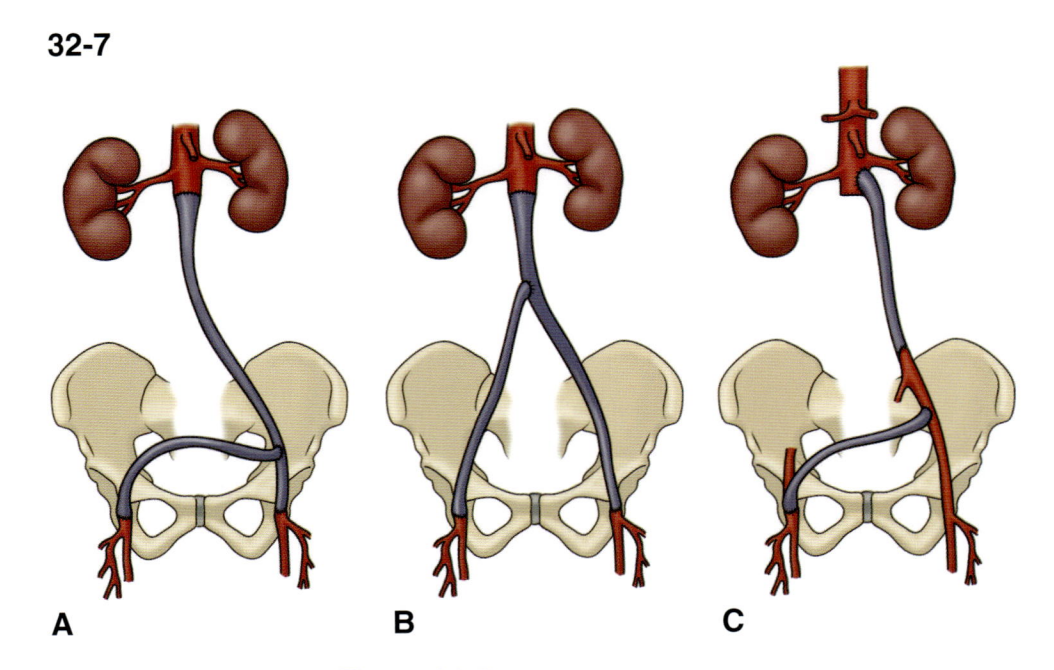

A   B   C

Figure 32-7 Graft configurations.

32-8

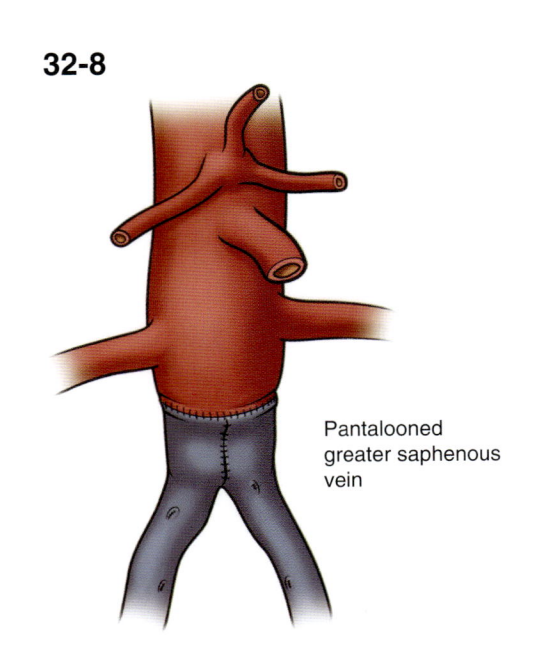

Pantalooned greater saphenous vein

Figure 32-8 Spliced greater saphenous veins.

32-9

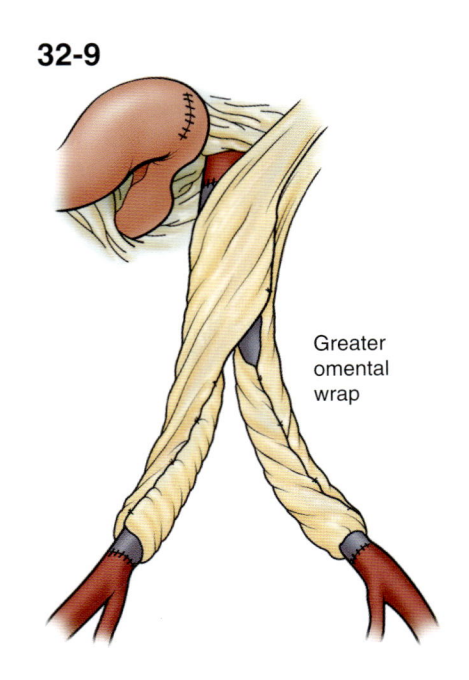

Greater omental wrap

Figure 32-9 Omental wraparound graft.

ENDOGRAFT EXPLANT

Murray Shames, MD • **Angelyn Thayer, MD**

INDICATIONS The rise of endovascular aneurysm repair (EVAR) for the treatment of abdominal aortic aneurysms (AAA) has resulted in a growing need for endovascular and open reinterventions. Endovascular techniques range from aortic cuff or iliac limb extensions and embolization to complex reinterventions such as graft relining, branch extensions, custom branched or fenestrated endografts, and physician-modified endografts. While endovascular reinterventions are often appropriate, there remain circumstances necessitating open surgical intervention with specific graft explantation and conventional repair. In the setting of any type of endoleak that has failed to resolve with endovascular intervention and that demonstrates evidence of ongoing aneurysm sac enlargement, the Society for Vascular Surgery (SVS) guidelines provide a strong recommendation for open repair with graft explantation. In the setting of a type II endoleak that has failed to resolve with endovascular intervention and demonstrates evidence of ongoing enlargement, the SVS guidelines provide recommendation (albeit weak) for open repair, often with sac exploration and ligation of lumbar vessels or the inferior mesenteric artery. Graft explantation may also be indicated in cases of late onset graft or iliac limb thrombosis, rupture anatomically unfit for endovascular repair, aortic graft infection, and secondary aortoenteric fistula. Historically, 30-day mortality rates for urgent and emergent open repair have been dismal with reported rates up to 40%, with improved outcomes for elective cases and at high-volume centers.

PREOPERATIVE CONSIDERATIONS Operative planning includes a thorough patient history and physical exam with attention to any previous abdominal procedures, including reviewing the operative notes. Computed tomographic angiography (CTA) is the most frequently used method of preoperative imaging; however, magnetic resonance angiography can also be helpful. Imaging is critical for operative planning, providing information as to the graft's proximal extent, fixation type, relation to the aortic wall, and aberrant anatomy. Visceral vessel locations and patency can also be discerned and are particularly important in the case of suprarenal, fenestrated, or branched device removal. Additionally, distal graft extent and iliac and femoral vessel patency can be assessed to plan for clamp placement and location of the distal anastomosis. If persistent endoleak can be confidently located on preoperative imaging, the operative plan may include only partial endograft removal, leaving components with adequate seal in-situ. In the case of suspected aortoenteric fistula, preoperative imaging may indicate need for additional surgical teams that can assist with bowel repair or resection. Preoperative esophagogastroduodenoscopy (EGD) can help diagnosis a proximal aortoenteric fistula. Finally, in cases of infected aortic endografts, preoperative axillary femoral bypass may be indicated. Additional preoperative workup for open aortic repair includes thorough cardiac, renal, and pulmonary evaluations. All patients should undergo an electrocardiogram and echocardiogram at baseline. While some routinely get chemical cardiac stress tests (CCST), in cases of dyspnea of unknown origin or worsening dyspnea, or in patients who are unable to complete four metabolic equivalents, CCST is mandatory. Pulmonary evaluation includes pulmonary function testing for preoperative baseline. Renal function should be considered, but renal dysfunction is not prohibitive to open repair. Judicious preoperative hydration should be considered in those at high risk for renal injury, including patients with preoperative hemoglobin <10 g/dL, eGFR <60 mL/min/1.73 m², decreased creatinine clearance, and those with a history of ischemic heart disease.

OPERATING ROOM CONSIDERATIONS: General anesthetic is administered with endotracheal intubation. An arterial line is placed for drawing intraoperative blood gas samples, activated clotting time following heparin administration, and continuous blood pressure monitoring. Central venous catheters are indicated for administration of fluids and vasoactive medications. Swan-Ganz catheters may be indicated for additional hemodynamic monitoring. Placement of a nasogastric tube, central venous access, two or more large bore peripheral IVs, and a Foley catheter are also standard. Transesophageal echocardiography capabilities may be useful in some situations. Cell-saver system utilization lessens the need for blood replacement products but should be avoided in cases of infected endografts.

OPERATIVE APPROACH SELECTION: Choice of operative approach is dependent on several patient factors as well as surgeon preference for a given exposure. The retroperitoneal (RP) approach provides excellent exposure of the paravisceral aortic segment without violating the peritoneal cavity, which is useful in patients with a hostile abdomen. The incision itself crosses fewer dermatomes, which allows for less postoperative pain. Additionally, studies have shown shorter ICU stays and faster return of bowel function. However, it is potentially more difficult to reconstruct the right iliac artery. In cases of aortic graft infection and suspected aortoenteric fistula or erosion, the transperitoneal (TP) approach is indicated for access to the viscera and duodenal mobilization. There has been ongoing debate for decades on whether the RP or TP approach is better tolerated in patients with pulmonary insufficiency.

TRANSPERITONEAL APPROACH

POSITIONING AND PREPARATION: The TP approach begins with the patient in supine position in slight Trendelenburg to aid with small bowel retraction from the lower abdomen. Arms are abducted and secured with adequate access to peripheral IVs and arterial lines. Pulses and/or Doppler signals should be marked and verified by the surgeon preoperatively. Hair should be clipped in standard fashion and the patient should be prepped from the nipples to knees bilaterally.

INCISION AND EXPOSURE: The TP approach allows for infrarenal aortic exposure, and when combined with medial visceral rotation, provides suprarenal exposure. A midline laparotomy incision is made extending from the xyphoid process to the symphysis pubis. The midline fascia is incised, the peritoneal cavity is entered, and the abdominal contents are inspected. For exposure of the infrarenal aorta, the omentum and transverse colon are retracted cephalad (**FIGURE 33-1**). The small bowel is packed either directly into the right hemi-abdomen or can be inserted into a plastic bowel bag and partially constricted with tape at the mouth of the bag and eviscerated. The ligament of Treitz is divided to allow for reflection of the 3rd and 4th parts of the duodenum to the right (**FIGURE 33-2**). Periaortic tissues are divided and encountered lymphatics are ligated. The inferior mesenteric vein is encountered during this portion of the dissection and should be treated with care but can be ligated to increase exposure. The posterior peritoneum covering the aorta is incised starting on the patient's left side near the ligament of Treitz, and then coursing right of the aortic midline to avoid the IMA, sigmoid mesentery, and autonomic plexus at the bifurcation.

Exposure of the pararenal aorta with planned suprarenal clamp necessitates additional proximal aortic exposure. The incision on the posterior peritoneum is extended to the level of the renal veins. On the left, the gonadal, adrenal, and lumbar veins may be divided to provide more proximal aortic exposure (**FIGURE 33-3A**). Alternatively, the left renal vein can be divided as close to the IVC as possible, and the other veins left intact to maintain venous drainage (**FIGURE 33-3B**). **CONTINUES ▶**

33-1

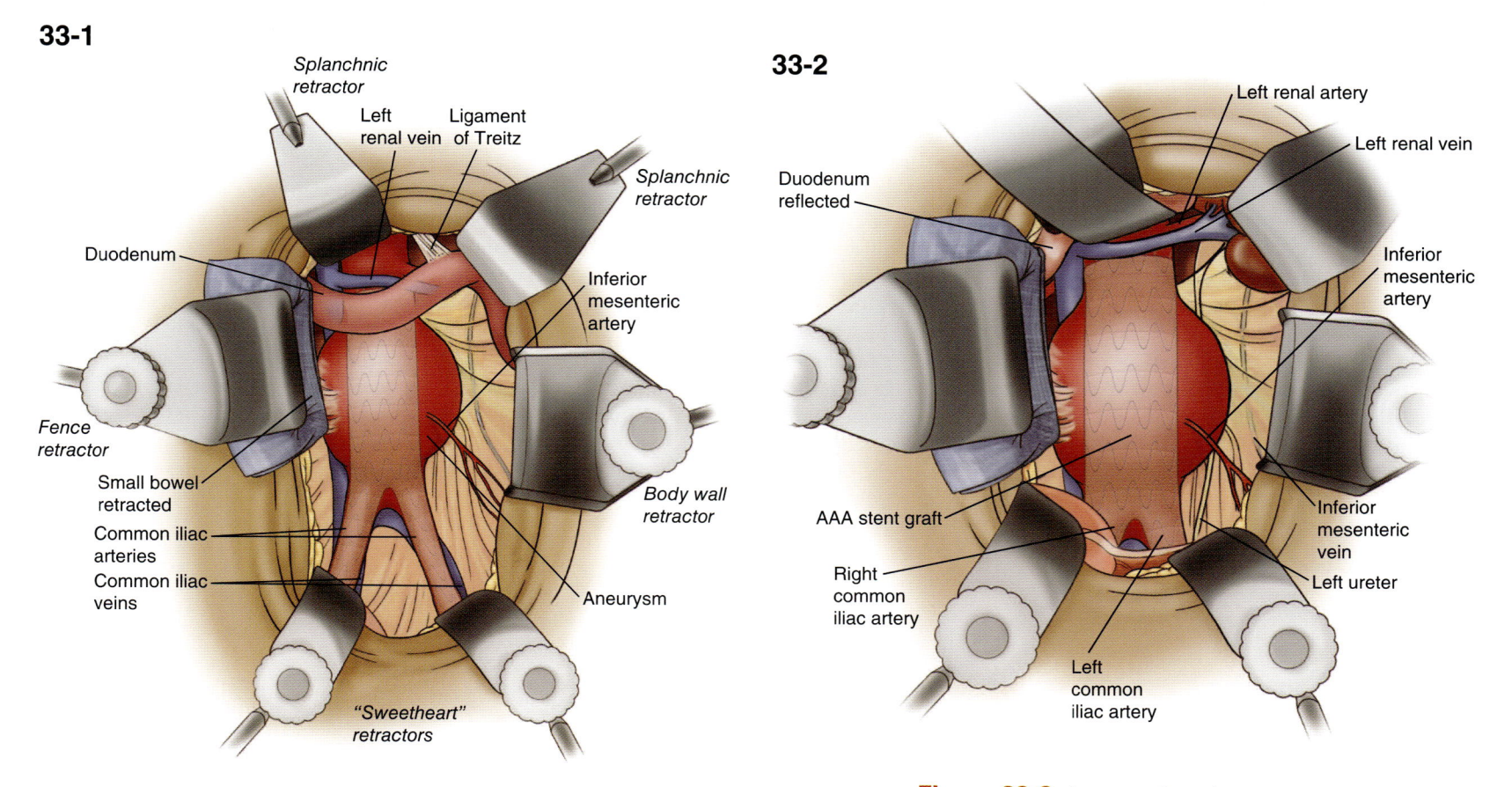

Figure 33-1 Exposure of infrarenal aorta.

Figure 33-2 Juxtarenal aortic exposure.

33-3

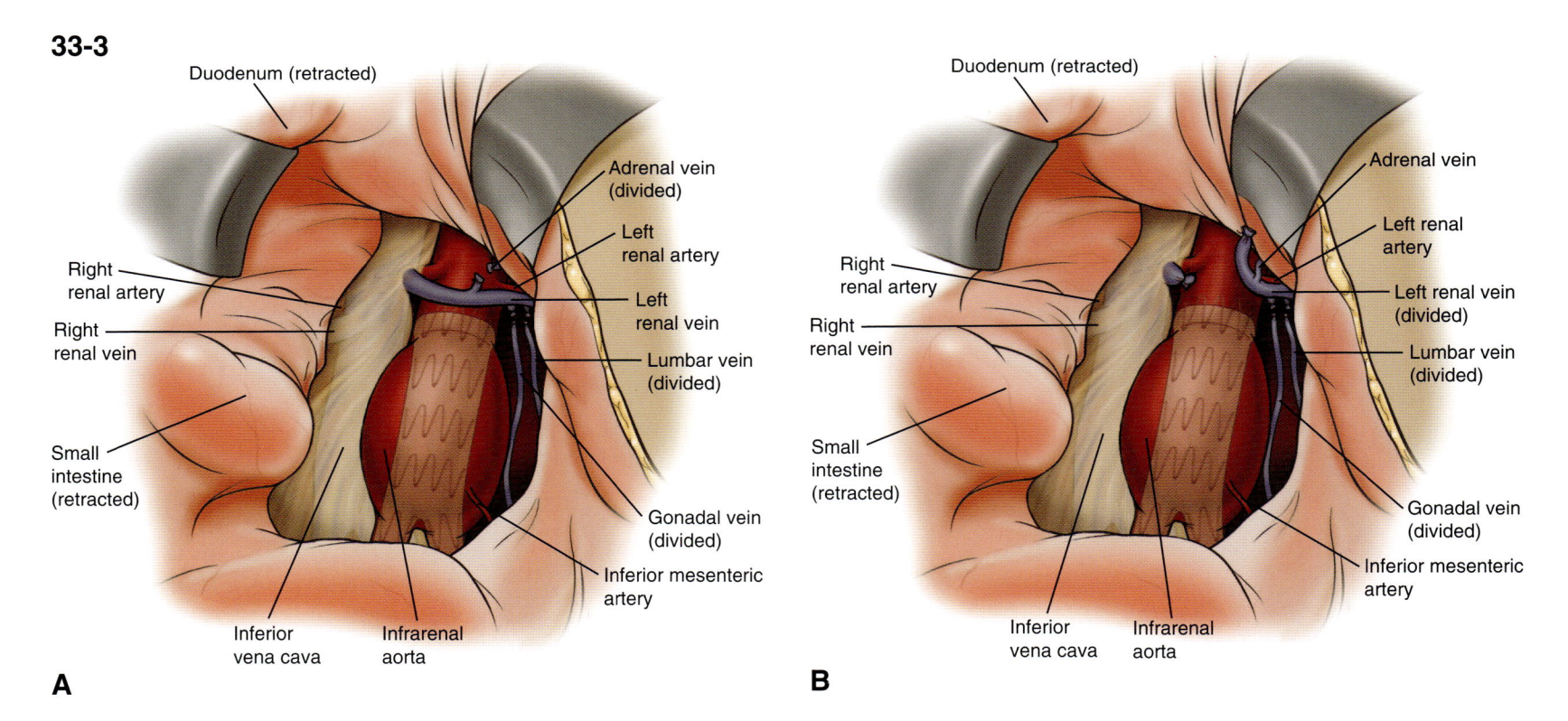

A

B

Figure 33-3 A. Mobilization of the left renal vein. B. Division of left renal vein with preservation of collaterals to expose peri renal aorta.

TRANSPERITONEAL APPROACH *INCISION AND EXPOSURE:*

◄ CONTINUED Exposure to the supraceliac aorta (see Chapter 30) involves division of the lesser omentum or gastrohepatic ligament. The right crus of the diaphragm may be divided along its fibers. If needed, the left lobe of the liver is mobilized by dividing the left triangular and coronary ligaments as well as the falciform ligament. A nasogastric tube helps to identify the esophagus, which is retracted with the stomach to the left to prevent inadvertent injury (FIGURE 33-4A). The dissection can then be carried to the celiac axis along the anterior aorta, avoiding the pancreas. If room allows for a suprarenal clamp instead if supraceliac clamp, the left renal vein can be divided to facilitate exposure (FIGURE 33-4B).

Although the RP approach may be more favorable, the left medial visceral rotation can be used for the TP exposure of the suprarenal visceral aorta. The posterior peritoneum is divided lateral to the line of Toldt and the left colon is then mobilized (FIGURE 33-5). The phrenicolic ligament is divided, and the incision is carried medially toward the aortic hiatus along the underside of the diaphragm allowing for the spleen to be mobilized superiorly and medially. The dissection continues posteriorly between the spleen and left kidney where the splenocolic and splenorenal ligaments will be encountered and are divided and ligated. Following the lateral curvature of the spleen, a plane is developed posterior to the pancreas. At this point the colon, spleen, left kidney, and pancreas can be mobilized off the retroperitoneum and medially to expose the suprarenal aorta. The left renal lumbar vein is ligated to prevent avulsion. This is a key gateway to find the left renal artery. The kidney may also be left in the renal fossa; the lienorenal and lienophrenic ligaments are divided, and a plane is developed between Gerota's fascia and the posterior surface of the colonic mesentery and pancreas. The retroperitoneal and periaortic fat are dissected. If more proximal exposure is needed, the left crus of the diaphragm may be divided along its fibers, as can the medial arcuate ligament for exposure of the celiac artery origin. This is a key gateway to the supraceliac aorta. Self-retaining or open-ringed retractors are used to optimize exposure.

RETROPERITONEAL APPROACH

POSITIONING AND PREPARATION: Positioning for a retroperitoneal (RP) approach begins with the patient in a modified right lateral decubitus position with the left shoulder rotated superiorly and to the right by 45 to 60 degrees (see Chapter 29). The left pelvis is angled slightly with hips rotated 20 to 30 degrees and the right leg partially flexed. A surgical bean bag is used to assist with positioning. The table may be broken at the level of the umbilicus such that the space between the left costal margin and iliac crest is maximized. Like the TP approach, pulses and/or Doppler signals should be marked and verified by the surgeon preoperatively. Hair should be clipped in standard fashion and the patient should be prepped from the nipples to knees bilaterally and posteriorly toward the spine. **CONTINUES ►**

33-4

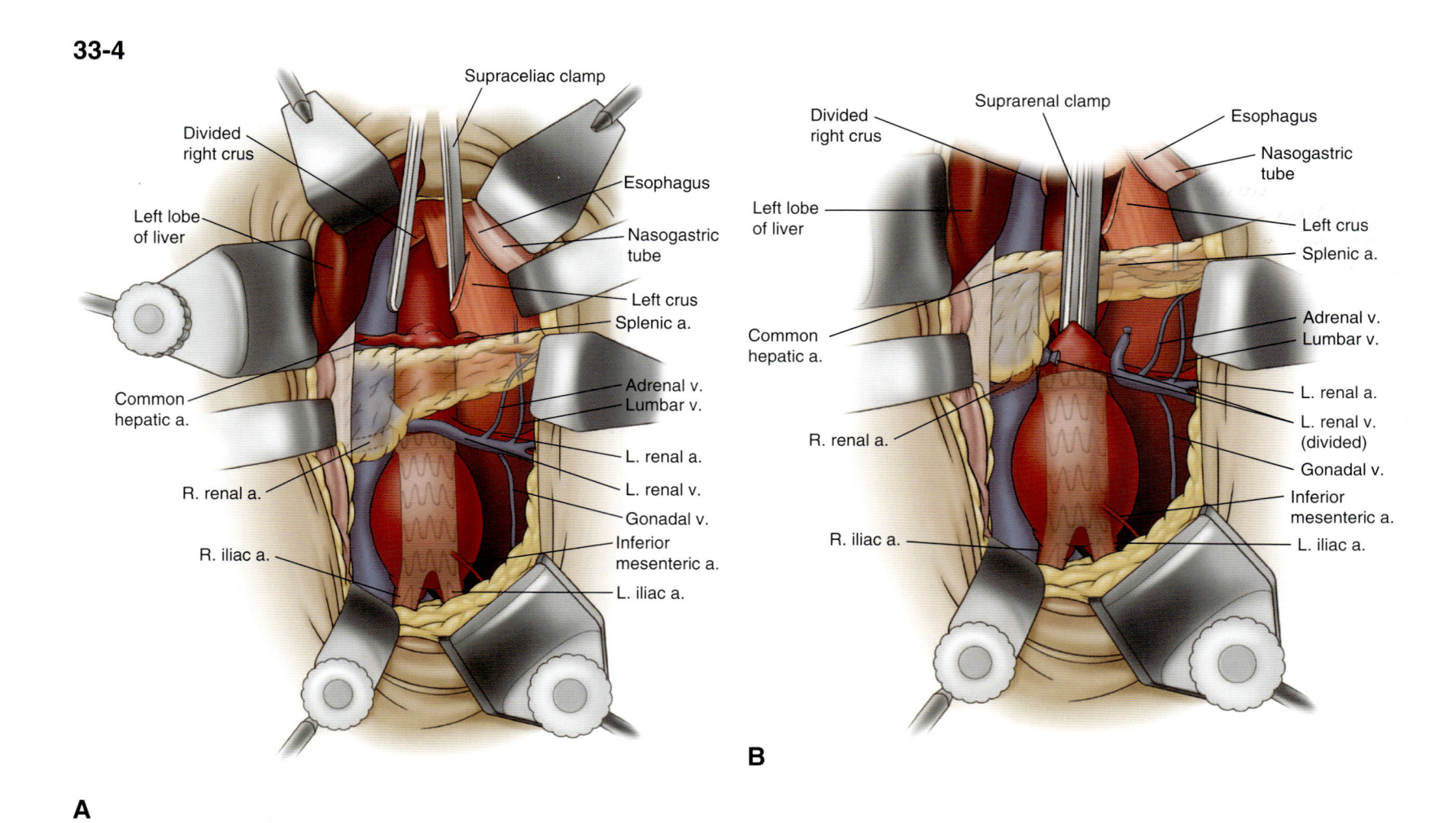

Figure 33-4 A. Supra celiac aorta exposure. B. Suprarenal exposure.

33-5

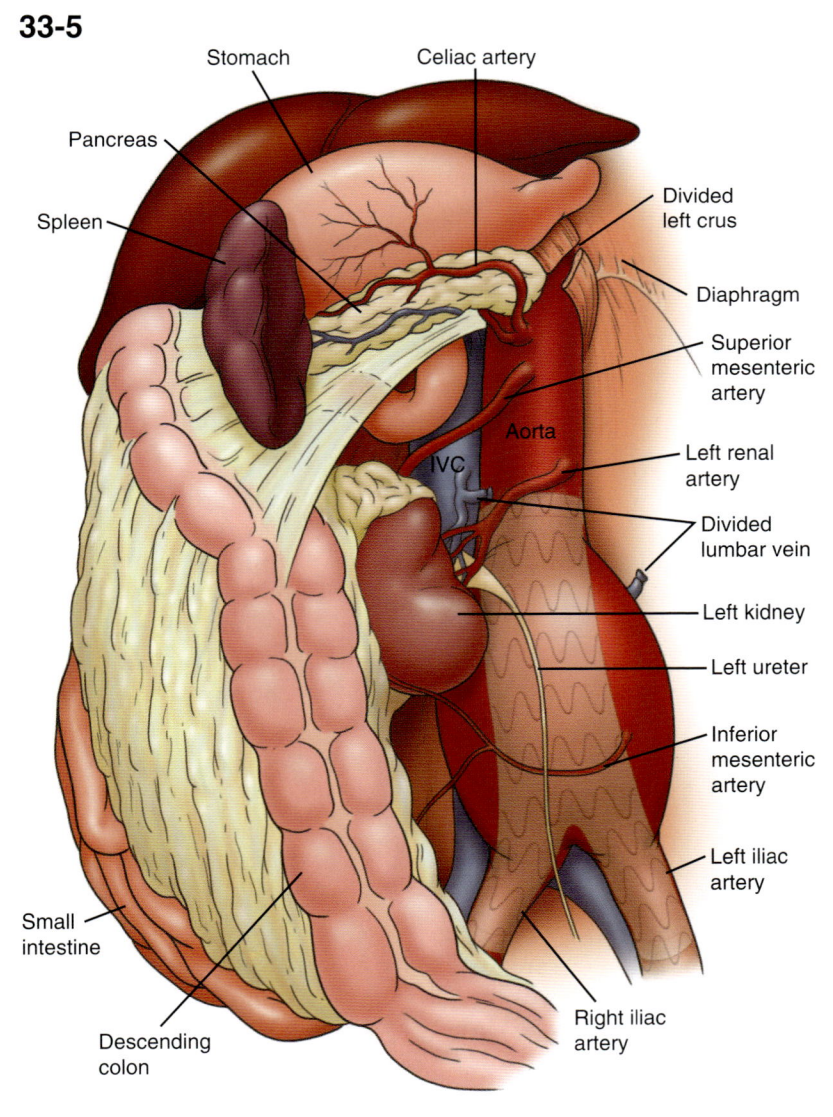

Figure 33-5 Medial visceral rotation.

RETROPERITONEAL APPROACH *INCISION AND EXPOSURE:* `CONTINUED` The RP incision is curvilinear, beginning at the midline between the umbilicus and the pubic symphysis, and is extended laterally to the 9th to 11th intercostal space. Electrocautery is used to deepen the incision along the lateral edge of the rectus abdominis muscle dividing the anterior layer of the rectus sheath. If right common iliac exposure is needed, the posterior rectus sheath can be divided as well, leaving the rectus muscle fibers intact. The RP plane is then developed moving the left kidney, ureter, pancreas, and spleen anteriorly. This plane may also be developed anterior to the kidney, leaving it in its dorsal position. The dissection proceeds into the preperitoneal space, anterior to the psoas muscle and medial. The renal lumbar vein is divided to allow for exposure of the left renal artery. For access to the suprarenal aorta, the left crus of the diaphragm is divided along the line of its fibers, like the TP exposure. The left ureter should be identified and protected in its position anterior to the aortal and left common iliac artery. Self-retaining or open-ringed retractors are used to optimize exposure. Once adequate exposure is obtained, the patient is heparinized. Silastic vessel loops are used to control the celiac, superior mesenteric, and renal arteries (FIGURE 33-6).

PROCEDURAL CONSIDERATIONS Ideally, operative planning includes imaging and knowledge of implant history to determine endograft type and relation to the aortic wall and branches (TABLE 33-1). It is also important to note the presence of any adjunctive devices such as endoanchors. Knowledge of proximal fixation extent and various graft removal techniques is particularly important for atraumatic removal of suprarenal devices. In cases of known endoleak location, partial stent graft removal and in situ reconstruction can be planned. One must decide whether to do partial or complete removal of the endograft. That decision is made in the operating room based on difficulty with removing the graft.

INFRARENAL FIXATION

Proximal Aorta The infrarenal aorta is prepared for cross-clamping in standard fashion. If there is no adequate space for proximal clamping, a suprarenal or supraceliac cross-clamp location can be prepared (see Chapter 30). Alternatively, an aortic occlusion balloon can be used, but this should have a buttress and needs continuous superior pressure by an assistant. The iliac arteries are also prepared for clamp placement distal to the level of the planned anastomosis, which will depend upon plan for full or partial stent graft removal. Consider using Fogarty insert clamps, which tend to be less traumatic when clamping the stent graft. Balloon occlusion of the iliac arteries or iliac graft limbs can also be used. Once proximal and distal control are obtained, in cases where there is no suspected type 1a or 1b endoleak, the aneurysm sac is then opened with a T-shaped longitudinal arteriotomy prior to proximal clamping, followed by removing all thrombus and debris (FIGURE 33-7). Back-bleeding lumbar and inferior mesenteric arteries are oversewed, which may be the only culprits responsible for the AAA sac growth. If a type 1a endoleak is incidentally discovered, the aorta is clamped above the endograft in a location safe to allow for sewing the proximal anastomosis (see FIGURE 33-4A and B). Next, in cases that are not type 1a, 1b, or II endoleaks, the initial clamps are placed on the body of the stent graft once the sac is opened (FIGURE 33-8); the iliac limbs are also clamped with Fogarty hydragrip clamps, which are then separated from the main body. `CONTINUES`

TABLE 33-1 AORTIC ENDOGRAFT DEVICES AND FEATURES

Manufacturer	Product Name	Fixation Location	Stent Type	Graft Material
Terumo Aortic	Treo Abdominal Stent-Graft	Suprarenal and infrarenal	Self-expanding Nitinol	Tightly woven polyester
Terumo Aortic	Aortic Cuff	Suprarenal and infrarenal	Self-expanding Nitinol	Tightly woven polyester
Cook Medical	Zenith Fenestrated (distal bifurcated body)	N/A	Stainless steel	Woven polyester
Cook Medical	Zenith Fenestrated AAA (one proximal seal stent)	Suprarenal	Self-expanding stainless steel	Woven polyester
Cook Medical	Zenith Fenestrated AAA (two proximal seal stents)	Suprarenal	Self-expanding stainless steel	Woven polyester
Cook Medical	Zenith Flex AAA	Suprarenal	Self-expanding stainless steel	Woven polyester
Cordis	INCRAFT AAA Stent Graft System	Suprarenal	Self-expanding Nitinol	Woven polyester
Endologix	AFX and AFX-2 bifurcated system	Bifurcation, infrarenal, suprarenal	Cobalt shromium alloy	DuraPly multilayer ePTFE
Endologix	Alto abdominal stent graft system	Suprarenal	Nitinol non-expensive polymer-filled ring	PTFE
Endologix	Ovation iX	Suprarenal	Nitinol non-expensive polymer filled ring	PTFE
Gore & Associates	Excluder Endoprosthesis C3	Infrarenal	Self-expanding Nitinol	ePTFE
Gore & Associates	Excluder Conformable Active Control	Infrarenal	Self-expanding Nitinol	ePTFE
Medtronic	Endurant II AAA	Suprarenal	Self-expanding Nitinol	Woven polyester
Medtronic	Endurant AUI	Suprarenal	Self-expanding Nitinol	Woven polyester
Medtronic	Endurant IIs AAA	Suprarenal	Self-expanding Nitinol	Woven polyester

33-6

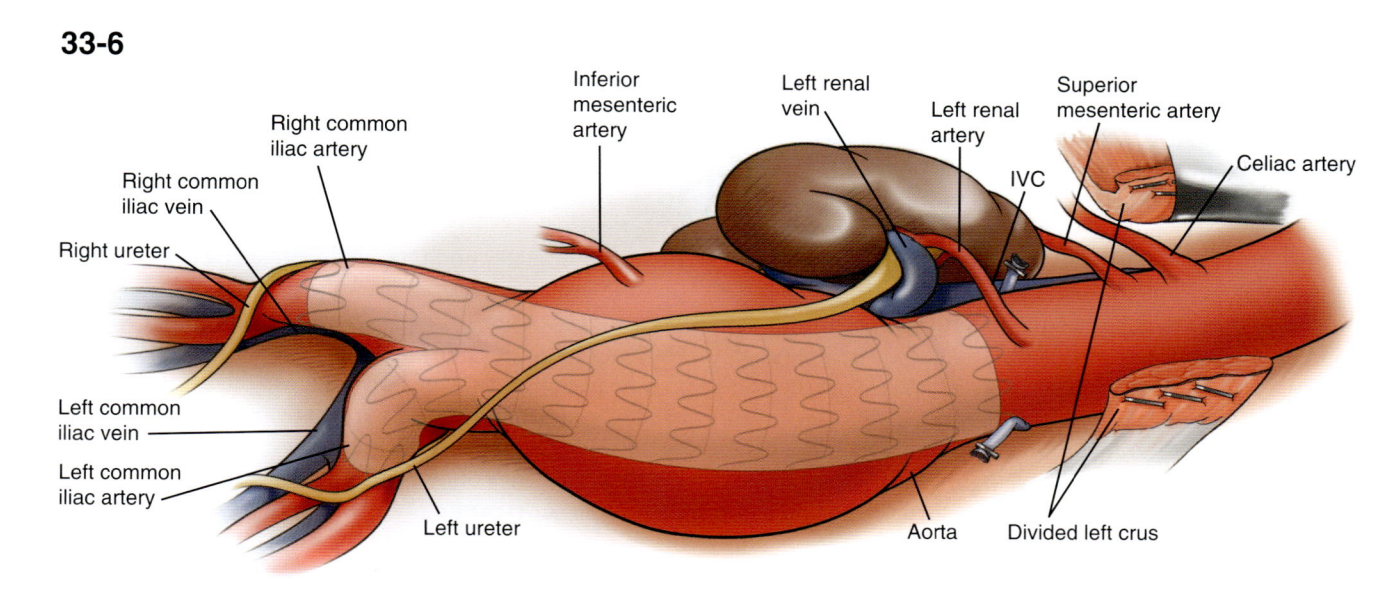

Figure 33-6 Retroperitoneal perivisceral exposure.

33-7

33-8

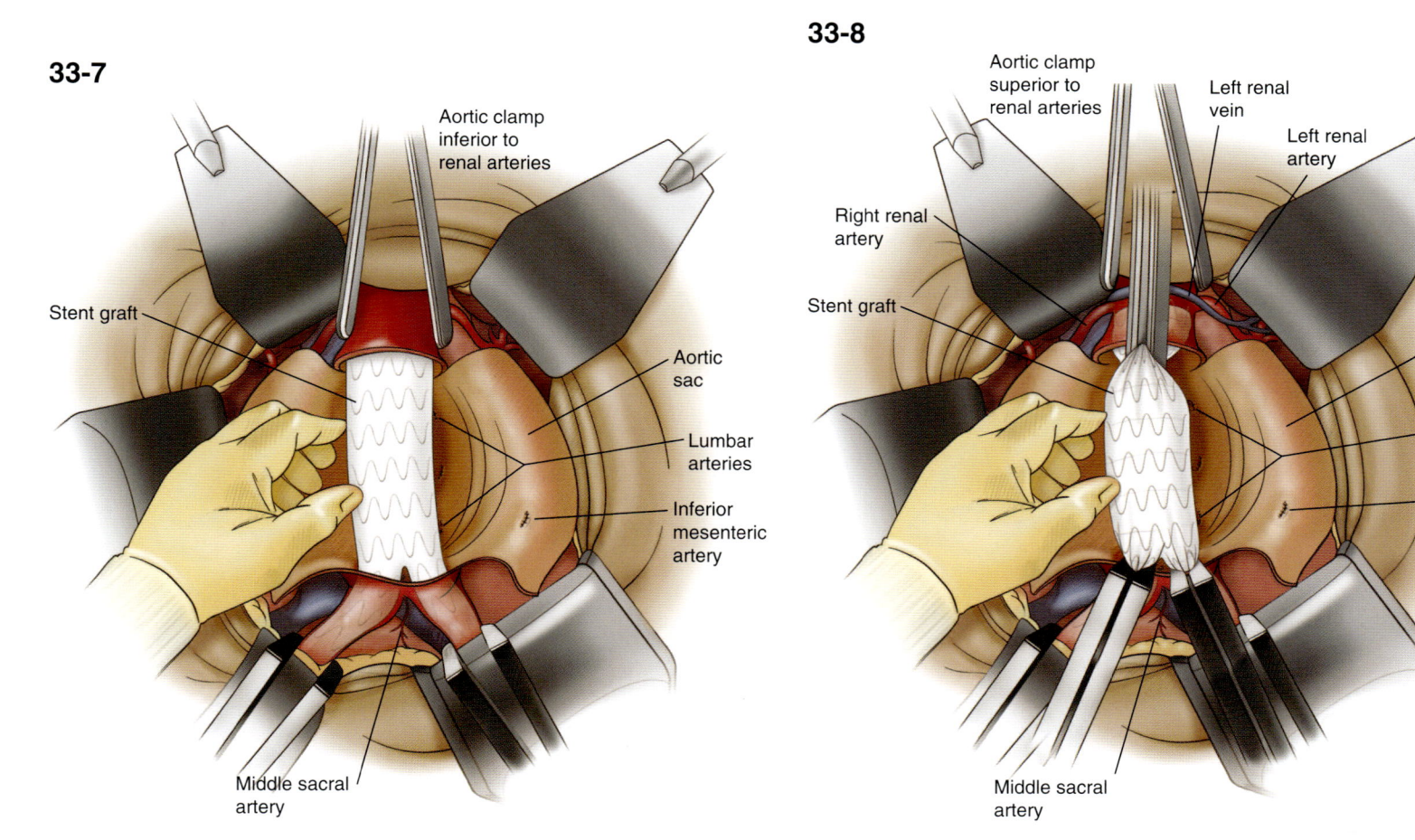

Figure 33-7 Opening AAA sac prior to clamp.

Figure 33-8 Clamp Stent graft proximal and distal after oversewing lumbars and/or removing damaged area of stent graft.

PROCEDURAL   CONSIDERATIONS *INFRARENAL   FIXATION Proximal Aorta* `CONTINUED` This is done for type III endoleaks. For endograft infection, the limbs generally can be extracted easily with retrograde traction and control of the iliac arteries gained with balloon occlusion or standard cross-clamping. Occasionally the proximal stent graft and/or distal stent graft will heal into the vessel. In this circumstance, it is frequently easier to sew the new graft with a direct anastomosis to the stent graft using a felt pledget to avoid tears in the graft, a key gateway to the procedure (FIGURE 33-9). Of note, late iliac artery degeneration leading to iliac rupture has been reported following endograft removal and is an important consideration when planning partial or full explant. Alternatively, the limbs can be left behind, transected, and oversewn at the orifice of the iliac bifurcation, taking care to avoid injury to the underlying iliac veins. The distal anastomosis is then done to normal native iliac vessels. We recommended including native tissue whenever possible to avoid late iliac degeneration and hemorrhage. More distal revascularization can then be undertaken to the external iliac arteries or femoral arteries as necessary.

If complete removal of the graft is known preoperatively (such as infection or type 1a endoleak), this will always be the first step. The proximal aorta above the stent graft is clamped (see FIGURE 33-4), and the sac opened (FIGURE 33-10). The sac is opened like above, and clamp placed on the main graft body. For some infrarenal devices (TABLE 33-1) there may exist adequate infrarenal space for aortic cross clamping and graft removal without readjusting. Some centers favor the use of an aortic occlusion balloon during graft removal as it avoids the extensive suprarenal dissection required for clamp placement, but keeping these in place without movement from forward blood pressure can be challenging. The balloon may be passed in the cranial direction into the aorta from within the stent graft or in the caudal direction via the axillary artery into the suprarenal aorta. The graft can usually be easily compressed and removed from the aorta, or the aorta can be transected above the area of fixation if adequate tissue is present. The endograft can be teased away with one's finger or constrained with Rommel tourniquets if necessary to remove it from the aortic wall.

SUPRARENAL FIXATION: For removal of pararenal devices with uncovered stents extending above the renal arteries, a suprarenal or supraceliac clamp placement may be used for a brief period while the device is extracted and replaced in the infrarenal location for creation of the proximal anastomosis to allow for quicker reperfusion. In the case of suprarenal fixation, care must be taken to avoid damage to the renal arteries and paravisceral aorta. There are several described techniques to remove barbed stent grafts with minimal damage to the aortic wall. The simplest is to advance the stent graft cranially and then gently crush the graft in a radial fashion such that the proximal fixation hooks and barbs dislodge from the aortic wall (FIGURE 33-11A). It is also possible to digitally push each barb away from the wall, and sometimes this makes it very simple, but a second or third glove may be necessary to avoid barb injury to one's finger. The proximal portion of stent graft can is then withdrawn from the aorta in the caudal direction. In the absence of a proximal endoleak or infection, the proximal portion of the stent graft may often be well incorporated and can be left in situ rather than removed (FIGURE 33-11B). In this case, the stent graft is transected between stents and the remaining stent graft components are incorporated with the aortic wall into the proximal anastomosis. Barbs in the way can be cut with a wire cutter, or circumferential release of stent barbs with a wire cutter can be done but can be time consuming. `CONTINUES`

33-9

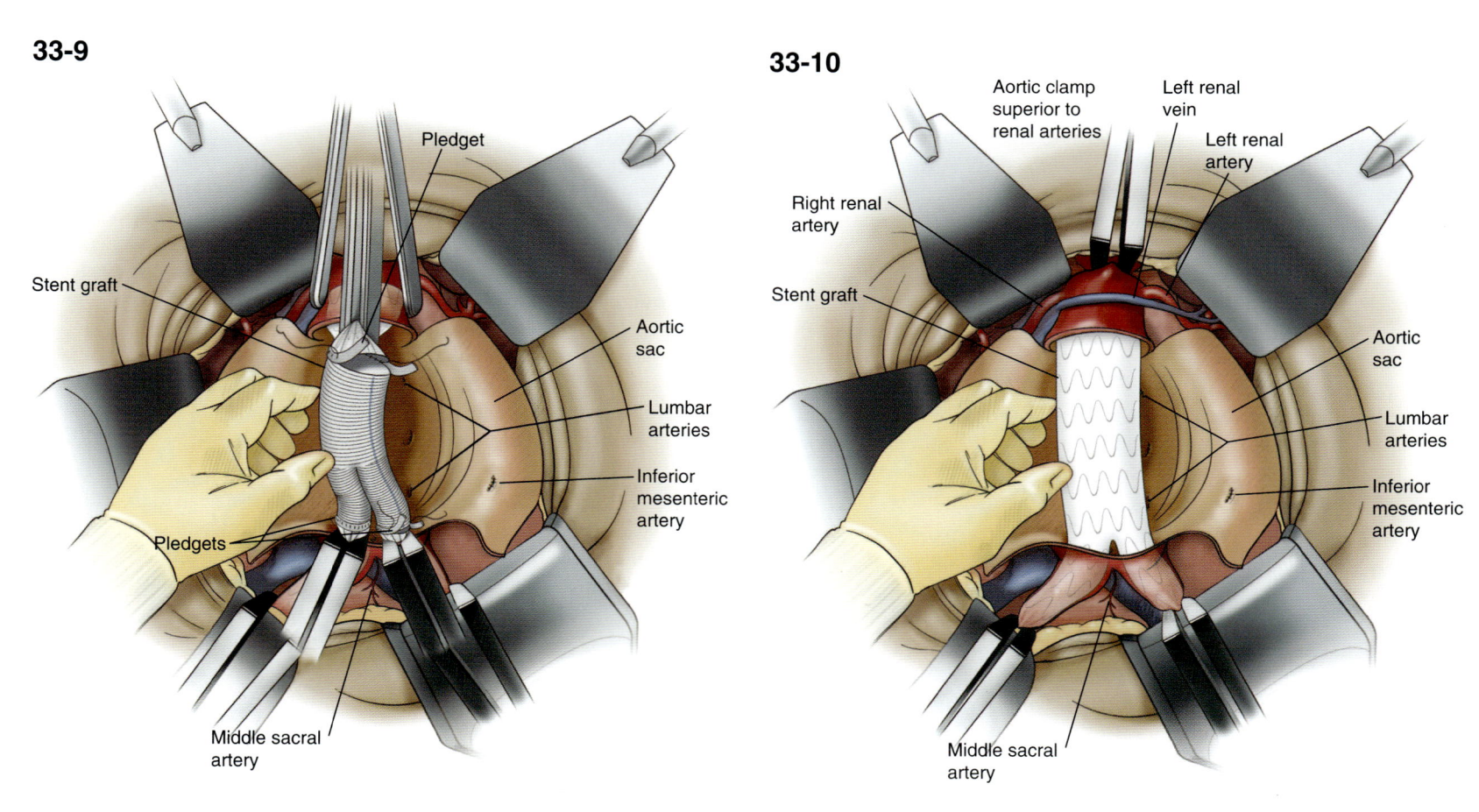

Figure 33-9 In situ repair to stent graft sewing new graft to remnant stent graft with pledget.

33-10

Figure 33-10 Suprarenal clamp showing stent graft not opposed causing a type 1 endoleak.

33-11

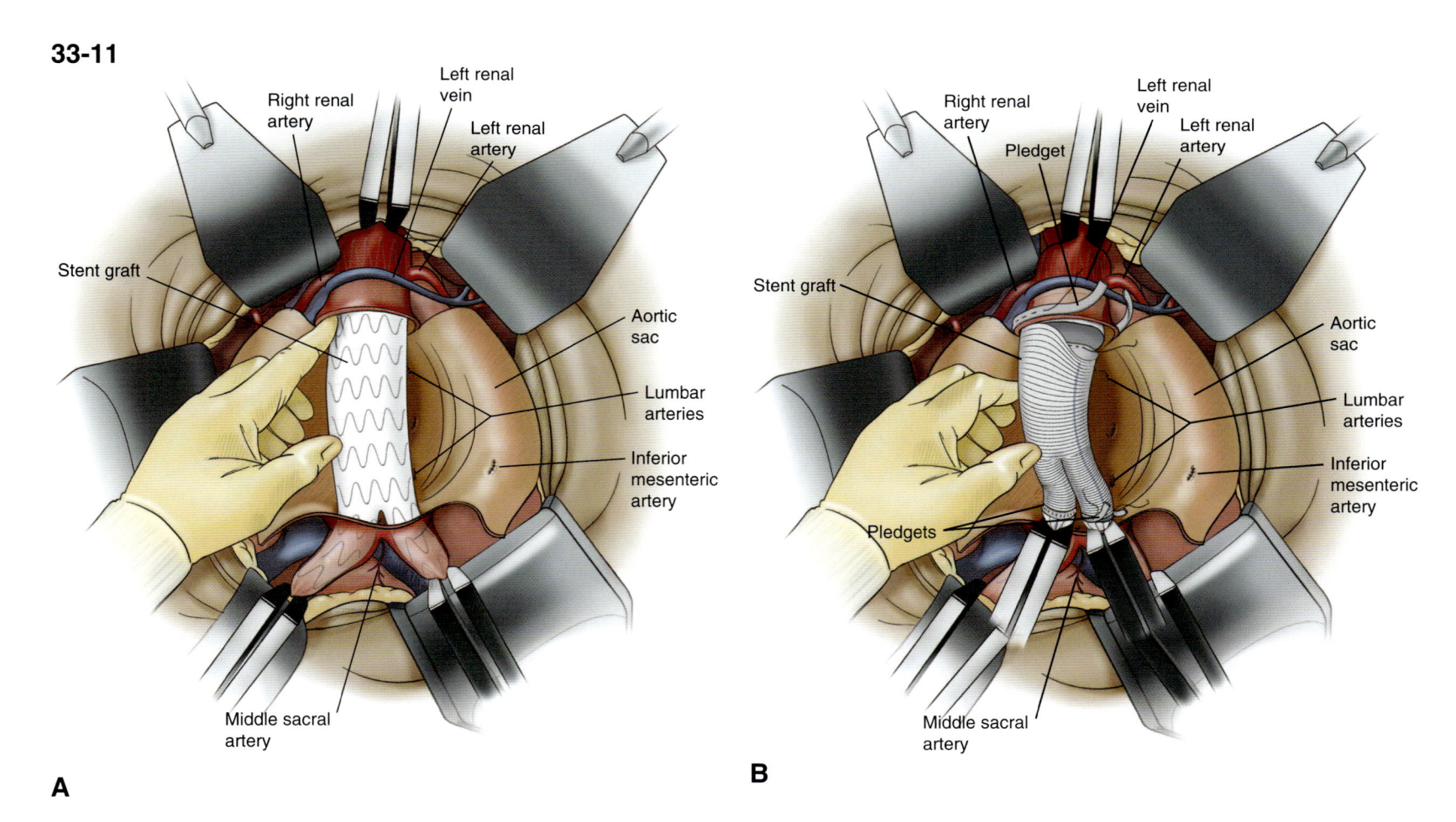

A

B

Figure 33-11 A. Index finger with digit aided removal of stent graft. B. Suprarenal clamp and sew to stent graft and aorta together.

PROCEDURAL CONSIDERATIONS *SUPRARENAL FIXATION:* `CONTINUED` While the cranial advancement and manual crush technique can be used in the case of suprarenal fixation as well, care must be taken in these cases to avoid damaging the pararenal aorta. Additional adjunctive techniques include using some type of constraining device to compress the stent graft in a radial fashion, thereby dislodging the barbs. Koning et al. first described a simple and inexpensive technique for removal of a Zenith endograft (Cook Medical) with suprarenal fixation using a 20-mL syringe. The device can be constructed by cutting off the tip of a 20-mL syringe and rounding off any sharp edges (FIGURE 33-12). Retraction tape is secured to the distal portion of the transected main body of the stent graft and fed through the cut syringe.

The retraction tape is then used to stabilize the stent graft as the syringe is advanced in a cranial direction, radially constricting the graft and disengaging the barbs from the aortic wall. The device can then be removed from the aorta in a caudal direction. Similar techniques have been described for device extraction, such as the use of a disposable proctoscope to re-sheath the device in the same fashion as the 20-mL syringe by Poppelwell et al. This technique is done to facilitate easy removal of the endograft, but if the endograft does not come out easily, one should abandon this and consider other approaches described.

EXPLANT OF ENDOVASCULAR ANEURYSM SEALING SYSTEM: The Nellix Endovascular Aneurysm Sealing (EVAS) System (Endologix Inc., Irvine, CA) has been associated with high long-term failure risk and open conversion rates of up to 13%. Its unique properties are important to be aware of. The system employs polymer-filled endobags to surround dual balloon expandable stents within the aortoiliac lumen with the goal of obliterating the flow lumen and theoretically preventing migration. While the endobag system avoids need for fixation barbs, allowing it to easily slide out from the aneurysm sac, their presence renders the sac noncompressible and has been reported to create significant periaortic inflammation seen during aortic mobilization. Additionally, the iliac component is a bare-stent configuration and has been reported to fracture upon removal. Care should be taken when removing this component to prevent intimal damage.

EXPLANT OF FENESTRATED ENDOVASCULAR GRAFTS: There are few reported cases of FEVAR explant; however, with the rise of custom-made fenestrated devices, experience with their removal will be valuable at select centers. Surgical techniques are like thoracoabdominal aortic repair and include sequential cross-clamping of branch vessels to minimize visceral ischemic time. In addition, to avoid removing the stent and damaging the artery, one can sew a new limb from the graft to a branched stent graft. Care must be taken during removal of bridging stents to ensure ostium are free of damage or dissection. Alternatively, vessels can be transected distal to the bridging stent and an aortovisceral bypass may be performed. With prolonged operative time and varying degrees of visceral ischemia time, these patients are apt to be at higher risk for morbidity and mortality than those undergoing infrarenal endograft explant.

Revascularization Plan Once the device is removed, in part or in full, revascularization is then performed. The configuration will depend on patient anatomy and reason for explant. With partial removal, consider using a felt strip as a buttress. Also use smaller needles, as the graft material in many instances is thinner than conventional open aortic grafts. Aortic graft infection warrants full device removal and either the construction of an extra-anatomic bypass or reconstruction with Rifampin-soaked Dacron Gelsoft (Terumo Inc., Somerset, NJ) or cryopreserved allograft. If the native aorta is not incorporated into the proximal anastomosis, the stump should be oversewn in two layers with a horizontal mattress stitch followed by a baseball stitch. This can be particularly challenging in the case of infection when tissue is friable; the use of an omental pedicle is often helpful. Hemostasis is obtained before moving on to closure.

CLOSURE For the TP approach, the aneurysm sac and posterior peritoneum are closed over the graft with a running absorbable suture. An omental flap may be utilized in cases with limited tissue. The additional layers of tissue coverage help to exclude the graft from the bowel and retroperitoneum. The bowel is then returned to its normal anatomic position and the anterior abdominal wall is closed according to surgeon preference.

For the RP approach, the peritoneal sac can be returned to its typical anatomic position. The peritoneum should be inspected, and any rents repaired with absorbable suture. If the peritoneum has not been violated the aneurysm sac does not need to be closed, as the contents remain separate from the graft. Once the operating table has been returned to the neutral position the incision is closed in multiple layers. The incorporation of ribs and diaphragm can add support to the closure of the transversus abdominus and internal oblique muscles. The authors prefer to close external oblique and its fascia with an interrupted fashion over this layer to provide additional strength to the closure.

The femoral vessels should be palpated, and pedal vessels auscultated with a Doppler prior to closure to verify patency. Pedal Doppler signals should also be obtained at the end of the case, and any changes can be investigated with angiography.

POSTOPERATIVE CARE Patients are typically transferred to the intensive care unit for the first 24 to 48 hours for close hemodynamic and respiratory monitoring. Hourly assessment of vital signs, urine output, and lower extremity neurovascular exams are important during the initial recovery period. Frequent lab studies monitoring renal function, acid-base balance, and hematologic status can be useful in guiding postoperative care. ■

SUGGESTED READINGS

Arnaoutakis DJ, Sharma G, Blackwood S, Shah SK, Menard M, Ozaki CK, et al. Strategies and outcomes for aortic endograft explantation. *J Vasc Surg.* 2019;69(1):80-85.

Chaikof EL, Dalman RL, Eskandari MK, Jackson BM, Lee WA, Mansour MA, et al. The Society for Vascular Surgery practice guidelines on the care of patients with an abdominal aortic aneurysm. *J Vasc Surg.* 2018;67(1):2-77.e2.

Jimenez JC, Moore WS, Quinones-Baldrich WJ. Acute and chronic open conversion after endovascular aortic aneurysm repair: a 14-year review. *J Vasc Surg.* 2007;46(4):642-647.

Koning OHJ, Hinnen J-W, Van Baalen JM. Technique for safe removal of an aortic endograft with suprarenal fixation. *J Vasc Surg.* 2006;43(4):855-857.

Lee CJ, Cuff R. Explanting the Nellix Endovascular Aortic Sealing Endoprosthesis for Proximal Aortic Neck Failure. *Ann Vasc Surg.* 2019;54:144 e1-e7.

Nonaka T, Kimura N, Hori D, Sasabuchi Y, Nakano M, Yuri K, et al. Predictors of acute kidney injury following elective open and endovascular aortic repair for abdominal aortic aneurysm. *Ann Vasc Dis.* 2018;11(3):298-305.

Perini P, Gargiulo M, Silingardi R, Piccinini E, Capelli P, Fontana A, et al. Late open conversions after endovascular abdominal aneurysm repair in an urgent setting. *J Vasc Surg.* 2019;69(2):423-431.

Popplewell MA, Garnham AW, Hobbs SD. A new technique to explant an infected aortic endograft. *J Vasc Surg.* 2015;62(2):512-514.

Singh AA, Benaragama KS, Pope T, Coughlin PA, Winterbottom AP, Harrison SC, et al. Progressive device failure at long term follow up of the Nellix EndoVascular Aneurysm Sealing (EVAS) system. *Eur J Vasc Endovasc Surg.* 2021;61(2):211-218.

Tang Y, Chen J, Huang K, Luo D, Liang P, Feng M, et al. The incidence, risk factors and in-hospital mortality of acute kidney injury in patients after abdominal aortic aneurysm repair surgery. *BMC Nephrol.* 2017;18(1).

Twine CP, Humphreys AK, Williams IM. Systematic review and meta-analysis of the retroperitoneal versus the transperitoneal approach to the abdominal aorta. *Eur J Vasc Endovasc Surg.* 2013;46(1):36-47.

33-12

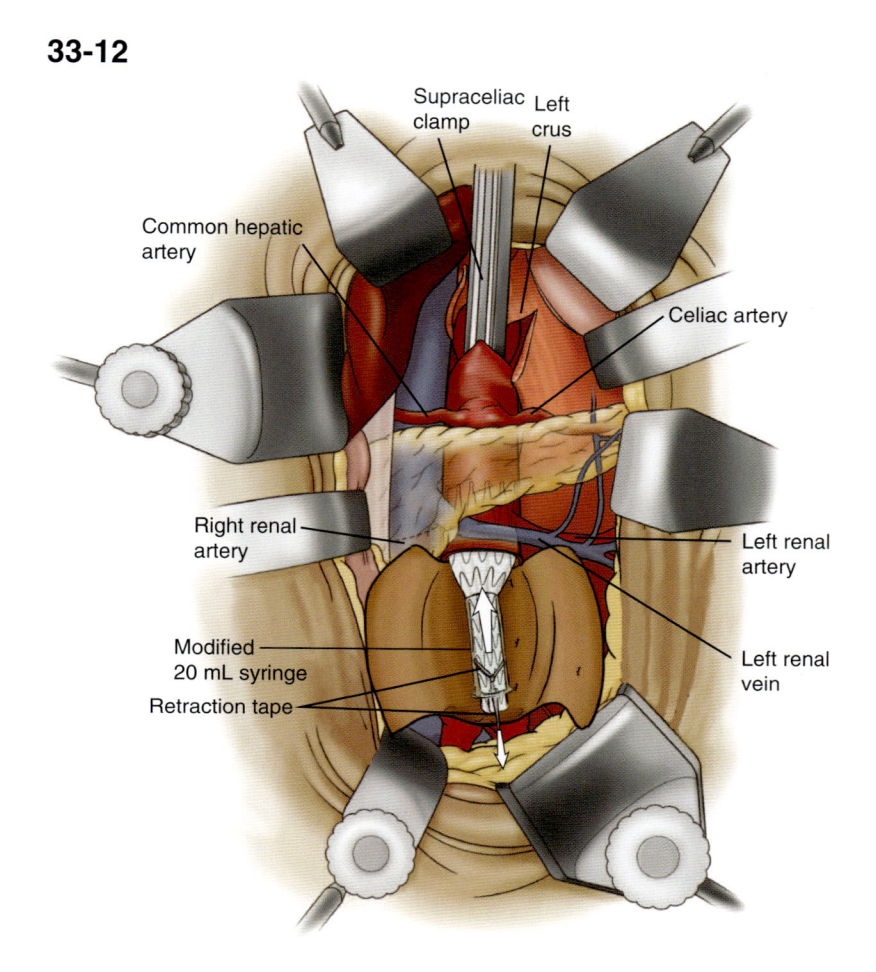

Figure 33-12 Supraceliac clamp with syringe aided removal of stent graft.

ABDOMINAL AORTA ENDOVASCULAR

EVAR: Suprarenal and Infrarenal Devices and Repair

Alan Dietzek, MD • Emilia Krol, MD

INDICATIONS The indications for treatment of abdominal aortic aneurysms (AAA) have evolved over the past 50 years. AAA repair, by open or endovascular means, is generally indicated in patients when an AAA meets criteria as set forth in one's corresponding major societal guidelines such as the European Society for Vascular Surgery or the Society for Vascular Surgery (SVS). According to the current SVS guidelines, elective repair for patients with low or acceptable surgical risk should be offered when the aneurysm size is equal to or greater than 5.5 cm in men and 5 cm in women. Other indications include aneurysms that rupture, symptomatic aneurysms, and rapidly expanding aneurysms with an increase in diameter greater than 0.5 cm over 6 months or 1 cm within 1 year. In addition, relative indications include patients who suffer distal embolism from the aneurysm or who have significant symptomatic concomitant aortoiliac occlusive disease. The discussion as to whether an open or endovascular repair should be performed in a particular patient is beyond the scope of this chapter. That said, patients who are considered for endovascular repair, unlike those considered for an open repair, must meet anatomic criteria that makes them suitable for this option. This will depend upon a combination of factors, such as which aortic stent graft devices are at a vascular surgeon's disposal, level of training and endovascular skill set, and most importantly, good judgement.

Initial evaluation of a patient's aortic aneurysm should begin with a duplex ultrasound of the aorta, preferably performed in an Intersocietal Accreditation Commission (IAC) accredited noninvasive vascular laboratory. This test provides reliable information regarding the size of the aneurysm, iliac extension, and usually can distinguish between an infrarenal and juxtarenal aneurysm. It is the test of choice for both the initial diagnosis and surveillance of AAA. Aneurysms 5 cm in size and greater should be further imaged with computed tomography angiography (CTA) to best determine a patient's anatomic suitability for EVAR.

Patients evaluated for AAA repair should undergo thorough physical examination, with specific consideration to femoral and popliteal arteries, as arteriopathy of those arteries is associated with AAA. Preoperative risk assessment should be performed in all patients, with particular attention to cardiac and renal function evaluation. Patients with impaired kidney function should be hydrated prior to intervention, with renal protective strategies implemented.

PREOPERATIVE SIZING AND DEVICE SELECTION Accurate preoperative sizing is a key factor for the success of any endovascular aneurysm repair. The aortic neck, also defined as the proximal landing zone, is the length of normal aorta, with parallel walls, below the level of renal arteries. The proximal aortic neck diameter at the level of the renal arteries and 10 and 15 mm below the renal arteries is obtained. In general, a neck length of less than 1 cm and neck diameter of greater than 32 mm preclude routine endovascular aneurysm repair. The distal landing zone is defined as the available length of iliac artery for which an adequate seal of 2 cm with the iliac stent graft limb can be achieved. The diameter of the stent graft is usually 10 to 20% larger than the landing vessel. Undersizing the graft can lead to graft migration and endoleaks, whereas oversizing can lead to graft infolding and consequent endoleaks and aortic injury. The presence of common and/or internal iliac artery aneurysms may also alter the selected distal landing zone. Preoperative planning will take into consideration the size of the iliac aneurysms, the maximum distal diameter of the iliac limbs for the selected stent graft device, and the need for internal iliac artery preservation. Additionally, for endovascular aneurysm repair, it is recommended that one hypogastric artery be patent or that an iliac branch device or hypogastric artery bypass be considered to minimize pelvic ischemia. Currently, only one device allows for treating iliac aneurysms with a hypogastric branch device (Gore, Flagstaff, AZ).

The key measurements for perioperative planning include:

- The total treatment length, defined as length from the most caudal renal artery to the aortic bifurcation and to each iliac bifurcation
- Diameter and length of the aortic neck
- Diameter and length of iliac landing zones or zones
- Diameter and patency of common femoral and iliac arteries used for vascular access

In patients with severe, common, or external iliac occlusive disease, iliac angioplasty and or stenting (endopaving) may be required for accommodation of aortic devices if the other external iliac artery cannot be utilized. An aorto-uni-iliac graft and femoral-femoral bypass should be considered if this strategy cannot be implemented or the external and/or common iliac arteries on one side are occluded. Patients who have external iliac and femoral arteries that are less than 7 mm in diameter may require an iliac conduit (to deliver the stent grafts). An iliac conduit is necessary to deliver an endograft when the external and/or common iliac arteries are too small to accommodate a large sheath. In this circumstance, an 8- or 10-mm Dacron graft is sewn to the common iliac bifurcation and the common femoral artery, providing a large vessel to deliver the stent graft. This may be necessary for patients with severe occlusive disease or vessel diameters of less than 6 to 7 mm.

In patients with an imperfect neck (short, conical, reverse conical, highly angulated, with abundant thrombus or extensive calcifications), the use of anchoring devices (i.e., Aptus Heli-FX EndoAnchor system; Medtronic Vascular, Santa Rosa, CA) may be beneficial. Alternatively, the use of a fenestrated graft should be considered if the aortic anatomy meets criteria for use. Finally, it is important to include the need for bridging/extension stent graft pieces. Devices currently available on the market differ slightly with regard to sizes and mechanism of action. The Excluder C3 device (W.L. Gore) requires a sheath for insertion. The device offers unique ability to reconstrain the main trunk in case of inaccurate deployment. The device does not have suprarenal fixation, has anchoring barbs, and is rapidly deployed by releasing the constraining sheath around the endograft by unscrewing and pulling a knob. The Endurant device (Medtronic Vascular, Santa Rosa, CA) is prepackaged with hydrophilic sheaths that require an 0.035 wire. The device is deployed by unsheathing it through handle rotation mechanism. The stent graft has suprarenal uncovered stent, and anchor pins for active fixation. It is approved for 10-mm neck, or 4-mm neck with additional anchor fixation, and its key feature is the M-Stent, which among many things offers conformability and superior seal. The Zenith device (Cook Medical) is prepackaged with hydrophilic sheaths on 0.035 wire. The device is deployed by manually unsheathing it in desired position. Proximal attachment consists of suprarenal Z stent with hooks. The Ovation Prime (Endologix, Irvine, CA) has a unique sealing mechanism of two polymer-filled sealing rings, thought to improve proximal seal zone in the non-ideal neck. The device uses the lowest profile available (14F) and is a valuable alternative in patients with poor iliac access. The Treo (Terumo Aortic Ltd, Renfrewshire, Scotland, UK) is prepacked with hydrophilic sheaths, on 0.035 wire, that can be then detached and left in place for further ballooning. The stent has suprarenal uncovered stent with fixation barbs. Also, there are fixation barbs on the limbs which prevent component separation with resultant type 3 endoleaks. The device profile ranges from 18F to 19F.

ANESTHESIA Anesthesia for endovascular aneurysm repair can be spinal, general, or local block. However, patients should be prepared for possible open conversion, so routine central venous line access and arterial line access are required.

POSITION The patient is placed on the operating table in supine position. Prior to draping, radiologic evaluation assures good visualization, without obstructing elements on the patient's lower chest, abdomen, and groin area.

OPERATIVE PREPARATION The hair at the operative sites is removed with clippers. Patients are placed in the supine position and should be prepped from the nipples to knees in the event conversion is required. The arterial line is usually placed on the patient's right side to allow for urgent left brachial artery access in case of emergency for gaining visceral/renal artery access.

INCISION AND EXPOSURE Traditionally, oblique groin incisions are made for endovascular aneurysm repair (**FIGURE 34-1**), but preclosure with two percutaneous Proglide devices is common. Incisions for endovascular aneurysm repair are made approximately 4 cm below and parallel to the inguinal ligament (anterior superior iliac spine to pubic tubercle.) This location allows for direct access to the femoral arteries and the bifurcation. It is also helpful to identify the femoral artery bifurcation with duplex ultrasound and the femoral head under fluoroscopy, which again provides a useful landmark (**FIGURE 34-2**). CONTINUES ▶

34-1

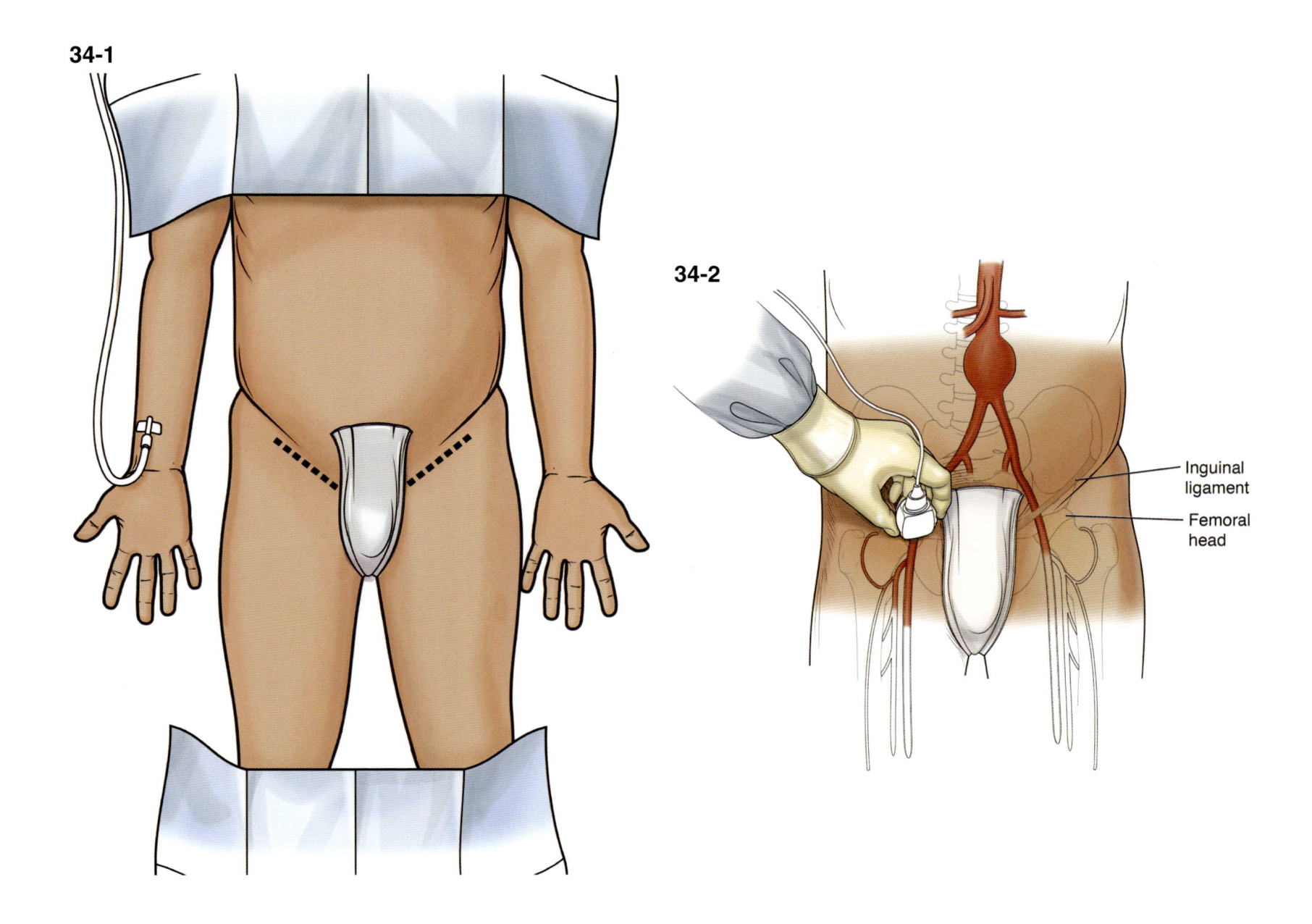

34-2

Inguinal ligament

Femoral head

INCISION AND EXPOSURE CONTINUED The pulse is palpated on the line connecting those two anatomic points. Duplex ultrasound is mandatory if considering a total percutaneous preclose technique. Open exposure of the common femoral arteries is made with either vertical or transverse skin incisions. The vertical incision is more commonly used for those patients with significant femoral artery occlusive disease; it should extend from below to above (1–3 cm) the groin crease to allow for proximal and distal control. If a transverse incision is used, it should be made above the groin crease and below the inguinal ligament and should be 2 to 5 cm in length, depending on the size and habitus of the patient (FIGURE 34-3). The authors prefer the latter incision, particularly in more obese patients, as it avoids crossing the groin crease and thus the greater possibility for skin maceration and wound infection postoperatively. Once through the subcutaneous tissues and fascia, the inguinal ligament marks the superior aspect of the exposure. The femoral sheath is then accessed, and the common femoral artery is dissected proximally and the profunda femoris and superficial femoral arteries distally. All are encircled with vessel loops for control.

Needle access (FIGURE 34-4) is obtained under direct ultrasound visualization, proximal to the femoral bifurcation. Percutaneous access for EVAR (PEVAR) has gained popularity in recent years. If that access is chosen, ultrasound guidance with the use of a sterilely prepped duplex probe is utilized to access the common femoral artery with a micropuncture needle, wire, and sheath. Wire position is checked with fluoroscopy prior to exchanging to an 0.035 wire and larger sheath sizes. Two Perclose ProGlide devices (Abbot Vascular, Redwood, CA) are now put in place in each common femoral artery and are left untied until the entire procedure is completed. Perclose devices perform poorly in heavily calcified arteries, and those patients are better suited for open surgical exposure for arterial access.

DETAILS OF PROCEDURE After obtaining needle access, an ipsilateral wire 0.035″ glidewire is then advanced into the ascending thoracic aorta distal to the aortic valve for the ipsilateral device. A second access site is obtained from the contralateral femoral artery, and a wire is placed in the upper abdominal aorta for the contralateral device. A measuring aortogram is done through the contralateral side (FIGURE 34-4) with a measuring catheter with multiple side holes. This allows for confirmation of preoperative measurements and identification of the renal arteries, which are usually located in the vicinity of the second lumbar vertebral body. The ipsilateral wire is then exchanged out over a catheter for a stiffer wire (e.g., Amplatz or Lunderquist) to allow for easy traceability of the main body of the device. Patients are given systemic heparin at 100 units/kg, and the activated clotting time is maintained at greater than 200 seconds.

A pigtail catheter is inserted on the contralateral side after the appropriately sized delivery sheath (usually 12–15F) is inserted over a stiff wire for arterial access. This may require the artery to be serially dilated. The appropriately sized ipsilateral sheath is done the same as above (14–22F sheath), as a stent graft device (if the sheath is a part of the device) or large delivery sheath are positioned into the distal abdominal aorta under direct fluoroscopic guidance. In general, the main body of the device is inserted on the right side and the contralateral limb from the left, but patient anatomic constraints (e.g., artery size and tortuosity) may dictate switching sides for the main body and contralateral limb. It is imperative that every maneuver be done under direct fluoroscopic visualization and deployed according to manufacturer's guidelines.

The main body of the device is then inserted over the wire under direct vision (FIGURE 34-5), orienting the contralateral gate marker to the opposite limb side. Occasionally, this marker may need to be oriented in the anterior or ipsilateral position to facilitate gaining access to the gate (FIGURE 34-6). A second measuring aortogram is taken with magnified views of the renal arteries. CONTINUES

34-3

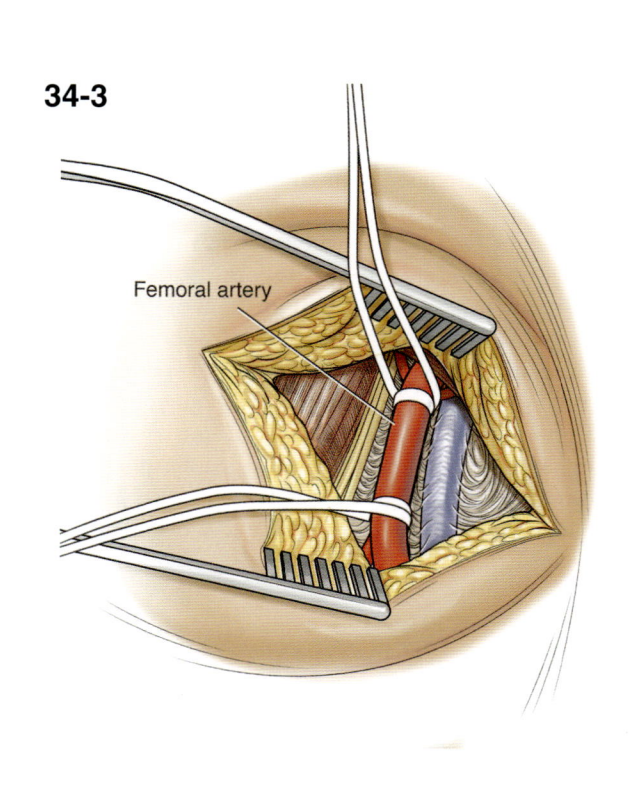

Femoral artery

34-4

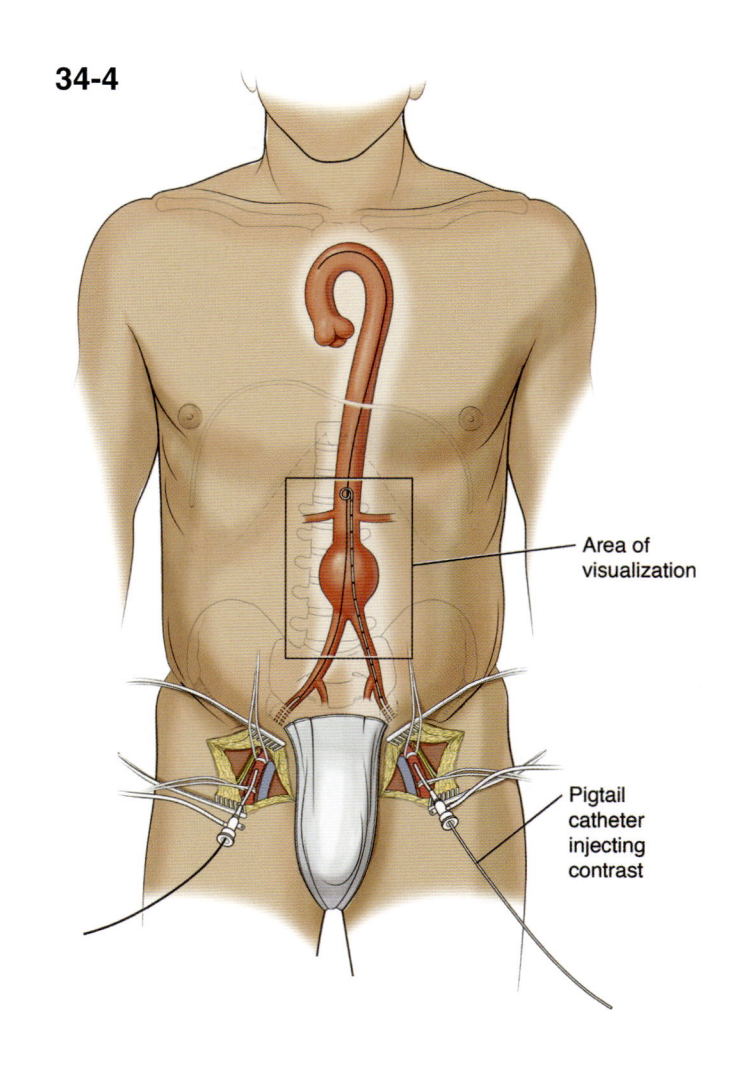

Area of visualization

Pigtail catheter injecting contrast

34-5

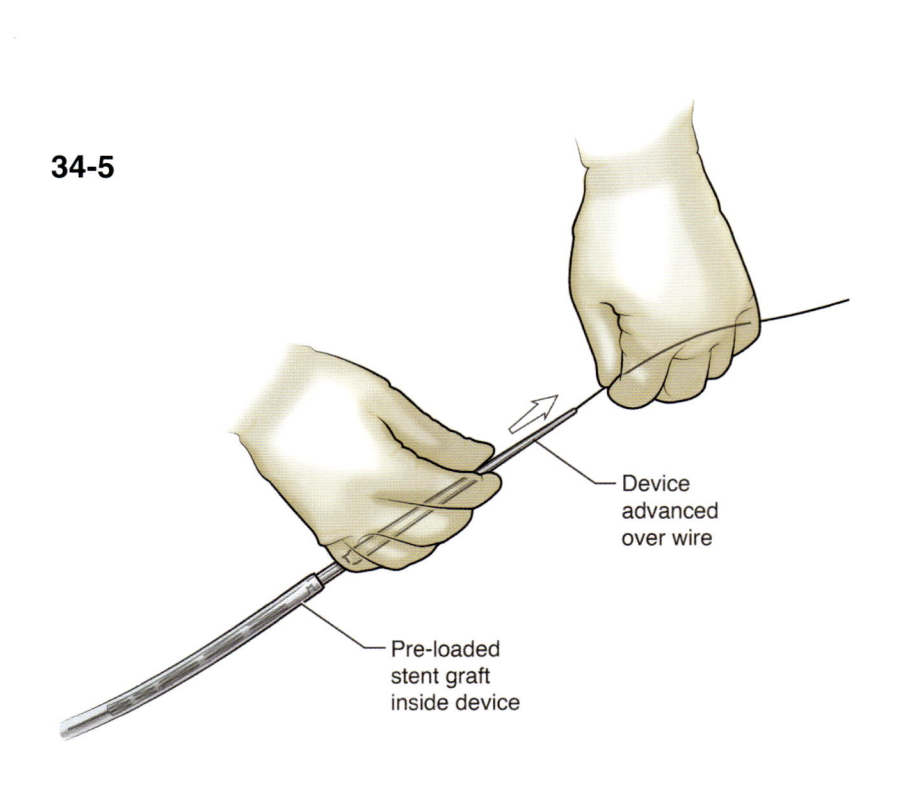

Device advanced over wire

Pre-loaded stent graft inside device

34-6

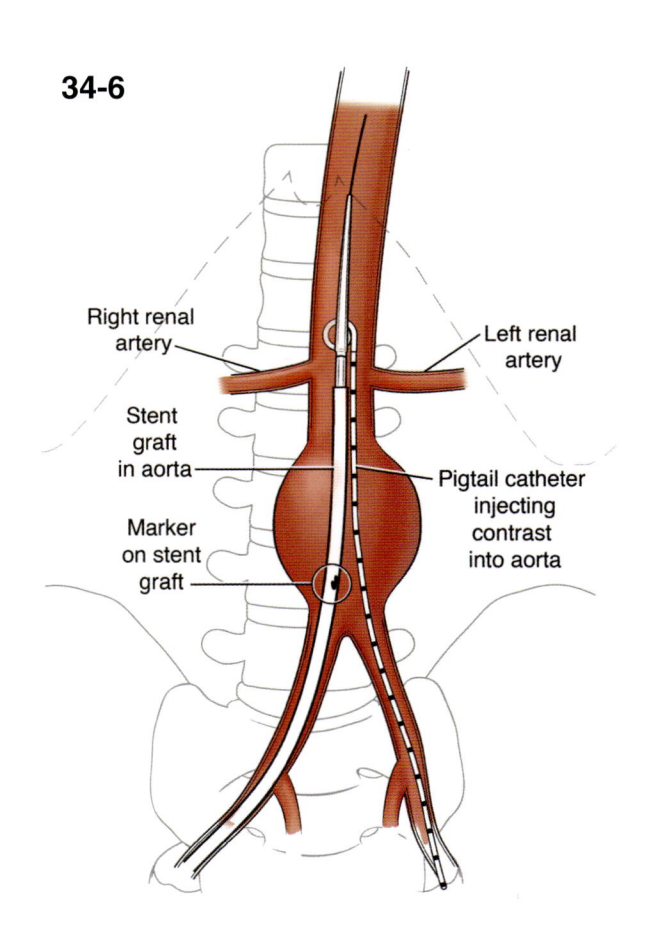

Right renal artery

Left renal artery

Stent graft in aorta

Marker on stent graft

Pigtail catheter injecting contrast into aorta

DETAILS OF PROCEDURE `CONTINUED` This may require tilting the image intensifier in the cranial caudal position to remove parallax and a right anterior oblique position to allow visualization of the renal arteries while removing the overlying superior mesenteric artery (FIGURE 34-7A). An angiogram is taken from the pigtail catheter on the contralateral side and an aortogram is performed noting the position of the renal vessels. The author's preferred approach is to then exchange Pigtail catheter over a Glidewire (Terumo Medical Corp., Somerset, NJ) for a SOS catheter, and the lowest renal artery is cannulated with Glidewire to mark the renal artery. The SOS catheter is positioned in the ostium of this renal artery to prevent inadvertent coverage (FIGURE 34-7B) . The main body of the device is deployed just below the renal arteries, paying attention not to cover the ipsilateral internal iliac artery (FIGURE 34-8). After the main body, proximal fixation, and the contralateral limb are fully deployed, the SOS catheter is removed.

The next step requires cannulation of the contralateral limb gate with the wire from the contralateral side. This may require adjusting the image intensifier angle to allow exposure of the gate. Once the contralateral gate limb is cannulated, it is imperative to confirm that you are inside the endograft. The contralateral gate is cannulated with a Glidewire and an angled catheter. If the gate is particularly difficult to access, a variety of shaped catheters can be utilized to achieve successful cannulation, and in extenduating circumstances one may need to come from the brachial artery and snare a wire. It is paramount to assure that proper gate cannulation has occurred prior to deploying contralateral limb, as failure to do so can have devastating consequences. One of the methods to assure that the wire is within the graft and not outside of it is to spin the reconformed pigtail catheter in the proximal seal zone of the graft. This can be done by placing a pigtail catheter in the endograft over the wire, removing the wire, and spinning it in the proximal portion of the endograft. If the catheter spins easily, it is not caught against the aortic wall outside the endograft, and this confirms intragraft placement (FIGURE 34-9). Another method involves placing a large compliant balloon (i.e., Medtronic Reliant, Cook Medical Coda) in the native aorta just proximal to the proximal end of the aortic stent graft. If the balloon can be gently brought down into the main body of the graft without difficulty and without deforming the graft, this indicates that the wire is intraluminal. Further confirmation can be obtained by bringing the balloon halfway down into the limb of the graft and inflating it. If it is within the graft, the distal half of the balloon will conform to the limb and the proximal end of the balloon will bulge into the main body of the graft. Other maneuvers include obtaining an angiogram, both of which allow visualization of the wire location. A stiff 0.035″ wire is then placed, and an angiogram is then taken with the image intensifier placed in a contralateral position to splay the external and internal iliac arteries. It is useful to do this through the sheath with a measuring catheter in place, which will adjudicate proper sizing. `CONTINUES`

34-7

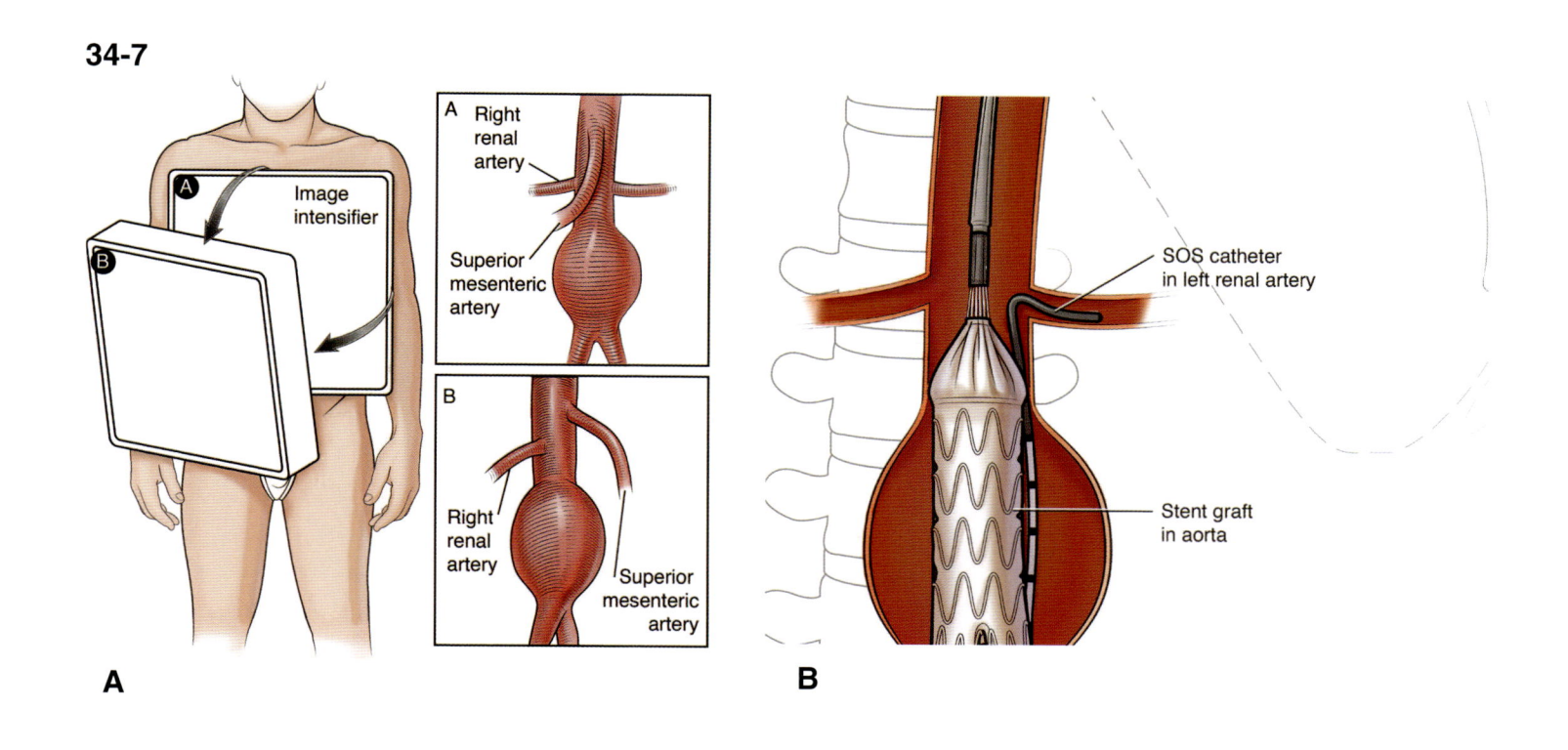

34-8

34-9

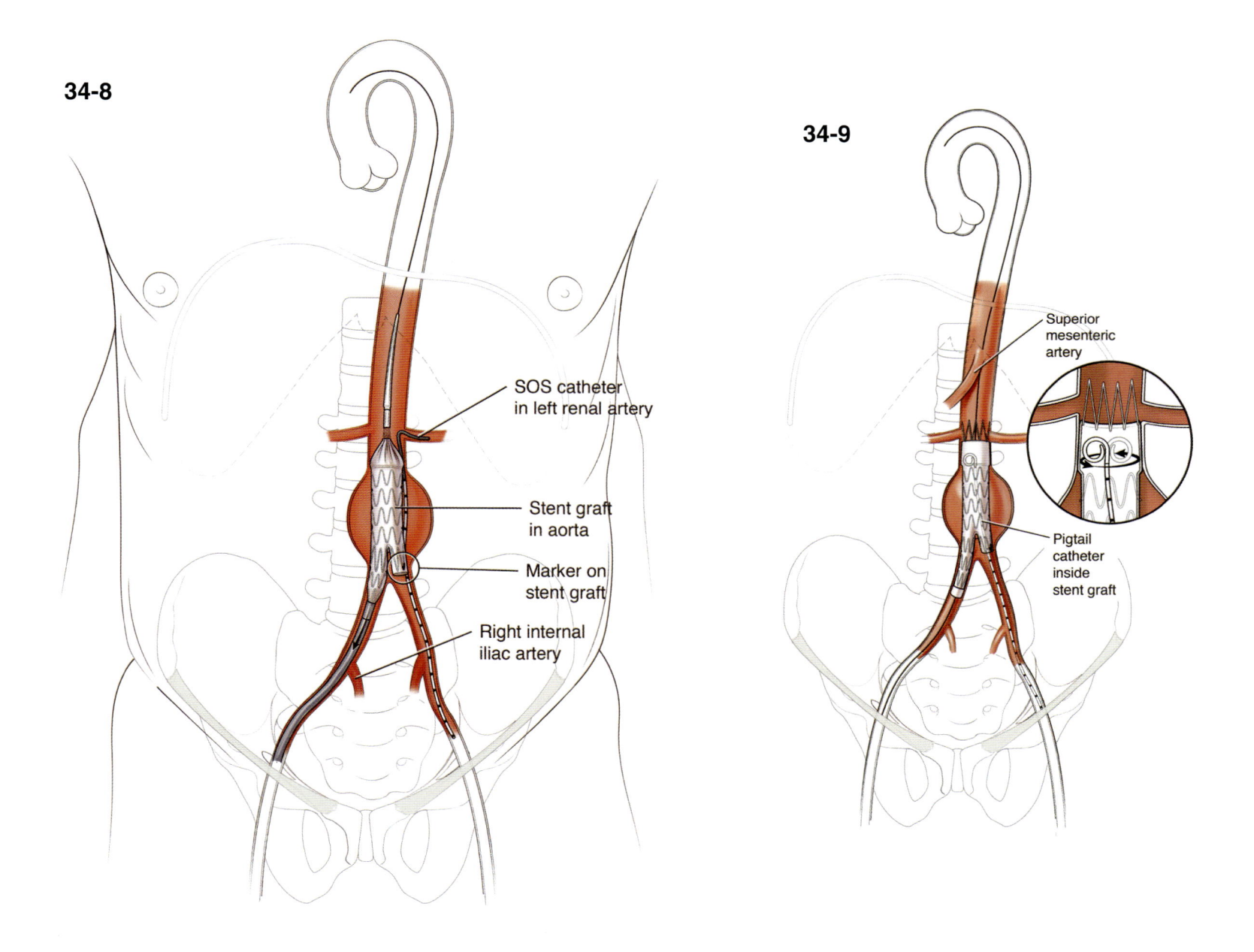

DETAILS OF PROCEDURE <CONTINUED> The contralateral limb is then deployed, paying attention to keeping the device above the internal iliac artery bifurcation (FIGURE 34-10). A second extension limb may be required for the ipsilateral side, and this is done in similar fashion to the contralateral limb.

Most if not all devices require post-implantation ballooning. This is done to ensure complete deployment and molding of the endograft to the aortic and iliac walls (FIGURE 34-11). It is NOT meant to act as an angioplasty balloon, but instead a molding balloon. Be careful not to overinflate or use it for angioplasty. The final step requires a completion angiogram to confirm proximal and distal placement of the endograft, to check for endoleaks, and to visualize the patency of the renal and iliac arteries (FIGURE 34-12). In most circumstances, type I and III endoleaks should be addressed prior to leaving the operating room.

CLOSURE After assuring appropriate exclusion of the aneurysm, all wires, catheters, and sheaths are removed. Pre-deployed closure devices are used to achieve hemostasis in the case of percutaneous access. In cases of open femoral exposure, the artery is repaired under direct visualization. The artery is then repaired with interrupted transverse 6-0 prolene sutures, and heparin is reversed with protamine sulfate. Subcutaneous tissue and skin are then closed in standard fashion. Protamine should be given depending on the initial heparin dose and length of the procedure.

POSTOPERATIVE CARE All patients require postoperative imaging with CT scanning to confirm that the endograft has properly excluded blood flow from the aneurysm sac and to identify endoleaks, with the usual first CT scan obtained at 1 month to include noncontrast, contrast, and delayed venous views. Type I (leak at the proximal or distal graft attachment site) and type III endoleaks (leak through a defect in the graft) are treated as soon as identified, whereas type II endoleaks (aneurysm sac filling through a branch vessel, usually a lumbar) are only treated if the sac enlarges more than 5 mm. Yearly imaging studies with either computed tomography scanning or duplex ultrasound are done for life to continue to monitor the size of the aneurysm and for any new endoleaks.

Immediately after completion of the procedure, the patient's peripheral perfusion must be assessed and should match that of the preoperative exam. It should not be assumed that a change in a patient's peripheral pulse exam following EVAR is the result of spasm and should almost always be addressed prior to leaving the operating room. The most common causes are injuries to the access arteries, distal embolization from the aneurysm resultant from wire and catheter manipulation, and misadventure with one or more of the closure devices.

Patients with a patent inferior mesenteric artery prior to EVAR should be monitored for colonic ischemia postoperatively. Any change in the patient's clinical exam such as abdominal pain and/or tenderness, bloody diarrhea, or an immediate postoperative bowel movement may indicate the presence of left colon/sigmoid ischemia and warrants that an immediate sigmoidoscopy be performed. ■

SELECTED READINGS

Chaikof EL, et al. The Society for Vascular Surgery practice guidelines on the care of patients with an abdominal aortic aneurysm. *J Vasc Surg.* 2018;67(1):2-77.e2.

Kratzberg JA, Golzarian J, Raghavan ML. Role of graft oversizing in the fixation strength of barbed endovascular grafts. *J Vasc Surg.* 2009 Jun;49(6):1543-1553. doi: 10.1016/j.jvs.2009.01.069. PMID: 19497518; PMCID: PMC3139438.

Sternbergh WC 3rd, Money SR, Greenberg RK, Chuter TA; Zenith Investigators. Influence of endograft oversizing on device migration, endoleak, aneurysm shrinkage, and aortic neck dilation: results from the Zenith Multicenter Trial. *J Vasc Surg.* 2004 Jan;39(1):20-26. doi: 10.1016/j.jvs.2003.09.022. PMID: 14718806.

34-10

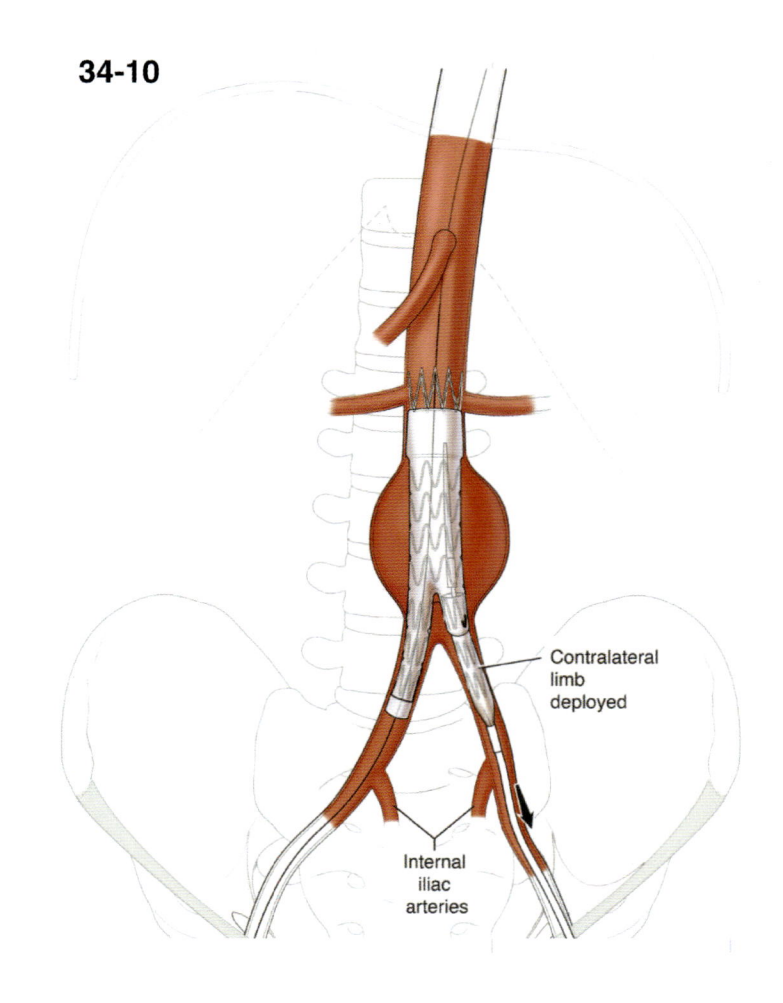

Contralateral limb deployed

Internal iliac arteries

34-11

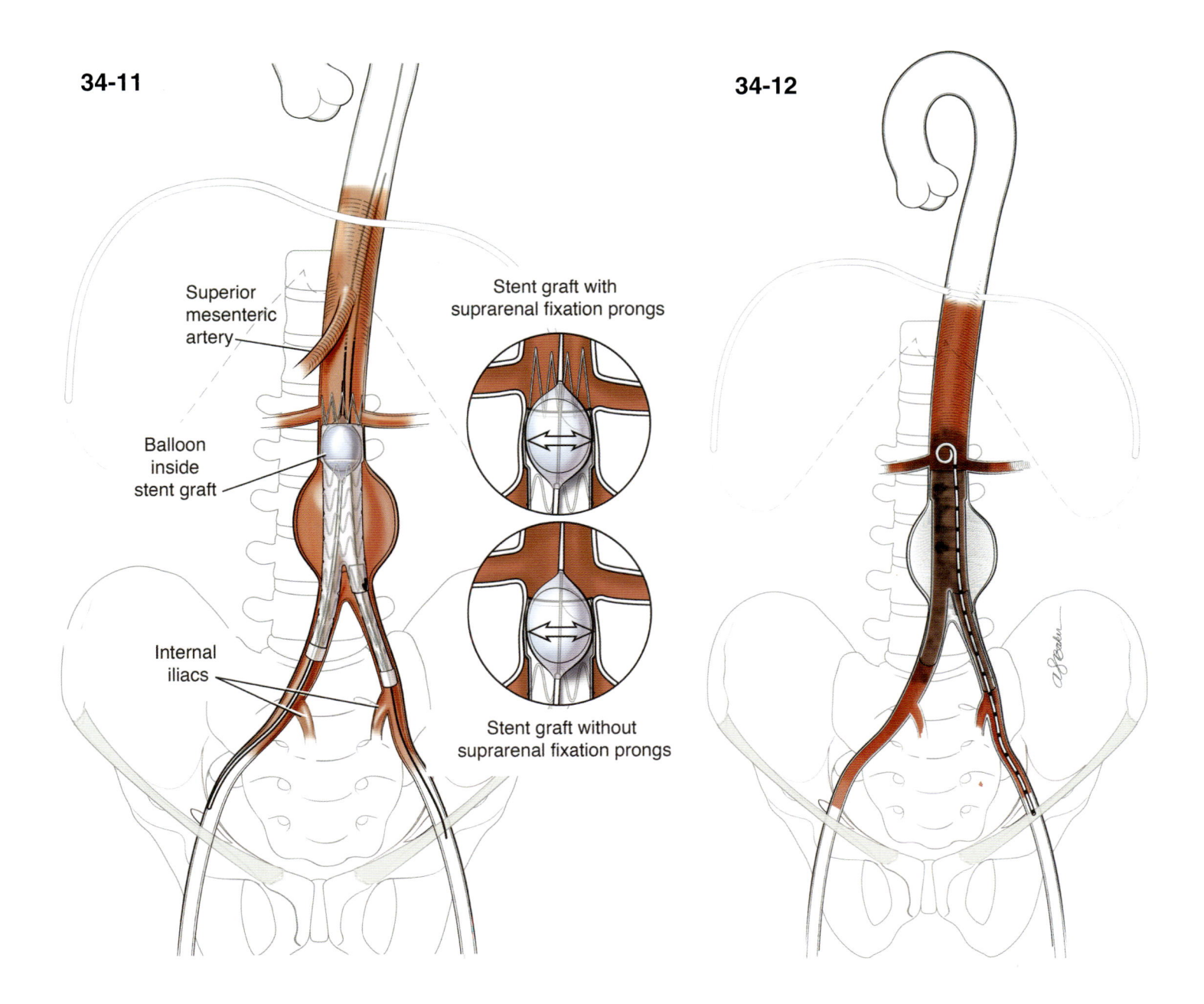

Superior mesenteric artery

Balloon inside stent graft

Internal iliacs

Stent graft with suprarenal fixation prongs

Stent graft without suprarenal fixation prongs

34-12

Iliac Branch for the Abdominal Aorta Endovascular

Javairiah Fatima, MD • Edward Woo, MD

INTRODUCTION Endovascular aneurysm repair (EVAR) is widely accepted as the first-line treatment of abdominal aortic aneurysms (AAA). However, 25 to 30% of them are associated with common iliac artery aneurysms (CIAA) that render the distal landing zone anatomically unfavorable for standard EVAR. Exclusion of the internal iliac artery (IIA) to extend the landing zone into the external iliac artery was initially adopted as the primary treatment for common iliac artery aneurysms (FIGURE 35-1A). While this is still a viable option, we quickly learned that these patients are susceptible to pelvic ischemia complications, notably gluteal claudication and erectile dysfunction, often resulting in significantly impaired quality of life. Other less frequent complications include gluteal or perineal necrosis, and ischemic colitis if bilateral IIA exclusion is attempted.

The iliac branch device (iliac branch endoprosthesis [IBE]) and the GREAT Registry data demonstrate that pelvic preservation can successfully be maintained with zero incidence of gluteal claudication and no new onset of erectile dysfunction. Internal iliac preservation using IBE is safe, effective, durable, and associated with high technical success rates. Iliac preservation, whenever possible, is the standard of care, and all anatomically eligible patients with common iliac artery aneurysms should be considered for treatment with an IBD. Pelvic preservation is particularly important to minimize spinal cord injury after endovascular treatment of thoracoabdominal aortic aneurysms and plays an integral role in multimodal spinal cord protection during fenestrated EVARs. Therefore, preservation of at least one if not both IIA is strongly recommended in clinical practice guidelines. Classic open repair of CIAA (FIGURE 35-1B) is technically challenging because of the deep pelvic location of the aneurysm, especially in the obese or hostile abdomen. Open repair carries significantly higher mortality and longer hospital stay compared to EVAR. CONTINUES ▶

35-1

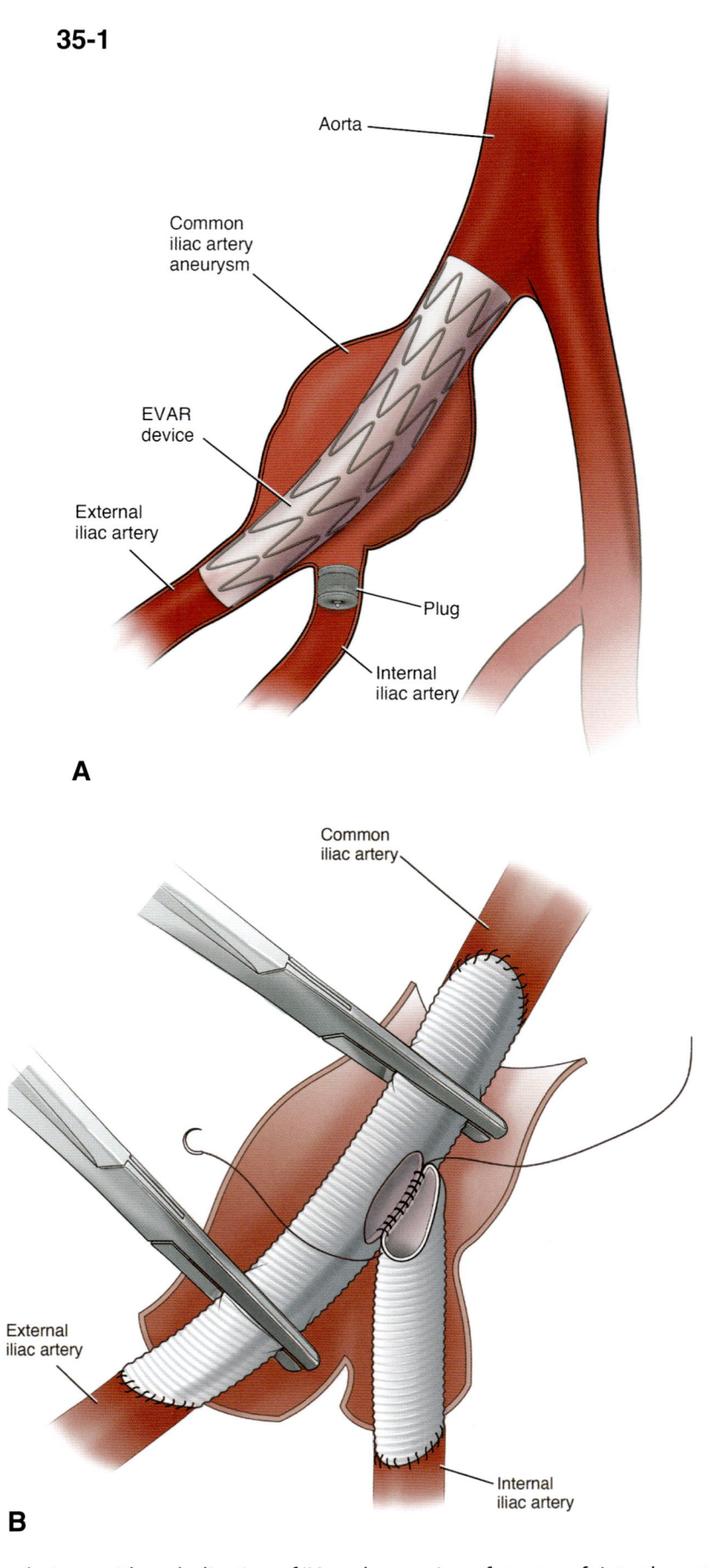

A

B

Figure 35-1 A. Coil and cover technique with embolization of IIA and extension of stent graft into the external iliac artery for exclusion of common iliac artery aneurysm. B. Open repair of common iliac artery aneurysm with bypass to the IIA.

INTRODUCTION `CONTINUED` Five configurations of iliac branch devices are made by three different manufacturers, but only one is commercially available in the United States. Cook has the straight, helical, and bi-branch (bif-bif) design (FIGURE 35-2A–D), Gore developed IBE (FIGURE 35-2E) with a separate internal iliac component, and the Jotec E-iliac system (FIGURE 35-2F) consists of a bifurcated graft including a main iliac limb with an additional reinforced stump for the IIA side branch. Gore is currently the only commercially available device in United States, and this chapter will focus on the technical conduct of its implantation.

PREOPERATIVE PREPARATION Computed tomographic angiogram (CTA) with 3-dimensional multiplanar reconstructions (MPRs) is used to create centerline of flow for obtaining precise measurements, which is a gateway key to determine anatomic feasibility of IBE use. Identification of factors that can constitute challenges or compromise repair is a critical step during preoperative assessment. Inadequate distal landing zone such as iliac tortuosity, calcifications, or stenosis affect the ability to introduce large-diameter sheaths and may predispose stent grafts to kinks or occlusion. Characteristics of landing zone within the IIA, such as aneurysmal involvement or poor runoff because of distal branch vessel disease, represent limitations to any technique of pelvic revascularization, open or endovascular.

Certain anatomic criteria need to be met prior to proceeding with IBE (FIGURE 35-3). The Gore IBE device Instructions for Use (IFU) requires the following anatomic criteria:

- Minimum lowest renal artery to IIA distance ≥165 mm in order to accommodate the main excluder device, IBE and all its components. One may still be able to use IBE if the length is shorter than 165 mm, but would require raising the bifurcation.

- Minimum CIA diameter of ≥17 mm at proximal implantation zone.
- Minimal diameter at iliac bifurcation should be ≥14 mm.
- External iliac artery diameter of 6.5 to 25 mm with at least 10-mm seal zone length.
- Internal iliac artery diameter of 6.5 to 13.5 mm with at least 10-mm seal zone length.
- Adequate anatomy to receive an EVAR stent graft.

  Ancillary tools needed:
- 12Fr, 45-cm DrySeal Flex Sheath and 16 to 20Fr, 33-cm DrySeal Sheath
- 0.038″ snare
- Catheters
  - KMP
  - VS1/SOS
  - Cobra (C2)
  - Angled glide catheter
  - VanSchie
  - Marker pigtail or Omniflush catheter
- Wires
  - 0.035″ 260-cm Glidewire
  - 0.035″ 260-cm Lunderquist
  - 0.035″ 480-cm Metro wire
  - 0.035″ 1-cm tip Amplatz wire
- 14 × 2 cm angioplasty balloon
- Gore MOB balloon, or Reliant (Medtronic, Santa Rosa, CA), or CODA (Cook Inc, Bloomington, IN)
- Advanced imaging system in a dedicated hybrid room or angiographic suite `CONTINUES`

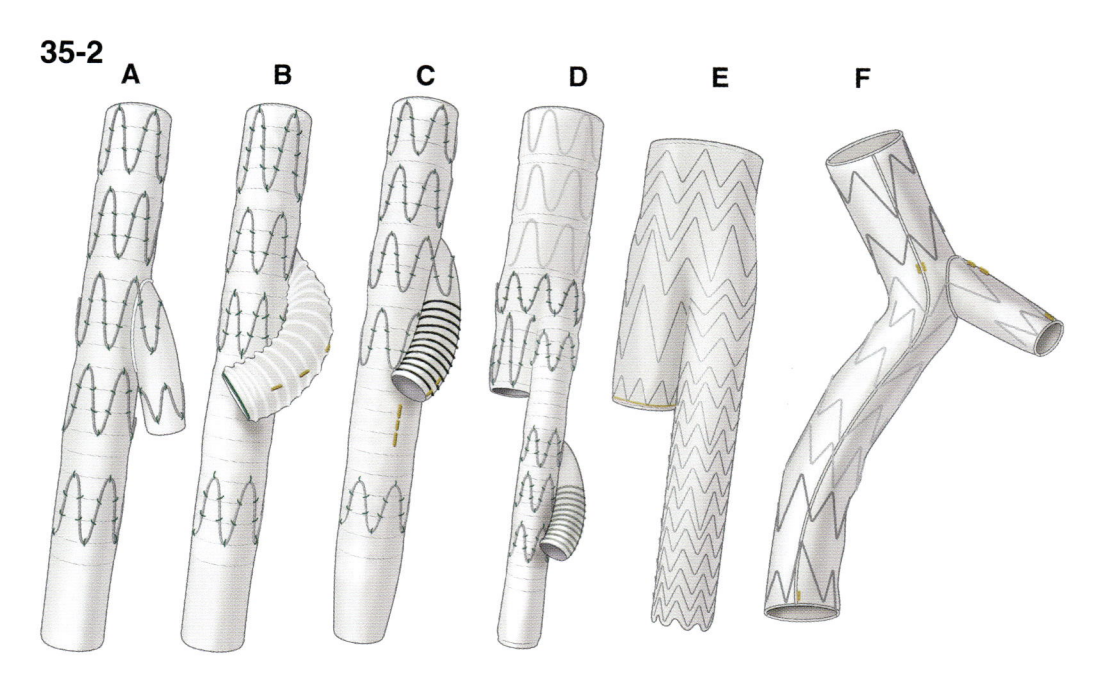

Figure 35-2 Five configurations of iliac branch devices including Cook straight (A), helical (B, C) and bi-branch design (D), Gore iliac branch endoprosthesis (IBE) (E) and Jotec E-iliac system (F).

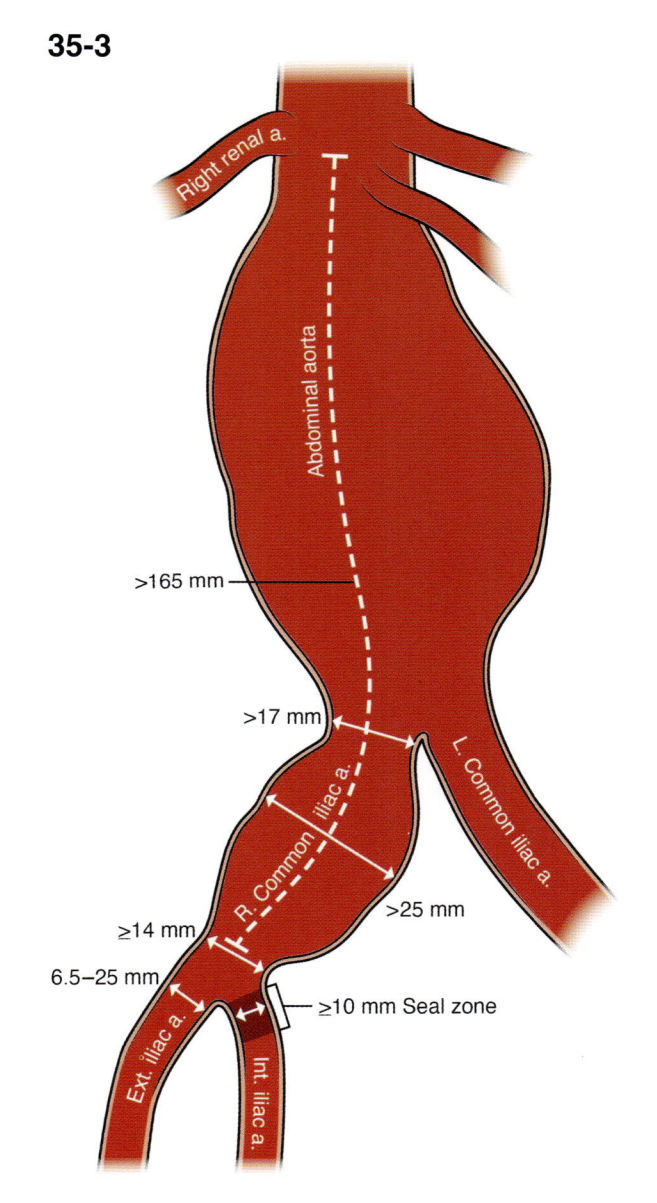

Figure 35-3 Anatomic criteria for suitability for Gore IBE device.

ANESTHESIA Preoperative anesthesia evaluation is commonly performed to prepare the patient for the procedure, including obtaining cardiac evaluation, basic labs including renal function assessment, and arrangement for perioperative hydration if deemed necessary. The procedure is most commonly performed under general anesthesia for the comfort of the patient and to limit their intraoperative mobility and therefore optimize the ability of the surgeon to utilize CT fusion and minimize contrast and radiation use. Alternatively, it can be performed under conscious sedation with close monitoring in appropriately selected cooperative patients. Large bore IV access and arterial line blood pressure monitoring, along with a Foley catheter are placed.

POSITION The patient is positioned supine on the operating table, and arms are tucked to the side or occasionally left out or raised above the head (if possible). The patient is prepped and draped in a sterile fashion from nipple to knees to have an adequately prepped field in case of an adverse event that could require conversion to open. The imaging gantry should be positioned from the head (least radiation) or from the left side while the surgeon, the first assist, and the scrub technician are positioned on the patient's right side (FIGURE 35-4). CONTINUES ▶

35-4

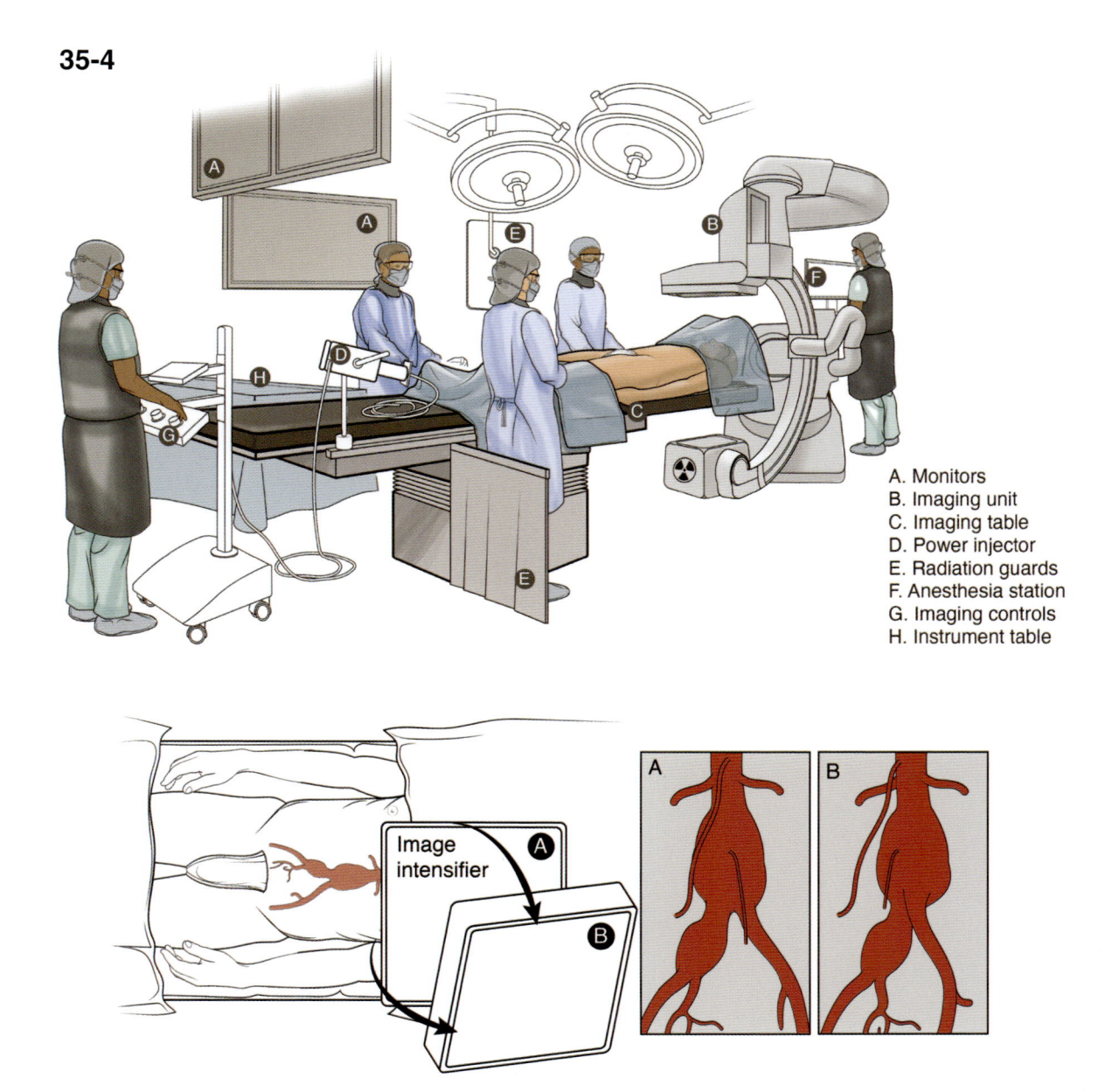

A. Monitors
B. Imaging unit
C. Imaging table
D. Power injector
E. Radiation guards
F. Anesthesia station
G. Imaging controls
H. Instrument table

Figure 35-4 Positioning of the patient, surgeons, and imaging unit.

PROCEDURE DETAILS Bilateral transfemoral access is obtained under ultrasound guidance using a 0.018″ micro-puncture set. A Glidewire is introduced into the aorta from bilateral access sites followed by use of pre-closure technique for placement of Perclose Proglide sutures, typically positioned at 2- and 10-clock positions (see Chapter 5). Short 8Fr sheaths are positioned at femoral access sites. The Glidewire is exchanged for a 0.035″ super-stiff wire such as Lunderquist, followed by upsizing the sheath to on the ipsilateral (IBE) side to a 16 or 18Fr Gore Dryseal sheath and a 12Fr Gore Dryseal Flex sheath on the contralateral side. Once the sheaths are in place, a snare is placed in the contralateral limb, which allows passing an ipsilateral 0.035″ Glidewire through the snare. The snare grasps the ipsilateral wire, which is then brought up and over the aortic bifurcation and out the contralateral femoral sheath (FIGURE 35-5A). This up-and-over wire is then loaded onto the removable guidewire tube on the ipsilateral IBE device, thereby pre-cannulating the internal iliac gate (FIGURE 35-5B, C).

CONTINUES ▶

35-5

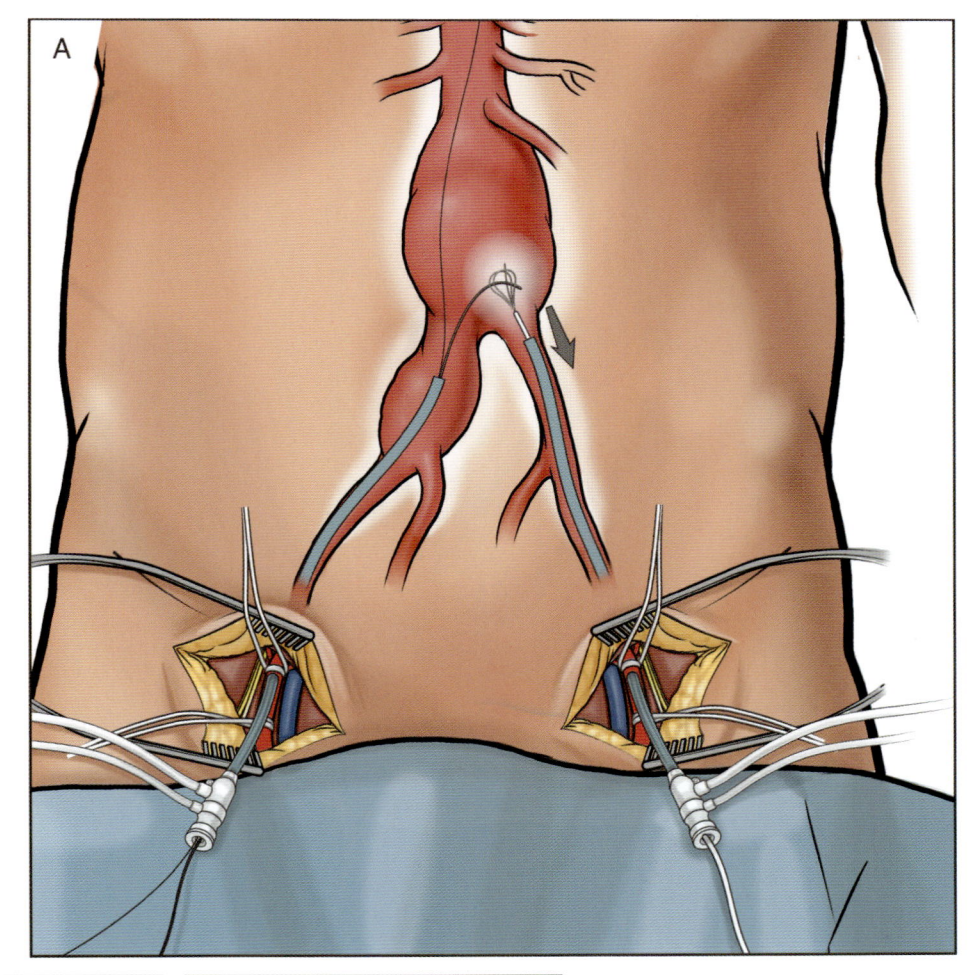

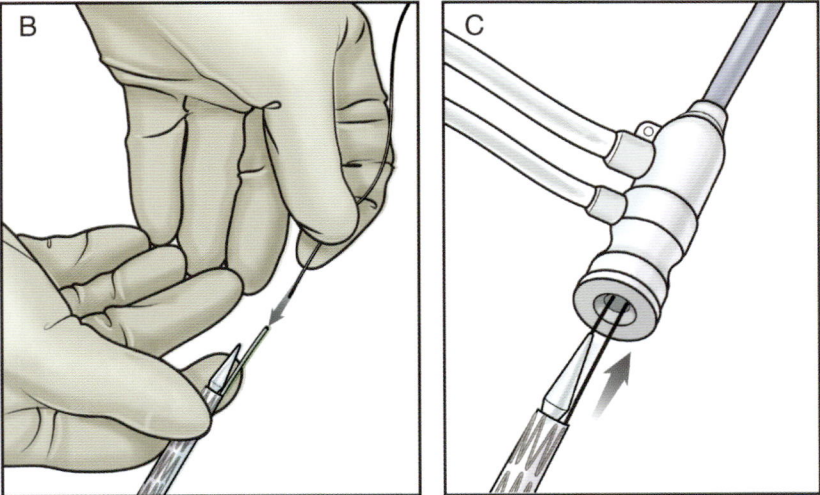

Figure 35-5 A, B. Gore IBE design to allow for precannulation of the up-and-over through-and-through guidewire via the guidewire tube.

PROCEDURE DETAILS ◄ CONTINUED The IBE device is then advanced over the main wire with the contralateral preload gate through the ipsilateral large sheath into the aorta and pulled back in position to take the slack out of the contralateral wire (FIGURE 35-5C). In doing so, both ends of the up-and-over wire should be kept taut, a key gateway to the procedure. Another key is to visualize and assure that the radio-opaque markers of the internal iliac limb are aligned to position it approximately 1 to 1.5 cm proximal to the ostium of the IIA. The IBD sheath is then withdrawn to partially deploy the device until the IIA gate opens (FIGURE 35-6). The contralateral 12Fr sheath is advanced over the bifurcation and into the internal iliac gate while maintaining tension on the through-and-through wires. Use the push-and-pull maneuver to allow the sheath to sit over the bifurcation, as shown in FIGURE 35-7. It is important to avoid wire wrap to facilitate smooth advancement the contralateral sheath up and over into the IIA gate. Additionally, the up-and-over wire should be exchanged for a 0.035″ Rosen wire or even Amplatz wire, which are stiffer and improve trackability for the large sheath. CONTINUES ►

35-6

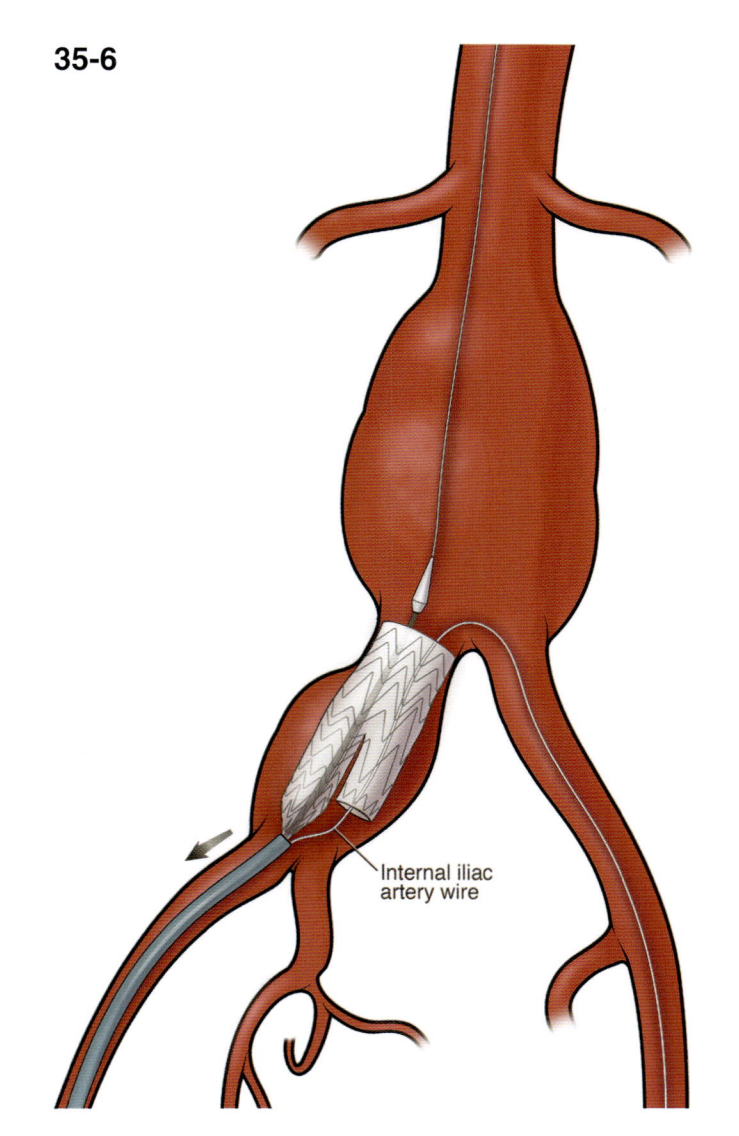

Figure 35-6 The contralateral 12Fr sheath is advanced over the bifurcation and into the internal iliac gate.

35-7

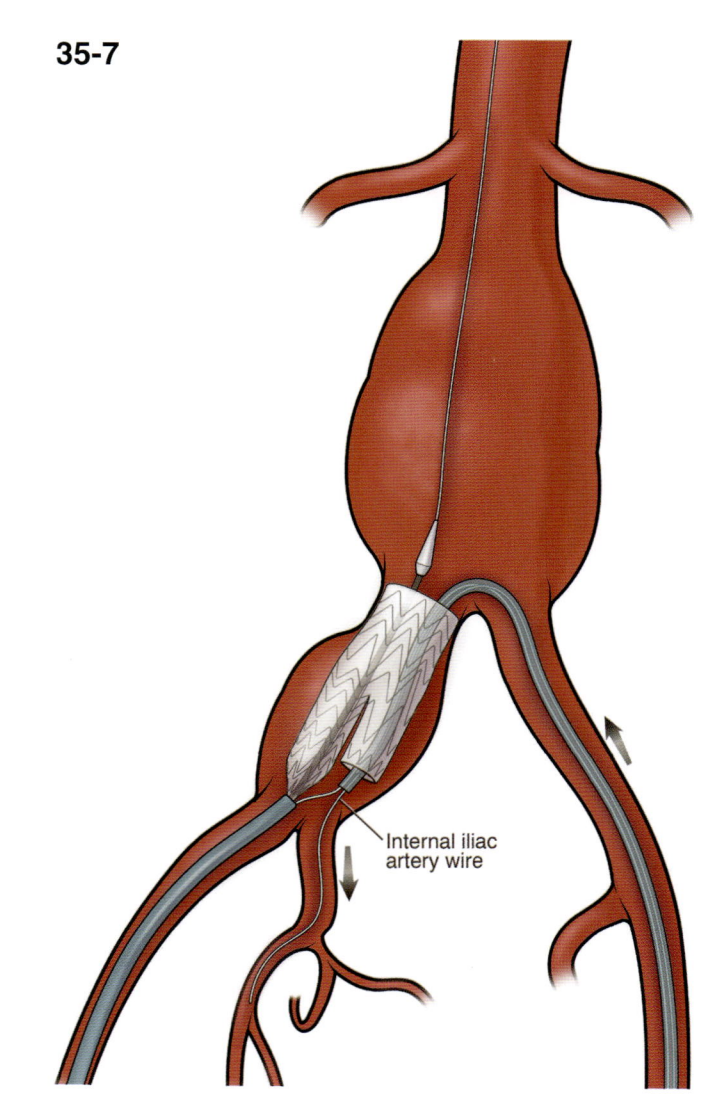

Figure 35-7 An 8Fr sheath is advanced through the 12Fr sheath over a buddy wire, which is used to catheterize the IIA.

PROCEDURE DETAILS `CONTINUED` It is very helpful to next obtain angiographic confirmation of device positioning above the iliac bifurcation. Next, optimize the C-arm angle to visualize the IIA orifice (usually angled opposite the side you are treating). An 8Fr sheath is advanced through the 12Fr sheath over a buddy wire which is used to catheterize the IIA.

Once the IIA is cannulated, a 0.035″ Glidewire is then passed into the IAA and is hubbed into the deepest branch to maximize wire purchase, while exercising caution to not perforate or dissect any outflow branches (FIGURE 35-8A). The Glidewire is then exchanged under the protection of the KMP catheter for a stiffer wire, such as the short (1 cm)-tipped Amplatz wire. Internal iliac stent graft is then advanced into the IIA through the 8Fr sheath, positioned at the intended landing zone and deployed. To ensure

adequate overlap, the short radio-opaque marker of the ipsilateral anatomic proximal end of the IIA stent graft should be directly aligned the the long radio opaque marker on the partially deployed iliac branch component (FIGURE 35-8B). If the IIA is stenotic, consider angioplasty prior to stent placement.

A 14-mm balloon is then used to reinforce the apposition of the IIA component to the iliac branch IIA gate proximal to the IIA. The distal end of the IIA stent graft should be ballooned with an appropriately sized balloon to ensure apposition of the stent graft to the IIA wall. The IBE deployment is completed with unsheathing the EIA stent graft. Kissing balloon angioplasty is then performed to ensure patency of both components (FIGURE 35-9). `CONTINUES`

35-8

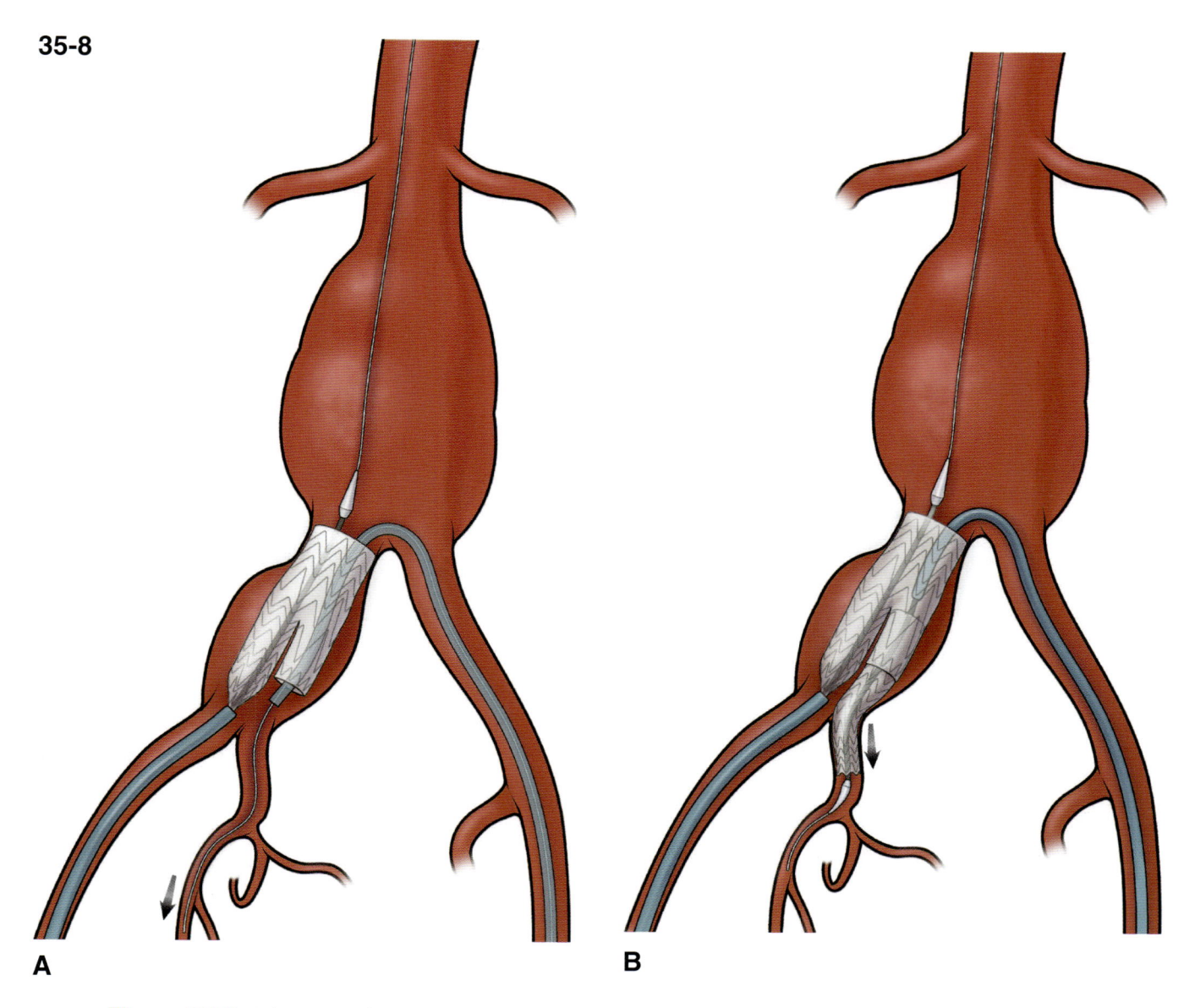

A   B

Figure 35-8 Selective catheterization of the IIA branch for deployment of the internal iliac component.

35-9

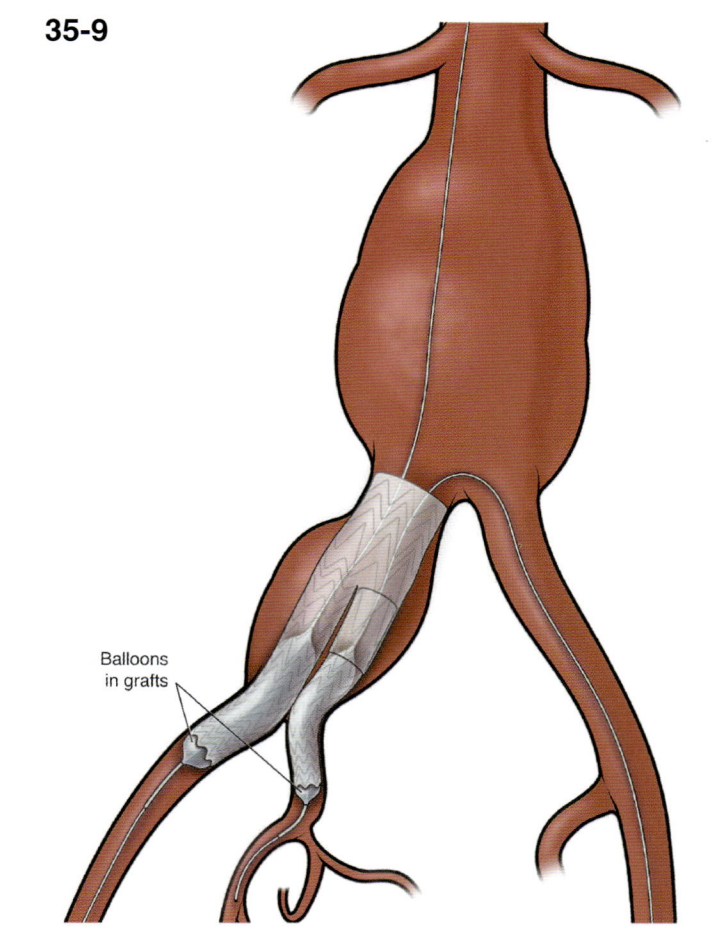

Balloons
in grafts

Figure 35-9 Kissing balloon angioplasty.

PROCEDURE DETAILS `CONTINUED` Once IBE deployment is complete, the EVAR device is then advanced over a Lunderquist wire to just caudal to the lowest renal artery and deployed. Steps of EVAR deployment have been detailed in Chapter 34. Once the main body is complete, advance and deploy the contralateral leg as bridging component (23- or 27-mm diameter) between the IBE and EVAR devices (**FIGURE 35-10**). A large molding balloon (Gore MOB, Medtronic Reliant, or Cook CODA) is then used to mold the stent graft to the aorta and iliac arteries, which assures excellent graft apposition to the aortic wall and/or other modular components of the graft system.

CHALLENGES AND ANATOMIC CONSTRAINTS

SHORT CIA: It is not uncommon to have anatomic constraints or challenges that need to be addressed. In the case of a short common iliac artery, data have shown that it is acceptable to land the proximal trunk of the IBE device above the aortic bifurcation without any sequelae. This will raise the bifurcation and will not impact technical success.

INTERNAL ILIAC ARTERY ANEURYSMS: In patients with IIA aneurysms where the distal landing zone of the internal iliac component is intended to be in the anterior or posterior division branch of the IIA, the safest strategy is to place the proximal stent within the main trunk and then extend the repair distally to avoid losing guidewire access into the target branch. A wide range of balloon expandable and self-expandable covered stents (BECS, SECS) can be deployed within the side branch. Alternatively, if there is a large-diameter discrepancy, one may deploy the distal stent first, and then bridge to the IBD. Other branches of the IIA are embolized prior to placing the stent graft in the anterior/posterior division of IIA to minimize risk of type II endoleaks (**FIGURE 35-11**). It is important to secure a wire in the designated outflow branch prior to losing all branches. When the repair is extended beyond the IIA bifurcation and more stents are necessary to bridge the longer distance to the distal landing zone, proximal SECS may be preferred to provide stability, while distal BECS may be selected to ensure flexibility.

BILATERAL COMMON ILIAC ARTERY ANEURYSMS: It is safe and feasible to do bilateral IBEs. In patients with bilateral CIA aneurysms, bilateral IBE devices can be deployed using an up-and-over technique, with caution to avoid dislodgement of the IBE components during sheath advancement, as that can lead to type III endoleaks. Alternatively, axillary/brachial access may be used for cannulation of the IIA gate and IIA stent graft deployment.

USE OF IBE WITH A PRIOR EVAR: A prior aortic endograft device can create a higher, acutely angled aortic bifurcation which can present a challenge to deployment of an IBE. The up-and-over technique with a flexible 12Fr sheath mated with a coaxial 8Fr sheath can provide a stable platform when used over a through-and-through wire. Alternatively, upper extremity (brachial/axillary) can be used. One may also consider using an ipsilateral single access approach. This approach has been used frequently by the authors in patients with prior FEVAR to prevent destabilization of the fenestrations or branches.

CLOSURE A completion angiogram is performed to confirm adequate stent graft placement and look for endoleaks, graft kinks, stenosis, or other technical concerns that may need immediate intervention. Intravascular ultrasound or a cone-beam CT may be used when indicated for final confirmation. Closure is performed by removal of wires, sheaths, and catheters, and Perclose sutures are cinched down to achieve hemostasis. In the case of standard open exposure, conventional transverse arteriotomy closure is done.

POSTOPERATIVE CARE Patients are usually extubated at the end of the procedure and then recovered in a post-anesthesia care unit for a brief period before being transferred to ward care where neurovascular checks should be performed at intervals. Most patients can be discharged after an overnight observation. A follow-up CTA scan is typically performed at 1 month to evaluate the repair, followed by routine surveillance at 6 and 12 months and annually thereafter. ■

SUGGESTED READINGS

Gore Bilateral IBE Study Group. *J Vasc Surg.* 2018 Jul;68(1):100-108.e3. doi: 10.1016/j.jvs.2017.12.043. Epub 2018 Mar 8.

Kalteis M, Gangl O, Huber F, Adelsgruber P, Kastner M, Lugmayr H. Clinical impact of hypogastric artery occlusion in endovascular aneurysm repair. *Vascular.* 2015;23(6):575-579.

Schneider D, Milner R, Heyligers JMM, Chakfe N, Matsumura J. Outcomes of the Gore Iliac Branch Endoprosthesis in clinical trial and real-world registry settings. *J Vasc Surg.* 2019:69(2);367-377.

Maldonado TS, Mosquera NJ, Lin P, Bellosta R, Barfield M, Moussa A, et al. Gore Iliac Branch Endoprosthesis for treatment of bilateral common iliac artery aneurysms. *J Vasc Surg.* 2018;68(1):100-108.e3.

Millon A, Della Schiava N, Arsicot M, De Lambert A, Feugier P, Magne JL, Lermusiaux P. Preliminary Experience with the GORE (®) EXCLUDER (®) Iliac Branch Endoprosthesis for Common Iliac Aneurysm Endovascular Treatment. *Ann Vasc Surg.* 2016 May;33:11-17. doi: 10.1016/j.avsg.2015.12.003. Epub 2016 Jan 22.

van Sterkenburg SM, Heyligers JM, van Bladel M, Verhagen HJ, Eefting D, van Sambeek MR, et al; Dutch IBE Collaboration. Experience with the GORE EXCLUDER Iliac Branch Endoprosthesis for common iliac artery aneurysms. *J Vasc Surg.* 2016 Jun;63(6):1451-1457. doi: 10.1016/j.jvs.2016.01.021

35-10

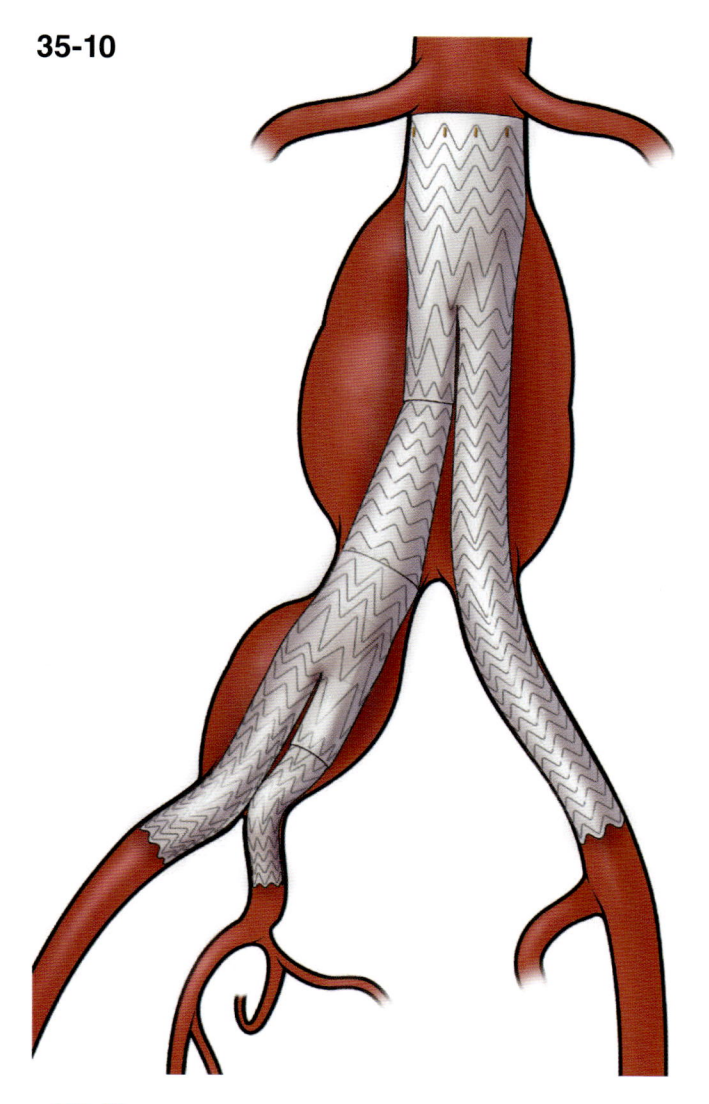

Figure 35-10 Advancement and deployment of the contralateral leg as bridging component between the IBE and EVAR devices.

35-11

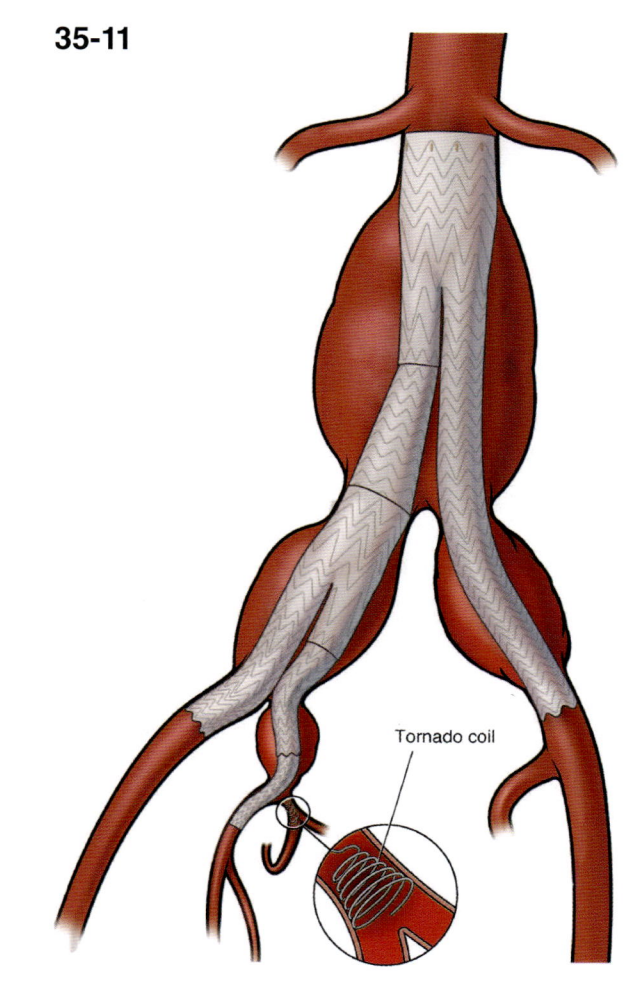

Figure 35-11 Selective catheterization of the designated IIA branch, usually the posterior division. Embolization of the IIA branches that are to be excluded.

EVAR FOR RUPTURE ANEURYSMS

Benjamin Starnes, MD

INDICATIONS The indications for treating a ruptured abdominal aortic aneurysm (AAA) are somewhat obvious to the layperson, as the mortality rate associated with this acute disease, if left untreated, approaches (but is not always) 100%. The intention of this emergent procedure is to prevent death and avoid major complications and/or a prolonged postoperative hospital course. Some authors have tried to implement risk scores (ex. Glasgow, Hardman index) that incorporate both preoperative and intraoperative variables. These risk scores are not helpful in that they all rely on the patient undergoing an operation. In 2007, the University of Washington implemented a strategy to manage all these patients with an endovascular-first strategy. If the patient was a candidate for endovascular aortic aneurysm repair (EVAR) based on preoperative computed tomography, they would undergo EVAR, with a preference for local anesthesia to start. If they were not a candidate, they would still have an aortic occlusion balloon placed prior to induction of general anesthesia and formal open repair, although this choice is operator dependent and in many cases it is not feasible. Our overall 30-day mortality rates using this approach dropped from 58% prior to the protocol to 35% after implementation. Furthermore, if the patient received EVAR as opposed to open repair, their 30-day mortality rate was only 18.5%, and others have had similar results.

POSITIONING Positioning for the endovascular repair of a ruptured abdominal aortic aneurysm (rEVAR) is critical, and use of a hybrid room has become standard at most institutions. If this is not available, a back-up strategy is to perform the rEVAR in any room using a portable C-arm. We perform all our rEVARs with the surgeons standing on the patient's right side and the imaging monitor to the patient's left (FIGURE 36-1). These patients are often very sick, and the anesthesia providers diligently work toward getting intravenous lines. As Stanley Crawford, MD, said, "the most important initial aspect of saving this patient's life is to get a clamp on the aorta (or in this instance an intra-aortic occlusion balloon)." This cannot happen until the patient is prepped and draped and the imaging equipment has been brought in from the patient's left side, or with some systems the head, if the imaging system reaches low enough. Therefore, the absolute very first step when placing the patient onto the imaging table is to determine where the image intensifier and source will come from, whether in a hybrid OR or any operating room with portable imaging. The left arm is tucked if the image intensifier comes from the left side, or it may be left extended out if concomitant visceral stenting is needed, as the left brachial may need to be accessed. The right arm can be extended out to the right side on an arm board for the anesthesia providers. A Foley is be placed if the patient is hemodynamically "stable," and the chest, abdomen, and both groins are widely prepped and draped. Even if intravenous lines and arterial lines for monitoring blood pressure have not yet been placed, the vascular surgeon should immediately scrub, as they can very efficiently place a femoral intravenous large bore sheath for rapid infusion and the sheath for the aortic occlusion balloon. The usual routine of checking and marking distal pedal pulses is a worthless exercise in this scenario in an unstable patient, and no time should be wasted on this. In addition, if radiolucent EKG wires and pads are not available, any lead or wire should be kept out of the imaging window.

OPERATIVE PREPARATION It is common at major academic centers for a patient to be diagnosed with a ruptured abdominal aortic aneurysm (rAAA) at an outside institution using cross-sectional CT imaging. These images are most often uploaded into a picture archive and communication system (PACS) or similar system prior to the patient arriving, and one can rapidly make measurements based on this imaging. The most important measurements are of the proximal aortic neck diameter and length, and the length from the lowest renal artery to the aortic bifurcation. This allows for selection of the main body bifurcated device. The other important measurement is diameter for access to the iliac arteries and evaluation for iliac artery calcification and tortuosity. The aortic occlusion balloon sheath is best placed from the least tortuous side if feasible. This is because it is easier to facilitate contralateral gate cannulation, which can often cause significant delay of case completion. Thus, when feasible the main-body device should be inserted from the most tortuous access side. Even patients who are not rEVAR candidates based on anatomy due to a low-lying "discrepant" renal artery can undergo successful endovascular repair using a physician-modified endograft and back-table placement of a single fenestration for the renal artery, or as more commonly done, chimney stent grafts. If the patient has a juxtarenal or thoracoabdominal aneurysm, plans can be considered for placement of an aortic occlusion balloon at the proper vertebral body level prior to induction of general anesthesia for a formal open repair, in this case at the T1L1 interspace. **CONTINUES ▶**

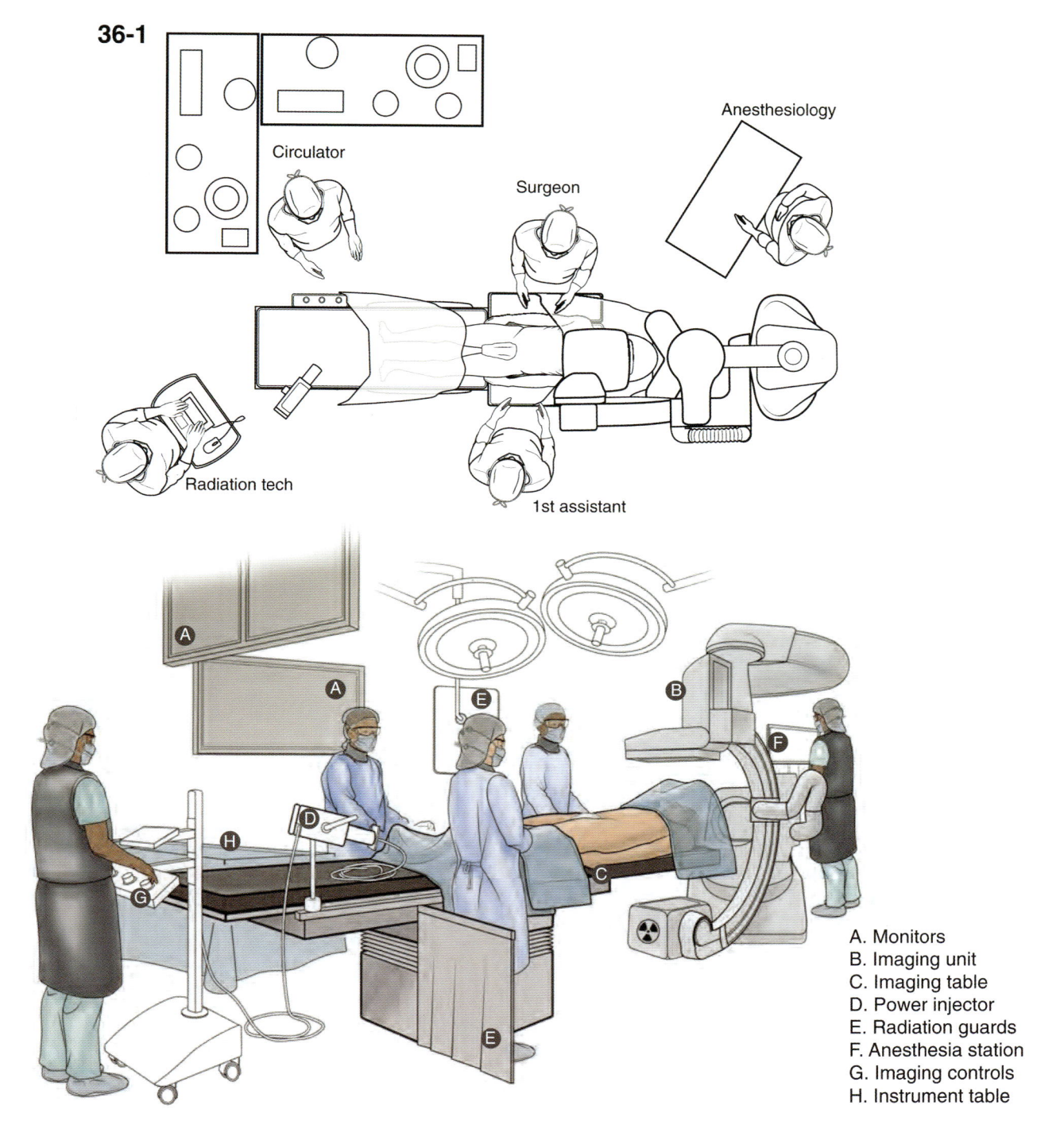

36-1

Circulator

Anesthesiology

Surgeon

Radiation tech

1st assistant

A. Monitors
B. Imaging unit
C. Imaging table
D. Power injector
E. Radiation guards
F. Anesthesia station
G. Imaging controls
H. Instrument table

Figure 36-1 Operating room setup for a rEVAR. Note the imaging equipment to the patient's left, with the left arm tucked. The operative team stands to the patient's right. A long three-sided sterile table with all catheters, guidewires, and devices resides behind the surgical team.

INCISION AND EXPOSURE B-mode ultrasound is used to gain percutaneous access to each common femoral artery, and placement of suture-mediated closure devices when the patient is hemodynamically stable. If they are hemodynamically unstable, straight percutaneous access using landmarks and palpation should be done, with the plan to cut down on the femoral arteries and repair them at the completion of the case. In some circumstances, it easier and faster to do a cutdown directly on the femoral artery (FIGURE 36-2A and B). CONTINUES

36-2

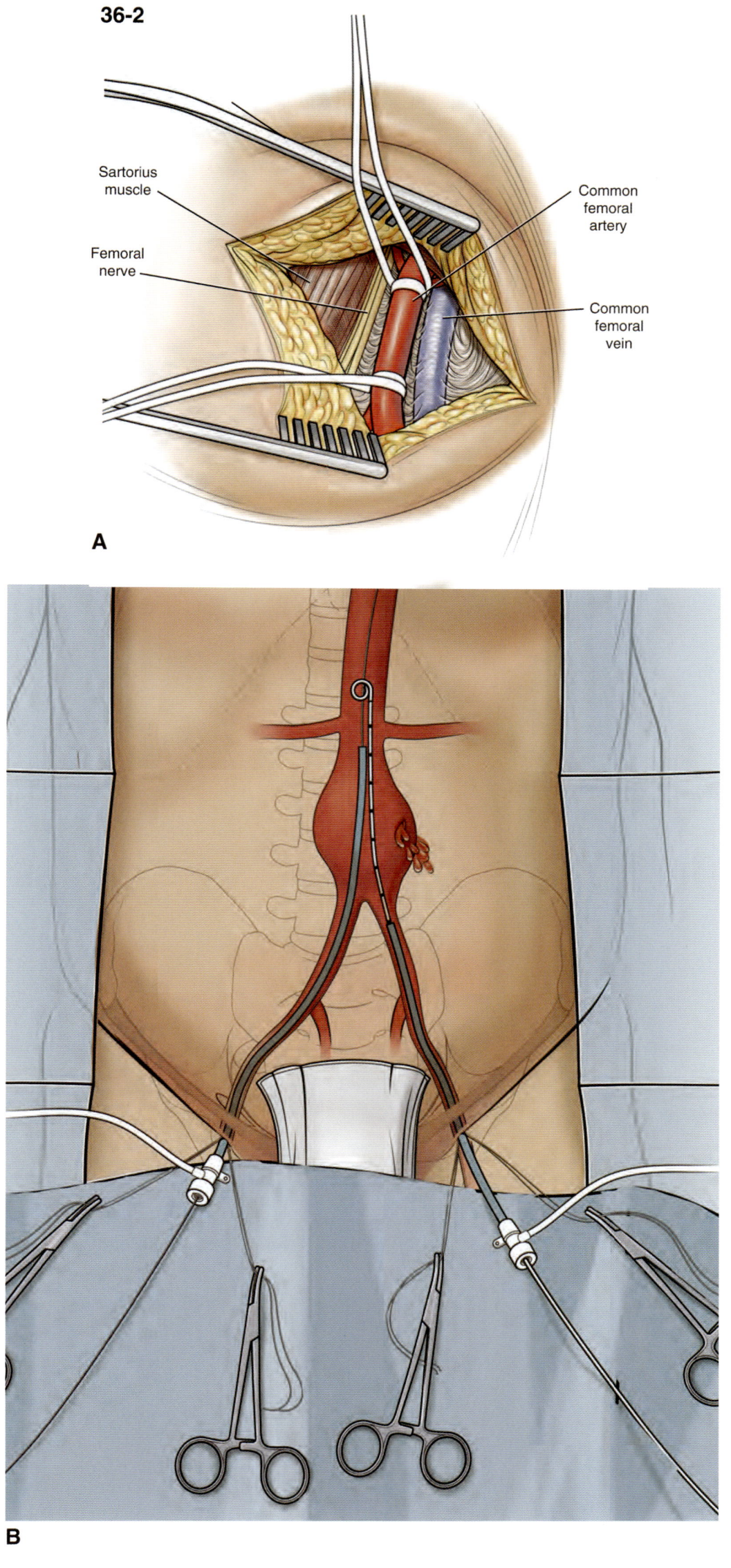

A

B

Figure 36-2 A. Transverse incision for open femoral artery exposure. B. Bilateral percutaneous access with placement of sheaths.

DETAILS OF THE PROCEDURE Most of these procedures can be performed just like any other standard EVAR, but there are some important differences. Once bilateral common femoral sheaths have been placed, it is important to place stiff 0.035″ wires to the level of the left subclavian artery on each side. One side is used to insert the main body of the EVAR device and the other side is used for the aortic occlusion balloon sheath (FIGURE 36-3A). In an unstable patient, it is important to place the aortic occlusion balloon first at the level of the 12th vertebral body on fluoroscopy. At minimum a 55 cm 12Fr sheath and CODA Balloon (Cook Incorporated; Bloomington, IN) or RELIANT Balloon (Medtronic Incorporated, Minneapolis, MN) works well for this purpose. The sheath should be kept adjacent to the occlusion balloon to serve as a buttress to prevent blood pressure from pushing the balloon down; this often requires an assistant to maintain firm superior pressure on the sheath (FIGURE 36-3B). CONTINUES ▶

36-3

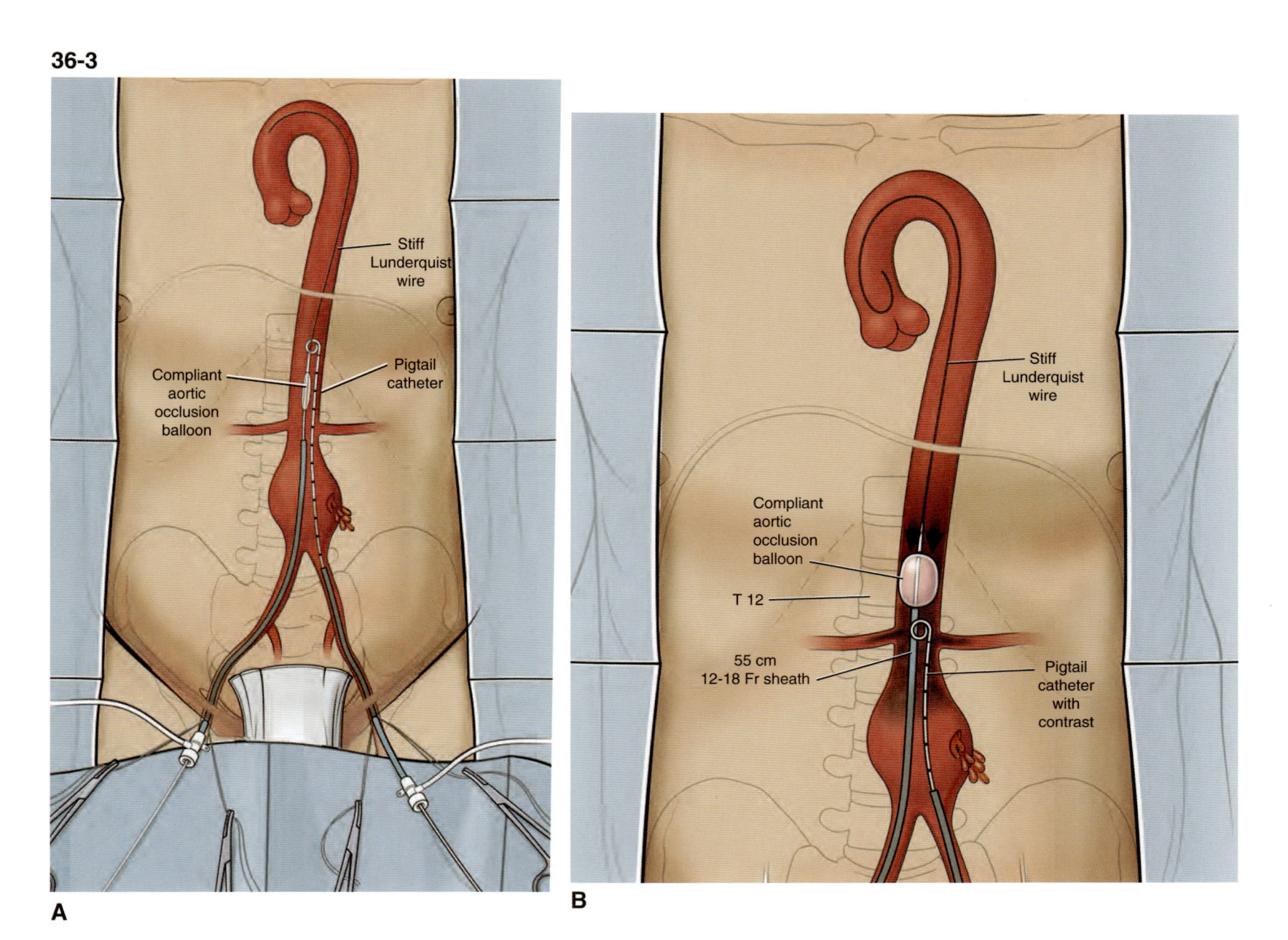

Figure 36-3 A. Placement of aortic occlusion balloon from the right and pigtail catheter from the left. B. Aortic occlusion balloon inflated at T12 and pigtail catheter immediately below.

DETAILS OF THE PROCEDURE CONTINUED The initial angiogram is easily done through the 12F sheath with the aortic occlusion balloon inflated and a hand injection of contrast to identify the lowest renal artery (FIGURE 36-4A). Occasionally, a patient will be "balloon dependent," meaning that every time the balloon is deflated, the blood pressure tanks. This can be remedied by using "tandem balloons." After marking the lowest renal artery, the initial aortic occlusion balloon can be partially deflated as the main body of the device is advanced past the balloon into position and fully deployed over the flexor sheath (FIGURE 36-4B). Using the wire of the main body device, a second balloon can then be advanced into the main body of the device and inflated while the initial balloon is removed through the flexor sheath (FIGURE 36-4 C, D). CONTINUES

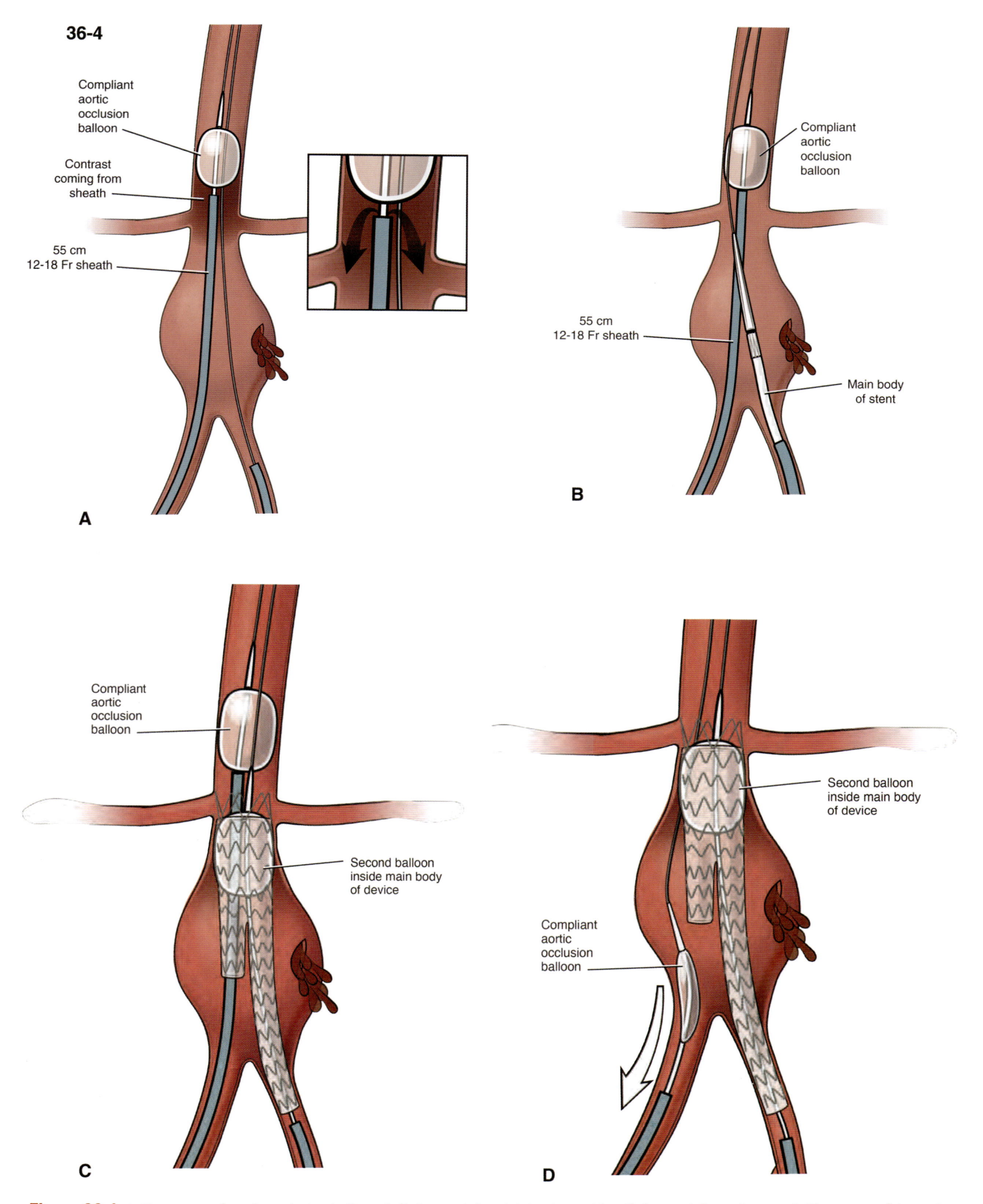

Figure 36-4 A. Placement of aortic occlusion balloon, inflation and sheath injection to identify lowest left renal artery. B. Placement of the main body EVAR device with balloon still inflated. C. "Tandem balloon" technique in an unstable patient. D. Withdrawal of initial balloon into flexor sheath along outside of the endograft.

DETAILS OF THE PROCEDURE ◄CONTINUED▶ In general, once the main body of the device has been deployed (FIGURE 36-5), even with the contralateral limb not yet implanted, this is the time when the patient appears to stabilize, and they may not require the aortic occlusion balloon any longer. The contralateral gate is then cannulated, and confirmation of entry is done with a pigtail catheter (FIGURE 36-6A). The contralateral limb is deployed above the hypogastric artery. It is imperative to preserve at least one hypogastric artery, as on occasion an iliac aneurysm may preclude placement of an extension limb in only the common iliac artery (FIGURE 36-6B). Once the remainder of the EVAR procedure is completed, it is important to rule out two things: a type 1A endoleak and development of abdominal compartment syndrome. Completion imaging must be performed in more than one view. We prefer intraoperative DYNA CT imaging but if using a portable C-arm, a 20-cc injection of 50/50 dilute contrast injected at 10 cc/sec in both a 30-degree LAO and RAO projection of the proximal aortic neck should suffice. Magnified views of the proximal and distal landing zones are important for completion angiograms. ◄CONTINUES▶

36-5

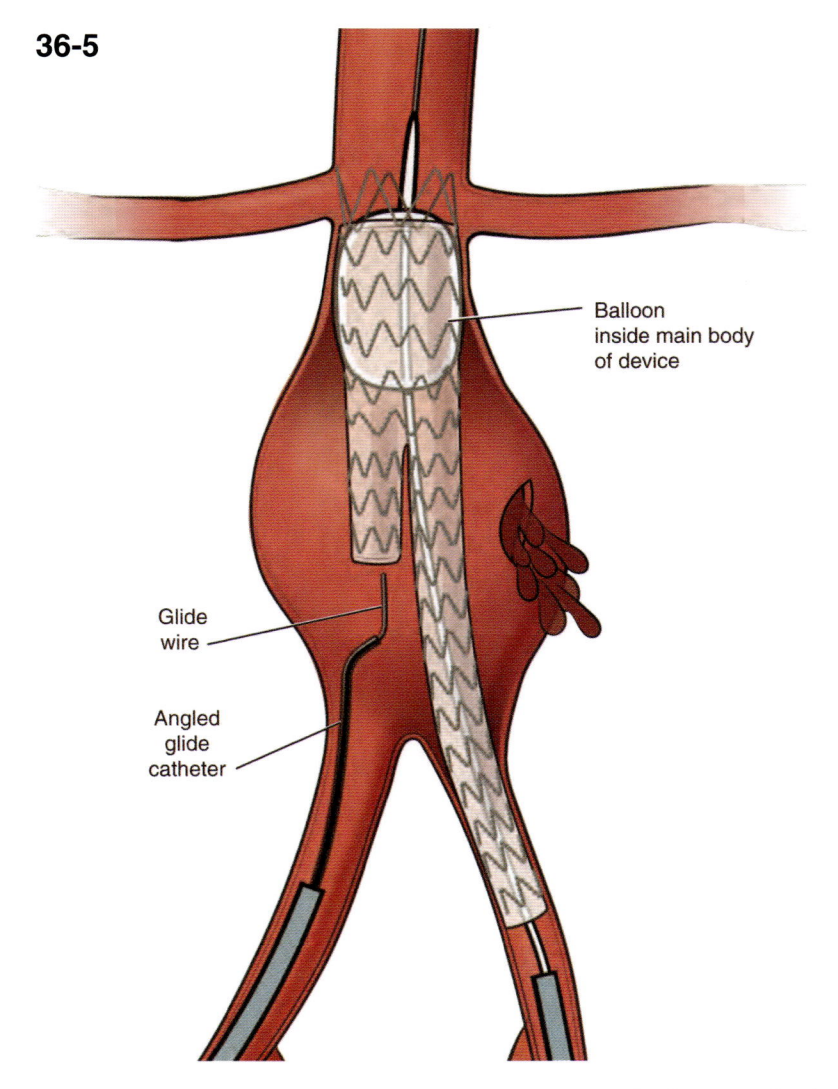

Figure 36-5 Aortic occlusion balloon inflated in proximal endograft after main body deployment.

36-6

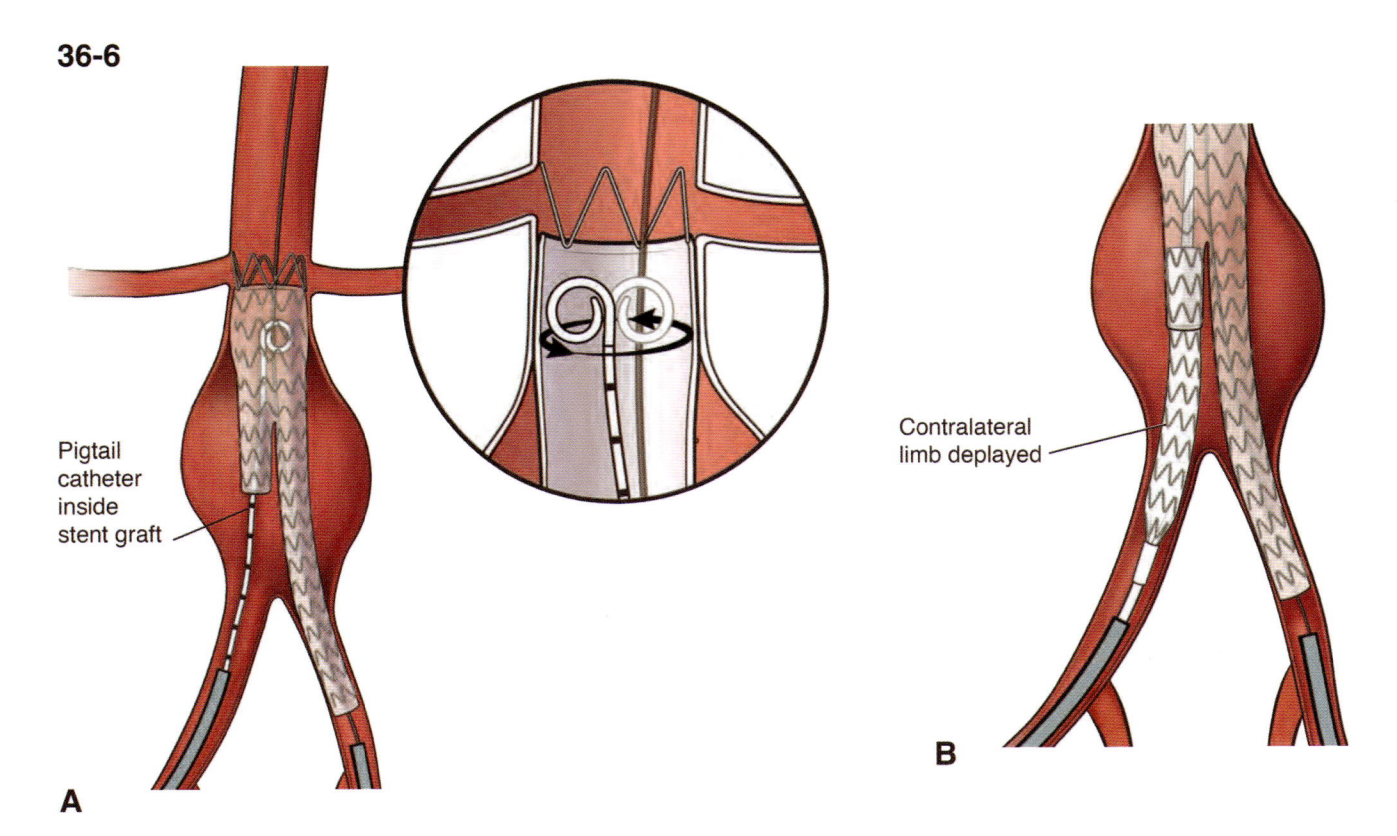

Figure 36-6 A. Pigtail catheter spinning in the main body of the proximal endograft after cannulatiion of the contralateral limb. This confirms you are not outside of the limb. B. Deployment of contralateral limb above the hypogastric artery.

DETAILS OF THE PROCEDURE `CONTINUED` Increased peak airway pressures and a firm, tense abdomen signifies abdominal compartment syndrome. There should be a low threshold for performing decompressive laparotomy in this setting. A midline incision is made, the abdomen entered, the bowel eviscerated, and all the blood evacuated. The retroperitoneum should not be entered in any way. Simply evacuating the blood, counting and placing dry laparotomy sponges along the peritoneal gutters and in the pelvis, and placing a temporary vacuum-assisted dressing is quick and will allow for rapid transport of the patient to the intensive care unit for further resuscitation (FIGURE 36-7). The abdomen can be closed 1 to 3 days later in an elective setting.

CLOSURE If the luxury of hemodynamic stability has allowed you to place suture-mediated closure devices at the onset of the procedure, these may be used to close the arteriotomies and then place dressings on each femoral wound. If no suture-mediated devices were used, oblique femoral cutdown incisions can be made with the sheaths left indwelling to allow for standard exposure of the common femoral arteries and direct arterial repair. We recommend using interrupted 5-0 Prolene sutures followed by closure of each wound in several layers with absorbable deep-dermal interrupted sutures and skin staples or subcuticular stitch.

POSTOPERATIVE CARE Contrary to popular belief, these patients that undergo rEVAR can be just as sick as those undergoing formal open repair and require ongoing resuscitation. In an intubated patient, pulse-pressure variability is the best method for resuscitating a patient with intravenous fluids and blood products. Serial laboratory measurements to include chemistries, coagulation profile, and serum lactate levels should all be checked every 2 to 4 hours and aggressively corrected as needed. Ischemic colitis still occurs in rEVAR patients, albeit with a much lower incidence than with open repair, and should be suspected if hematochezia occurs or the lactate fails to clear. ■

SUGGESTED READINGS

Desikan SK, Singh N, Steele SR, et al. The incidence of ischemic colitis after repair of ruptured abdominal aortic aneurysms is decreasing in the endovascular era. *Ann Vasc Surg.* 2018;47:247-252.

Sarac, TP, Bannazadeh M, Flynn A, et al. Comparative predictors of mortality for endovascular and open repair of ruptured abdominal aortic aneurysms. *Ann Vasc Surg.* 2011;25(4):461-468.

Schermerhorn ML, Buck DB, O'Malley AJ, et al. Long-term outcomes of abdominal aortic aneurysm in the medicare population. *N Engl J Med.* 2015;373:328-338.

Starnes BW, Quiroga E, Hutter C, et al. Management of ruptured abdominal aortic aneurysm in the endovascular era. *J Vasc Surg.* 2010 Jan;51:9-18.

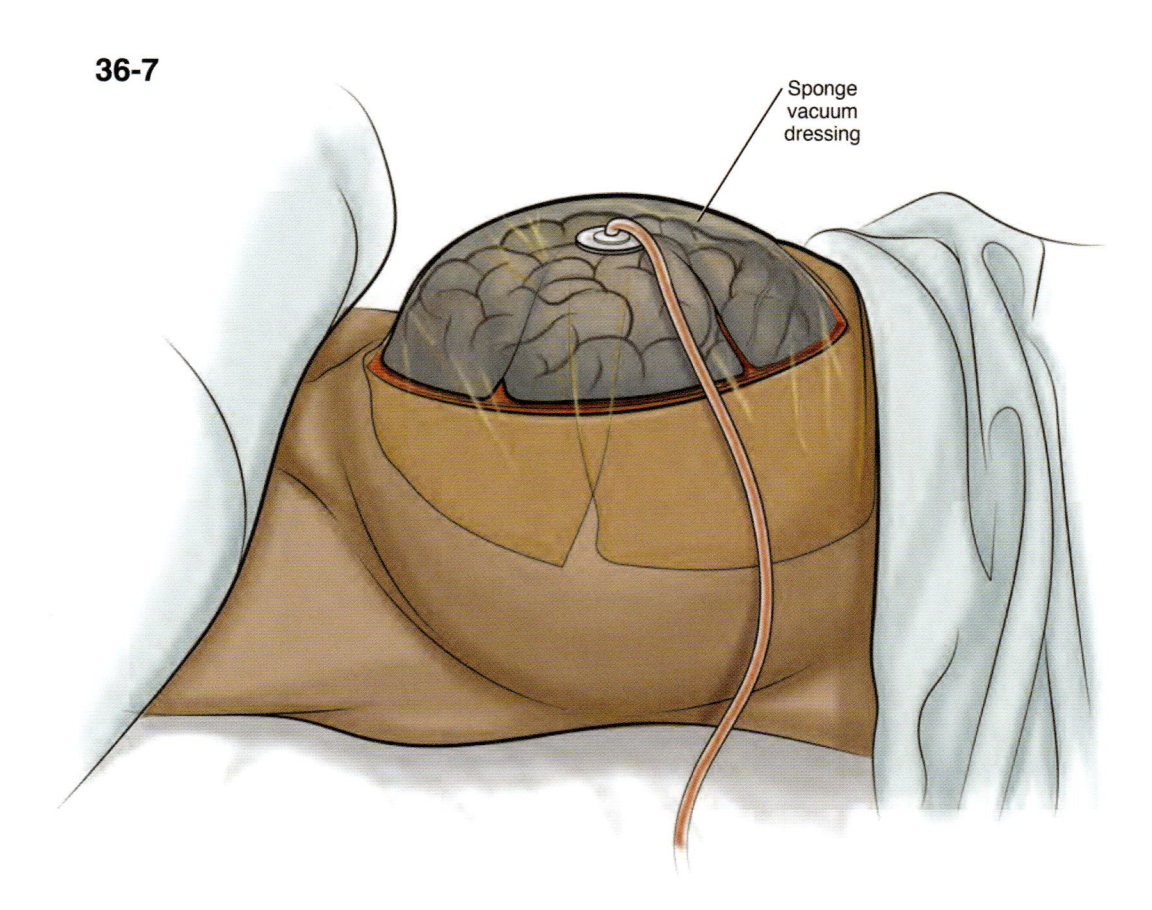

36-7

Sponge
vacuum
dressing

Figure 36-7 rEVAR patient with an abdominal compartment syndrome after decompressive laparotomy and temporary vacuum-assisted
dressing.

Section VIII
Thoracic Aorta-Open

EXTENT II AND III THORACOABDOMINAL AORTIC ANEURYSM OPEN REPAIR

Christopher McQuinn, MD • John Bozinovski, MD, MSc

INDICATIONS Repair of thoracoabdominal aortic aneurysm (TAAA) is a technically challenging intervention that is physiologically stressful on the patient. The benchmark outcomes from the center with the greatest volume of cases finds a morality rate in elective cases of 6% and paralysis or paraplegia risk of 5%. TAAAs are classified by the extent of their involvement. Extent II aneurysms involve the proximal descending thoracic aorta (DTA) (above the level of the 6th thoracic vertebrae [T6]) to below the renal arteries, while extents III involve the DTA below T6 and proceed into the abdomen. The most common etiology for TAAA is degenerative. These patients more commonly have advanced pulmonary, renal, and cardiovascular comorbidities increasing their perioperative risk. Aneurysms can also be secondary to heritable aortopathy. Repair in these patients can be difficult due to friability of the tissue. Other causes include dissection, trauma, vasculitis and mycotic etiologies. The size at which repair is recommended is 6 cm due to the risk of rupture. Patient age, comorbidities, presence of aortic dissection, occlusive disease or aneurysms of the branch vessels, patient values and preferences, and alternative interventions should be factored into the decision of when to operate.

POSITION On a table that allows for anteflexion at the waist between the anterior superior iliac spine and the 12th rib, the patient is positioned in right lateral decubitus position on a vacuum-assisted bean bag with optional padding under the right axilla and along each bony landmark. The shoulders are angled 30°, and the pelvis 60° from vertical allowing for access to the left and right femoral vessels. The right hip is flexed 30° and the knee 90°, and the leg padded before the extended left leg is rested upon it. This also allows for checking pulses at the completion before moving the patient (**FIGURE 37-1**). The left arm is extended anteriorly and the patient is secured to the bed and padded. The cerebrospinal fluid (CSF) drainage catheter must be secured to the patient outside of the operative field. Defibrillator pads are placed over the sternum, and superiorly on the back to capture the heart between them.

OPERATIVE PREPARATION CSF drains are generally placed the day prior to surgery. An arterial line is placed in the right radial artery. Central venous access to allow for rapid infusion of shed/washed blood is required along with consideration for a pulmonary artery catheter. A double lumen endotracheal tube or a single lumen tube with an endobronchial blocker is placed and its position confirmed after repositioning in the right lateral decubitus position. Transesophageal echocardiography (TEE) is usually used. Moderate systemic hypothermia (31–34°C) for a clampable proximal aorta, and deep hypothermia for an unclampable proximal aorta, is used to prolong end-organ ischemic tolerance. Bypass circuits are discussed below, but a separate circuit to allow for warm or cold renal perfusion via 9 Fr perfusion catheters is also utilized.

INCISION AND EXPOSURE The surgeon operates from the left side of the operative table with the first assistant on the right side and a second assistant moving into position as needed. The incision starts below the level of the umbilicus, parallel and displaced left lateral to midline, and travels obliquely in a curvilinear manner across the costal margin. It continues along the desired rib interspace, typically the 6th for extent II aneurysms and 7th or 8th for extents III, ending in a superiorly directed curve between the inferior lateral margin of the left scapula and vertebral prominence, if needed for extents II (**FIGURE 37-2A** and **B**). The anterior portion of the latissimus overlying the inferior border of the scapula is incised as is the serratus over the rib inferior to the scapula. The plane between the scapula and ribs is developed with the surgeon's right hand. This blunt dissection is taken in a posterior direction superiorly to the first rib, identified by its flat surface. The index finger is then flexed, hooking the posterior scalene insertion onto the 2nd rib, allowing one to count down the ribs to the desired interspace. The left lung is deflated and the intercostal muscle is separated from the inferior rib and taken down with cautery posteriorly and anteriorly, coming across the costal margin. The distal left internal mammary artery posterior to the cartilage is doubly clipped and transected. **CONTINUES ▶**

37-1

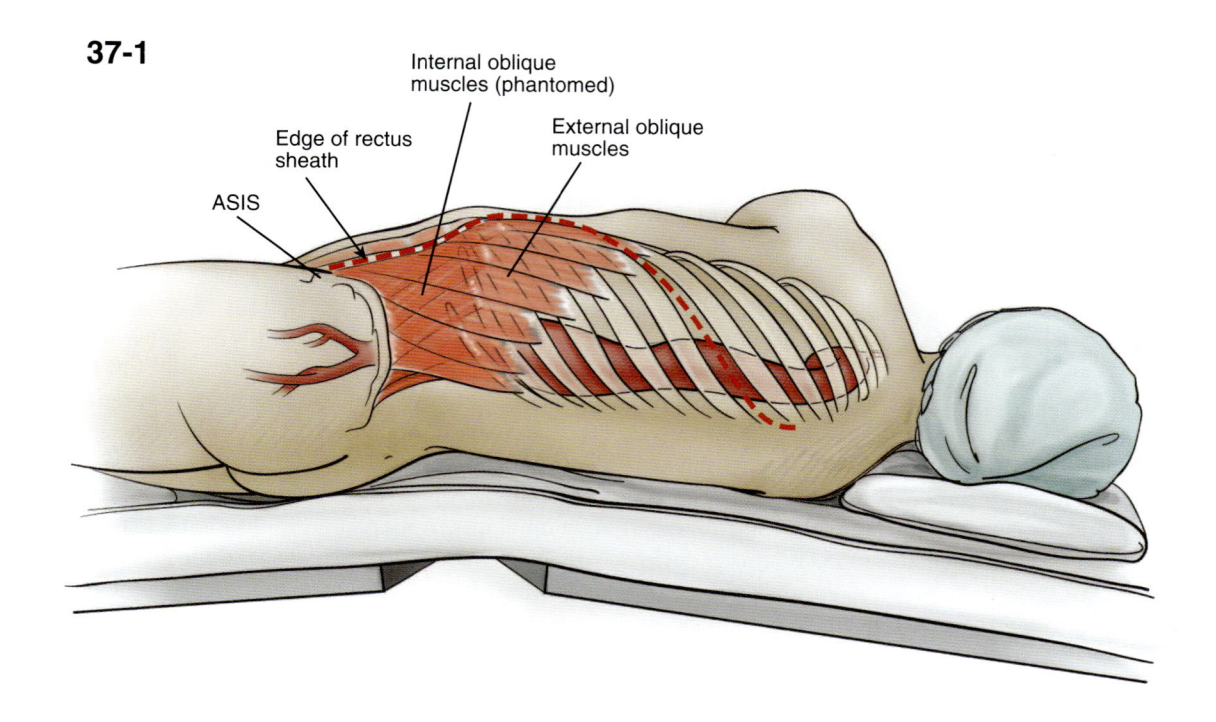

37-2

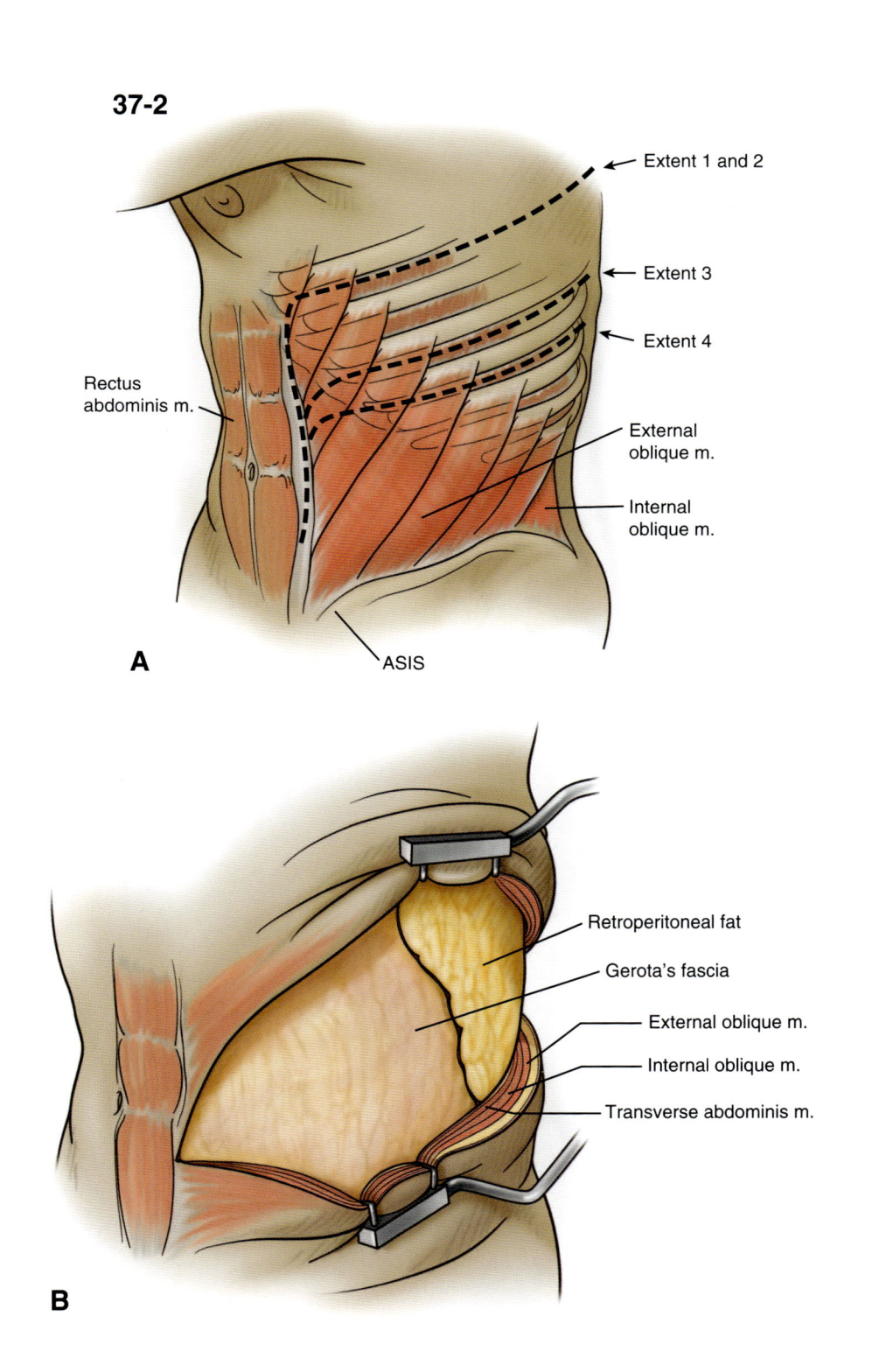

INCISION AND EXPOSURE CONTINUED We prefer to avoid taking this incision into the peritoneum and do a complete retroperitoneal dissection starting the plane at the costal margin, and bluntly develop this plane posteriorly over the psoas muscle, anterior to the aorta, and along the inferior side of the left hemidiaphragm. Preference is given to sparing the diaphragm, but if needed a partial incision laterally displaced from the tendinous portion of the diaphragm is made leaving a generous rim attached to the chest wall to allow for a tension-free repair. If the diaphragm is divided, we use a GIA stapler, which allows easy identification of margins at the time of closure, and a buttressed repair. An Omni or ringed retractor is then secured to the bed to retract the peritoneal cavity anteriorly, the rib superiorly, and the flank posteriorly (FIGURE 37-3). It is sometimes helpful to resect a rib to facilitate exposure.

Proximal exposure of the aorta depends on the proximal aortic clamp placement. For extent II aneurysms, determine whether the aorta can be clamped to fashion the anastomosis. If it cannot be clamped because of size, adhesions, infection, or preference for an open anastomosis, a path down hypothermic circulatory arrest (HCA) is then followed. For the vast majority of time it can be clamped, but often the clamp needs to be applied in zone 2 between the left common carotid artery (LCCA) and left subclavian artery (LSCA). Placing the patient in a head-down position rotated to the right facilitates this part of the dissection. The pleural adventitia overlying the aortic arch can be developed to allow retracting the phrenic and vagus nerves anteriorly, or develop the space between them and separate them avoiding their injury. The recurrent laryngeal nerve lying posterior to the ligamentum arteriosum is also spared by identifying and avoiding it during aortic clamping (FIGURE 37-4). Dividing the ligamentum facilitates more complete aortic arch exposure. The superior intercostal vein crosses the arch here and it is ligated. The LSCA is encircled with an umbilical tape, again taking care to avoid the vagus nerve running along the anterior surface. To expose the LSCA, the surgeon's left hand over a sponge, with controlled force, can compress medially the proximal aneurysmal DTA, bringing the LSCA into view. Placing the right index finger between the LCCA and LSCA and the thumb along the lesser curvature to encircle the arch, it is bluntly dissected on the posteromedial side, completing the arch dissection. A practice passage of a non-applied clamp is made to satisfy clamp-ability. If a decision to do an open anastomosis is made, this arch dissection can be avoided, or abandoned if too difficult. For those extents II that allow for a clamp distal to the LSCA, the nerves need to be addressed as above but the arch and LSCA encirclement and ligamentum ligation are unnecessary. For extents III where the proximal clamp will be much lower in the chest, all of this not applicable. CONTINUES

37-3

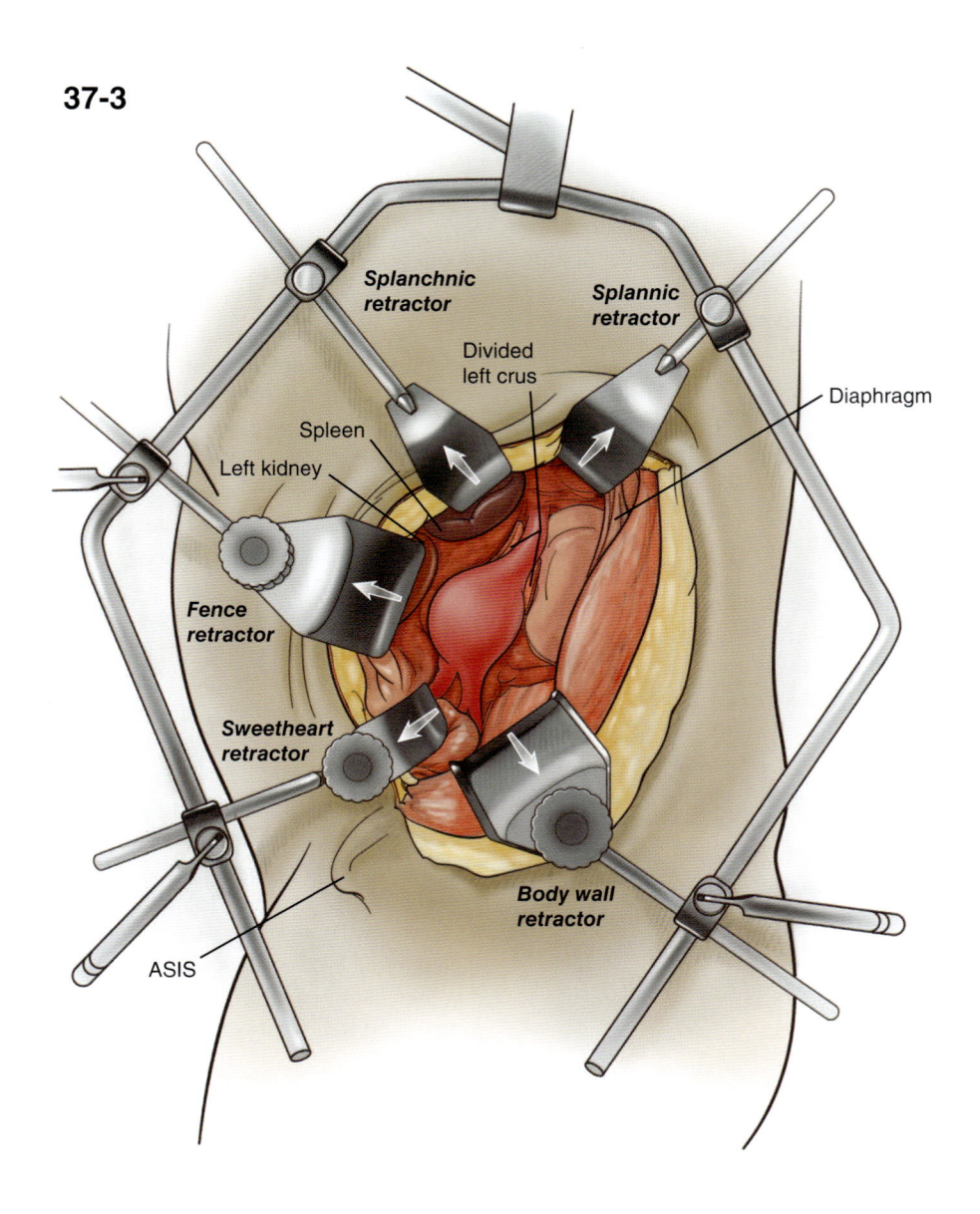

37-4

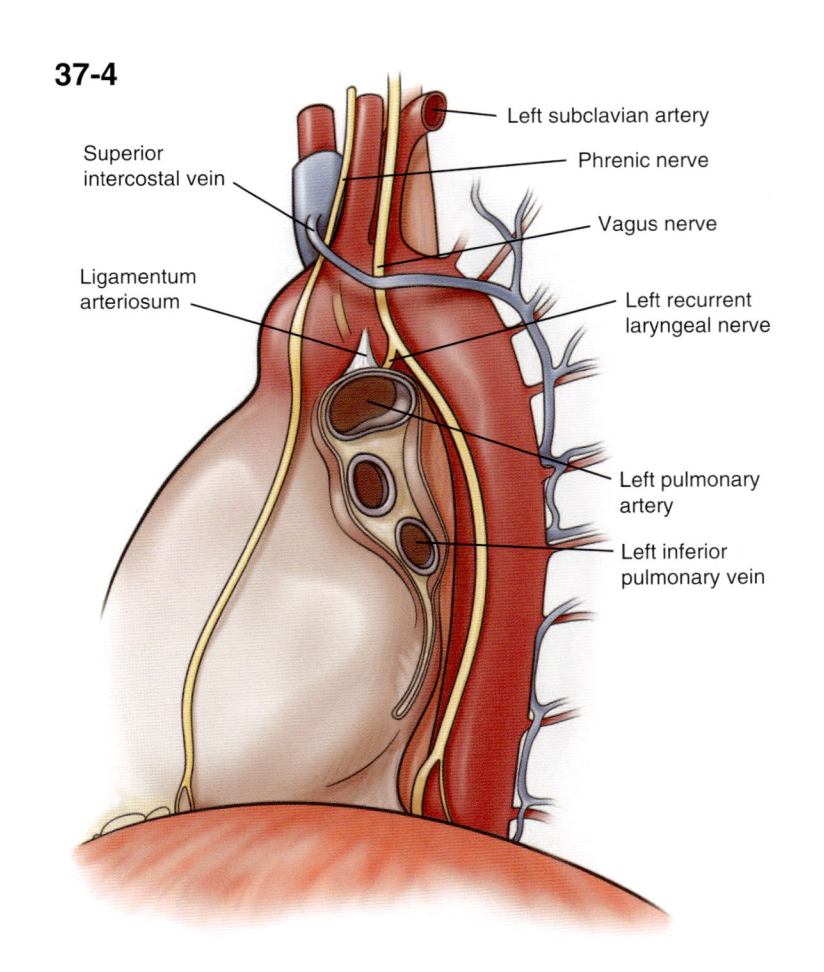

INCISION AND EXPOSURE `CONTINUED` A place to apply a distal clamp for extents II, or the proximal clamp in extents III, is found around the level of T6. The aorta here is dissected free circumferentially, taking care to separate it from the esophagus (which can be palpated by feeling the TEE probe or NG tube), and to not avulse intercostal vessels. The same thing is done further along to clamp the distal DTA for extents III. More discetion and ligating intercostal arteries (ICAs) here is unwarranted but not absolutely prohibited. The artery of Adamkevitz lies between T7 and L2 95% of the time. In this region, the ICA should be preserved for reimplanation of a short "bucket-handle graft." The lung is then retracted posteriorly and the pericardium overlying the left inferior pulmonary vein (LIPV) is incised, exposing the vessel, and a purse-string suture is placed in the vessel.

The next gateway is exposing the retroperitoneum in the abdomen, in an envelope type fashion. The costal margin is transected and a plane is developed between Gerota's fascia and the retroperitoneum (see **FIGURE 37-2**). The spleen is taken down from the diaphragm as described in Chapter 29, and the left crus of the diaphragm (the gateway to the immediate supra-celiac aorta) (**FIGURE 37-5**) is divided to expose the aorta. The gateway to the left renal artery (LRA) is usually a large lumber vein that is identified by visualization or palpation of the origin off the aorta. It is not necessary but is helpful to also dissect free the celiac and superior mesenteric artery, which lie immediately cephalad to the LRA, and control them with vessel loops (**FIGURE 37-5A**). Remaining posterior to the LRA, the tissue covering the aorta is dissected free inferiorly to the iliac arteries (**FIGURE 37-5B**). Anterior retraction of the peritoneal contents takes the ureter with it to lie anterior to the aorta. It needs to be identified to avoid injury. A soft spot is identified to clamp the aorta above the aotic bifurcation and below the renal arteries. Pay careful attention to preserve the middle sacral artery. Look for an anomalous retroaortic left renal vein on preop imaging. It can be preserved by leaving the kidney down during dissection, but occasionally warrants division and reattachment.

DETAILS OF PROCEDURE The conduct of the operation differs for an open proximal anastomosis utilizing full cardiopulmonary bypass (CPB) with HCA from that for a clampable aorta utilizing left heart bypass (LHB). These will be discussed separately.

FOR A CLAMPABLE PROXIMAL AORTA: Intravenous (IV) heparin (100 units/kg) is given to achieve an activated clotting time (ACT) over 280 seconds. The left femoral artery (LFA) is cannulated (15–19 Fr) in all patients to allow for distal perfusion during the repair. The arterial limb of the bypass circuit is split to allow for visceral perfusion via a second arterial limb when the abdominal aorta is opened. The LIPV is cannulated for LHB. LHB is initiated at 500 mL/min and systolic blood pressure should be <100 mm Hg to accommodate increased afterload upon proximal aortic clamping. A second more distal clamp is then applied while manually compressing the aorta between the clamps to evacuate blood (**FIGURE 37-6**). If there is rapid refilling of the aorta between the clamps, incomplete clamping has occurred. Once the aorta is completely clamped, the aneurysm between the clamps is opened. LHB flow and pharmacologic agents are adjusted to keep right radial artery–monitored mean arterial pressure 70 to 90 mm Hg. Any ICA encountered here is oversewn with 2-0 braided suture. The DTA is transected circumferentially at the site for your proximal anastomosis, taking care on the posterior side to lift the aorta and not injure the esophagus. The aortic diameter is sized and a four-branched polyester TAAA graft is bought into the field. Holding with forceps the branch corresponding to the celiac artery at the celiac artery, the proximal part of the graft is stretched to the proximal aortic anastomotic site and the graft is cut at the proximal end to this length. Paying attention to the orientation of the graft for the visceral attachments, the proximal anastomosis to the aorta is fashioned with 3-0 or 4-0 monofilament suture or, in the case of very friable tissue, interrupted pledgetted 2-0 braided suture with the pledget outside the aorta. The graft is then clamped and the proximal aortic clamp is released, allowing assessment and hemostatic attention to the anastomosis. `CONTINUES`

37-5

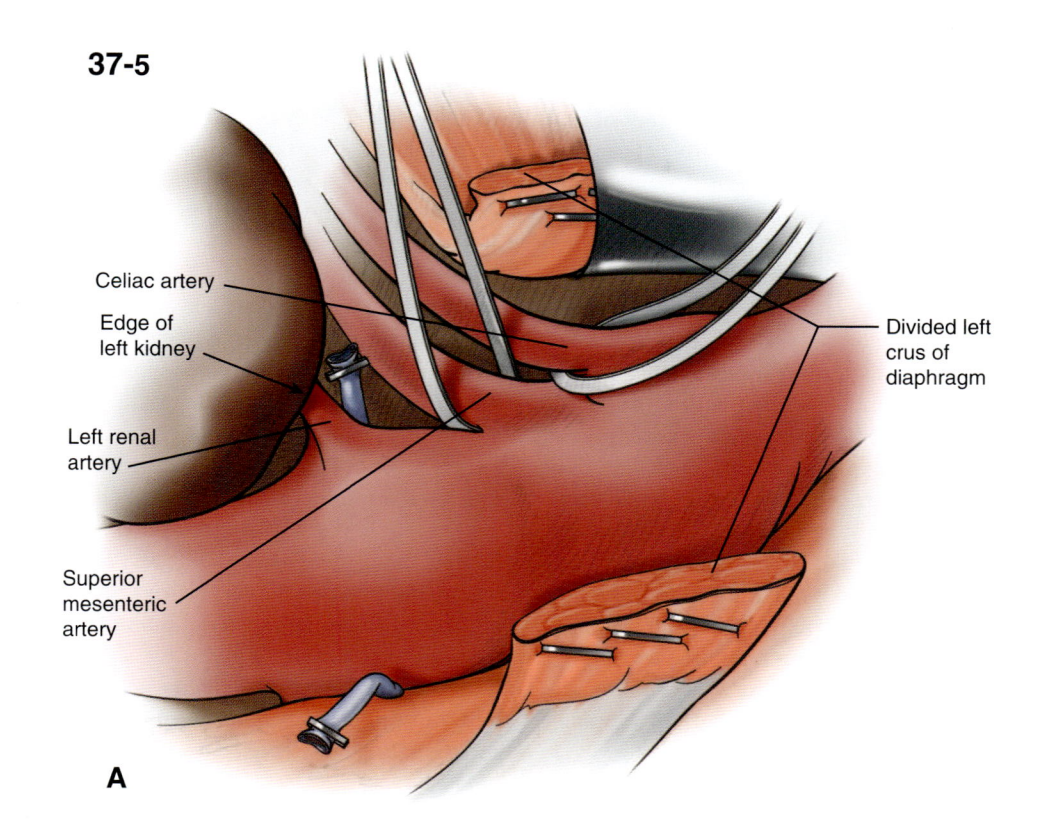

Celiac artery

Edge of
left kidney

Left renal
artery

Superior
mesenteric
artery

Divided left
crus of
diaphragm

A

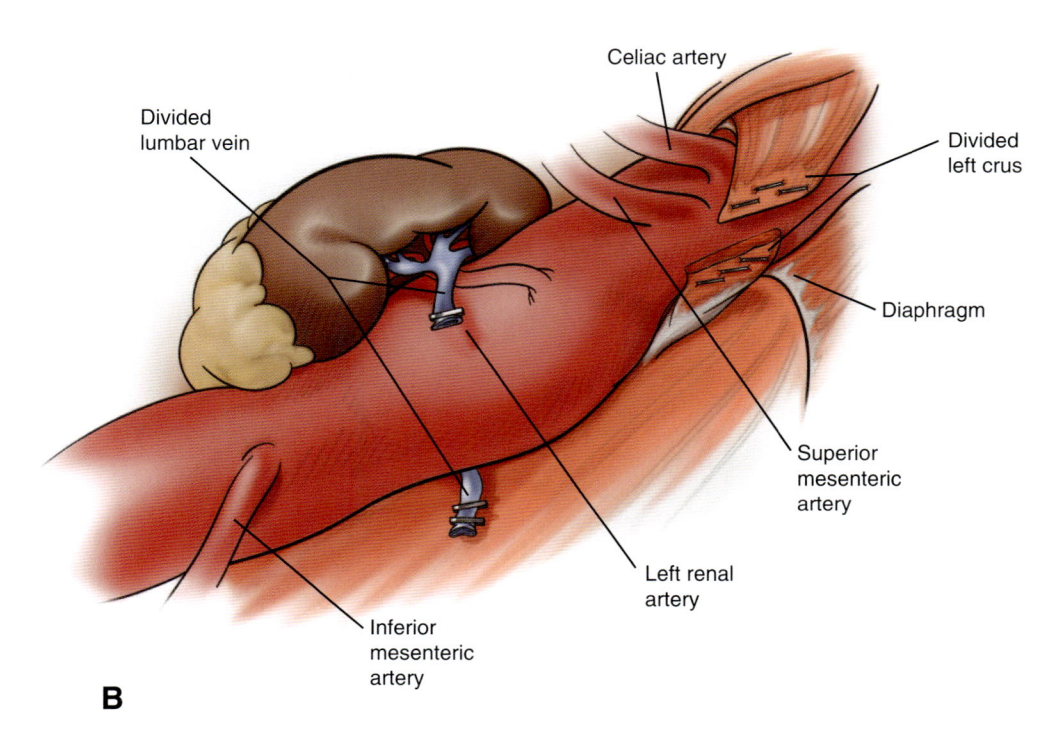

Divided
lumbar vein

Celiac artery

Divided
left crus

Diaphragm

Superior
mesenteric
artery

Left renal
artery

Inferior
mesenteric
artery

B

37-6

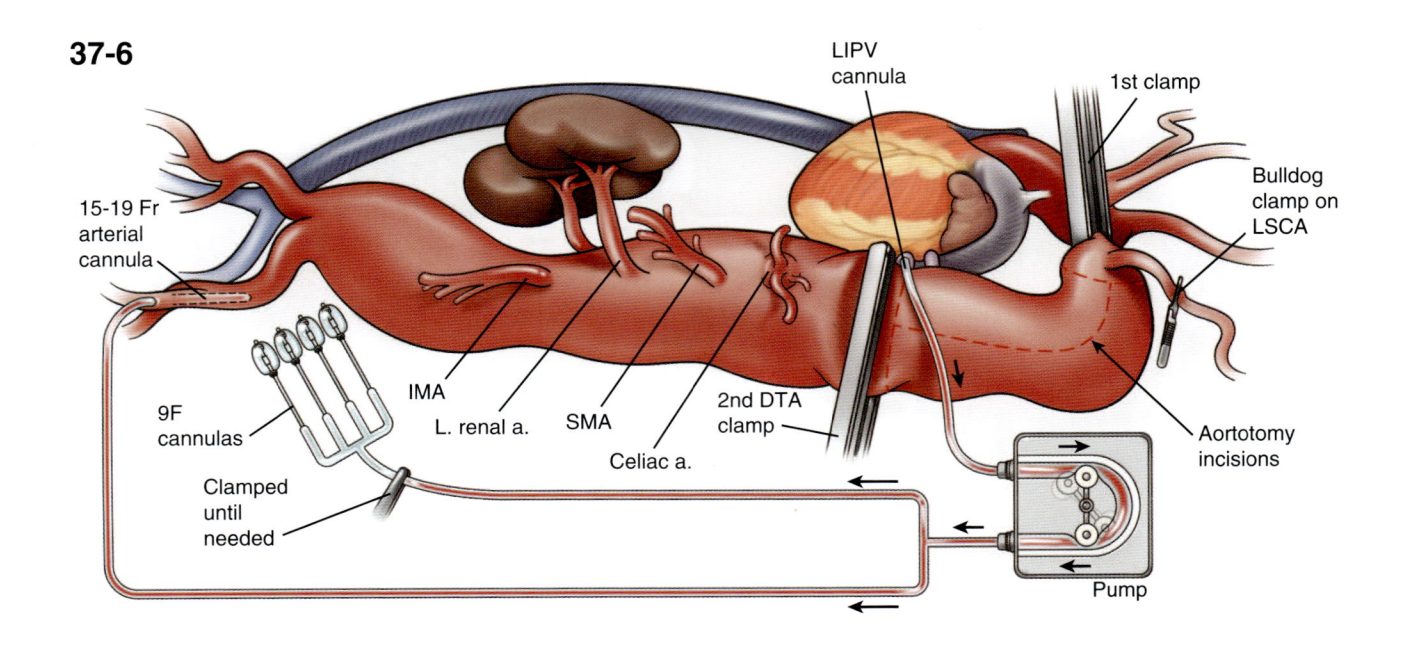

LIPV
cannula

1st clamp

Bulldog
clamp on
LSCA

15-19 Fr
arterial
cannula

9F
cannulas

Clamped
until
needed

IMA

L. renal a.

SMA

Celiac a.

2nd DTA
clamp

Aortotomy
incisions

Pump

DETAILS OF PROCEDURE *FOR A NON-CLAMPABLE PROXIMAL AORTA*: **CONTINUED** IV heparin (300 units/kg) is given to achieve an ACT over 400. The LFA is cannulated (17–21 Fr). The venous limb of the bypass circuit is spliced in two for dual drainage and the arterial limb is spliced twice to allow for three-arterial inflow. The LIPV is cannulated to vent the fibrillating left heart during cooling. A multiport venous cannula is inserted in the left femoral vein resting the tip in the right atrium under TEE guidance. CPB and cooling to 18°C can begin. Once at target temperature, the aorta is clamped at T6, the LSCA is clamped, and the aorta is opened and transected circumferentially at the proximal anastomotic site. A 30-cc Foley inserted via the open arch to sit in the ascending aorta can be inflated and used to instill a dose of cardioplegia into the root. Any ICA encountered here is oversewn. A side-armed polyester graft is used for the proximal anastomosis. Thereafter, the side arm can be cannulated with one of the arterial limbs of the bypass circuit restoring flow to the upper body (FIGURE 37-7). Lower body flow can also be restored via the LFA limb of the circuit if it was interrupted during this part of the operation. If the anastomosis was proximal to the LSCA it will need to be reattached to the main body of the graft, but not necessarily now. Rewarming to 37°C can begin. A suitably matched four-branched polyester TAAA graft is tailored for length, as described above, and sewn to the proximal end of the side-armed graft that will need to be shortened to allow for proper lie and length of the four-branch graft.

Hereafter, conduct of the operation is similar. The aorta between the iliac bifurcation and the renal arteries is clamped, adjusting flows as necessary to maintain upper body MAP 70 to 90 mmHg. The second DTA clamp is now released and the aorta is splayed open inferiorly to the distal clamp, making sure to remain posterior to the LRA. If not using full CPB, shed blood is collected, washed, and returned to the patient with a rapid infuser. If ICA reimplantation is planned, these vessels should be identified, typically between T8 and L2, and controlled with occlusion catheters. The remaining intercostal and lumbar vessels are expeditiously oversewn to minimize blood loss and maximize collateral perfusion. Any dissection flap present is completely resected, and laminated clot is scraped off to reveal branch vessels that are otherwise obscured and are potential sources of postop bleeding. The four visceral vessels are identified and cannulated with 9 Fr perfusion catheters. Buttons of aorta around the ostia of these vessels are fashioned. The renal arteries are perfused with either cold crystalloid or blood similar to the celiac and superior mesenteric artery (SMA). If cold renal perfusate is desired, using the separate dedicated circuit, the renals are perfused at either 400 mL intermittently every 10 to 15 minutes or via continuous infusion at 15 mL/min. The available arterial limb of the bypass circuit is used to provide continuous perfusion of blood at 500 mL/min to the celiac artery and SMA (FIGURE 37-8), and bilateral renal arteries. If desired, ICAs can be implanted into the graft as a patch, using an 8-mm ringed ePTFE graft, or as a button, and the clamp repositioned to restore flow to the ICAs. **CONTINUES**

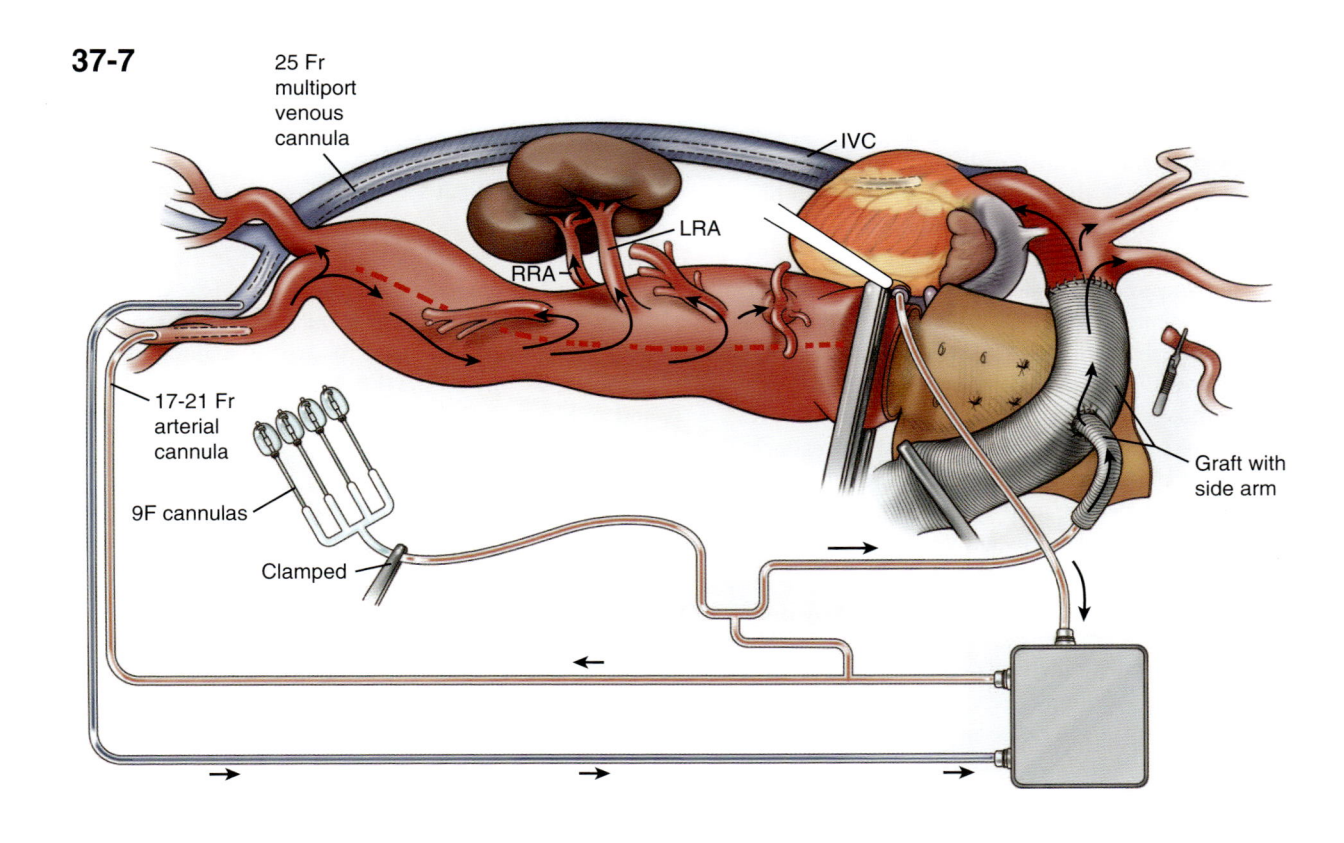

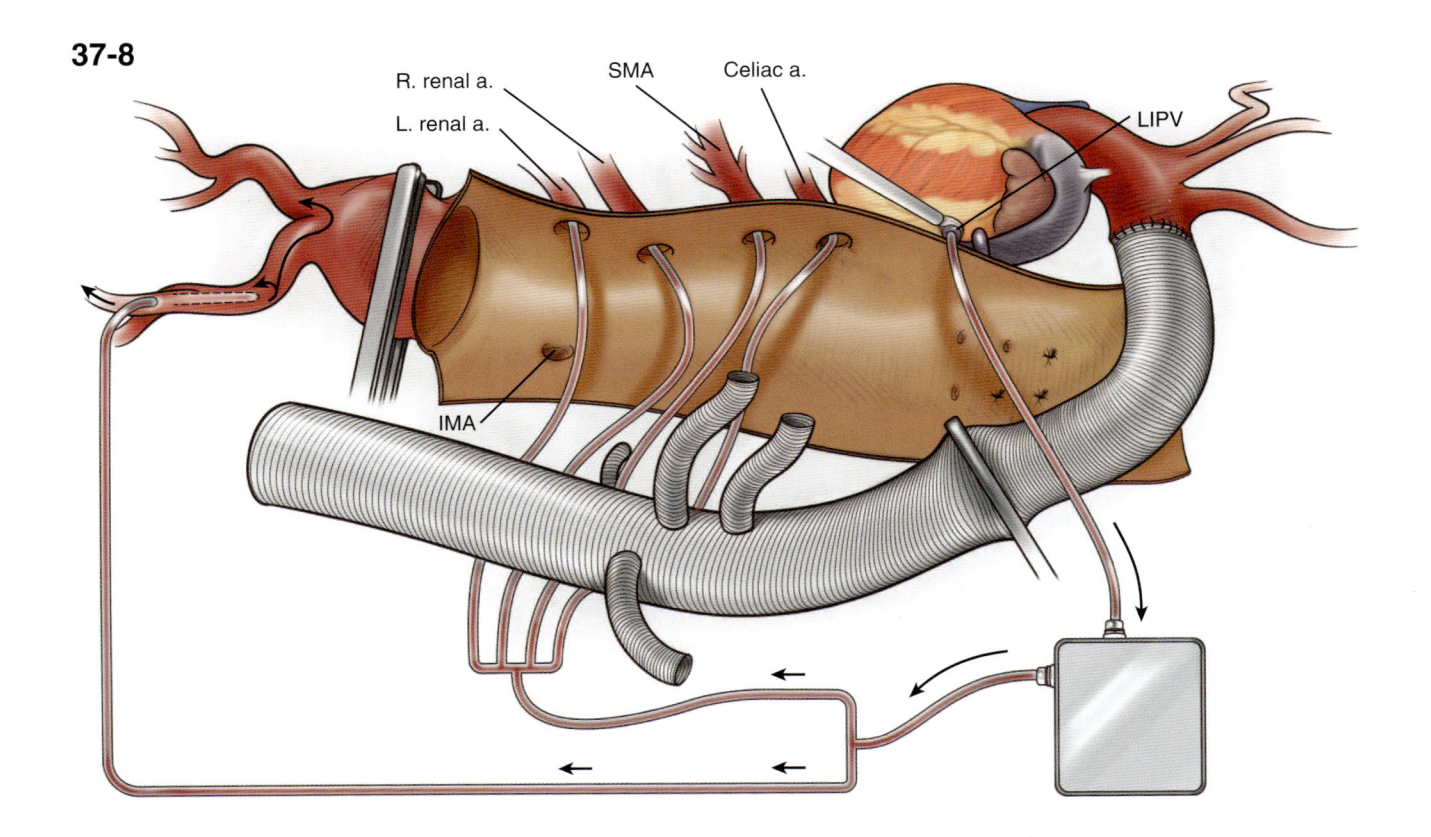

DETAILS OF PROCEDURE *FOR A NON-CLAMPABLE PROXIMAL AORTA*: **CONTINUED** The graft is passed through the open aorta/diaphragmatic hiatus. While it is the surgeon's preference which vessel to bypass first, some choose sequential anatomic bypasses from proximal to distal. However, this author's preference is to bypass the right renal artery (RRA) as the first of the four visceral arteries to be anastomosed, using 4-0 monofilament to the corresponding 8-mm limb of the four-branched graft that is trimmed to length. The perfusion catheter is removed with the last few stitches, and renal perfusate flow is adjusted for the single vessel. After the distal graft and three other branches are clamped, the clamp on the proximal graft is removed, restoring RRA flow. This is followed by the celiac artery button anastomosis to the 10-mm branch, then the SMA to the other 10-mm branch, and finally the LRA to the other 8-mm branch, sequentially restoring flow to each vessel as its anastomosis is completed. Flow into the LFA is stopped and the clamp on the distal aorta is released, allowing for an open distal anastomosis if needed (**FIGURE 37-9**). Instead, in patients with iliac involvement, a bifurcated graft can be sutured to the distal portion of the four-branch graft and the limbs sutured to the iliac arteries. Flow is restored to the LFA de-airing the aorta/graft, and the clamp on the distal part of the graft is released.

If needed, a separate interposition graft can be used to reattach the LSCA to the neo-aorta or, if a side-armed graft was used, the side arm can be uncoupled from the bypass circuit and used to attach to the LSCA (**FIGURE 37-10**). The heart can be more consistently defibrillated with success once rewarmed to above 29°C. Flow is confirmed in all bypasses and in the dorsalis pedis via hand-held ultrasound.

CLOSURE Hemostasis is pursued with focused determination. In the case of LHB, protamine is given and the lung is retracted posteriorly, exposing the LIPV cannula for removal. In the case of full CPB, protamine is reserved until the femoral venous cannula is also removed, waiting until core temperature is above 36°C before separation from CPB. Blood in the CPB circuit is returned to the LFA. If anatomy allows, the aneurysmal aorta is loosely wrapped and tacked around the graft in places. We do not routinely drain the retroperitoneum. Two 32 Fr chest tubes are placed in the left pleural space. The diaphragm, if transected, is reconstructed with running #2 monofilament suture, taking care to avoid tearing the muscular diaphragm. The ribs are reapproximated with multiple figures-of-eight #5, nonabsorbable braided sutures, avoiding injury to the intercostal neurovascular bundles. The soft tissues are reapproximated in multiple layers using absorbable suture, paying attention to bring corresponding fascia together.

POSTOPERATIVE CARE The importance of postoperative care is not subordinate to that of the operation itself. Comprehensive suggested readings are found below. Patients are taken to the ICU, intubated, and ventilated until they are rewarmed, as they often arrive fairly hypothermic. Strict maintenance of MAP over 80 is maintained with volume and pharmacologic agents. Coagulopathy is corrected and blood provided to keep hemoglobin above 10 g/L. A priority is placed on transiently holding sedation to do a rudimentary assessment of motor function in the lower limbs upon arrival in the ICU. Spinal fluid drainage is continued to maintain CSF pressure <10 cm H_2O for a few days until a consistent neurologic exam is established. Interventions are pursued in the event of diminished motor function; MAP is driven above 90 mm Hg, CSF is drained more aggressively, a naloxone infusion is initiated, and steroids are provided. Bedrest with elevation of the head to <30° is maintained until the CSF drain is removed, usually on the third or fourth day postop, and then mobilization and ambulation is encouraged. ∎

SUGGESTED READINGS

Chatterjee S, Casar JG, LeMaire SA, Preventza O, Coselli JS: Perioperative care after thoracoabdominal aortic aneurysm repair: The Baylor College of Medicine experience. Part 2: Postoperative management. *J Thorac Cardovasc Surg.* 2021;161:699-705.

Coselli JS, de la Cruz KI, Preventza O, LeMaire SA, Weldon SA: Extent II thoracoabdominal aortic aneurysm repair: how I do it. *Semin Thoracic Surg.* 2016;28:221-237.

Coselli JS, LeMaire SA, Preventza O, de la Cruz KI, Cooley DA et al: Outcomes of 3309 thoracoabdominal aortic aneurysm repairs. *J Thorac Cardovasc Surg.* 2016;151:1323-1338.

Oderich GS, Ribeiro M, Reis de Souza L, Hofer J, Wigham J, Cha S: Endovascular repair of thoracoabdominal aortic aneurysms using fenestrated and branched endografts. *J Thorac Cardiovasc Surg.* 2017;153:S32-S41.e7.

Tanaka A, Estrera AL, Safi HJ: Open thoracoabdominal aortic aneurysm surgery technique: how we do it. *J Cardiovasc Surg (Torino).* 2021 Feb 15: doi 10.23736/S0021-9509.21.11825-7. Online ahead of print.

37-9

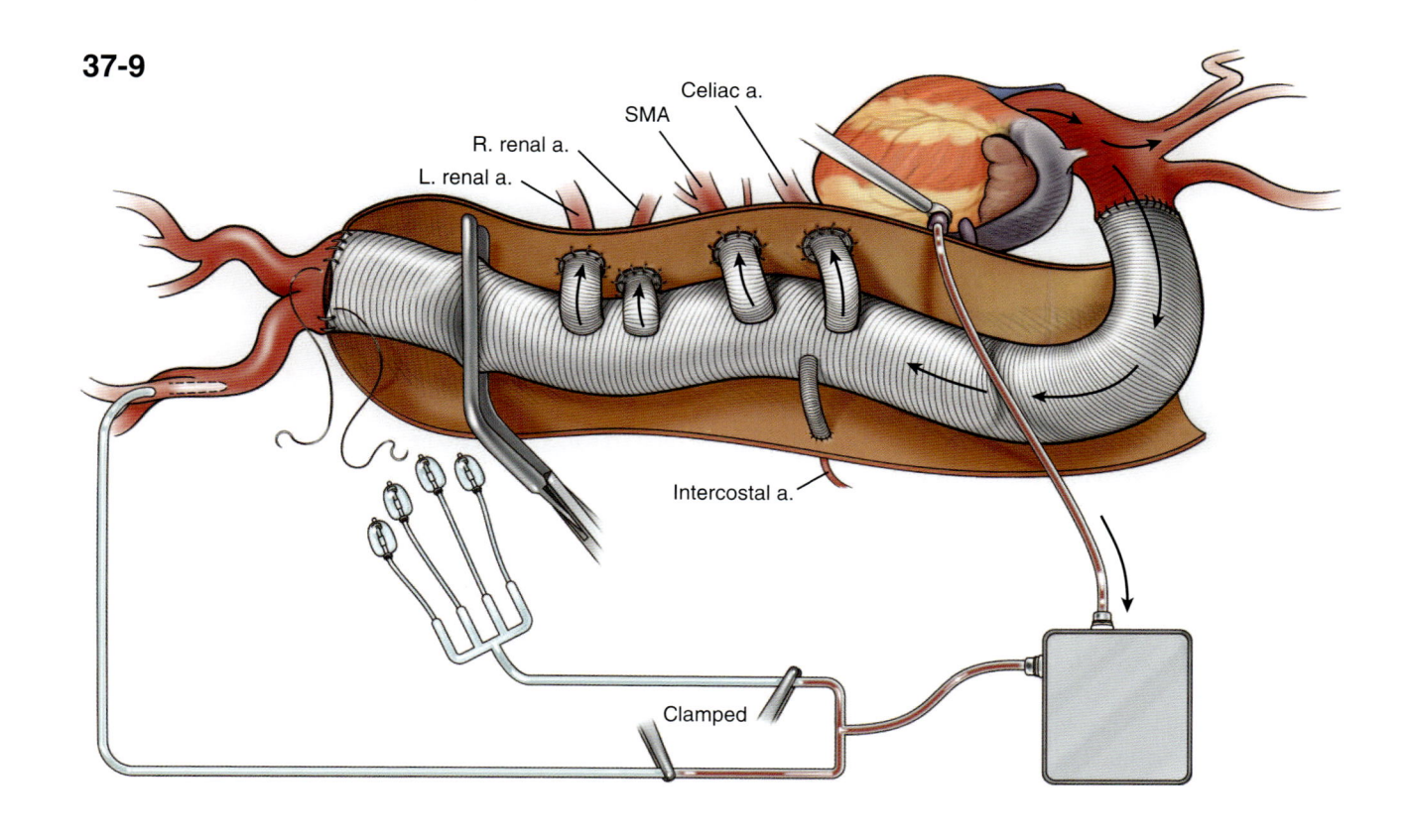

37-10

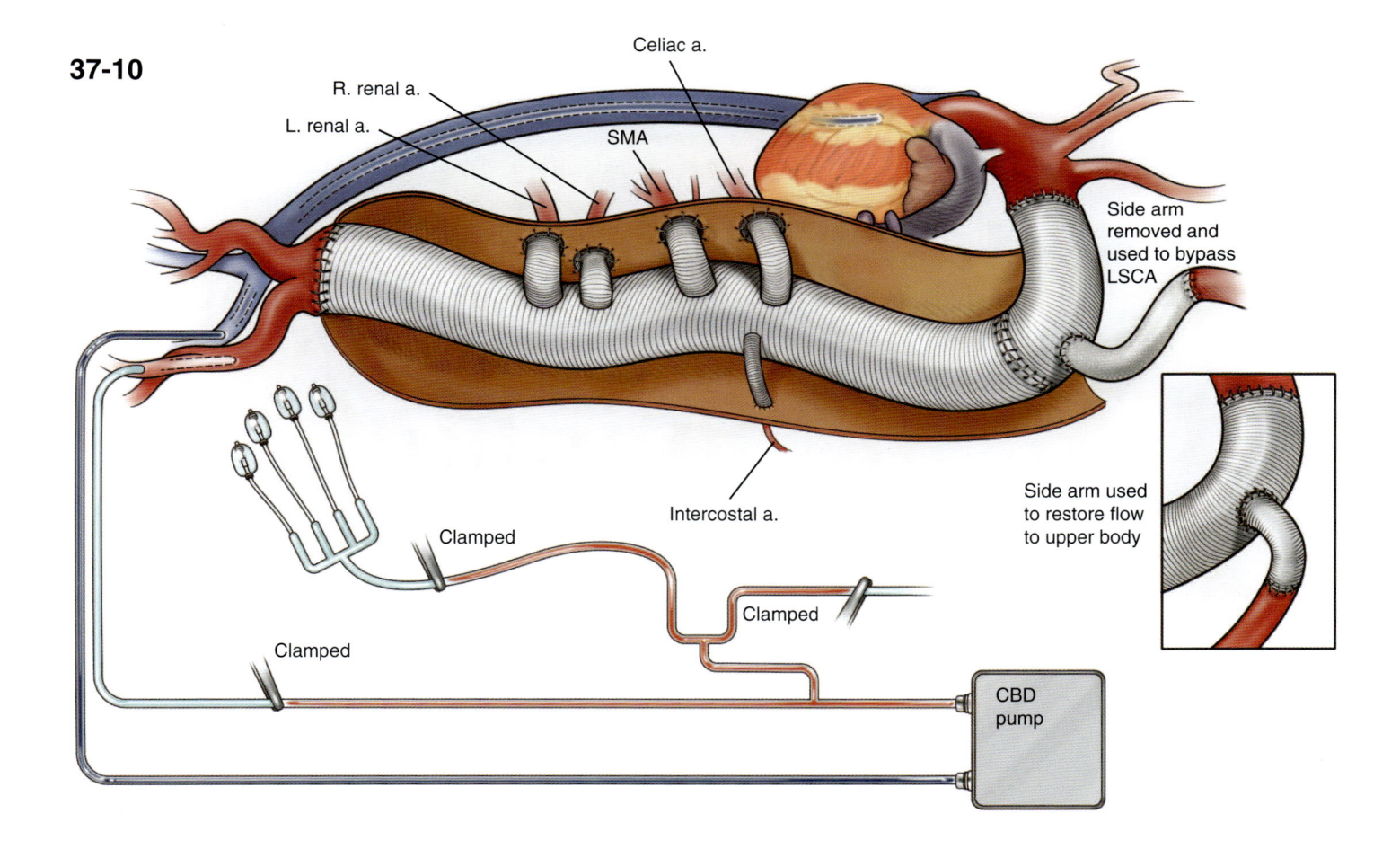

CRAWFORD TYPE IV THORACOABDOMINAL AORTIC ANEURYSM

Kristine Orion, MD • Kara Hessel, DO • Timur P. Sarac, MD

INDICATIONS The Crawford system for outlining thoracoabdominal aortic aneurysms (TAAA) was developed in the 1970s. The classification system outlines four types of TAAA. Types I through III are described in the preceding chapters. Type IV TAAA begins at the aortic hiatus of the diaphragm and extends to the aortic bifurcation. Nevertheless, the techniques described here can be very useful for most pararenal/suprarenal abdominal aortic aneurysms, as sewing to poor tissue can cause not only intraoperative difficulties, but also long-term recurrence rates can be higher. The surgical approach to each TAAA differs and the potential complications differ as a result of the extent of the dissection and aortic replacement necessary. Type IV TAAAs make up 20% of TAAAs. Indications for intervention for type IV TAAA most commonly include aneurysm size greater than 5.5 cm in men and 5 cm in women or rapid growth (greater than 0.5 cm in 6 months or 1 cm in 1 year). Smaller size aneurysms are often repaired in patients with family history of aortic rupture or those with a known connective tissue disorder. Symptomatic aneurysms should proceed with urgent repair. Additionally, those patients with persistent back or abdominal pain of unexplained etiology in the setting of a moderate sized aneurysm should be considered for repair. Inflammatory or infectious aneurysms should similarly be intervened upon expeditiously.

ANESTHESIA We recommend the surgical team confer directly with the anesthesia team in preparation for an open thoracoabdominal aortic repair. This early discussion can avoid last-minute pitfalls on the day of surgery. Good communication between the two teams generally involves the following considerations.

Preoperative consideration of postoperative pain control should be explored. Patients can have both an epidural and a lumbar drain placed for these cases. A high thoracic epidural can often facilitate good pain control in the postoperative period. General anesthetic should be administered for open aortic intervention. Because repair of type IV TAAA usually requires entry into the left chest for exposure and proximal clamping, the anesthesia team must be adequately prepared to provide single lung ventilation in this instance. This can be accomplished with either a dual lumen tube or a bronchial blocker. Two 18-gauge or larger peripheral IVs and large bore central access should be obtained to facilitate massive transfusion, fluid resuscitation, or vasopressor administration. An arterial line for close monitoring of hemodynamics should also be placed, preferably in the radial artery or brachial.

Some patients may also benefit from intraoperative transesophageal echocardiography (TEE) monitoring of cardiac activity. This may allow for early identification of cardiac instability with cross-clamping and assist in guiding volume resuscitation. However, nasogastric decompression is important to limit the spleen being pushed out by the stomach when exposing the supraceliac aorta, and this should be placed first a priori, as a Swan-Ganz catheter can take the place of TEE temporarily. It is very unusual for left heart bypass or pelvic shunting to be needed, but if the circumstance arises where prolonged visceral ischemia (celiac and SMA longer than 40 minutes), then LHP should be considered (see Chapter 37). The renal arteries are cooled by instilling 200 cc of "kidney cocktail," which consists of a mixture of mannitol, Lasix, and prednisone, in 1 L of lactated Ringer's.

Alternatively, an additional limb can be sewn onto the bypass graft for anastomosis to the left external iliac artery prior to aortic cross-clamp. Following cross-clamp, the proximal anastomosis is sewn and, on completion, flow is restored through the pelvis to the graft. The proximal clamp is placed distal to the takeoff of this shunt to allow for completion of the remaining renovisceral anastomoses. This technique is particularly useful if the aortic cross-clamp can be placed below the diaphragm, limiting chest dissection. The anatomy of the aneurysm dictates the best option for visceral, renal, and pelvic perfusion throughout the course of the operation and consideration should be given to all techniques based on the anatomy and the surgeon's expertise with each technique.

POSITION AND OPERATIVE PREPARATION The patient is initially placed in the supine position on the table with underlying bean bag (FIGURE 38-1). Once general anesthesia has been induced and appropriate lines and monitoring devices have been placed, positioning may commence. The break in the bed should be placed midway between the left 12th rib and the left anterior superior iliac spine. This allows for flexion of the bed and increases the working space in the retroperitoneum. The patient, once positioned correctly over the break, should be rotated on the bean bag into a semi-right lateral decubitus position. The shoulders are generally at a 60-degree angle from the bed, while the hips are slightly less at 30 degrees. This allows adequate exposure to both groins. All bony prominences should be padded, an axillary roll may be placed but is not imperative, and the left arm draped across the patient on an arm board or pillows. Great care should be taken to avoid pressure on the brachial plexus to avoid inadvertent injury. The bottom leg should be bent and the top leg kept straight. Ample pillows or padding should be used in between the knees and under both ankles. If able, we recommend securing the patient at two points, usually thigh and high chest, with Underwriting Labs (UL)–rated safety straps and 3-inch silk tape (FIGURE 38-2). CONTINUES ▶

38-1

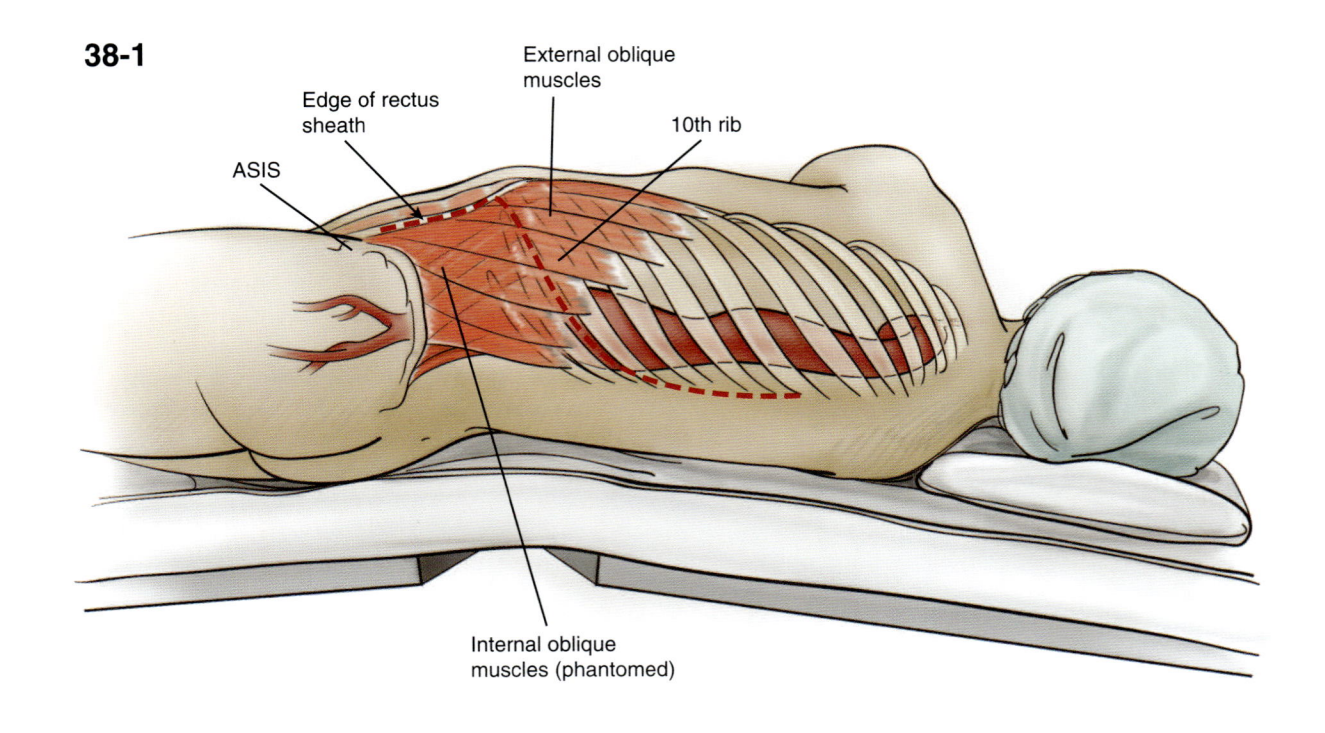

ASIS

Edge of rectus sheath

External oblique muscles

10th rib

Internal oblique muscles (phantomed)

38-2

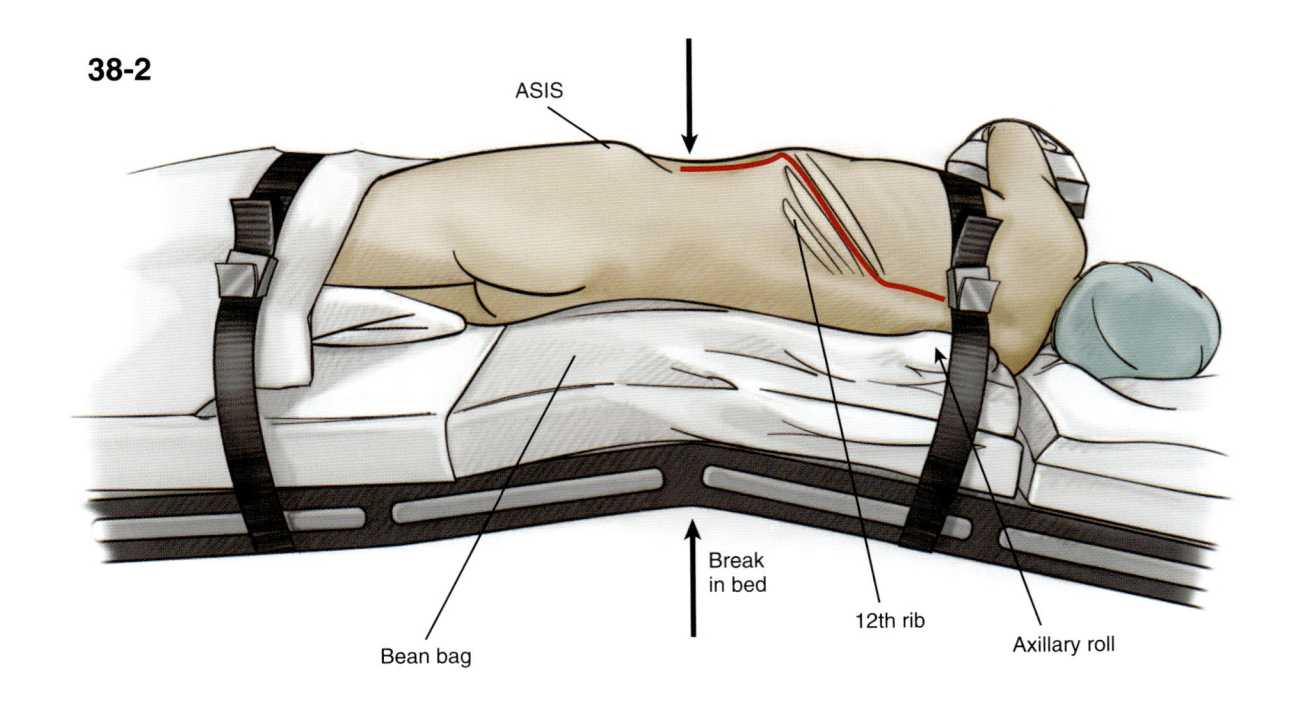

ASIS

Break in bed

Bean bag

12th rib

Axillary roll

INCISION AND EXPOSURE   The chosen incision varies based on the level at which the aortic cross-clamp will be placed. For TAAA IV, we prefer an incision along superior border of the 10th rib, or the 9th intercostal space. The 10th rib is easily palpated as the lowest rib still attached to the costal margin. The skin incision is carried along the distal aspect of the rib and then directed toward the pelvis while staying lateral to the rectus abdominis, termed the Risberg incision (FIGURE 38-3 anterior view). The retroperitoneal space is most readily entered by dividing the costal margin (see Chapter 31). The underlying retroperitoneal fat will be apparent, and this space is dissected using a combination of blunt, sharp, and electrothermy away from Gerota's fascia. The dissection is done gently so as to not violate the peritoneal sac, which can be onerous if peritoneal contents are released into the surgical field. Once the retroperitoneum is entered, the peritoneal contents are retracted to the patient's right. When the psoas muscle is identified, the ureter should be sought, protected, and swept up with the peritoneal sac, leaving the psoas fascia in place. If the ureter is adhered to the iliac artery, separation should be taken sharply rather than with electrocautery. Superiorly, the dissection can be carried out either posterior or anterior to the kidney. The left kidney can either be left down or can be swept up medially with the peritoneum. In most cases, we reflect the kidney medially. Leaving the kidney down allows for more distal access of the SMA as well as some exposure of the origin of the right renal artery (FIGURE 38-4 kidney up; see Chapter 31 for kidney down).   CONTINUES▶

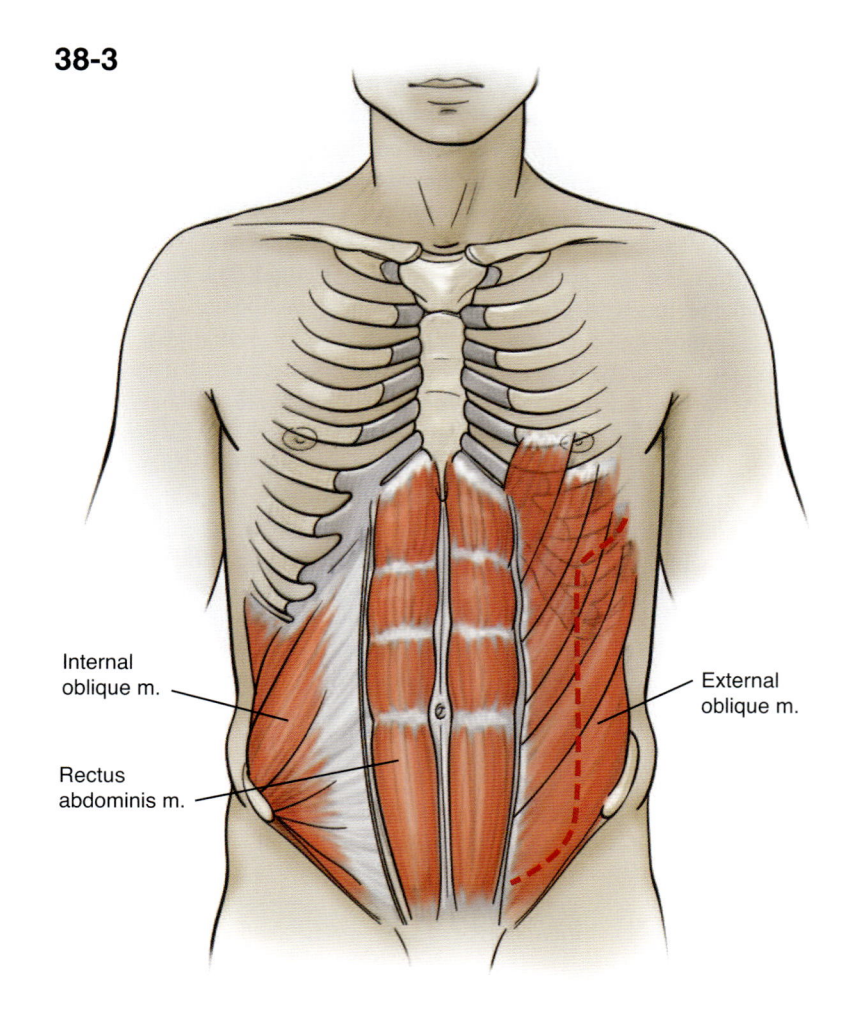

38-3

Internal oblique m.

External oblique m.

Rectus abdominis m.

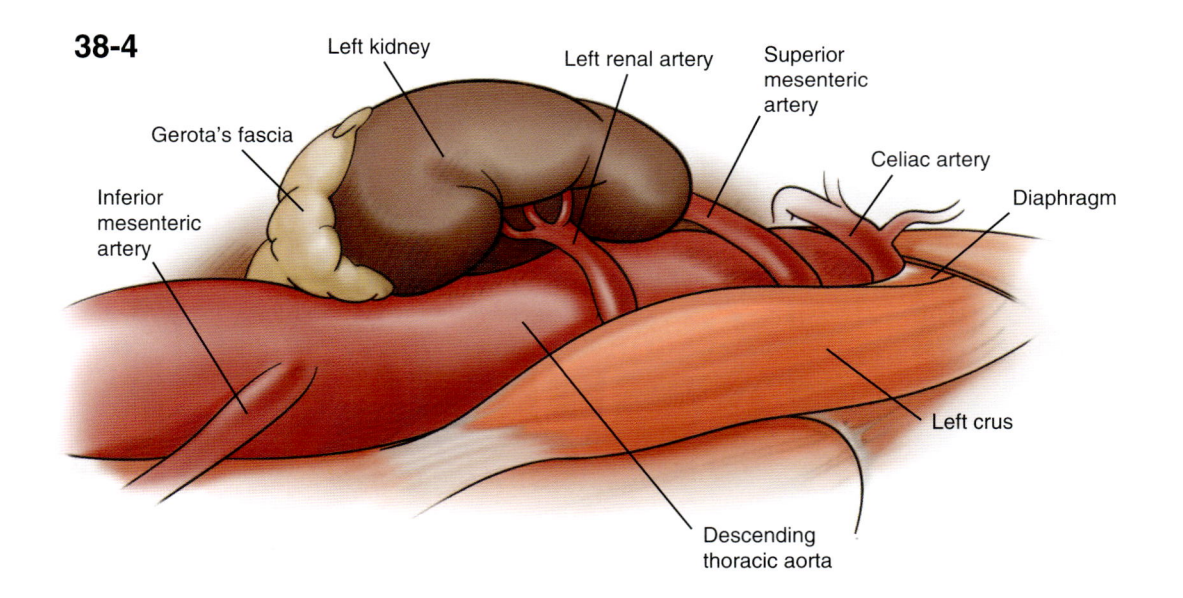

38-4

Left kidney

Left renal artery

Superior mesenteric artery

Celiac artery

Diaphragm

Gerota's fascia

Inferior mesenteric artery

Left crus

Descending thoracic aorta

INCISION AND EXPOSURE CONTINUED When exposing the retroperitoneal diaphragm, caution should be taken as there are significant attachments that should be identified and are subsequently discussed. An important gateway to the retroperitoneal aorta is mobilizing the spleen from the diaphragm (see Chapter 31). This can be accomplished sharply, with electrocautery dissection, or bluntly, using a sponge stick. The spleen is gently teased away from the diaphragm and carefully positioned medially. There is often a phrenic vein near the splenophrenic ligament that needs to be divided. When retractors are placed, laporotomy pads should be used between the retractor and the spleen to prevent injury. If an injury is encountered, we have low threshold for splenectomy at the conclusion of the case. Once the retroperitoneum is largely exposed, a large self-retaining retractor is placed. We prefer the Omni retractor system, though a Bookwalter or Thompson can also be utilized (FIGURE 38-5).

If the chest is to be entered for exposure and cross-clamping, the incision is extended up onto the chest wall. When entering the chest for clamping, single lung ventilation is optimal to avoid injury to the pleura. The incision is carried along the superior edge of the 10th rib to avoid the neurovascular bundle of the 9th rib. The rib can either be left in place or can be resected to allow for visualization. If the latter is preferred, a bone cutter is utilized and the intercostal artery is oversewn utilizing a permanent suture. Gentle dissection is carried out around the aorta, palpating for the esophagus to ensure that only the aorta is cross-clamped, and an umbilical tape is placed to facilitate circumferential control should immediate cross-clamping become necessary. Exposure may be limited by the diaphragm. Great care should be undertaken with either technique to avoid injury to the phrenic nerve, which generally enters at the dome of the diaphragm.

DETAILS OF PROCEDURE Once the retroperitoneal space is exposed and the peritoneum reflected to the right medial aspect of the abdomen, dissection over the aorta can be undertaken. It is helpful to start distally at the left common iliac to identify the correct plane and follow it proximally. Optimally, the iliac arteries are circumferentially controlled, but this may not be possible if there is extensive inflammation in the pelvis. Care should be taken to not injure the iliac veins throughout the course of the dissection.

It is essential that one comes down directly onto the aorta: "get on the aorta and stay on the aorta." This not only decreases operative time but avoids injury to parallel venous structures, lumbar arteries, and the 3rd/4th portion of the duodenum. When the left kidney is rotated medially, the left renal vein is not visible in the surgical field unless there is a retroaortic left renal vein. The gateway to the left renal artery is usually a large lumbar vein, which should be ligated and divided. It is then easily palpated and dissected free, and should be encircled with vessel loops (FIGURE 38-6). There should be no major structures on this plane of the aorta as one carries the remainder of the aortic dissection to the crus. The left crus of the arcuate ligament of the diaphragm is the gateway to the supraceliac aorta, and its most inferior portion identified by a white central tendon band. It is then divided to expose the supraceliac aorta (particularly if this should be the chosen site for cross-clamp). This can be accomplished with the Bovie or sharply.

Once proximal and distal aortic exposure are obtained, the visceral arteries are sought. The celiac and superior mesenteric artery can be found on the right medial aspect of the exposed aorta and either circumferentially controlled or clamped. If the left kidney is rotated up during aortic exposure, the right renal artery origin is not readily accessible from the left retroperitoneum and will need control from within the aorta. The left renal artery should be controlled circumferentially.

The patient is then systemically heparinized. When ready to proceed, the distal aorta or iliacs are clamped first, followed the by branch vasculature and then the proximal aorta. This is vital to protect the viscera and kidney from microemboli during the proximal aortic clamp. The aneurysm sac is then opened in the infrarenal segment. Thrombus is extracted and any bleeding lumbar vessels are suture ligated with permanent suture. This step can be a period of significant blood loss, so effective communication with the anesthesia team is vital. Cold renal perfusate is instilled. This solution consists of 25 grams of mannitol and 1 gram of methylprednisolone in 1 L Lactated Ringer's cooled to 4°C, for a total volume of approximately 200 cc per kidney. The right renal artery is often controlled with either a Pruitt or Fogarty occlusion balloon. If the inferior mesenteric artery (IMA) is patent, it should be controlled with a vessel loop, and decide on reimplantation toward the end of the case. CONTINUES

38-5

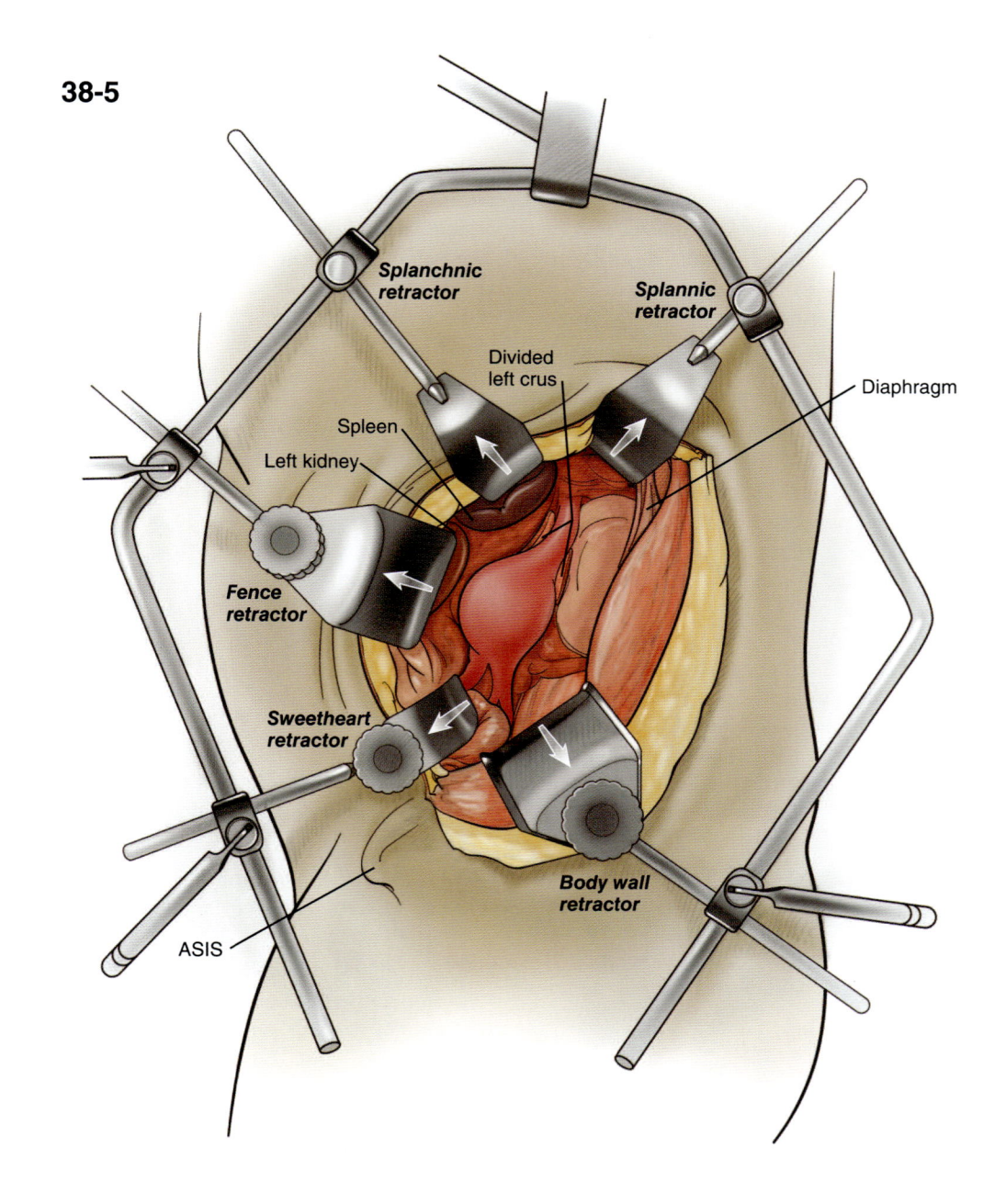

38-6

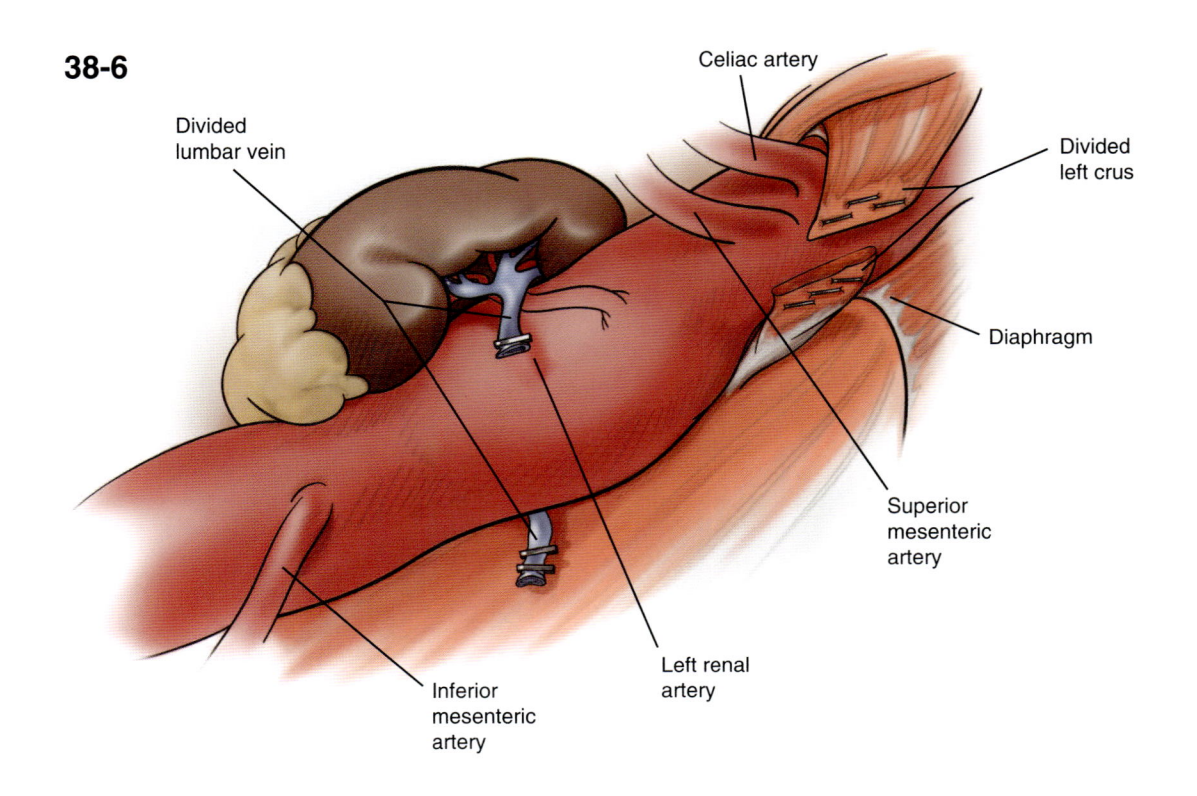

DETAILS OF PROCEDURE CONTINUED The choice of graft is determined by the diameter of the proximal aortic rim. The anatomy of the aneurysm will dictate the degree to bevel the proximal anastomosis (FIGURE 38-7). In general, the right renal artery, superior mesenteric artery, and the celiac artery can be incorporated into the beveled anastomosis (FIGURE 38-8). The left renal artery usually will require reimplantation or a short bypass with a ringed ePTFE heparin-bonded graft, which helps eliminate kinking of the anasatmosis. Once the proximal and left renal artery anastomoses are completed, the distal anastomosis is completed with either a tube or bifurcated graft. The IMA may be reimplanted if it was not previously thrombosed and demonstrates poor back-bleeding. In most cases, it can be ligated if pulsatile back-bleeding is present.

CLOSURE All vessels, including the legs, are checked for patency, and then the patient is reversed with protamine sulfate, and appropriate blood products are given as necessary. It is essential to double check for small lumbars within the sac once perfusion to the pelvis has been restored. When hemostasis has been achieved, the peritoneal sac is allowed to fall back into the abdomen. Inspection of the bowel and spleen through the peritoneal sac should be undertaken to ensure no intraperitoneal catastrophe, and the left renal artery is reinspected to ensure it lays correctly.

If the chest has been entered, chest tubes should be placed at the time of closure. Take care to insert the chest tube on patient's anterior axillary line; in this exposure, chest tubes can erroneously placed laterally, which will result in the patient laying on the tube. If divided, the diaphragm should be reapproximated utilizing permanent suture. Once this is completed, the rib space can be brought together utilizing large caliber semipermanent suture in an interrupted, figure-of-eight fashion. Chest tubes should be secured with nylon or silk suture and placed to wall suction initially.

The abdominal wall can be closed in one or two layers, most often utilizing a running semipermanent monofilament suture. The subcutaneous tissue is reapproximated using an absorbable, braided suture. Skin is generally closed using staples, though can also be closed with absorbable, monofilament, or braided suture.

POSTOPERATIVE CARE/FOLLOW-UP Postoperatively, patients require aggressive pulmonary hygiene, particularly if a thoracotomy has been performed. Patients are initially taken to the ICU. Frequent lab monitoring, including lactate levels, transaminase levels, and creatinine is initiated. Urine output is also closely monitored. If a lumbar drain is used, the drain is kept at 10 cm of water, and neuro exams are performed hourly until 24 hours post drain removal. Drain levels can generally be raised on postoperative day (POD) 1 to 2 and then removed on POD 3 after a short clamp trial between 6 and 24 hours, assuming no lower extremity neurologic deficits develop. As stated above, aggressive pain control measures should also be undertaken, as this has previously been demonstrated to improve respiratory outcomes. Chest tubes should be transitioned to water seal and then removed when output reaches physiologic levels.

Potential postoperative complications are extensive and include respiratory failure, renal failure, mesenteric ischemia, hepatic failure, lower extremity paralysis, stroke, myocardial infarction, coagulopathy, and death. The risk of composite cardiac event, including atrial fibrillation and MI, is 22%, while the risks of respiratory and renal failure are 8% and 5.7%, respectively. Significant predictors of perioperative mortality include age over 70 years, preoperative coronary artery disease, chronic kidney disease, and visceral lesions (Kieffer). A large series out of Baylor Houston reported long-term survival at 83% at 1 year, 63% at 5 years, 36% at 10 years, and 18% at 15 years, demonstrating the overall poor health of patients with TAA.

Outpatient follow-up should include close monitoring of all wounds as well as lab work. Postoperative visits should include a visit within 2 to 4 weeks and then can be spaced out to every 3 months for the first year, followed by every 6 months for the second year and yearly following that. This monitoring is necessary, as late graft complications such as anastomotic pseudoaneurysm, branch occlusion, or graft infection present in 14% of patients at 5 years. Postoperative monitoring and related imaging should also continue of any other aneurysmal disease in the standard timeframe based on Society for Vascular Surgery guidelines. ■

SUGGESTED READINGS

Chiesa T, Melissano G, Civilini E, Liberato M, Carozzo A, Zangrillo A. Ten years experience of thoracic and thoracoabdominal aortic aneurysm surgical repair: Lessons learned. *Annals of Vascular Surgery*. 2004;18:514-520.

Coselli JS, et al. Outcomes of 3309 thoracoabdominal aortic aneurysm repairs. *The Journal of Thoracic and Cardiovascular Surgery*. 2016;151(5):1323-1338.

Kieffer E, et al. Type IV thoracoabdominal aneurysm repair: Predictors of postoperative mortality, spinal cord injury, and acute intestinal ischemia. *Annals of Vascular Surgery*. 2008;22:822-828.

Latz C, et al. Durability of open surgical repair of type IV thoracoabdominal aortic aneurysm. *Journal of Vascular Surgery*. 2019;661-670.

Svensson L, Hess K, Coselli JS, Safi H, Crawford ES. A prospective study of respiratory failure after high-risk surgery on the thoracoabdominal aorta. *Journal of Vascular Surgery*. 1991;14(3):271-282.

Wahlgren CM, Wahlberg E. Management of thoracoabdominal aneurysm type IV. *European Journal of Vascular and Endovascular Surgery*. 2005;29:116-123.

38-7

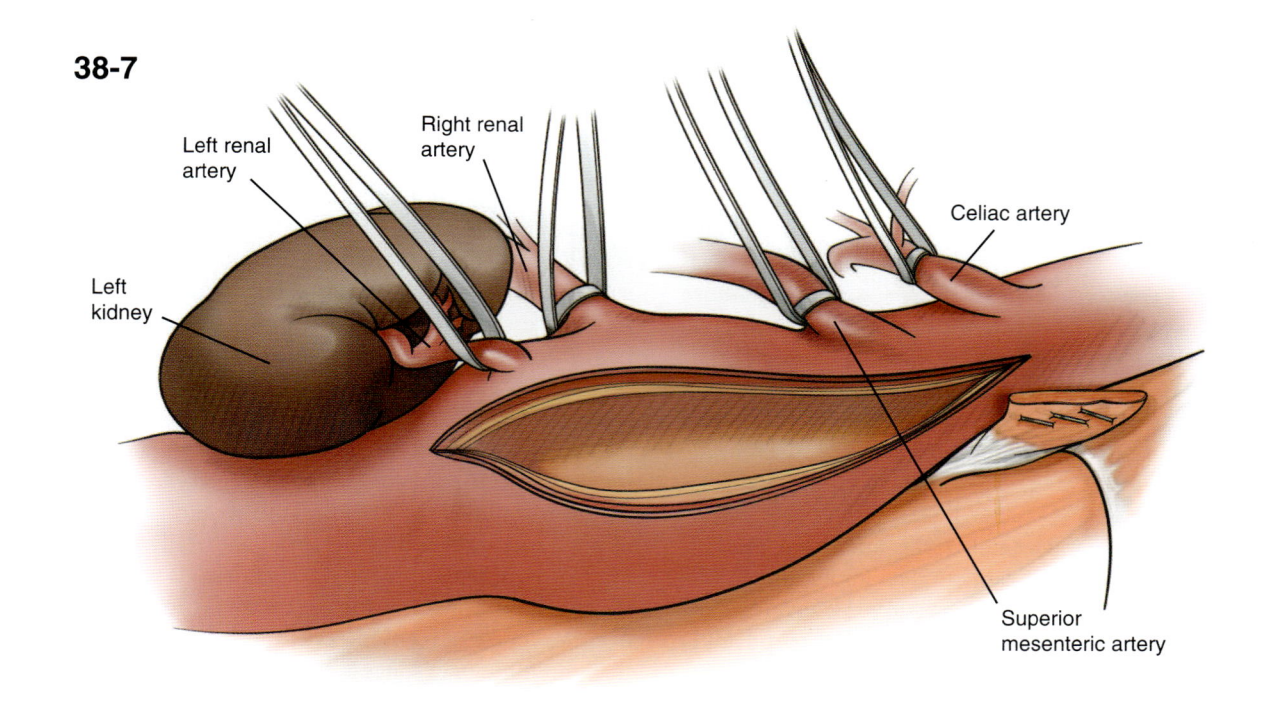

38-8

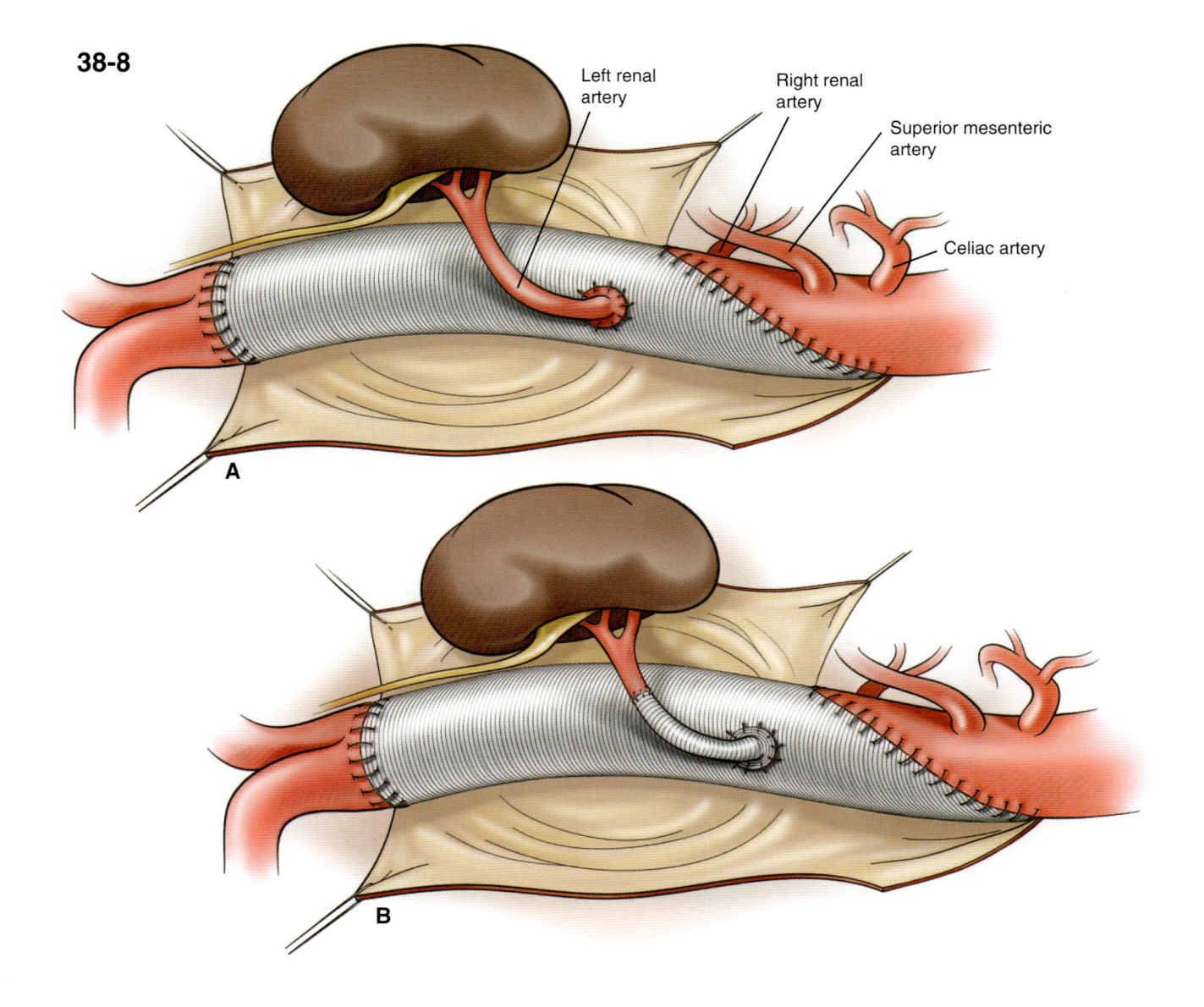

REPAIR OF THORACOABDOMINAL AORTIC ANEURYSMS SECONDARY TO CHRONIC AORTIC DISSECTION

James H. Black III, MD

INDICATIONS The surgical threshold to consider aortic replacement for chronically dissected aortic segments is 5.5 to 6.0 cm in size. Rapid enlargement of an aortic segment, 0.5 cm in 6 months or 1 cm in 1 year, is also an indication for surgical replacement in selected patients. An aneurysm below the 5.5 cm threshold can be considered for surgical repair when those aneurysms become symptomatic. For patients with underlying connective tissue disorders, consideration is given to surgical replacement of the thoracoabdominal aorta when the aneurysm reaches between 5 and 5.5 cm in size, depending upon the patient's personal history of fragility with aortic tissues, family history of rupture or dissection, and the expertise of the surgical team involved.

PREPARATION Repair of thoracoabdominal aortic aneurysm secondary to chronic aortic dissection is a significant surgical undertaking, thus attention should be paid to optimizing the patient's preoperative cardiac, pulmonary, and renal comorbidities. For patients with a history of COPD or emphysema, pulmonary function tests should be performed to assess the patient's vital capacity and determine if single lung isolation, as part of a thoracoabdominal exposure, will be physiologically tolerated. Cardiac reserve can be assessed by echocardiography. It is of particular importance to determine if the patient has any underlying aortic valve abnormalities. Patients with aortic stenosis may not tolerate partial bypass techniques where left ventricular end-diastolic volume will be reduced as part of distal perfusion. Additionally, aortic regurgitation may present significant problems for deep hypothermic circulatory arrest, as an incompetent aortic valve will lead to increased left ventricular pressure during systemic hypothermia, producing fatal subendocardial myocardial ischemia that will prevent separation from bypass. Patients with significant renal insufficiency deserve special consideration. Even with robust distal perfusion techniques and systemic hypothermia, renal complications are not uncommon in thoracoabdominal aortic replacement. Therefore, patients with compromised renal function may not recover from the operation without need for hemodialysis.

ANESTHESIA Close communication between an experienced anesthesia team and an experienced surgical team is mandatory for good outcomes after thoracoabdominal aortic surgery. Before surgical positioning, large bore intravenous and central vein access is obtained. Placement of a transesophageal echocardiogram probe may also be helpful for assessment of cardiac performance during periods of hypotension. It may also aid confirmation of placement of the partial bypass inflow cannula from the inferior pulmonary vein into the left atrium, and confirm the cannula does not reside in the appendage, does not cross into the left ventricle, and does not abut and damage the mitral valve leaflets.

Placement of a lumbar catheter for drainage of cerebrospinal fluid during thoracoabdominal aortic surgery has been proven to reduce the risk for spinal cord injury. This catheter can be placed on the day of the operation;

the author's preference is to place the catheter on the day prior to the operation, for fear that injury to the lumbar vein plexus during placement could increase the risk for epidural hematoma during mandatory systemic anticoagulation or aortic surgery. During thoracoabdominal aortic replacement surgery, drainage from the lumbar catheter should be monitored closely to avoid excessive drainage which would place the patient at risk for subdural hematoma. The drainage system should be zeroed against the left earlobe, keeping the drainage level set at 10 cm of water as a general rule.

Intraoperative assessment of motor evoked potentials (MEPs) using transcranial stimulation may be helpful to guide intraoperative decision-making regarding intercostal patch replacement and spinal cord ischemia. In this technique, the anesthesia team and surgical teams must avoid use of paralytics during the operation. Generally, a twitch monitor maintaining two twitches during a "train of four" is necessary to have stable MEP monitoring throughout the operation. Three successive MEP assessments over the course of 15 minutes demonstrating a greater than 50% decrease in the amplitude may suggest a dominant blood supply to the spinal cord is present within the isolated surgical segment.

POSITION AND PREPARATION The patient is positioned in a right lateral decubitus position and the left arm is extended and lifted cephalad to mobilize the scapula laterally across the left chest wall (FIGURE 39-1A). The table should be flexed to facilitate opening the distance between the iliac crest and the lowest rib. The patient is prepped and draped to allow access to the entire left chest, left flank, and the left groin. Cell-Saver for intraoperative salvage of red blood cells during aortic exposure, aortic opening, and aortic replacement, is mandatory to reduce the need for allogeneic blood transfusions.

INCISION AND EXPOSURE A surgical incision is chosen to facilitate exposure of the aortic segment planned for replacement. Exposure of the thoracoabdominal aorta, in and of itself, is a major surgical operation which should be performed rapidly to reduce body heat losses from convection and radiation into the operating room. As many patients with chronically dissected thoracoabdominal aortic aneurysms will have significant dilation of the distal aortic arch or proximal descending thoracic aorta, a two intercostal incision approach through a single skin incision may be helpful to facilitate exposure of the aortic arch for mobilization and clamping. An incision placed in the fourth intercostal space allows easy inspection of the distal aortic arch, mobilization of the aortic arch by dividing the ligamentum arteriosum, placement of a tourniquet on the left subclavian artery for additional vascular control, and cross-clamping of the mid-aortic arch (FIGURE 39-1B). Alternatively, a single thoracoabdominal incision placed in the sixth intercostal space with resection of the sixth rib along its entire length may also provide suitable access to the proximal descending thoracic aorta; however, mobilization of the aortic arch will be appreciably more difficult. **CONTINUES** ▶

39-1

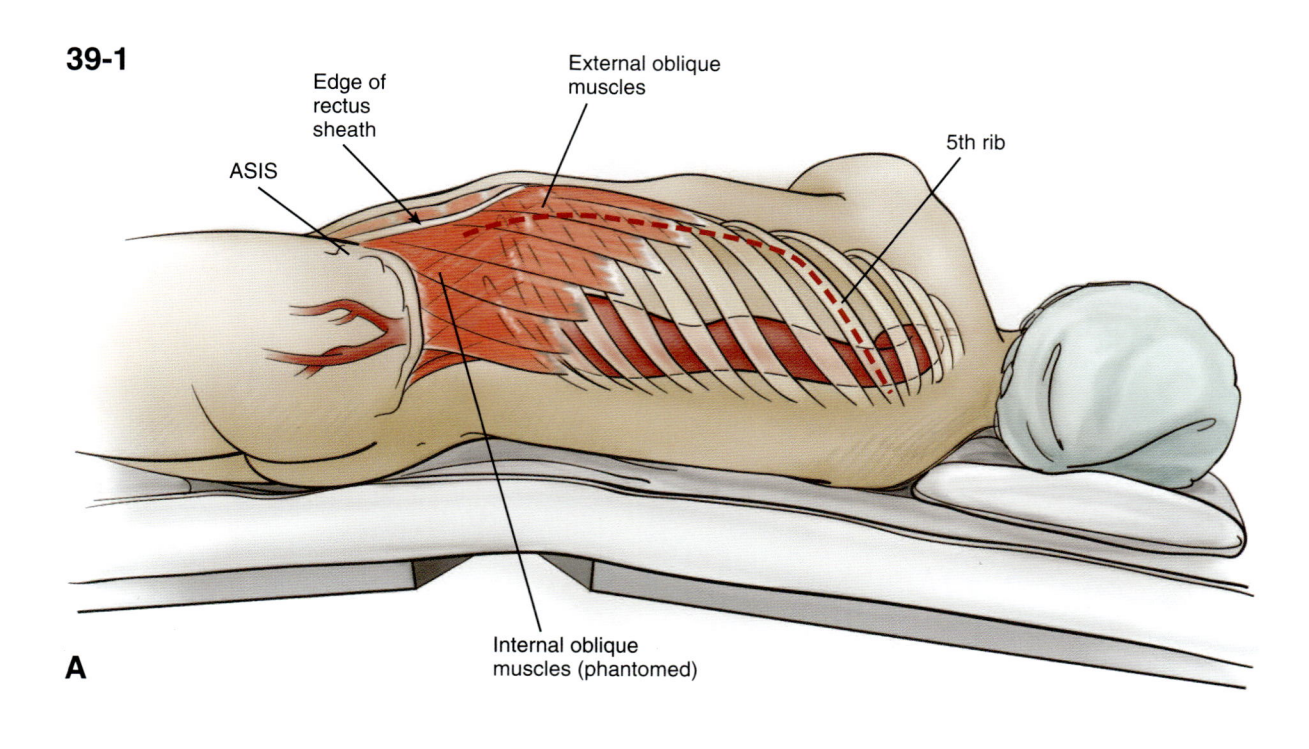

A

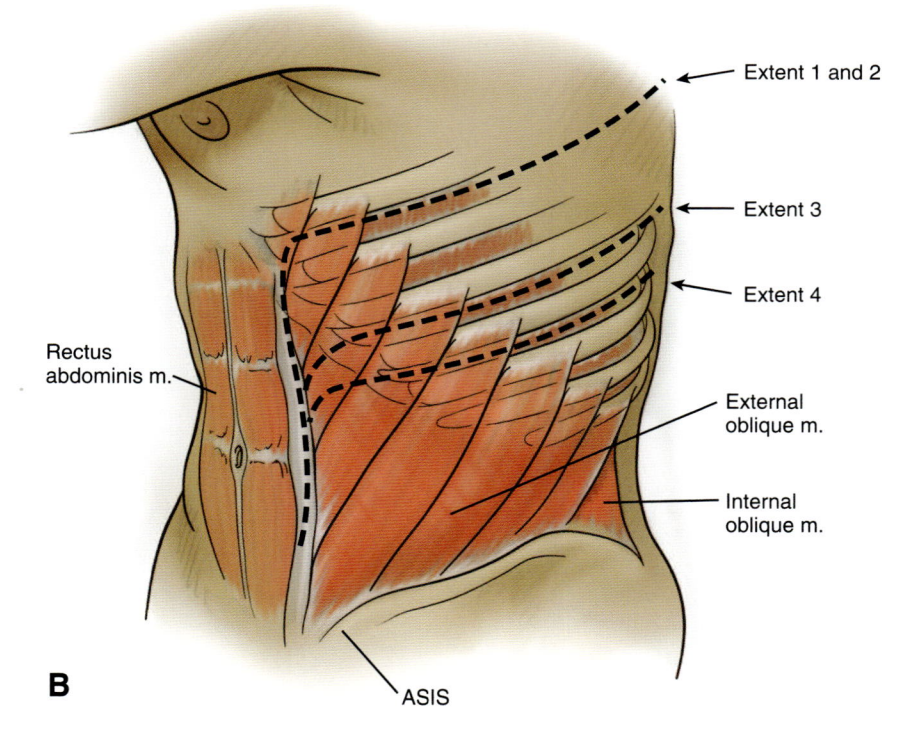

B

INCISION AND EXPOSURE `CONTINUED` Exposure of the distal thoracic aorta, visceral segment of aorta, and abdominal aorta will require division of the diaphragm. A seventh intercostal space incision is most advantageous for this exposure. Preservation of the diaphragm in its anatomic position is not necessary to preserve its postoperative function. The diaphragm can be mobilized circumferentially off the chest wall, leaving the central tendon and the phrenic innervation intact, by leaving a cuff of 3 cm laterally for approximation (**FIGURE 39-2**). It may be advantageous to divide the diaphragm with a gastrointestinal anastomosis to facilitate closure. Additionally, mobilizing the peritoneal sac off the undersurface of the diaphragm is not necessary. The diaphragm can be left on top of the peritoneal sac as the left retroperitoneum is entered; this facilitates approximation of the diaphragm at the final closure of the operation.

DETAILS OF PROCEDURE

PARTIAL BYPASS TECHNIQUE: A partial left heart bypass technique for distal aortic perfusion during the thoracoabdominal surgery has the advantage of providing oxygenated blood to the lower extremity directly through an extracorporeal pump without use of an oxygenator, thus only moderate levels of anticoagulation are required (ACT: 225–300 seconds). A separate circuit may also be added with branches to perfuse the visceral vessels (see Chapter 37). A 20 to 24 French venous cannula is placed into the inferior pulmonary vein under direct venotomy through a purse-string suture and used as inflow for the bypass circuit. Identification of the inferior pulmonary vein is achieved by dividing the inferior pulmonary ligament up to the level of the hilum. It is not necessary or advisable to mobilize inferior pulmonary vein circumferentially, as superior and medial to the inferior pulmonary vein resides the fragile pulmonary artery and left mainstem bronchus (**FIGURE 39-3**). Distal perfusion support for the partial bypass technique is achieved by placing an 8-mm Dacron graft in end-to-side fashion on the left common femoral artery or left external iliac artery, depending upon the extent of distal aortoiliac exposure planned. This 8-mm Dacron graft allows antegrade perfusion down the left leg as well as retrograde perfusion into the aortoiliac system for end-organ support. Importantly, maintaining left-leg antegrade circulation allows for continuous assessment of MEPs, without an occlusive arterial cannula producing distal limb ischemia that may be misinterpreted as spinal cord injury under MEP monitoring. `CONTINUES`

39-2

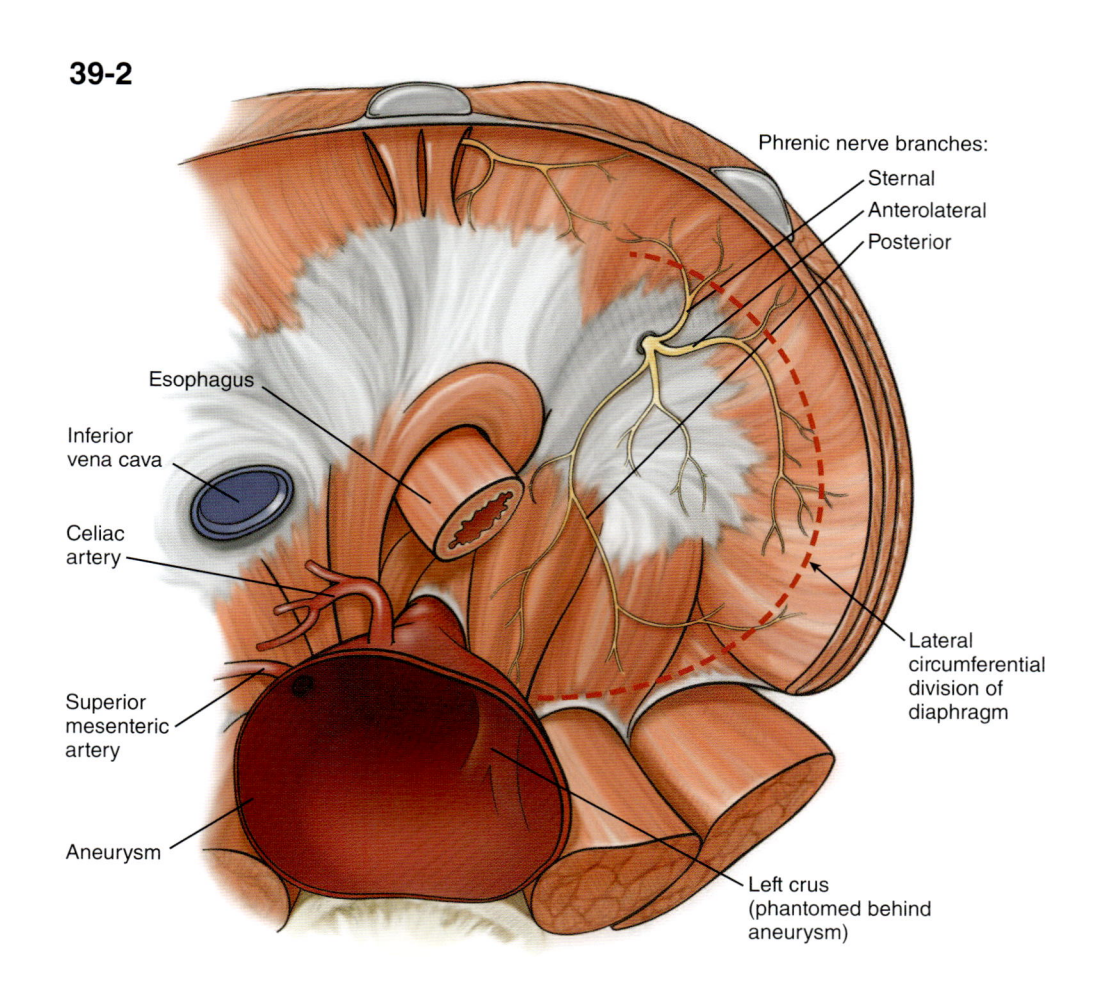

39-3

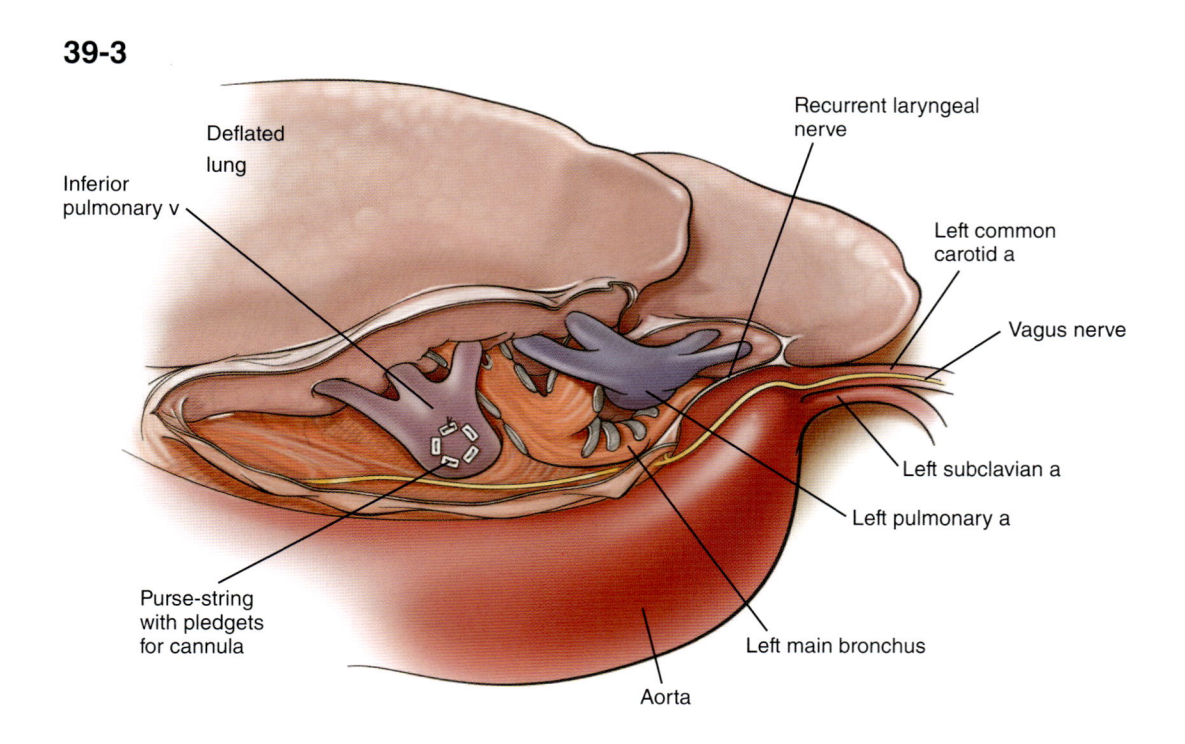

DETAILS OF PROCEDURE *SEQUENTIAL AORTIC CROSS-CLAMPING:* CONTINUED Identification of cross-clamp sites extending through the thoracoabdominal aorta is an advantageous gateway during aortic replacement surgery to reduce blood loss from intercostal bleeding, identify aortic segments that may contribute to spinal cord circulation under MEP monitoring, and foster hemodynamic instability (FIGURE 39-4). In patients with chronic aortic dissections and extensive thoracoabdominal aortic aneurysms, it is not uncommon that control of the distal aorta requires two aortic cross clamps—one may provide initial aortic control of the true lumen, and a second clamp for additional compression of thin-walled false lumen. A proximal cross-clamp site may be placed on the distal aortic arch or proximal descending thoracic aorta, inclusive of underlying chronic aortic dissections, even when present in the aortic arch. Anesthesia teams should maintain a proximal aortic pressure of 90 to 100 mmHg to reduce risk of clamp injury or new retrograde dissection. A second cross-clamp is placed in the region of the sixth thoracic vertebrae. This length of aortotomy allows a comfortable anastomosis, while the bypass circuit maintains distal perfusion. Once the proximal anastomosis is completed, a clamp is placed on the distal thoracic aorta, isolating the T7 to T10 region. During 10 to 15 minutes of aortic cross-clamping, MEPs are closely watched. A rapid decrease in the amplitude of the MEPs suggests that dominant circulation to the spinal cord is present in this area, and an intercostal inclusion patch is mandatory (FIGURE 39-5). The next sequential aortic cross-clamp site is considered below the renal vessels. This allows opening of the visceral segment of aorta, excision of the dissection flaps, ligation of lumbar arteries, and placement of a surgical graft to re-perfuse the critical visceral and renal branches. Individual "octopus" branches are placed for perfusion in each vessel. The last aortic cross-clamp site is placed at the aortic bifurcation or the bilateral common iliac arteries to facilitate the distal anastomosis at that level; this allows a suitable length of proximal aorta.

ANASTOMOTIC TECHNIQUE FOR AORTIC DISSECTION: Patients with acute aortic dissections or patients with chronic aortic dissection with underlying connective tissue disorders may have significant tissue fragility that produces surgical bleeding with simple needle penetration of the tissues as part of routine anastomotic technique. The proximal aorta is mobilized circumferentially for a distance of 2 or 3 cm. The dissection flap present within the aortic lumen is cut back to the level of the proximal aortic clamp and a 1-cm strip of Teflon felt is laid underneath the posterior aspect of the mobilized aorta (FIGURE 39-6). CONTINUES

39-4

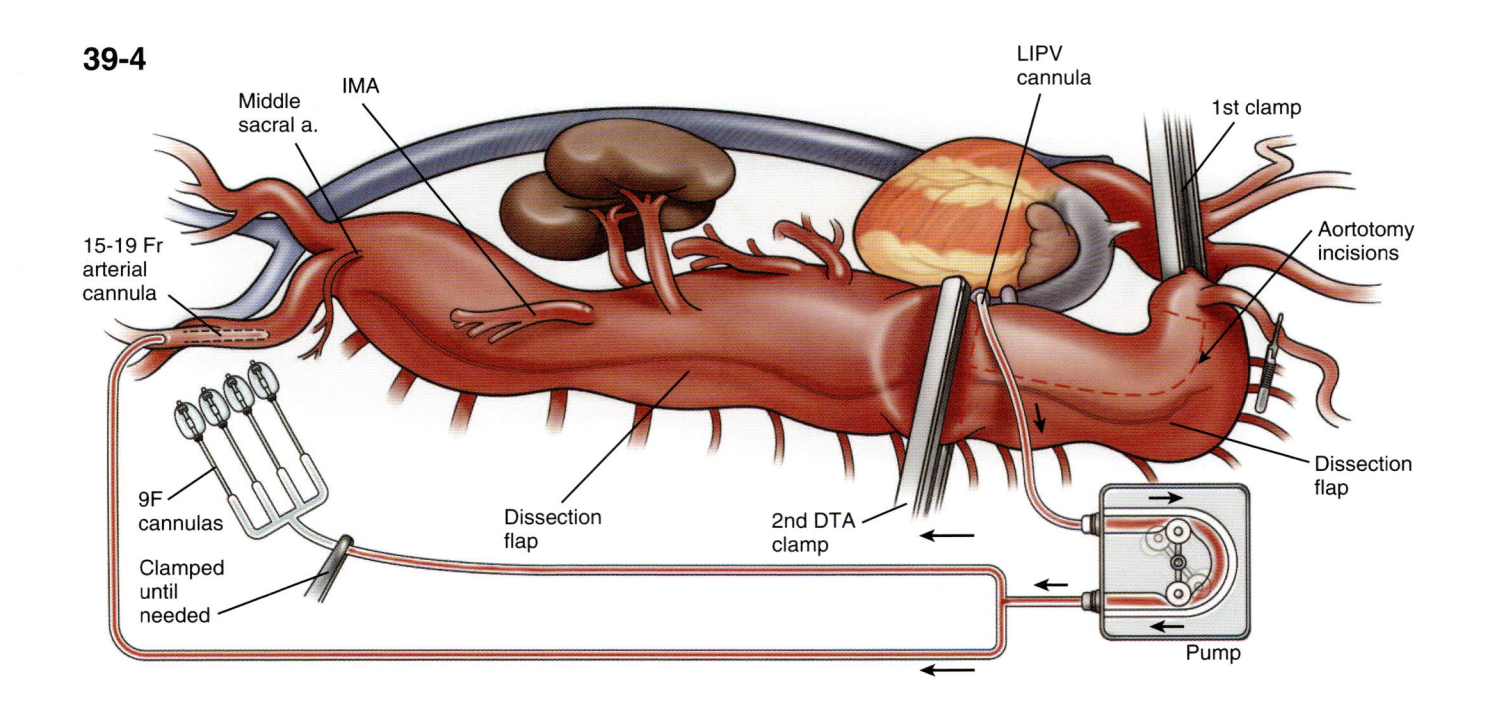

39-5

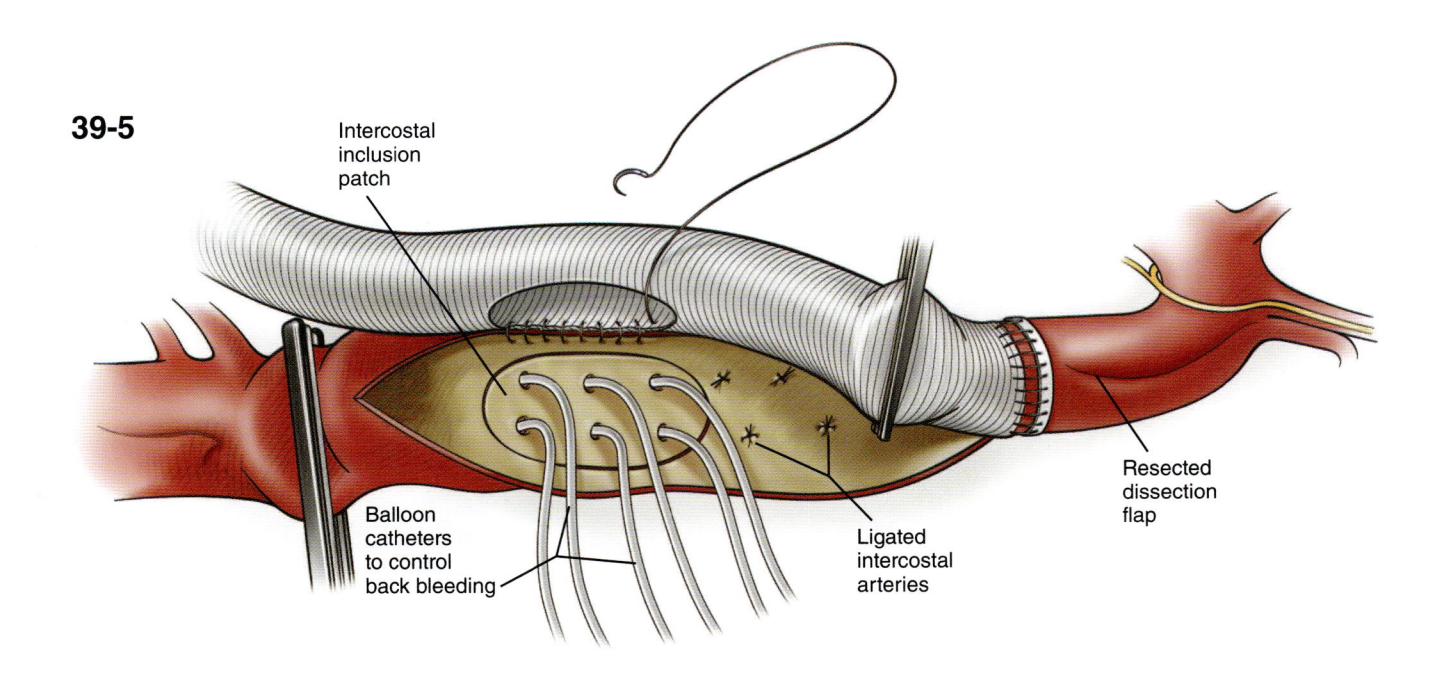

39-6

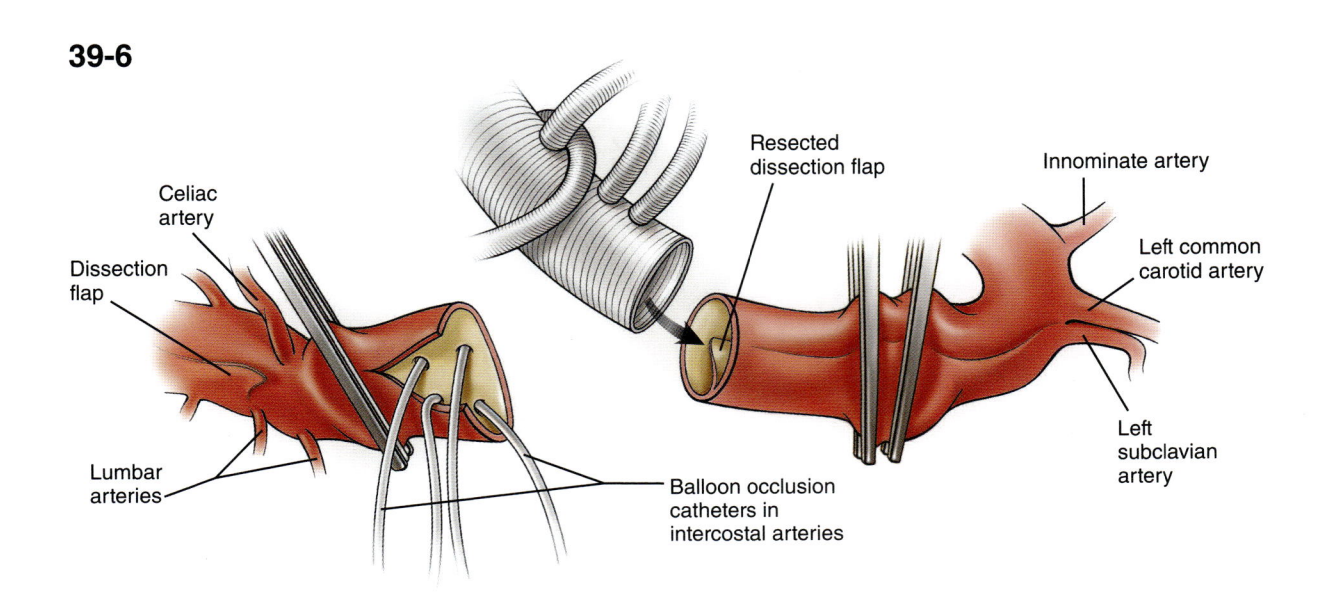

DETAILS OF PROCEDURE *ANASTOMOTIC TECHNIQUE FOR AORTIC DISSECTION:* ◀CONTINUED A key technical point is that the surgical suture should be passed through the leading edge of the Teflon strip, and the native tissue should be sutured 1 or 2 cm proximally (**FIGURE 39-7A** and **B**). This allows the surgical felt to be pulled proximally, away from the anastomosis, sandwiching the aortic tissue between the felt strip and the Dacron graft seated in the aortic lumen. Circumferential reinforcement of an end-to-end surgical anastomosis with felt is a technique that is optimal and a special gateway for such patients. If sewing to a stent graft, it is often helpful to have a second layer of felt on the inside of the graft. If the needle passes through the deep edge of the Teflon felt in error, the felt strip will be pulled across the aortic edge, obscuring the interface between the aortic graft and the native artery native aortic lumen.

INTERCOSTAL PATCH TECHNIQUE FOR AORTIC DISSECTION: Patients with extensive aortic dissections and chronic thoracoabdominal aortic aneurysms may have robust intercostal collaterals along the vertebral column which maintain spinal cord function despite intercostal origin ligation. Intraoperative assessment of MEPs is helpful to identify these patients who do not require intercostal patch reimplantation. *Performance of an intercostal inclusion patch may be one of the most difficult surgical anastomoses in all of aortic surgery.* The quality of the mid-thoracic aorta in most patients with chronic aortic dissections and thoracoabdominal aneurysms is suspect and fragile. In this regard, placement of a long inclusion patch is likely to present a significant hazard for surgical bleeding. If confronted with loss of MEPS during thoracoabdominal aortic surgery, the surgeon should choose to implant a pair of T8 or T9 intercostal vessels, as this is a likely location of dominant spinal cord circulation on anatomic studies. A thin and/or calcified false lumen wall should *not* be chosen for suturing. To construct an intercostal inclusion patch of a pair of intercostal arteries, pledgeted 3-0 prolene sutures are taken in a horizontal mattress fashion circumferentially around the intercostal vessels (**FIGURE 39-8A** and **B**). CONTINUES▶

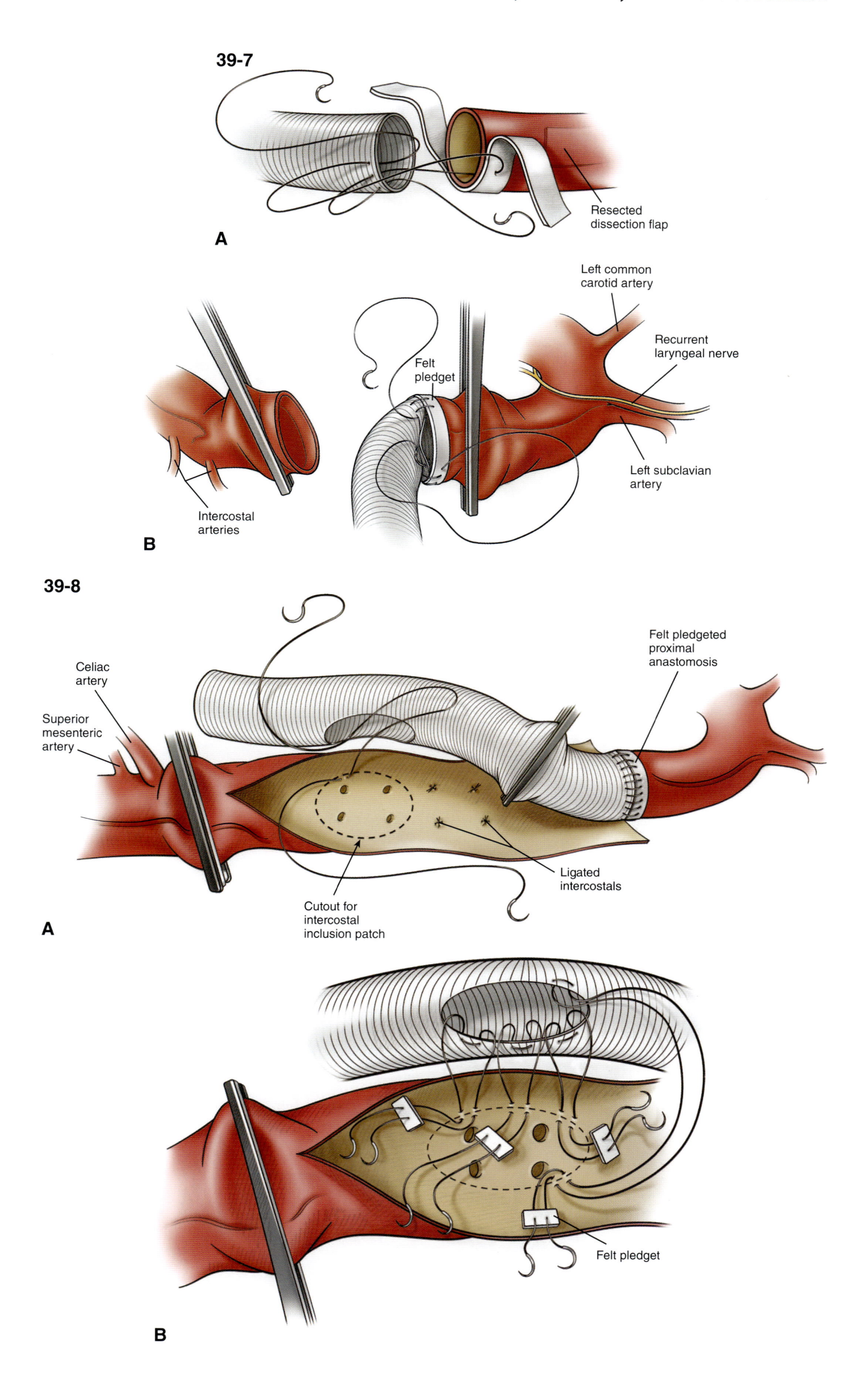

39-7

Resected
dissection flap

A

Left common
carotid artery

Recurrent
laryngeal nerve

Felt
pledget

Left subclavian
artery

Intercostal
arteries

B

39-8

Celiac
artery

Superior
mesenteric
artery

Felt pledgeted
proximal
anastomosis

Ligated
intercostals

Cutout for
intercostal
inclusion patch

A

Felt pledget

B

DETAILS OF PROCEDURE *INTERCOSTAL PATCH TECHNIQUE FOR AORTIC DISSECTION:* **CONTINUED** It is important to maintain a 1- to 2-cm margin around the individual intercostal artery origin to prevent occlusion of the intercostal artery as it courses posterior to the aorta. Make certain you are sewing to the true lumen of the intercostals and not the false lumen. This is a key gateway, as not recognizing there are two lumens can lead to sewing to the wrong spot (FIGURE 39-9).

ABDOMINAL AORTIC RECONSTRUCTION: It is not uncommon for chronic aortic dissections to have significant involvement of the visceral and renal vessels of the abdominal aorta. The dissection flaps present within the abdominal aorta or branches should be cut back to the aortic wall or branch origin prior to attempt of reconstruction of the visceral and renal branches. For patients with underlying connective tissue disorders or young patients with chronic dissections, a branched surgical Coselli graft (FIGURE 39-9) may be preferable to an inclusion patch technique for the visceral arteries (FIGURE 39-10A and B) to reduce the risk for late inclusion patch aneurysm. Similarly, involvement of the iliac vessels by the dissection may produce significant aneurysms requiring additional surgical graft replacement. **CONTINUES**

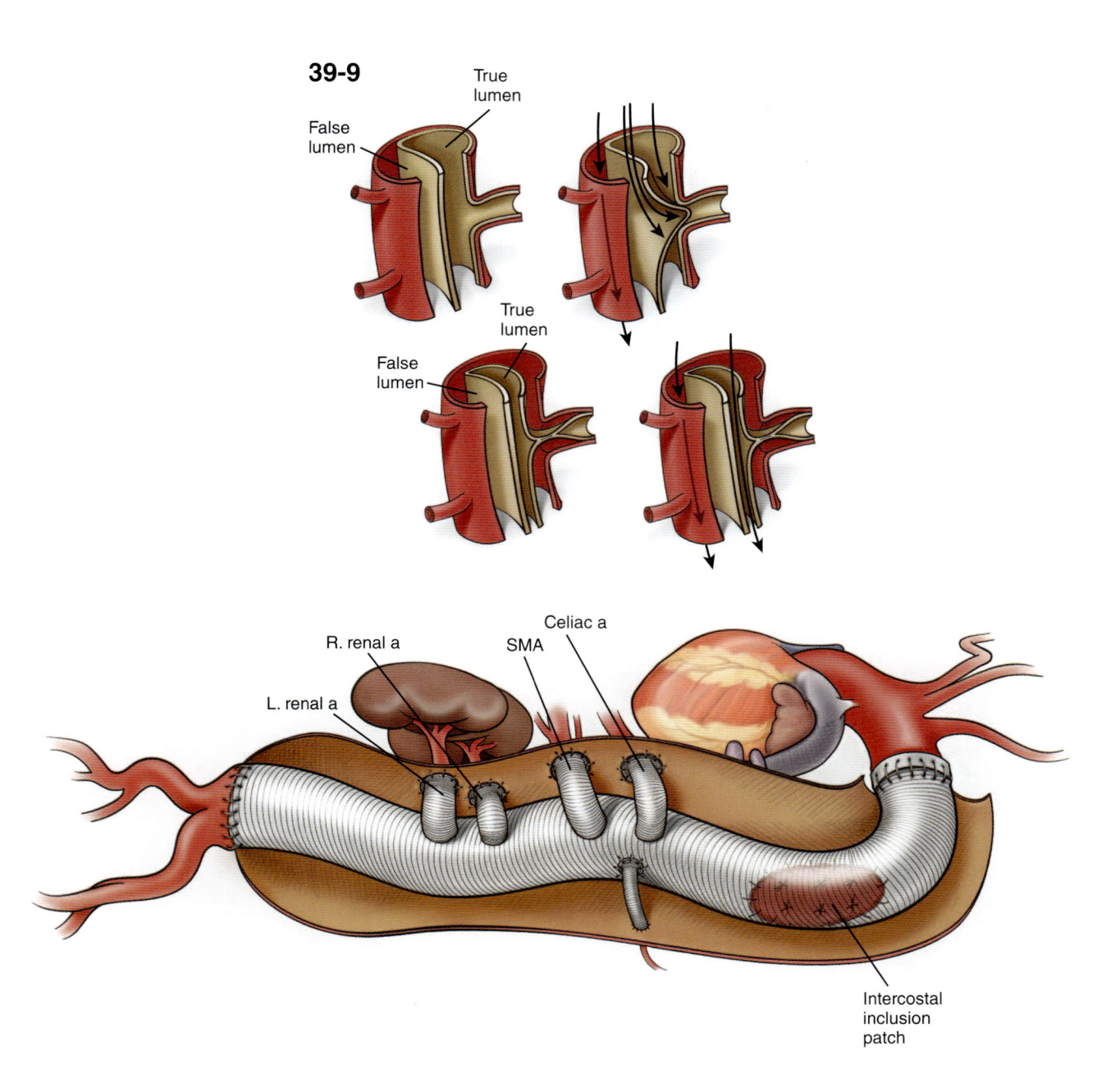

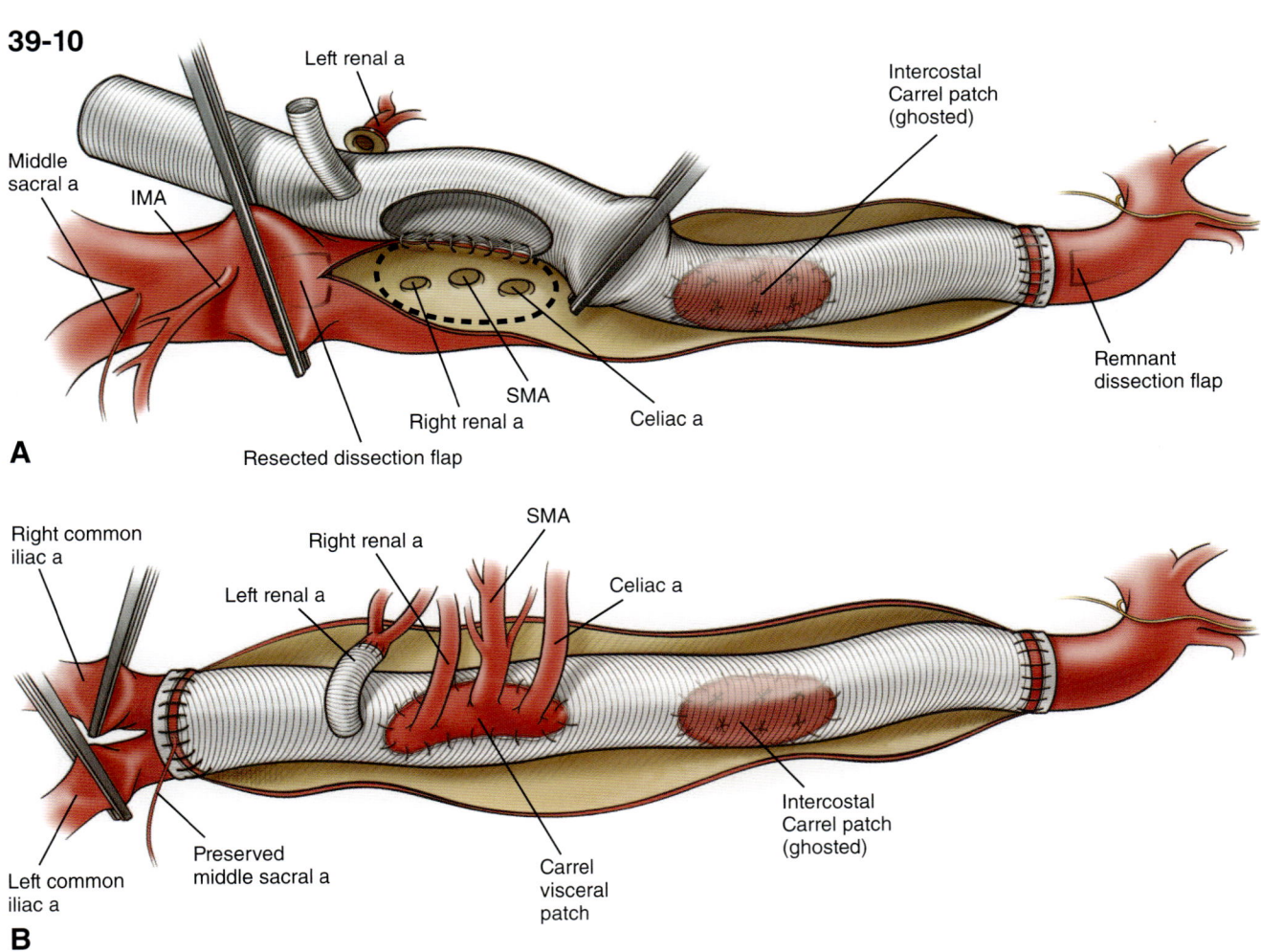

DETAILS OF PROCEDURE *ABDOMINAL AORTIC RECONSTRUCTION:* **CONTINUED** The surgeon should not be constrained to the standard bifurcated grafts; use of a large diameter 16- to 20-mm surgical graft into an iliac aneurysm is usually the safest course of action for direct reconstruction (**FIGURE 39-11**). Every attempt should be made to preserve the middle sacral artery and nearby lumbar arteries, which are key blood supply to the spinal cord, if possible.

POSTOPERATIVE CARE Postoperative management of patients who undergo extensive thoracoabdominal aortic replacement surgery for chronic aortic dissections requires vigilant management of expected postoperative coagulopathy, labile hemodynamics, and serial examination for surgical bleeding from indwelling chest and retroperitoneal drains. Intensive blood pressure management for a target systolic blood pressure of 90 to 140 mmHg is appropriate for most patients. At this level of blood pressure, end-organ function should be preserved and spinal cord circulation should be maintained. Maintenance of lumbar drainage of cerebrospinal fluid should be maintained for 48 to 72 hours. At that point the catheter can be removed and lower extremity neurologic function can be assessed daily. Late onset spinal cord dysfunction should be treated with reinsertion of a lumbar catheter for spinal drainage and pharmacologically induced hypertension (mean arterial pressure 110–130 mmHg) to promote collateral perfusion to ischemic spinal neurons. ■

SUGGESTED READINGS

Black JH. Technique for repair of suprarenal and thoracoabdominal aortic aneurysms. *J Vasc Surg.* 2009:50(4):936-941.

Coselli JS, Bozinovski J. Hypothermic circulatory arrest: safety and efficacy in the operative treatment of descending and thoracoabdominal aortic aneurysms. *Ann Thorac Surg.* 2008;85:956-964.

Coselli JS, Lemaire SA, Koksoy C, Schmittling ZC, Curling PE. Cerebrospinal fluid drainage reduces paraplegia after thoracoabdominal aortic aneurysm repair: Results of a randomized clinical trial. *J Vasc Surg.* 2002;35;631-639.

Hicks CW, Lue J, Glebova NO, Ehlert BA, Black JH 3rd. A 10 year institutional experience with open branched graft reconstruction of aortic aneurysms in connective tissue disorders versus degenerative disease. *J Vasc Surg.* 2017 Nov;66(5):1406-1416. Jun 22 (epub).

39-11

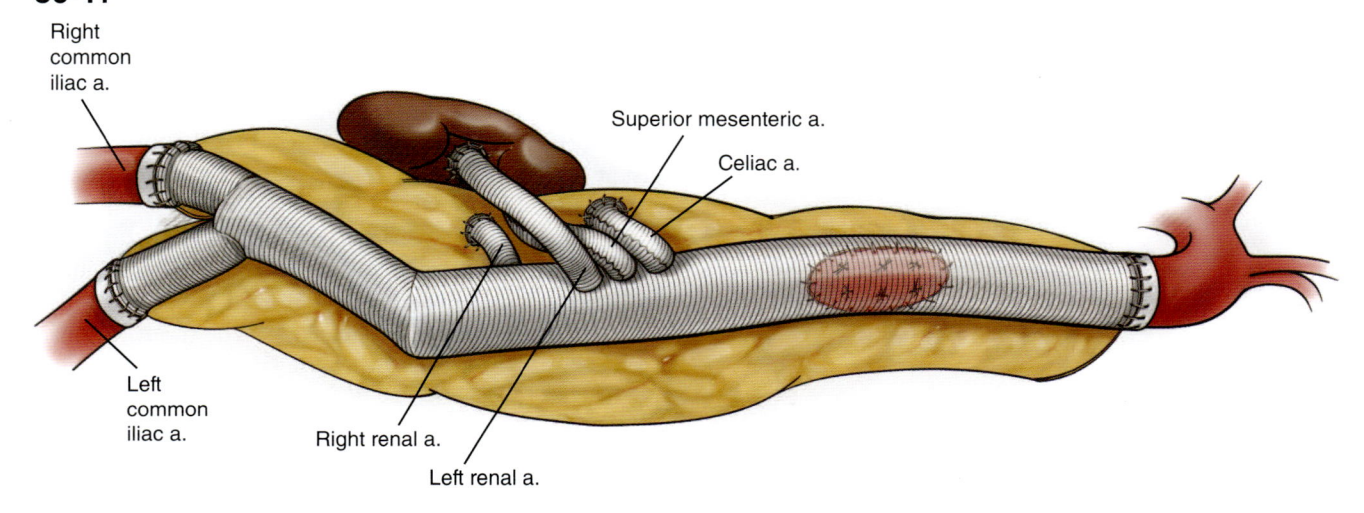

Right common iliac a.

Superior mesenteric a.

Celiac a.

Left common iliac a.

Right renal a.

Left renal a.

Veno-Arterial Bypass and Hybrid Thoracoabdominal Aortic Aneurysm Repair

Amanda C. Filiberto, MD • Gilbert R. Upchurch Jr, MD

INDICATIONS Untreated extensive thoracoabdominal aortic aneurysms (TAAAs) have mortality rates as high as 75% at 2 years, with most deaths attributed to rupture. Traditional open TAAA repair can be performed with acceptable results at high-volume aortic centers; however, mortality rates of 10 to 40% remain nationally. Thoracic endovascular aneurysm repair (TEVAR) has decreased aneurysm repair-related mortality and morbidity compared with open surgery for isolated thoracic aortic aneurysms. Given the high mortality and complication rates, especially associated with renal failure and paraplegia/paraparesis, hybrid approaches to TAAA repair emerged.

The early hybrid approach was first described as an open operation in which the visceral segment of the abdominal aorta was debranched via extra-anatomic bypass grafts originating from the distal abdominal aorta or iliac arteries to provide a distal seal zone for subsequent second-stage placement of a thoracic endograft (see Chapter 32). Comparative analysis of intermediate-term outcomes found this approach to be associated with a higher risk for early morbidity and a higher risk for reoperation when compared with open TAAA repair. Thus, we sought to describe a "staged hybrid" approach in which the endovascular portion of the procedure was performed first, allowing conversion of type II and III into type IV TAAAs, thereby lowering the accompanying mortality and morbidity. Comparative recent analyses documented that a staged hybrid approach that starts with the endovascular repair followed by open TAAA repair is associated with a lower composite measure of death, spinal cord ischemia, and renal failure. This approach is therefore a suitable therapeutic option, particularly in those considered high risk for standard open type II and III repair, including those with TAAAs associated with aortic dissections.

PREOPERATIVE PREPARATION Patients present either as an emergency after acute type B dissection or as an elective case for chronic TAAA evaluation. Elective patients should undergo a full preoperative workup, including risk factor modification and medical optimization. Adequate imaging with computerized tomographic angiography (CTA) scanning with thin cuts (1 mm or less) of the entire thoracic and abdominal aorta down through the femoral arteries is mandatory for sizing an endograft. After careful review of the patient's comorbidities, TAAA etiology, and anatomic appropriateness, a staged hybrid repair with TEVAR of the proximal aorta followed by open surgical repair of the distal aorta may be considered first-line treatment.

If the origin of the dissection flap is <2 cm of the origin of the left subclavian artery, a left common-to-left subclavian artery bypass should be performed prior to TEVAR to extend the proximal landing zone. Typically, the left subclavian artery is not ligated during the carotid-to-subclavian bypass to allow possible left brachial artery access to guide TEVAR placement. In general, coiling of the proximal left subclavian artery is performed at the time of TEVAR.

OPERATIVE PREPARATION AND POSITION

STAGE 1. ENDOVASCULAR TECHNIQUE: Patients are placed in the supine position and should be prepped from nipples to knees in the event conversion to an open procedure is required. A spinal drain is typically placed the day before, given the extent of aneurysm being treated is associated with the highest paraplegia risk. Routine central venous line access and arterial line access are required. An arterial line should be placed on the patient's right side to allow for access to the left brachial artery. See Chapter 42 for detailed description of TEVAR.

STAGE 2. OPEN DISTAL TAAA REPAIR TECHNIQUE: Spinal drains should be placed prophylactically for cerebrospinal fluid drainage. Typically, a right femoral arterial line is placed under sterile conditions while in the supine position using ultrasound prior to positioning and prepping the patient. This allows the perfusionist to better monitor flows on the bypass circuit. The patient is positioned in a partial right lateral decubitus position with left side up to allow for thoracoabdominal and left groin exposure (see Chapters 37 and 39). Patients may undergo either left-sided heart cardiopulmonary bypass with inflow from the left inferior pulmonary vein or left atrium and outflow to the left femoral artery. Another option is partial cardiopulmonary bypass with inflow from the right atrium via a left femoral venous cannula and outflow into the left femoral artery. Individual perfusion cannulas coming off the bypass circuit can be inserted into the visceral, renal, and spinal arteries upon opening the TAAA visceral segment. While percutaneous approach is always feasible, it is best to perform a cutdown for both the left femoral artery and vein to allow safe and simple closure at completion. The sizes of these cannulas vary based on the size of the native arteries, and can range from 12 to 26 F, typically bigger in the vein than the artery. Each individual cannula is removed as the anastomosis of each branch artery nears completion to minimize ischemia reperfusion time. While we have used circulatory arrest in some of these complex patients, especially with previous visceral patch aneurysms or complex dissections, in general when femoral artery and vein bypass is used, standard cardiopulmonary doses of heparin can be decreased.

DETAILS OF THE PROCEDURE

STAGE 1. ENDOVASCULAR TECHNIQUE: TEVAR is performed in the standard fashion often requiring multiple stent grafts (see Chapter 44). Access may be obtained via percutaneous, open femoral, or open iliac. The goal of TEVAR coverage should be as extensive as possible, with approximate aortic coverage from the level of the left subclavian artery origin to just above the level of the celiac artery. The stent graft should be oversized proximally 10 to 20% to achieve a proximal seal. The distal size should be based on the distal aortic true lumen size, which is determined using a curved line measurement of the ellipsoid of the true lumen aortic circumference just proximal to the origin of the celiac artery. It is important to note that the endograft distally needs to be sized such that it is compatible with the open graft that it will be sewn on to after performing a septotomy.

STAGE 2. OPEN DISTAL TAAA REPAIR TECHNIQUE: After dissecting the distal thoracic, visceral, and aortic segments via a thoraco-retroperitoneal exposure, control of the celiac, super mesenteric, and left renal artery is obtained with vessel loops (**FIGURE 40-1**). Heparin is given, and the midthoracic aorta and underlying endovascular stent are occluded with a Fogarty hydrogrip aortic clamp(s) (**FIGURE 40-2**). Be prepared to have two large Fogarty hydrogrip clamps available, as the first may not be 100% occlusive. The infrarenal aorta/iliac arteries are then clamped, and the lower half of the body is perfused via bypass (see Chapters 37 and 39). The aortic aneurysm sac is entered, and the visceral arteries are cannulated with individual catheters from the bypass system to allow visceral perfusion during prolonged aortic occlusion. If the infrarenal abdominal aorta is not severely diseased, the distal aortic clamp may be initially placed across the supraceliac aorta, allowing retrograde visceral perfusion from the bypass circuit to the visceral and renal arteries as well as the arteries supplying the spinal cord. At the time of the distal anastomosis, the clamp should be temporarily moved to the infrarenal aorta with minimal visceral ischemic time. **CONTINUES** ▶

40-1

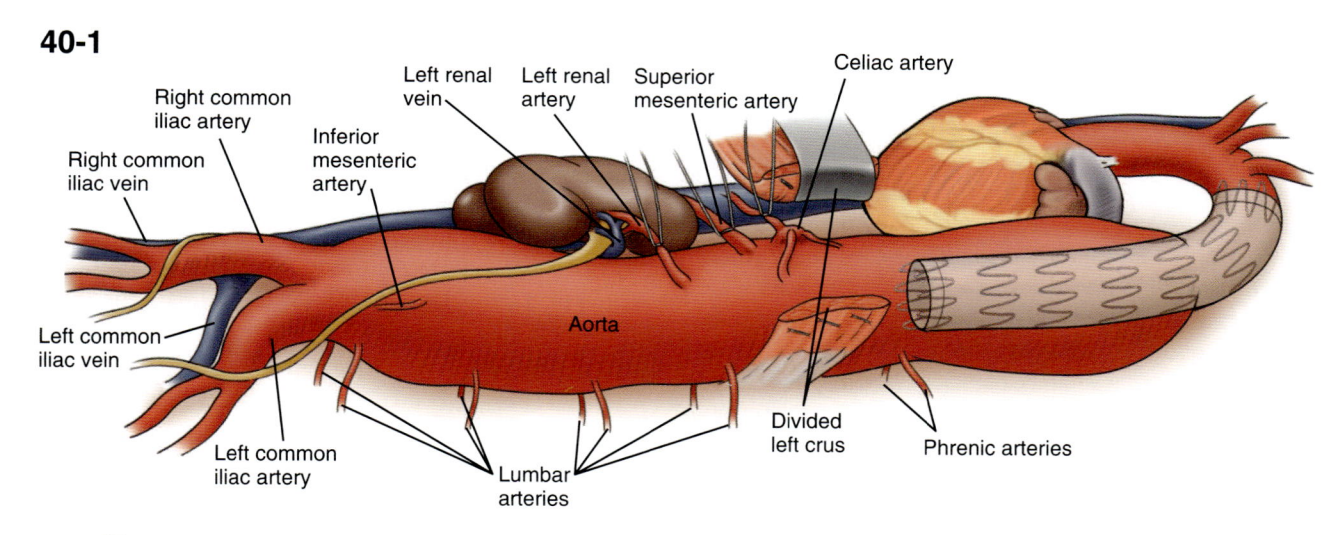

Figure 40-1 Type II thoracoabdominal aneurysm with initial thoracic aorta stent graft placed (TEVAR).

40-2

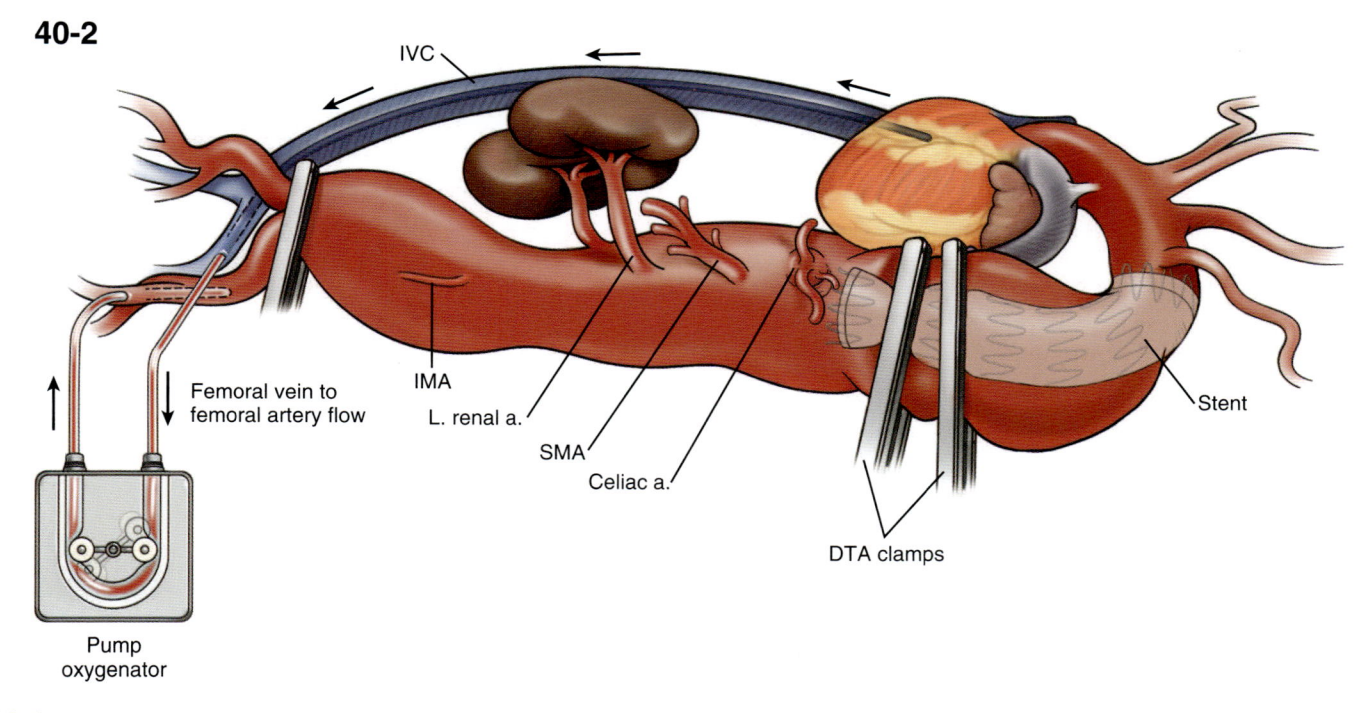

Figure 40-2 Partial cardiopulmonary bypass initiated after the aorta is clamped with two Fogarty hydrogrip clamps proximally and the native aorta at the bifurcation.

DETAILS OF THE PROCEDURE *STAGE 2. OPEN DISTAL TAAA REPAIR TECHNIQUE:* **CONTINUED** The thoracic aorta and underlying endograft are divided together; wire cutters may be required to divide the endograft (**FIGURE 40-3**). The aortic lumen is cleared of thrombus and debris, and the dissection septum is divided proximally for approximately 3 to 5 cm to allow full endograft expansion. The thoracic aorta is tapered to closely approximate the endograft diameter (**FIGURE 40-4**). The proximal anastomosis is performed, attaching the new Dacron graft directly to the endograft, tapered aortic wall, and circumferential outer wall felt reinforcement. It can be beneficial to use both an inner and outer layer of felt to minimize leakage from needle holes through the stent graft. The involved visceral vessels are anastomosed end-to-end with graft branches from a multibranch aortic graft or as an inclusion patch to the main aortic graft (see Chapters 37 and 39). The visceral segment is reconstructed by either: (1) a beveled anastomosis that incorporates the origin of the visceral arteries, (2) an aortic patch for celiac, superior mesenteric artery, and right renal arteries with a separate anastomosis for the left renal artery, or (3) using a multibranch graft with separate anastomoses for each visceral vessel. Performance of the right renal artery anastomosis first, followed by the left renal, the superior mesenteric artery, the celiac, and finally the distal aortic anastomosis, is our sequence of repair. Large intercostal vessels, when identified, are preserved and reimplanted into the graft or bypassed with a short 6-mm Dacron graft or ringed ePTFE attached to the aortic graft (**FIGURE 40-5**). The timing of this is somewhat controversial, with a recent move to performing this early in the sequence of the operation. Universally, when the aorta is dissected or when performing the staged hybrid repair in patients with connective tissue disease, an end-to-end graft to each visceral and renal artery is preferred.

POSTOPERATIVE CARE After major aortic surgery, patients should be recovered in a dedicated ICU familiar with spinal drains, and subsequently transferred to a dedicated cardiovascular ward to be actively monitored. Generally, the individual surgeon's discretion determines timing of care transition and discharge based on patient factors. Patients typically remain in the ICU for at least 48 to 72 hours and may be transferred to the ward after remaining hemodynamically stable without need for vasoactive agents, have acceptable pain control to ensure mobility, and have adequate urine output with normal renal biochemistry and a stable hematocrit.

SURVEILLANCE: Patients should undergo CT angiography (CTA) of the chest, abdomen, and pelvis between day one and five after stent placement to evaluate stent position, endoleaks, and aortic dimensions. It is best to fix any undiscovered issues especially related to type 1A endoleaks at this time. Patients following the second stage of the staged hybrid repair should then be monitored closely in the clinic, with visits every 3 to 6 months and CTA performed at 1 month, 6 months, 1 year, and then annually. ■

SUGGESTED READING

Hawkins RB, Mehaffey JH, Narahari AK, et al. Improved outcomes, and value in staged hybrid extent II thoracoabdominal aortic aneurysm repair. *J Vasc Surg.* 2017 Nov;66(5):1357-1363. doi:10.1016/j.jvs.2017.03.420. Epub 2017 May 31. PMID: 28579290; PMCID: PMC5654680.

Jain A, Flohr TF, Johnston WF, et al. Staged hybrid repair of extensive thoracoabdominal aortic aneurysms secondary to chronic aortic dissection. *J Vasc Surg.* 2016 Jan;63(1):62-69. doi: 10.1016/j.jvs.2015.08.060. Epub 2015 Oct 1. PMID: 26432283.

Johnston WF, Upchurch GR Jr, Tracci MC, et al. Staged hybrid approach using proximal thoracic endovascular aneurysm repair and distal open repair for the treatment of extensive thoracoabdominal aortic aneurysms. *J Vasc Surg.* 2012 Dec;56(6):1495-1502. doi: 10.1016/j.jvs.2012.05.091. Epub 2012 Jul 24. PMID: 22832268; PMCID: PMC3508078.

Kabbani LS, Criado E, Upchurch GR Jr, et al. Hybrid repair of aortic aneurysms involving the visceral and renal vessels. *Ann Vasc Surg.* 2010 Feb;24(2):219-224. doi: 10.1016/j.avsg.2009.08.007. Epub 2009 Nov 25. PMID: 19932951.

Patel HJ, Upchurch GR Jr, Eliason JL, et al. Hybrid debranching with endovascular repair for thoracoabdominal aneurysms: a comparison with open repair. *Ann Thorac Surg.* 2010 May;89(5):1475-1481. doi: 10.1016/j.athoracsur.2010.01.062. PMID: 20417763.

Patel R, Conrad MF, Paruchuri V, et al. Thoracoabdominal aneurysm repair: hybrid versus open repair. *J Vasc Surg.* 2009 Jul;50(1):15-22. doi: 10.1016/j.jvs.2008.12.051. PMID: 19563950.

Quiñones-Baldrich WJ, Panetta TF, Vescera CL, et al. Repair of type IV thoracoabdominal aneurysm with a combined endovascular and surgical approach. *J Vasc Surg.* 1999 Sep;30(3):555-560. doi: 10.1016/s0741-5214(99)70084-4. PMID: 10477650.

40-3

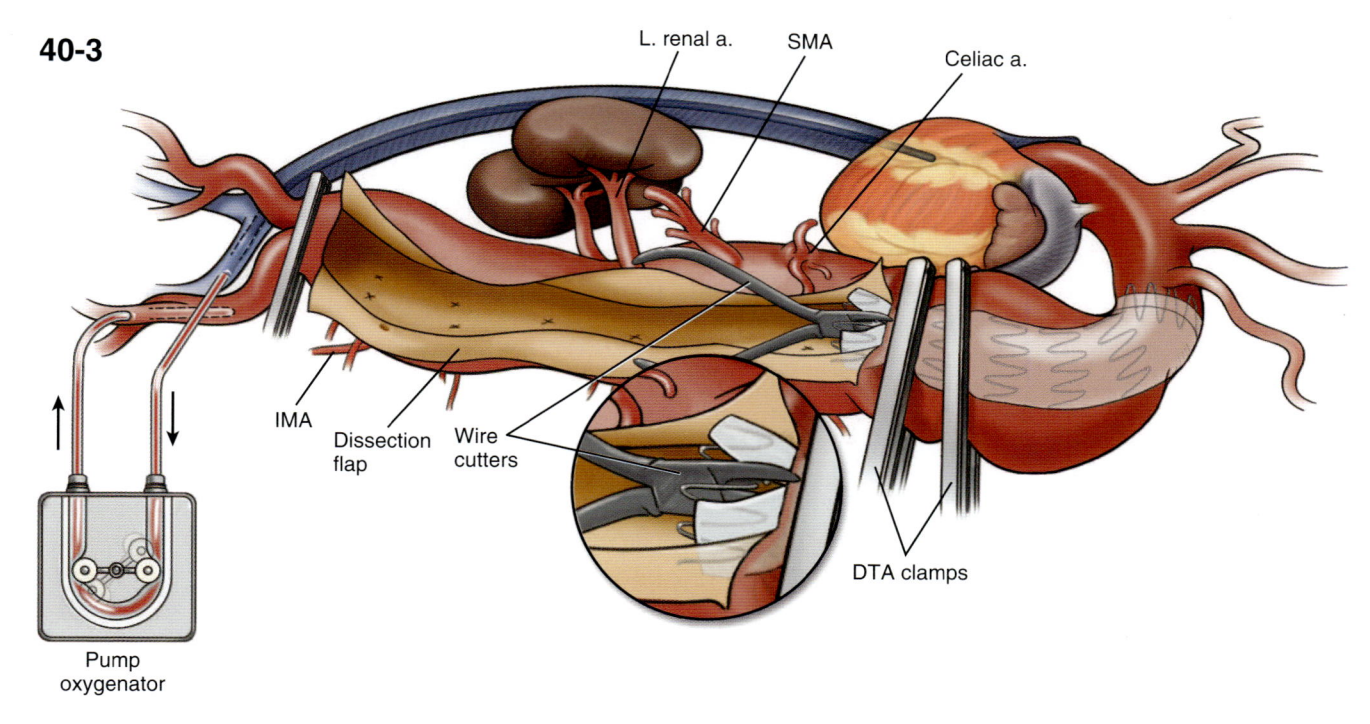

Figure 40-3 Once the aorta is cross-clamped, the TAA sac is incised. Thrombus/debris is removed from the false lumen, the dissection septum is divided, and the aortic wall is cut and tapered. Wire cutters are used to cut part of stent graft.

40-4

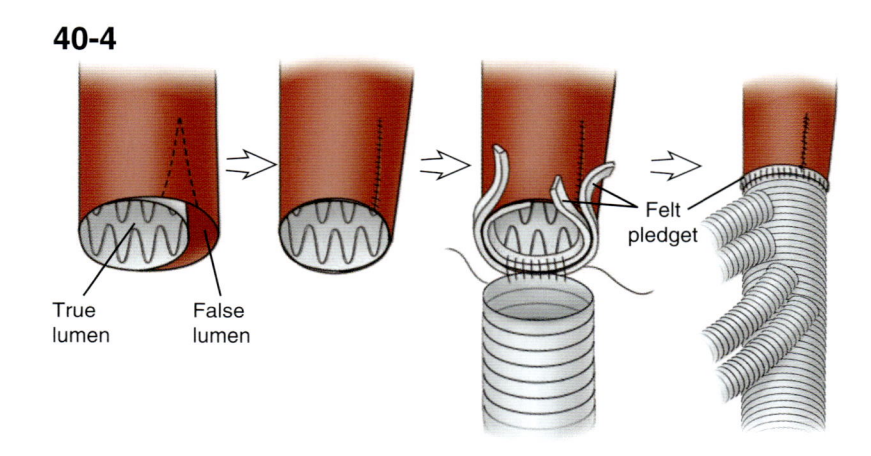

Figure 40-4 The proximal anastomosis is created with a felt pledget after fashioning the aortic fall.

40-5

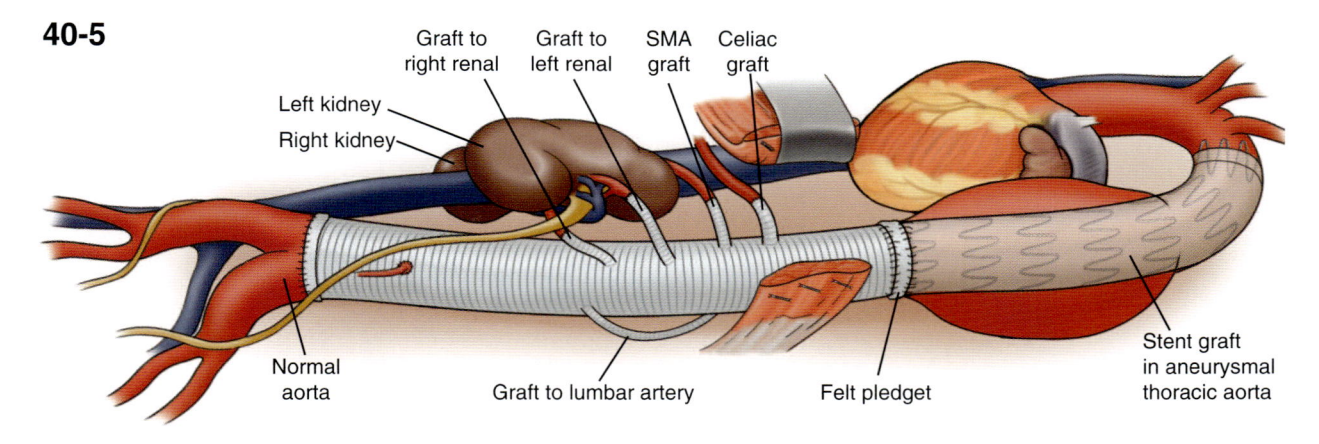

Figure 40-5 The intercostal branch bypass and four-vessel visceral bypasses completed, followed by the distal aortic anastomosis.

VENO-VENOUS AND VENO-ARTERIAL ECMO

Asvin M. Ganapathi, MD • Matthew C. Henn, MD

INDICATIONS Extracorporeal membrane oxygenation (ECMO) is a life-saving therapy for patients with end stage cardiac and/or pulmonary failure. The indications can be either acute or chronic heart or lung failure, but in all cases ECMO serves as a bridge to a more definitive therapy, which can include: (1) transplantation, (2) ventricular assist device for cardiac failure, or (3) medical recovery. Patients with isolated pulmonary failure are typically placed on veno-venous (VV) ECMO (FIGURE 41-1A), while patients also requiring hemodynamic support require veno-arterial (VA) ECMO (FIGURE 41-1B).

ECMO is a summation of multiple parts. Cannulas, which for adults typically range in size from 15 to 31 french (Fr) in diameter, are connected to a pump, which is typically centrifugal in nature. The cannulas provide drainage (deoxygenated venous blood taken to the pump) and then return to patient (oxygenated blood returned to the patient) of blood. Additionally, an oxygenator is part of the system which serves for gas exchange of oxygen and carbon dioxide. Most circuits will also have a heat exchanger to allow for temperature control of the patient due to heat transfer outside the body. Finally, all these components are regulated by a central unit controller that provides key information about function and allows for changes to be made, and includes temperature, flow rate, oxygenation, and mean blood pressure.

Because ECMO is a temporary support for patients, a thorough evaluation of the potential for an "exit" strategy is necessary. Patients in whom there is no potential recovery, but who are not candidates for more durable or long-term therapies, are not appropriate candidates. However, a large proportion of patients placed on ECMO are done so emergently, which precludes preoperative workup. In the urgent setting, ultrasound to evaluate venous patency as well as computed tomography to evaluate for evidence of peripheral vascular disease can be useful to help delineate the appropriateness of the access points for ECMO.

POSITION Patients are placed in the supine position on a bed that will allow for fluoroscopy. If access involves the internal jugular (IJ) vein, a Trendelenburg position may be useful, and if access through the axillary artery or subclavian vein is planned, then a shoulder roll will aid in exposure.

OPERATIVE PREPARATION Following routine prepping of the skin with chlorhexidine or betadine, the appropriate body areas are draped into the field. If the groin is to be used exclusively, drapes are placed to the mid-thigh, umbilicus, and laterally over the anterior superior iliac spine. A towel is placed over the genitals such that it does not extend laterally past the pubic symphysis. If the IJ vein is to be utilized, the drapes are placed superiorly to the level of the mandible and inferiorly to the level of the clavicle. CONTINUES ▶

41-1

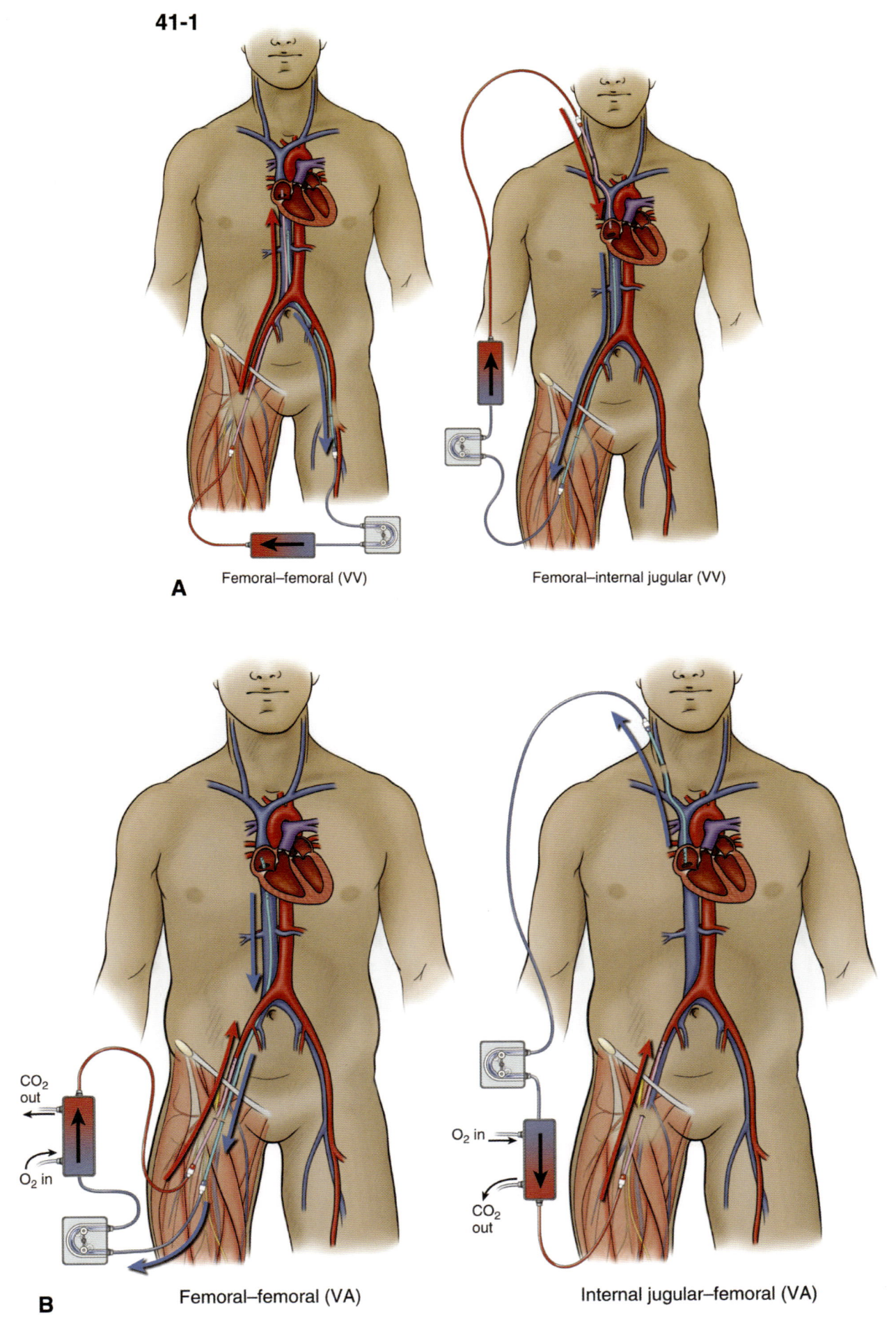

A   Femoral–femoral (VV)   Femoral–internal jugular (VV)

B   Femoral–femoral (VA)   Internal jugular–femoral (VA)

Figure 41-1 A. VV ECMO configurations. B. VA ECMO configurations.

OPERATIVE PREPARATION CONTINUED Cannula selection is also of importance. For VV ECMO; typically a 21/23 Fr or a 19 Fr cannula are selected for the patient return cannula for femoral vein or internal jugular vein cannulation, respectively. The drainage cannula will typically be a 25 Fr multistage cannula that allows for multiple side ports (FIGURE 41-2). For VA ECMO the drainage is the same as previously described, and the return is typically a 15/17/19 Fr short cannula, while the distal perfusion catheter (DPC) can range from 6 to 10 Fr depending on the vessel size and cannulation technique.

INCISION AND EXPOSURE

PERCUTANEOUS CANNULATION: Using an ultrasound (FIGURE 41-3), an introducer needle is placed in the vessel of choice. For femoral venous access, a long (0.035 inches [in] × 180 or 260 centimeters [cm]) stiff wire with a soft distal end (short tip Amplatz) should be placed into the superior vena cava (SVC) with the aid of transesophageal echocardiography (TEE) or fluoroscopy. For IJ venous access a long (0.035 in−180 or 260 cm) stiff wire is placed into the inferior vena cava (IVC) or preferably an iliac vein.

In the case of VA ECMO, if time permits it would be prudent to place a wire into the common femoral artery (CFA) both retrograde into the iliac vessel and antegrade into the superficial femoral artery (SFA). The DPC is essential in cases of cannulation of the femoral artery, as lack of a DPC has been associated with high rates of limb ischemia and potential for limb loss (FIGURE 41-4). This is typically accomplished with the Micropuncture Introducer Set (Cook Medical, Bloomington, IN). In the case of emergent cannulation, access is only retrograde through the CFA with a wire into the iliac vessel. Once the patient's circulation has been restored with ECMO, then access for a DPC is gained antegrade into the SFA with the use of ultrasound and a Micropuncture kit. If available, fluoroscopy is utilized to confirm placement of these wires.

OPEN CANNULATION FOR VA ECMO: Access for all cannulas is accomplished through either the right or left groin. The femoral pulse, or presumed area of the femoral pulse in cases of a patient who is coding, is identified. A transverse incision is made 1 to 2 cm below the inguinal ligament that is centered over the location of the femoral artery (FIGURE 41-5). Dissection is carried down through subcutaneous tissue and fascia, and the CFA down through the SFA/profunda bifurcation is identified. The CFA is then encircled with vessel loops. CONTINUES

41-2

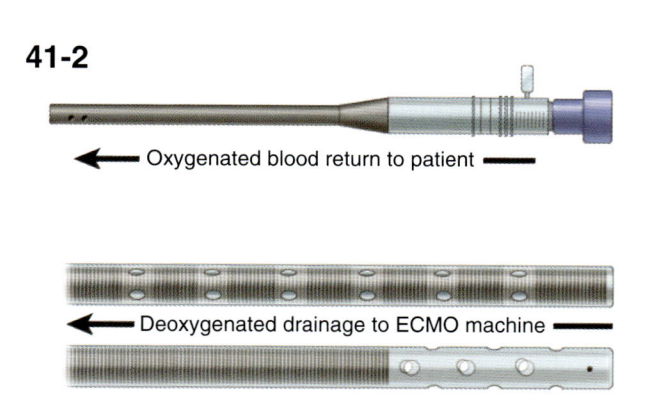

Figure 41-2 ECMO return and drainage cannulas.

41-3

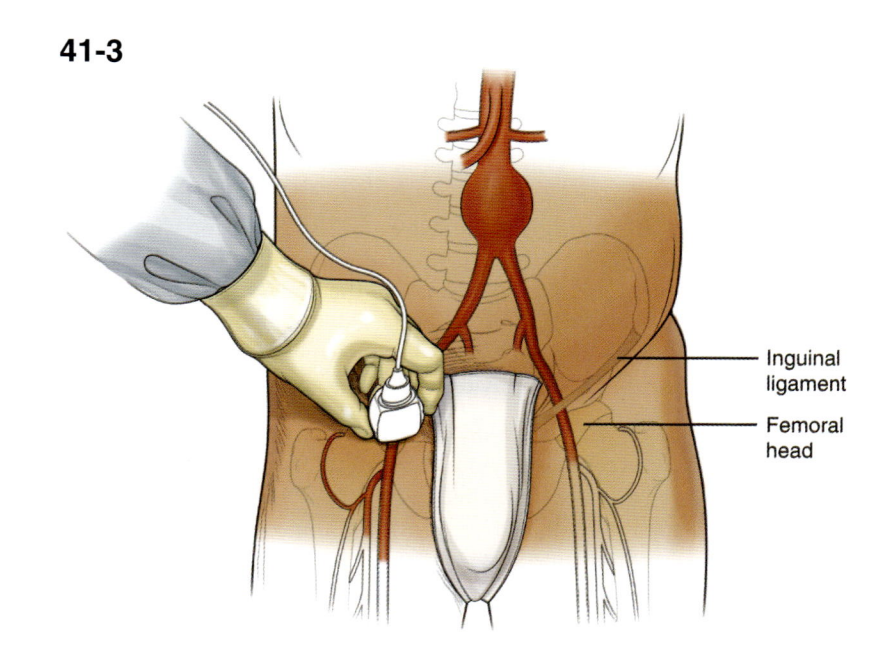

Figure 41-3 Ultrasound-guided femoral artery and vein access.

41-4

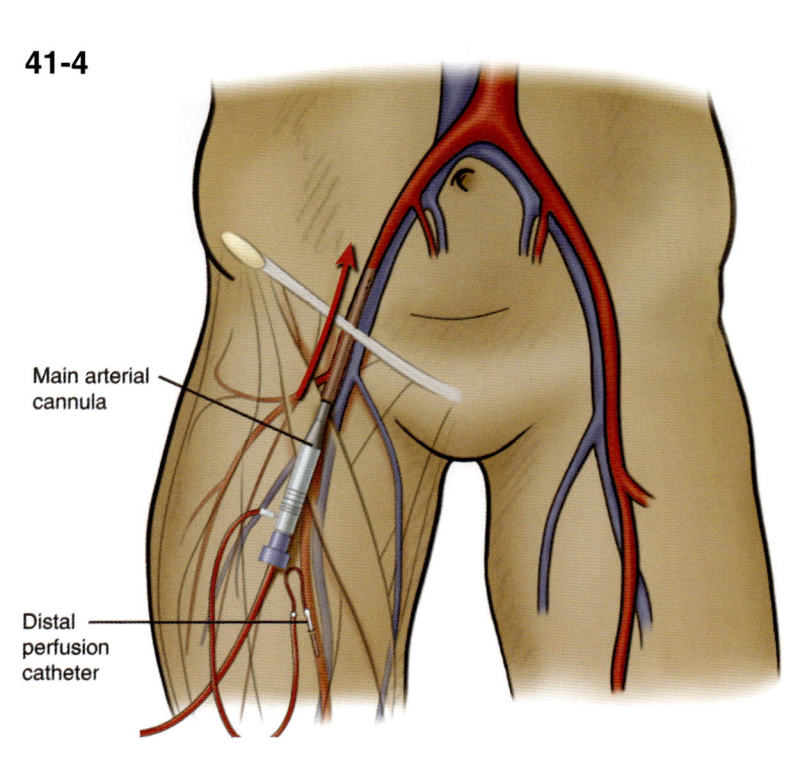

Figure 41-4 Superficial femoral artery distal perfusion cannula.

41-5

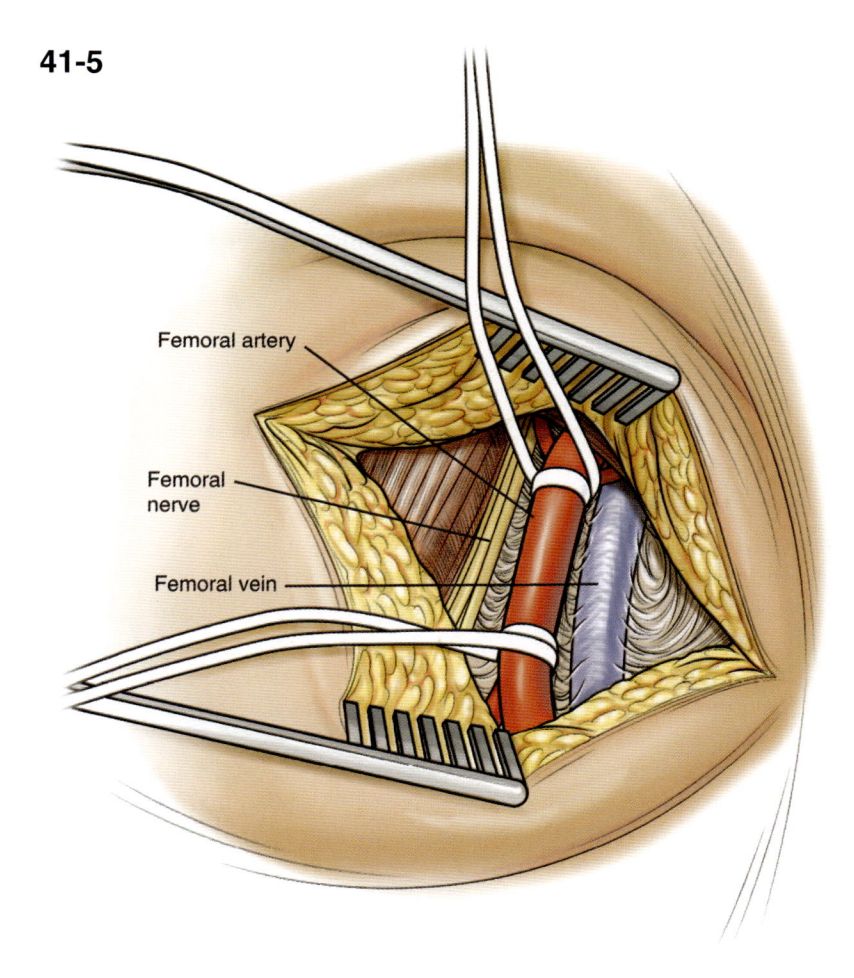

Figure 41-5 Open femoral artery exposure for cannula access.

DETAILS OF PROCEDURE

VENO-VENOUS ECMO

Femoral/Femoral Cannulation Next to the existing wires in the femoral veins bilaterally, an 11 blade is used to make a small skin incision to accommodate the cannulas. It can be helpful to use a tonsil clamp to dilate this tract through the subcutaneous tissue down to the vessel prior to any use of dilators. At this point 2500 or 5000 units of heparin is administered. The tract is then sequentially dilated with accompanying dilators and the wire is routinely checked with TEE and ultrasound to ensure that it remains in the SVC. The return cannula is then placed (typically on the right side), and using fluoroscopy or TEE the cannula is advanced and confirmed to be in the right atrium or SVC. Next multistage, drainage cannula is then placed into distal IVC typically at the right atrial/IVC junction with ideally at least 5 cm of separation between the two cannulas. The cannulas are then flushed with heparinized saline. The lines for the ECMO circuit are passed onto the field and the arterial limb is connected to the return cannula and the venous limb to the drainage cannula following appropriate deairing. ECMO is then initiated and slowly titrated to the appropriate flow.

Femoral/Internal Jugular Cannulation The drainage cannula is placed and heparin administered as previously described. A skin incision is made over the existing wire in the IJ vein and the tract dilated with a tonsil clamp. The tract is sequentially dilated using the Seldinger technique and the return cannula is placed into the right atrium with fluoroscopic or TEE guidance. Again, adequate separation of the return and drainage cannula must be achieved.

Dual Lumen Internal Jugular Single Cannula Dual lumen cannulas are specifically designed such that a single cannula contains the return and drainage. Side holes that will end up in the SVC and IVC will serve as the drainage, while a single side hole that is in the right atrium serves for return. Additionally, the side hole that is in the right atrium is directed at the tricuspid valve to allow for ease of flow through the heart. All side holes are also marked by radiopaque markers (**FIGURE 41-6**). It is imperative that the wire be in the distal IVC or ideally the iliac vein to ensure the tip of the cannula does not travel into a hepatic or renal vein. A skin incision is made to accommodate the cannula, which may range in size from 24 to 32 Fr, and heparin is administered. The tract is sequentially dilated using the dilators included with cannula, and the cannula is then oriented with the right atrial side hole facing the patient's left side and then inserted such that the radiopaque markers designating the appropriate side holes are in the SVC, right atrium, and IVC. The lines from the ECMO circuit are then connected to the return and drainage following deairing maneuvers. Notably, if the right IJ vein is not an option for access, the left subclavian or in certain cases right subclavian can be used for access with a similar percutaneous technique.

VENO-ARTERIAL ECMO

Percutaneous Femoral Cannulation The venous drainage cannula is placed after heparin is administered as previously described. Notably, it can be placed with the tip into the right atrium or SVC given that the return is on the arterial side. A small skin incision is made over the femoral artery for the wire placement. Percutaneous needle access is obtained, and the wire is placed retrograde into the iliac/abdominal aorta. The common femoral artery is then serial dilated over the wire, followed by placing a perfusion cannula. The cannula is placed such that the tapered part is hubbed against the skin, typically leaving the cannula in the distal abdominal aorta. For the DPC, percutaneous access is obtained with ultrasound and a wire that is placed antegrade into the SFA, dilated, and the DPC is placed. A bifurcation "Y" is added to the arterial limb of the ECMO circuit and then connected to the two cannulas following deairing.

Open Femoral Cannulation Following exposure of the femoral artery and vein, there are two methods for cannulation. The first is a hybrid open/percutaneous approach. Purse-string sutures are placed on the CFA (two for the return cannula and one for the DPC, typically) and common femoral vein (one) with 5-0 Prolene. Rommel tourniquets are applied to all purse strings and heparin administered. Counter-incisions are made on the skin outside the incision and wires are placed into the vessel inside the appropriate purse strings and positioned as previously described. These tracts are then dilated with the Seldinger technique and the cannulas placed in the appropriate position. The Rommel tourniquets are tightened and tied to the cannulas within the incision to secure all cannulas in place, and then the ECMO circuit lines are connected to the cannulas.

An alternative to the hybrid open/percutaneous approach is the use of a graft to provide flow to the femoral artery. In this scenario a site on the CFA is chosen for the graft, and following administration of heparin the proximal and distal CFA are clamped. The artery is opened longitudinally. A 6- or 8-millimeter (mm) graft is then beveled and sewn end-to-side on the CFA using 5-0 or 6-0 prolene. A counter-incision is made outside the transverse incision and the graft tunneled out inferiorly. The graft is then deaired and connected to the arterial limb of the ECMO. The venous cannula is placed as described in the hybrid approach.

CLOSURE For VV ECMO or VA ECMO that is done percutaneously, typically a purse string using a 0-silk suture (or other thick braided suture) is placed around the entry site of the cannula and then secured to the cannula. Additionally, at least two other securing stitches for the cannula are placed. In the case of an open femoral cannulation, following hemostasis, the existing rommel tourniquets are placed below the skin edges and the skin is closed with a running 2-0 nylon suture. This is done as the incision is only temporary and will need to be reopened at the time of decannulation.

POSTOPERATIVE CARE Following initiation of ECMO, the patient is transported to the appropriate intensive care. While there, the patient should undergo frequent vascular checks, particularly if VA ECMO is employed, to ensure no limb ischemia is present. Continuous heparin should be initiated as soon as possible and titrated to a goal-activated partial thromboplastin time (PTT) of approximately 50 to 80 to prevent/minimize clot formation in the cannulas/oxygenator. Additionally, as the DPC is more susceptible to thrombosis, heparin and/or nitroglycerin can be administered directly into the DPC to help prevent these issues. Patients with VV ECMO must also be monitored for mixing if the cannulas are not adequately separated, and if this is to occur the cannula may need to be repositioned. Finally, there may be bleeding around the cannulas, which typically can be temporized with pausing the heparin or placing a purse string around the skin entry site for the cannulas. However, in cases of more significant bleeding operative exploration is mandatory. ∎

SUGGESTED READINGS

Brogan TV, Lequier L, Lorusso R, MacLaren G, Peek G, eds. *Extracorporeal Life Support: The ELSO Red Book.* 5th ed. 2019. Extracorporeal Life Support Organization, Ann Arbor, MI.

Gaffney AM, Wildhirt SM, Griffin MJ, Annich GM, Radomski MW. Extracorporeal life support. *BMJ.* 2010 Nov 2;341:c5317.

Juo YY, Skancke M, Sanaiha Y, et al. Efficacy of distal perfusion cannula in preventing limb ischemia during extracorporeal membrane oxygenation: a systematic review and meta-analysis. *Artif Organs.* 2017; 41:E263–E273.

Makdisi G, Weng I. Extra Corporeal Membrane Oxygenation (ECMO) review of a lifesaving technology. *J Thorac Dis.* 2015;7:E166-E176.

Pavlushkov E, Berman M, Valchanov K. Cannulation techniques for extracorporeal life support. *Ann Transl Med.* 2017;5:70.

Reeb J, et al. Vascular access for extracorporeal life support: tips and tricks. *J Thorac Dis.* 0216;8:S353-363.

Ventetuolo CE, Muratore CS. Extracorporeal life support in critically ill adults. *Am J Respir Crit Care Med.* 2014;190:497-508.

Yau P, et al. Factors associated with ipsilateral limb ischemia in patients undergoing femoral cannulation extracorporeal membrane oxygenation. *Ann Vasc Surg.* 2019;54:60-65.

41-6

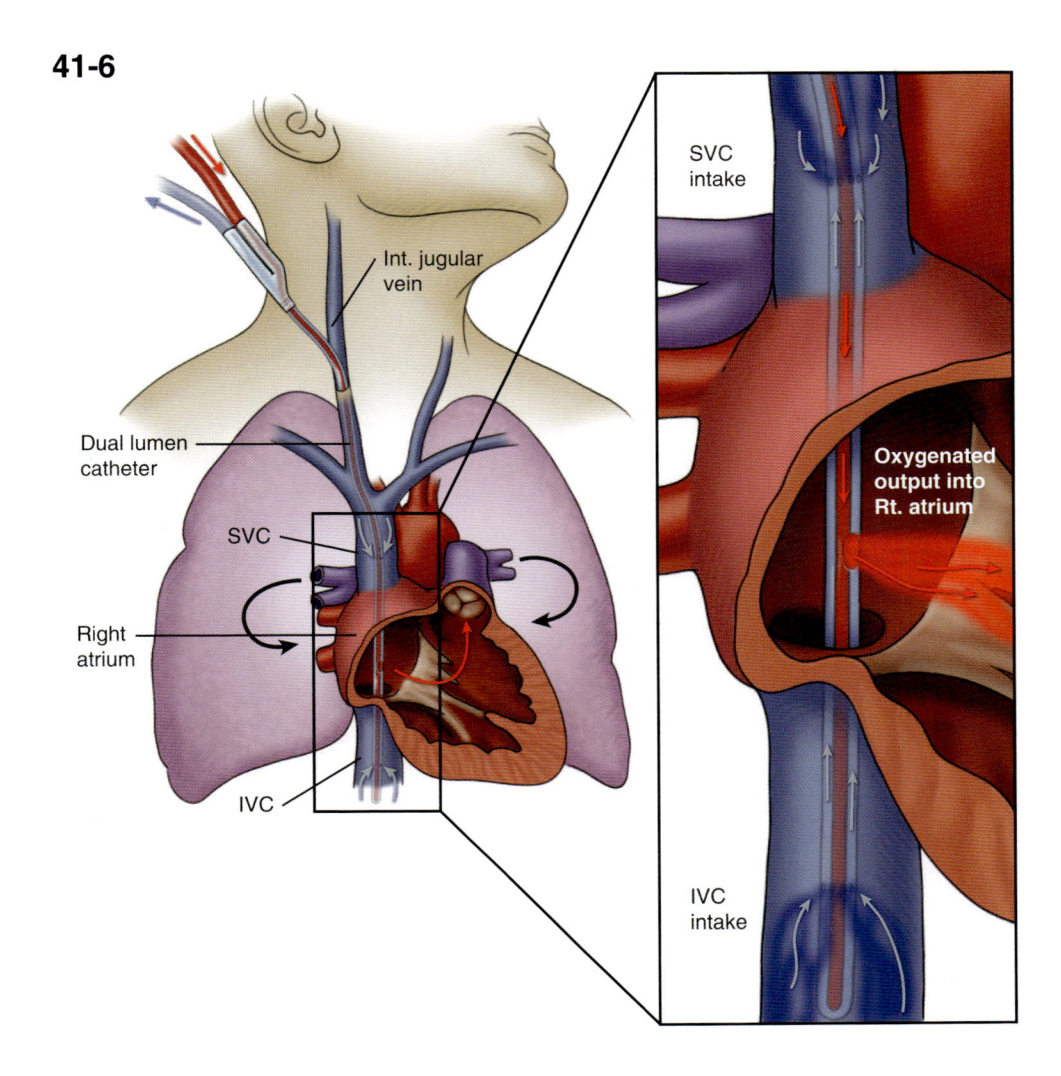

Figure 41-6 Single catheter dual lumen access.

THORACIC ENDOVASCULAR AORTIC REPAIR

Rae S. Rokosh, MD • Patric Liang, MD • Melinda S. Schaller, MD • Elliot L. Chaikof, MD, PhD

INDICATIONS Thoracic endovascular aortic repair (TEVAR) has quickly supplanted open repair as the preferred approach for both elective and emergent repair of complex thoracic aortic pathologies due to its minimally invasive nature and lower associated morbidity and mortality. The most common pathology treated with TEVAR is aneurysmal disease. A descending thoracic aneurysm meets the threshold for repair if symptomatic, saccular in nature, or if the aortic diameter exceeds 5.5 cm in asymptomatic patients deemed low risk for intervention, with a higher diameter threshold deemed more appropriate for high-risk patients.

TEVAR is also accepted as a first-line therapy for complicated Stanford type B aortic dissections (TBAD) with superior aorta-specific survival and favorable aortic remodeling in the stented segment as compared to medical management alone. Given the high incidence of aneurysmal degeneration associated with conservative management of uncomplicated TBAD patients, recent evidence suggests that TEVAR may also have potential benefit for those patients presenting with anatomic criteria indicative of a high risk of late aortic expansion. TEVAR may also have a role as a temporizing measure for patients presenting with a mycotic aneurysm of the thoracic aorta and may be used for patients with lower diameter penetrating aortic ulcers (PAU), and collagen vascular disease in the appropriate settings.

Additional acute aortic syndromes for which TEVAR is also recommended include symptomatic intramural hematoma (IMH) and PAU. In the event of an asymptomatic lesion, the decision to intervene is individualized. Thresholds for repair include an IMH wall thickness greater than 10 mm or PAU that exceed 10 mm in depth or 20 mm in diameter. However, indications for intervention remain unsettled without well-defined parameters in current clinical practice guidelines.

TEVAR is also indicated for treatment of traumatic thoracic aortic injury (types II to IV) (**FIGURE 42-1**), as well as during a hybrid approach to repair a Kommerell diverticulum, a bulbous origin of an aberrant subclavian artery that exceeds 30 mm in diameter, or associated with aneurysmal degeneration of the adjacent descending thoracic aorta greater than 5 cm. Relative contraindications to TEVAR may include an inadequate proximal or distal endograft seal zone or the need for complex aortic arch reconstruction. In addition, given limited long-term data regarding the durability of repair, the appropriateness of elective TEVAR as first-line therapy in young patients with a progressive connective tissue disorder should be carefully considered and is generally considered second-line therapy.

OPERATIVE PREPARATION Preoperative planning should entail fine-cut (<1 mm) computed tomography angiography (CTA) of the chest, abdomen, and pelvis to capture the aortic arch through the femoral access vessels, with subsequent analysis using three-dimensional image reconstruction software, such as TeraRecon (TeraRecon Inc., Durham, NC). Magnetic resonance angiography, though it provides lower quality spatial resolution compared to CTA, is a viable alternative for pregnant patients or those with severe allergy to iodinated contrast. Appropriate assessment of the great vessel arch anatomy, particularly the origin of the vertebral arteries, is required to minimize the risk of cerebral ischemic complications. Proximal and distal endograft landing zones must be at least 2 cm in length in healthy aorta to ensure appropriate seal. In addition, an ideal landing zone should exhibit minimal tapering (<15%), tortuosity, and angulation, and contain minimal thrombus or calcification.

Under the most ideal anatomic circumstances, the proximal landing zone is located distal to the left subclavian artery (SCA) Zone 2 (**FIGURE 42-2**). However, in the presence of a limited landing zone distal to the left subclavian, the endograft may cover the origin of the left SCA to achieve appropriate proximal endograft fixation. In such instances, left SCA revascularization should be performed prior to endograft placement, most achieved by left SCA transposition or a carotid-SCA bypass. Coverage of the left SCA has been associated with an increased risk of spinal cord ischemia and posterior circulation stroke. Therefore, indications for

preoperative or concomitant left SCA revascularization include the presence of (i) a left internal mammary artery coronary artery bypass graft to avoid coronary ischemia; (ii) a left upper extremity arteriovenous fistula to facilitate adequate dialysis without a risk of arm ischemia; (iii) a dominant left vertebral artery where compromised flow could lead to posterior cerebral ischemia or spinal ischemia; or (iv) other factors that increase the risk of paraparesis or paraplegia, such as the need for extensive (>15 cm) coverage of the descending thoracic aorta, preexisting or planned hypogastric artery occlusion, or prior history of infrarenal aortic repair with limited lumbar artery collateral flow. In emergent situations, left SCA revascularization can be performed selectively following TEVAR. Should the need for an adequate landing zone require TEVAR coverage of the left common carotid artery (Zone 1), preoperative carotid-carotid and carotid-subclavian bypasses or branched or fenestrated grafts would be required for adequate revascularization (**FIGURE 42-3**). Alternative endovascular revascularization strategies include in situ needle or laser fenestration of the thoracic endograft with placement of a stent graft, or parallel branch vessel endografting using a "chimney" or "snorkel" technique via brachial or carotid artery access.

With respect to the distal landing zone, the celiac artery can be covered to attain adequate seal if sufficient collaterals are established between the celiac and superior mesenteric arteries (SMA) on preoperative imaging or intraoperative selective SMA angiography. When deploying a graft that may encroach on the mesenteric arteries, it is important to first cannulate and leave a wire down the SMA or celiac artery to have access to the artery after graft deployment. Transient balloon occlusion of the celiac artery can be considered to assess collateral flow if standard imaging is equivocal. In the event of inadequate collateral circulation, the distal seal zone can be extended by performing an iliohepatic bypass or through use of chimney/snorkel stenting or endograft fenestration. In the presence of >50% SMA stenosis, a balloon-expandable stent can be deployed to ensure vessel patency.

Adequate preoperative imaging of the pelvic circulation is imperative to characterize the quality of the intended iliofemoral access route. In the presence of small (<8 mm), excessively tortuous, or heavily calcified iliac arteries, access can be achieved by retroperitoneal (RP) exposure of the common iliac artery with placement of an end-to-side 10-mm Dacron graft as an access conduit. Such a strategy minimizes the risk of vessel rupture or dissection during the placement or removal of a large delivery sheath. As an alternative approach, 10-mm self-expanding stent grafts have been deployed within a smaller iliac artery followed by balloon dilation to create an endoluminal conduit. Left carotid or axillary artery access represent other nontraditional access sites if iliofemoral access is not feasible. Likewise, concomitant repair of the aortic arch and the descending thoracic aorta may entail access via a midline sternotomy for conventional proximal aortic arch replacement with antegrade delivery of an endograft through the transected arch during circulatory arrest as a "frozen elephant trunk." All told, an appropriate inventory of covered stents should be available for emergent repair of an inadvertently disrupted access artery.

Accurate preoperative device selection that accounts for the unique anatomic features of an individual patient is required to ensure a successful outcome. Commercially available endografts vary in size, shape, radial force, conformability, bare-metal versus covered proximal component, precision of deployment under varying anatomic constraints, as well as size of delivery sheath. Typically, an endograft diameter is oversized 10 to 20% of the intended aortic landing zone for treatment of aneurysmal disease and minimal or no oversizing for acute aortic dissection or aneurysm secondary to a connective tissue disorder. Thus, optimal oversizing varies by device, intended site of placement, and underlying pathology. While undersizing can result in type I endoleak or device migration, oversizing can lead to retrograde dissection, device infolding, and, in the presence of significant arch angulation, bird-beaking with risk of endograft collapse (**FIGURE 42-4**). CONTINUES ▶

42-1

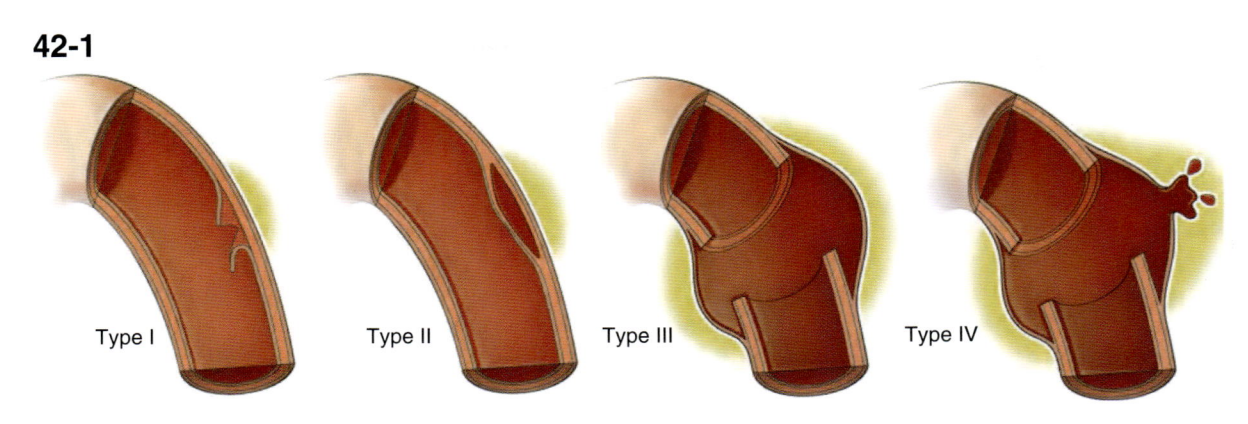

Type I   Type II   Type III   Type IV

Figure 42-1 Classification of traumatic aortic injury types. (Reproduced with permission from Azizzadeh A, Keyhani K, Miller III C, et al. Blunt traumatic aortic injury: Initial experience with endovascular repair. *J Vasc Surg.* 2009;49(6):1403-1408.)

42-2

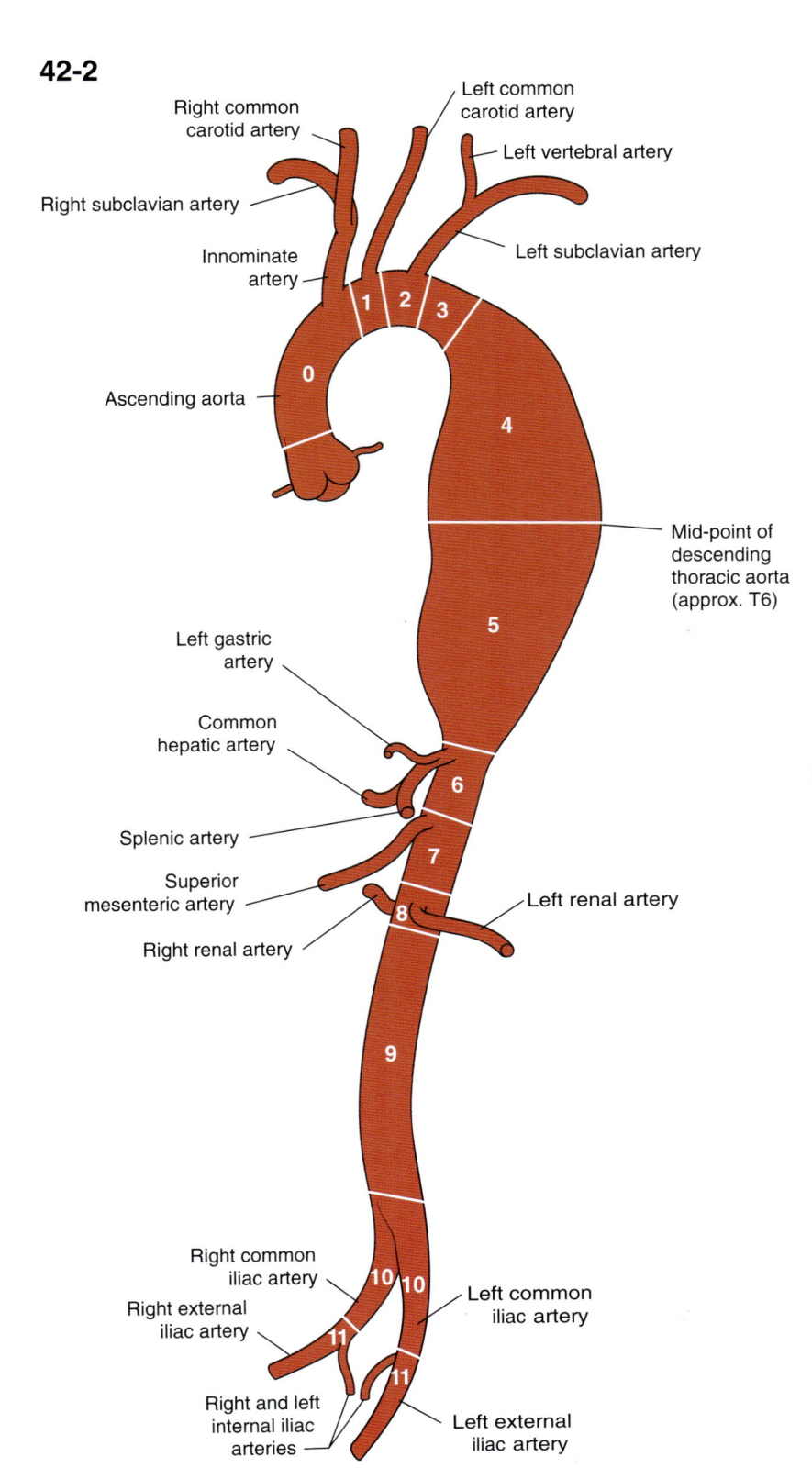

Figure 42-2 Aortic zones of attachment. (Reproduced with permission from Fillinger MF, Greenberg RK, McKinsey JF, Chaikof EL and Society for Vascular Surgery Ad Hoc Committee on TRS. Reporting standards for thoracic endovascular aortic repair (TEVAR). *J Vasc Surg.* 2010;52:1022-1033.)

42-3

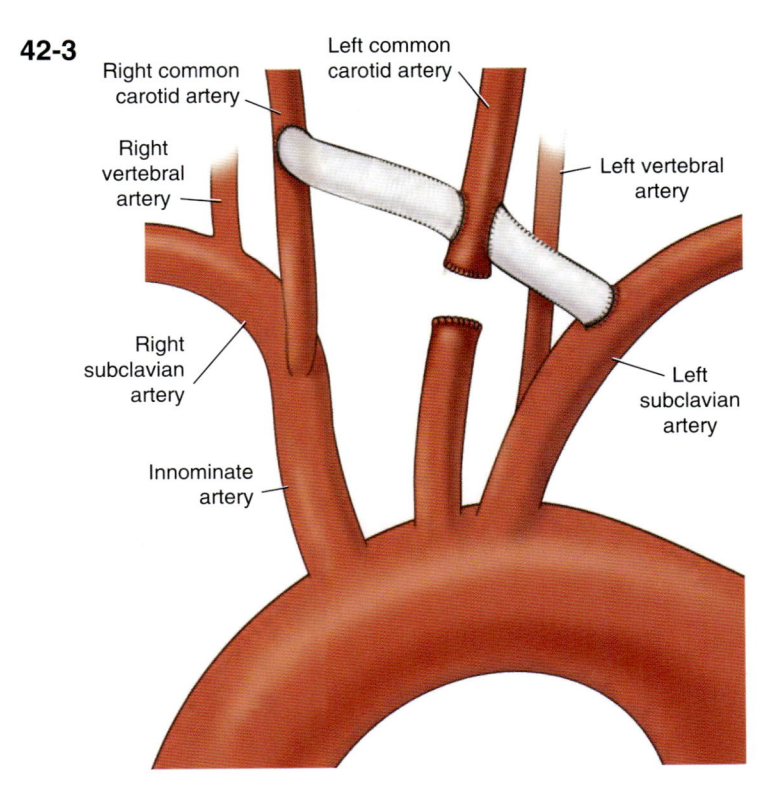

Figure 42-3 Right common carotid to left common carotid bypass, and left common carotid artery to subclavian artery bypass with over-sewing proximal left common carotid artery.

42-4

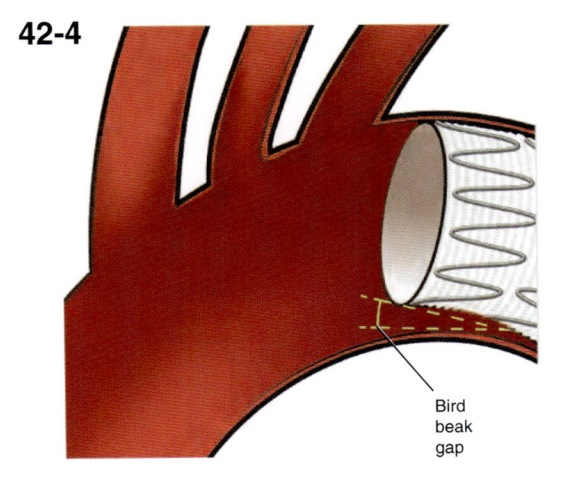

Figure 42-4 Bird beak configuration after TEVAR on postoperative computed tomography angiography (CTA). (From Kudo T, Kuratani T, Shimamura K, Sawa Y. Determining the optimal proximal landing zone for TEVAR in the aortic arch: comparing the occurrence of the bird-beak phenomenon in Zone 0 vs Zones 1 and 2. *J Endovasc Ther.* 2020;27(3):368-376.)

OPERATIVE PREPARATION `CONTINUED` Preoperative placement of a lumbar cerebrospinal fluid (CSF) drain, an arterial line, central venous access, and a Foley catheter are case specific and dependent on anticipated case complexity, blood loss, and known risk factors associated with spinal cord ischemia (SCI). These include prior infrarenal aortic repair, planned extended coverage of the thoracic aorta (>15–20 cm), coverage of the distal descending thoracic aorta in the region of the artery of Adamkiewicz within 5 cm or less above the celiac artery (T8-L1 vertebral segments), bilateral hypogastric artery occlusion, or left SCA coverage. Evidence for prophylactic lumbar drain placement is largely based on open surgical experience, with no definitive evidence that routine use with TEVAR leads to a reduction in SCI. CSF drains are associated with a low but non-negligible rate of complications, including subdural and epidural hematoma, spinal headache, and meningitis. As a result, implementation varies widely by institution. Similarly, somatosensory or motor-evoked potentials are not commonly used with routine TEVAR. Blood products, additional TEVAR devices, as well as an aortic occlusion balloon should be readily available.

ANESTHESIA AND POSITIONING Although TEVAR can be performed under general anesthesia or sedation with local anesthesia, general anesthesia is preferred, with evidence comparing the two anesthetic techniques lacking. The patient is positioned supine with arms tucked or with both arms extended above the head to facilitate fusion imaging, unless brachial access is anticipated. Some prefer to routinely use the left brachial artery as the portal for aortic arch imaging. Pedal pulses or Doppler signals should be marked preoperatively. After routine skin preparation from sternum to knees, the operative field is draped to expose bilateral groins. Preoperative antibiotics are administered.

INCISION AND EXPOSURE Access for TEVAR can be obtained percutaneously (`FIGURE 42-5A`) if anatomically suitable or via open femoral exposure (`FIGURE 42-5B`). The preferred route for delivery of the main body of the endograft, whether via right or left femoral artery access, is determined based on preoperative assessment of the dimensions and tortuosity of the iliofemoral vessels. `CONTINUES`

42-5

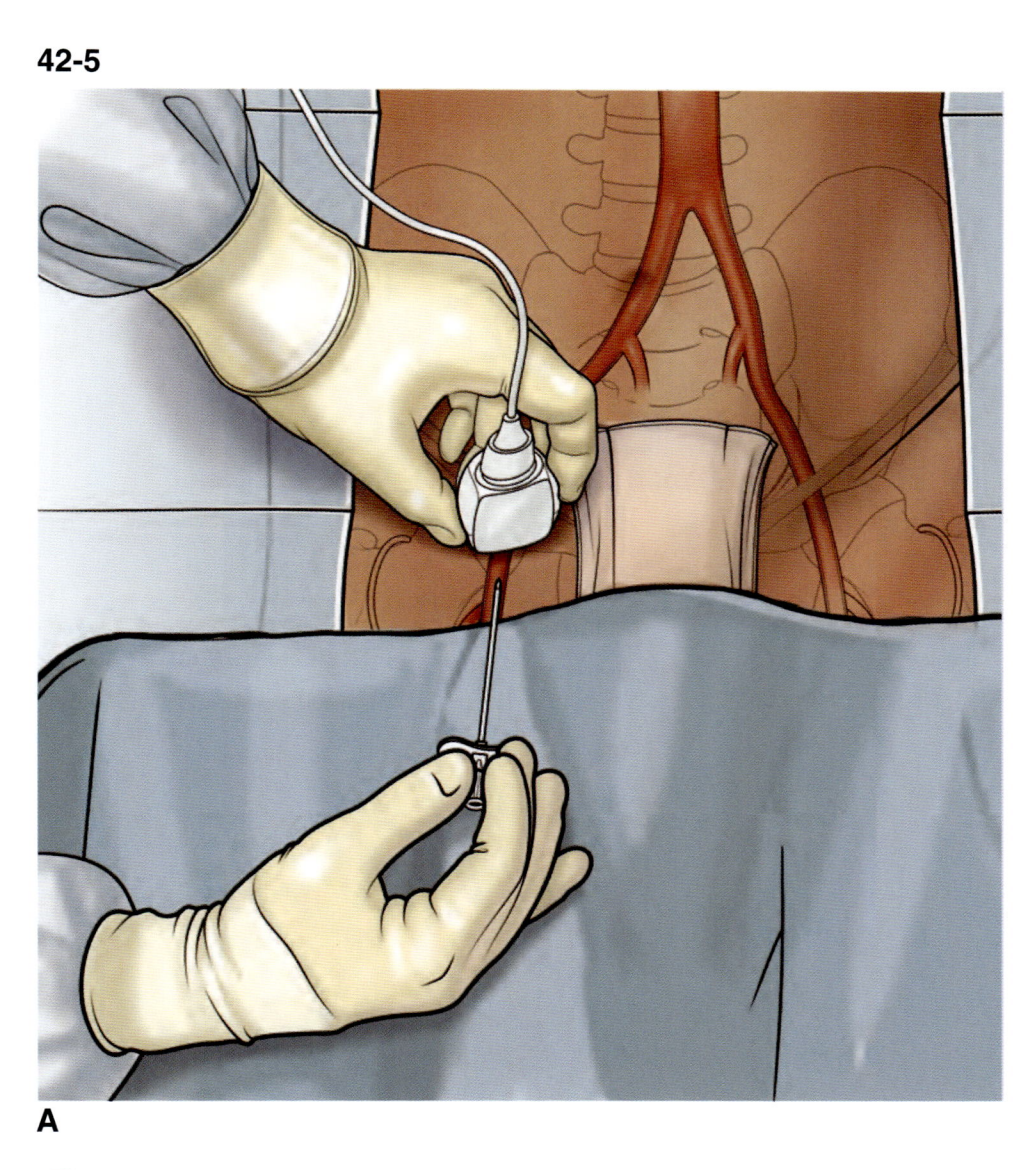

A

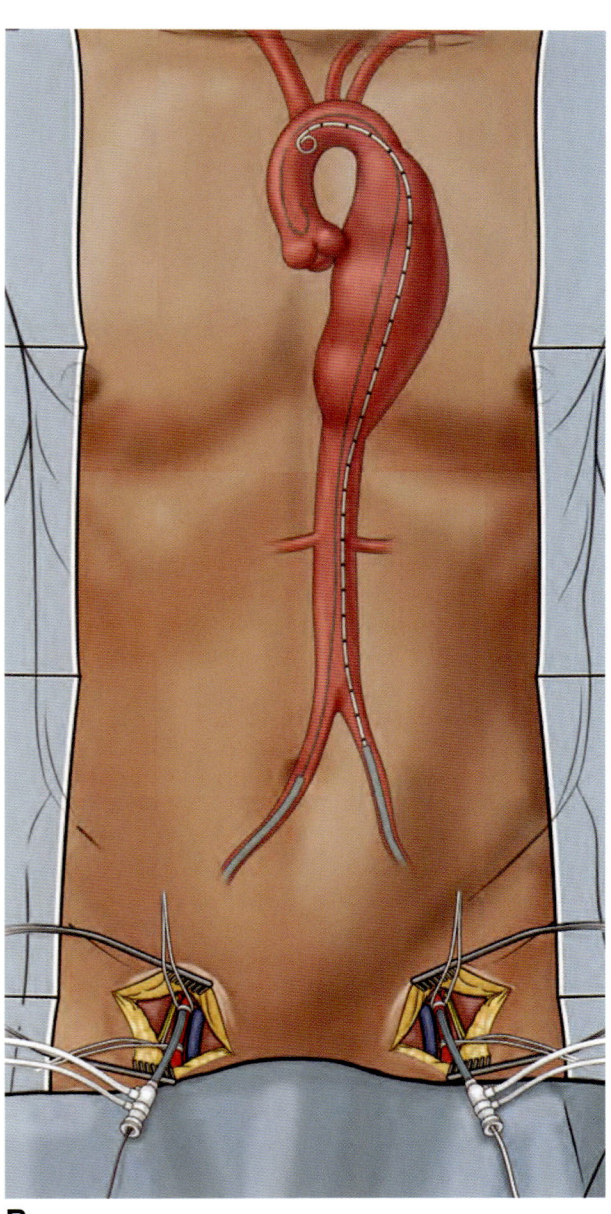

B

Figure 42-5 A. Percutaneous ultrasound guided femoral artery access. B. Bilateral femoral artery cut down for femoral artery access.

INCISION AND EXPOSURE *PERCUTANEOUS COMMON FEMORAL ACCESS:* ◂CONTINUED Under duplex ultrasound guidance, the CFA chosen for main body delivery is accessed using a micropucture kit. After placing an 0.035″ starter wire, the arteriotomy is dilated using the inner dilator of a 7-Fr sheath. Using a pre-close technique, two percutaneous Perclose ProGlide closure devices are placed followed by upsizing to a 9-Fr or 10-Fr sheath. In a similar manner, the contralateral side is often accessed percutaneously with placement of a 5-Fr sheath to facilitate advancement of nonselective angiographic catheters, although TEVAR can be performed successfully via a unilateral approach. Many surgeons prefer accessing the left brachial artery for arch imaging and possible later subclavian embolization if a carotid subclavian bypass is done (FIGURE 42-6). If 0.035″ intravascular ultrasound (IVUS) is anticipated, the diagnostic side sheath can be upsized to a minimum 9-Fr so IVUS can be delivered directly though the larger main body side sheath. IVUS can be used for further assessment of the landing zones or branch vessels or in an effort to minimize contrast use. IVUS is particularly useful for assessment of aortic diameter in the young patient presenting with traumatic aortic injury, where initial CT imaging may reflect pre-resuscitation status, as well as to identify the location of a proximal entry tear and help differentiate between a true and false lumen in a patient with an aortic dissection (FIGURE 42-7).

OPEN COMMON FEMORAL EXPOSURE: Should percutaneous access not be considered feasible, the CFA is exposed, controlled proximally and distally with vessel loops, and access obtained with an 18-gauge needle and an 0.035″ guidewire, followed by placement of a sheath. Percutaneous femoral access is obtained in the contralateral groin, if needed, for passage of a diagnostic catheter or IVUS. CONTINUES▸

42-6

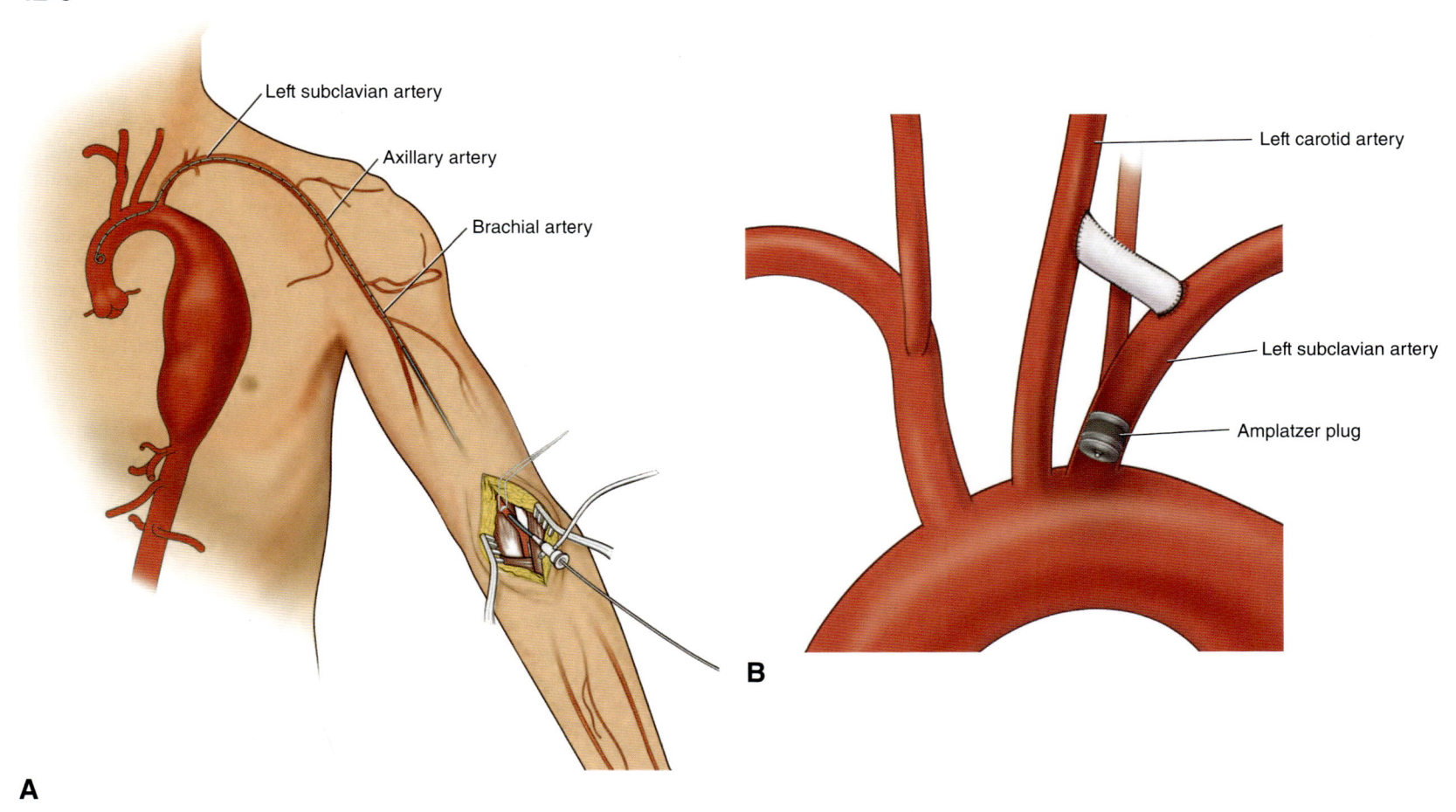

Figure 42-6 A. Left brachial artery access via cut down. B. Placement of proximal amplatzer plug after carotid subclavian artery bypass to prevent retrograde endoleak.

42-7

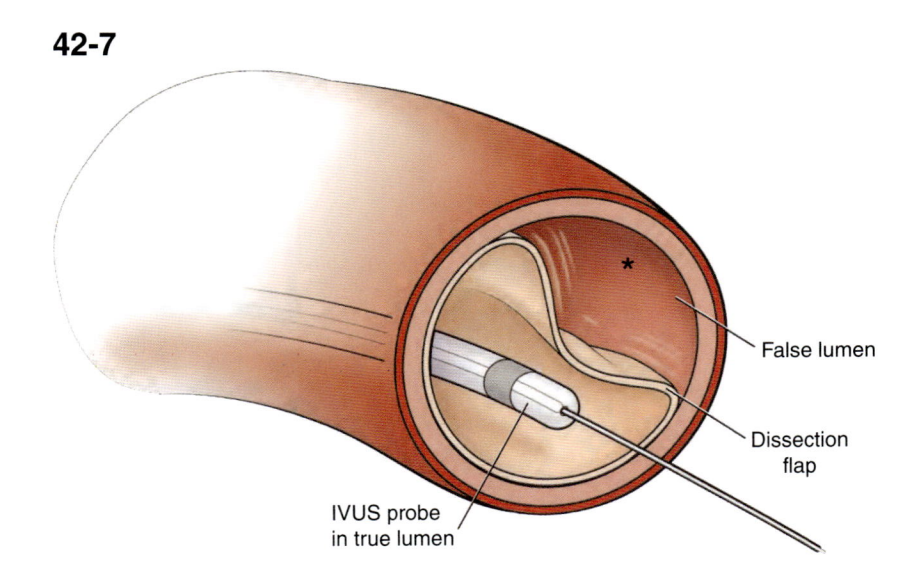

Figure 42-7 IVUS catheter within true lumen with asterisk denoting false lumen.

DETAILS OF PROCEDURE Following initial sheath placement, the patient is systemically heparinized with a goal of an activated clotting time (ACT) >250 seconds. Systemic heparinization is required to prevent thrombosis when using a large caliber sheath, and to reduce thromboembolic events associated with aortic arch manipulation. A lower dose of systemic anticoagulation or forgoing anticoagulation may be considered in the patient with traumatic aortic disruption and other concomitant injuries.

On the main body side, a 0.035″ wire is inserted under direct fluoroscopic visualization into the ascending aorta. Special attention is required in the setting of an aortic dissection to ensure the wire remains within the true lumen—this is best ascertained with IVUS. The wire is then exchanged to a stiff 0.035″, 300-cm length Lunderquist, Amplatz, or Meier wire via an exchange catheter. Stiff wires facilitate subsequent delivery of large devices through tortuous or calcified aortic segments. If needed, the sheath is upsized to permit delivery of the selected endograft, with visualization under fluoroscopy as the sheath is advanced.

On the diagnostic side, a 0.035″ wire is introduced and a nonselective diagnostic catheter positioned for aortic angiography and to identify the location of aortic arch vessels. As previously indicated, this can be done through the left femoral approach or a left brachial approach. The left brachial approach has the advantage of giving precise location to the left subclavian artery, and also allows for delivery of a plug or coils in the circumstance where this is necessary following subclavian artery bypass and TEVAR for dissection to prevent retrograde pressure on the diseased tissue.

To obtain adequate views of the arch, a left anterior oblique projection is employed (FIGURE 42-8A). For visceral segments, lateral or oblique views permit appropriate visualization of the superior mesenteric and celiac artery orifices (FIGURE 42-8B). The cranial-caudal projections are used for the renal orifices. Branch vessel involvement is reevaluated, proximal and distal landing zones assessed, and device sizing confirmed. Fusion imaging technology, such as Vessel-Navigator (Phillips Healthcare, Best, Netherlands), is a powerful adjunct that facilitates anatomic accuracy and precision with device deployment. This technology combines preoperative CTA with live intraoperative fluoroscopy to provide a dynamic, real-time three-dimensional roadmap overlay. Application of this software has been associated with significant reductions in radiation exposure, contrast use, fluoroscopy, and operative times.

Prior to angiographic aortic arch images or insertion of devices, all sheaths and catheters should be carefully de-aired to reduce the risk of air embolization. Some have advocated flushing with angiographic-grade CO_2. The endograft is introduced through the sheath with the tip of the device advanced proximal to the landing zone. A key gateway to successful outcome is that the device is withdrawn from the desired level prior to deployment, and then advancing again while allowing acquired torque or other forces that may have built up during advancement of the device through the aorta to dissipate. A strategy of slight restrained withdrawal of the device during deployment limits inadvertent forward movement of the endograft. Adjunctive systemic measures are another gateway to excellent outcomes to assist with accurate device deployment. These include transient reduction of cardiac output or flow arrest by adenosine boluses, prolonged Valsalva maneuvers, and rapid ventricular pacing. It is helpful to have the systolic blood pressure reduced to 80 mmHg to reduce wind-socking.

If more than one endograft component is required to treat the underlying aortic pathology, adequate device overlap is required to avoid a type III endoleak and consideration is required as to the proper sequence of device deployment, dependent upon the size of the selected endografts. In general, 5-cm overlap is a minimum starting point. For example, treatment of an aortic dissection requires initial deployment of the proximal component to minimize the risk of retrograde extension, while an extensive thoracic aneurysm requiring multiple components may require initial placement of proximal and distal graft segments followed by a bridging segment. Additionally, tapered TEVAR devices may be needed to account for the size discrepancies of the treated aortic segments. In the treatment of thoracic aneurysms, seal zones are typically molded with a compliant balloon after device deployment, with concurrent implementation of aforementioned impulse control adjuncts to prevent distal endograft displacement while ballooning. However, balloon molding should be avoided altogether after device placement for thoracic dissection or traumatic aortic injury to avoid aortic disruption. Following device deployment, the large delivery sheath can be pulled back into the external iliac to decrease the associated risk of SCI associated with hypogastric occlusion. **CONTINUES ▶**

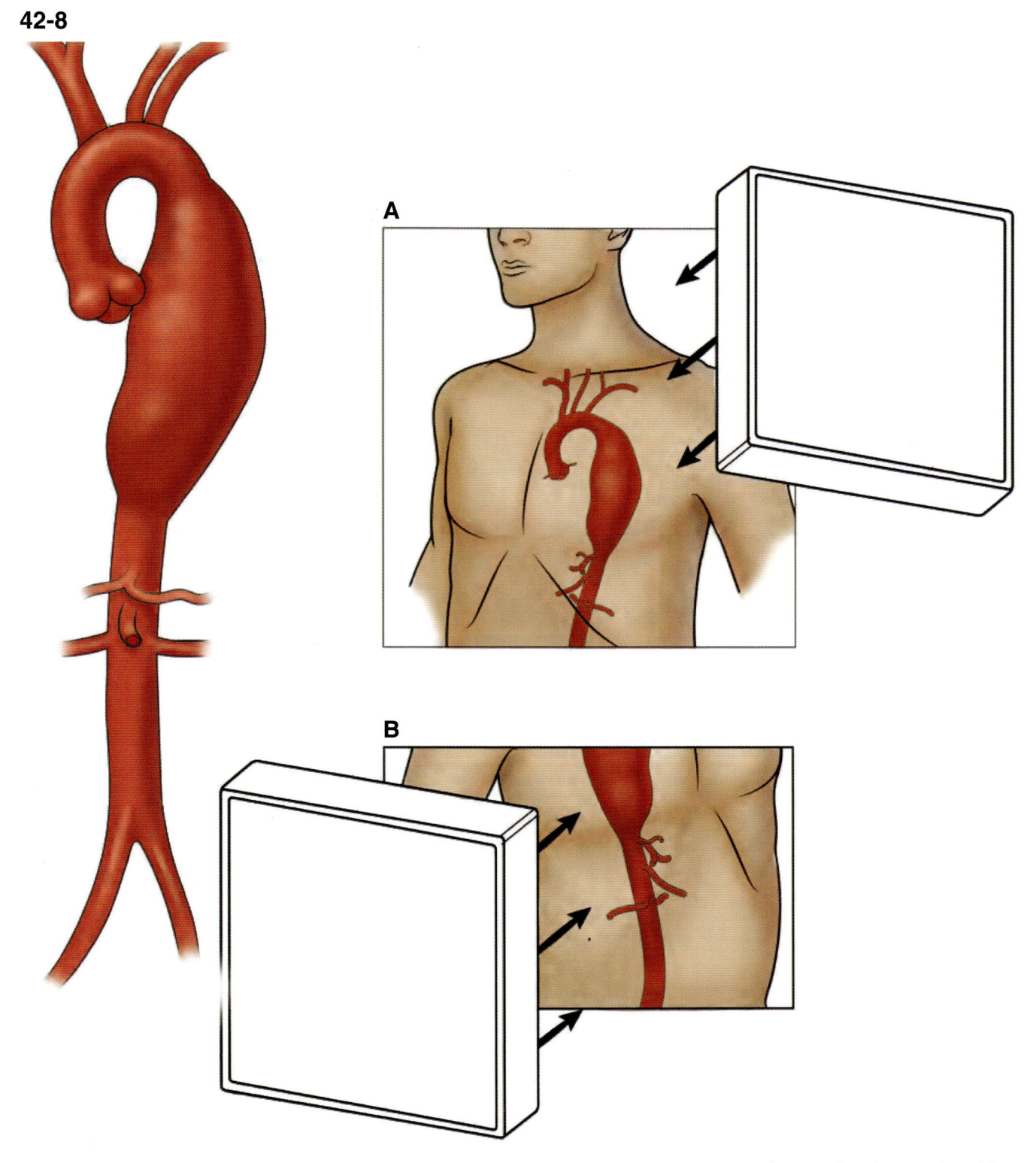

Figure 42-8 A. Arch angiogram done with left anterior oblique view. B. Mesenteric angiogram done with right anterior oblique view.

DETAILS OF PROCEDURE **CONTINUED** At the conclusion of the procedure, a completion angiogram is performed with magnified views both proximally and distally to assess for appropriate deployment within target landing zones, type I or III endoleak, patency of adjacent branch vessels, and absence of device deformation, such as bird beaking or graft infolding (FIGURE 42-9). If a type I endoleak is identified, balloon molding, placement of a proximal or distal extension cuff, or use of endoanchors may be required to achieve an adequate seal. All sheaths are flushed with 0.9% normal saline to auto transfuse blood.

CLOSURE Protamine sulfate is administered to reverse procedural heparinization. For percutaneous access on the main body side, the sheath is withdrawn, and the two pre-close suture knots placed at the beginning of the case are tightened. The 0.035″ wire can be left in while pulling up on the Perclose sutures should additional Perclose devices be needed for hemostasis. If contralateral access was obtained, the 0.035″ starter wire is introduced, the sheath removed, the percutaneous closure device deployed, and direct pressure held. For open femoral exposure, the sheath and wire are withdrawn and the arteriotomy closed with 5-0 monofilament polypropylene suture. The subcutaneous tissue is closed in two layers with 3-0 absorbable suture and skin edges approximated with a 4-0 subcuticular suture and a topical skin adhesive or skin staples. The presence of baseline pedal pulses or Doppler signals is confirmed prior to extubation and patient transfer to the post-anesthesia care unit. If there is a concern of an access-related complication, on-table evaluation using an ultrasound is recommended.

POSTOPERATIVE CARE Hemodynamic and neurological status as well as lower extremity perfusion are closely monitored during the postoperative period. The spinal drain is leveled at the tragus and kept at 10 mm H_2O, and can be capped and removed within the first 24 hours if no neurologic changes are noted. Discharge home can be anticipated in 1 to 3 days for an uncomplicated procedure.

COMPLICATIONS TEVAR can be performed safely and effectively for a variety of complex aortic pathologies; however, no procedure is without inherent risk. TEVAR is associated with a 3% risk of stroke, which is predominately attributed to atheroembolism due to wire manipulation in a diseased aortic arch. Less common etiologies of stroke include air embolism or cerebral hypoperfusion if a critical arch vessel is occluded without revascularization. Left SCA coverage without revascularization may be associated with left upper extremity ischemia and vertebrobasilar insufficiency. Given a requirement for a large sheath, the incidence of access-related complications is 3 to 4%, which includes iliac artery dissection, perforation, avulsion, or rupture. As discussed earlier, a conduit should be considered for those patients with diminutive and calcified vessels.

SCI with transient or permanent paraparesis or paraplegia is a devastating complication, with a reported incidence of approximately 2 to 8% depending on the extent of aortic coverage. Given the lack of robust evidence to support routine prophylactic CSF drain placement, guidelines suggest selective placement for patients considered high risk for SCI. However, varied definitions of "high risk" exist. A standard postoperative protocol in those with evidence of SCI includes hourly neurologic assessment, controlled elevation of mean arterial pressure (MAP >90 mmHg) to encourage perfusion of spinal collaterals, maintenance of oxygen saturation >99%, transfusion to a target hemoglobin of 10 to 12 mg/dL, and CSF drainage to maintain cerebrospinal pressure <10 mmHg. The drain remains in place from 24 to 72 hours postoperatively depending upon the extent of thoracic coverage, risk of SCI, and neurologic exam.

FOLLOW-UP Postoperative surveillance should entail contrast-enhanced imaging at 1 and 12 months after TEVAR, followed by annual imaging for life, with consideration of more frequent imaging in the event of a detected endoleak or other concerning abnormality. ∎

SUGGESTED READINGS

Buth J, Harris PL, Hobo R, van Eps R, Cuypers P, Duijm L, et al. Neurologic complications associated with endovascular repair of thoracic aortic pathology: incidence and risk factors. a study from the European Collaborators on Stent/Graft Techniques for Aortic Aneurysm Repair (EUROSTAR) registry. *J Vasc Surg.* 2007;46(6):1103-1110.

Jones DW, Stangenberg L, Swerdlow NJ, Alef M, Lo R, Shuja F, et al. Image fusion and 3-dimensional roadmapping in endovascular surgery. *Ann Vasc Surg.* 2018;52:302-311.

Keith CJ Jr., Passman MA, Carignan MJ, Parmar GM, Nagre SB, Patterson MA, et al. Protocol implementation of selective postoperative lumbar spinal drainage after thoracic aortic endograft. *J Vasc Surg.* 2012;55(1):1-8.

Lee WA, Matsumura JS, Mitchell RS, et al. Endovascular repair of traumatic thoracic aortic injury: clinical practice guidelines of the Society for Vascular Surgery. *J Vasc Surg.* 2011;53(1):187-192.

Lombardi JV, Hughes GC, Appoo JJ, Bavaria JE, Beck AW, Cambria RP, et al. Society for Vascular Surgery (SVS) and Society of Thoracic Surgeons (STS) reporting standards for type B aortic dissections. *J Vasc Surg.* 2020;71(3):723-747.

Nelson PR, Kracjer Z, Kansal N, Rao V, Bianchi C, Hashemi H, et al. A multicenter, randomized, controlled trial of totally percutaneous access versus open femoral exposure for endovascular aortic aneurysm repair (the PEVAR trial). *J Vasc Surg.* 2014;59(5):1181-1193.

Swerdlow NJ, Wu WW, Schermerhorn ML. Open and endovascular management of aortic aneurysms. *Circ Res.* 2019;124(4):647-661.

Tsilimparis N, Debus S, Chen M, Zhou Q, Seale MM, Kolbel T. Results from the Study to Assess Outcomes After Endovascular Repair for Multiple Thoracic Aortic Diseases (SUMMIT). *J Vasc Surg.* 2018;68(5):1324-1334.

Upchurch GR Jr., Escobar GA, Azizzadeh A, et al. Society for Vascular Surgery clinical practice guidelines of thoracic endovascular aortic repair for descending thoracic aortic aneurysms. *J Vasc Surg.* 2021;73(1S):55S-83S.

Wong CS, Healy D, Canning C, Coffey JC, Boyle JR, Walsh SR. A systematic review of spinal cord injury and cerebrospinal fluid drainage after thoracic aortic endografting. *J Vasc Surg.* 2012;56(5):1438-1447.

42-9

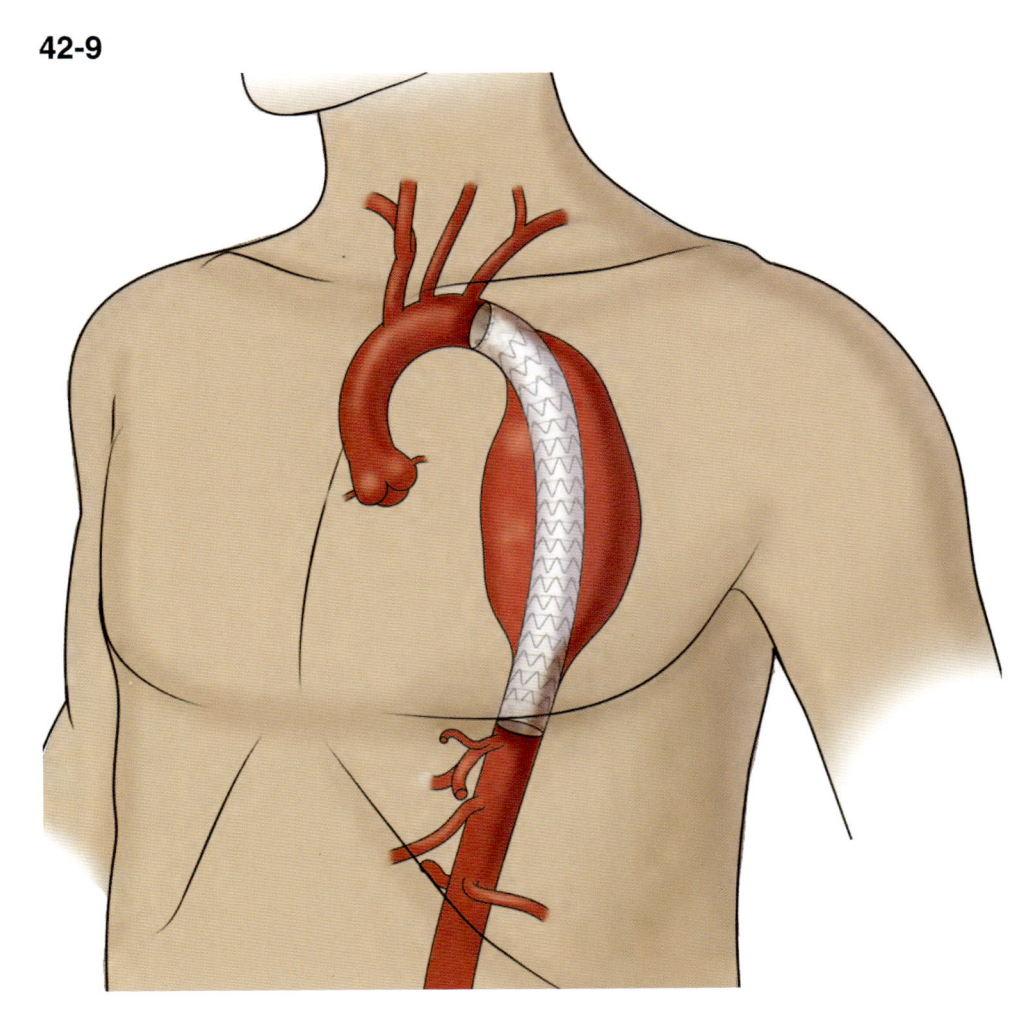

Figure 42-9 Completion angiogram.

CHAPTER 43

TEVAR for Aortic Dissection

Joseph V. Lombardi, MD • Katherine K. McMackin, MD

INDICATIONS Thoracic endovascular aortic repair (TEVAR) for dissection is performed to treat malperfusion or ruptured dissecting aortic aneurysms and can serve as a preventative prophylactic measure to in the setting of high-risk features which predispose to rupture. For patients presenting with malperfusion, a proximal TEVAR serves to maximize true lumen flow while decompressing the false lumen, and also treats dynamic obstructions of visceral, limb, or spinal vessels. Those patients with high-risk features include refractory pain, uncontrollable hypertension, hemorrhagic pleural effusion, large aortic diameter (>40 mm), asymptomatic severe radiographic only malperfusion from true-lumen compression, lesser curve location entry tear, or false lumen diameter >22 mm. In these circumstances, TEVAR can prevent conversion to a complicated dissection in the subacute phase as well as prevent late aneurysmal degeneration.

Preoperative CT angiogram should be performed with both an arterial phase and a venous phase to allow for late opacification of the false lumen. On occasion, the left subclavian artery may need to be covered. While carotid subclavian bypass is strongly advocated in an elective setting, this is not always feasible in emergent situations. If this is necessary, the patient's spinal cord, upper extremity, and vertebrobasilar circulation should be monitored and postoperative revascularization done if there is any sign of ischemia. Additionally, imaging of the contralateral vertebral artery for size and disease should be done before covering the left subclavian artery. Oversizing of the aorta should be kept to 10 to 15% of the healthy proximal aorta to prevent infolding or induce proximal dissection. A proximal landing zone requires 2 cm of healthy aorta, free of dissection, intramural hematoma, or penetrating atherosclerotic ulcers. Iliac and femoral vessels should be evaluated to assure adequate caliber for TEVAR pieces to pass through. In addition, for dissections ending in zone 10 and above (FIGURE 43-1), this serves as identifying an entry point known to be true lumen. Finally, consideration of deploying a dissection-specific uncovered stent graft (Cook Inc., Bloomington, IN) for long-term remodeling is at the discretion of the surgeon (FIGURE 43-2). Preoperative consent should include the possibilities of complications, including paralysis, retrograde dissection, and stroke.

POSITION The patient is placed supine on the operating table with the arms tucked. The arterial line should be placed on the right side as the left subclavian may be either therapeutically or unintentionally covered during the procedure or used for access. General anesthesia should be used to allow for angiogram with ventilator cessation ability during digital subtraction angiography (DSA). **CONTINUES**

43-1

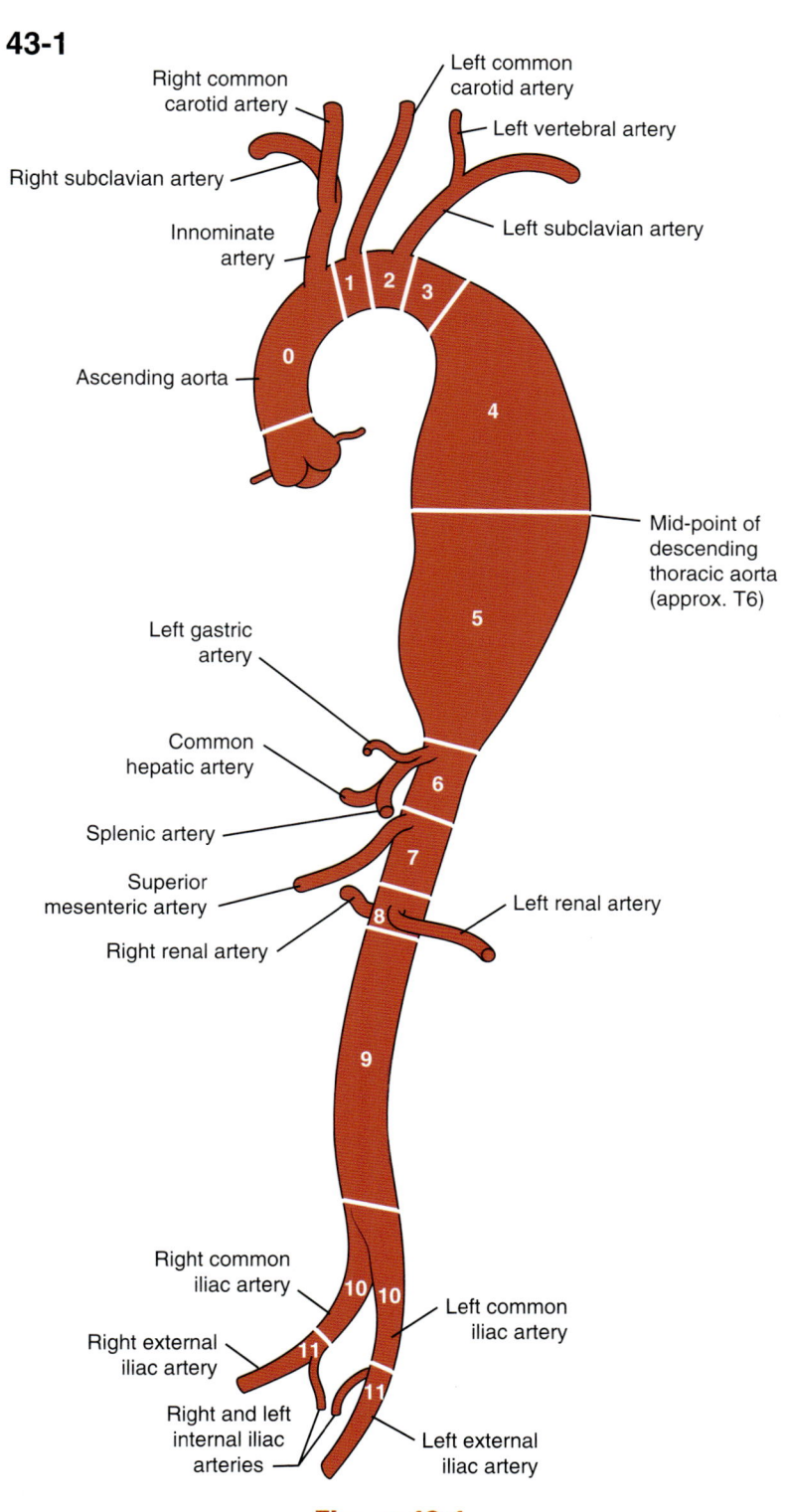

Right common carotid artery

Left common carotid artery

Left vertebral artery

Right subclavian artery

Innominate artery

Left subclavian artery

Ascending aorta

Mid-point of descending thoracic aorta (approx. T6)

Left gastric artery

Common hepatic artery

Splenic artery

Superior mesenteric artery

Left renal artery

Right renal artery

Right common iliac artery

Left common iliac artery

Right external iliac artery

Right and left internal iliac arteries

Left external iliac artery

Figure 43-1

43-2

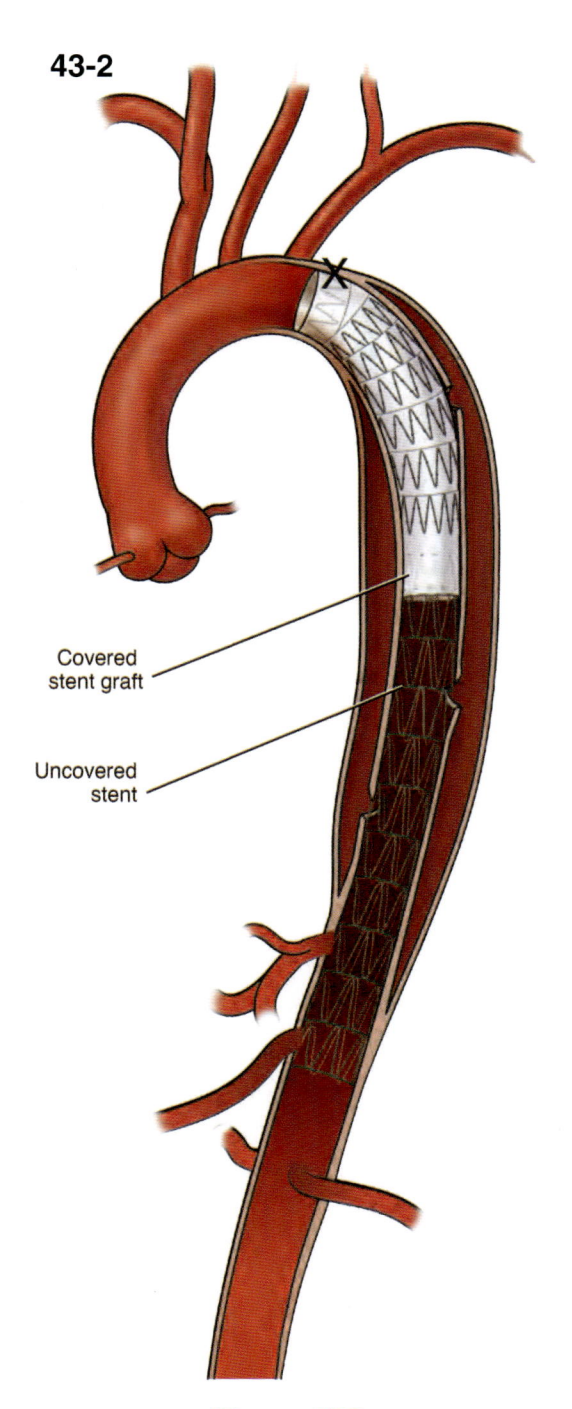

Covered stent graft

Uncovered stent

Figure 43-2

OPERATIVE PREPARATION Perioperative antibiotics are administered. Skin prep is applied from the level of the sternal notch to the knees, and the patient is draped to allow for access to the thoracic or abdominal aorta if necessary.

INCISION AND EXPOSURE

PERCUTANEOUS FEMORAL APPROACH: A time-out is performed confirming identity, laterality, and procedure. Using the ultrasound, the right common femoral artery is assessed and noted to be patent and suitable for access. Under ultrasound-guided direct visualization, the common femoral artery is accessed with a micropuncture kit and an access image is obtained in the oblique position to confirm site of entry. The same is repeated for the contralateral common femoral artery (FIGURE 43-3), and the sheath is upsized over a 0.035" Bentson wire (Boston Scientific, Marlborough, MA) to a 7 French. On the contralateral side (usually the left side), the microsheath is upsized to a 5 French sheath over a Bentson wire. After this, two Perclose ProGlide sutures are placed bilaterally (Abbott Laboratories, Plymouth, MN) and deployed sequentially at 10 o'clock and 3 o'clock positions (FIGURE 43-4). Their external suture ends were secured with rubber shods and tucked under a blue towel. The patient was systemically heparinized. CONTINUES ▶

43-3

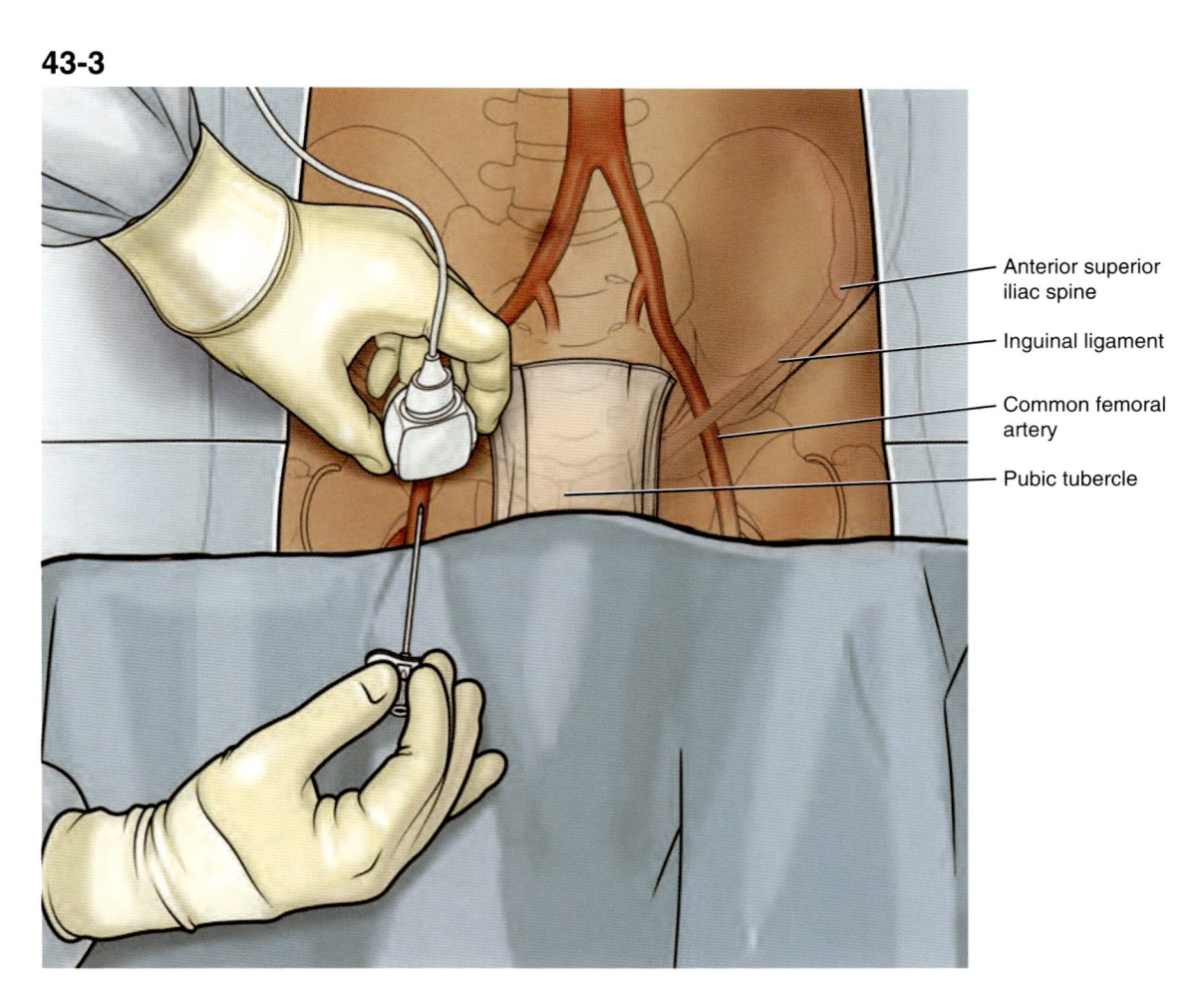

Figure 43-3 Femoral artery oblique access picture—RAO for splaying vessels.

43-4

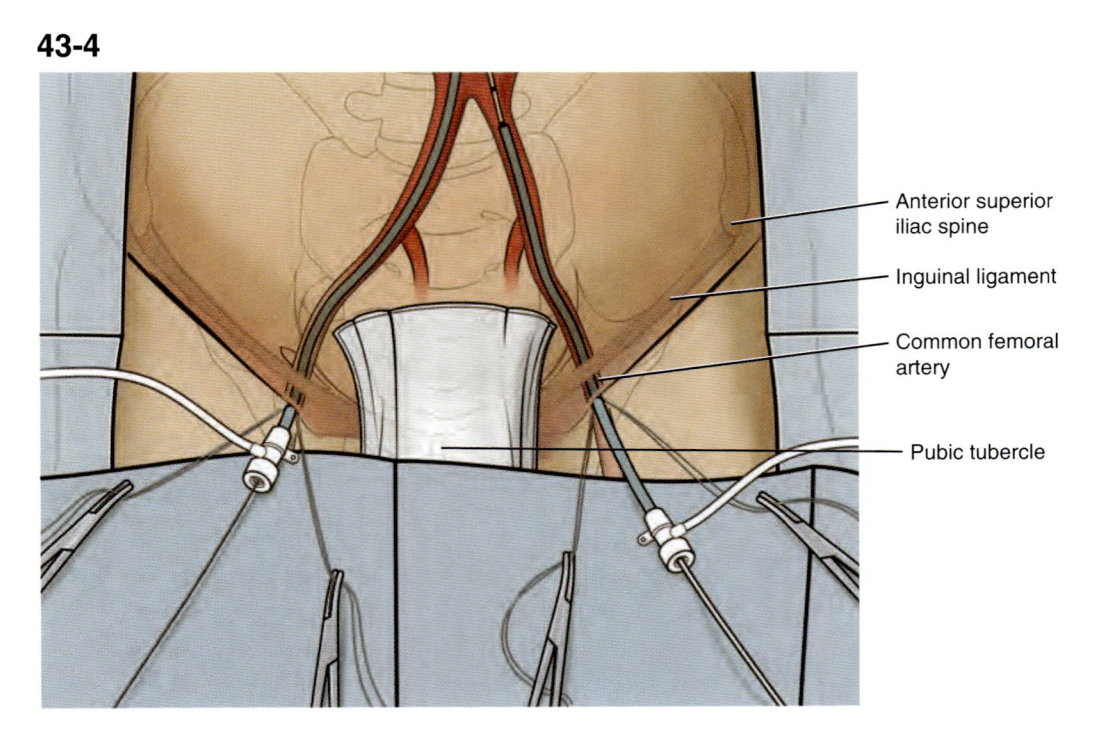

Figure 43-4 Preclose pictures: see Chapter 34.

INCISION AND EXPOSURE *ALTERNATIVE OPEN FEMORAL APPROACH:* **CONTINUED** The anterior superior iliac spine and pubic tubercle are marked bilaterally to define the inguinal ligament. On the right side, 2 cm inferior to the ligament, a 4-cm transverse incision is made over the palpable femoral pulse (**FIGURE 43-5**). Dissection is carried down through the soft tissue with electrocautery. Care is taken to ligate all crossing lymphatic channels. Upon entry to the femoral sheath, Metzenbaum scissors are used to sharply dissect the common femoral arteries for a length of 5 cm. The artery is encircled with two vessel loops proximally and distally. This is repeated on the contralateral side. Under direct visualization, bilateral common femoral arteries are cannulated with a micropuncture kit while gentle traction is performed with the distal vessel loop. The sheath is upsized over a Bentson wire to a 7 French sheath. On the contralateral side, the microsheath is upsized to a 5 French sheath over a Bentson wire. The patient is then systemically heparinized to maintain the ACT greater than 250 seconds.

DETAILS OF PROCEDURE In general, if the dissection flap anatomy is favorable, the right side is used to deliver the device. A multipurpose A (MPA) catheter is brought up over the Bentson wire to the ascending thoracic aorta and exchanged for a double curved Lunderquist wire through the MPA. The wire is seated adjacent to the aortic valve (**FIGURE 43-6**). A key gateway is to confirm the presence of the wire in the true lumen with intravascular ultrasound (IVUS). The wire should sit on the concave portion of the true lumen and the pulsations are noted to be in an outward direction from the lumen of the wire (**FIGURE 43-7**). **CONTINUES**

43-5

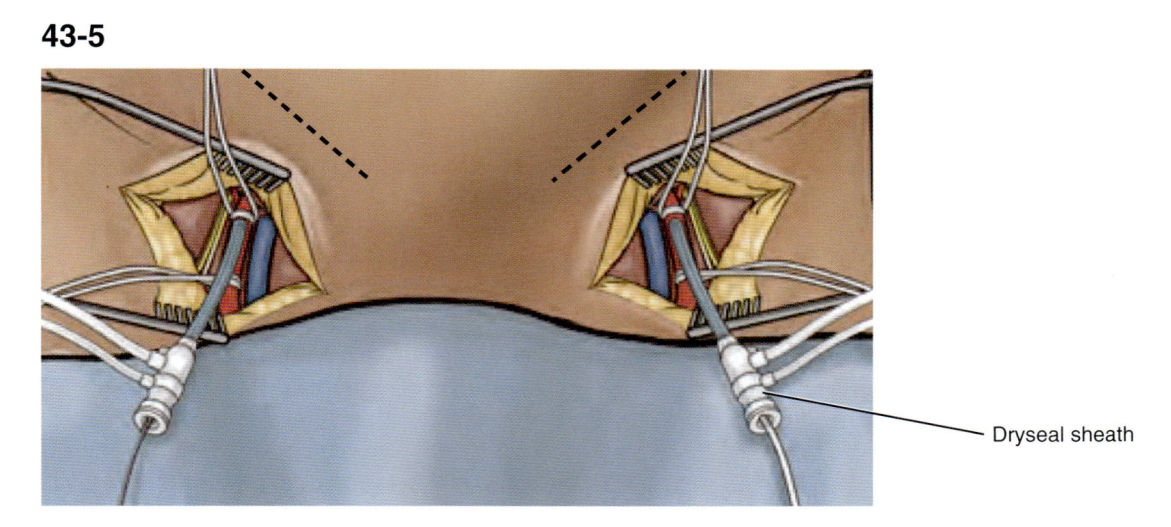

Dryseal sheath

Figure 43-5

43-6

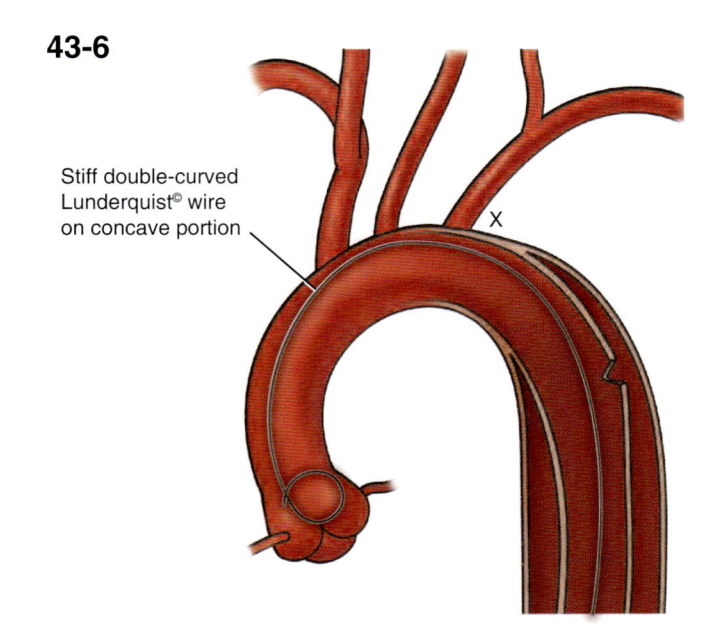

Stiff double-curved
Lunderquist© wire
on concave portion

X

Figure 43-6 Angiogram of thoracic aorta with double curved Lunderquist wire on aortic valve (star) with true and false lumen opacifying.

43-7

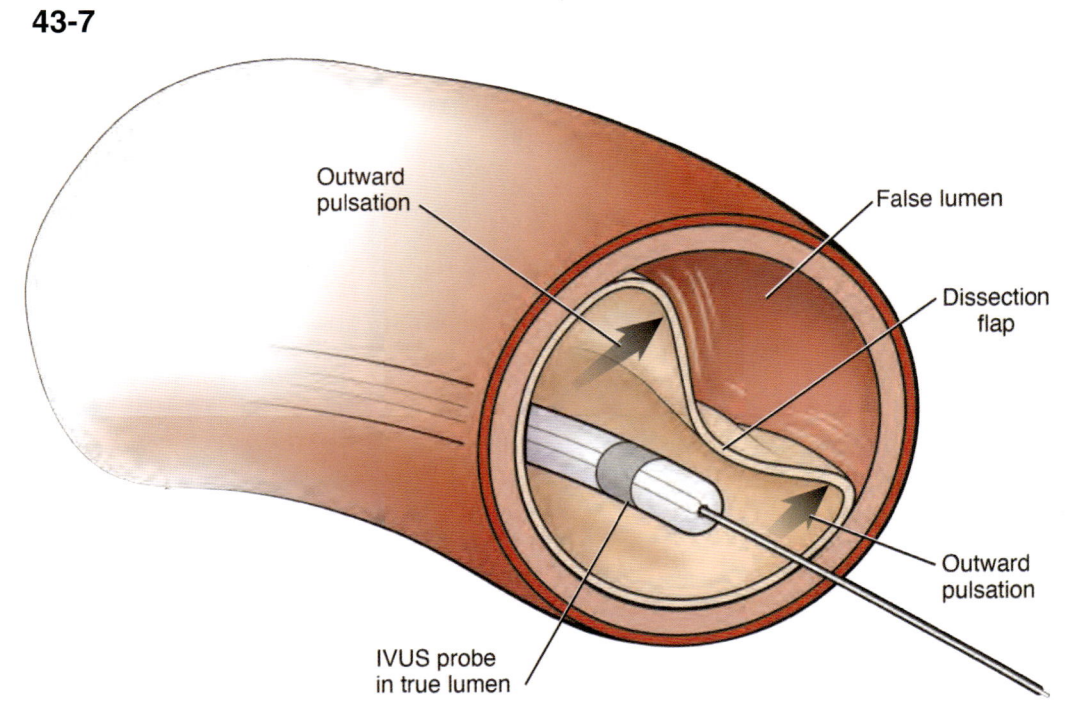

Outward
pulsation

False lumen

Dissection
flap

Outward
pulsation

IVUS probe
in true lumen

Figure 43-7 IVUS.

DETAILS OF PROCEDURE **CONTINUED** As with thoracic aneurysms, the left brachial artery is also helpful in catheter access to the aortic arch for imaging and delivering an Amplatzer plug or coils to the subclavian artery if a carotid subclavian bypass is needed. Via the left side or left brachial artery, a Bentson wire is extended to the level of the aortic arch. A marked pigtail catheter is brought up over this wire, and this catheter is used to identify the angle at which the arch of the catheter is maximally splayed out to minimize angiographic overlap of the great vessels, usually through a 45-degree left anterior oblique (LAO) projection of the image intensifier. The device delivery side wire is again confirmed in the true lumen with the IVUS probe. After holding respirations, an angiogram is performed marking the origin of the innominate, left carotid, and left subclavian arteries with vessels at the bottom of the screen. Next, the thoracic endograft device is brought up to the level of planned deployment (FIGURE 43-8). If a large sheath is not part of the device, the next step will be to pass sequentially larger dilators and then the delivery sheath, usually 20 to 22 Fr. Manual forward tension should be kept on the stiff wire to ensure the wire hugs the greater curve of the arch. There should be minimal adjustments once the endograft is at the level of the arch to minimize sheering forces of the endograft on the aortic wall. Excessive scraping of the endograft along the aortic arch can lead to a shower effect, as platelets may aggregate (inflammation of newly dissected aorta) and can be freed from the wall, resulting in a stroke. Another key gateway is that prior to deployment, the endograft should be released from the hands of the surgeon to see if without tension the endograft has developed unreleased torque. While this is performed, gentle forward tension should be maintained on the stiff wire to keep it adjacent to the outer aortic curvature.

At the very least, prior to deployment the systolic blood pressure should be reduced to 80 mmHg pre-deployment to prevent pushing the device inferiorly. Rapid ventricular pacing or adenosine can be used to decrease cardiac output for tenuous or very proximal deliveries. Deployment should be slow and methodical to ensure proper proximal placement. Once the first two proximal stent rings are deployed, the rest of the graft should be deployed with pace to ensure that a "windsock" effect does not displace the intended proximal seal zone.

Determining the extent of distal seal zone has been the subject of debate. Most now agree that enough of the descending thoracic aorta should be treated to assure adequate expansion of the true lumen to maintain branch vessel perfusion and prevent late degeneration. If possible, the entire dissection flap down to the celiac artery should be considered for coverage and true lumen expansion for the distal landing zone. This is because degeneration of the rest of the aorta into an aneurysm occurs in up to 50% of patients. The downside is this potentially increases the risk of paraplegia. After the first piece is deployed, the left femoral pigtail catheter is advanced through the endograft for angiographic visualization of the distal landing zone of the celiac artery and superior mesenteric artery, often best seen through a right anterior oblique view (FIGURE 43-9). The distal extension is then deployed similar to the proximal stent graft. If there are large intercostal arteries in this region, attempts should be made not to cover them. **CONTINUES**

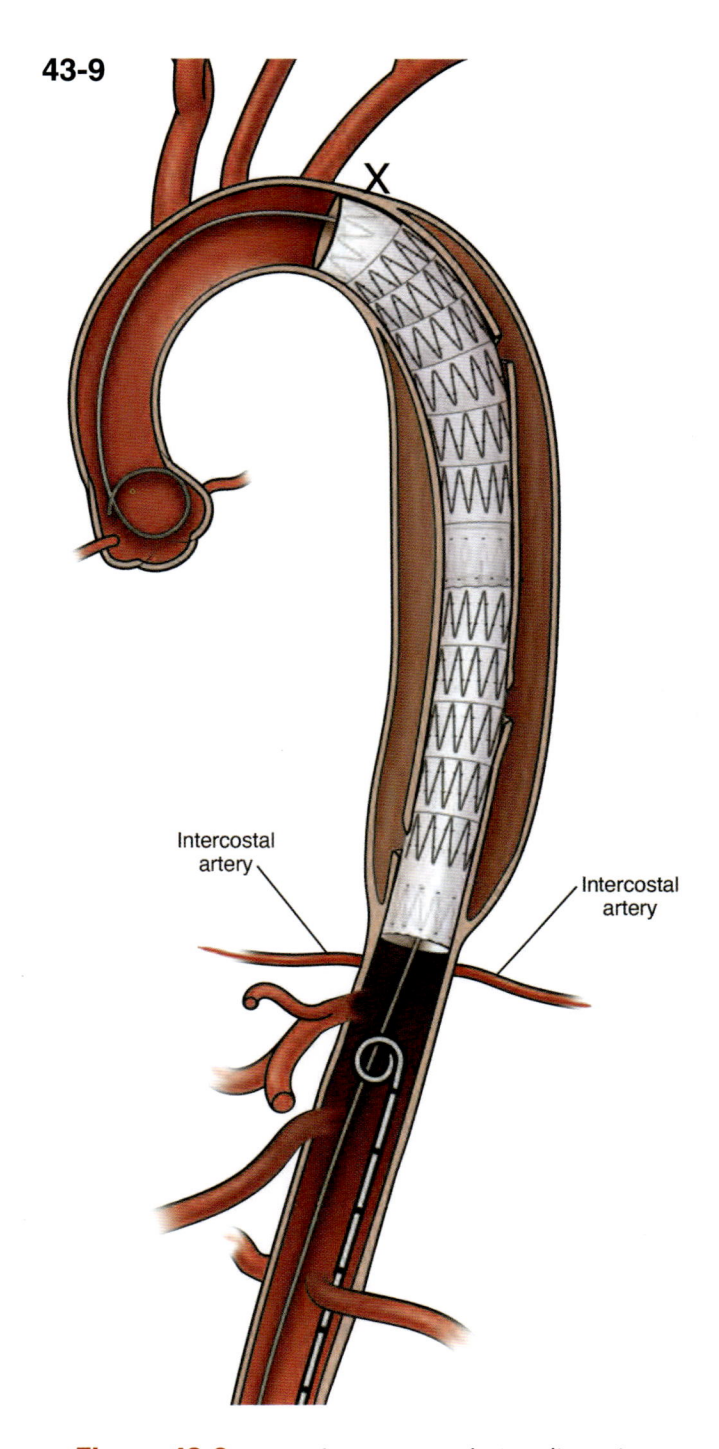

43-9

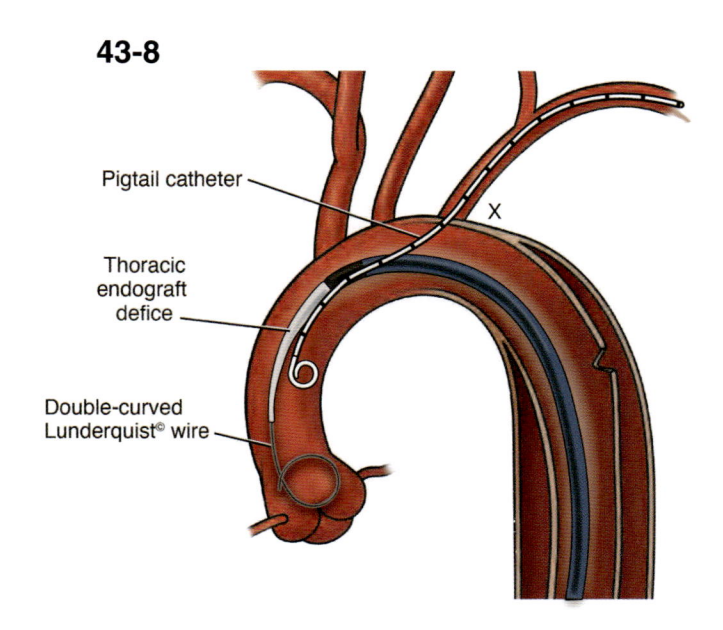

43-8

Pigtail catheter

Thoracic
endograft
defice

Double-curved
Lunderquist© wire

Intercostal
artery

Intercostal
artery

Figure 43-8 Angiogram of thoracic aorta with thoracic endograft covering the proximal entry tear. Flow is only seen in the true lumen after deployment.

Figure 43-9 Visceral angiogram during dissection.

DETAILS OF PROCEDURE `CONTINUED` Determining distal perfusion of the celiac artery, superior mesenteric artery, and bilateral renal arteries is the next important step. Both the true and false lumen can cause static (**FIGURE 43-10A**) and dynamic compression of the visceral arteries (**FIGURE 43-10B**). If the celiac or SMA has significant narrowing (particularly the SMA), and if the main body of the graft does not improve perfusion, a peripheral stent may be appropriate. In this case, selective angiography is imperative to confirm you are in the true lumen, and peripheral stenting should be done expeditiously (**FIGURE 43-11**).

BRANCH VESSEL PERFUSION: If there is concern for proximal displacement of the endograft during deployment, potentially covering the left carotid or innominate, the pigtail should not be retracted. It can be used for an angiogram, which if confirms unintentional coverage of cerebral perfusion can be used to exchange for a wire and balloon. When inflated, the balloon will push the endograft away from the lumen of the arch, allowing for cerebral perfusion as rescue maneuvers, extra atomic cerebral bypasses, or parallel grafting through a retrograde approach. Completion angiogram should evaluate for entry flow. Type 1B, II, and re-entry flow can be surveilled, except in the setting of rupture. Type 1A entry flow, with perigraft flow allowing antegrade flow into the false lumen, may require a second, more proximal endograft piece to be placed. Ballooning of the endograft after deployment, even in the setting of persistent entry flow, should not be performed due to the risk of inducing a retrograde dissection.

CLOSURE

PERCUTANEOUS FEMORAL APPROACH: All catheters and sheaths are removed and bilateral femoral arteries are repaired using the knot pushers to tie down the previously placed Prolene Perclose ProGlides. Palpable pulses distal to this repair and signals in the feet should be evaluated. We find it helpful to place a single interrupted subcuticular stich, although some prefer a Steri-Strip and skin glue application to the percutaneous access sites.

ALTERNATIVE OPEN FEMORAL APPROACH: All catheters and sheaths are removed and bilateral femoral arteries repaired with interrupted 6-0 Prolene sutures. Prior to tying down the last knot, the arteries are forward- and back-flushed to ensure there are no residual particles or air. Soft tissue is closed in three layers of 3-0 Vicryl, the first two as a figure-of-eight and the final as a running deep dermal layer. A 4-0 Monocryl is used for the skin in a subcuticular fashion. The wound is sterilely draped. Palpable pulses distal to this repair are noted.

POSTOPERATIVE CARE Spinal ischemia leading to paralysis may occur secondary to coverage of intercostal or lumbar arteries and can be exacerbated if there is coverage of the left subclavian artery. The patient should remain on every-hour neurovascular checks for the first 24 hours along with monitor for hematoma and access complications. The neurovascular checks should include monitoring pulses, and the patient must be able to lift their legs off the bed. Mean arterial pressure should be maintained above 90 to assist with spinal perfusion. The patient must be able to ambulate after mean arterial goals have been normalized prior to discharge. If the patient develops paraplegia or paraparesis postoperatively and a spinal drain is not in place, one should be immediately placed and maintained at 20 cc/drainage per hour until neuro function is restored, then at 10 cc/hour for the next 24 hours. Mean arterial pressures are first liberalized and then the spinal drain is placed to monitor (never "capped") to ensure the catheter is still indwelling during cessation of drainage. If the patient remains neurologically intact for 24 hours, the drain can then be removed. ■

SUGGESTED READINGS

Lombardi JV, Hughes GC, Appoo JJ, Bavaria JE, Beck AW, Cambria RP, Charlton-Ouw K, Eslami MH, Kim KM, Leshnower BG, Maldonado T, Reece TB, Wang GJ. Society for Vascular Surgery (SVS) and Society of Thoracic Surgeons (STS) reporting standards for type B aortic dissections. *J Vasc Surg.* 2020 Mar;71(3):723-747.

Lombardi JV. Type B aortic dissections-making the case for "practical" clinical practice guidelines. *J Vasc Surg.* 2022 Dec;76(6):1429-1431.

Lombardi JV, Gleason TG, Panneton JM, Starnes BW, Dake M, Haulon S, Mossop PJ, Segbefia E, Bharadwaj P, STABLE II investigators. Five-year results of the STABLE II study for the endovascular treatment of complicated, acute type B aortic dissection with a composite device design. *J Vasc Surg.* 2022 Nov;76(5):1189-1197.

Nienaber CA, Kische S, Rousseau H, Eggebrecht H, Rehders TC, Kundtn K, Glass A, Scheinert D, Czerny D, Kleinfeldt T, and for the INSTEAD-XL trial. Endovascular Repair of Type B Aortic Dissection Long-term Results of the Randomized Investigation of Stent Grafts in Aortic Dissection Trial. *Circulation: Cardiovascular Interventions.* 2013;6:407–416.

Ryan C, Vargas L, Mastracci T, Srivastava S, Eagleton M, Kelso R, Clair D, Sarac TP. Progress in management of malperfusion syndrome from type B dissections. *J Vasc Surg.* 2013 May;57(5):1283-90; discussion 1290.

Subramanian S, Roselli EE. Thoracic aortic dissection: long-term results of endovascular and open repair. *Semin Vasc Surg.* 2009 Jun;22(2):61-68.

43-10

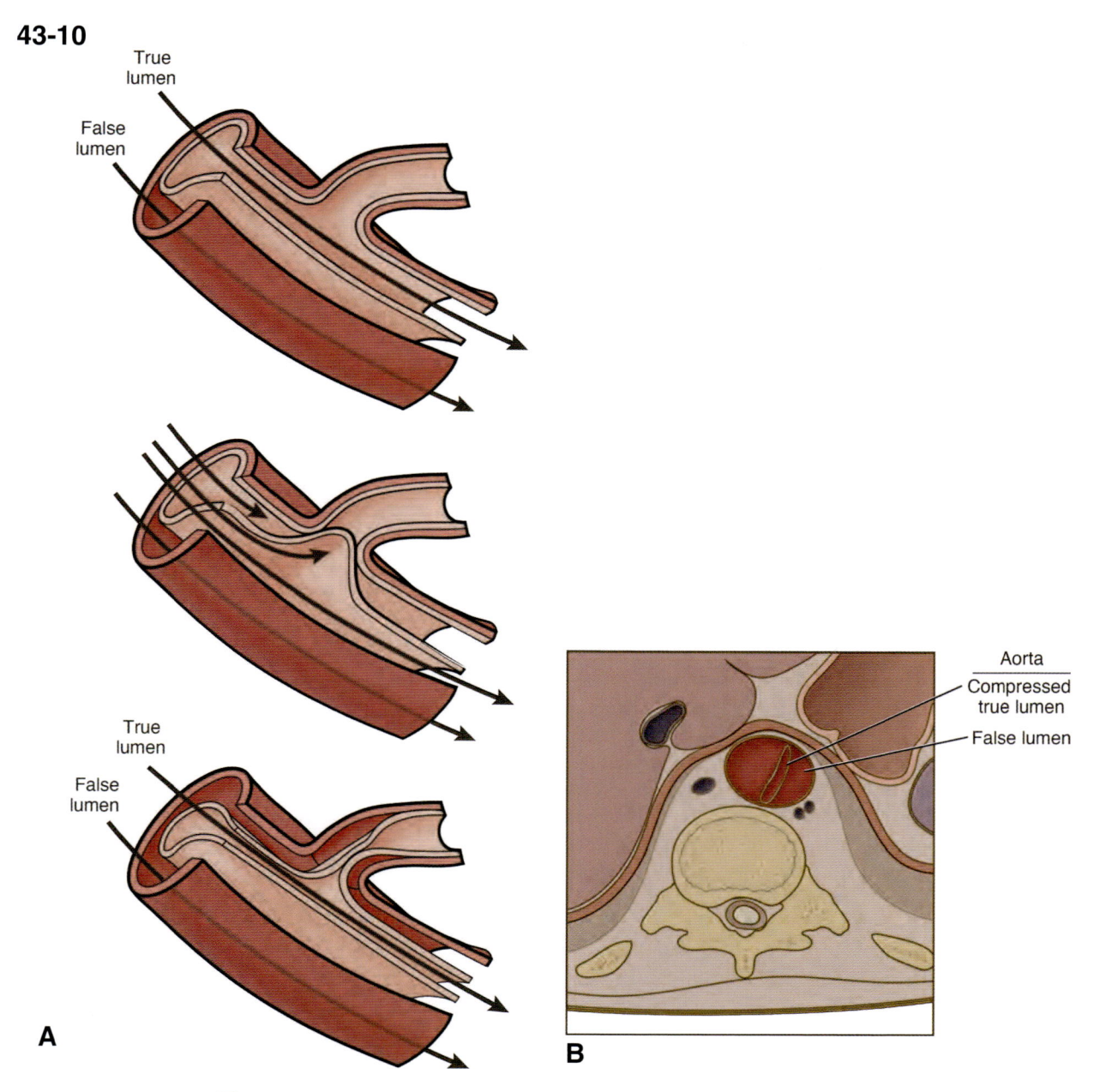

Figure 43-10 A. Dynamic obstruction. B. Compressed true lumen.

43-11

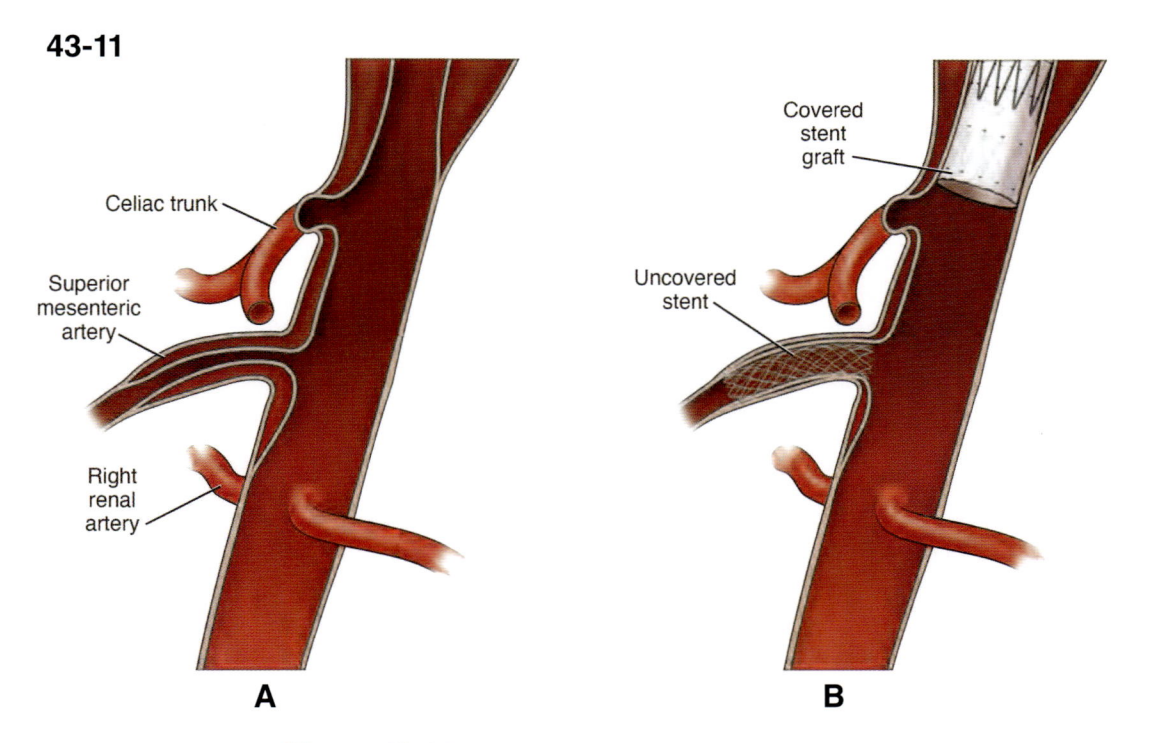

Figure 43-11 Brachial access with dissection flap.

Fenestrated Endovascular Aortic Aneurysm Repair

Jessica P. Simons, MD, MPH • Andres Schanzer, MD, FACS, DFSVS

INDICATIONS Patients with thoracoabdominal aortic aneurysms (TAAA) measuring 6.0 cm or greater in maximal diameter meet size criteria for repair for prevention of rupture. Both open and complex endovascular (fenestrated/branched endovascular aneurysm repair [FB-EVAR]) options may be considered, factoring in anatomic features and perioperative risk to a shared decision-making approach. The aneurysm extent must be classified; the Crawford or Safi classification systems are most commonly applied. The decisions that go into graft planning are the first of the gateway steps, as the design is absolutely critical to the success of the operation, but these considerations are beyond the scope of this chapter. Instead, the focus herein will be limited to steps for devices with ≥1 fenestration(s) for incorporation of target arteries (see Chapters 45 and 46 for discussion of branched devices). For those devices that will extend >4 cm above the celiac artery, consideration should be given to the placement of a lumbar drain for reduction of spinal cord ischemia (SCI) risk. Consideration should also be given for staging the procedure for more extensive TAAA to reduce SCI risk. For example, a TEVAR (with or without left carotid subclavian bypass) can be performed as a first stage, allowing time for adjustment of collateral flow to the spinal cord, followed by the second stage fenestrated endovascular aortic repair (FEVAR) approximately 2 to 4 weeks later, with a lumbar drain used at that operation.

POSITIONING Whenever possible, patients should undergo general endotracheal anesthesia, and the case should be conducted in a hybrid operating room with a fixed x-ray unit capable of fusion imaging. The patient should be placed supine with the arms either tucked or over the head to facilitate necessary imaging before and during the case. In most cases, sleds or armboards must be avoided, as they will obstruct the gantry. Once the patient is positioned, but prior to prepping, a cone beam computed tomography (i.e., 3D spin) should be performed to facilitate fusion with the preoperative computed tomography angiography images. The fusion image should be processed to include markers at the origins of the target vessels and the aortic bifurcation (FIGURE 44-1). The patient may be prepped and draped after the spin, taking care not to move the patient, which could disrupt the alignment of the fused images.

OPERATIVE PREP The patient should be prepped with a chlorhexidine and alcohol-based solution from the xiphoid to the knees. This permits laparotomy in the case of an emergency as well as adequate exposure of the femoral vessels. In cases where branches are planned, the chest/axilla, and or arm may be prepped but that will be covered elsewhere (Chapters 45 and 46).

A schematic of the device and any details about the planned operative steps and anticipated bridging stent grafts should be made in advance of the procedure. We favor displaying this on the lead shield in the room, under a clear sterile cover, for easy reference.

INCISION AND EXPOSURE Access can be obtained percutaneously to the femoral arteries in most cases. Ultrasound guidance is used to place the puncture in a healthy segment of common femoral artery; percutaneous sutures are deployed at the 10 o'clock and 2 o'clock positions in a pre-close fashion. The knots are tied down at the end of the procedure.

When open exposure is required, a transverse skin incision is preferred. The exposure is reoriented in a vertical fashion at the level of the fascia. The common femoral, superficial femoral, and profunda arteries are dissected sharply and encircled with vessel loops. The puncture is placed in a healthy segment of the common femoral artery.

An 18-gauge access needle and standard J-tip wire are advanced into the artery and then a 6 French sheath is placed. When using the Perclose technique, the sutures are next deployed and maintained on hemostats; an 8 French sheath is then placed.

DETAILS OF PROCEDURE Once 8 French sheaths are in place in both femoral arteries, systemic heparin is administered to achieve an activated clotting time goal of >300 seconds. A pigtail catheter is used to exchange out for stiff wires on both sides. The sheath on the side contralateral to intended device delivery side is upsized to the diameter necessary for accessing the target arteries and ultimately deploying bridging stent grafts. This diameter is dictated by the number of target arteries that will be cannulated from the contralateral side but is generally between 12 and 18 French.

The fusion marks at the origins of each target artery should be confirmed and adjusted based on angiography, intravascular ultrasound, or target artery selection. We prefer using a hydrophilic wire and directional catheter to select one of the target arteries, typically a renal artery. The fusion marks are used to guide initial cannulations, and then can be adjusted according to the demonstrated path of this marking wire once cannulation has been verified.

The next step involves orienting the device under fluoroscopy prior to inserting it. This is an absolutely critical step since failure to understand the marks on the device can result in unsheathing the device 180 degrees opposite the target vessels, making cannulation difficult and/or impossible. The graft must be carefully examined under fluoroscopy to clearly understand which side is anterior and which side is posterior (e.g., the superior mesenteric artery [SMA] fenestration must be at 12 o'clock rather than at 6 o'clock). This can be done by clearly identifying a fenestration, then verifying that it rotates in the anticipated direction when the device is slowly rotated away from the surgeon and back toward the surgeon (FIGURE 44-2). This orientation step also includes assessing for any twisting of the device within the sheath. For example, on a Cook device (Cook Medical, Bloomington, IN), there are three vertically aligned marks at the top and at the bottom of the device; if these are not aligned, it indicates some degree of twisting of the device within the sheath. Depending on the specific device being used and its marker scheme, various methods can be used to confirm the desired orientation for delivery. It is critically important to understand what each marker on a given device indicates. In general, the alignment of the SMA is the priority. Once it is determined how to rotationally align the SMA fenestration outside of the patient under fluoroscopy, a mental note is made of a landmark on the device sheath handle. It is important to choose a part that does not move. For example, with the SMA fenestration in the proper orientation under fluoroscopy, that may correspond to the sidearm on the sheath being oriented at 3 o'clock.

At this point, the device can be carefully inserted over the wire, with the sidearm in the appropriate rotational orientation. As the device is advanced, the focus must be maintained on (1) rotational clock face alignment and (2) longitudinal proximal-distal alignment relative to the fusion marks. The device must be advanced under fluoroscopic guidance the whole time. Ultimately, the alignment of the SMA is the most critical and will serve as the key reference for unsheathing.

Fenestrations should be aligned essentially at the level of the target artery origins, perhaps 1 to 2 mm proximal, as the device may tend to move slightly distally as it is unsheathed. Unsheathing should be done slowly, pausing to assess rotational clock face orientation and proximal-distal longitudinal alignment of the fenestration marks with the fusion marks (FIGURE 44-3). Small degrees of misalignment can be tolerated, since the diameter-reducing ties will pull the fenestrations slightly posteriorly; but the SMA remains the priority for alignment overall.

Once the device is unsheathed, if preloaded wires are included, these should be used to exchange for sheaths at this time. Care must be taken to leave several centimeters of an 0.018 wire advanced out the fenestration so the sheath can be advanced a few millimeters out the fenestration.

CONTINUES ▶

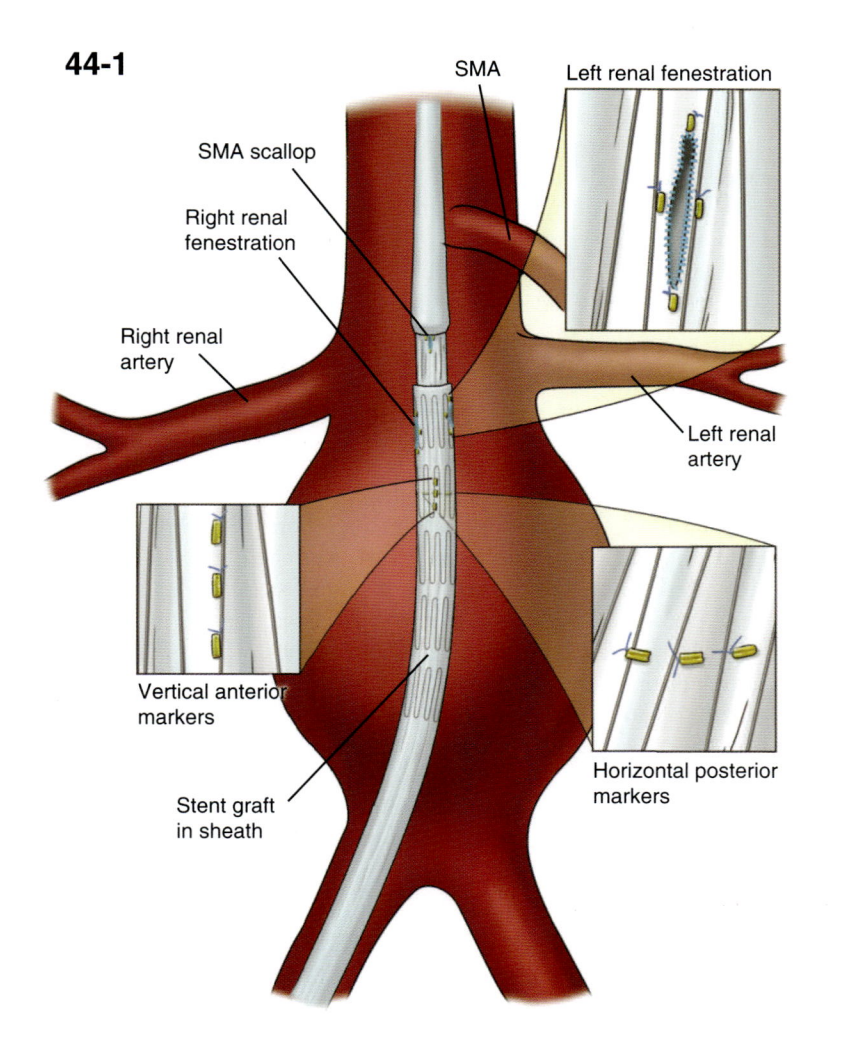

Figure 44-1 Fusion imaging to create a 3-dimensional model with marks for the origins of the target arteries and the aortic bifurcation.

Figure 44-2 Orienting the device under fluoroscopy, verifying the fenestration marks rotate in the anticipated direction.

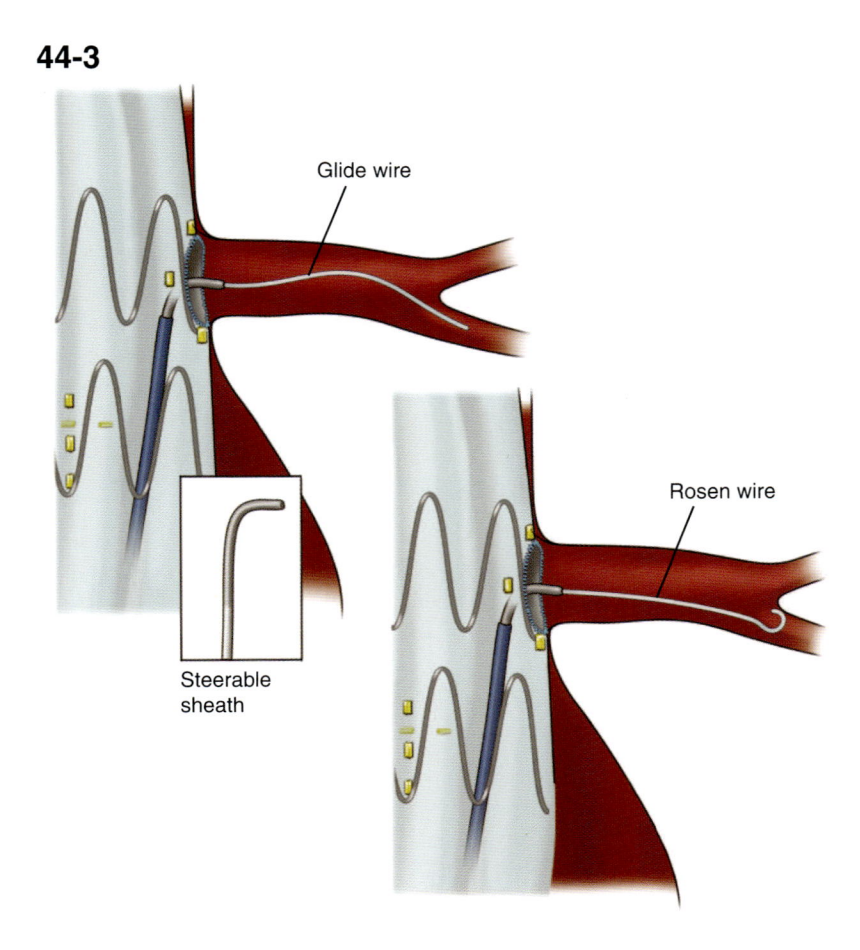

Figure 44-3 Gradual unsheathing under fluoroscopy, verifying clock face orientation and proximal-distal alignment of the fenestration marks with the fusion marks.

DETAILS OF PROCEDURE CONTINUED Cannulation of the target arteries is next performed from the contralateral sheath. First, wire access inside the fenestrated component must be verified. Then a steerable sheath is introduced over an exchange-length, hydrophilic, angled-tip wire and used to select the SMA fenestration. Once the sheath has selected the fenestration, the wire can be used to cannulate the target artery. Several centimeters of purchase are generally sought, then a crossing catheter is placed to facilitate exchange for an intermediate-stiffness J-tip wire (e.g., Rosen wire). A selective angiogram is performed to verify the target vessel. The steerable sheath is withdrawn over the wire and then reinserted parallel to the wire in the contralateral sheath. The same general steps are followed to cannulate the celiac artery, ultimately leaving an intermediate stiffness wire in place. Care must be taken to ensure that each wire is adequately controlled once multiple wires/sheaths are inserted in a parallel fashion; movement of one will translate to the others otherwise.

The renal arteries are next cannulated, either through the contralateral sheath or using a bi-port handle design with preloaded wires. Once intermediate stiffness wires are in place in all the target arteries, diameter reduction is removed (**FIGURE 44-4**). The proximal and distal fixation wires are released as well, signifying the complete dis-attachment of the fenestrated component from the delivery system. In general, the bridging stent grafts can next be advanced into the target arteries in any order; however, if any of the cannulations seems particularly less stable than another, it may be advantageous to treat that target artery first. The overall device alignment also tends to improve with each subsequent bridging stent graft deployment.

Deployment of the bridging stent grafts requires advancing a sheath over the wire into the target artery origin. The stent graft is advanced, then unsheathed, with approximately 2 to 3 mm of fabric extending into the lumen of the aortic device. It is inflated to profile, and as it is deflated, the sheath is advanced over it into the target artery again. A 10-mm × 2-cm balloon is used to flare the aortic portion of the stent graft, creating a tight seal with the fenestration itself (**FIGURE 44-5**). A selective angiogram is performed, assessing for any endoleak at the distal extent of the stent graft (type Ic) or at the fenestration (type IIIc), or evidence of distal dissection of the target artery.

Once all bridging stent grafts are completed, the bifurcated device can be advanced in the standard manner as for an infrarenal EVAR. The wires may be left in place in the target arteries as the bifurcated device is delivered but must be removed prior to unsheathing the bifurcated device. In the case of fenestrated repair, care must be taken to ensure a minimum of two-stent overlap between the fenestrated component and the bifurcated component. At this time, the goal for heparinization may be liberalized to an activated clotting time of >220 seconds. While complete details of EVAR deployment are covered elsewhere, in brief, the device is opened to the level of the contralateral gate. The gate is cannulated, and an intra-graft cannulation is confirmed. A limb extension is placed. The remainder of the ipsilateral side of the bifurcate is deployed, and a limb extension is placed.

A compliant balloon is used for molding each of the overlap zones, including that between the fenestrated component and the bifurcated component, and the distal seal zones. Care must be taken to ensure that the compliant balloon does not interfere with the target artery bridging stent grafts.

Either a completion 2-D aortogram or cone-beam CT, with or without contrast, can be performed to assess the architecture of the repair. In general, endoleaks seen on this completion imaging are not addressed unless the source is obvious (e.g., type 1a or 1b) since each target artery was already interrogated with a selective angiogram.

CLOSURE The sheaths are removed from each groin, maintaining wire access initially. The percutaneous sutures are tied down, ultimately removing the wire once hemostasis is achieved, prior to cinching them completely. Manual pressure is held while protamine is administered. The puncture sites are approximated with cyanoacrylate skin glue.

In the case of an open exposure, the sheaths and wires are removed, and the vessels are clamped. The intima is inspected to ensure it is incorporated into closure of the puncture as a transverse arteriotomy, using interrupted monofilament sutures. The wounds are irrigated and closed in multiple layers.

POSTOPERATIVE CARE Patients are monitored closely in the postoperative period for any signs of SCI. Lumbar drains, when present, are managed with a standardized protocol to keep intracranial pressures less than 10 to 12 cm H2O. These patients with coverage extensive enough to warrant lumbar drain placement are also managed with a mean arterial pressure goal of >90 mm Hg and hematocrit goals of >30%. Antihypertensive medications are held and only gradually resumed over time. Dual antiplatelet therapy is initiated on postoperative day 7.

Computed tomography angiography of the chest, abdomen, and pelvis is performed at the 1-month postoperative timepoint. It is repeated at 6 and 12 months, then annually thereafter for life. In some cases, a noncontrast scan can be coupled with a duplex of the fenestrated vessels and the aneurysm sac. ∎

SUGGESTED READINGS

Antoniou GA, Juszczak MT, Antoniou SA, Katsargyris A, Haulon S. Fenestrated or branched endovascular versus open repair for complex aortic aneurysms: meta-analysis of time to event propensity score matched data. *Eur J Vasc Endovasc Surg.* 2021 Feb;61(2):228-237.

Katsargyris A, Marques de Marino P, Verhoeven EL. Graft design and selection of fenestrations versus branches for renal and mesenteric incorporation in endovascular treatment of pararenal and thoracoabdominal aortic aneurysms. *J Cardiovasc Surg (Torino).* 2019 Feb;60(1):35-40.

Mirza AK, Tenorio ER, Kärkkäinen JM, Hofer J, Macedo T, Cha S, Ozbek P, Oderich GS. Learning curve of fenestrated and branched endovascular aortic repair for pararenal and thoracoabdominal aneurysms. *J Vasc Surg.* 2020 Aug;72(2):423-434.e1.

Oderich GS, Forbes TL, Chaer R, Davies MG, Lindsay TF, Mastracci T, Singh MJ, Timaran C, Woo EY. reporting standards for endovascular aortic repair of aneurysms involving the renal-mesenteric arteries. *J Vasc Surg.* 2021;73:4S-52S.

Timaran CH, Oderich GS, Tenorio ER, Farber MA, Schneider DB, Schanzer A, Beck AW, Sweet MP; Aortic Research Consortium. Expanded use of preloaded branched and fenestrated endografts for endovascular repair of complex aortic aneurysms. *Eur J Vasc Endovasc Surg.* 2021 Feb;61(2):219-226.

44-4

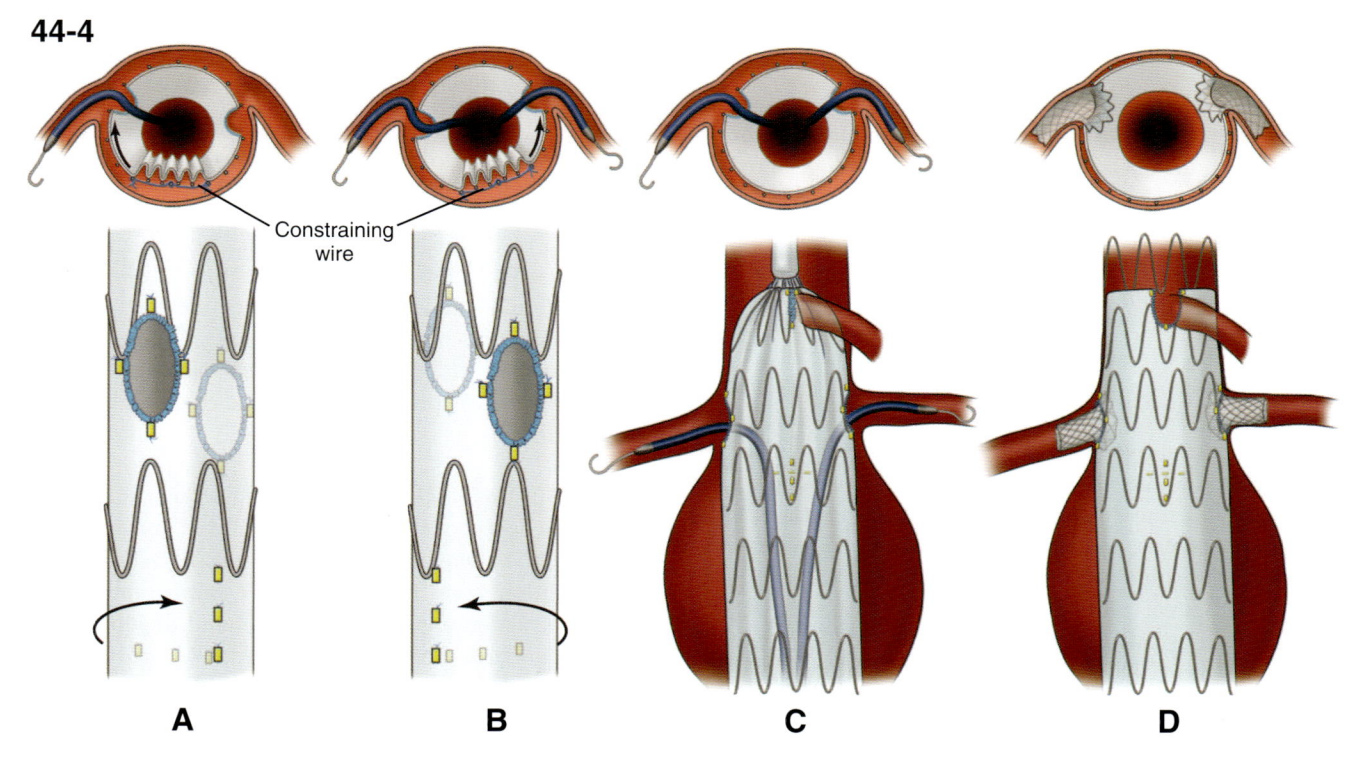

Constraining wire

A   B   C   D

Figure 44-4 Once all target arteries are cannulated, diameter reduction is removed.

44-5

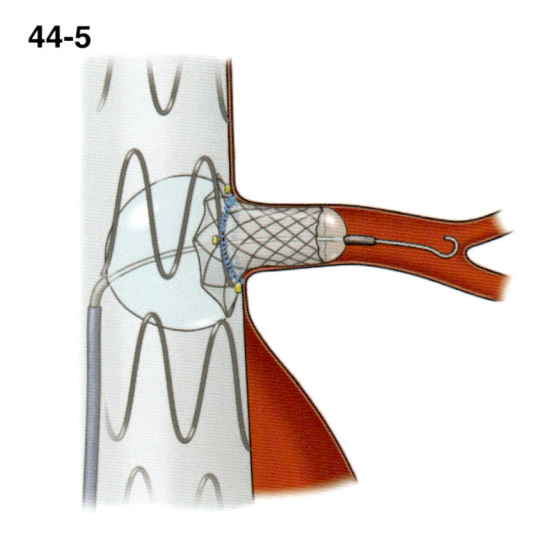

Figure 44-5 Flaring of the bridging stent graft at the fenestration using a balloon that is larger in diameter than the fenestration.

BRANCHED ENDOVASCULAR AORTIC ANEURYSM REPAIR

Emanuel R. Tenorio, MD, PhD • Gustavo S. Oderich, MD

INDICATIONS The majority of patients with thoracoabdominal aortic aneurysms (TAAAs) are asymptomatic and are diagnosed incidentally. Recent SVS guidelines recommend thoracic endovascular aortic repair (TEVAR) for patients with aneurysms larger than 5.5 cm. Because the morbidity of endovascular TAAA repair is higher, a minimum diameter threshold of 6 cm is recommended to indicate repair. Treatment is also indicated in patients with symptoms, rupture, or rapid aneurysm expansion, defined as enlargement of >5 mm in 6 months. A lower size threshold to recommend repair is reasonable in patients with saccular aneurysms, pseudoaneurysms, and aneurysms involving anastomotic suture lines. A higher threshold is advised in higher risk patients with advanced age, severe comorbidities, sarcopenia, and frailty.

PREOPERATIVE EVALUATION Patients evaluated for elective TAAA repair undergo a comprehensive clinical and anatomical evaluation. Clinical assessment focuses on cardiac, pulmonary, renal, and neurological risks. Medical genetic evaluation is considered in patients age <50 years old at presentation and in those with family history or phenotypic features of Marfan, Loyes-Dietz, or other syndromes.

A computed tomography angiography (CTA) is essential for planning endovascular aortic repair providing accurate assessment of extent of disease, involvement of side branches, adequacy of femoral and brachial access vessels, and presence of other extravascular conditions that might affect treatment selection and approach. The CTA should assess the chest, abdomen, and pelvis extending from the innominate to femoral artery bifurcation with 1- to 2-mm cuts for assessment in workstations and 1-mm cuts for three-dimensional (3D) reconstructions. A single-phase arterial study is adequate for preoperative assessment and three-phase studies (noncontrast, arterial, and delayed) are obtained for postoperative surveillance.

Assessment of disease extent requires analysis of presence of arterial wall abnormalities such as calcium, thrombus, debris, or thickening, as well as changes in the aortic diameter using centerline of flow (CLF) measurements. Selection of the proximal and distal landing zones is the most important strategic decision for planning any endovascular aortic repair. The ideal proximal landing zone should be >20 mm in length with diameter of 18 to 42 mm in the thoracic aorta. Each renal and mesenteric artery should be evaluated for suitability of endovascular incorporation. Minimum requirements are diameters from 4 to 11 mm and absence of early vessel bifurcation, defined by <15 mm length from the origin to the first branch.

PATIENT SELECTION: Patients with anticipated survival of at least 2 years with TAAAs ≥6 cm are considered for elective open or endovascular repair. The most important determinants for branched endovascular aortic repair (BEVAR) candidacy are presence of suitable landing zones, absence of severe atherosclerotic debris ("shaggy aorta") in the arch and thoracoabdominal aorta, and suitable renal and mesenteric targets. Among patients with involvement of the aortic arch, total arch replacement using frozen elephant trunk technique or cervical debranching may be needed.

SPINAL CORD INJURY PREVENTION: Spinal cord injury (SCI) is the most devastating complication of open or endovascular TAAA repair, with estimated risk of 5 to 20%. Patients with poor collateral network circulation due to chronic occlusion of the hypogastric and/or vertebral arteries have higher risk of SCI. Staging has been widely utilized as a strategy to reduce risk of SCI. Although multiple strategies have been described, we recommend that patients with Extent I to II TAAAs be treated with proximal TEVAR from Zone 3 to Zone 5, leaving an intentional Type IB endoleak (FIGURE 45-1). A second-stage BEVAR is done with 1 week between the two stages. Among patients treated with patient-specific devices, wait periods of >6 to 8 weeks are required for device manufacturing.

The need for prophylactic cerebrospinal fluid (CSF) drainage remains controversial. Although we initially used it routinely, we currently avoid prophylactic drainage because of risk of hemorrhagic intracranial and spinal complications. Our protocol evolved to use of therapeutic or rescue CSF drainage, which is needed in approximately 10% of TAAA patients who develop postoperative SCI. Spinal fluid pressure is set in a closed, pressure-controlled system at a baseline of 10 mmHg. The spinal drain is kept clamped for 45 minutes and opened for 15 minutes of every hour to drain a maximum of 20 mL per hour at 10 mmHg, after which the drain is clamped again for the remainder of the hour.

Intraoperative neuromonitoring with motor evoked potential (MEP) and somatosensory evoked potential (SSEP) is used to identify early signs of SCI and allow rescue maneuvers to increase mean artery pressure (MAP) and restore pelvic and lower extremity perfusion. In patients with persistent changes in neuromonitoring despite the maneuvers, temporary aneurysm sac perfusion (TASP) is performed by leaving one of the directional branches or the contralateral iliac limb gate unstented with intentional endoleak.

PERIOPERATIVE MEASURES: Patients with stage IIIB or IV chronic kidney disease are admitted prior to the operation for intravenous hydration and oral acetyl-cysteine. Acetyl-salicylic acid (325 mg/day) is continued perioperatively, but clopidogrel and oral anticoagulants are discontinued because of potential placement of a CSF drain. Beta-blockers and statins are continued on the day of the operation with sips of clear fluids. Vasodilator antihypertensive medications are decreased or discontinued starting the week prior to the operation in order to keep a systolic blood pressure >140 mmHg and <160 mmHg. All patients are instructed to shower with Hibiclens liquid skin cleanser (chlorhexidine gluconate 4%) the day prior to the procedure to reduce bacterial counts. Gentle bowel preparation with magnesium citrate is recommended. Perioperative antibiotics are administrated intravenously prior to incision and re-dosed up to 24 hours after the procedure.

HYBRID ROOM SETUP Complex endovascular aortic procedures are performed in a hybrid operating room with fixed imaging and advanced applications such as two- and three-dimensional (2D)/3D onlay CTA fusion, high-definition cone beam computed tomography (CBCT), rotational digital subtraction angiography (DSA), and digital zoom. The principles of "as low as reasonably achievable" (ALARA) radiation exposure should be applied, including operator shields, reduced frame rates (7.5 fps), fluoroscopic pedal at the control of the most senior operating surgeon, image collimation, and avoidance of DSAs and excessive gantry angulations (>30°).

A wide range of catheters, wires, and stents is needed during these procedures to deal with potentially unanticipated problems. The endovascular inventory should be kept in close proximity to the hybrid operating room and should be managed by a coordinator who is familiar with device technology, manufacturer, clinical need, in-service training, and cost. In addition to having the proper tools, physicians performing these procedures need to master endovascular skills and often use their creativity on how to further simplify steps of the operation.

PATIENT POSITION AND ARTERIAL ACCESS Patients are positioned supine with both arms raised overhead to optimize imaging from lateral and oblique views (FIGURE 45-2). The imaging gantry is oriented from the head of the table. The EKG leads, urinary catheter, and monitoring cables and lines are secured away from the field of view and from the path of the x-ray beam and C-arm gantry. The chest, axilla, upper arm, abdomen, and both thighs are prepped and draped in the usual sterile fashion.

Percutaneous femoral approach is used whenever possible, unless there is a high femoral bifurcation, dense calcification, or anterior plaque. Using duplex ultrasound guidance, the femoral artery is punctured with a stiff 0.018-inch Micropuncture needle. The 0.018-inch stiff introducer guidewire is exchanged for a 0.035-inch Benson guidewire and a 6Fr sheath. A small oblique incision is made and the dermis and subcutaneous tissue are dilated circumferentially. Each femoral puncture is pre-closed with a two Perclose ProGlide closure devices (Abbott Vascular, Santa Clara, CA) oriented at 1:30 and 10:30 o'clock position. Once pre-closure is completed, an 8Fr sheath is advanced to the external iliac arteries and the patient is systemically heparinized with intravenous bolus of heparin (80–100 units/kg). A target activated clotting time (ACT) >250 seconds is maintained during the procedure. Continuous heparin (500–1000 units/hour) infusion is started and diuresis is induced with intravenous mannitol. If brachial access is needed, our preference is to use the right side in patients with Type I arch and absence of atheromatous debris. A small incision is done at the level of the anterior axillary line, and the brachial artery is circumferentially dissected for access with Micropuncture set. **CONTINUES ▶**

45-1

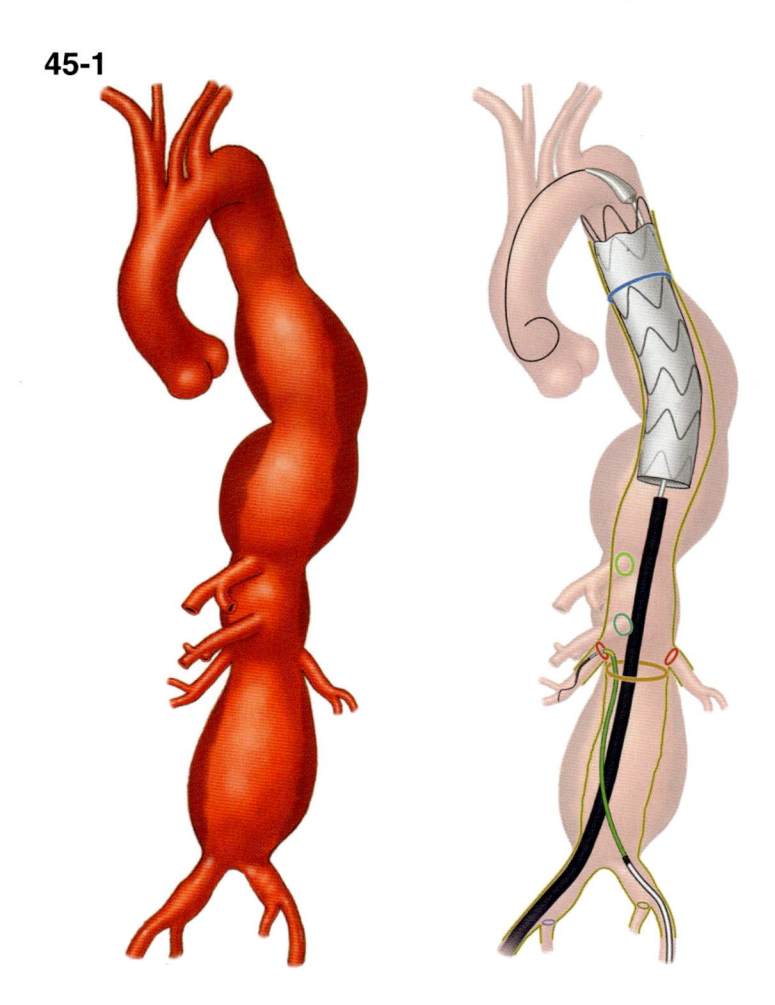

Figure 45-1 First stage TEVAR. (Reproduced with permission from Dr. Gustavo S. Oderich. University of Texas Health Science at Houston for Medical Education and Research.)

45-2

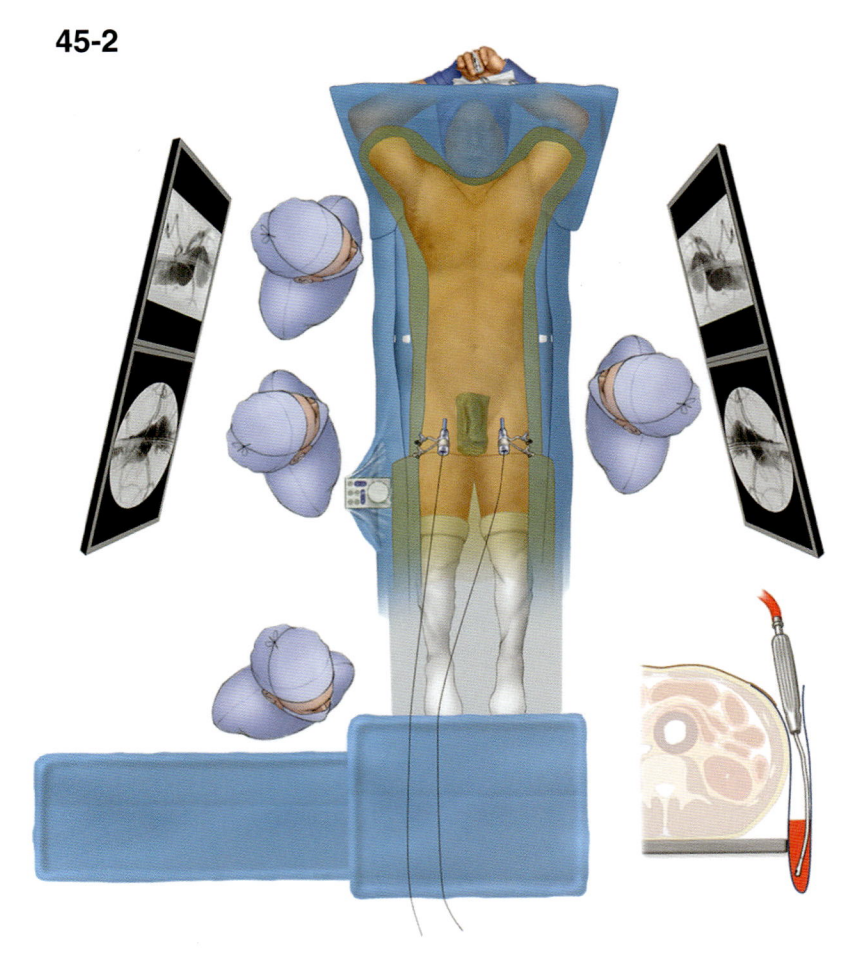

Figure 45-2 Patient position with overhead arm setup. (Reproduced with permission from Dr. Gustavo S. Oderich. University of Texas Health Science at Houston for Medical Education and Research.)

DETAILS OF THE PROCEDURE Variations in BEVAR technique include choice of brachial-femoral versus total femoral approach, use of preloaded systems, or staggered stent deployment techniques. The latter are used preferentially in patients with narrower aortic diameters, such as patients with chronic dissections and compressed true lumen to facilitate branch vessel catheterization. The off-the-shelf Gore TAMBE has preloaded wires for selective branch vessel catheterization and a staged device deployment. The most common techniques are summarized below.

STANDARD MULTIBRANCHED TECHNIQUE (BRACHIAL AND FEMORAL APPROACH): The extent of repair varies depending on the proximal extension of aneurysm within the thoracic aorta. The standard brachial and femoral approach is the most frequently used technique for multibranch stent-grafts (e.g., t-Branch stent-graft, Cook Medical, Bloomington, IN) and other investigational and patient-specific devices. Bilateral femoral and upper brachial approach is obtained. A 12Fr DrySeal flex sheath is introduced via the right brachial artery into the descending thoracic aorta over an Amplatz wire (Boston Scientific, Bloomington MN). Our preference is to obtain brachial-femoral through-and-through access, which is done by snaring a 0.035-inch 480-cm Tracer Metro Direct Wire Guide (Cook Medical, Bloomington IN). In general, the repair starts with deployment of a proximal thoracic stent-graft aiming for a distal stent-graft diameter of 30 to 34 mm. Precatheterization of one of the renal arteries is performed using a 7Fr LIMA guide catheter and 4Fr Berenstein catheter to calibrate the onlay fusion CT. Once the onlay fusion is calibrated, the t-Branch device is oriented extracorporeally and introduced via the through-and-through guidewire. Although the implantation does not need to be done with extreme precision, it is important to ensure proper orientation of the branch device and placement of each directional branch proximal to the intended target vessel. The directional branches are ideally deployed 1.5 to 2.0 cm above the intended target vessels and there should be a minimum internal aortic diameter of 25 mm to allow space for catheter manipulations (**FIGURE 45-3A**). After the branched device is deployed, the distal bifurcated component and ipsilateral iliac limb are placed, and the attachments and landing zones are dilated with coda balloon. The large 22Fr sheath is then removed, and flow is restored to the lower extremity while guidewire access is maintained with through-and-though wire. The contralateral gate is not completed at this stage, allowing access into the aneurysm sac if needed for possible "snare-ride" technique and the option of TASP in patients who develop changes in neuromonitoring.

The 12Fr DrySeal sheath is advanced inside the t-Branch stent-graft and positioned in the distal descending thoracic aorta. The through-and-through brachial-to-femoral artery wire provides support for advancement of the bridging stents. Each side branch is individually catheterized in a sequential fashion, usually starting with the lowest renal artery and moving cranially toward the celiac axis (**FIGURE 45-3B**). A 5Fr MPA or Kumpe catheter (Cook Medical, Bloomington, IN) is used to access the directional branch and target vessel. Once the vessel is catheterized, the soft Glidewire is exchanged for a stiff guidewire. In general, a Rosen guidewire is used for the renal arteries and short-tip Amplatzer for the superior mesenteric artery and celiac axis. The bridging stent-graft is oversized by 1 to 2 mm to the nominal vessel diameter and should be landed at least 2 cm distal to the target vessel origin, and should extend 2 to 5 mm proximal to the directional branch. Choice of bridging stent includes Viabahn self-expandable stent-grafts for renal branches and VBX balloon-expandable stent-grafts for renal and mesenteric branches (**FIGURE 45-3C**). If the patient has no changes in MEP, the aneurysm sac is closed by placement of the contralateral iliac limb extension (**FIGURE 45-3D**). Final completion rotational DSA and CBCT are obtained. **CONTINUES ▶**

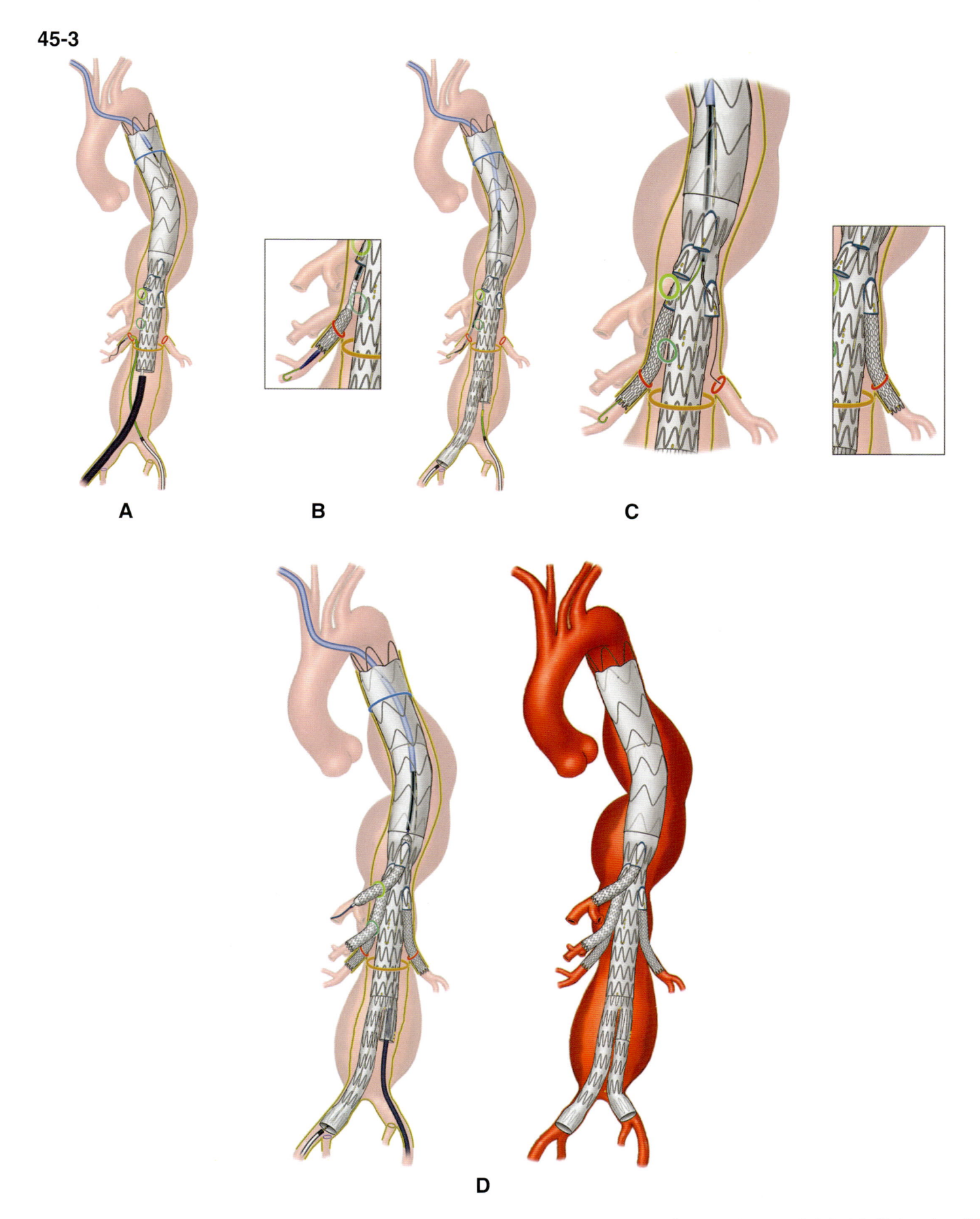

Figure 45-3 Standard t-Branch technique brachial and femoral. (Reproduced with permission from Dr. Gustavo S. Oderich. University of Texas Health Science at Houston for Medical Education and Research.)

DETAILS OF THE PROCEDURE *SEQUENTIAL OR STAGGERED MULTIBRANCHED TECHNIQUE (BRACHIAL AND FEMORAL APPROACH):* CONTINUED The staggered technique is a variation recommended in patients with limited luminal space from a narrow aortic segment or compressed true lumen due to chronic dissection. In these cases, complete release of the multibranch device and diameter-reducing ties may limit workspace for vessel catheterization. Instead, a staggered deployment is used and vessel catheterization is done from proximal to distal, starting first with the celiac axis branch. Once arterial access is obtained as previously described, the t-Branch stent-graft is oriented extracorporeally, introduced via the femoral access, and partially deployed releasing only the first directional branch (FIGURE 45-4A). The gold knob of the diameter-reducing tie is removed and partially deployed, followed by removal of the black knob, which releases the proximal fixation stent. This allows access into the t-Branch stent-graft from the brachial sheath (FIGURE 45-4B). Using a Kumpe catheter, the celiac axis directional branch and celiac axis are selectively catheterized, followed by placement of a 0.035-inch Amplatz guidewire. The same steps are repeated for the SMA and renal arteries (FIGURE 45-4C, D). The t-Branch stent-graft is fully deployed, followed by placement of the distal universal bifurcated stent-graft and ipsilateral iliac limb extension (FIGURE 45-4E). Once flow is restored to the lower extremity, the renal arteries, SMA, and celiac axis are sequentially stented (FIGURE 45-4F, G). The contralateral iliac limb extension is placed, followed by completion CBCT. CONTINUES

45-4

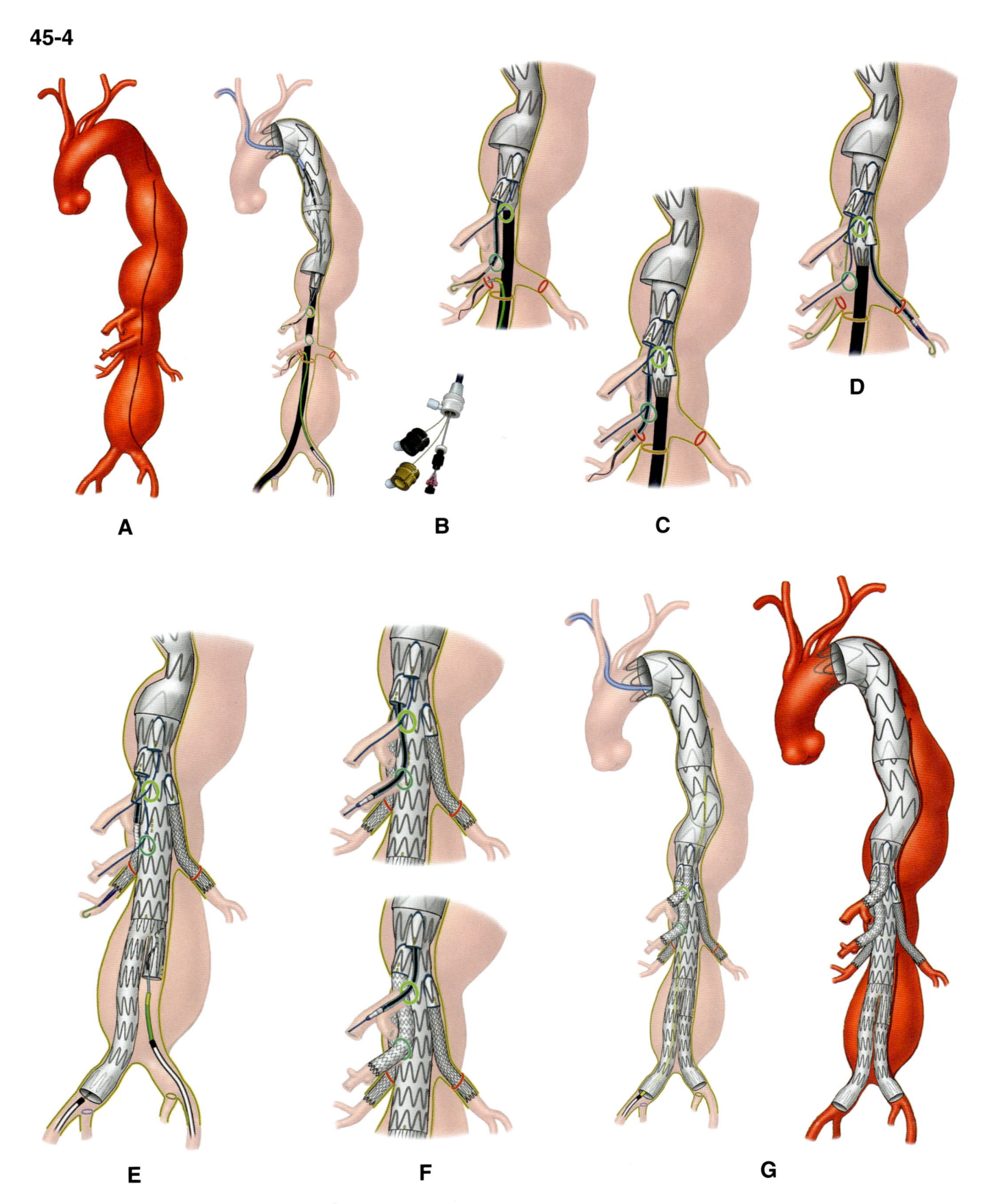

Figure 45-4 Sequential t-Branch technique brachial and femoral. (Reproduced with permission from Dr. Gustavo S. Oderich. University of Texas Health Science at Houston for Medical Education and Research.)

DETAILS OF THE PROCEDURE *TOTAL FEMORAL MULTIBRANCHED TECHNIQUE USING STEERABLE SHEATH*: **CONTINUED** The total transfemoral technique was championed by the Hamburg group and gained widespread popularity. The technique avoids use of brachial access, which may help reduce risk of cerebral embolization. The technique uses a steerable sheath system to provide support for catheterization and stenting of the directional branches and target vessels using the femoral approach. In these cases, the axilla is prepped into the surgical field, but open access is not obtained. Using the technique already described, the t-Branch stent-graft, universal bifurcated stent-graft, and ipsilateral iliac limb extension are sequentially deployed. The 22Fr sheath is downsized into a 12Fr (33-cm) DrySeal sheath, which is advanced as high as possible into the thoracic aorta. The steerable sheath setup is prepared using an 8.5Fr 55-cm usable length steerable sheath. A 0.014-inch 190-cm wire is loaded through the valve of the 8.5Fr sheath and looped outside of the sheath. A 6Fr 90-cm shuttle sheath is introduced through the 8.5Fr sheath and used as a coaxial system, which is loaded via the aortic guidewire through the 12Fr DrySeal sheath (FIGURE 45-5A). Once the 8.5 and 6Fr sheaths are advanced into the thoracic aorta just above the most proximal directional branch, the aortic wire and dilator of the 6Fr sheath are removed. The 6Fr sheath is partially withdrawn and the 8.5Fr steerable sheath is formed. A Kumpe catheter is used for selective catheterization of the directional branch (FIGURE 45-5B).

The first directional branch is selectively catheterized with Glidewire, and the 6Fr shuttle sheath is advanced through the directional branch. The target vessel is then catheterized using Glidewire and Kumpe catheter. Once the vessel is catheterized, the 6Fr sheath is used for selective angiography. The 6Fr sheath is removed over the wire and a VBX stent-graft is advanced into the target vessel without sheath support. The 0.014-inch wire provides enough support for safe advancement without change in the steerable sheath shape. Once the bridging stent is deployed and post-dilated, the 6Fr sheath is readvanced for final angiography. The same steps are repeated for the contralateral renal artery, SMA, and celiac axis (FIGURE 45-5C). The procedure is finalized with catheterization and stenting of the contralateral iliac limb extension and CBCT.

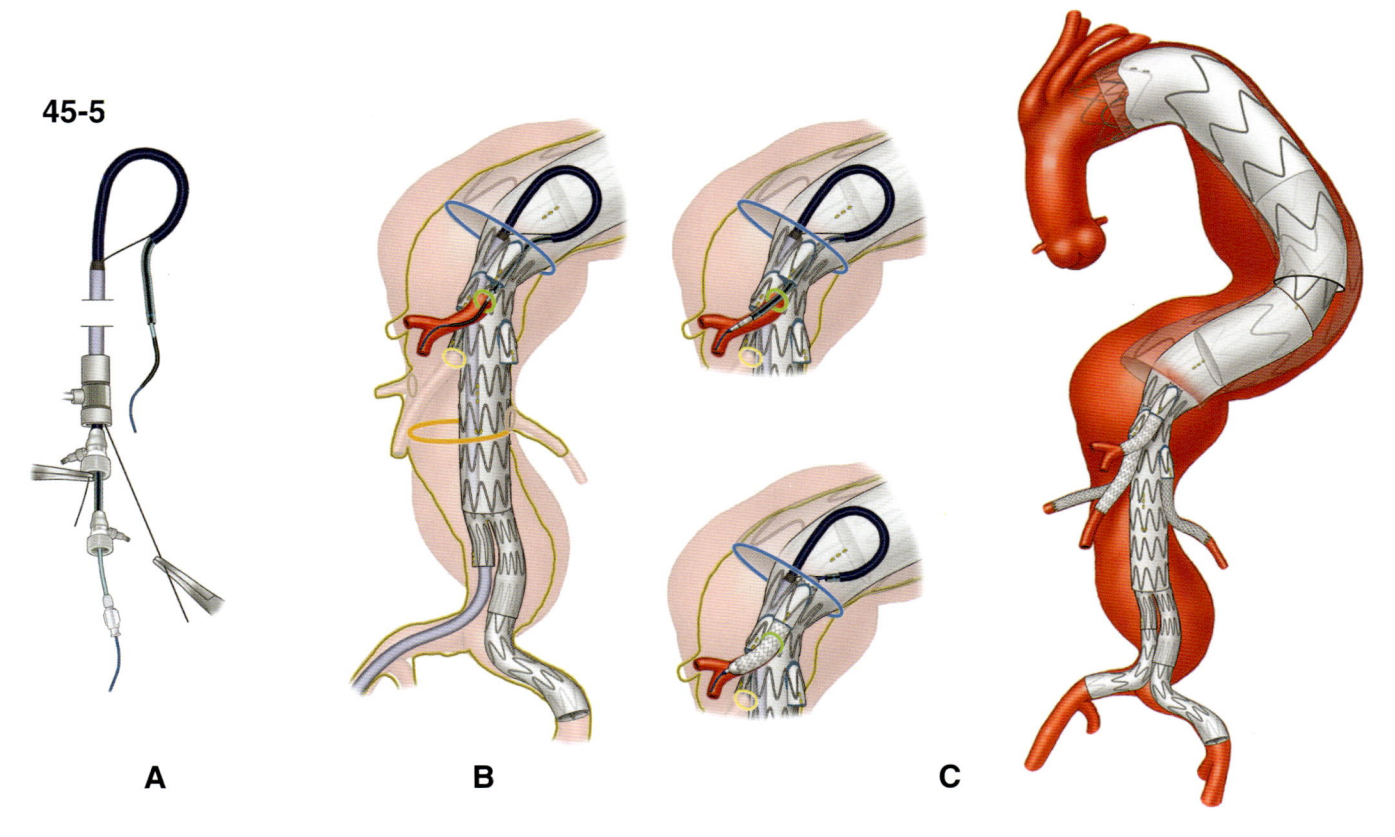

45-5

A   B   C

Figure 45-5 Total femoral t-Branch technique. (Reproduced with permission from Dr. Gustavo S. Oderich. University of Texas Health Science at Houston for Medical Education and Research.)

DETAILS OF THE PROCEDURE *INTENTIONAL DIRECTIONAL BRANCH OCCLUSION*: CONTINUED Patients with variations of the normal four-vessel renal and mesenteric anatomy due to chronic occlusion of one of the vessels or congenital or surgical absence of kidney may require occlusion of one or more directional branches (FIGURE 45-6). The technique is also applicable to patients in whom target vessel catheterization was not feasible. In these cases, the branches intended to be stented are completed first. Once this is done, the directional branch to be occluded is extended distally using a balloon expandable covered stent-graft followed by placement of an endovascular occlusion plug.

POSTOPERATIVE CARE Meticulous postoperative care is needed to prevent major adverse events and decrease the risk of SCI. Significant clinical events that result in systemic hypotension such as hemorrhagic, infectious, or respiratory complications may lead to decrease in spinal cord perfusion and delayed ischemia. Intracranial and spinal hemorrhagic complications are also a concern in patients who underwent placement of CSF drains. The length of stay averages 1 or 2 days in the intensive care unit, with total hospital stay of 2 to 3 days for Extent IV and 4 to 5 days for Extent I through III repairs. The first 24 to 48 hours are critical for hemodynamic support. We recommend maintaining a MAP >80 mmHg, systolic blood pressure >130 mmHg, hemoglobin >10 g/dL, and normal coagulation profile. Patients with Extent I through III TAAA are placed on strict bed rest with maximum of 30-degree elevation to decrease hydrostatic venous pressure in the first 36 hours. If a prophylactic CSF drain is placed, this is discontinued on postoperative day 2 after a 6-hour clamp trial and documentation of normal coagulation profile. Oral diet is resumed with clear liquids the day after the operation for uncomplicated cases requiring four fenestrations, but it is typically withheld for 1 or 2 days for difficult cases or those with extensive aortic coverage. A CTA is obtained prior to dismissal if there is clinical concern or if CBCT was not obtained during the procedure, but otherwise can be omitted. Patients are maintained on aspirin indefinitely. Clopidogrel is recommended for patients with renal directional branches but is otherwise not necessary. However, clopidogrel is not initiated until 2 weeks after the operation because of risk of deployed SCI and hemorrhagic brain complications. Follow-up includes clinical examination and imaging (CTA and ultrasound or renal and mesenteric stents) in 6 to 8 weeks, every 6 months during the first year, and yearly thereafter. ∎

SUGGESTED READINGS

Eilenberg W, Kölbel T, Rohlffs F, Oderich G, Eleshra A, Tsilimparis N, et al. Comparison of transfemoral versus upper extremity access to antegrade branches in branched endovascular aortic repair. *J Vasc Surg.* 2021 May;73(5):1498-1503.

Ferreira M, Katsargyris A, Rodrigues E, Ferreira D, Cunha R, Bicalho G, et al. "Snare-Ride": a bailout technique to catheterize target vessels with unfriendly anatomy in branched endovascular aortic repair. *J Endovasc Ther.* 2017 Aug;24(4):556-558.

Hiratzka LF, Bakris GL, Beckman JA, Bersin RM, Carr VF, Casey DE Jr, et al. 2010 ACCF/AHA/AATS/ACR/ASA/SCA/SCAI/SIR/STS/SVM Guidelines for the diagnosis and management of patients with thoracic aortic disease. A Report of the American College of Cardiology Foundation/American Heart Association Task Force on Practice Guidelines, American Association for Thoracic Surgery, American College of Radiology, American Stroke Association, Society of Cardiovascular Anesthesiologists, Society for Cardiovascular Angiography and Interventions, Society of Interventional Radiology, Society of Thoracic Surgeons, and Society for Vascular Medicine. *J Am Coll Cardiol.* 2010;55(14):e27-e129.

Oderich GS, Forbes TL, Chaer R, Davies MG, Lindsay TF, Mastracci T, et al; Writing Committee Group. Reporting standards for endovascular aortic repair of aneurysms involving the renal-mesenteric arteries. *J Vasc Surg.* 2021 Jan;73(1S):4S-52S.

Oderich GS, Tenorio ER, Mendes BC, Lima GBB, Marcondes GB, Saqib N, et al. Midterm outcomes of a prospective, non-randomized study to evaluate endovascular repair of complex aortic aneurysms using fenestrated-branched endografts. *Ann Surg.* 2021 Jun 16.

Tenorio ER, Kärkkäinen JM, Mendes BC, DeMartino RR, Macedo TA, Diderrich A, et al. Outcomes of directional branches using self-expandable or balloon-expandable stent-grafts during endovascular repair of thoracoabdominal aortic aneurysms. *J Vasc Surg.* 2020 May;71(5):1489-1502.e6.

Tenorio ER, Oderich GS, Sandri GA, Ozbek P, Kärkkäinen JM, Vrtiska T, et al. Prospective nonrandomized study to evaluate cone beam computed tomography for technical assessment of standard and complex endovascular aortic repair. *J Vasc Surg.* 2020;71(6):1982-1993.e5.

Tenorio ER, Ribeiro MS, Banga PV, Mendes BC, Kärkkäinen J, DeMartino RR, et al. Prospective assessment of a protocol using neuromonitoring, early limb reperfusion, and selective temporary aneurysm sac perfusion to prevent spinal cord injury during fenestrated-branched endovascular aortic repair. *Ann Surg.* 2021 Jan 7.

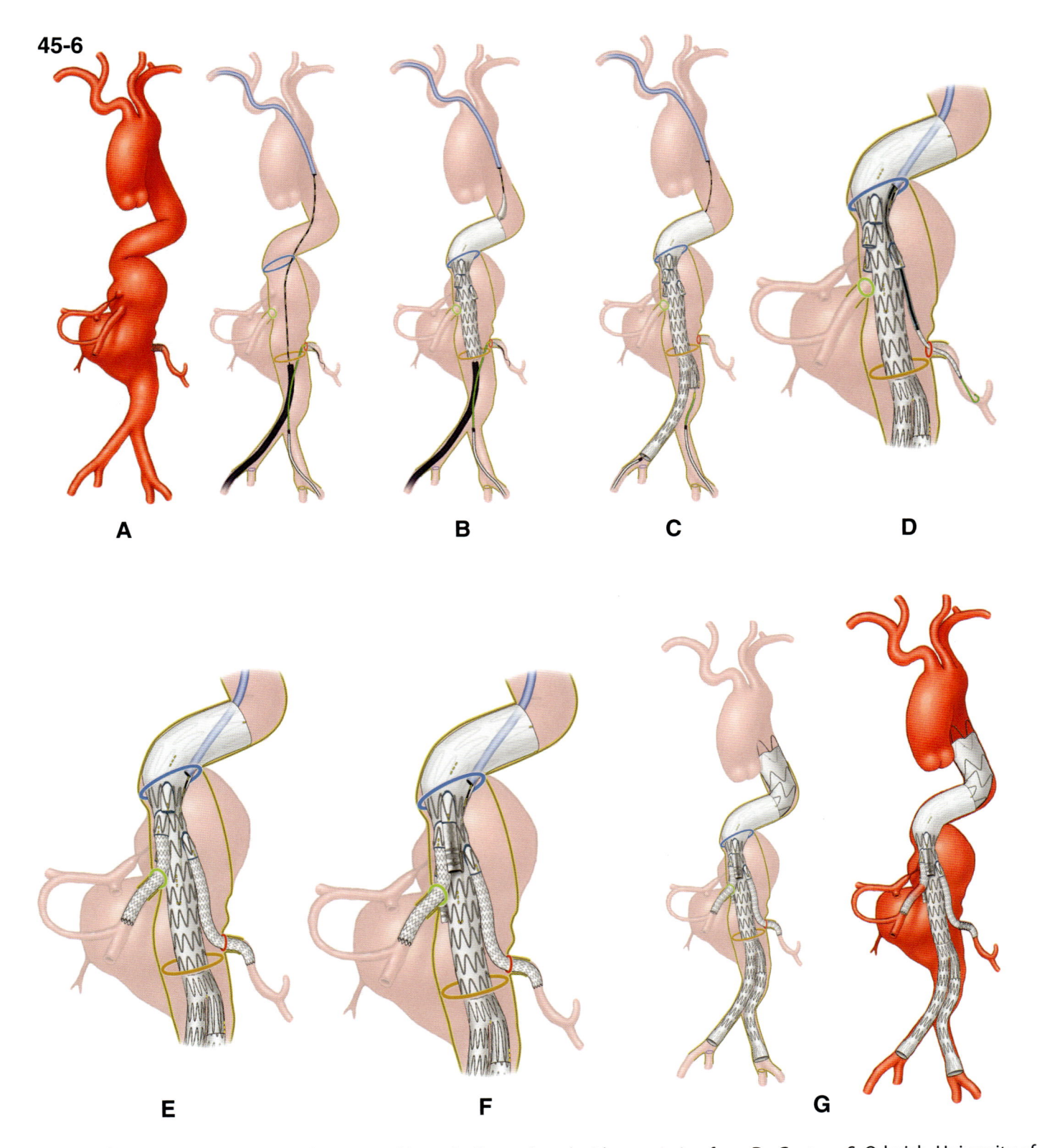

Figure 45-6 Intentional occlusion of directional branch. (Reproduced with permission from Dr. Gustavo S. Oderich. University of Texas Health Science at Houston for Medical Education and Research.)

PARALLEL STENT GRAFTS: THE CHIMNEY TECHNIQUE

Ross Milner, MD • Angela Giese, MD

PARARENAL AND JUXTARENAL AORTIC ANEURYSMS

INTRODUCTION Parallel grafts can be used for thoracoabdominal aortic aneurysms (TAAA), pararenal aortic aneurysms, or juxtarenal aortic aneurysms. Pararenal aortic aneurysms are morphologically defined as an abdominal aortic aneurysm (AAA) that includes the origin of the renal arteries. This is in distinction from juxtarenal AAA that encroaches the renal arteries but does not include their orifice. Parallel grafting is a technique that encompasses a range of deployment configurations in which peripheral stent grafts are placed extending from the aortic branches in a parallel fashion into the thoracic or abdominal aorta to both maintain visceral artery perfusion and treat the aortic aneurysm. This technique is used when coverage of an aortic branch is planned in order to extend the proximal seal zone. When deployed, parallel grafts (PGs) lie parallel to the aortic graft.

Various configurations of parallel grafting exist and are referred to in the literature as follows. The terms "chimney" and "snorkel" have become synonymous and are defined as parallel grafts that extend *proximal* to the aortic graft and perfuse via antegrade flow (FIGURE 46-1A). Conversely, the periscope configuration describes a parallel graft that extends *distal* to the aortic graft and perfuses via retrograde flow (FIGURE 46-1B). Given the nature of these configurations, a covered peripheral stent graft is necessary for parallel grafting to avoid gutter leaks. It should be noted that in the United States, these grafts are used "off-label" when traditional surgery is not possible.

INDICATIONS Chimney endovascular aortic repair (ChEVAR) is indicated for patients with TAAs, pararenal aortic aneurysms, and juxtarenal abdominal aortic aneurysms >5.5 cm for men and >5 cm for women. The standard indications for EVAR apply to this subgroup as well, including appropriate use for patients with ruptured or symptomatic aneurysms, and patients with rapid aneurysmal growth. Patients with saccular morphology should be considered for repair at smaller size criteria. Additionally, patients with previous EVAR who have developed a type 1a endoleak may be considered for ChEVAR. The patient's anatomy should be evaluated and meet the standard criteria necessary for endovascular aortic repair. It should not be discounted that open surgical repair remains a good option.

Currently, there are no commercially available endovascular devices to treat pararenal and thoracoabdominal aneurysms in the United States. Treatment of these complex aneurysms requires the use of either a branched or fenestrated device, which can take weeks to make, and branched devices need to be part of a clinical trial. The ChEVAR technique is a safe and effective alternative for patients in whom branched/fenestrated grafts are not readily available, although it is still considered "off-label" use by the FDA. It allows the use of off-the-shelf devices for urgent endovascular repair in patients with challenging aortic neck anatomy, inadequate fixation zones for traditional EVAR, or who have the above with compromised physiology. Several series have demonstrated the equivalent effectiveness of the chimney technique with fenestrated endografts.

PREOPERATIVE CONSIDERATIONS The procedural goal is to exclude the aneurysm while preserving visceral branch perfusion. An aortic neck sealing length of at least 2 cm is recommended, but for visceral stent sealing, having a length greater than 5 cm can cut down on gutter leaks. We recommend aortic stent graft oversizing by 20 to 30% for the chimney technique. Parallel grafts should be oversized no more than 10%, which can often be achieved with 1:1 sizing and post dilation. We also recommend avoiding more than two chimney grafts through any seal zone, but this is not always feasible. CT angiography and centerline with 3D reconstruction provides the most accurate measurements of the aorta and its visceral branches. We recommend at least 2 cm of purchase of the peripheral stent into the renal arteries to achieve maximal seal (FIGURE 46-2). An aortic neck sealing length of at least 2 cm is recommended, though some do advocate for longer lengths to reduce the rate of gutter leaks.

The authors prefer right axillary access as opposed to left, as ergonomically it is more comfortable to operate on the patient's right side and avoid competing for space with the image intensifier. However, this is surgeon dependent and many still use the left, as there is less sheath coverage of the great vessels. Literature from the author's institution supports the safe use of right axillary access and does not portend a higher risk of stroke compared to left upper extremity access. Sterile preparation is more facile with an axillary exposure, which avoids the circumferential arm preparation with brachial access. This also allows anesthesia to use both forearms for IV access during the procedure. While brachial access is a reasonable alternative, brachial artery diameter and sheath length can be an issue, and the arm must be positioned out instead of tucked; this can make lateral imaging challenging. Single-side access can be performed with direct access, a conduit with multiple sheaths, or via a buddy wire technique.

POSITIONING AND PREPARATION The patient is positioned supine. Both arms are tucked, and a vertical shoulder roll is placed between the scapula to facilitate axillary exposure. The chest, abdomen, and bilateral axillary and groin sites are sterilely prepped. The patient is then draped in the usual manner and the access sites are covered with Ioban drape (3M Corp, St. Paul, MN).

DETAILS OF THE PROCEDURE

PARARENAL, JUXTARENAL, AND PARAVISCERAL AORTIC ANEURYSMS: The procedure is initiated with either a right or left axillary cutdown depending on the surgeon's preference, and is done before systemic heparinization. Once the axillary artery dissection is completed, one or two pledgeted purse-string sutures can be placed at the intended arterial access sites to facilitate hemostatic closure upon removal. Some prefer to access all branches through the axillary artery, but we recommend no more than two sheaths placed directly into the axillary artery (FIGURE 46-3). If three or more vessel cannulations are planned, we advocate the use of a conduit for multiple sheath access. Vessel loops are used to encircle each sheath to prevent bleeding. **CONTINUES** ▶

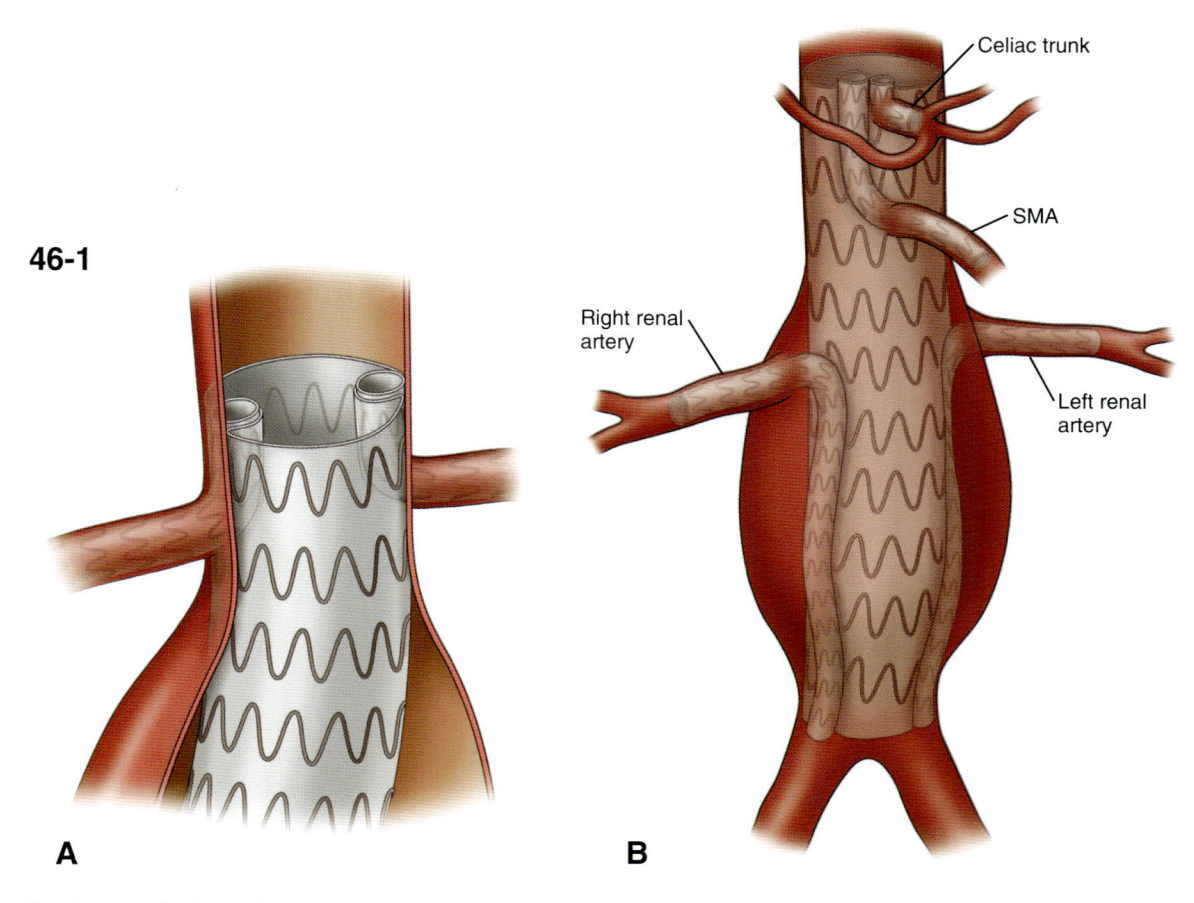

Figure 46-1 A. Illustration of bilateral renal chimney grafts in a ChEVAR. B. Two chimneys (celiac and SMA above) and two periscopes (bilateral renals below) in ChEVAR.

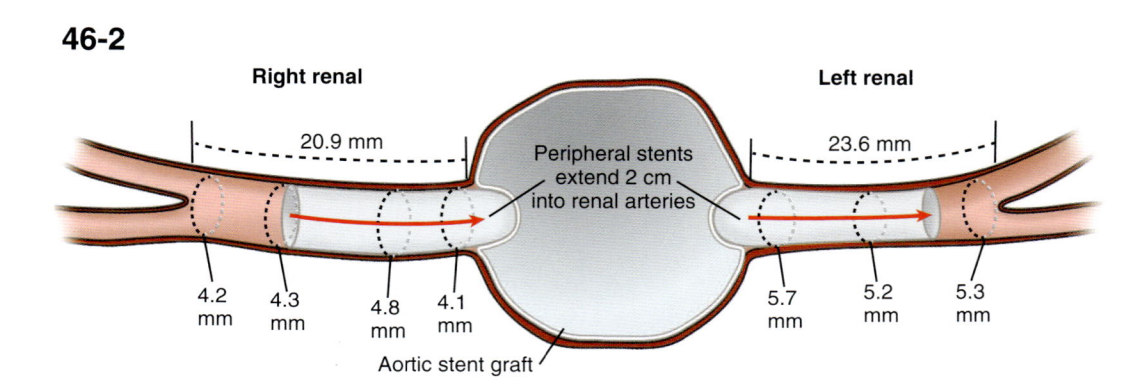

Figure 46-2 Conformation of ChEVAR and renal artery stents; bilateral renal artery length, and diameter measurements.

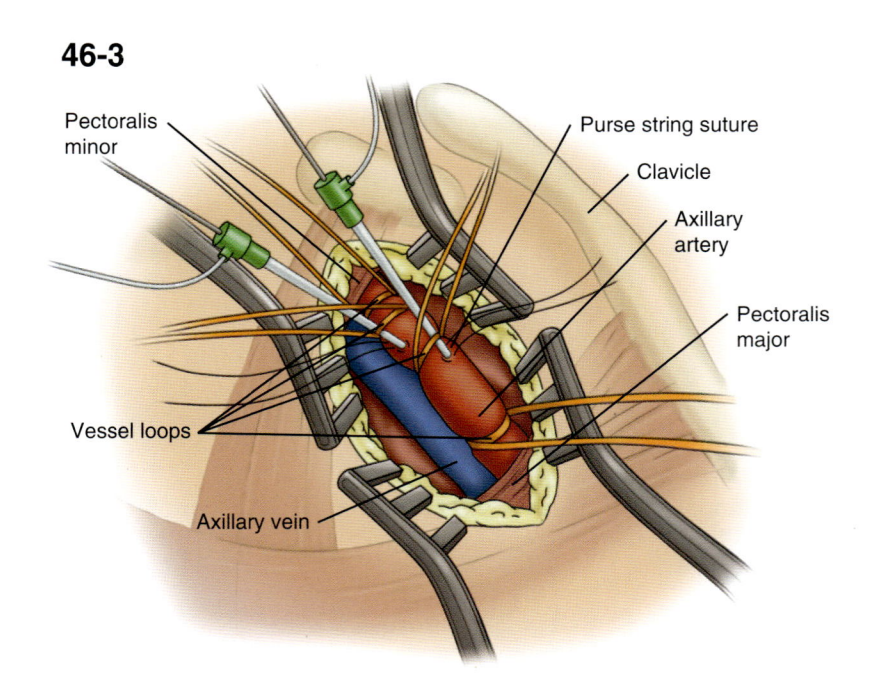

Figure 46-3 Axillary artery exposure with cannulation. Vessel loop shown here for proximal control around the axillary artery and sheaths.

DETAILS OF THE PROCEDURE *PARARENAL, JUXTARENAL, AND PARAVISCERAL AORTIC ANEURYSMS*: CONTINUED Either open exposure or bilateral common femoral artery percutaneous access is performed under ultrasound guidance utilizing a Micropuncture Access Kit (Cook Medical, Bloomington, IN). Perclose ProGlide suture-mediated closure devices (Abbott Inc, Minneapolis, MN) are deployed to facilitate femoral artery closure at the end of the case. Access sites are then serially dilated over a stiff 0.035" wire until the appropriate sheath size is reached. The patient is then systemically heparinized with 80 to 100 units/kg of heparin. Throughout the procedure, an activated clotting time of >250 seconds is advised. It is our preference to re-dose heparin every 45 minutes after the procedure begins.

We prefer to use a 7Fr Tour-Guide 90 cm (Medtronic) or a 70 cm/90 cm Ansel/Raabe sheath (Cook Medical) for upper extremity access. Axillary sheaths are introduced and guided across the arch under fluoroscopic visualization to their intended targets. A key gateway is that all entry points should be equally spaced circumferentially around the axillary artery or conduit (FIGURE 46-4).

The renal arteries, celiac artery, and superior mesenteric artery (SMA) are cannulated, and selective angiogram of each target vessel is performed to confirm the appropriate vessel cannulation and outflow. Preoperatively-planned gantry angles are used to optimize visibility of target branches. Some prefer to retrograde pre-canulate the renal arteries to facilitate antegrade cannulation. Balloon-expandable stent grafts are placed through the sheaths prior to placement of the endograft (FIGURE 46-5).

At least 2 cm of purchase into the renal arteries is recommended. Depending on chimney graft length, we prefer to use either Viabahn VBX stent grafts (WL Gore, Flagstaff, AZ) or iCAST stent grafts (Atrium Medical Corp) for our chimney grafts. A recent report shows equivalent patency outcomes using balloon-expandable stents without an increase in type 1A endoleaks.

Next, the main body endograft is prepared. A stiff wire is advanced up the ipsilateral groin into the aortic arch, and a pigtail catheter is placed through the contralateral groin. The aortic endograft is then advanced into the aorta. A lateral projection aortogram is performed to evaluate the distance from the SMA and/or celiac artery to the proximal landing zone at least 2 cm above the aneurysm, and preferably 5 cm above the beginning of the seal zone. The level of the origin of the SMA is marked and the aortic endograft is deployed. We then advocate for rotating back into an AP view or your preferred gantry angle for optimal visualization of the renal arteries. In this view, the renal chimney grafts are sequentially deployed. The contralateral gate of the aortic endograft is cannulated and bilateral iliac limbs are completely deployed.

A pigtail catheter and a compliant balloon are advanced transfemorally. Bilateral renal arteries and the aortic endograft are ballooned simultaneously in a "kissing" fashion (FIGURE 46-6). When additional chimney grafts are needed for the mesenteric vessels, they too should undergo simultaneous ballooning with the aortic endograft (see below). We recommend deflating the aortic balloon first, then deflating the balloon-expandable chimney stent grafts to maximize chimney graft patency. Completion aortogram is then performed to evaluate for endoleaks. In a similar fashion, for those presenting with a type 1A endoleak after EVAR, a ChEVAR may be performed. Utilizing an EVAR or TEVAR extension cuff and axillary access for bilateral renal stents, suprarenal fixation can be obtained. CONTINUES

46-4

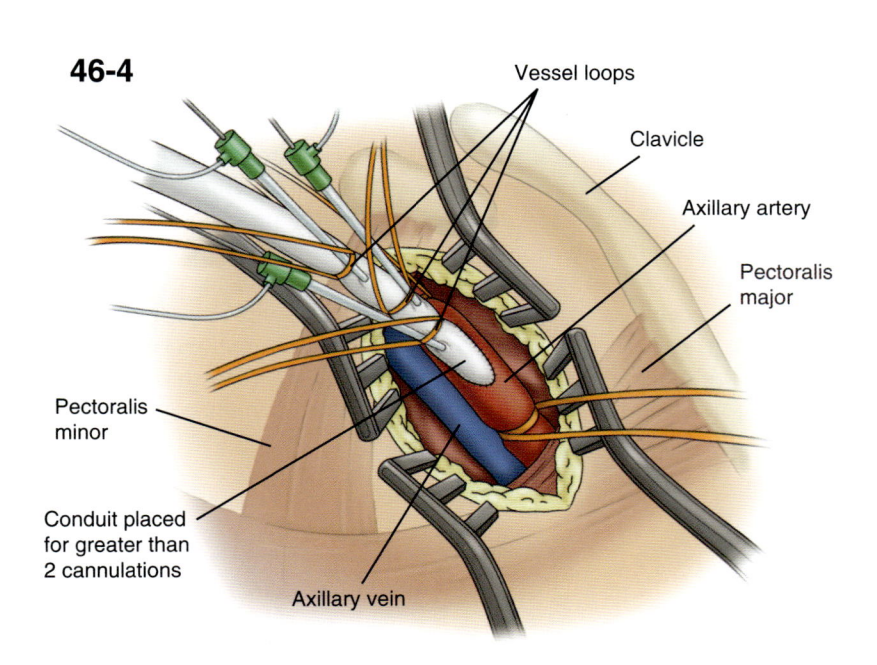

Vessel loops

Clavicle

Axillary artery

Pectoralis major

Pectoralis minor

Conduit placed for greater than 2 cannulations

Axillary vein

Figure 46-4 Axillary conduit for multi-sheath access.

46-5

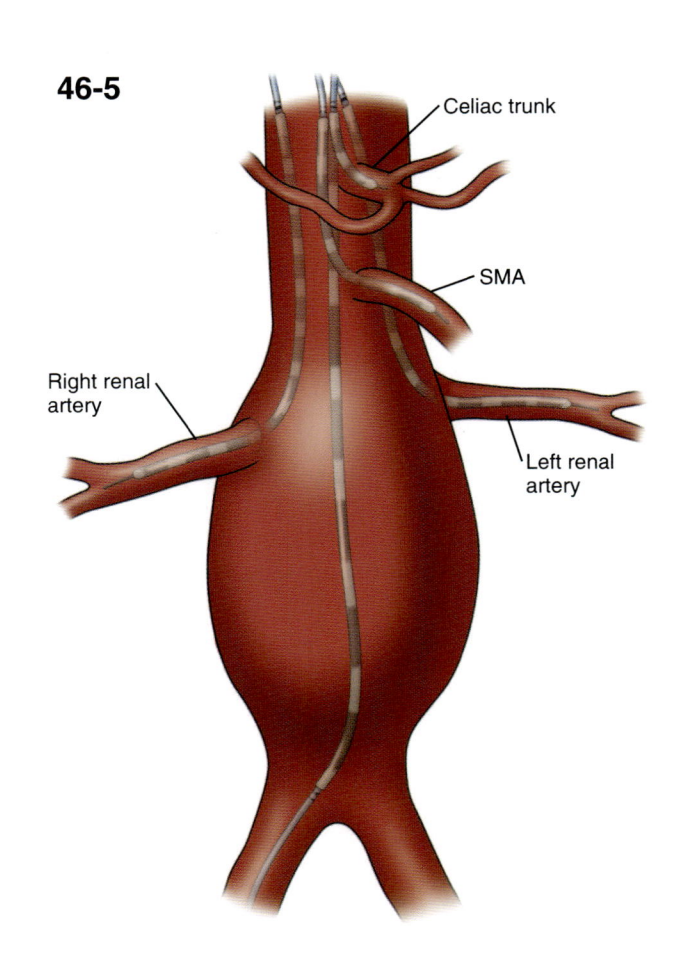

Celiac trunk

SMA

Right renal artery

Left renal artery

Figure 46-5 Placement of all stent grafts prior to deployment.

46-6

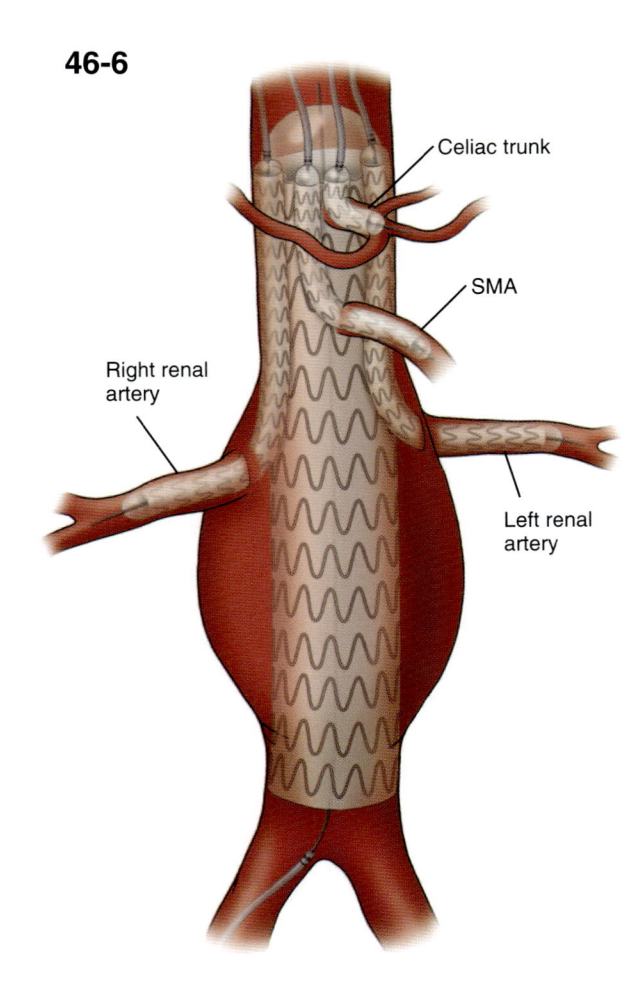

Celiac trunk

SMA

Right renal artery

Left renal artery

Figure 46-6 Depiction of simultaneous balloon molding within the main aortic graft, celiac artery, SMA, and bilateral renal arteries.

THORACOABDOMINAL AORTIC ANEURYSMS

INTRODUCTION Thoracoabdominal aortic aneurysms (TAAAs) are aneurysms that span both the thoracic and abdominal cavities. The Crawford classification breaks them up into five distinct types. TAAAs can also be treated via parallel grafting. Given the increased complexity of TAAAs, several modifications to the previously described pararenal ChEVAR technique are recommended. One such consideration is the use of the "sandwich" technique, in which parallel grafts are placed between two aortic endograft components. This essentially "sandwiches" them together while allowing them to extend beyond the inner aortic graft (FIGURE 46-7). This extends the landing zone for the chimneys, reducing the length of the peripheral stent grafts. The goal in these cases is to exclude the aneurysm, incorporate the necessary renal and visceral branches, and minimize paraplegia risk.

PREOPERATIVE CONSIDERATIONS

MANAGEMENT OF THE CELIAC AXIS: The celiac axis may potentially be safely covered without revascularization in patients with patent SMA collateral supply via the gastroduodenal artery. A review of the literature shows a relatively low rate (~7%) of foregut ischemia associated with celiac artery coverage. Additionally, patients with a replaced right hepatic artery or pre-existing celiac stenosis tolerate celiac coverage well. Spinal fluid drainage should be considered for any patient with planned extensive aortic repair or in patients with previous aortic coverage. Placement of a lumbar

drain preoperatively can assist with maintaining spinal fluid pressures <10 mm Hg. In combination with maintaining high mean arterial pressures (>90 mm Hg), spinal cord perfusion can be optimized and the paraplegia risk reduced. Further benefits may be provided by staging the patient's aortic coverage, especially for those with Crawford type II TAAAs.

DETAILS OF THE SANDWICH PROCEDURE
After the appropriate upper extremity and femoral access is obtained, we start at the proximal seal zone. The proximal thoracic endograft is deployed at least 5 cm above the celiac artery to leave enough room to manipulate catheters which will cannulate the peripheral vessels. We then address the distal sealing zone by deploying a bifurcated abdominal aortic device distal to the renal arteries. Be certain there is at least 5 cm of overlap for the sealing zone of the bridging stent. The axillary approach is used to establish access into the celiac and/or the superior mesenteric arteries as preoperatively planned. The renal arteries can be cannulated via the axillary above or femoral artery approach below. After the initial proximal thoracic stent graft and infrarenal stent grafts are placed, all renal and visceral arteries are cannulated, sheaths advanced, and stent grafts placed as discussed above. A second thoracoabdominal aortic bridging stent graft is advanced into the aorta. (FIGURE 46-8)

This device is placed to overlap with the proximal and distal aortic components and deployed. We typically oversize the bridging component by 20 to 30%. The chimney and periscope parallel grafts are then sequentially deployed. A compliant aortic balloon is inflated simultaneously with the opposing parallel grafts to maintain patency and minimize gutter leaks. Completion aortogram is done. **CONTINUES ▶**

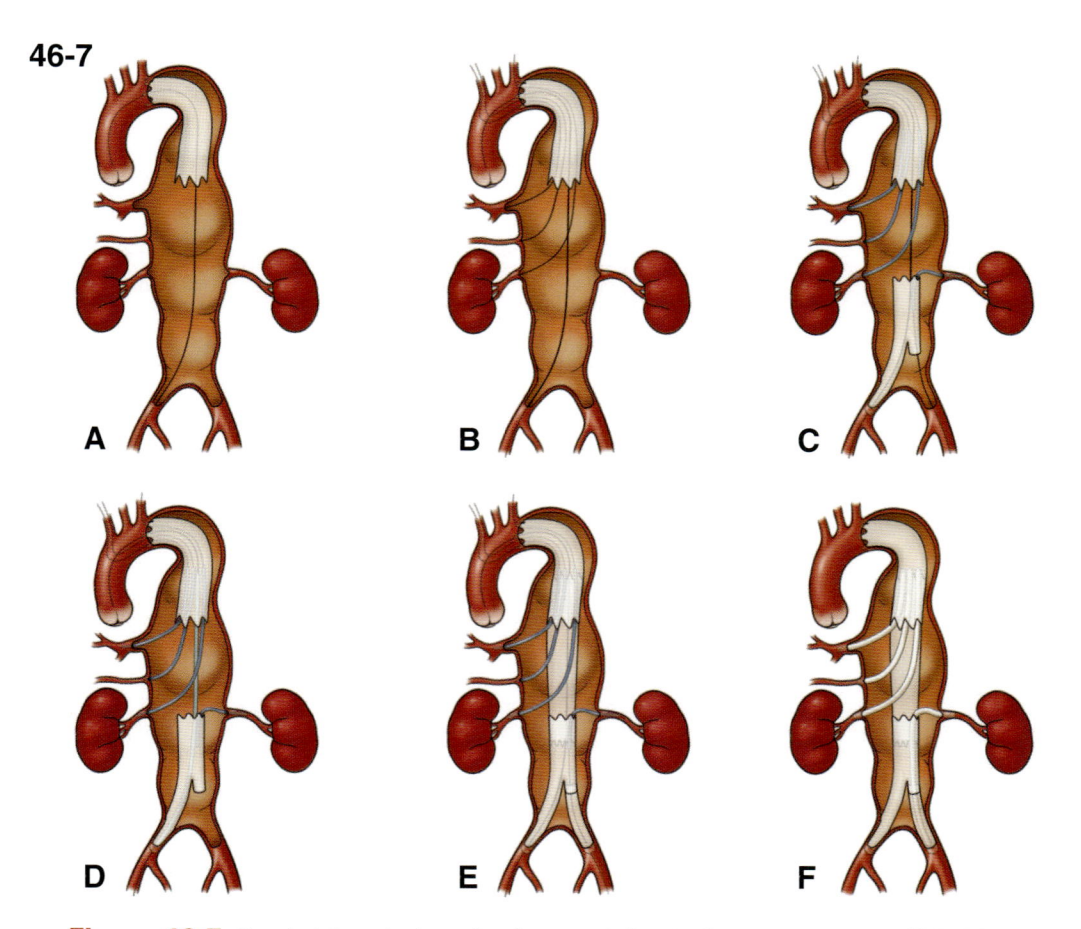

Figure 46-7 Sandwich technique for thoracoabdominal aortic aneurysm ChEVAR.

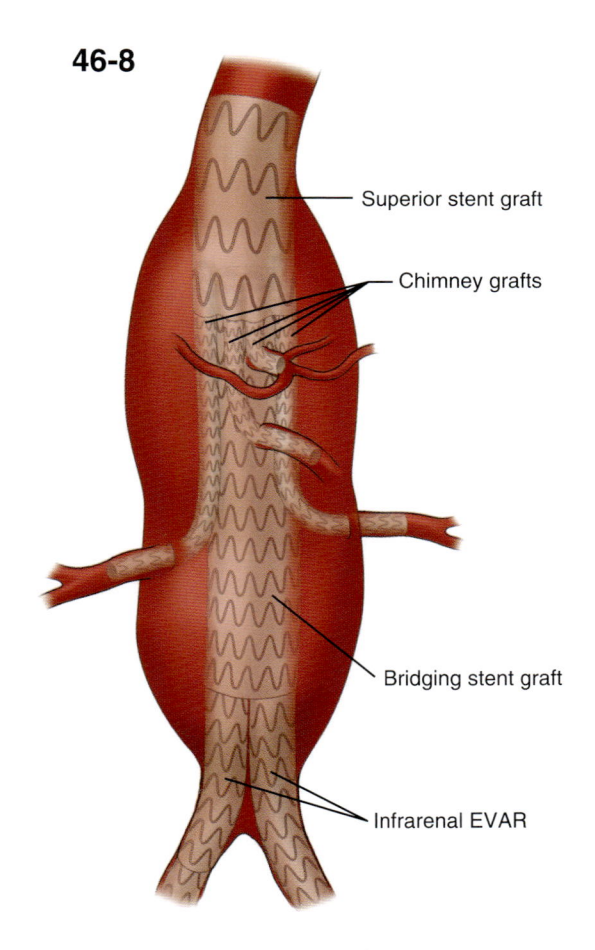

Figure 46-8 Completed ChEVAR sandwich with celiac, SMA, bilateral renal arteries.

AORTIC ARCH & THORACIC AORTIC ANEURYSMS

INTRODUCTION Endovascular debranching with the chimney technique can be used for aortic arch aneurysms and TAAs for arch deployment in zones 1 and 2 (FIGURE 46-9). This technique may be combined with a hybrid technique when more than one supra-aortic branch is covered. Parallel grafts can be placed in both an antegrade (chimney) or retrograde (periscope) configuration. When utilizing the periscope configuration, the authors recommend using a flexible stent that comes in a variety of longer lengths, such as the Viabahn self-expanding stent graft (Gore). The proximal chimney graft should extend at least 1 cm proximal to the aortic endograft. Recall that most TEVAR devices typically require 10 to 20% oversizing. For parallel grafting in the arch, we recommend aortic endograft oversizing of 15 to 20%. It is our experience that higher rates of gutter leaks are seen with double PGs as compared to a single PG when this technique is used in the arch. Thus, we try to design our repairs with the intent to implant a single chimney graft and perform an extra-anatomic bypass as necessary, such as carotid-to-carotid and carotid-to-subclavian artery bypass.

The involvement of zone 0 pathology is often managed with open aortic arch debranching through a median sternotomy and then TEVAR.

INDICATIONS The indications are similar to those listed previously for TEVARs. In general, asymptomatic TAAs with diameters >5.5 to 6.5 cm should be considered for repair. Symptomatic aneurysms or TAAs that are rapidly growing >1.0 cm/year or >0.5 cm/6 mo should undergo repair.

The decision to proceed with endovascular repair necessitates detailed imaging and procedural planning. 3D reconstructions with centerline technology should be performed and precise measurements obtained. Other preoperative considerations should include aortic arch anatomy, appropriate landing zone lengths of at least 2 cm, interpretation of aortic angulation, and access vessel diameter/quality. Caution is advised in patients with hostile necks, either from radiation exposure or previous surgery, which preclude the ability to safely debranch the arch.

PREOPERATIVE CONSIDERATIONS

MANAGEMENT OF THE LEFT SUBCLAVIAN: Guidelines from the Society of Vascular Surgery recommend preoperative revascularization of the left subclavian artery (L SCA) if coverage is planned. Several studies have shown a higher complication rate of arm ischemia and posterior circulation infarcts with L SCA coverage compared to preservation of perfusion. The Eurostar review showed that coverage of L SCA without revascularization was an independent predictor of spinal cord ischemia with an odds ratio of 3.49. This is thought to be in part due to the prevalence of left vertebral artery dominance in ~60% of the population. Typically, revascularization is performed first with either a left subclavian-to-left common carotid bypass or a left subclavian transposition onto the left common carotid artery. The appropriate revascularization procedure is individualized to each patient. Special consideration should be given to those patients that cannot withstand any interruption in subclavian perfusion, such as those with LIMA grafts. Those patients cannot be treated with transposition and must be bypassed. Mandatory left subclavian revascularization should be planned for those with left arm arteriovenous fistulas, LIMA grafts, dominant left vertebrals and/or absent or diminutive right vertebral arteries, and aberrant right subclavian arteries.

DETAILS OF THE PROCEDURE

ZONE 2 DEPLOYMENT: Left upper extremity access is obtained. Heparin is administered and the sheath is advanced into the proximal L SCA. The image intensifier is placed in the optimal positioning for arch views, LAO ~30 to 60 degrees. The thoracic endograft is advanced from a femoral access site and deployed in zone 2, distal to the left common carotid artery (L CCA). The L SCA stent graft is then deployed and both stent grafts are ballooned in a kissing fashion. Care should be taken to minimize aortic ballooning in the aortic arch.

ZONE 1 DEPLOYMENT: For deployment in aortic zone 1, left axillary access as well as L CCA open surgical access is obtained. Prior preoperative planning should address the management of the L SCA either via reconstruction with a bypass or transposition. Sheath and stent are then advanced into the proximal L CCA. The aortic graft is then advanced into the thoracic aorta and positioned distal to the innominate artery in zone 1.

The authors find that the application of steady forward pressure on the wire helps to pin the endograft against the aortic outer curve during deployment. This reduces the windsock effect and helps avoid distal migration. The aortic endograft is deployed. The left common carotid stent is deployed, and both are ballooned in a kissing fashion. The excluded proximal L SCA is then managed with proximal coils to avoid a type II endoleak if bypassed.

If the placement of two endografts is necessary for coverage, then the smaller device is deployed first. Overlap should be at least 5 cm or per instructions for use (IFU). If the devices are equivalent sizes, then an increased overlap zone is necessary, typically ~10 cm or per IFU. ∎

SUGGESTED READINGS

Buth J, Harris PL, Hobo R, et al. Neurologic complications associated with endovascular repair of thoracic aortic pathology: incidence and risk factors. A study from the European Collaborators on Stent/Graft Techniques for Aortic Aneurysm Repair (EUROSTAR) registry. *J Vasc Surg*. 2007;46:1103-1110.

Cires G, Noll RE Jr, Albuquerque FC Jr, Tonnessen BH, Sternbergh WC 3rd. Endovascular debranching of the aortic arch during thoracic endograft repair. *J Vasc Surg*. 2011 Jun;53(6):1485-1491.

Clark EC, Babrowski TA, Milner R. Outcomes of chimney and fenestrated endografting using Viabahn VBX and atrium iCAST stents. *J Cardiovasc Surg*. 2021 Apr;62(2):136-145.

Cooper DG, Walsh SR, Sadat U, et al. Neurological complications after left subclavian artery coverage during thoracic endovascular aortic repair: a systematic review and meta-analysis. *J Vasc Surg*. 2009;49:1594-1601.

Donas KP, Criado FJ, Torsello G, Veith FJ, Minion DJ; PERICLES Registry Collaborators. Classification of chimney EVAR-related endoleaks: insights from the PERICLES Registry. *J Endovasc Ther*. 2017 Feb 1;24(1):72-74.

Donas KP, Lee JT, Lachat M, Torsello G, Veith FJ. Collected world experience about the performance of the snorkel/chimney endovascular technique in the treatment of complex aortic pathologies: the PERICLES Registry. *Ann Surg*. 2015; 262:546-553.

Donas KP, Torsello GB, Piccoli G, et al. The PROTAGORAS study to evaluate the performance of the Endurant stent graft for patients with pararenal pathologic processes treated by the chimney/snorkel endovascular technique. *J Vasc Surg*. 2016 Jan;63(1):1-7.

Donas KP, Usai MV, Taneva GT, et al. Impact of aortic stent-graft oversizing on outcomes of the chimney endovascular technique based on a new analysis of the PERICLES Registry. *Vascular*. 2019 Apr;27(2):175-180.

Huynh TT, et al. Determinants of hospital length of stay after thoracoabdominal aortic aneurysm repair. *J Vasc Surg*. 2002;35(4).

Maximus S, Long K, Babrowski T, Park J, Milner R. Right-sided upper extremity access for patients undergoing parallel graft placement during endovascular aortic repair is not associated with increased neurologic events when compared with left upper extremity access. *Ann Vasc Surg*. 2021 May;73:37-42.

Mehta M. Is coverage of the celiac artery without revascularization acceptable? *Endovasc Today*. 2015;14(11):85-88.

Ohrlander T, Sonesson B, Ivancev K, Resch T, Dias N, Malina M. The chimney graft: a technique for preserving or rescuing aortic branch vessels in stent-graft sealing zones. *J Endovasc Ther*. 2008 Aug;15(4):427-432.

Peterson BG, Eskandari MK, Gleason TG, et al. Utility of left subclavian artery revascularization in association with endoluminal repair of acute and chronic thoracic aortic pathology. *J Vasc Surg*. 2005;43(3):433-439.

Planer D, Elbaz-Greener G, Mangialardi N, et al. NEXUS Arch. *Ann Surg*. 2021 March 04.

Reece TB, Gazoni LM, Cherry KJ, et al. Reevaluating the need for left subclavian artery revascularization with thoracic endovascular aortic repair. *Ann Thorac Surg*. 2007 Oct;84(4):1201-1205.

Scali ST, Beck AW, Torsello G, et al. Identification of optimal device combinations for the chimney endovascular aneurysm repair technique within the PERICLES Rgistry. *J Vasc Surg*. 2018 Jul;68(1):24-35.

Taneva GT, Criado FJ, Torsello G, et al. Results of chimney endovascular aneurysm repair as used in the PERICLES Registry to treat patients with suprarenal aortic pathologies. *J Vasc Surg*. 2020 May;71(5):1521-1527.

Taneva GT, Lee JT, Tran K, et al. Long-term chimney/snorkel endovascular aortic aneurysm repair experience for complex abdominal aortic pathologies within the PERICLES Registry. *J Vasc Surg*. 2021 Jun;73(6):1942-1949.

46-9

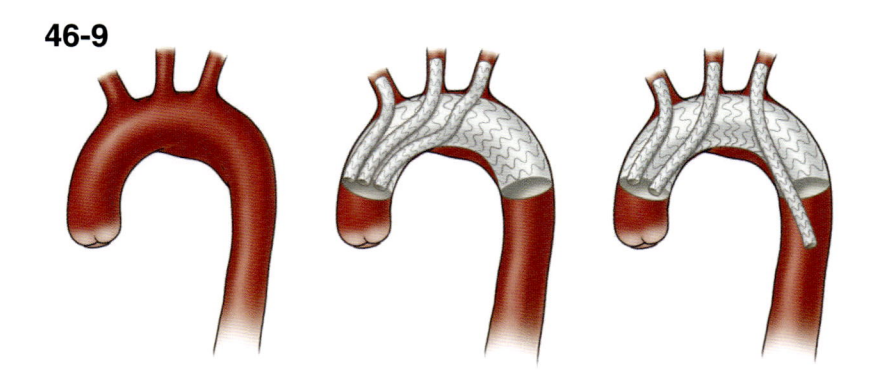

Figure 46-9 Aortic ach parallel grafting configuration.

SECTION X

MESENTERIC AND RENAL OPEN AND ENDOVASCULAR REPAIR

OPEN MESENTERIC BYPASS, EMBOLECTOMY AND ENDARTERECTOMY

Timur P. Sarac, MD • **Thomas Forbes, MD**

INDICATIONS Both acute and chronic mesenteric ischemia (CMI) are life-threatening conditions and should be treated expeditiously. Treatment options include endovascular, open, and hybrid surgery. While the endovascular minimally invasive approach has become first-line therapy, open revascularization is still common, as patients often have disease progression and anatomic limitations which will preclude an endovascular approach. For CMI, the patient may be cachectic but will not have enough time or hepatic reserves to be improved with total parenteral nutrition. Like CMI, expeditious treatment of acute mesenteric ischemia is imperative, as time is of the essence.

CHRONIC MESENTERIC ISCHEMIA: Patients with symptomatic chronic mesenteric artery occlusive disease typically present with postprandial pain that begins 20 to 60 minutes after ingestion of a meal, often termed mesenteric angina; this is not absolute, as the pain onset can be variable. They develop a fear of food and can have significant weight loss and bowel dysfunction, with constipation or diarrhea. The etiology of CMI in most patients is atherosclerotic occlusive disease. Other cause include vasculitis, chronic dissection, and fibromuscular dysplasia. For CMI, the indications for revascularization are symptoms with known stenosis greater than 50%, which specifically includes two of the three visceral vessels. Most commonly, the superior mesenteric artery (SMA) is involved, and if this is the only vessel that is occluded or stenotic, selective celiac and inferior mesenteric artery (IMA) angiography should be done to demonstrate the presence of collaterals as patients can get CMI with only the SMA diseased if there are poor collaterals, or if the patient had a previous bowel operation with disruption of collaterals. Imaging studies consist of mesenteric duplex and CT angiogram, where both axial and sagittal views are necessary for CTA, and demonstration of meandering mesenteric artery is pathopneumonic.

ACUTE MESENTERIC ISCHEMIA: Patients with acute mesenteric ischemia usually present with progressive abdominal pain, which is not often detected by physical exam alone, often described as pain out of proportion to physical findings. If lactic acidosis is present, they are usually far into the process, and a high lactate is not needed to diagnose acute mesenteric ischemia in the early stages. The most common etiology of acute mesenteric ischemia is usually due to embolism from atrial fibrillation, followed by acute occlusion of a chronic lesion, aortic dissection, and nonocclusive

mesenteric ischemia. While it almost always involves the SMA, on occasion it can include an isolated celiac or IMA (resulting in ischemic colitis). The diagnosis historically is made by clinical exam with diagnostic angiography; however, CT angiography is now the most common imaging modality used.

POSITION The patient is placed in a supine position for most bypasses and right lateral decubitus position for an endarterectomy.

OPERATIVE PREPARATION Large bore IV access including central access and arterial line blood pressure monitoring are imperative. Cell saver should be made available, and the patient should be monitored postoperatively in the surgical intensive care unit. After routine skin preparation, the operative field is draped from nipples to knees in case a vein is needed.

INCISION AND EXPOSURE The author's preference is a chevron incision when a bypass is planned, and longitudinal midline for embolectomy. The inferior abdominal wall is retracted inferiorly for the chevron incision (**FIGURE 47-1**), and the abdomen explored. The conduit of choice is Dacron or Rifampin soaked Gelsoft graft (Terumo Medical, Somerset, NJ); however, if there is perforation and gross spillage, then vein conduit should be used. In general, both the celiac and SMA are revascularized with a bifurcated graft. Additionally, the preferred inflow source is the surpaceliac aorta; however, if this is too diseased or the patient's physiologic status is compromised, then either the infrarenal aorta or an iliac artery can be used. On rare occasions, the ascending aorta may need to be used.

DETAILS OF PROCEDURE

CHRONIC MESENTERIC ISCHEMIA: After the initial incision, the abdomen is thoroughly explored. It is not uncommon to have a chronically ischemic gallbladder, and this may need to be addressed at the completion. If there is spillage of enteric contents, this should be controlled first. We prefer to revascularize *both* the celiac and SMA, and usually use the common hepatic as the outflow for the celiac artery revascularization. The preferred approach is antegrade revascularization using the supraceliac aorta. This is exposed by mobilizing the left lobe of the liver and dividing coronary and triangular ligaments (**FIGURE 47-2**). **CONTINUES ▶**

47-1

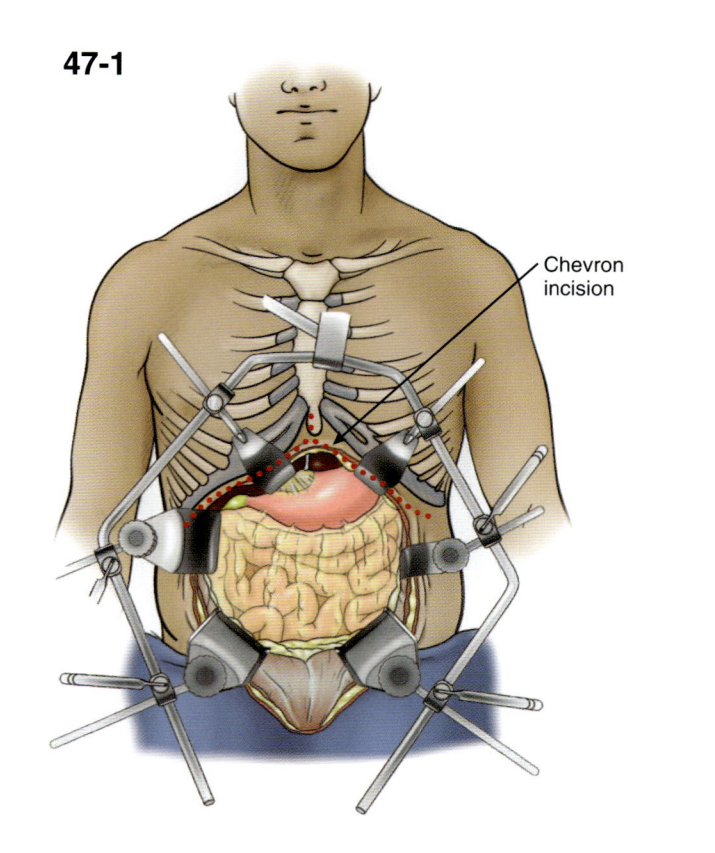

Figure 47-1 Open abdomen chevron with Omni retractor.

47-2

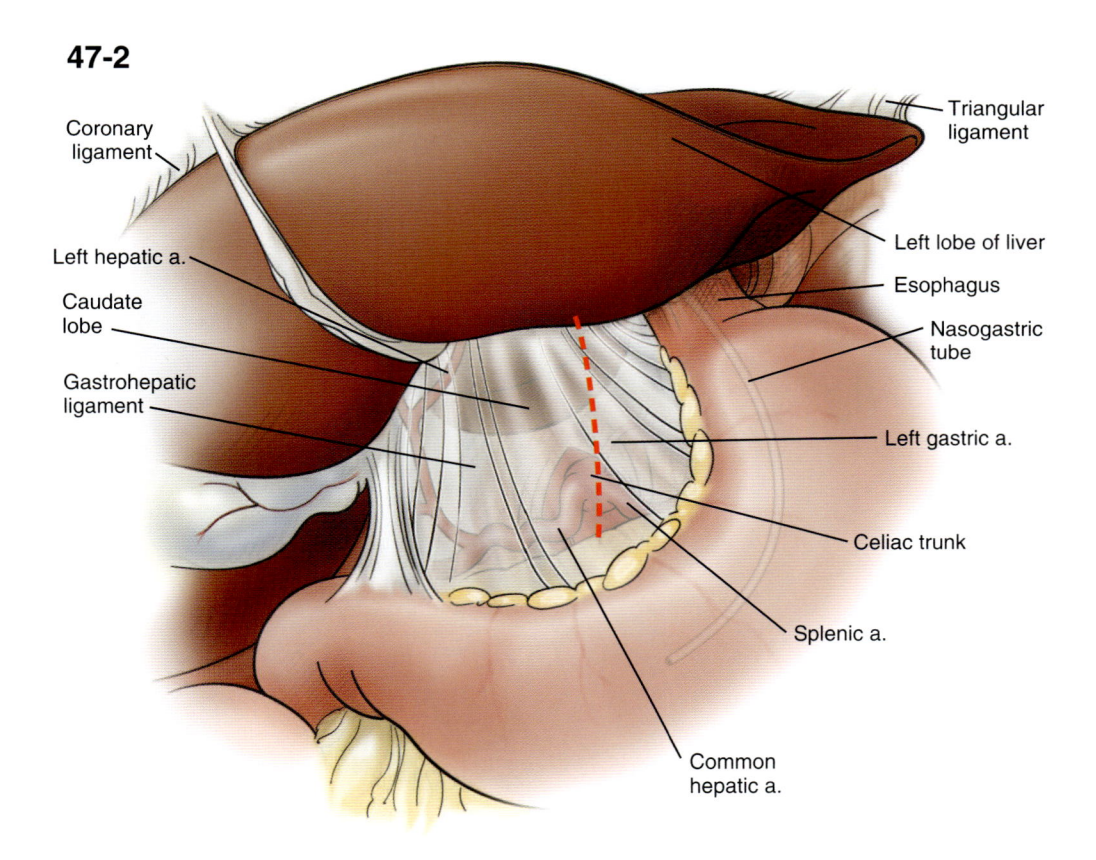

Figure 47-2 Dissecting the sura celiac aorta through the gastrohepatic ligament.

DETAILS OF PROCEDURE *CHRONIC MESENTERIC ISCHEMIA*: **CONTINUED** Next, the gastrohepatic ligament is divided (and retractors are placed on the left lobe of the liver, and esophagus) (**FIGURE** 47-3). In a small percentage of patients, an aberrant left hepatic artery runs through the gastrohepatic ligament, and this should be preserved. For the left lobe of the liver, be careful not to retract too hard, as the caudate lobe of the liver can be injured. The esophagus is easily identified by feeling for the NG tube, and is retracted to the patient's left with a self-retaining renal vein retractor attached to an Omni retractor. The stomach, greater omentum, and transverse colon are retracted inferiorly. The crus of the diaphragm are taken down on both the left and right (**FIGURE** 47-4). Be careful not to go too lateral, as the pleura can be entered; however, enough aorta must be cleared to accommodate a side-biting Lambert K or Satinsky clamp. Additionally, there are lumbar arteries in this region, and one should avoid circumferential dissection of the aorta. **CONTINUES**

47-3

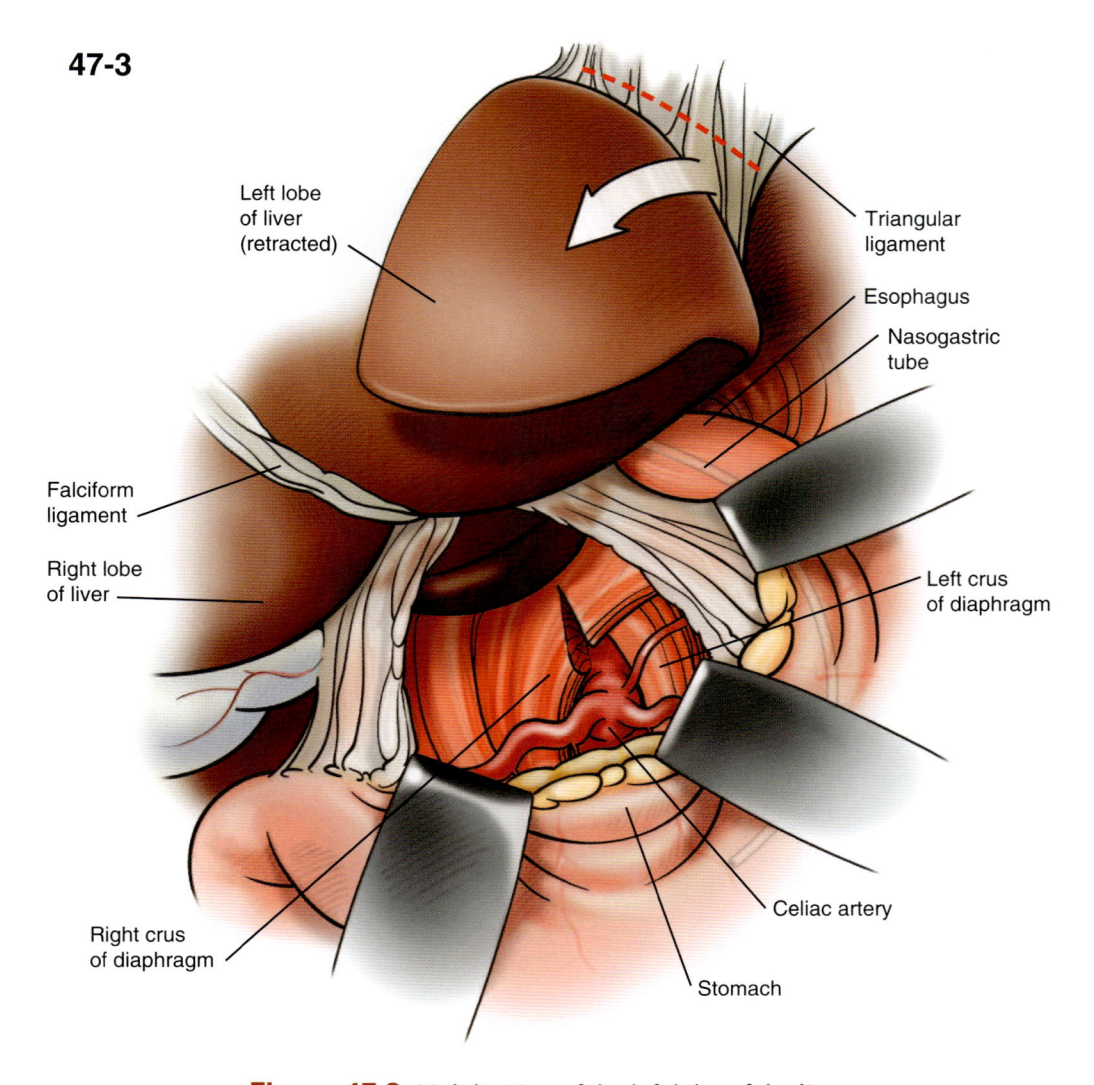

Figure 47-3 Mobilization of the left lobe of the liver.

47-4

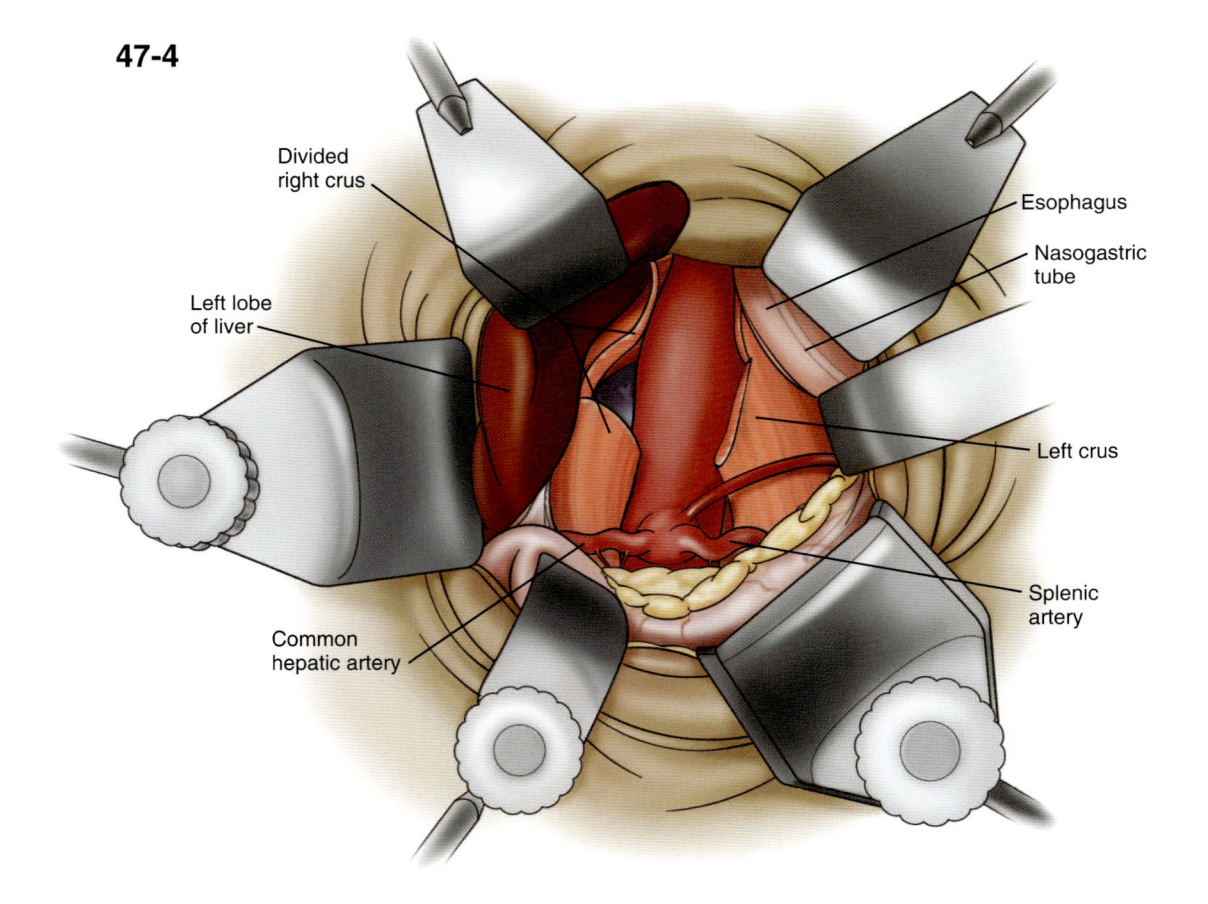

Figure 47-4 Dissection of the supraceliac aorta.

DETAILS OF PROCEDURE *CHRONIC MESENTERIC ISCHEMIA:* **CONTINUED** The hepatic artery and the SMA are then mobilized. The hepatic artery is identified in the porta hepatis and dissected past the gastroduodenal artery (FIGURE 47-5). If one has trouble identifying it, the splenic artery can be traced medially, as it is noted just superior to the pancreas, and auscultating with a continuous handheld Doppler may be beneficial. The SMA is the most difficult artery to dissect free, and a tedious dissection using patience and persistence is paramount. The SMA is dissected by entering the lesser sac between the stomach and transverse colon (FIGURE 47-6A). This location is chosen depending on the side of the SMA. The pancreas is identified and gently retracted in a superior direction. The next step is tedious and involves dividing the fatty tissue to identify the superior mesenteric vein (SMV). The key gateway here is to find the SMV, which can be found by elevating the transverse colon and tracing the middle colic vein in the transverse mesocolon cephalad to the SMV (FIGURE 47-6B). The SMA lies just medial and posterior (deep) to the SMV. Small venous tributaries are often encountered and divided on the way with a bipolar cautery. After the SMA is dissected free, the last step before performing the bypass is creating a retropancreatic tunnel between the pancreas and splenic vein. **CONTINUES**

47-5

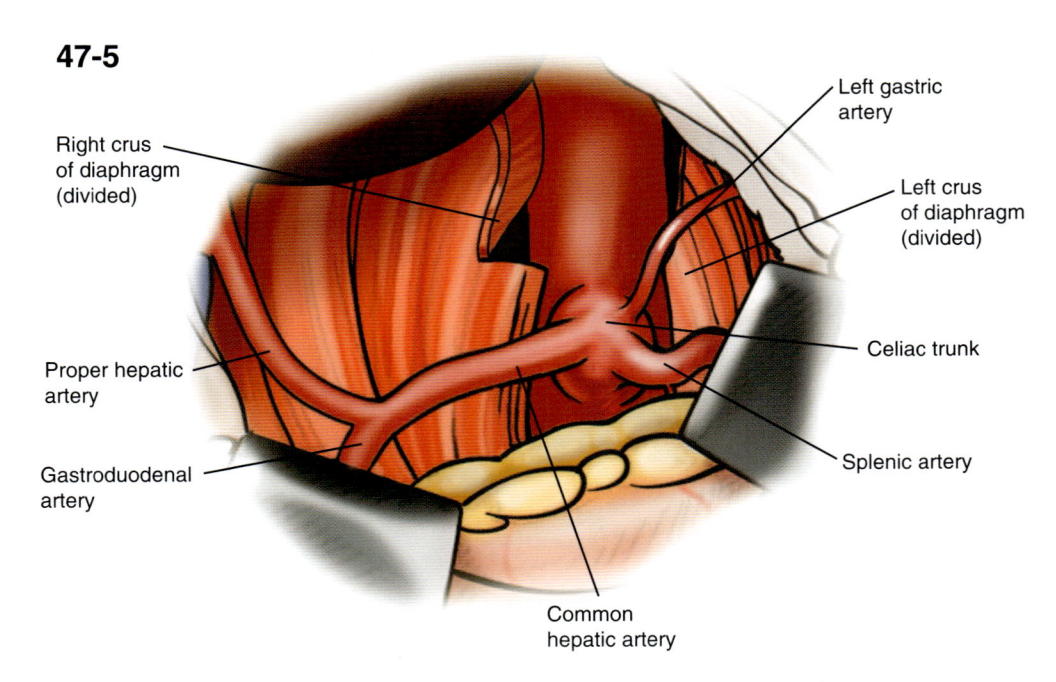

Figure 47-5 Dissection of the hepatic and gastroduodenal arteries.

47-6

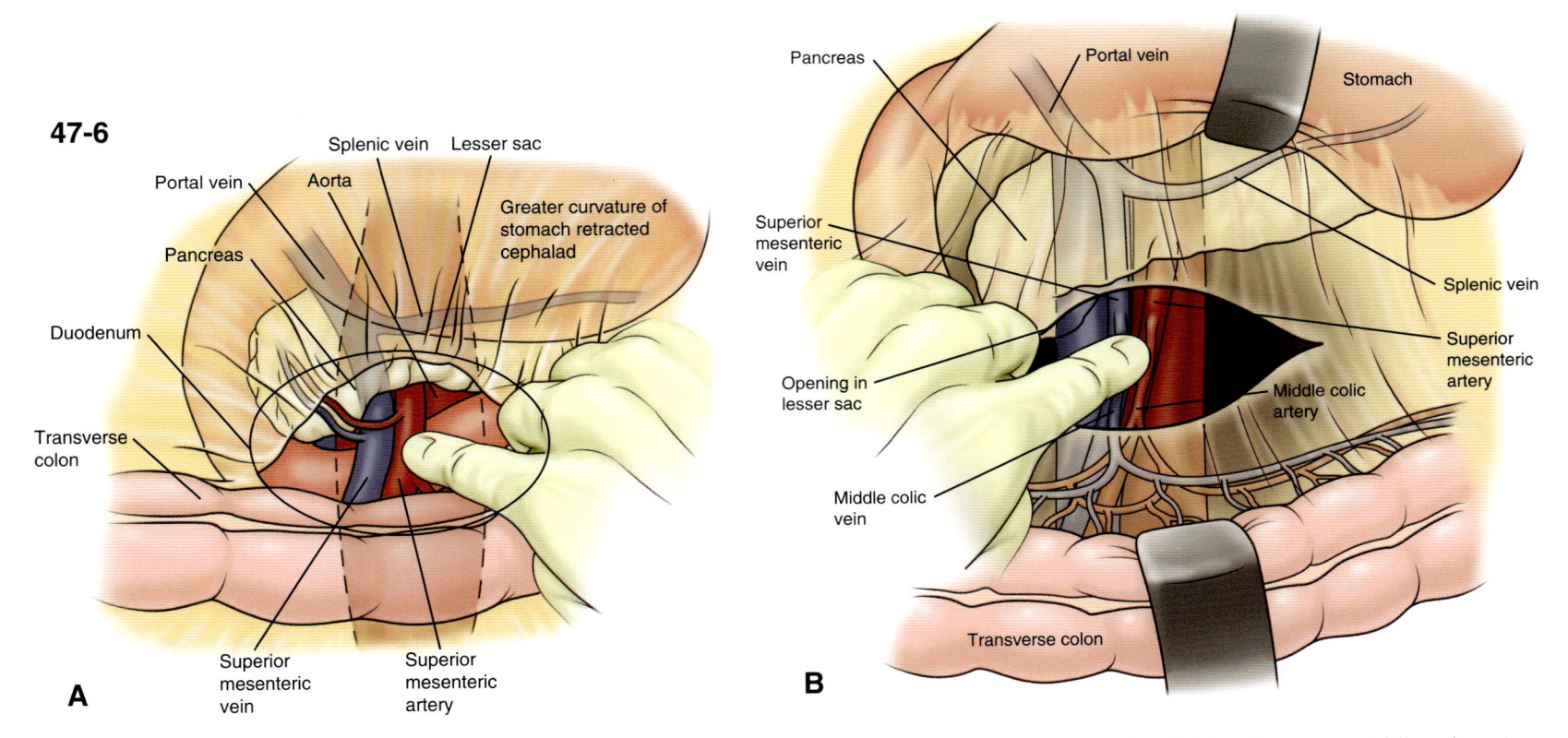

Figure 47-6 A. Dissection of the SMA—entering the lesser sac between the stomach and transverse colon. B. Identifying the middle colic vein and arteries to help find the SMV and SMA.

DETAILS OF PROCEDURE *CHRONIC MESENTERIC ISCHEMIA:* CONTINUED There are often small venous tributaries that need to be divided. A tonsil clamp then is passed from inferior to superior, anterior to the splenic vein and posterior to the pancreas, and an umbilical tape is passed to preserve the tunnel (FIGURE 47-7).

The patient is systemically heparinized, a side-biting clamp is placed in the supraceliac aorta, and an arteriotomy is made. Careful attention is paid to be certain the clamp occludes flow and there is enough room to perform the anastomosis. Usually, a 14 × 7 or 16 × 8 bifurcated graft is placed in the AP orientation and anastomosed to the surpaceliac aorta in an end-to-side

fashion using 4-o Prolene suture (FIGURE 47-8). The anterior limb is then anastomosed to the common hepatic artery in an end-to-side fashion with 6-o Prolene suture. A tonsil clamp is then used to grasp the umbilical tape and recreate the tunnel, and the posterior limb of the bifurcated graft is grabbed by the tunnel and passed between the pancreas and splenic vein. The distal anastomosis is then done to the superior mesenteric artery in an end-to-side fashion with 6-o Prolene suture (FIGURE 47-9). Protamine is then used to reverse the heparin, and the lesser sac is closed with absorbable suture. CONTINUES

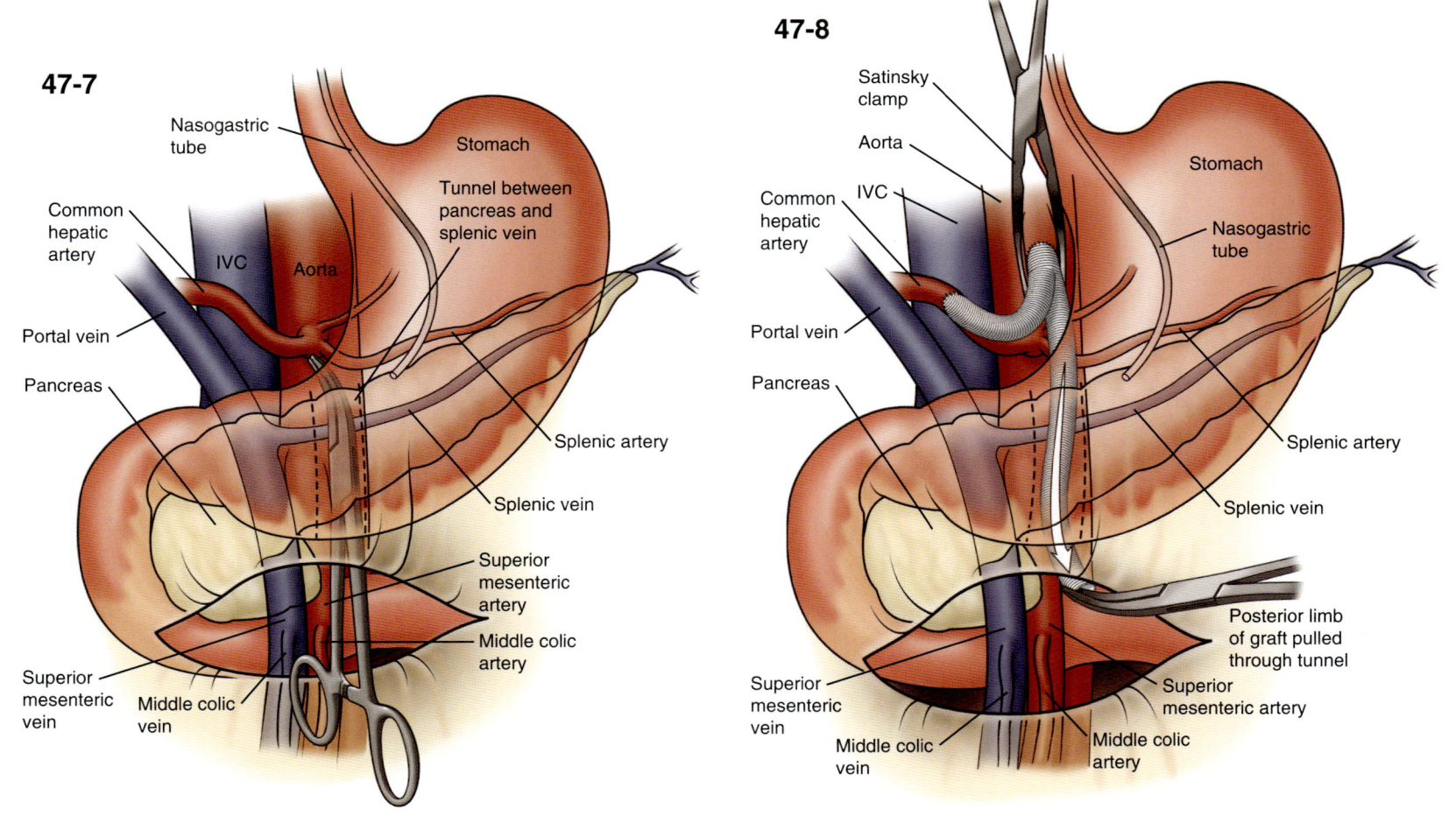

Figure 47-7 Creation of retropancreatic tunnel.

Figure 47-8 Configuration of bifurcated graft with anterior limb to the hepatic artery and posterior limb to the SMA.

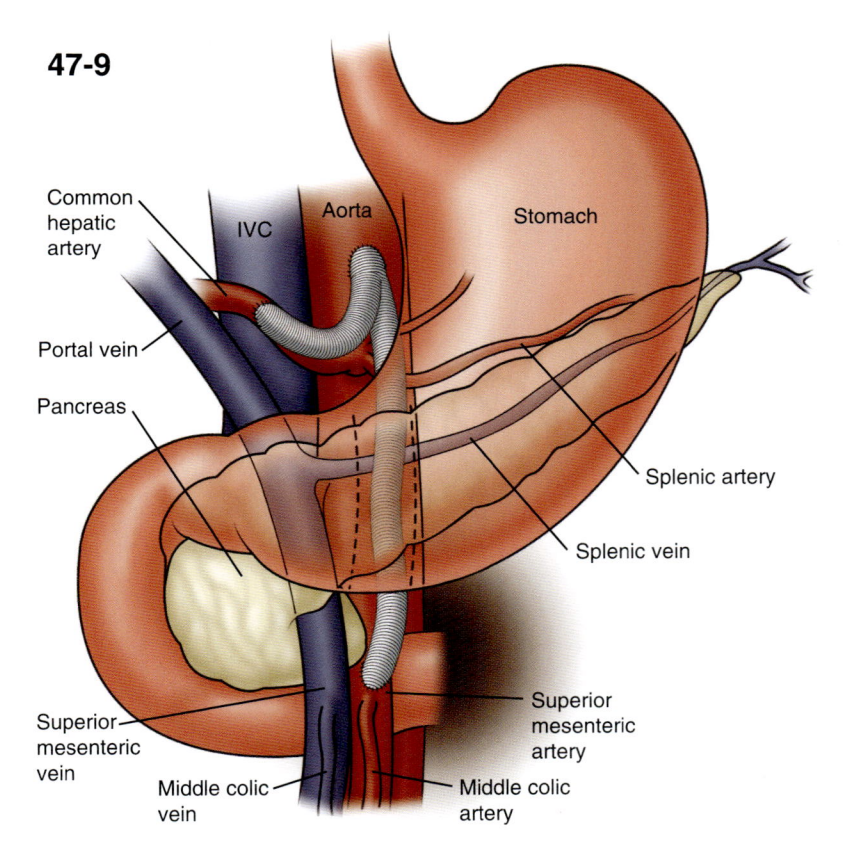

Figure 47-9 Final bypass graft with anastomoses.

DETAILS OF PROCEDURE *CHRONIC MESENTERIC ISCHEMIA:* **CONTINUED** For patients in whom a retrograde approach is taken, it has previously been described to perform the proximal anastomosis off the iliac artery or aorta and creating a gentle C loop so as not to kink the graft (FIGURE 47-10A). However, the author has found that coming straight on is adequate (FIGURE 47-10B). Here the graft is tunneled through the transverse mesocolon, or alternatively it can be done to the SMA inferior to the mesocolon, but the vessel is much smaller here. The mesentery is closed over the limbs of the graft.

The last technique to revascularize the visceral arteries is a retroperitoneal approach with a trap-door endarterectomy This method is chosen when the patient has orifice lesions of the celiac and SMA (and renal arteries) and a coral reef plaque also producing lower extremity ischemic rest pain. The traditional retroperitoneal aorta and celiac, SMA, and renal artery exposure is done (FIGURE 47-11) (see Chapter 29 for details of exposure). **CONTINUES**

47-10

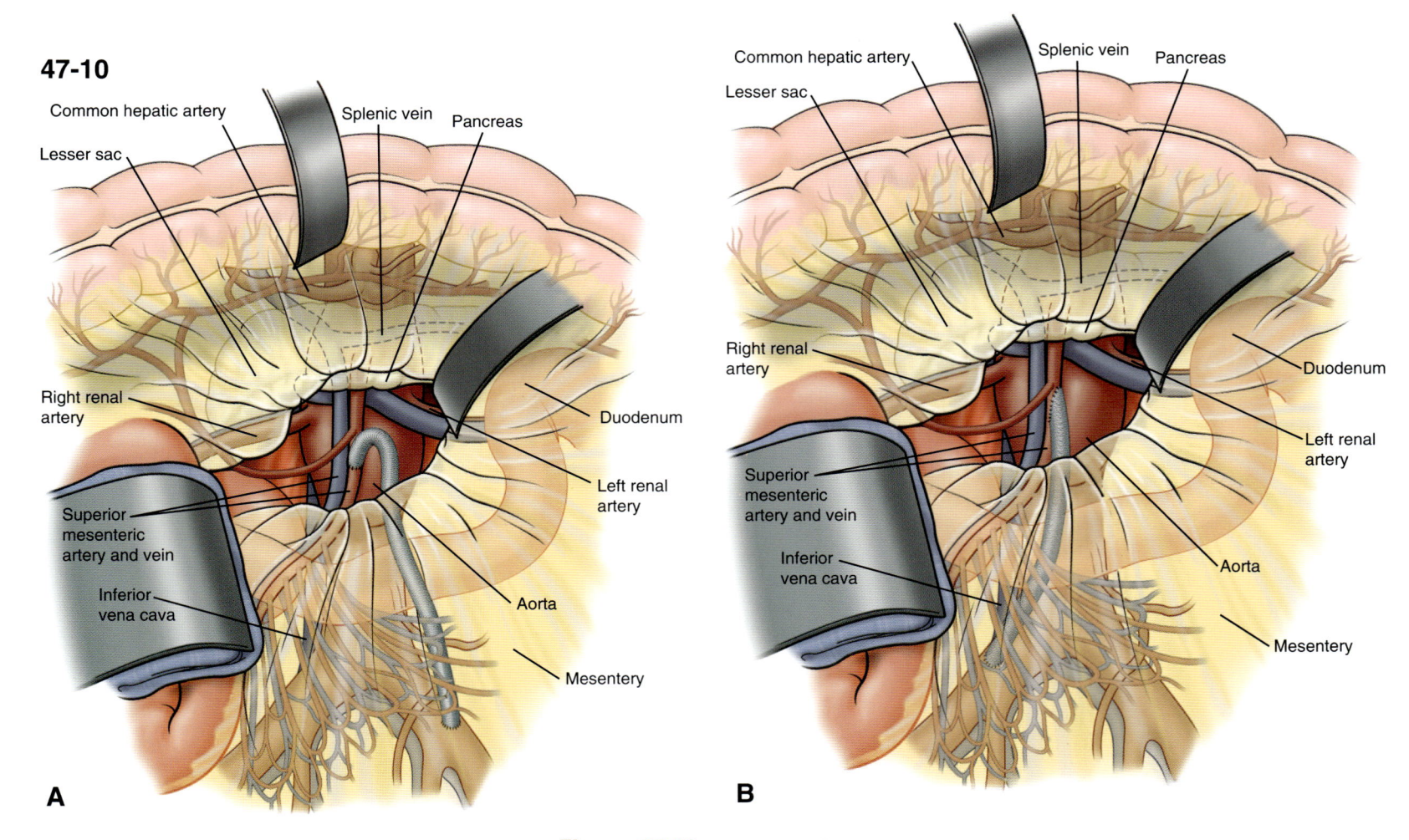

Figure 47-10 Iliac to SMA bypass.

47-11

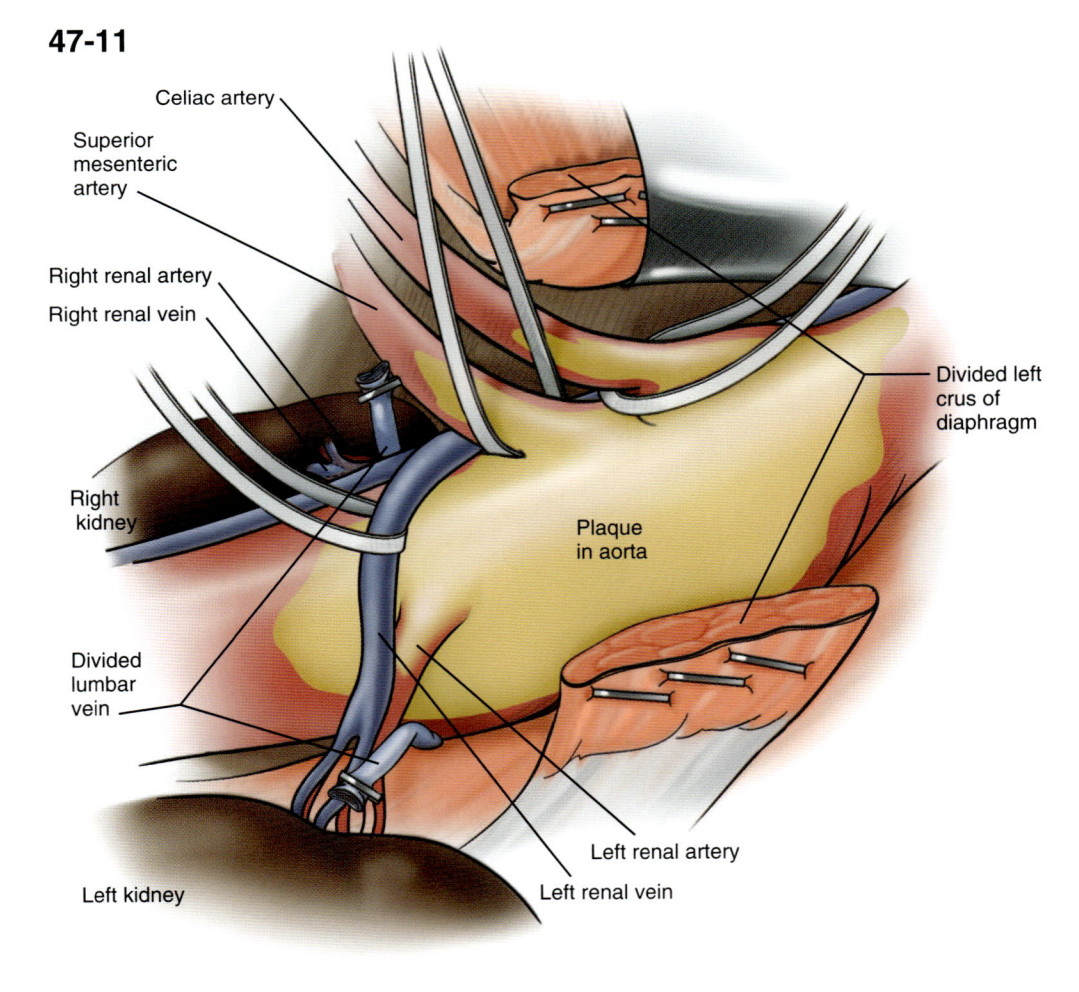

Figure 47-11 Retroperitoneal approach for trapdoor aortic endarterectomy.

DETAILS OF PROCEDURE *CHRONIC MESENTERIC ISCHEMIA:* **CONTINUED** After heparinization, the aorta is clamped above and below, a trap-door incision is made extending above and below the plaque, and endarterectomy plane is created to remove the plaque (**FIGURE 47-12**). The celiac, SMA lesions, and renal plaque are removed through an eversion technique (**FIGURE 47-13**). Intimal endpoints are tacked down with 4-50 Prolene suture and the arteriotomy closed using 4-0 Prolene suture.

ACUTE MESENTERIC ISCHEMIA: If the patient has acute onset CMI, if open surgery is necessary, a bypass is chosen and performed as described above. If the patient has an embolism, the SMA can also be exposed as described above, preferably through an infra-mesocolic approach if distal embolectomy is needed (**FIGURE 47-14**). For a proximal clot just beyond the orifice, it may be easier to expose the SMA just above the duodenum. This is done by retracting the abdominal contents like open abdominal aneurysm repair, and then mobilizing the duodenum (**FIGURE 47-15**). The SMA will lie cephalad in the mesentery, and water hammer pulse can be heard with a continuous handheld Doppler and palpated in the root of the mesentery. **CONTINUES**

47-12

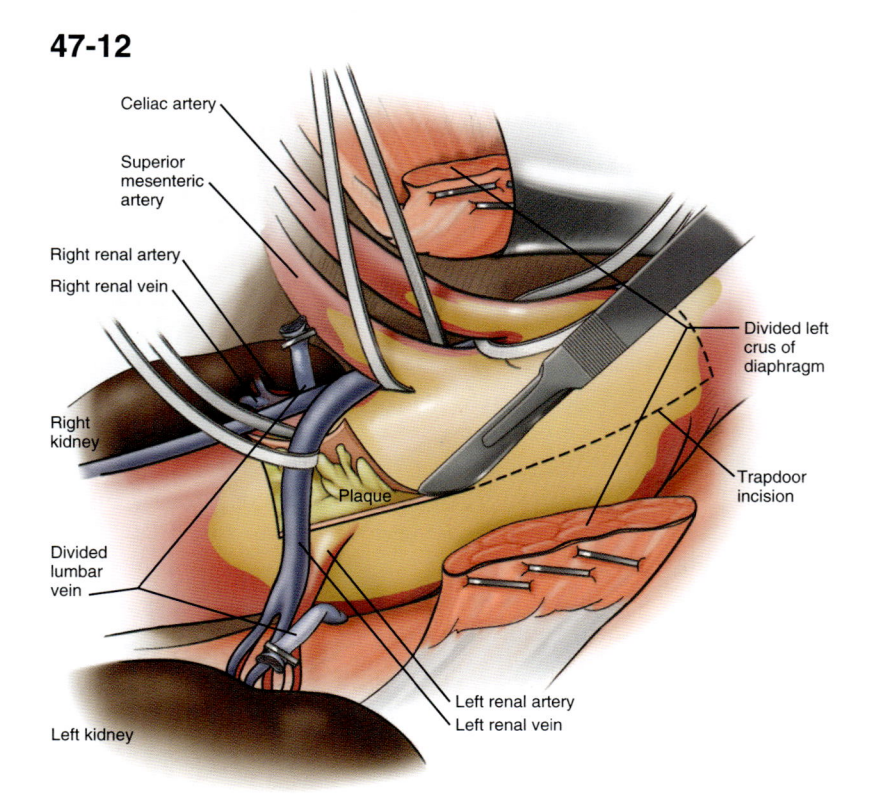

Figure 47-12 Vessels exposed leaving left kidney in situ and trap door aortotomy.

47-13

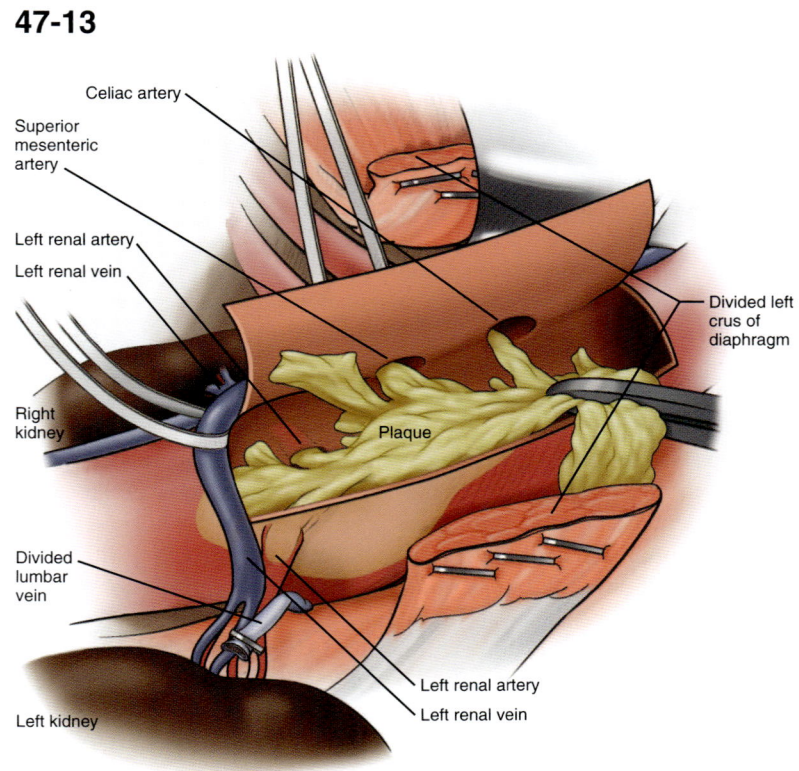

Figure 47-13 Enbloc aorta and branch vessel endarterectomy with branch vessel eversion endarterectomy.

47-14

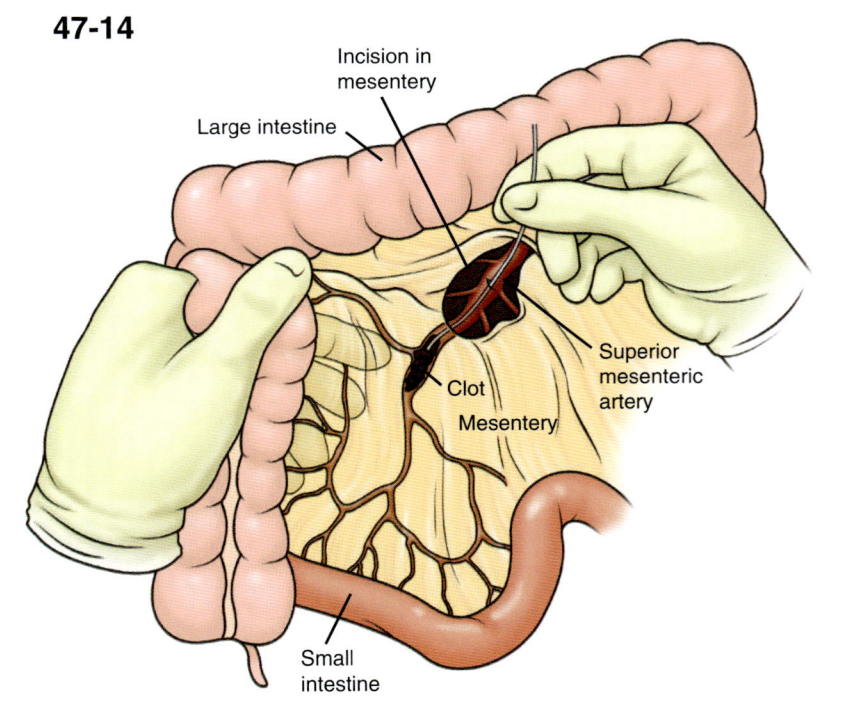

Figure 47-14 SMA embolectomy inframesocolic through mesentery.

47-15

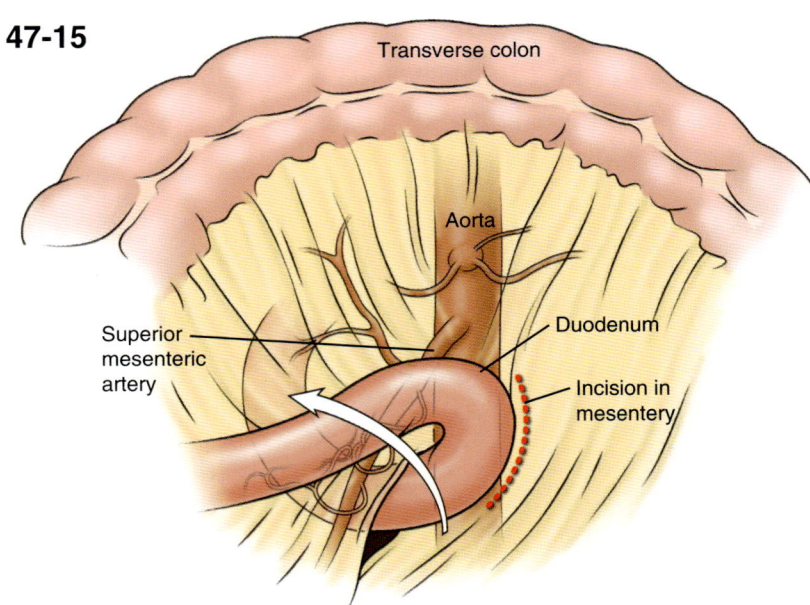

Figure 47-15 Proximal SMA exposure superior to duodenum.

DETAILS OF PROCEDURE *ACUTE MESENTERIC ISCHEMIA*: **CONTINUED** The artery is exposed, and here a transverse arteriotomy is made after proximal and distal control (FIGURE 47-16). If there is significant SMA plaque noted, a longitudinal arteriotomy is made and patch angioplasty with a bovine pericardium may be necessary. A Fogarty type embolectomy catheter is used to extract the clot, and the arteriotomy is closed with interrupted 6-0 Prolene sutures.

CLOSURE For the transverse incision, the fascia is closed in closed in two layers using #1 double-looped PDS, subcutaneous tissue is closed using a 2-0 absorbable suture, and the skin is closed with clips.

POSTOPERATIVE CARE All patients should be admitted to the intensive care unit after surgery. There can be significant third spacing, so aggressive fluid resuscitation is warranted. In patients with embolic acute mesenteric ischemia, intravenous heparin should begin as soon as possible. Frequent laboratory evaluation of serum lactate is imperative. Delayed reperfusion injury is common and can manifest as an inflammatory reaction with acute lung injury, transaminitis, and thrombocytopenia, which may not present until postoperative day 2 or 3. The patient's graft should be monitored for patency and stenosis with duplex ultrasound every 3 months for the first year and every 6 months thereafter. Additionally, for patients with CMI, the viscera myenteric plexus also has been ischemic, and prolonged ileus is common. Advancing to oral intake should be done slowly, and offering six small meals per day is often helpful. ■

SELECTED READINGS

Arthurs ZM, Titus J, Bannazadeh M, Eagleton MJ, Srivastava S, Sarac TP, Clair DG. A comparison of endovascular revascularization with traditional therapy for the treatment of acute mesenteric ischemia. *J Vasc Surg.* 2011;53(3):698-704.

Gentile AT, Moneta GL, Taylor LM Jr, Park TC, McConnell DB, Porter JM. Isolated bypass to the superior mesenteric artery for intestinal ischemia. *Arch Surg.* 1994 Sep;129(9):926-931.

Jimenez JG, Huber TS, Ozaki CK, Flynn TC, Berceli SA, Lee WA, Seeger JM. Durability of antegrade synthetic aortomesenteric bypass for chronic mesenteric ischemia. *J Vasc Surg.* 2002 Jun;35(6):1078-1084.

Mell MW, Acher CW, Hoch JR, Tefera G, Turnipseed WD. Outcomes after endarterectomy for chronic mesenteric ischemia. *J Vasc Surg.* 2008 Nov;48(5):1132-1138.

Oderich G, Fatima J, Clair DG, Sarac TP. Outcomes of re-interventions done in failing or failed open mesenteric reconstructions *J Vasc Surg.* 2014 Dec;60(6):1612-1619.

Sarac TP, Altinel O, Kashyap VS, Bena J, Lyden S, Srivastava S, Eagleton M, Clair D. Endovascular treatment of stenotic and occluded visceral arteries for chronic mesenteric ischemia. *J Vasc Surg.* 2008;47:485-491.

47-16

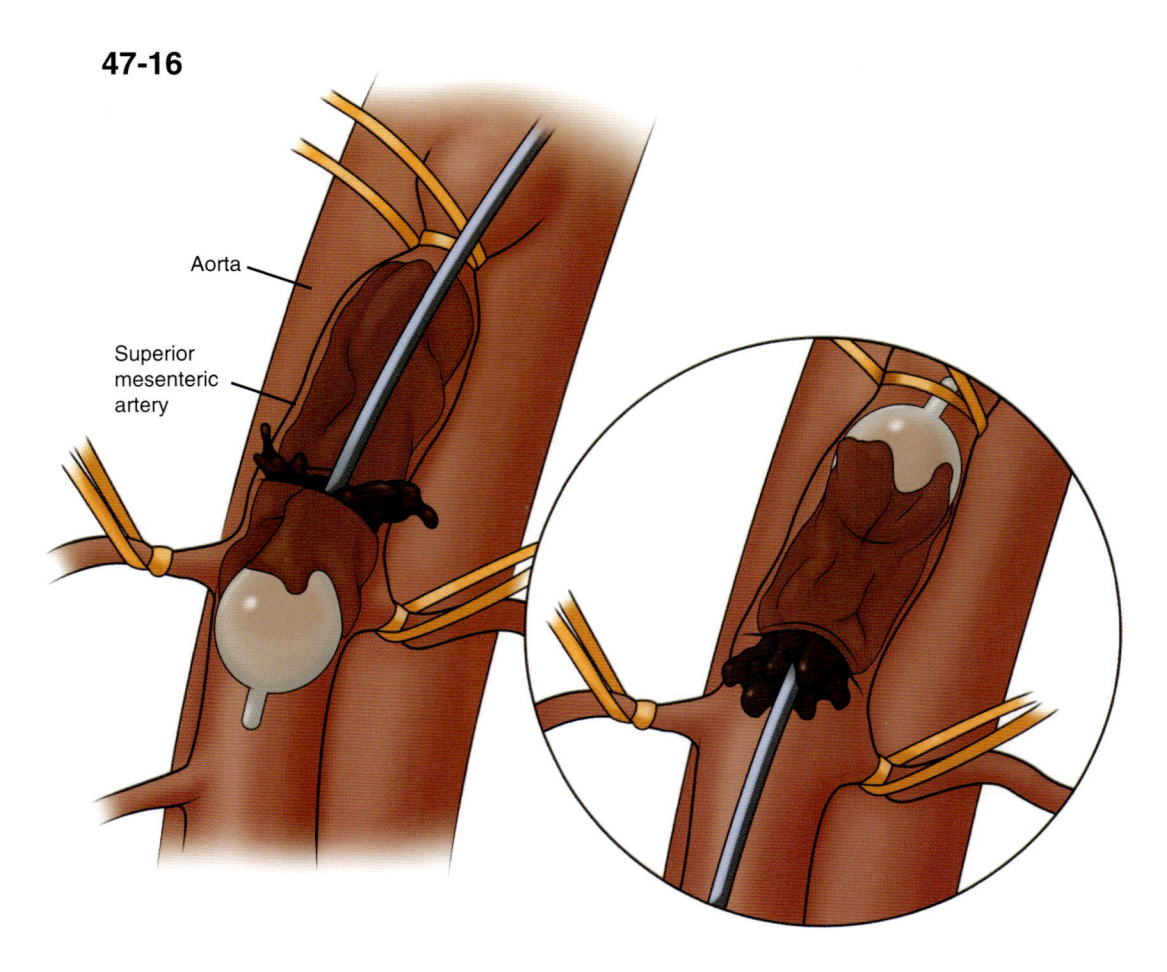

Aorta

Superior
mesenteric
artery

Figure 47-16 SMA embolectomy.

RENAL ARTERY ANEURYSM RESECTION AND BYPASS

Drew J. Braet, MD • Dawn M. Coleman, MD

INDICATIONS Renal artery aneurysms (RAAs) are rare, with an incidence that approximates 1% (1, 2). Most RAAs are asymptomatic, and thus are diagnosed incidentally. However, RAAs are thought to contribute to hypertension, which may be present in up to 70 to 75% of patients with a RAA (3–5). Symptoms rarely associated with RAAs include flank pain, abdominal pain, and hematuria (6, 7). Although RAA can rupture, most studies agree that rupture rarely occurs, especially when the aneurysms are symptomatic (5, 8, 10). Multiple studies suggest that rupture rates are below 3%, with some reporting rates as much as tenfold lower (9, 10).

Most RAAs are saccular in nature but can be fusiform or intralobar. Rundback et al. classified RAA into three categories: type 1, saccular aneurysms arising from the main renal artery; type 2, fusiform aneurysms; and type 3, intralobar aneurysms arising from small segmental arteries or accessory arteries (11). RAAs occur more commonly on the right side (61%) with the most common location being the renal bifurcation, followed by the renal pelvis, the distal renal artery, the mid renal artery, and rarely the proximal renal artery (5, 10).

Although most RAAs are identified incidentally on imaging obtained for other reasons, computed tomography angiogram (CTA) remains the diagnostic tool of choice for RAAs (12). If available, CTA with short (1 mm or less) cuts should be favored for better anatomic definition, and three-dimensional (3D) reconstitution can allow for a better representation of all involved branches. In patients with compromised renal function, noncontrast enhanced MRA can be used. Additionally, preoperative catheter-based angiography can help for operative planning and allow for assessment of anatomic association of multiple renal arteries. In cases of concomitant hypertension, renal vein renin sampling can also be of utility. Patients should be screened for fibromuscular dysplasia, which is associated with RAAs in up to 68% of cases, as well as concomitant aortic, visceral, and iliac arterial aneurysms, which can be present in up to 30% of cases (12). Patients not undergoing intervention should have annual CTA surveillance imaging, and if two consecutive studies are stable imaging this may be extended to every 2 to 3 years. MRA can be used for routine surveillance in younger patients in order to decrease the malignancy risk with cumulative radiation exposure (12).

Indications for aneurysm repair should be individualized to consider patient age and gender, perioperative risk and comorbidities, anticipated (or potential) pregnancy in female patients, aneurysm morphology and complexity, and size. Historical guidance supported repair of asymptomatic aneurysms >2 cm in maximum diameter and those associated with symptoms, hypertension, and rupture. However, recent guidelines support a more conservative size threshold for treatment, including repair of asymptomatic aneurysms greater than 3.0 cm (10, 12). While most data support that repair is unnecessary for aneurysms <2.0 cm, rupture of smaller aneurysms has been reported (9, 13–17). As such, patients with risk factors for rupture, including pregnancy, connective tissue disorders, and other autoimmune disorders like polyarteritis nodosa, should be carefully considered as candidates for operative repair at smaller sizes (11, 18). Pregnancy is a notable risk factor for rupture secondary to increased vascular flow and weakening of the vessel wall. A review of ruptured renal artery aneurysms revealed that 81% occurred in women, and about half of the women with ruptured RAA were pregnant (19). Furthermore, rupture of renal artery aneurysms in pregnant women has been associated with maternal mortality of 55% and fetal mortality of 85% (20). Aneurysm calcification has not consistently been associated with risk of growth or rupture (21, 22). Additional indications for repair of RAAs include symptoms (pain, hematuria) and medically refractory hypertension (4). Emergent intervention is indicated

for aneurysm rupture. In these circumstances, nephrectomy is frequently required given the limited time available to salvage the ischemic kidney.

RAA can be treated by a variety of endovascular, laparoscopic, and open surgical methods. While endovascular therapy has gained recognition and utility in the management of RAAs, only a subset of patients fit the anatomic criteria to undergo this therapy, which is beyond the scope of this chapter (23). Open surgical treatment for RAAs most often includes in-situ reconstruction, including resection and reanastomosis, interposition grafting, or bypass. The tailoring technique, which includes a partial resection of the aneurysm with direct suture of the remaining arterial wall, has been proposed as an additional open option (24). Ex-vivo repair with or without auto transplantation of the kidney remains an alternative approach, of particular use in those patients requiring complex or distal reconstructions (25). Few studies are available to compare surgical techniques for repair of renal artery aneurysms directly, and careful attention to anatomy and location should be considered to create individualized treatment plans. This chapter will focus specifically on renal artery aneurysm resection, bypass, and auto transplant.

POSITION The patient is placed in a supine position with the arms out. A lumbar roll should be placed to accentuate lumbar lordosis, allowing for easier renal exposure.

OPERATIVE PREPARATION An epidural helps with postoperative pain control. An arterial and central venous line should be considered for hemodynamic monitoring and support, the former also facilitating easy phlebotomy to monitor intraoperative anticoagulation, and a Foley catheter should be placed. After routine skin preparation, the operative field is draped to expose the entire abdomen down to at least the knees.

INCISION AND EXPOSURE The incision can be made subcostal for unilateral aneurysms, transverse supra-umbilical, or midline incision. Midline incisions are specifically useful in cases where proximal (supraceliac) aortic control is required, while a subcostal or transverse incision facilitates wide retroperitoneal exposure for distal renal anatomic exposure and mobilization. Medial visceral rotation facilitates exposure of the kidney and renal vasculature, including the proximal renal artery (classically located posterior to the vein) and its branches beyond the aneurysm, which then should be meticulously dissected. Of note, if the RAA affects the posterior branch of the renal artery, further mobilization of the kidney from the retroperitoneum may be needed.

The specifics of the exposure following surgical incision are as follows. The fascia is entered followed by sharply entering the peritoneum. An ipsilateral medical visceral rotation is then performed by dividing the avascular "white line of Toldt." From there, the ipsilateral colon is mobilized medially. A key gateway is to leave both the kidney and ureter in situ. If exposing the right renal vasculature, the right line of Toldt is mobilized with the right colon and appendix from lateral to medial (**FIGURE 48-1**). Care is taken to identify and avoid the ureter. It is also helpful to mobilize the duodenum from lateral to medial (Kocher maneuver). The IVC is identified and dissected on its lateral border to facilitate mobilization and visualization of the proximal right renal artery, aorta and bilateral renal vein (**FIGURE 48-2**).

The artery is most cases sits posterior to the vein. If exposing the left renal artery, the left colon is mobilized medially up to the splenic flexure along with the duodenum, pancreas, and spleen (**FIGURE 48-3A**). The renal vein is encircled with silastic loops for retraction, the aorta is exposed anteriorly (**FIGURE 48-3B**), and the left renal artery is in view. **CONTINUES** ▶

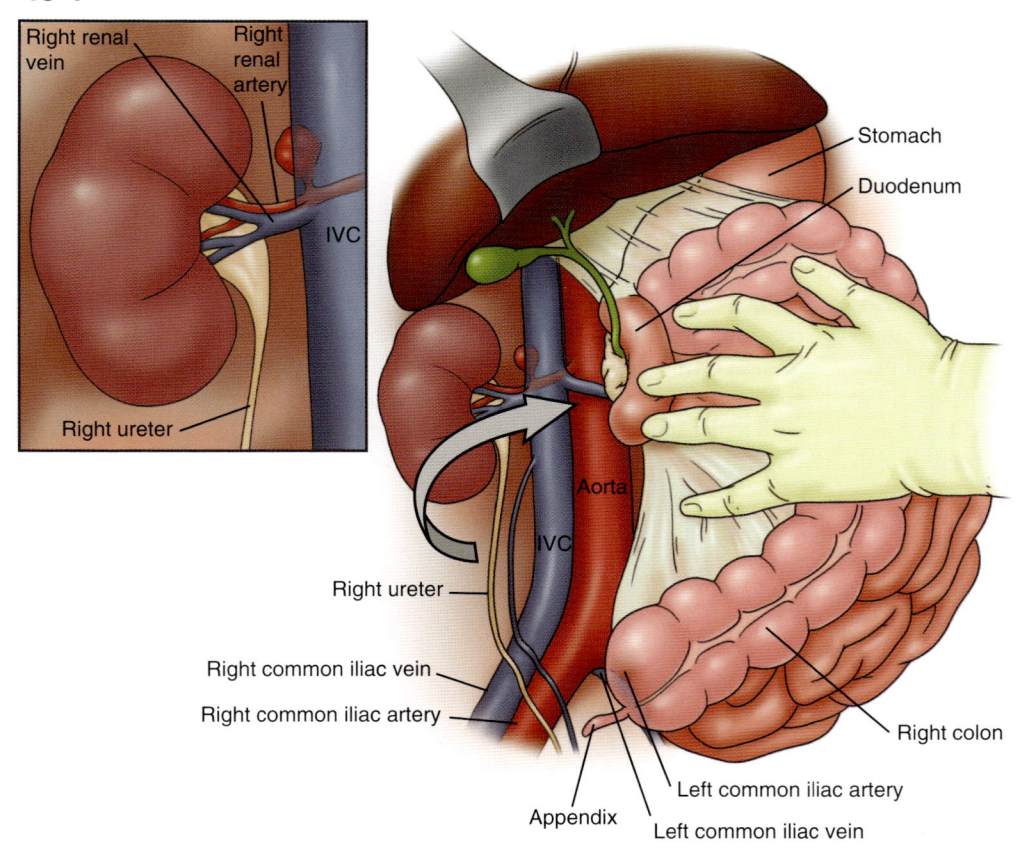

48-1

Figure 48-1 Right medial rotation.

48-2

Figure 48-2 Exposure of IVC and right renal vein to facilliatae renal artery exposure.

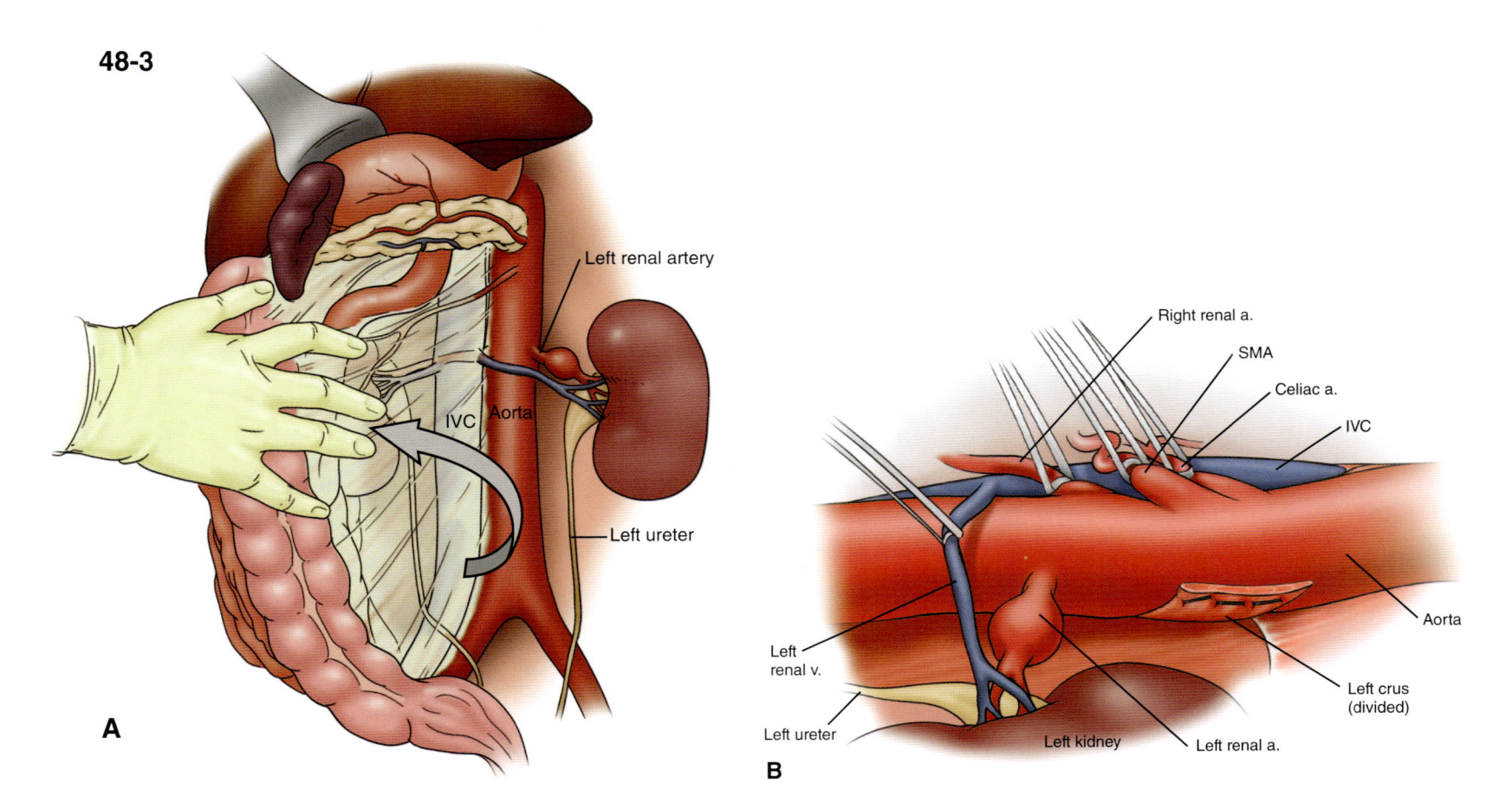

Figure 48-3 A. Left medial visceral rotation leaving kidney down. B. Retroperitoneal exposure of left renal artery.

DETAILS OF THE PROCEDURE With exposure secured, the patient is systemically anticoagulated with 100 to 150 units/kg of intravenous (IV) heparin to maintain the activated clotting time goal of greater than 250 seconds, which should be re-dosed and maintained for the entire repair. Two hundred cc of cooled (4°C) hypertonic renal perfusate (lactated Ringer's and 25 grams of mannitol) are administered directly into the renal artery immediately after cross clamping and arteriotomy to protect against acute tubular necrosis (9, 26, 27). All efforts should be made to limit total warm renal ischemia time to less than 30 minutes. If more than 30 minutes of ischemic time is anticipated for surgical reconstruction, repeat dosing of cooled renal perfusate or prostaglandin E can be administered (28). Intravenous mannitol should be considered at 0.5 grams/kg before clamping to facilitate an osmotic diuresis. Distal control of renal vasculature is obtained, often with Heifitz or any small atraumatic vascular clamps. Caution: simply "tightening" silastic loops can injure the artery, and they are in place as a precautionary measure. Pulling on them forcefully may avulse fragile small branches and risk endothelial damage leading to dissection and possible neointimal hyperplasia. Following proximal control of the artery, in a similar fashion, the aneurysm is opened sharply. Subsequently, the reconstruction proceeds with complete aneurysm resection or sharp excision of the anterior wall of the aneurysm.

Saccular aneurysms of the main renal artery are best treated with excision and primary repair if adequate length can be mobilized (**FIGURE 48-4**) (4). In fact, some authors use this technique in up to one-third of their repairs (15, 29, 30). Aneurysms that are located at primary branch points can be excised longitudinally and closed via patch angioplasty or in a transverse fashion, thus preventing luminal narrowing (**FIGURE 48-5**) (4). Another common technique is an end-to-side anastomosis of a small renal artery branch to the main renal artery, or a side-to-side anastomosis of multiple small renal arteries (i.e., syndactylization) to create a one-inflow channel with larger diameter, which can then be anastomosed to the more proximal renal artery or aorta (**FIGURE 48-6**) (4). **CONTINUES ▶**

48-4

48-5

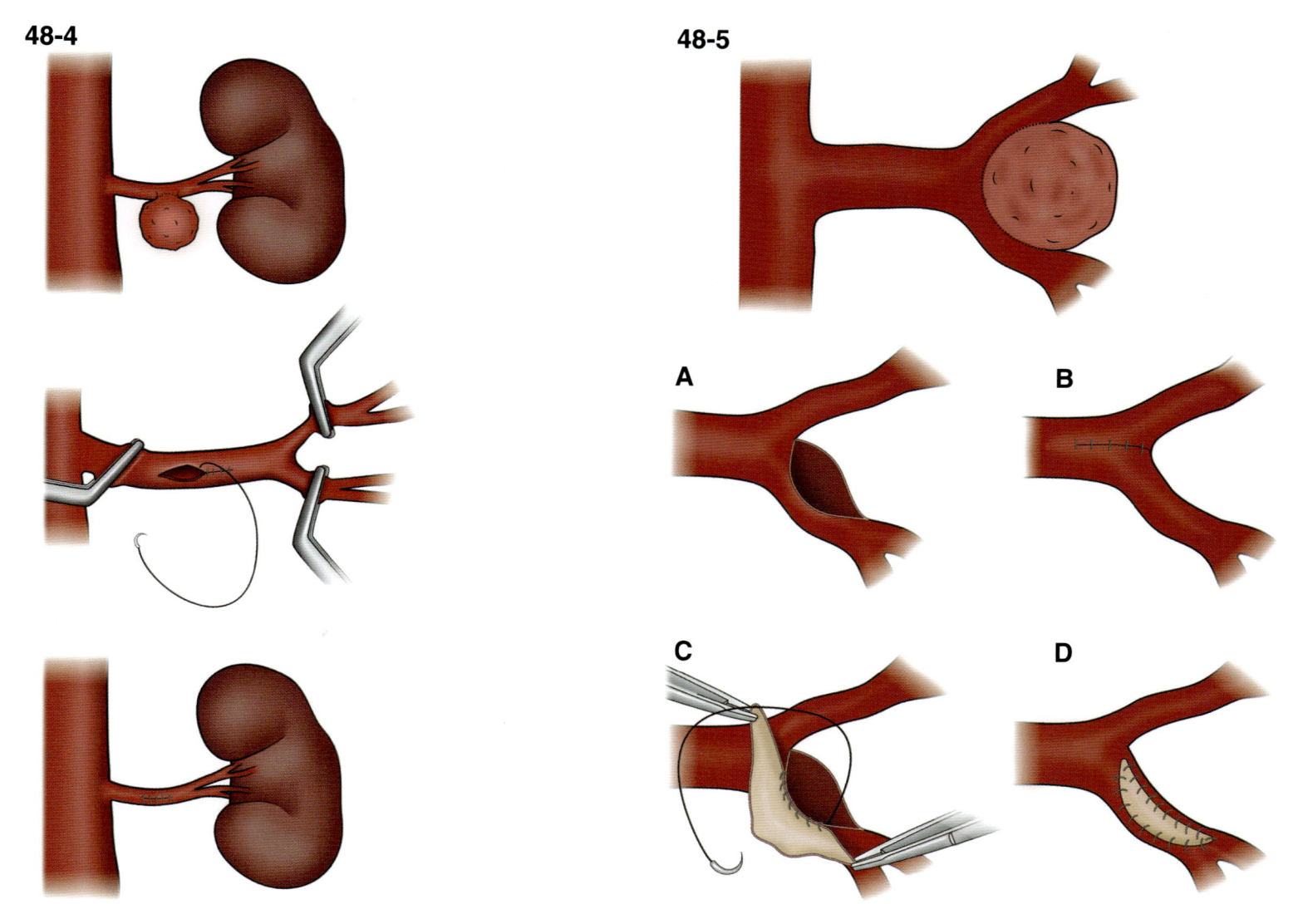

Figure 48-4 Sacuular aneurysm primary repair.

Figure 48-5 Branch point aneurysm repair. Following the longitudinal excision of a large saccular aneurysm located at the primary branch point (A), primary angioplastic closure of the defect in a transverse fashion (B), or patch angioplasty (C and D) may be considered.

48-6

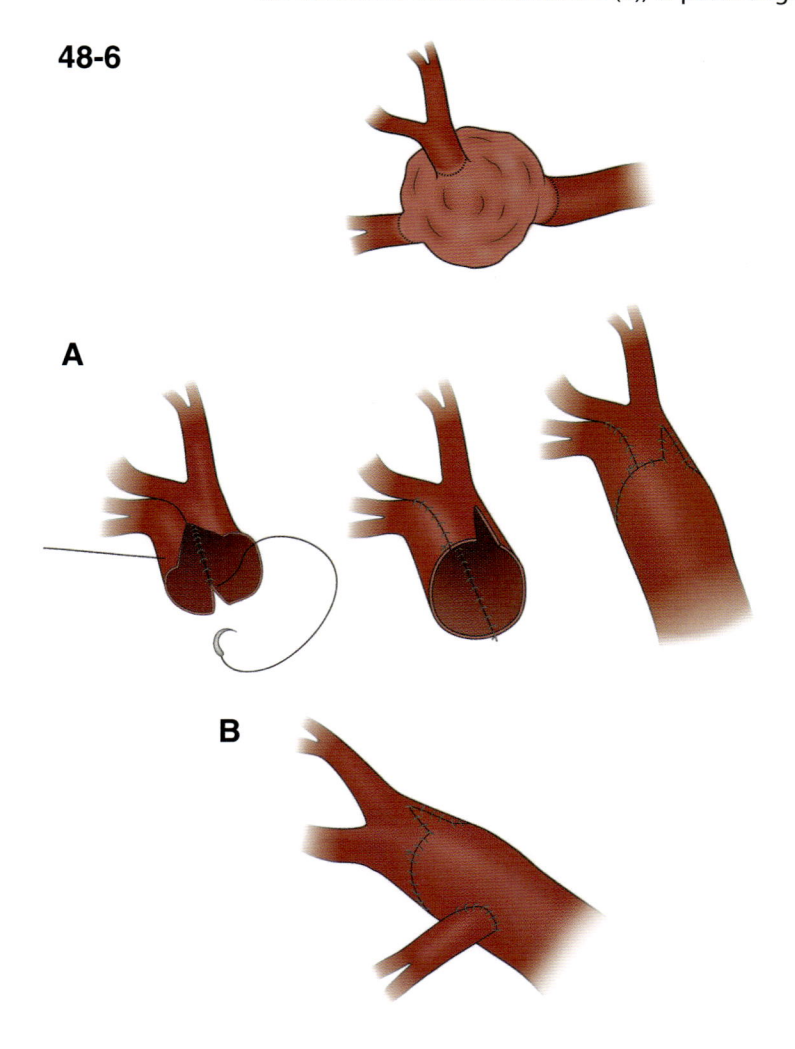

Figure 48-6 Aneurysms may have several outflow vessels of variable caliber. A. These vessels may be spatulated together to provide a common outflow target for a bypass graft; or B, branch vessels may require separate reimplantations onto the graft.

DETAILS OF THE PROCEDURE `CONTINUED` Other in situ reconstructions include interposition bypass (**FIGURE 48-7**), where the aneurysm is resected and an interposition vein graft is sewn end-to-end between the two artery segments. For distal or segmental renal artery aneurysms and those involving small branches of the main renal artery, aorto-renal bypass can be used (4). Aortic inflow is preferred over extra-anatomic sources (i.e., hepatic or splenic artery). Retrograde inflow from the iliac artery is another alternative when requisite. On the right side, the medial edge of the IVC should be mobilized, and the bypass graft tunneled underneath the IVC. When doing this, caution should be taken to avoid avulsing the posterior lumbar veins (**FIGURE 48-8**).

Autogenous conduit (reversed saphenous vein) is preferred to prosthetic; 6-mm ringed ePTFE should be considered only as an option for those renal arteries measuring greater than 6 mm in diameter. The use of a branched conduit (i.e., internal iliac artery) can also be considered for distal reconstructions that require revascularization of multiple segmental branches (31). In cases where the artery is of small diameter or feeds a small area, an end-to-end anastomosis with pantaloon, side-to-end anastomosis, or branch ligation can be used (4, 32).

In cases of rupture, the abdomen is often packed initially to control hemorrhage, and the supraceliac aorta may require clamping. If the patient is hemodynamically stable and warm ischemia duration is permissible, reconstruction should be considered. However, in most cases nephrectomy is required. On a similar note, if the renal ischemic time is expected to exceed 60 minutes, extracorporeal or bench surgery may be required (33, 34). In these cases, nephrectomy followed by hypothermic perfusion of the kidney may be required. The kidney can then be auto-transplanted to its original bed or the iliac fossa (**FIGURE 48-9**) (35, 36).

Before the anastomosis is completed, all branches should be vented to de-air and vent any debris or thromboembolic source. The kidney is then reperfused with release of vascular clamps. Doppler insonation of the reconstructed artery, renal hilum, and parenchyma should be used to confirm restoration of flow. If the kidney appears slow to re-perfuse and/or the Doppler has concerning signals, technical problems or vasospasm should be suspected. Vasospasm, which is common in young patients, can be addressed with subadventitial injection of papaverine or nitroglycerin. If there is still no improvement, a technical issue should be suspected and there should be a low threshold for revision. Intraoperative duplex is another useful adjunct for confirming patency.

CLOSURE Hemostasis must be achieved to prevent hematoma formation. Protamine sulfate is used to reverse anticoagulation. The wound is irrigated and then closed in a multilayer fashion. The skin is closed with clips or 4-0 Monocryl, and skin adhesive and a sterile dressing are applied. `CONTINUES`

48-7

48-8

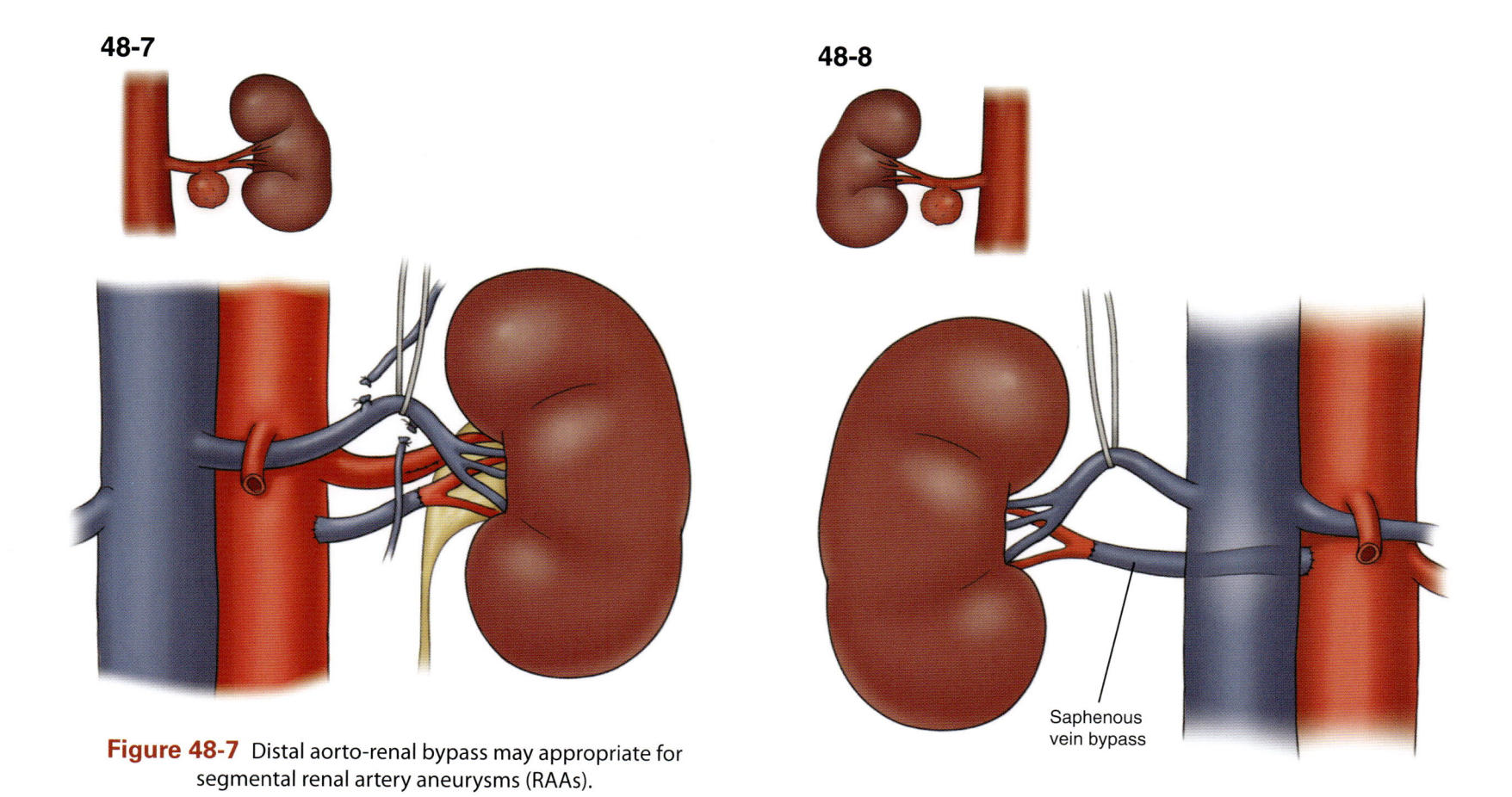

Figure 48-7 Distal aorto-renal bypass may appropriate for segmental renal artery aneurysms (RAAs).

Saphenous vein bypass

Figure 48-8 Aorta to right renal artery vein bypass tunneled underneath IVC.

48-9

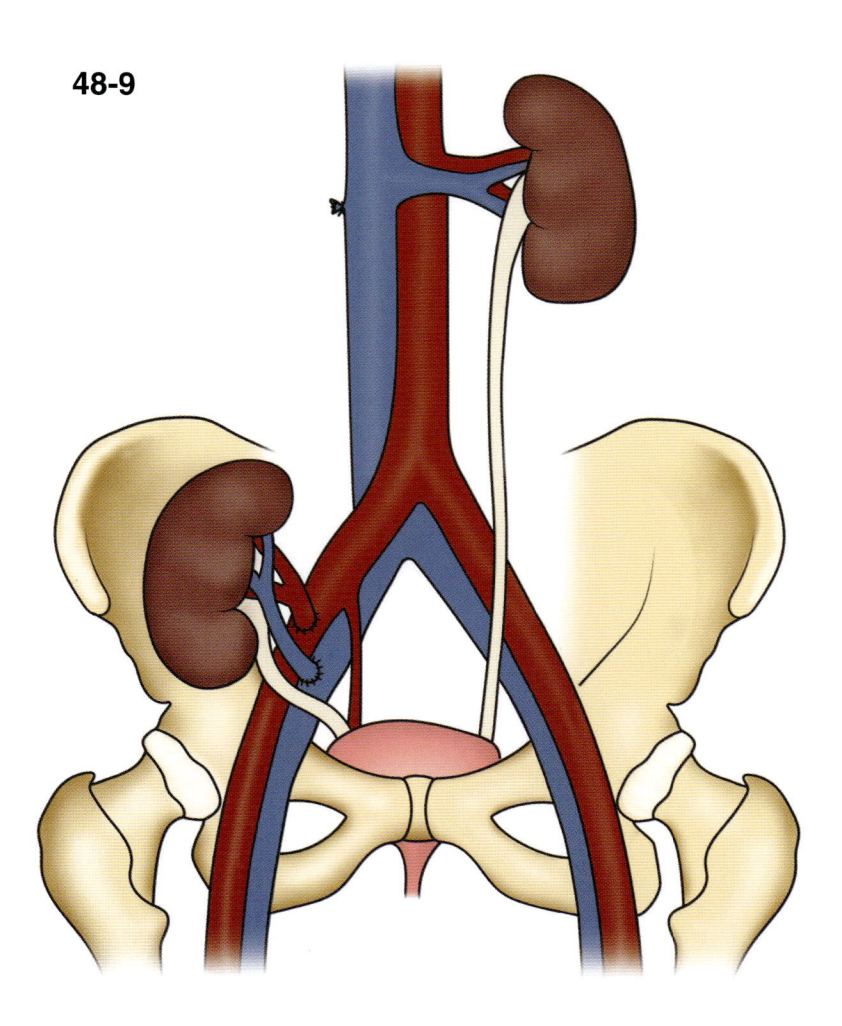

Figure 48-9 Right kidney auto transplanted into the pelvis.

POSTOPERATIVE CARE Patients typically require 5 to 10 days of inpatient care following open RAA repair. Perioperative complications following such may include hemorrhage, renal thrombosis, acute kidney injury, deep venous thrombosis, pneumonia and other pulmonary complication requiring reintubation, third-degree heart block, pancreatitis, prolonged postoperative ileus, and infection. A completion study postoperatively is imperative, and these authors favor angiogram on approximately postoperative day 5, which coincides with resolution of postoperative acute tubular necrosis and acute kidney injury and decreases the risk of further injury (through contrast-induced nephropathy). This study will detect technical problems that might benefit from early corrective therapy and serve as a new baseline to which surveillance studies will be compared. Antiplatelet therapy (i.e., aspirin 81 mg daily) is prescribed for at least 6 weeks, and often extended indefinitely (12).

Postoperative surveillance includes monitoring of blood pressure, renal function, and kidney perfusion/size. Patients are encouraged to maintain a blood pressure log, and are seen at 1 month, 6 months, and 12/18/24 months with serology (creatinine) and renal duplex. Thereafter follow-up every year is advised (9, 12). Late complications such as stenosis, conduit degeneration and aneurysm, and graft thrombosis may threaten patency and renal function. All efforts and reintervention to ensure preserved primary and secondary patency should be employed, to include anastomotic angioplasty, reoperation for graft thrombosis, revision of bypass grafts for aneurysmal degeneration, and percutaneous embolization of stenotic segmental branches. Patients with worsening hypertension, declining renal function, or abnormal duplex findings should be studied with catheter-based selective angiogram.

In summary, open surgery may remain the gold standard technique for RAA, especially when aneurysm anatomy and patient risk factors preclude endovascular repair. Most retrospective studies comparing open and endovascular repair of RAA have demonstrated no significant difference in mortality, postoperative complications, or change in renal function (10, 37, 38). However, some studies have suggested that open repair is associated with higher rates of cardiac and infectious complications, while endovascular repair has higher hemorrhagic complications as well as a shorter length of stay (39). Open repair for RAA remains a viable and durable option with low mortality and morbidity and a 1-year survival of nearly 90% (40). ◼

REFERENCES

1. Orion KC, Abularrage CJ. Renal artery aneurysms: movement toward endovascular repair. *Semin Vasc Surg.* 2013;26(4):226-232.

2. González J, Esteban M, Andrés G, Linares E, Martínez-Salamanca JI. Renal artery aneurysms. *Curr Urol Rep.* 2014;15(1):376.

3. Titze N, Ivanukoff V, Fisher T, Pearl G, Grimsley B, Shutze W. Surgical repair of renal artery aneurysms. *Proc (Bayl Univ Med Cent).* 2015;28(4):499-501.

4. Coleman DM, Stanley JC. Renal artery aneurysms. *J Vasc Surg.* 2015;62:779-785.

5. Brownstein A, Erben Y, Rajaee S, Li Y, Rizzo J, Mojibian H, et al. Natural history and management of renal artery aneurysms in a single tertiary referral center. *J Vasc Surg.* 2018;68(1):137-144.

6. Stanley JC, Rhodes EL, Gewertz BL, Chang CY, Walter JF, Fry WJ. Renal artery aneurysms. Significance of macroaneurysms exclusive of dissections and fibrodysplastic mural dilations. *Arch Surg.* 1975;110:1327-1333

7. Klausner JQ, Harlander-Locke MP, Plotnik AN, Lehrman E, DeRubertis BG, Lawrence PF. Current treatment of renal artery aneurysms may be too aggressive. *J Vasc Surg.* 2014;59:1356-1361

8. Calligaro KD, Dougherty MJ. Renovascular disease: aneurysms and arteriovenous fistulae. *Rutherford's Vascular Surgery.* 8th ed. Philadelphia, Saunders. 2014:2326-2334.

9. Henke PK, Cardneau JD, Welling TH, Upchurch Jr G, Wakefield TW, Jacobs LA, et al. Renal artery aneurysms: a 35-year clinical experience with 252 aneurysms in 168 patients. *Ann Surg.* 2001;234:454-462.

10. Klausner JQ, Lawrence PF, Harlander-Locke MP, Coleman DM, Stanley JC, Fujimura N, et al. The contemporary management of renal artery aneurysms. *J Vasc Surg.* 2015;61:978-984.

11. Rundback JH, Rizvi A, Rozenblit GN, Poplausky M, Maddineni S, Crea G, et al. Percutaneous stent-graft management of renal artery aneurysms. *J Vasc Interv Radiol.* 2000;11(9):1189-1193.

12. Chaer RA, Abularrage CJ, Coleman DM, Eslami MH, Kashyap VS, Rockman C, et al. The Society for Vascular Surgery clinical practice guidelines on the management of visceral aneurysms. *J Vasc Surg.* 2020;72:3S-39S.

13. Bastounis W, Pikoulis E, Georgopoulos S, Alexiou D, Leppaniemi A, Boulafendis D. Surgery for renal artery aneurysms: a combined series of two large centers. *Eur Urol.* 1998;33:22-27.

14. Lumsden AB, Salam TA, Walton KG. Renal artery aneurysm: a report of 28 cases. *Cardiovasc Surg.* 1996;4:185-189.

15. Dzsinich C, Gloviczki P, McKusick MA, Pairolero PC, Bower TC, Hallett JW, et al. Surgical management of renal artery aneurysm. *Cardiovasc Surg.* 1993;1:243-247.

16. Reiher L, Grabitz K, Sandmann W. Reconstruction for renal artery aneurysm and its effect on hypertension. *Eur J Endovasc Surg.* 2000;20:454-456.

17. Hupp T, Allenberg JR, Post K, Roeren T, Meier M, Clorius JH. Renal artery aneurysm: surgical indications and results. *Eur J Surg.* 1992;6:477-486.

18. Cura M, Elmerhi F, Bugnogne A, Palacios R, Suri R, Dalsaso T. Renal aneurysms and pseudoaneurysms. *Clin Imaging.* 2011;35(1):29-41.

19. Turpin S, Lambert R, Querin S, Soulez G, Leveille J, Taillefer R. Radionuclide captopril renography in postpartum renal artery aneurysms. *J Nucl Med.* 1996;37:1368.

20. Cohen JR, Shamash FS. Ruptured renal artery aneurysms during pregnancy. *J Vasc Surg.* 1987;6:51.

21. Poutasse EF. Renal artery aneurysms. *J Urol.* 1975;43:113.

22. Hidai H, et. al. Rupture of renal artery aneurysm. *Eur Urol.* 1985;11:249.

23. Duran M, Hausmann D, Grabitz K, Schelzig H, Simon F, Sagban T. Reconstruction for renal artery aneurysms using the tailoring technique. *J Vasc Surg.* 2015;65(2),438-443.

24. Ham S, Weaver F. Ex vivo renal artery reconstruction for complex renal artery disease. *J Vasc Surg.* 2014;60(1):143-151.

25. Jibiki M, Inoue Y, Kudo T, Toyofuku T. Surgical procedures for renal artery aneurysms. *Ann Vasc Dis.* 2012;5(2):157-160.

26. Pfeiffer T, Reiher L, Grabitz K, Gunhage B, Hafele S, Voiculescu A, et al. Reconstruction for renal artery aneurysm: operative techniques and long-term results. *J Vasc Surg.* 2003;37:293-300.

27. Miller CL, Myers BD. Pathophysiology and preservation of acute renal failure associated with thoracoabdominal or abdominal aortic surgery. *J Vasc Surg.* 1987;5:518-523.

28. English W, Pearce J, Craven T, Wilson D, Edwards M, Ayerdi J, et al. Surgical management of renal artery aneurysms. *J Vasc Surg.* 40(1):53-60. doi: 10.1016/j.jvs.2004.03.024

29. Martin RS, Meacham PW, Ditesheim JA, Mulherin JL, Edwards WH. et al. Renal artery aneurysm: selective treatment for hypertension and prevention of rupture. *J Vasc Surg.* 1989;9:26.

30. Panayiotopoulos YP, Assadourian R, Taylor PR. Aneurysms of the visceral and renal arteries. *Ann R Coll Surg Engl.* 1996;78:412-419.

31. Jibiki M, Inoue Y, Kudo T, Toyofuku T. Surgical procedures for renal artery aneurysms. *Ann Vasc Dis.* 2012;5(2):157-160.

32. Brayman KL, Gincherman Y, Levy MM, et al. Ex vivo reconstruction of the renal artery for aneurysm and other abnormalities of renal vascular anatomy.

33. Calligaro KD, Dougherty MJ, Dean RH. *Modern Management of Renovascular Hypertension and Renal Salvage.* Baltimore. Williams & Wilkins. 1996.

34. Dubernard JM, Martin X, Gelet A, Mongin D. Aneurysms of the renal artery: surgical management with special reference to extracorporeal surgery and auto transplantation. *Eur Urol.* 1985;11:26-30.

35. Dean RH, Meacham PW, Weaver WA. Ex vivo renal artery reconstructions: indications and techniques. *J Vasc Surg.* 1986;4:546-552.

36. Crutchley TA, Pearce JD, Craven TE, Edwards MS, Dean RH, Hansen KJ. Branch renal artery repair with cold perfusion protection. *J Vasc Surg.* 2007;46:405-412.

37. Cochennec F, Riga CV, Allaire E, Cheshire NJ, Hamady M, Jenkins MP, et al. Contemporary management of splanchnic and renal artery aneurysms: results of endovascular compared with open surgery from two European vascular centers. *Eur J Vasc Endovasc Surg.* 2011;42:340-346.

38. Tsilimparis N, Reeves JG, Dayama A, Perez SD, Debus ES, Ricotta JJ. Endovascular vs open repair of renal artery aneurysms: outcomes of repair and long-term renal function. *J Am Coll Surg.* 2013;217:263-269.

39. Hislop SJ, Patel SA, Abt PL, Singh MJ, Illig KA. Therapy of renal artery aneurysms in New York State: outcomes of patients undergoing open and endovascular repair. *Ann Vasc Surg.* 2009;23:194-200.

40. Steuer J, Bergqvist D, Björck M. Surgical renovascular reconstruction for renal artery stenosis and aneurysm: long-term durability and survival. *Eur J Vasc Endovasc Surg.* 2019;57(4):562-568.

TRANS FEMORAL AND TRANSBRACHIAL ACCESS FOR VISCERAL INTERVENTIONS

Elizabeth Chou, MD • **Sunita D. Srivastava, MD**

INDICATIONS The treatment of mesenteric occlusive disease has shifted from open surgical therapy to a primarily endovascular approach. Transcatheter therapy as a first-line treatment for symptomatic mesenteric disease is justified based on the ease of access to the lesion via percutaneous route, avoidance of laparotomy, faster revascularization of ischemic bowel, and proven patency over time. While bare metal stenting was initially favored, recent studies have demonstrated superior patency of covered balloon expandable stents in these vascular beds.

Access to the mesenteric vessels has traditionally been via the femoral arteries. The factors favoring femoral access include ease of access to all vascular regions and effortless operator position regardless of hand dominance as well as radiation safety considerations such as distance from radiation source, image intensifier, and accessible use of lead shields. Hostile femoral access is related to previous femoral surgery with or without prosthetic conduit or patch presence, occlusive disease resulting in unfavorable conditions such as plaque, dissection, and lack of femoral pulse as well as the scarring from such conditions which make the insertion of needles, sheaths, and subsequent closure devices challenging.

Transbrachial access has evolved as the preferred point of entry given unfavorable femoral characteristics and the growing use of transradial/transulnar approaches in coronary interventions. The use of brachial access entry has been reported with consistent technical success and minimal complications. In addition, with the growth of aortic endovascular therapies such as fenestrated/branched/hypogastric branch endografting, chimney and snorkel techniques as well as adjunctive therapies such as anchors, cuffs, and embolization, the brachial and axillary arteries are essential additional points of entry. Typically, the axillary artery is used for larger device sizes while the brachial artery can accommodate up to 7F sheaths. Anything above a 6F sheath will usually need a brachial artery cutdown. This is done by making a longitudinal incision over the artery approximately 2 cm proximal to the antecubital fossa. The brachial sheath is then incised, and the median nerve is usually encountered. This is then gently retracted, and the brachial artery is deep (**FIGURE 49-1**).

Imaging is critical in the decision of access site entry for mesenteric stenoses. The overall tortuosity of the arch, descending thoracic and infrarenal aorta, angles of take-off of the visceral vessels, and presence of subclavian and iliac occlusive disease are variables to consider when assessing for retrograde brachial or femoral approach. The selection of sheath properties, French size, and catheters are impacted by the anatomy of the visceral entry. Computed tomography to include the arch, thoracic, and abdominal aorta is useful, as is baseline duplex of the brachial and femoral arteries. The measurement of bilateral upper extremity blood pressures can reveal a proximal subclavian stenosis, while the performance of an Allen test and insonation of audible radial/ulnar and palmar signals relays important perfusion information. Pressure volume measurements or ankle brachial indices also assist in preprocedural decision-making.

POSITION The patient is placed in a supine position with the head toward the imaging system. Typically, the left upper extremity is selected to avoid traversal of hardware across the right carotid ostia with a right brachial approach. Consideration for preexisting hemodialysis access site, history of mastectomy and axillary node dissection as well as previous extremity surgery play roles in selection. The arm is placed on an arm board with the entire extremity placed palmar side up. A Kerlix or roll of gauze is placed in the palm and tape is used to secure the palm to the arm board. The radial, ulnar, and palmar signals are marked with a surgical marker.

For transfemoral access, the side that is selected is based on axial imaging and the absence of proximal iliac occlusive disease, strongest pulse palpation, or duplex insonation demonstrating the least amount of plaque or calcium. Distal pedal signals are insonated and marked. Some operators prefer to use duplex imaging prior to prep and drape to isolate the more favorable access side. In the obese patient with a significant pannus, upward taping of the additional skin and fat is accomplished with linen tape and benzoin application.

OPERATIVE PREPARATION After routine skin preparation of the upper arm, antecubital fossa, and upper forearm, the drapes are placed to permit access to the brachial artery. Occasionally, adhesive barriers such as an iodine-impregnated plastic is placed to assure the sterility of the field and drapes.

A pediatric laparotomy sheet is then used lengthwise and cut to permit access to the sterile field. A moist towel can be placed along the forearm portion of the draped field to permit a nonstick surface for hydrophilic wires and catheters. This can transition to the procedural table that is in line with the upper extremity. The image intensifier is typically positioned at the patient's head and used to transition from upper chest and arm imaging to the abdomen. Lead shield can be brought from the front or overhead for protection.

For femoral access, bilateral groins are typically prepped if both sides are equally accessible. Site of puncture is based on operator hand dominance and preference.

The groin is covered with a towel, and square draping of the infraumbilical and groin regions is used. Adhesive barriers can be used as in the arm approach.

INCISION AND EXPOSURE Entry in both femoral and brachial (if smaller sheath) access is performed with ultrasound guidance and needle access via Seldinger technique. Direct visualization of the needle entry in the anterior surface of the artery is key to avoid back wall puncture and extreme angles of entry that can make sheath traversal and closure device use challenging. For the femoral artery, common femoral puncture at the level of the inferior femoral head and below the inguinal ligament is advised. Brachial access is performed in the antecubital fossa and elbow joint. The bony landmarks in both approaches permit compression against the humeral or femoral head for successful hemostasis if manual pressure is used. Mid-vessel punctures and avoidance of the region above the vessel bifurcations can assist in avoidance of compromising distal perfusion if complications from the access or closure device deployment occur. High brachial or femoral bifurcations can result in inadvertent radial and superficial femoral artery punctures if duplex imaging is not carefully assessed.

DETAILS OF PROCEDURE The anatomy of the proximal access vessels should be evaluated for occlusive disease, dissection, or aneurysms, as additional complications can arise from negligent manipulation of endovascular hardware in these areas. The operator must be prepared to address preexisting disease or subsequent complications from the delivery of sheaths and deployment of stent delivery systems and balloon catheters. Micropuncture 4/5 French (Cook Inc, Bloomington, IN) or starter needle and wire are used to access the entry vessel. A short length (7- to 10-cm) sheath is placed to ensure access for the diagnostic portion of the case. Active fluoroscopic imaging of the wire and hardware along the access vessels to the target area is critical to avoid mishap. Selection of the appropriate type of wire, sheath, and catheter to facilitate access into the visceral region for diagnostic and subsequent therapeutic intervention is key. Lengths and diameters of endovascular tools should be based on patient body habitus, access vessel sizes, vessel tortuosity, and diameters of targeted mesenteric vessels. When coming from the axillary or brachial artery, an LAO projection allows better visualization of where the arch of the aorta lies (**FIGURE 49-2**). A curved C2 or similar catheter can help manipulate the wire into the descending thoracic aorta.

Once the paravisceral aorta is reached with the wire, a nonselective multi-side hole flush catheter is placed, and diagnostic imaging is performed in multiplanar views to identify the mesenteric vessels, extent, and length of stenosis(es) and best angles to enter selectively (**FIGURE 49-3**).

Measurements are taken off the diagnostic runs with calibration of the vessel diameter and length of stenoses visualized. Preliminary review for the need of preemptive balloon angioplasty balloon length and diameters as well as for stent dimensions are done at this time. Inventory is brought to the attention of the operator for review. The next step is variable and operator dependent. Some operators at this junction will place the working sheath of selected French size needed based on intended stent delivery size in the vicinity of the target visceral vessel to access. A selective catheter will then be placed within the sheath to cannulate the visceral vessel. Other operators prefer to access the targeting mesenteric vessel first with a selective end hole catheter and hydrophilic wire of choice (**FIGURE 49-4**).

At this point heparin is given intravenously, based on body weight, by the monitoring anesthetic team at the proceduralist's discretion. Activated clotting times are used to monitor heparin dosing and appropriate levels of anticoagulation. Aspirin and/or Plavix are not held preoperatively.

CONTINUES ▶

49-1

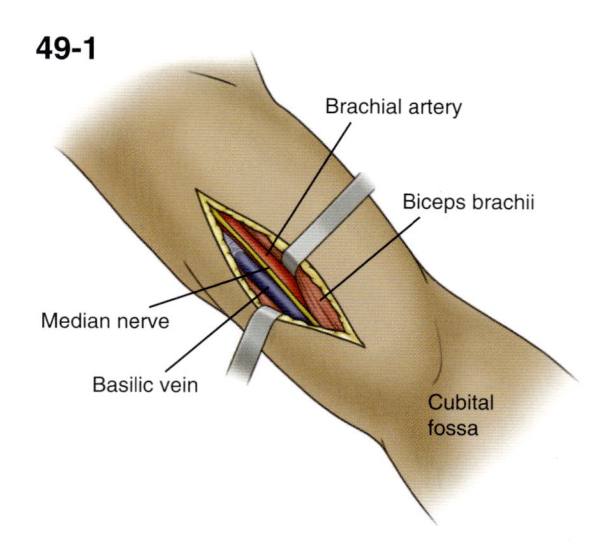

Figure 49-1 Left brachial artery exposure.

49-2

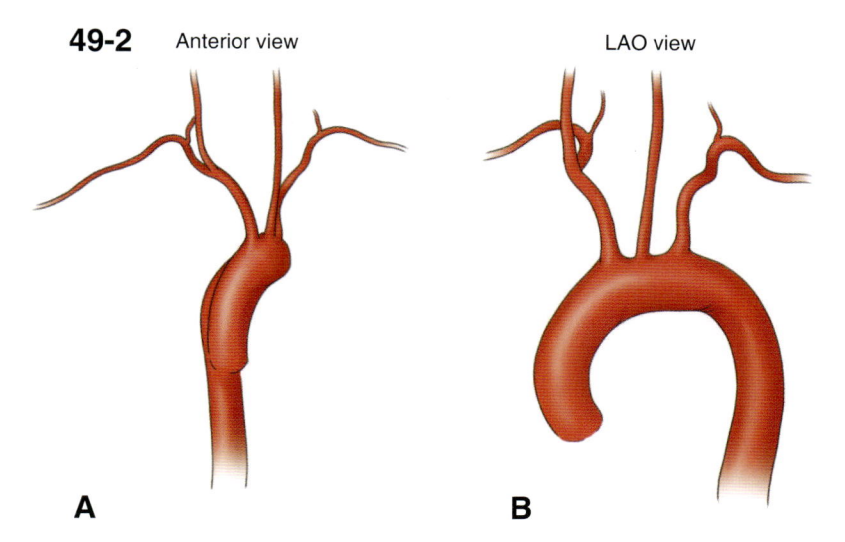

Figure 49-2 Arch aortogram for transbrachial access. A. Anterior image intensifier position B. Left anterior oblique (LAO) image intensifier position. Branch vessels are best seen in the LAO projection.

49-3

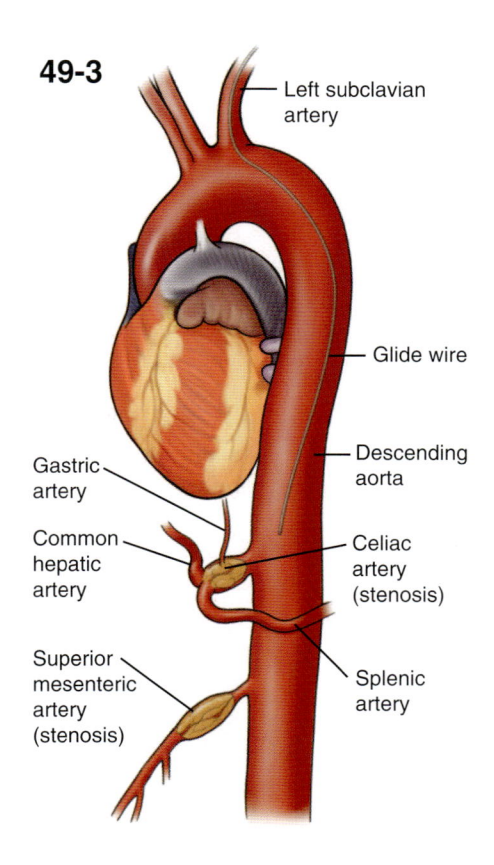

Figure 49-3 Visceral stenoses on lateral/sagittal view.

49-4

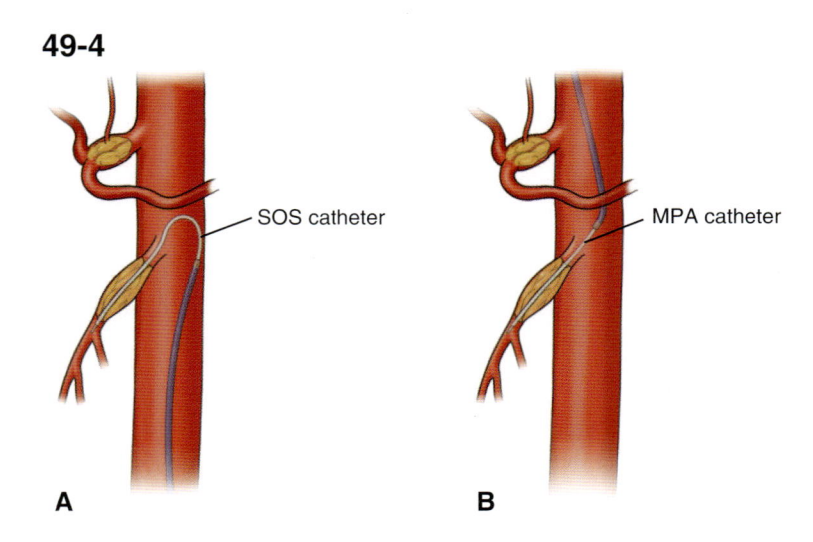

Figure 49-4 Femoral and brachial approach with selective cannulation of stenotic SMA with SOS (A) or MPA (B) catheter.

DETAILS OF PROCEDURE CONTINUED Once the stenotic vessel is entered, the wire is placed safely in the ileocolic branch of the superior mesenteric artery or the splenic artery branch of the celiac vessel. Vigilant fluoroscopy to follow wire entry and passage into the second- or third-order branch is essential to avoid distal dissection and perforation. The end hole catheter is placed into the branch vessel and the hydrophilic wire is exchanged out for a more robust (Rosen 0.035″) wire to facilitate sheath entry. The catheter is either removed to allow placement of the sheath dilator or remains and serves as the dilator to permit sheath placement across the stenosis. This will enable the safe delivery of the balloon and stent catheters.

The lesion may not permit safe traversal of the selective catheter or the working sheath. A microcatheter system can be used within the selective catheter or sheath to navigate a subocclusive lesion. Placement of the catheter may follow if the path is not subintimal and is verified to be in the true lumen of the visceral vessel. Passage of an 0.14 or 0.18 wire into the secondary branch vasculature follows.

Preemptive balloon dilation in these cases is necessary (FIGURE 49-5). Typically a 3- to 4-mm balloon is employed for predilation and based on the wire platform system that is currently across the lesion. Once balloon angioplasty is performed, the sheath can be moved forward while the balloon is deflated to allow passage. A more conservative and safe technique is to remove the balloon and place the dilator within the sheath to advance across the lesion without the risk of snowplowing the freshly dissected plaque.

At all points, selective imaging is performed to assure location of the catheters and wires in the true lumen as well as vessel status. Pre- and post-balloon angioplasty/stent delivery of vasodilators such as nitroglycerin or papaverine intravenously into the selected visceral vessel may assist in avoiding elastic recoil of the vessel, flow limiting dissection, and enhancing visualization of the distal outflow. Aliquots of 200 to 300 mcg of nitroglycerin are given at intervals through the sheath or catheter based on operator preference and vessel characteristics. Communication with the anesthetic monitoring team at these times assures safe patient management practices during the procedure.

Once the lesion has been crossed safely (with or without predilation with the tip of the dilator/sheath system or formal balloon angioplasty), selective imaging in the best angle to visualize the lesion is performed. Final calibrations of lesion dimensions are measured, and the stent delivery system is selected as well as a post-stent balloon for flaring of the ostia as needed.

The ACT is measured prior to stent placement and if the patient is awake, discussion of pain on balloon inflation, breath holding, and lack of movement is discussed with them and the sedation team.

The endoflation system is filled with a mix of contrast and saline per operator preference (typically one-third contrast/two-thirds saline). The characteristics of the stent, including the nominal and burst atmospheres, are reviewed with the operating team. Typically balloon expandable stents are used in this location, and data from the Mayo Clinic suggests that ePTFE covered balloon expandable stents have better patency (FIGURE 49-6). Additional maneuvers include nitroglycerin administration within the vessel, patient blood pressure parameters, and the discussion of optimal deployment techniques. Using last image saved, fluorofade or road mapping techniques may assist in accurate device deployment. The use of magnification, collimation, and filters to reduce the bowel gas imaging as well as glucagon administration may assist in eliminating distractions of bowel peristalsis and gas. The location of key bony landmarks with respect to the visceral vessel and lesion may assist in preliminary stent traversal and placement. Using short bursts of hand-delivered contrast, real-time imaging can assist in stent placement prior to inflation. If the vessel is impacted by the respiratory cycle of the patient, a breath hold or suspension of respiration in an intubated patient may assist in accurate placement and deployment. Once the balloon of the covered stent is inflated, the assistant is ready to capture the balloon on deflation by moving the sheath forward into the deployed stent. This will ensure that the sheath is within the stent and aid in imaging and delivery of the post-stent angioplasty balloon for ostial inflation into the aorta. A limited hand injection to evaluate the stent position is done and if an additional stent is needed proximally or distally, it can be selected. Administration of an additional dose of nitroglycerin may assist in distal visualization and treatment of spasm from the manipulation. The selected imaging and medication delivery should be done with measured and slow delivery to prevent additional vasospasm and possible embolization of debris. Aspiration of the sheath prior to injections may be helpful to prevent sheath thrombosis and distal embolization.

Post-stent balloon is delivered and positioned halfway between the proximal stent and aorta. The stent is then flared under direct fluoroscopic guidance at the discretion of the operator. The sheath is again used to recapture the balloon for safe removal and for further imaging.

The final imaging consists of a selective angiogram of the entire stented vessel and runoff to evaluate for flow limitation, dissection, and embolization. If vasospasm is seen, additional nitroglycerin should be injected. The sheath is then pulled back into the aorta and a multiside flush catheter is placed to assure antegrade flow through the stent and vascular bed. This can also be performed through the sheath in the aorta and vigorous hand injection.

Following completion of the intervention, the ACT is drawn and based on the level of anticoagulation, protamine dosing and administration is done at the discretion of the operating and anesthetic team. Additional imaging of the access site and its runoff can also be performed. This is useful to document patency and issues with the access vessel that may not have been apparent in the beginning. Additionally, the location of the access and patency of the distal outflow can be visualized.

CLOSURE Once the ACT is normalized, selection of closure method is discussed. Manual pressure remains the basic form of access site hemostasis, and with the advent of novel low profile stent systems, a 5 or 6 French sheath site can be successfully managed with this technique. Other mechanisms of suture- versus nonsuture-mediated closure can be employed based on operator preference and experience. Additional manual pressure is used even in these situations to assure hemostasis. A dry sterile dressing is applied, and the limb is assessed for perfusion and embolization. The Doppler probe is used to evaluate the presence of absence of signals. Careful examination of the limb for discoloration, cyanosis, and impaired capillary refill is performed. Pulse oximetry in the hand can be measured and the patient is questioned for symptoms of vascular insufficiency, such as motor or sensory impairment, pain, and paresthesias.

If closure has been unsuccessful, whether due to failure of manual compression or closure device, open surgical cutdown can be performed. The operative team, including anesthetic monitoring and nursing, should be prepared for a limited exposure under deeper sedation, general anesthesia, or additional local anesthetic administration. Evacuation of hematoma, rapid proximal access, and clamp placement to identify the site of vessel entry and placement of 6-0 polypropylene suture should be performed.

POSTOPERATIVE CARE Bleeding from the access site can occur as well as postoperative hematoma, pseudoaneurysm, and acute limb ischemia. The patient should remain under physiologic and vascular monitoring during the postoperative period in the recovery unit. The site should be inspected regularly for bleeding and hematoma development. Sometimes extreme pain at the site or in the limb can be a sign of rapid nerve compression from hematoma formation, especially in the upper extremity, where the median nerve can be compressed with minimal hematoma presence. ■

SUGGESTED READINGS

Huber TS, Björck M, Chandra A, Clouse WD, Dalsing MC, Oderich GS, Smeds MR, Murad MH. Chronic mesenteric ischemia: Clinical practice guidelines from the Society for Vascular Surgery. *J Vasc Surg.* 2021 Jan;73(1S):87S-115S. doi:10.1016/j.jvs.2020.10.029. Epub 2020 Nov 7. PMID: 33171195.

Oderich GS, Erdoes LS, Lesar C, Mendes BC, Gloviczki P, Cha S, Duncan AA, Bower TC. Comparison of covered stents versus bare metal stents for treatment of chronic atherosclerotic mesenteric arterial disease. *J Vasc Surg.* 2013 Nov;58(5):1316-1323. doi:10.1016/j.jvs.2013.05.013. Epub 2013 Jul 1.

Sarac TP, Altinel O, Kashyap V, Bena J, Lyden S, Srivastava S, Eagleton M, Clair DJ. Endovascular treatment of stenotic and occluded visceral arteries for chronic mesenteric ischemia. *J Vasc Surg.* 2008 Mar;47(3):485-491. doi:10.1016/j.jvs.2007.11.046.

49-5

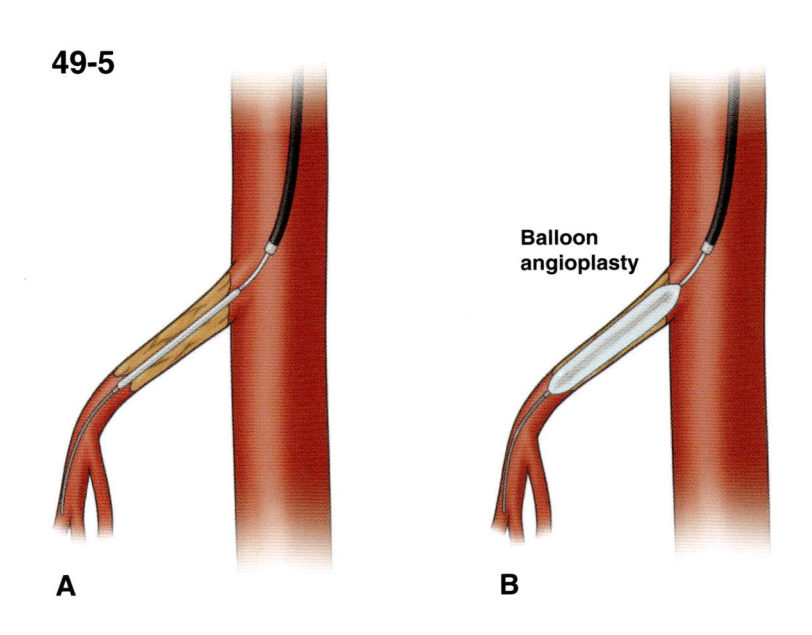

Figure 49-5 A. Small balloon advanced across lesion. B. Predilatation balloon angioplasty to allow passage of stent graft.

49-6

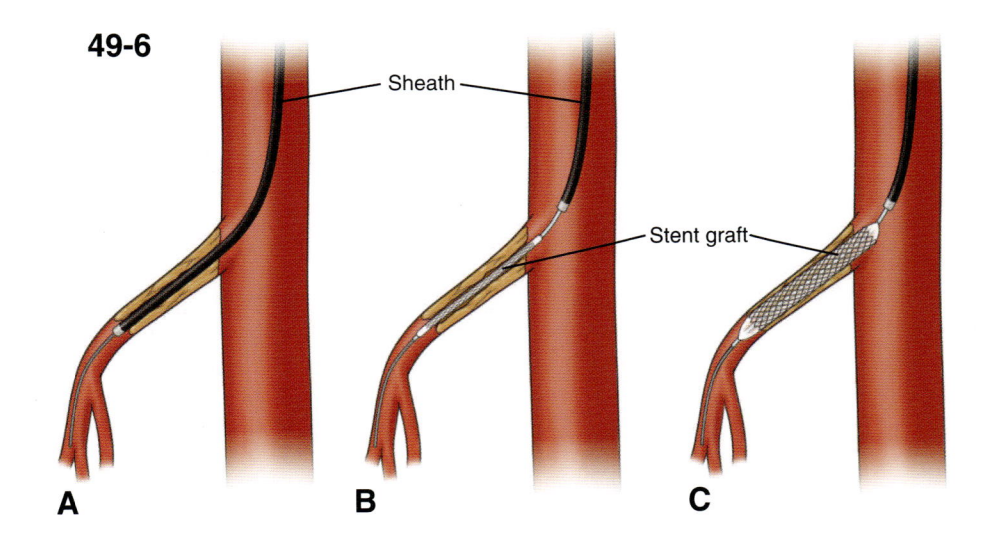

Figure 49-6 A. 7F sheath advanced across the lesion. B. Stent placed followed by withdrawal of sheath. C. Covered stent graft deployment.

RETROGRADE OPEN MESENTERIC STENTING

Jesse Chait, DO • Manju Kalra, MBBS

INDICATIONS First described by Milner et al. in 2004 and subsequently adopted and popularized by Wyers and colleagues in 2006, retrograde open mesenteric stenting (ROMS) is an ideal first-line approach for mesenteric revascularization in the setting of acute mesenteric ischemia (AMI) where exploratory laparotomy is deemed necessary for evaluation of the bowel for viability. When peritonitis, gangrene, or bowel perforation are present or suspected, percutaneous therapies are time consuming, unnecessary, and may delay adequate source control. Furthermore, ROMS allows for prompt revascularization when bowel ischemia is discovered intraoperatively.

From a technical perspective, ROMS may be preferable to an antegrade approach in the setting of acute-on-chronic and chronic mesenteric ischemia (CMI) when treating flush superior mesenteric artery (SMA) occlusions at the level of the aorta, long calcific occlusions, and lesions that have failed prior antegrade attempts.

ROMS does not require a robust endovascular inventory or hybrid operating room, as most lesions can be revascularized in a retrograde fashion with a single wire, catheter, sheath, and stent with fluoroscopic imaging provided by a mobile C-arm. This approach allows for quick and effective revascularization in resource-limited institutions without expertise in mesenteric bypass or advanced endovascular techniques. It allows for more expedient treatment without the need for transfer to a higher-level facility.

PREOPERATIVE PREPARATION All patients with suspected or known mesenteric ischemia should undergo computed tomography angiography (CTA) of the chest, abdomen, and pelvis to assess lesion etiology, character, extent, and amenability to different repair methods. Bowel viability and areas of ischemia can also be appreciated with CT imaging. Care should be taken to assess for variant anatomy, such as a replaced right hepatic artery. Axial imaging also allows for device sizing. Evaluation of the iliofemoral segments and upper extremities via physical examination and radiographic imaging guides decision making for adjunctive antegrade or retrograde endovascular access. Simultaneous resuscitation with intravenous crystalloid, broad-spectrum antibiosis, and appropriate analgesia should be administered during radiographic evaluation.

All patients should undergo near uninterrupted gastric decompression from the time of diagnosis well into the postoperative period. In certain patients, vasopressors may be required to maintain adequate end organ perfusion. Due to the selective effect on splanchnic vasculature, vasopressin should be avoided if possible.

If possible, patients with AMI should be managed in a hybrid operating room. Room setup should allow for operators to be on both sides of the patient without interruption, and this typically involves floor-mounted imaging to come from above the patient's head.

ANESTHESIA General endotracheal anesthesia, bladder, arterial and central venous catheterization for the purposes of resuscitation are recommended.

INCISION AND EXPOSURE In cases without a definitive diagnosis of AMI, diagnostic laparoscopy allows for assessment of bowel viability without a large surgical incision. In cases with high clinical suspicion, primary midline, transperitoneal laparotomy incision allows for complete assessment of the intraabdominal viscera and allows access to the mesenteric vasculature as well as several reliable inflow sources.

Should intraabdominal contamination, bowel gangrene, or impending intestinal rupture be recognized, prompt source control should be performed prior to assessment of the mesenteric vasculature. Otherwise, marginally viable bowel should be left in situ and reassessed following revascularization in an immediate and delayed (24–48 hours) fashion.

Adequate and reliable exposure is paramount to success for any mesenteric revascularization. Our institution prefers the Omni-Tract self-retraction system, preferably with radiolucent blades. Exposure of the SMA is typically obtained from an anterior approach but may also be obtained laterally.

There are two ways to expose the SMA from an anterior approach (see Chapter 47 for details). (1) To identify the SMA at the root of the mesentery, the transverse colon and small bowel are retracted cephalad and caudad, respectively. The root of the mesentery is exposed, allowing for palpation of either a pulsatile or calcified vessel along the inferior margin of the pancreas (**FIGURE 50-1A**). (2) Some operators prefer to expose the SMA through the lesser sac (**FIGURE 50-1B**), although it also may be found at the root of the mesentery (**FIGURE 50-2**). Dissection may prove difficult secondary to significant edema and often a lack of pulsatility. Herein, several landmarks may prove useful in identification of the SMA. The middle colic artery is typically easily identified in the transverse mesocolon and can be traced proximally to its origin from the SMA. The superior mesenteric vein lies to the right of the SMA; however, small venous tributaries are delicate and must be ligated with care. Doppler insonation may also be helpful. Once identified, the overlying peritoneum is incised at the base of the transverse mesocolon.

Similarly, small, delicate jejunal branches must be preserved. These do not need to be dissected circumferentially and can be controlled atraumatically with small Sugita or bulldog clamps to avoid traction injury from silastic vessel loops. **CONTINUES ▶**

50-1

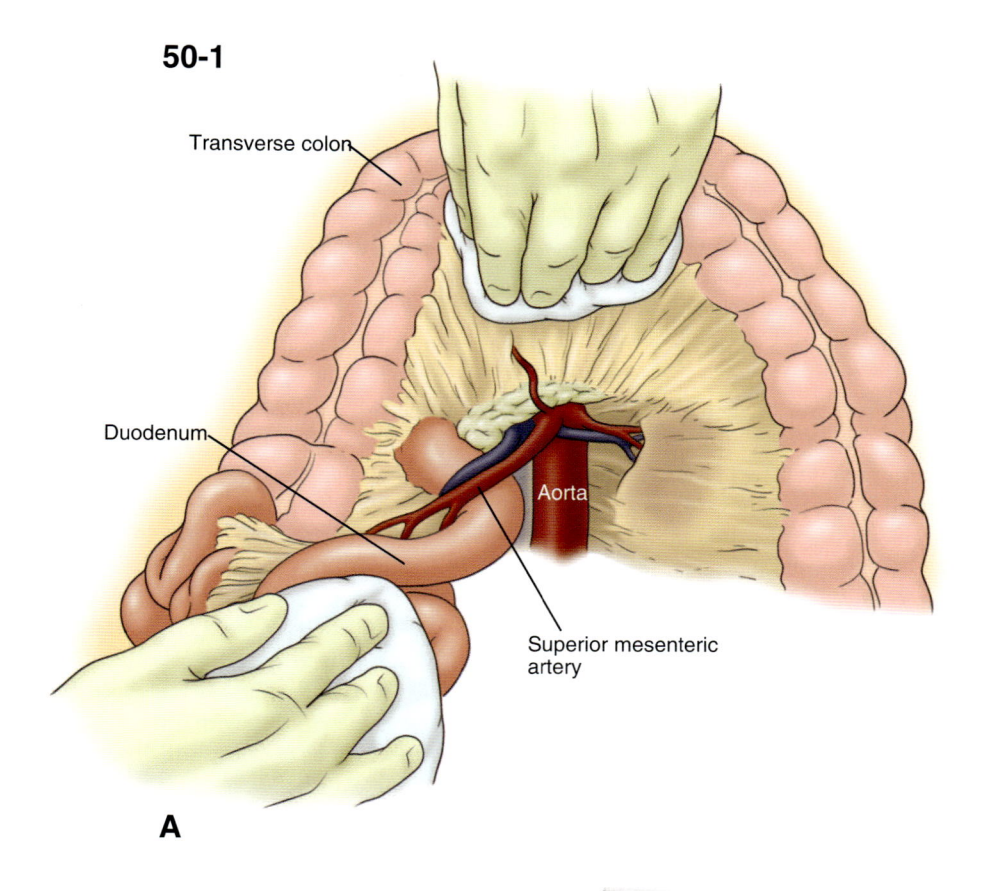

Transverse colon

Duodenum

Aorta

Superior mesenteric artery

A

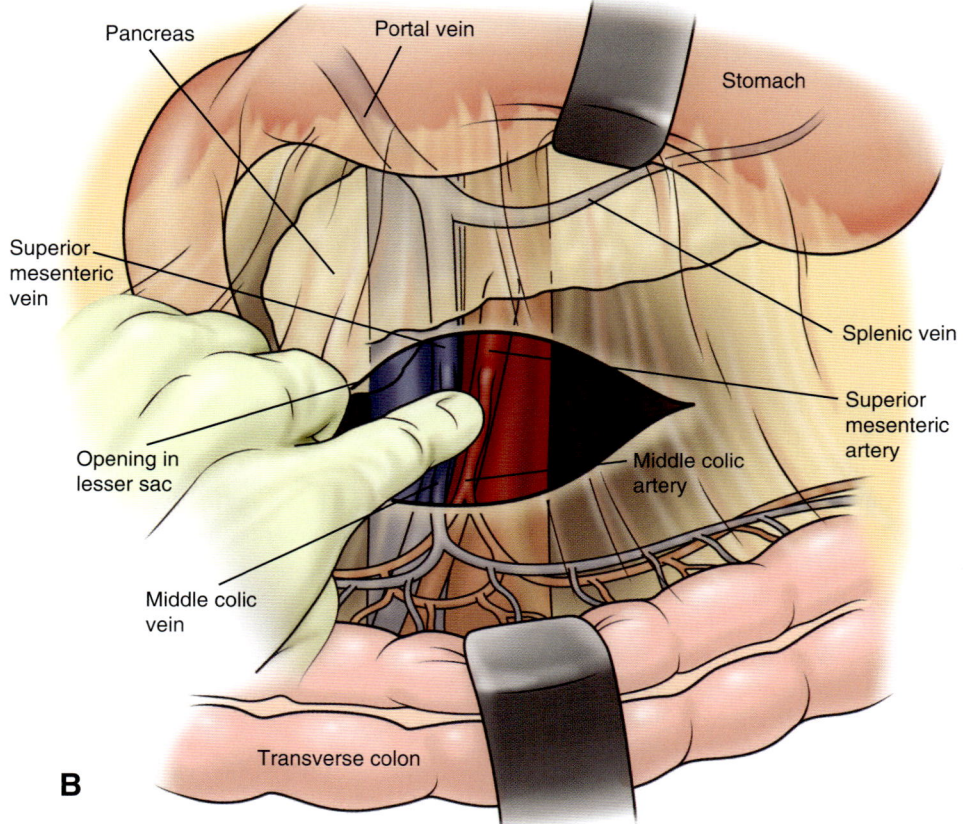

Pancreas

Portal vein

Stomach

Superior mesenteric vein

Splenic vein

Superior mesenteric artery

Opening in lesser sac

Middle colic artery

Middle colic vein

Transverse colon

B

50-2

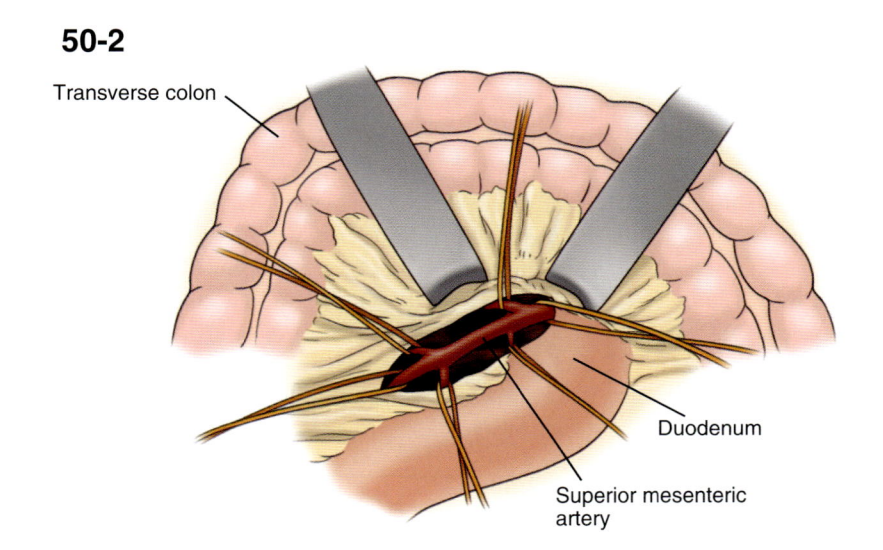

Transverse colon

Duodenum

Superior mesenteric artery

INCISION AND EXPOSURE CONTINUED From a lateral approach (FIGURE 50-3), the ligament of Treitz is taken down and the small bowel is retracted to the patient's right. The mesentery is then incised approximately 2 cm to the left of the ligament, allowing access to a significant length of the SMA. Access to small jejunal branches is often not feasible from this approach but allows for proximal revascularization. The extent of dissection is dictated by distribution of the causative lesion. An acute-on-chronic ostial in-situ thrombosis with chronic, distal disease does not mandate complete skeletonization of the SMA. However, to allow enough working length for stent placement, we typically prefer a more distal exposure.

TECHNIQUE All patients should be systemically heparinized with a bolus prior to obtaining occlusive control of any aspect of the SMA—main trunk or branches. A soft spot on the artery should be identified via palpation. The choice of arteriotomy is dictated by the patient's anatomy and the clinical scenario. Transverse arteriotomies allow for primary closure in healthy segments of large-caliber vessels. A longitudinal arteriotomy is preferably used for diseased or small-caliber vessels requiring endarterectomy and patch angioplasty. The choice of patch material is dependent on the level of contamination—bovine pericardium is readily available, but a vein patch may be preferred in the setting of gross spillage of intestinal contents. Intraluminal access to the SMA may also be obtained directly via the Seldinger technique: a silastic vessel loop is utilized to stretch and stabilize the distal aspect of the artery prior to proximal introduction of a Micropuncture needle to its anterior surface. Retrograde access to the aortic true lumen is typically obtained with a soft, straight-tipped guidewire (FIGURE 50-4A) and proper positioning should confirmed angiographically before upsizing to 45-cm sheath with a radiolucent tip (FIGURE 52-4B). Longer sheaths allow for the operators to avoid direct radiation while staying productive within the surgical field. Crossing of long, calcified SMA occlusions is much more likely to be achieved successfully and rapidly from this retrograde fashion compared to an antegrade approach. In the rare circumstance where recanalization is not possible from a retrograde mesenteric approach, alternative access sites such as the common femoral, brachial, and radial arteries may be utilized to cross antegrade and obtain through-and-through wire access (FIGURE 50-5). However, in the authors' experience, most SMA lesions are amenable and easily crossed in a retrograde fashion. This is corroborated by a high rate of technical success (98%) in a 2018 multicenter study examining the role of ROMS.

Retrospective studies have suggested that chronic mesenteric arterial lesions should be preferentially treated with balloon-expandable covered stents, owing to lower rates of restenosis, recurrence, and reintervention compared to bare metal stents. A contaminated intraoperative field is a relative contraindication to covered stent placement. Regardless of composition, stents may act as a nidus for infection. Any operative bed with hollow viscus contamination or recent bowel manipulation should be thoroughly irrigated, with sterile instruments exchanged. All members of the operative team should re-scrub with new gowns and gloves.

Prior to angioplasty and stenting, distal branches should be occluded with loops or microclips to prevent embolization. Balloon predilatation may be necessary prior to stent placement. Typically, mesenteric stents should be 6 mm or greater in diameter. Stent placement should be performed under direct fluoroscopic visualization with 2 to 4 mm of stent protruding into the aortic lumen (FIGURE 50-6).

The intra-aortic portion of the stent is then flared with an oversized balloon to 2 mm above profile. Angiographic evaluation of the treated artery should be confirmed adequate prior to removal of wires, catheters, and sheaths. Should there be concern for proximal thrombus or distal embolization beyond the stented portion of artery, an embolectomy catheter may be passed proximally and through distal branches. Once closed, either primarily or with a patch, the SMA should be palpated distal to stent placement and the mesenteric and antimesenteric borders should be palpated and assessed with Doppler insonation to ensure treatment success. Repeat angiography can be performed with either a Micropuncture sheath placed proximally to the arteriotomy closure or via existing antegrade access.

The abdomen should be temporarily closed, allowing for a "second look" of bowel viability within 24 to 48 hours of revascularization. This allows time for intra-abdominal viscera to declare themselves prior to definitive closure. In our single institution experience, we have observed a significant decrease in mortality when our practice evolved to make second-look laparotomies a standard of care.

Postoperatively, dual antiplatelet therapy should be initiated with a loading dose of a P2Y12 inhibitor. Intestinal discontinuity is not an absolute contraindication to oral antiplatelet use should there be a sufficient length of intact, viable proximal small bowel. Should enteral access be deemed high risk, intravenous heparin and rectal aspirin offer a reliable substitute. Duplex ultrasound (performed while fasting) and CTA are primarily used to surveil mesenteric stents.

OUTCOMES Technical success has been reported to be upward of 90% in most series. Primary patency rates range between 75% and 85% at 1- and 2-year follow-up intervals. Reinterventions, however, are not uncommon following ROMS and are typically driven by clinically apparent restenosis or asymptomatic, high-grade, impending occlusive lesions. Most often percutaneous endovascular reinterventions such as angioplasty and stenting are successful, but a small percentage may require conversion to open revascularization. There have been no randomized controlled trials to date comparing ROMS and other mesenteric revascularization techniques; however, several single- and multicenter reports demonstrate similar technical and mortality-related outcomes between bypass and retrograde stenting.

Our institution has evolved to consider ROMS the first-line approach for AMI and acute-on-CMI, as it allows for evaluation of bowel and prompt revascularization with outcomes comparable to open bypass. Furthermore, ROMS does not preclude or complicate future open bypass should stenting fail. Nevertheless, AMI carries a high mortality, upward of 40%, and morbidity rate regardless of the approach to revascularization.

CONCLUSION There are many advantages of a retrograde approach to SMA revascularization. Exploratory laparotomy provides immediate evaluation of bowel and source control of potential intra-abdominal contamination. Direct access to the SMA allows for prompt revascularization via angioplasty and stenting, which allows the operating surgeon to avoid dissection of an inflow source for bypass, vein harvesting, and obviates the use of a prosthetic conduit which may act as a nidus for infection. ROMS carries a high rate of technical success and can be performed safely at most institutions with minimal endovascular equipment. A second-look laparotomy should be considered in all patients undergoing revascularization.

Despite concerted efforts at earlier detection and improved endovascular and hybrid techniques of mesenteric revascularization, AMI remains a highly morbid and fatal disease process that warrants prompt recognition and management. ■

SUGGESTED READINGS

Andraska E, Haga L, Li X, Avgerinos E, Singh M, Chaer R, et al. Retrograde open mesenteric stenting should be considered as the initial approach to acute mesenteric ischemia. *J Vasc Surg*, 2020 Oct;72(4):1260-1268.

Blauw JTM, Meerwaldt R, Brusse-Keizer M, Kolkman JK, Gerrits D, Geelkerken RH, et al. Retrograde open mesenteric stenting for acute mesenteric ischemia. *J Vasc Surg*, 2014;60(3):726-734.

Milner R, Woo EY, Carpenter JP. Superior mesenteric artery angioplasty and stenting via a retrograde approach in a patient with bowel ischemia—a case report. *Vasc Endovasc Surg*. 2004;38:89-91.

Oderich GS, Erdoes LS, Lesar C, Mendes BC, Gloviczki P, Cha S, et al. Comparison of covered stents versus bare metal stents for treatment of chronic atherosclerotic mesenteric arterial disease. *J Vasc Surg*, 2013;58(5):1316-1323.

Oderich GS, Macedo R, Stone DH, Woo EY, Panneton JM, Resch T, et al. Multicenter study of retrograde open mesenteric artery stenting through laparotomy for treatment of acute and chronic mesenteric ischemia. *J Vasc Surg*, 2018;68:470-480.

Roussel A, Della Schiava N, Coscas R, Pellenc Q, Boudjelit T, Goëau-Brissonnière O, et al. Results of retrograde open mesenteric stenting for acute thrombotic mesenteric ischemia. *J Vasc Surg*, 2019;69(4):1137-1142.

Ryer EJ, Kalra M, Oderich GS, Duncan A, Gloviczki P, Cha S, et al. Revascularization for acute mesenteric ischemia. *J Vasc Surg*, 2012;55:1682-1689.

Wyers MC, Powell RJ, Nolan BW, Cronenwett JL. Retrograde mesenteric stenting during laparotomy for acute occlusive mesenteric ischemia. *J Vasc Surg*. 2007;45(2):269-275.

50-3

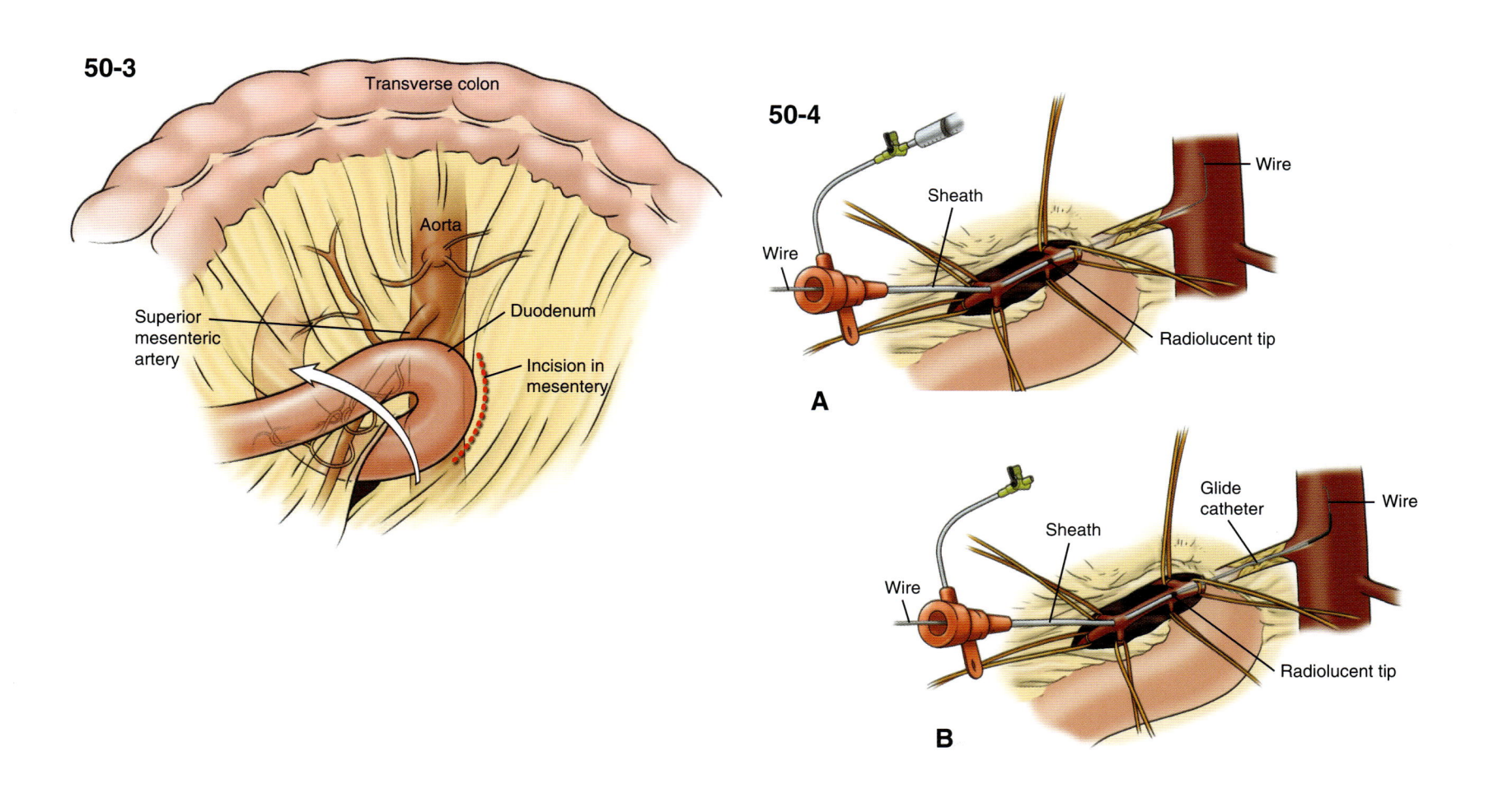

Transverse colon

Aorta

Superior mesenteric artery

Duodenum

Incision in mesentery

50-4

Sheath

Wire

Wire

Radiolucent tip

A

Glide catheter

Sheath

Wire

Wire

Radiolucent tip

B

50-5

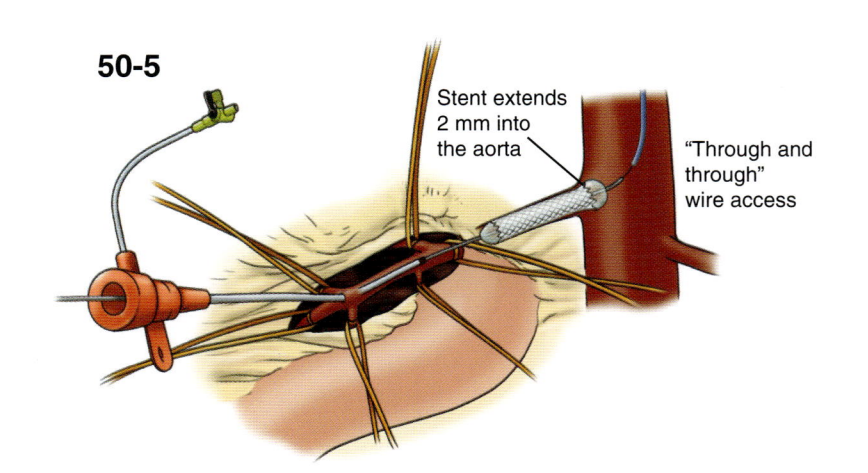

Stent extends 2 mm into the aorta

"Through and through" wire access

50-6

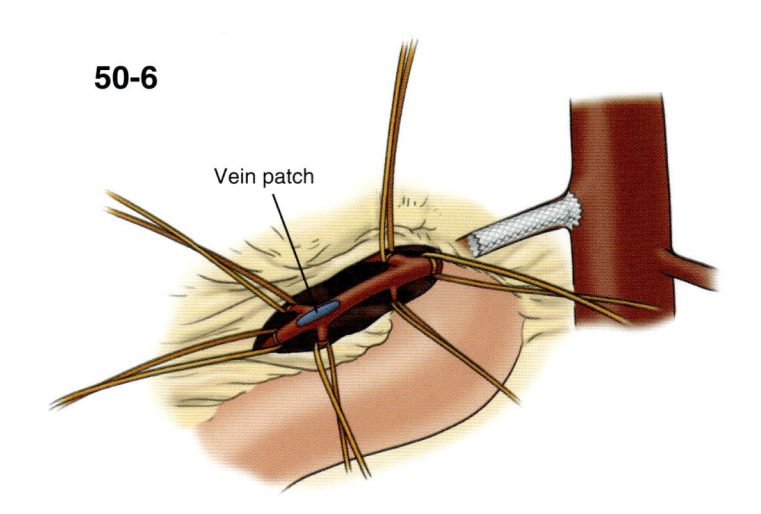

Vein patch

SECTION XI
AORTO-ILIAC OCCLUSIVE DISEASE OPEN AND ENDOVASCULAR

AORTOBIFEMORAL BYPASS

W. Darrin Clouse, MD

INDICATIONS Aortobifemoral bypass (ABF) is most commonly done for aortoiliac occlusive disease (AIOD), but in some circumstances, it is chosen for aortic aneurysm repair in patients with concomitant AIOD. There are three distinct patterns of AIOD: type 1 involves the distal abdominal aorta and the common iliac arteries (CIA) only; type 2 disease adds involvement of the iliofemoral segment, and type 3 comprises these along with infra-inguinal disease. AIOD can be asymptomatic, cause claudication, or lead to chronic limb-threatening ischemia (CLTI) with tissue loss or rest pain, particularly with type 3 disease. Indications for intervention in AIOD include lifestyle-limiting claudication failing conservative management, atheroembolism, CLTI, and occasionally acute limb ischemia (ALI) due to acute aortoiliac occlusion. Endovascular or hybrid iliofemoral procedures are held to be first-line treatments today as minimally invasive approaches are generally better tolerated, cause less physiologic stress, and offer reasonable results in the aortoiliac segment. When cardiopulmonary comorbidities are prohibitive, extra-anatomic axillary bifemoral bypass also may be useful. While these other therapies provide meaningful treatment of AIOD, ABF remains the most durable revascularization procedure generally affording the best hemodynamic results. This is related to its excellent long-term patency and direct anatomic in-line perfusion which translates into symptom relief. Nevertheless, both endovascular and open therapies for AIOD do fail, and failed prior treatment is an indication to consider ABF.

Along with the shift toward endovascular and hybrid therapies, ABF technical complexity has increased over the last two decades. Twenty-five percent of those undergoing ABF today have had at least one prior aortoiliac endovascular intervention, and up to 10% have already had some type of aortoiliac open operation. Concomitant lower extremity revascularization with bypass or endovascular intervention is performed in up to 25% of patients, mostly for tissue loss. Furthermore, proximal aortic anastomotic cuff thromboendarterectomy and femoral outflow adjuncts such as endarterectomy are commonplace, each needed in up to 40 to 50%, respectively. Renal or mesenteric operations are performed concurrently in up to 16%. Rarely, in patients needing renal or visceral artery revascularization with significant concomitant aortic disease or occlusion, ABF can be performed to provide an inflow source for open reconstruction. It is not surprising that aortic clamping above the renal arteries is needed in 30% of contemporary cases. A minority will have combined aneurysm and occlusive disease, which may be an indication for ABF. Rarely, disease may dictate considering thoracobifemoral bypass. Arterial noninvasive studies including ankle-brachial indices with segmental pressures, and aortoiliac and lower extremity duplex ultrasound can define the degree of perfusion reduction with initial anatomic disease localization. Computed tomography arteriography (CTA) of the aorta and lower extremities is today's standard to define disease extent, clamp sites, distal targets, needed inflow and outflow adjuncts, and proximal reconstruction methodology.

POSITION ABF is largely performed via standard transperitoneal, inframesocolic exposure with the patient in the supine position and a gentle lumbar break or roll to extend the lumbar spine and abdominal contents. This allows for supraceliac control if needed. Suprarenal clamping can also be performed from this positioning. Retroperitoneal ABF can also be accomplished. This requires the torso positioned left side up 45 degrees on bean bag or padding with the pelvis rotated back to allow left aortic approach and bilateral femoral exposure. It is helpful in patients with prior laparotomies, stomas, and need for more proximal renal-visceral reconstruction, but difficult to reach right-sided structures. Laparoscopic and robotic ABF for the abdominal component is described, but is not mainstream. The remainder of this section will focus on the supine transperitoneal operation.

OPERATIVE PREPARATIONS Routine skin preparation is performed from the mid-chest to toes bilaterally, allowing medial exposure of the popliteal artery and insonation of pedal pulses when done with the femoral anastomoses. Exposed skin is covered with antimicrobial draping. Autotransfusion blood salvage is planned, and arterial monitoring and venous access are achieved. Intravenous prophylactic antibiotics are given. Prior to induction, unless contraindicated due to spine morbidity or antithrombotic medications, an epidural catheter is placed to assist with anesthesia and postoperative analgesia.

INCISION AND EXPOSURE Bilateral longitudinal groin incisions are made, and the common femoral, superficial femoral, and profunda femoral arteries exposed. Frequently the pulse is not palpable. A key gateway to deciding where to make the proper longitudinal incision over the femoral artery is to either localize it with an ultrasound or manually roll one's fingers side to side, which allows detection of a tubular structure. When difficult, marking the saphenofemoral junction two fingers lateral and two fingers inferior to the pubic tubercle can be helpful. The type of femoral reconstruction required will dictate extent of femoral exposure (**FIGURE 51-1**). The common femoral (CFA), superficial femoral (SFA), and profunda femoris (PFA) arteries are controlled circumferentially. When anastomoses are needed to the mid-portion of the PFA, the crossing lateral femoral circumflex and occasionally profunda femoral vein should be doubly ligated and divided. The key gateway here for adequate exposure of the profunda is to mobilize the proximal SFA and retract it medially, which then opens a door to excellent visualization of the proximal profunda. The second key gateway is to ligate and divide the lateral femoral circumflex vein which usually crosses over the proximal profunda. The distal external iliac artery (EIA) anterior surface is skeletonized, and the deep circumflex iliac vein is doubly ligated and divided. Digital dissection along the anterior surface of both EIAs is carried well up into the pelvis to begin wide tunneling for the graft limbs.

Midline laparotomy is then performed, and self-retaining retractors placed. Aortic exposure is purposed to expose and clamp disease-free aorta. Standard inframesocolic aortic exposure is developed by mobilization of the duodenum, evisceration or retraction of the small bowel to the right, and ligation of the inferior mesenteric vein. The anterior surface of the aorta is exposed (**FIGURE 51-2**). The extent of aortic dissection necessary for safe and complete control during planned proximal anastomosis and adjuncts is performed. Circumferential infrarenal control is obtained at the level of the renal vein. In general, the infrarenal aorta just below the renal arteries has less plaque burden and is good proximal anastomosis of the graft. Occasionally, supraceliac or suprarenal control is necessary (see Chapter 28). **CONTINUES**

51-1

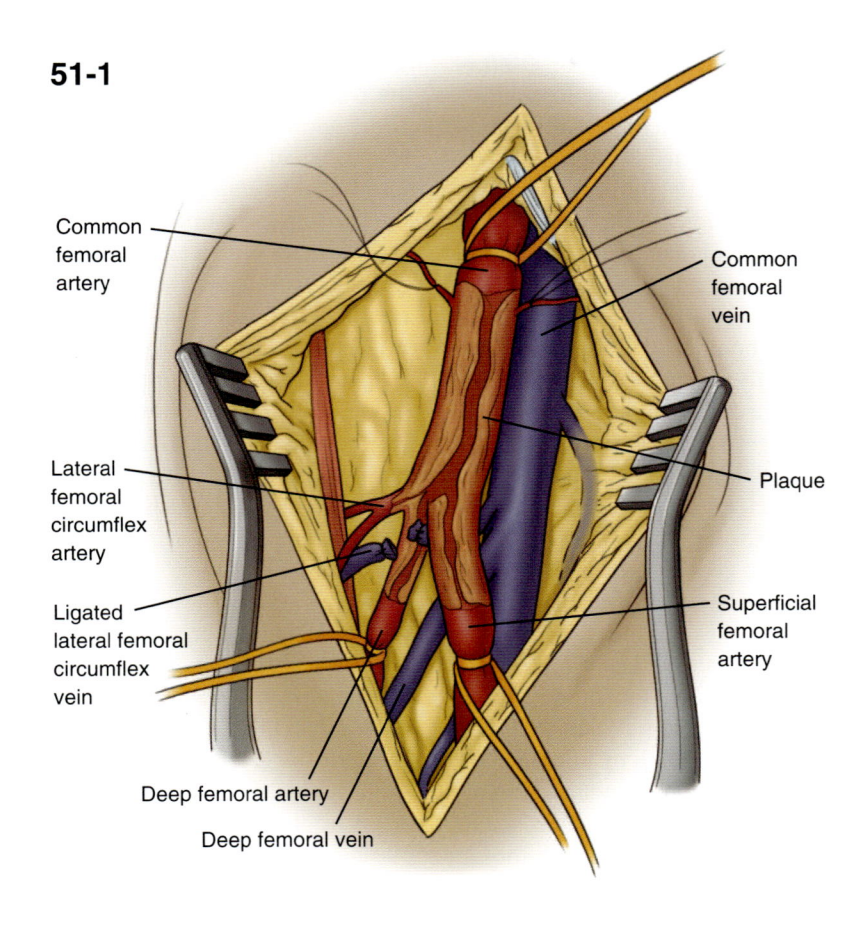

Figure 51-1 Femoral artery exposure with longitudinal incision.

51-2

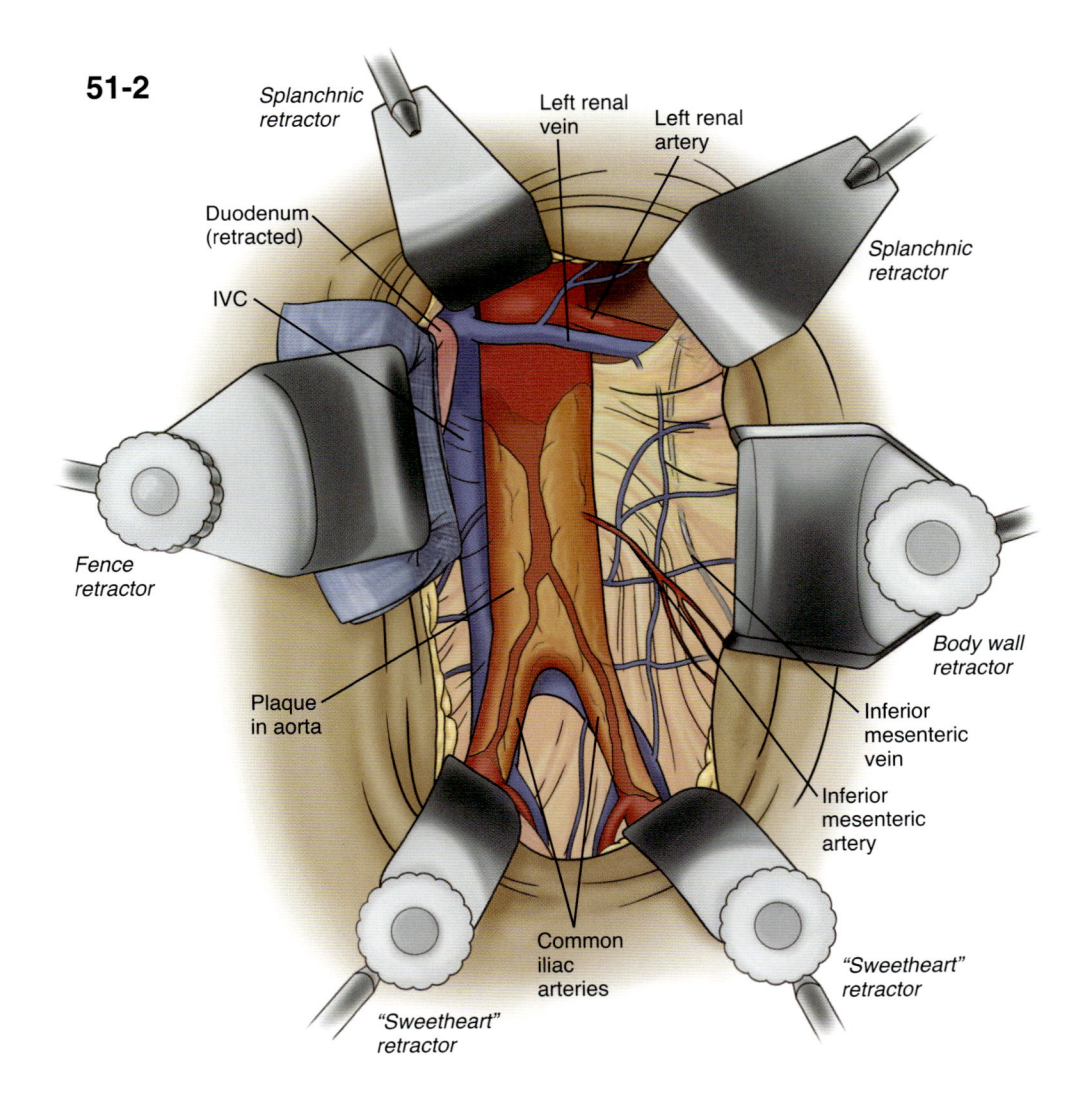

Figure 51-2 Aortic exposure.

INCISION AND EXPOSURE CONTINUED Distally, the aorta is fully dissected to the level of the inferior mesenteric artery (IMA). The aortic bifurcation is identified, and a distal aortic clamp site created. Along the anterior wall of both CIA digital tunneling is initiated. From each groin a finger is placed in the previous inferior tunnel, and this is married to a simultaneous finger in the tunnel from the abdomen staying directly on the iliac arteries sweeping the ureters anteriorly (**FIGURE 51-3A**). Most do this posterior to the ureter, although it is not required. A key component is following the artery along its anterior surface. Once completed, a large DeBakey aortic clamp is directed from the groin with the curve toward the back to take the tunnel course and meet the finger from the abdomen. The clamp is then flipped tip-up, and the tip delivered against the cephalad finger into the abdomen, taking the course directly on the iliac system and never passed bluntly without being against the upper finger (**FIGURE 51-3B**). If resistance is encountered, one should stop and attempt again through a freer plane, and this may require dissecting the iliac arteries for a greater length inferiorly. Penrose drains or umbilical tapes are placed in each tunnel and secured with a Kelly clamp. They are retracted gently anteriorly allowing full inspection of the tunnels digitally, facilitating later graft limb placement.

DETAILS OF PROCEDURE The patient is systemically heparinized, and the aorta clamped initially distally and then proximally. Depending on disease extent and patency of the iliofemoral segment, the femoral arteries may be clamped prior to aortic clamping to minimize risk of atheroembolization. If an extended proximal cuff or pararenal thromboendarterectomy is planned, then the renal arteries are controlled before proximal aortic clamping. The author generally prefers end-to-end proximal anastomoses as they are more hemodynamically normal, more cephalad in less diseased aorta usually, sit more anatomically natural in the aortic bed, reducing anterior bulging and possibly risk of duodenal fistulazation and minimizing later atheroembolization risk (**FIGURE 51-4A**). End-to-side anastomoses (**FIGURE 51-4B**) should be considered when there are accessory renal arteries, visceral artery disease with a large patent IMA (in this case the visceral arteries can be stented preop), or normal inline flow to the internal iliac arteries where end-to-end anastomosis might then require a bypass to an internal iliac artery to maximize pelvic blood flow. This occurs in those with isolated extensive bilateral EIA disease, minimal common iliac disease, and direct hypogastric inflow from above. For end-to-end anastomoses, the aorta is transected several centimeters below the renal arteries to allow enough room for the clamp and normal tissue for sewing. Lumbar arteries are ligated as needed and the proximal aorta is fashioned or crafted to facilitate an easy sewing ring. Adjunctive thromboendarterectomy can be accomplished but one should be certain not to thin the aortic wall and disrupt the strong adventitial layer. Most prefer a bifurcated Dacron prostheses but ePTFE grafts can also be used. The author sizes the main body at or a few millimeters smaller than the aorta owing to Dacron's tendency to chronically dilate 20% and avoid grafts smaller than 16 × 8 mm unless driven by diminutive femoral arteries. If the common femoral arteries are small, a patch angioplasty is recommended. Smaller aortic size is a known predictor of ABF occlusion. In the past, the graft body was trimmed to only a few centimeters for longer, straighter limbs. Today the body should be trimmed twice as long (at least 5 cm) to allow potential later endovascular options. Anastomosis is performed with running 3-0 Prolene suture, and felt strips may be helpful to minimize suture bleeding. Should the aorta be particularly fragile, an interrupted, pledgeted anastomosis can be invaluable. Once complete, the anastomosis can be checked for leakage by instilling under mild pressure heparinized saline into the graft limbs. The aortic clamp is released, flushing through both limbs to rinse debris, and hydrogrip clamps placed on both. If the renal arteries are also clamped, they are released after graft flushing to minimize air and debris, and checked with continuous-wave Doppler. A 2- to 5-cm segment of the distal aorta is resected, and plaque removed, associated lumbar arteries ligated, and the distal aortic stump over-sewn doubly suture ligated with 3-0 Prolene. When the cross-clamp is infrarenal, this can be done prior to proximal anastomosis, but afterward when a complex higher clamp used.

One surgeon now lifts on the prior Penrose drain in one of the limb tunnels. The DeBakey clamp is replaced from the groin into the abdomen. The respective graft limb, taking note of the premarked line, is secured in the clamp and withdrawn into the femoral exposure assuring no limb twisting or kinking. The limb should be secured at the groin, and the contralateral side now performed similarly. Penrose drains are removed from the groin incision in the direction of limb. The abdominal self-retraining retraction is now loosened. Retraction is readjusted in both groin incisions preparing for each femoral anastomosis. These may be sequentially or simultaneously performed as follows. The limb is withdrawn into the groin until gentle traction is seen in the entire graft in the abdomen. The limb is then allowed to relax 1 centimeter and this level is marked at the inguinal ligament for reference. Clamps are placed on the femoral arterial complex. Arteriotomy is created in the desired distal anastomotic configuration. Adjuncts such as femoral endarterectomy, profundaplasty, and bovine patch angioplasty are performed. Even when direct profunda femoris artery reconstruction is not necessary, most prefer to hood the limb over the profunda femoral artery origin, as the SFA is the most diseased artery in the body. When limb outflow is largely via the PFA, it should be interrogated to determine its robustness and likelihood to support limb patency if not clear on CTA. A quick but imprecise tool is to gently pass a #3 Fogarty and 4-mm vessel dilator. If the PFA will accept the Fogarty catheter to 15 cm and the 4 mm dilator for its length, there is good prospect of limb outflow patency support. If not, PFA reconstruction by endarterectomy and patch angioplasty may be warranted. Also, we have recently shown a Society for Vascular Surgery femoral runoff score ≥6 portends worse limb-based patency. This may be considered in decision-making for concomitant lower extremity revascularization, in addition to the presence of tissue loss. After oblique beveling of the limb, distal anastomosis is performed with 5-0 running Prolene suture. I prefer to use three interrupted 5-0 Prolene mattress sutures at the toe for visualization, running one strand from each of the side sutures. Prior to completion, standard flushing maneuvers are performed to protect the major limb outflow, which is back-flushed last and opened last. Initial unclamping of the limb in the abdomen is performed in conjunction with unclamping the proximal CFA or EIA clamp, allowing retrograde flushing into the pelvis followed by establishing antegrade flow into the extremity. On-table continuous-wave Doppler is performed. If concern for limb outflow is present, duplex and distal pulse and signal examination can be performed. Pre- and post- on-table pulse volume recordings can be performed when available. The IMA should be interrogated during the conduct of operation. With pulsatile back-bleeding or known occlusion, the IMA is ligated. If it is patent but has poor back-bleeding, there are occluded hypogastric arteries, there is concern due to other mesenteric artery disease, or surgeon preference, it should be revascularized either through reimplantation into the graft or rarely, via bypass. Back-pressure of less than 40 mmHg correlates to poor colon perfusion. I prefer selective revascularization and use a wide patch of the aortic wall around the IMA origin for reimplantation anastomosis, preferably to the graft body. CONTINUES

51-3

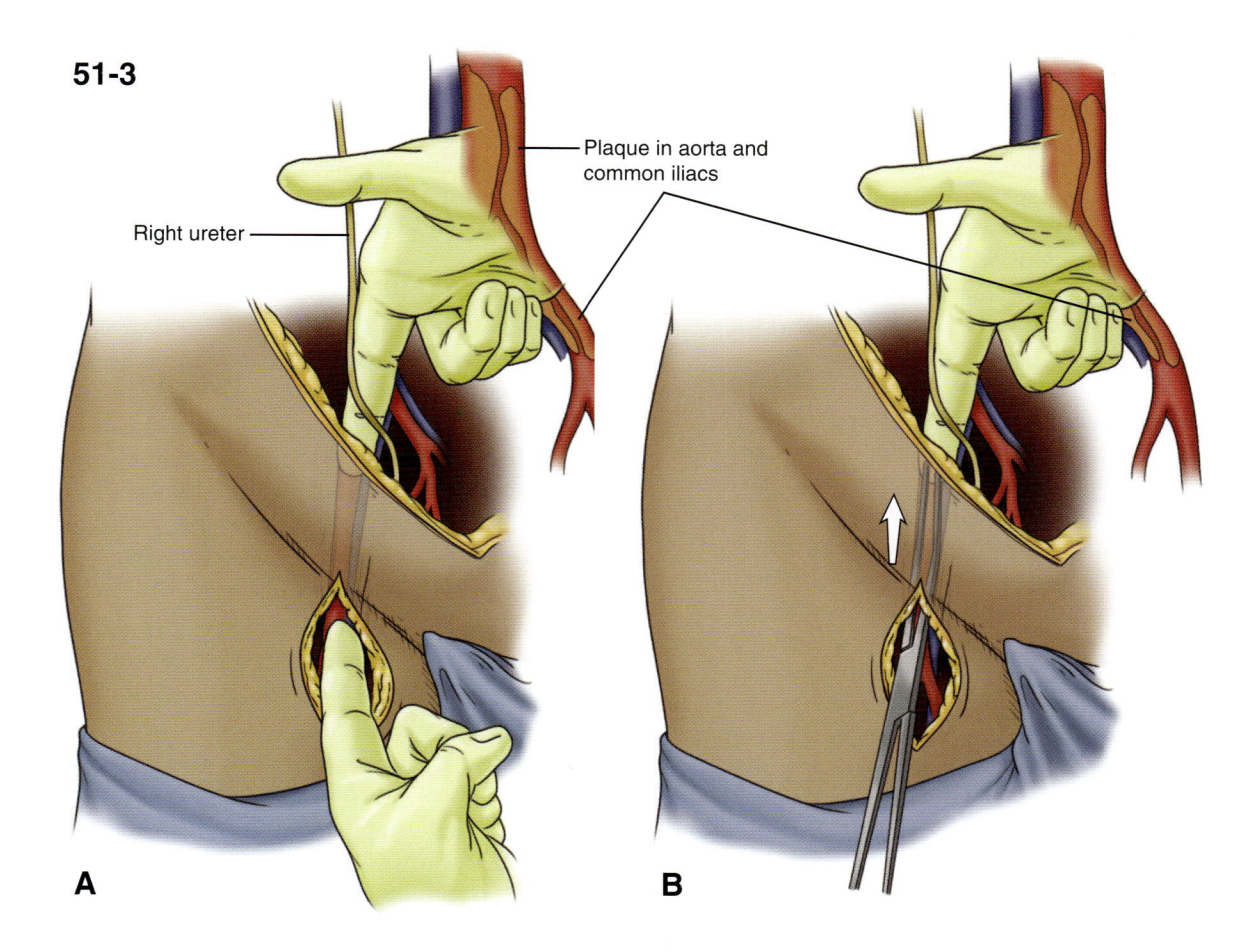

Plaque in aorta and common iliacs

Right ureter

A

B

Figure 51-3 A. Digitally, tunnels are created with fingers placed from the abdomen and from the groin gently bluntly tunneling directly on the iliac arterial system. B. Once open, a tunneling clamp is placed tip-down from the groin to meet the upper finger. The clamp is then flipped tip-up and brought into the abdomen against the upper finger at all times directly on the iliac arteries.

51-4

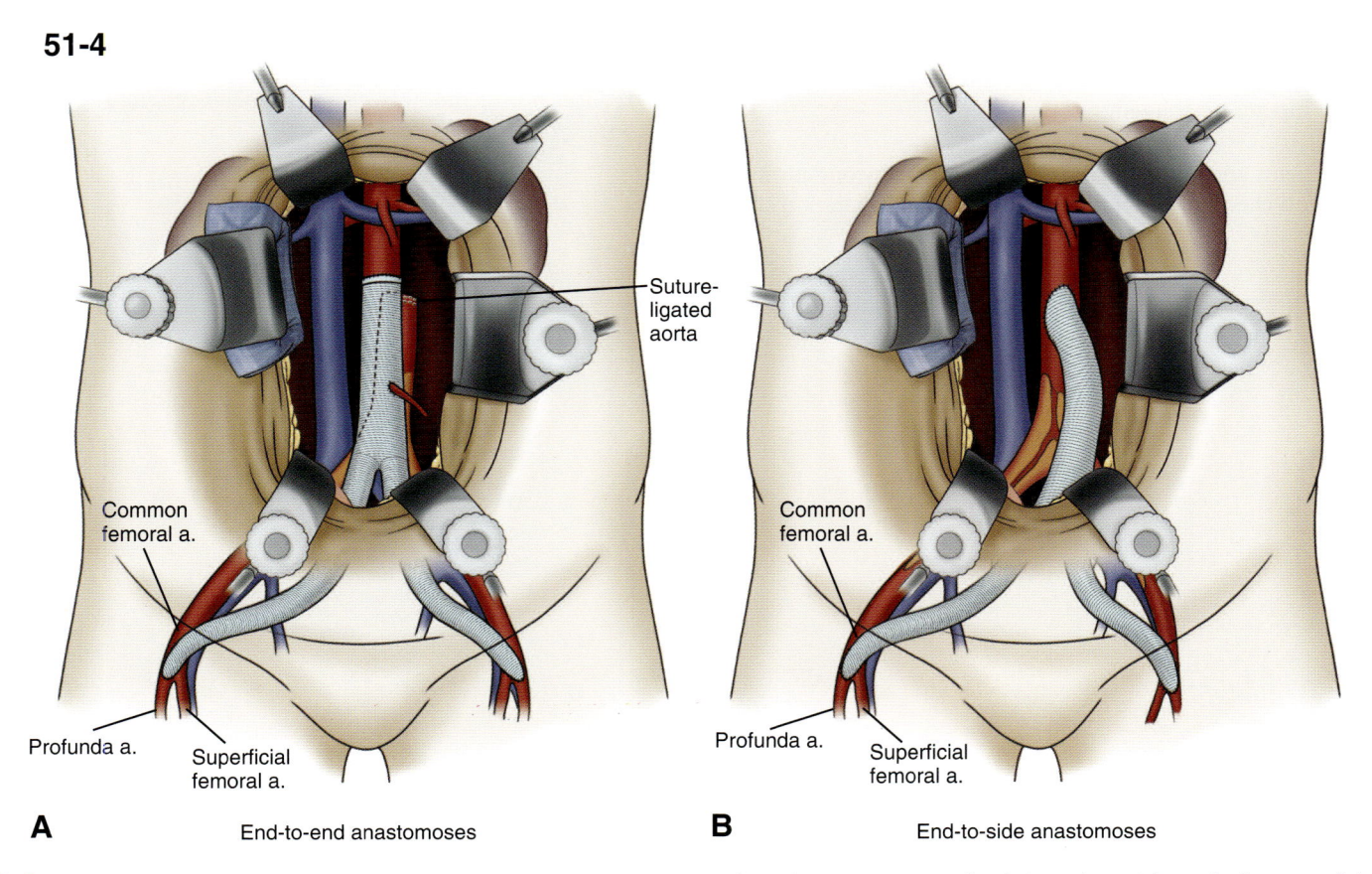

Suture-ligated aorta

Common femoral a.

Common femoral a.

Profunda a.

Superficial femoral a.

Profunda a.

Superficial femoral a.

A End-to-end anastomoses

B End-to-side anastomoses

Figure 51-4 A. End-to-end technique with aortic transection/resection. Graft in the native aortic bed. B. End-to-side technique useful to maintain accessory renal arteries, mandatory inferior mesenteric perfusion, and/or inline pelvic flow with heavily diseased external iliac arteries.

CLOSURE Once the graft is implanted, adjuncts considered, and the reconstruction deemed acceptable, heparin is reversed. The abdomen and the groins are washed, and further hemostasis achieved. The retroperitoneum is closed over the graft using Vicryl suture (**FIGURE 51-5**). Lack of tissue coverage may require omental flap. The abdomen is closed after final full inspection. The author uses #1 single strand PDS on the fascia and skin surgical clips. Once adequate groin hemostasis is present, they are closed in layers and the skin closed. I use interrupted 2-0 and 3-0 Vicryl suture and 4-0 Monocryl subcuticular skin closure. I do not leave closed suction drains unless large areas of flap or dead space are present. With redo operations or difficult groins, drainage, Sartorius muscle flaps, and negative pressure dressings are considered particularly with coverage concerns. Before leaving the OR, the team discusses and documents what the distal pulse or Doppler signal surveillance plan is for the graft based upon revascularization and residual disease.

POSTOPERATIVE CARE The patients are usually cared for in the ICU the night of surgery and transferred to floor status on postoperative day 2 or 3. Graft surveillance is documented twice daily. Intravascular volume is kept normalized. Blood products are transfused on a case-by-case basis but are generally not needed, particularly with autotransfusion use. Intravenous antibiotic prosthetic prophylaxis is continued for 24 hours postoperatively. With complex aortic clamping, particularly supraceliac, a nasogastric tube is kept in place until bowel sounds or function are present but is not required if standard infrarenal clamping is performed. Bowel function prior to postoperative day 3 should trigger concern for colon ischemia. The patient is kept in mild reverse Trendelenburg position with minimal hip flexion overnight, and in the afternoon of postoperative day 1, allowed to ambulate and sit in a chair. Pulmonary toilet maneuvers, such as coughing, and incentive spirometry begin as soon as possible. Physical therapy begins assessments and treatment on postoperative day 2. On postoperative day 2 or 3, the intravenous fluid is stopped and with evidence of fluid mobilization, diuresis is started and usually takes place over several days, depending upon the patient's oxygenation and fluid status. Usually on postoperative day 3 to 4, the epidural catheter is removed. Oral intake is allowed once bowel sounds or function are present. It has been our experience that patient's bowel function after ABF takes some time for re-coordination, so we usually start slowly with liquids and once proven tolerant, advance rather rapidly. Once ambulating or with a physical therapy rehabilitation plan, on a reasonable analgesia regimen, and tolerating food, patients are discharged. Most patients can be discharged home but some, particularly those older, living alone, or with preoperative need for functional support, may benefit from further rehabilitation stay.

FOLLOW-UP Patients are seen at 2 weeks after discharge by our advanced providers for wound check and overall functional and recuperation status update. At 6 weeks after ABF, we obtain new noninvasive studies, including ABIs and PVRs along with a graft duplex and select lower extremity duplex scans. This is done every 6 months for 18 to 24 months. Barring any problems or concerns, annual surveillance visits are scheduled with these noninvasive studies. In those with normal renal function, I obtain CTA of the graft and lower extremities at 6 to 12 months for baseline anatomic graft imaging. Patients are continued on antiplatelet and high-intensity statin medications. They are encouraged to continue scheduled walking exercise. Smoking cessation and available resources are emphasized throughout. Surveillance is important, as patients may not only have graft-related problems but nongraft laparotomy- or groin-related complications long-term. ■

SUGGESTED READINGS

Back MR, Johnson BL, Shames ML, et al. Evolving complexity of open aorto-femoral reconstruction done for occlusive disease in the endovascular era. *Ann Vasc Surg.* 2003;17(6):8.

Burke CR, Henke PK, Hernandez R, et al. A contemporary comparison of aorto-femoral bypass and aortoiliac stenting in the treatment of aortoiliac occlusive disease. *Ann Vasc Surg.* 2010;24(1):4-13.

DeCarlo C, Boitano LT, Schwartz SI, et al. Operative complexity and prior endovascular intervention negatively impact morbidity after aortobifemoral bypass in the modern era. *Ann Vasc Surg.* 2020;62:21-29.

DeCarlo C, Boitano LT, Schwartz SI, et al. Laparotomy- and groin-associated complications are common after aortofemoral bypass and contribute to reintervention. *J Vasc Surg.* 2020;72:1976-86.

DeCarlo C, Boitano LT, Schwartz SI, et al. Society for Vascular Surgery femoral runoff score is associated with limb-based patency after aortofemoral bypass. *J Vasc Surg.* 2021;74(1):124-133.e3.

DeCarlo C, Latz C, Boitano LT, et al. An endovascular-first approach for aortoiliac occlusive disease is safe: prior endovascular intervention is not associated with inferior outcomes after aortofemoral bypass. *Ann Vasc Surg.* 2021;70:62-69.

Prendiville EJ, Burke PE, Colgan MP, et al. The profunda femoris: a durable outflow vessel in aortofemoral surgery. *J Vasc Surg.* 1992;16(1):7.

Reed AB, Conte MS, Donaldson MC, et al. The impact of patient age and aortic size on the results of aortobifemoral bypass grafting. *J Vasc Surg.* 2003;37(6):1219-1225.

Sharma G, Scully RE, Shah SK, et al. Thirty-year trends in aortofemoral bypass for aortoiliac occlusive disease. *J Vasc Surg.* 2018;68(6):1796-804.

Tanaka A, Sandhu HK, Perlick A, et al. Superficial femoral artery occlusion reduces aortofemoral bypass graft patency. *Eur J Vasc Endovasc Surg.* 2019;57(5):650-657.

51-5

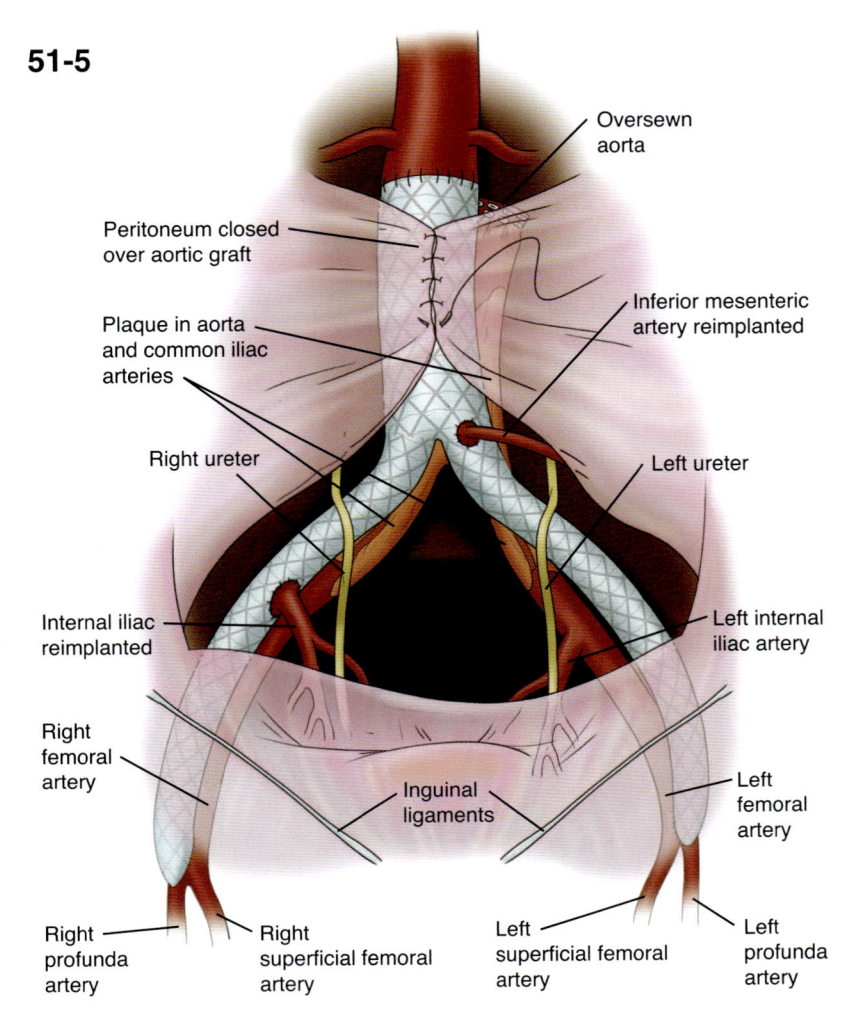

Oversewn aorta

Peritoneum closed over aortic graft

Plaque in aorta and common iliac arteries

Right ureter

Inferior mesenteric artery reimplanted

Left ureter

Internal iliac reimplanted

Left internal iliac artery

Right femoral artery

Inguinal ligaments

Left femoral artery

Right profunda artery

Right superficial femoral artery

Left superficial femoral artery

Left profunda artery

Figure 51-5 Completed bypass with reapproximation of peritoneum over the prosthetic graft.

Aortoiliac Endarterectomy

Michael J. Cheng, MD • Kaushal Patel, MD

INDICATION First popularized by Stoney, aortoiliac endarterectomy was the standard treatment for aortoiliac occlusive disease in the 1950s and 1960s prior to the widespread availability of prosthetic graft material for aortobifemoral bypass. Now in the modern era with aortobifemoral bypass further supplemented with endovascular techniques, the number of patients appropriate for aortoiliac endarterectomy continues to diminish.

Currently, aortoiliac endarterectomy is indicated for the select patients with focal aortoiliac occlusive disease limited to the distal aorta and common iliac arteries. While many of these patients are candidates for endovascular techniques, certain anatomic features such as small vessel diameter or unfavorable plaque morphology may make these less attractive options. More commonly, patients have occlusive disease that is more extensive and involves the external iliac arteries, in which case alternative treatments such as surgical bypass are recommended. One important advantage to aortoiliac endarterectomy is that the operation can be performed without the use of prosthetic graft material, which is advantageous in patients with high infectious risks. In this circumstance, a bovine patch may be useful. Another similar situation is patients with an infected aortobifemoral bypass that requires explantation. Aortoiliac endarterectomy can be used to help restore distal flow without complex aortoiliac reconstruction and avoiding femoral artery incisions. Special consideration is also made for symptomatic patients with high-grade ostial stenosis of the internal iliac arteries, as these lesions can often be addressed during the endarterectomy.

Evaluation of aortoiliac occlusive disease involves a thorough history and physical exam, with special attention to the presence of buttocks or thigh claudication, diminished femoral pulses, and erectile dysfunction in males (i.e., Leriche syndrome). Ankle-brachial indices are useful to obtain and are typically reduced in these patients. Computed tomography angiography (CTA), magnetic resonance angiography (MRA), and standard angiography are used to visualize the aortoiliac vasculature and characterize the extent and degree of stenosis. Overall, the outcomes after surgery are quite favorable. Despite the relative rarity of aortoiliac endarterectomy in practice today, multiple studies have reported excellent long-term durability with up to 90% patency rates at 5 years.

POSITION The patient is placed in a supine position.

OPERATIVE PREPARATION After routine skin preparation, the operative field is prepped and draped to expose bilateral groins and the entire abdomen up to the level of the xiphoid.

INCISION AND EXPOSURE The aortoiliac vessels can be approached via a transperitoneal or retroperitoneal approach. For a transabdominal approach, a midline incision is made, and the abdomen is explored for unexpected pathology (see Chapter 28 for details of this exposure). The retroperitoneal approach is done by placing the patient in a right lateral decubitus position (see Chapter 31 for details of this exposure). A left-sided flank oblique incision is commenced from the lateral edge of the rectus abdominus muscle and directed superiorly and posteriorly toward the costal margin. In cases of aortoiliac occlusive disease with a normal juxtarenal and suprarenal aorta, the incision can be extended more inferiorly toward the 11th to 12th interspace. The ureter is identified and brought medially with the peritoneum. The retroperitoneal plane is developed and carried toward the anterior surface of the psoas muscle. Medially the infrarenal aorta and aortic bifurcation can be visualized. A self-retaining retractor system is used to aid in visualization. The aorta is exposed as proximally as necessary for aortic cross-clamping. The left kidney can be either retracted anteriorly and medially with the abdominal contents to gain better exposure to the suprarenal aorta, or it can be left in its posterior position.

DETAILS OF PROCEDURE Once the retractors are in place, the infrarenal aorta and the common iliac bifurcation are exposed (**FIGURE 52-1**). During exposure of the infrarenal aorta, the lumbar arteries are identified and controlled to minimize bleeding. If the aortic endarterectomy needs to be extended proximally, dissection is carried proximally to the level of the aorta, where a proximal aortic cross-clamp can be safely placed. The inferior mesenteric artery should be identified and preserved. It is unusual to go up to the renal arteries, but they should be isolated and controlled depending on the level of aortic endarterectomy required. Dissection of the aortic bifurcation and the common iliac arteries is performed. Special care must be taken to avoid injury to the iliac veins which lie posterior to the aortic bifurcation. In addition, if possible, in men, preserve the pelvic nerves (nerves ergentes) on the aortic bifurcation to avoid retrograde ejaculation in men, which can occur up to 25% of the time. The main hypogastric autonomic nerve plexus lies anterior to the iliac vein; it should be left intact during dissection to avoid postoperative neurological complications. The bilateral common iliac arteries should be carefully isolated and controlled distal to where the aortoiliac endarterectomy will be performed to facilitate distal clamping. Umbilical tapes can be passed circumferentially around the aorta and bilateral iliac arteries to facilitate circumferential dissection. However, if there are clean anterior, medial, and lateral planes around the iliac arteries which will allow safe occlusive clamp placement, some surgeons prefer not to get circumferential control to avoid inadvertent iliac vein injury. Once proximal and distal controls are obtained, systemic heparin is administered to the patient by the anesthesia team and allowed to circulate prior to clamping the aorta. The anesthesia team should be prepared for any hemodynamic changes that may occur with cross-clamping of the aorta.

Once the patient is adequately heparinized and the proximal aorta and iliac arteries are clamped, a longitudinal arteriotomy is made on the anterior wall of the aorta with a #11 blade. The arteriotomy is carried sharply toward the aortic bifurcation with Potts scissors. The arteriotomy is then extended over both common iliac arteries, depending on the extent of disease and whether a counter-incision is planned for the contralateral iliac artery (**FIGURE 52-2**). **CONTINUES ▶**

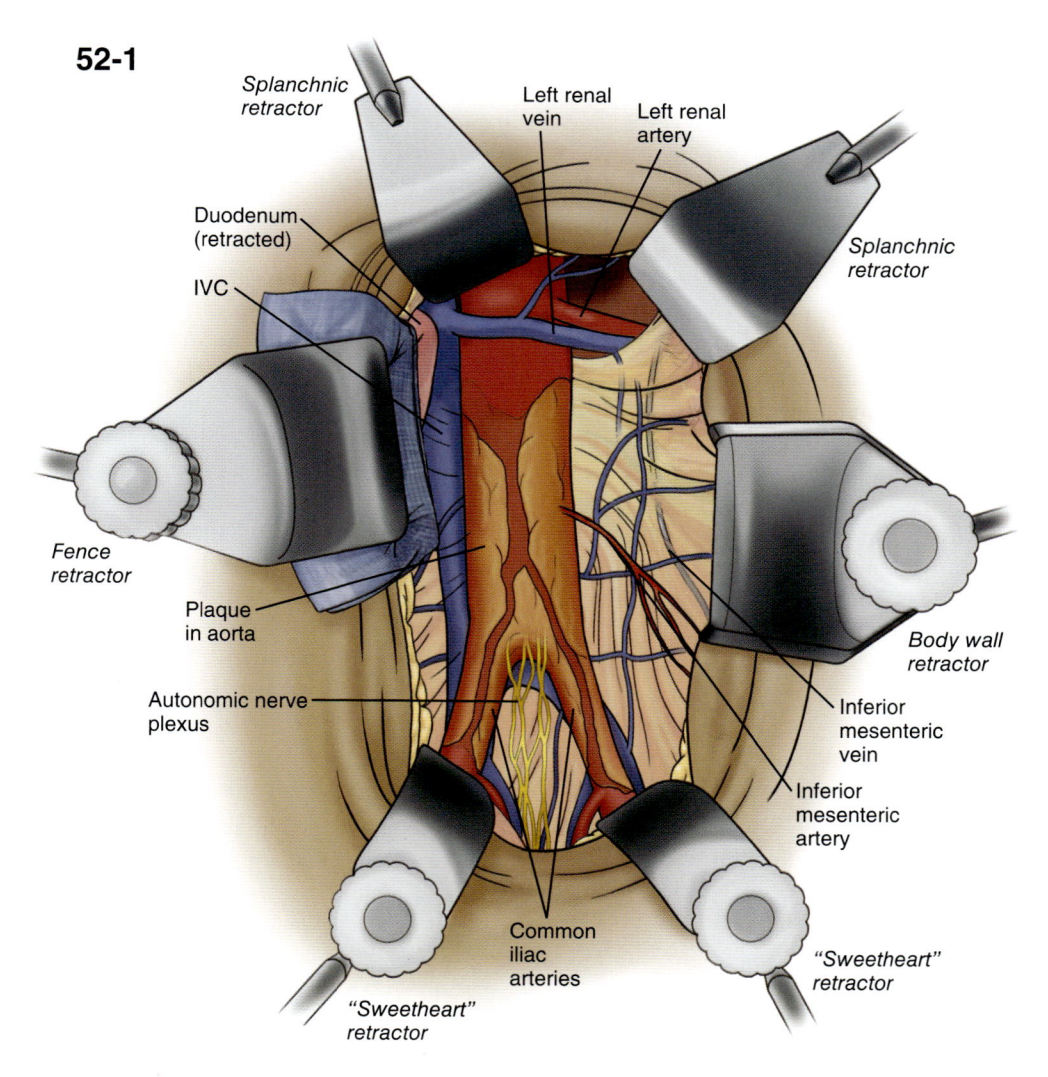

Figure 52-1 Exposure of the aorta and iliac arteries.

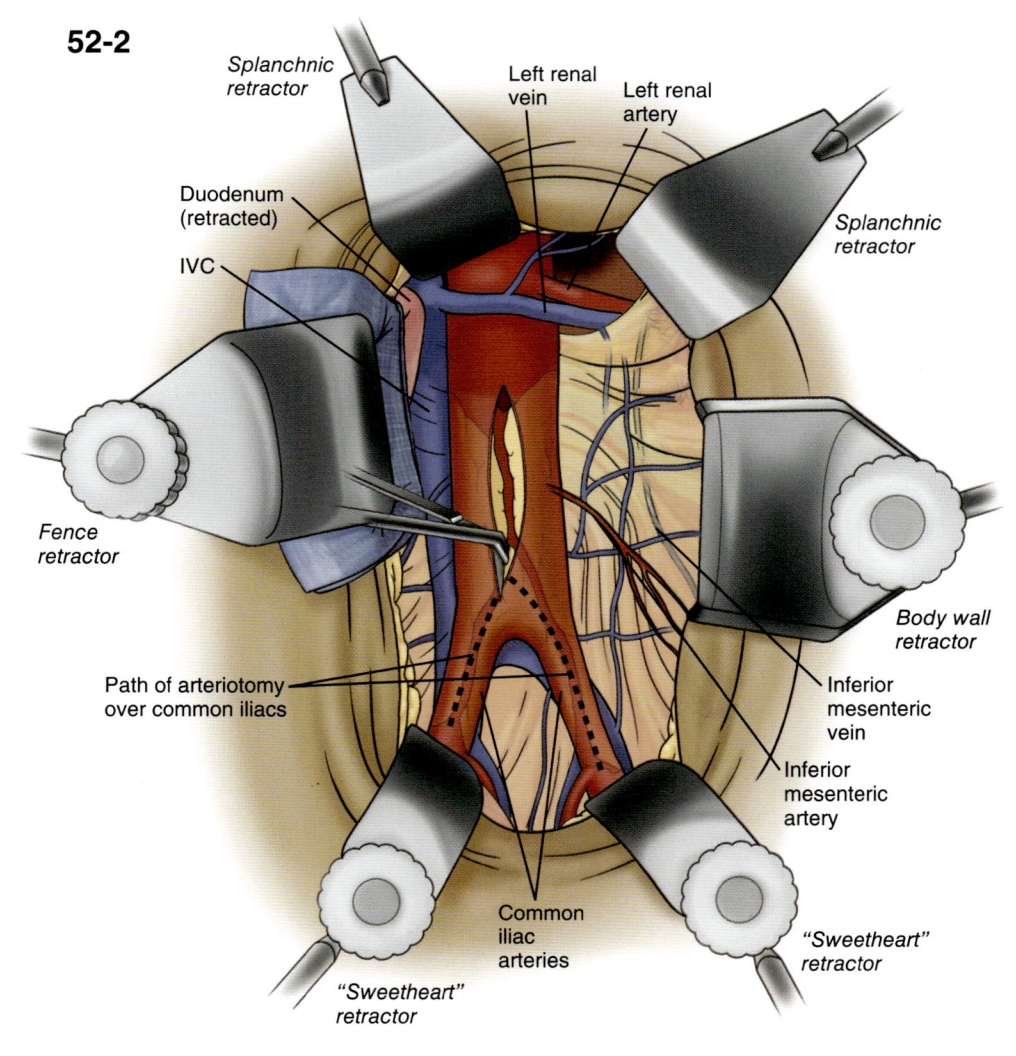

Figure 52-2 Aortotomy extending from above the plaque through the iliac arteries.

DETAILS OF PROCEDURE CONTINUED The endarterectomy is then performed with a dissecting spatula. Care must be taken to ensure that the correct plane is developed during the endarterectomy to avoid entering the adventitia (FIGURE 52-3) when removing the plaque. The endarterectomy is performed from the proximal extent of the aortic plaque toward the distal common iliac artery. Stenosis of the hypogastric artery ostia can be addressed with a long and narrow clamp. Care must be taken near the origin of the external iliac artery to avoid dissection flaps. While the endarterectomy should typically be performed to a smooth endpoint on the distal vessel, some surgeons prefer to secure the distal endpoint with interrupted 5-0 or 6-0 polypropylene "tacking" sutures. These sutures should be carefully placed in an "inside-out" fashion. For situations with aortic plaque that extends predominantly into a unilateral common iliac artery, this may be sufficient. If the native aorta and common iliac artery are of adequate size, the arteriotomy can be closed primarily with a running 5-0 polypropylene suture. However, we recommend a patch closure. This can be performed with a large bovine pericardial or prosthetic patch, which can be fashioned and sewn using a running 5-0 polypropylene suture (FIGURE 52-4). The aorta and iliac arteries should be allowed to flush antegrade and retrograde, to clear any residual debris or thrombus from the arterial system prior to securing the final suture line. The anesthesia team should be aware when the aortic cross clamp is removed and the extremity is reperfused, as there may be some transient hypotension.

Care is taken with regard to the origin of the hypogastric artery and external iliac artery to avoid dissection flaps. If the aortoiliac plaque extends beyond the common iliac artery into the external iliac artery, the patient is likely better suited with an aortofemoral or aortobifemoral bypass procedure. A strong pulse should be appreciated in bilateral external, internal iliac, and femoral arteries after completion, and a handheld Doppler should be used to interrogate pedal pulses to confirm patency.

CLOSURE Meticulous hemostasis is achieved. Any gaps in the suture lines should be repaired carefully with additional polypropylene sutures.

Thrombin-soaked gel foam or other various hemostatic agents can be used to help with minor bleeding. Heparin can be reversed with protamine if needed. Surgical drains are placed at the discretion of the surgeon. Once hemostasis is achieved, the self-retaining retractor is removed and the abdominal contents are allowed to return to their anatomic location. The anterior fascia is the primary strength layer of the closure, so the anterior rectus sheath is carefully closed with a running 1-0 or 0-0 monofilament suture. The subcutaneous and deep dermal layers are closed with sutures. The skin is closed with either a running subcuticular suture or skin stapler. If a separate infra-inguinal incision was used to facilitate external iliac endarterectomy, the incision should also be closed in several layers.

POSTOPERATIVE CARE The patient should be monitored closely for any hemodynamic, cardiac, respiratory, or renal function changes. Vital signs and urine output should be frequently assessed. Patient should ideally remain normotensive in the postoperative period. Distal pulses should be checked frequently in the lower extremities. A regular diet is slowly introduced to the patient, as typically patients who undergo retroperitoneal exposures have less postoperative ileus compared to transperitoneal incisions. Repeat ankle brachial indices should be obtained postoperatively to establish a new baseline. ∎

SUGGESTED READINGS

Brewster OC, Darling RC. Optimal methods of aortoiliac reconstruction. *Surgery*. 1978;84:739-748.

Leriche R, Morel A. The syndrome of thrombotic obliteration of the aortic bifurcation. *Ann Surg*. 1948;127:193-206.

Stoney J, Reilly LM. Endarterectomy for aortoiliac occlusive disease. In: Ernest CB, Stanley JC, eds. *Current Therapy in Vascular Surgery*. Philadelphia. Decker. 1987:157-160.

Wylie EJ. Thromboendarterectomy for arteriosclerotic thrombosis of major arteries. *Surgery*. 1952;32:275-292.

52-3

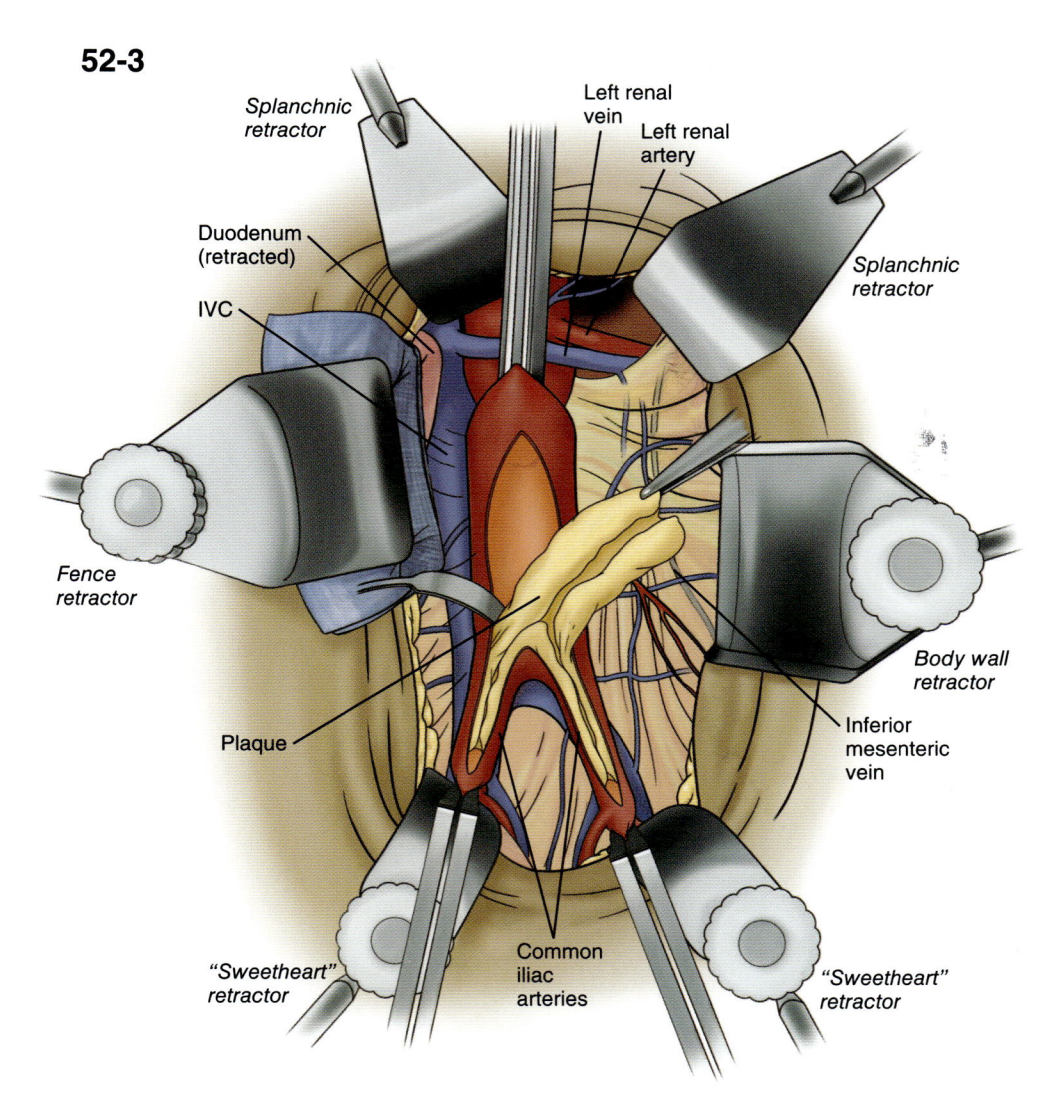

Figure 52-3 Endarterectomy with plaque removal.

52-4

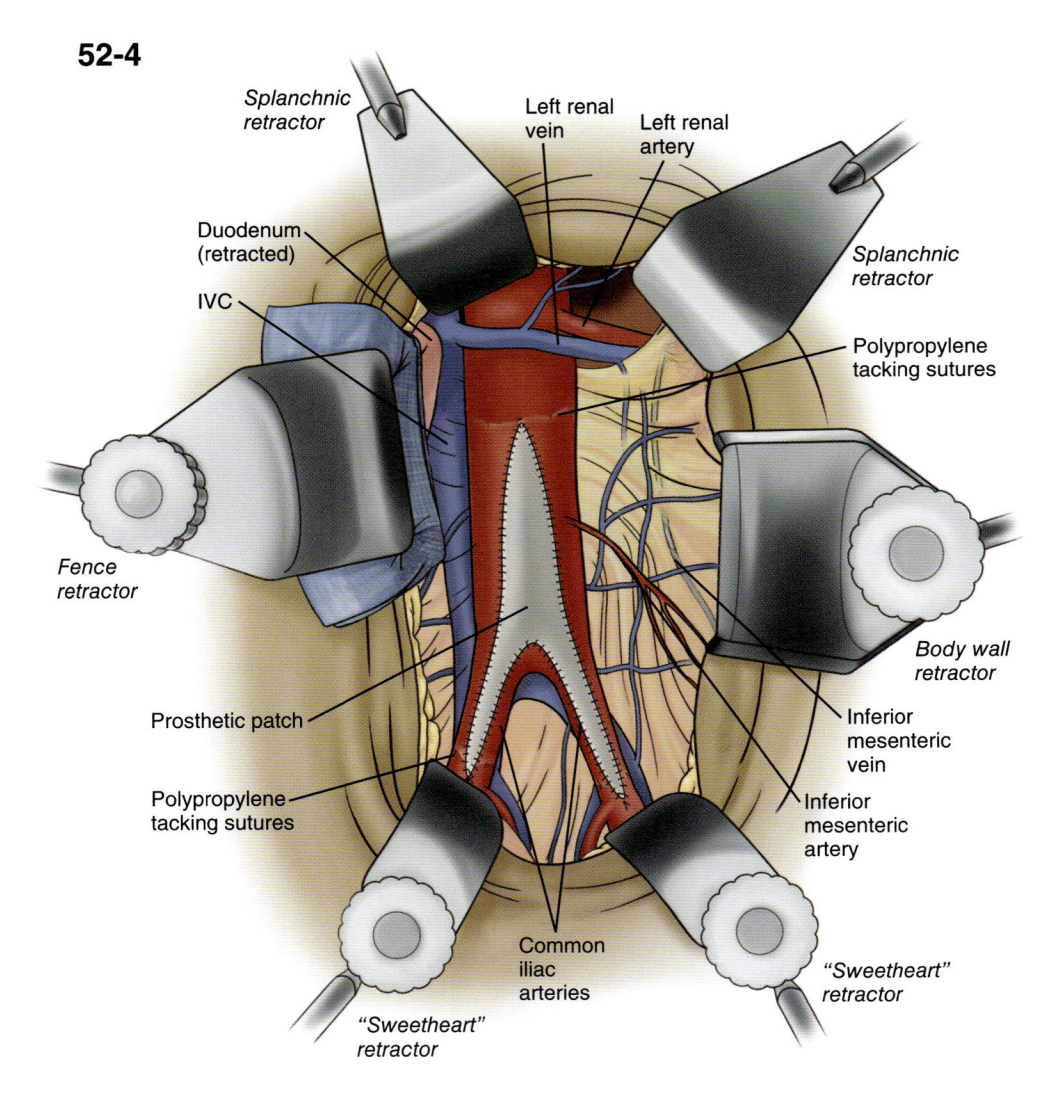

Figure 52-4 Bovine pericardial patch closure.

THORACOFEMORAL BYPASS

Martin R. Back, MD, MS, FACS • Mathew Wooster, MD, MBA, FACS

INDICATIONS Thoracobifemoral bypass (TBF) generally serves a tertiary role in supra-inguinal revascularization for patients presenting with lower limb ischemic symptoms (intermittent claudication, rest pain, tissue loss) due to aortoiliac occlusive disease. Aortobifemoral (ABF) and axillo-bifemoral (AxBF) are the preferred open surgical options when endovascular interventions have failed or are not indicated for severely diseased aortoiliofemoral segments. The ABF is the traditional open in-line reconstruction (midline transabdominal or left retroperitoneal), associated with reasonable perioperative risks and excellent long-term patency and limb preservation durability. AxBF bypass is acceptable in patients with severe medical comorbidities who are deemed at high risk for complication or death after an open abdominal aortic procedure. Given recent reports with heparin bonded ePTFE ringed grafts having patency rivaling ABF, AxBF is now an acceptable front-line therapy. TBF alternatively can be used in specific anatomical and pathological scenarios in modest medical risk patients considered fit enough to undergo a major cavitary operation. These factors include patients with "hostile" abdomens due to multiple transabdominal operations or ostomies, prior failed ABF, failed AxBF, prior aortic graft repair for aneurysm, severe paravisceral occlusive disease, de novo juxtarenal aortic occlusion, or prior infrarenal aortic ligation for infected pathologies. The relative contraindications to TBF are in patients with prior left retroperitoneal procedures (e.g., left nephrectomy, prior ABF, or aortic reconstruction), left hemidiaphragm division, prior left lung resection or severe pulmonary disease, and those with extensive circumferential calcification of the supraceliac/distal descending thoracic aorta.

The distinct advantages of TBF over redo ABF is avoidance of transperitoneal lysis of abdominal wall and bowel adhesions and tedious pararenal aortic dissection through scarred tissue planes. Via a first-time left thoracoretroperitoneal approach, exposure of the typically minimally diseased supraceliac aorta is straightforward and serves as proximal anastomotic site for TBF. The left renal, superior mesenteric (SMA), and celiac arteries are easily accessible for bypass or endarterectomy of occlusive lesions. The left TBF limb in the left retroperitoneum and the right limb in a preperitoneal (i.e., over the bladder) plane can be tunneled safely under direct vision.

Two variations of TBF can be utilized based on left chest and left retroperitoneal presenting anatomy. The original TBF procedure describes a left anterolateral thoracotomy exposure of the distal descending thoracic aorta and proximal anastomosis (**FIGURE 53-1A**). Prior scarring in the left retroperitoneum and diaphragm (e.g., prior left retroperitoneal aortic exposure) can be avoided with this thoracic cavity aortic exposure. "Blind" tunneling of the bypass limbs through the posterior left hemidiaphragm and through the left retroperitoneum is required from the thoracotomy to groin femoral exposures with possible injury to the spleen, kidney, and colon. When this approach is used, some favor a counter-incision into the lower left retroperitoneum for safe limb passage. Also, a unilateral thoracic aorta to left femoral bypass can be done with a left to right cross-femoral graft in a suprapubic, subcutaneous plane to minimize unsafe cross-pelvic tunneling. Our TBF technique preferred at the University of Florida instead avoids the left hemithorax and focuses the visceral aortic exposure at the level of or just below the left diaphragm through a retroperitoneal plane (**FIGURE 53-1B**).

Aortofemoral limb tunneling is then done under more direct vision in the left retroperitoneum. A scarred left chest (e.g., from prior thoracotomy, lung resection, or inflammatory pulmonary process) is avoided with this surgical exposure. Two potential pitfalls of this approach are higher risk of splenectomy from capsular avulsion occurring while left upper quadrant intraperitoneal organs are swept off the left hemidiaphragm, and dissecting through reoperative fields.

PREOPERATIVE PLANNING Operative planning requires high resolution, thin axial slice (1- to 2-mm cuts) CT arteriography ideally with coronal and sagittal reconstructions and interpretive attention to paravisceral/descending thoracic aortic clamping sites for proximal anastomotic construction of the TBF, visceral branch disease, hypogastric and distal iliofemoral patency, possible limb tunneling planes, adjunctive femoral arterial reconstruction, and any venous anomalies (e.g., retro-aortic left renal vein, and inferior vena cava anomalies). Our preferred medical optimization for patients undergoing TBF includes preoperative resting echocardiography (LVEF, valve disease), daily use of bronchodilator inhalers for active

smokers, appropriate cessation of antiplatelet agents 7 days prior (except aspirin 81 mg qd) and anticoagulants 3 to 5 days prior, alcohol-based skin prep starting 3 days prior (chlorhexidine) and renal protection measures (overnight IV hydration for chronic kidney disease and intraoperative mannitol and furosemide). Stress cardiac imaging and pulmonary function testing are selectively done in patients with more advanced cardiopulmonary disease and significantly abnormal results possibly precluding TBF and instead indicating need for a less invasive Ax-BF.

General endotracheal anesthesia is used without epidural or spinal anesthetic adjuncts. Due to short clamp times of the supraceliac aorta, prophylactic lumbar cerebrospinal fluid drainage is not needed. Central venous access and cell-saver collection system with re-transfusion is recommended with intraoperative maintenance of hemoglobin levels over 8 mg/dL. Normothermia is maintained during the procedure with upper body (over left upper chest, arms, and head) and lower body (below thighs) "bear hugger" warming blankets.

PATIENT POSITIONING Correct patient positioning is critical to optimizing ease of aortic exposure and TBF. The patient should be positioned on a bean bag with the anterior superior iliac crest at the level of break in the table. The left shoulder should be rotated 30 degrees to the right (45 degrees for anterolateral thoracotomy approach for TBF) with the left arm immobilized on a rest above the right arm and shoulder. The hips should be kept as flat as possible (see Figures 38-1 and 38-2). The bed is then retroflexed at its break to increase the distance between the anterior iliac crest and the costal margin and increase exposure of the left thoraco-retroperitoneal surgical site. The bed is then tilted to the right to bring the left retroperitoneal region anteriorly. Adjustment of bed into a reverse Trendelenburg position is done to level the position of the head above the level of the feet. Chlorhexidine skin prep is done "table to table" of the groins, anterior thighs, abdomen, and left chest with Ioban plastic skin coverage applied before draping. The inflated bean bag should keep this position throughout the operation. Exposure to the right groin in obese patients can be difficult and can be improved with upward traction to the right lower quadrant abdominal pannus with 4-inch-wide cloth strapping tape before skin preparation.

SURGICAL DETAILS Groin incisions and femoral artery exposures are performed first to minimize the time the retroperitoneum and chest are open. If limited femoral occlusive disease is present, some prefer an oblique incision above the inguinal crease and exposure of the common femoral and origins of the superficial and profunda branches. However, convention is to hood the graft over the profunda, and this is best accomplished with routine longitudinal incisions to allow full profunda exposure. This is especially true in redo and de novo cases where concomitant femoral endarterectomy with profundaplasty is anticipated. Hooding of femoral anastomoses into the SFA or PFA (when the SFA is diseased) should always be performed for inflow bypasses done for occlusive disease.

For the left anterolateral thoracotomy version of the TBF, more right lateral decubitus positioning (45-degree torsion of the upper trunk relative to flat hips) and more left chest exposure and skin prep is required. A 6th intercostal space thoracotomy is done with a rib-spreading retractor and superior mobilization of the left lung. A dual lumen endotracheal tube can be helpful for single (right) lung ventilation in patients with less severe obstructive lung disease. Exposure of the distal descending thoracic aorta above the diaphragm allows a proximal end-to-side anastomosis. A key step is mobilizing the inferior pulmonary ligament and manual palpation of the esophagus with the nasogastric tube in, which aids exposure (**FIGURE 53-2**). A left retroperitoneal tunnel is made through the outer margin of the posterolateral diaphragm (sometimes made safer with a counter-incision in the left flank) and the aortofemoral graft brought to the left groin incision (**FIGURE 53-3**). Our preferred alternative approach to the TBF focuses on paravisceral/supraceliac aortic exposure and only minimal left hemithorax violation through partial left hemidiaphragm division. The abdominal incision is started at mid-distance between umbilicus and pubis, kept horizontal across the left rectus abdominis muscle (can be preserved or divided), and continued vertically in an "S" shape in the left flank and across the 8th (in obese patients) or 9th intercostal space (see Chapters 37 and 38). **CONTINUES** ▶

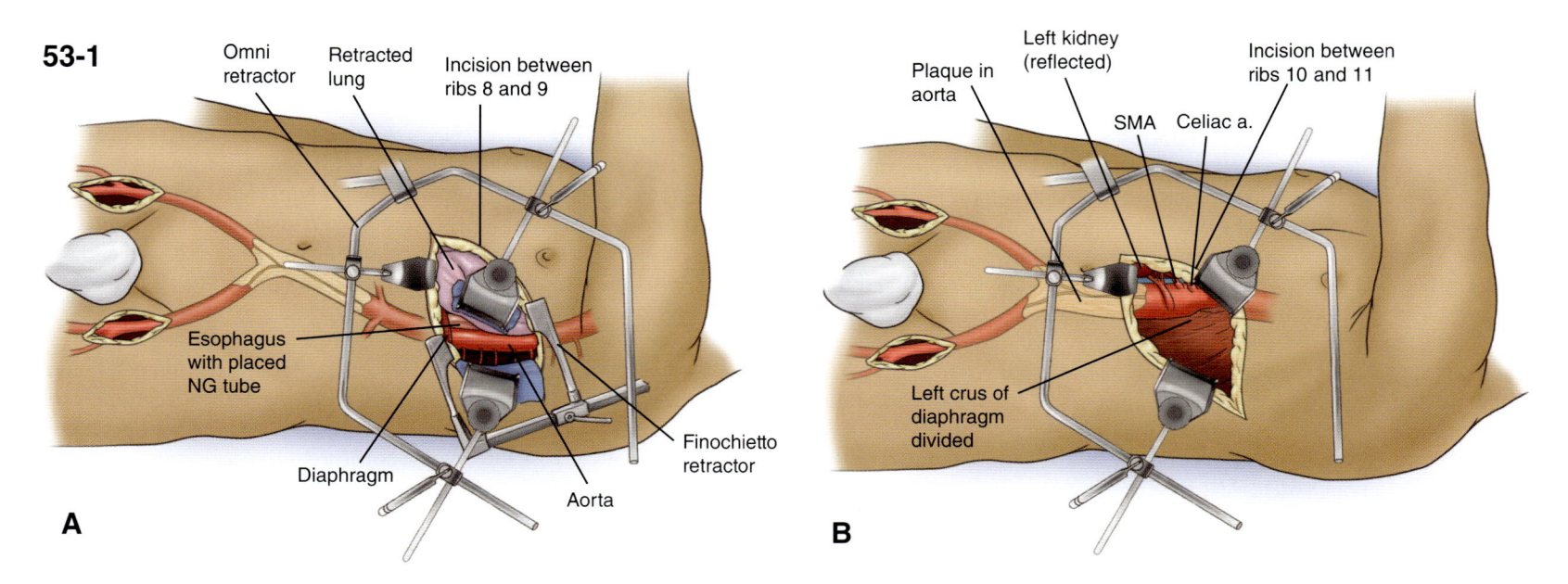

Figure 53-1 A. Eighth to ninth rib space for thoracic incision. B. Tenth to eleventh rib space for retroperitoneal incision.

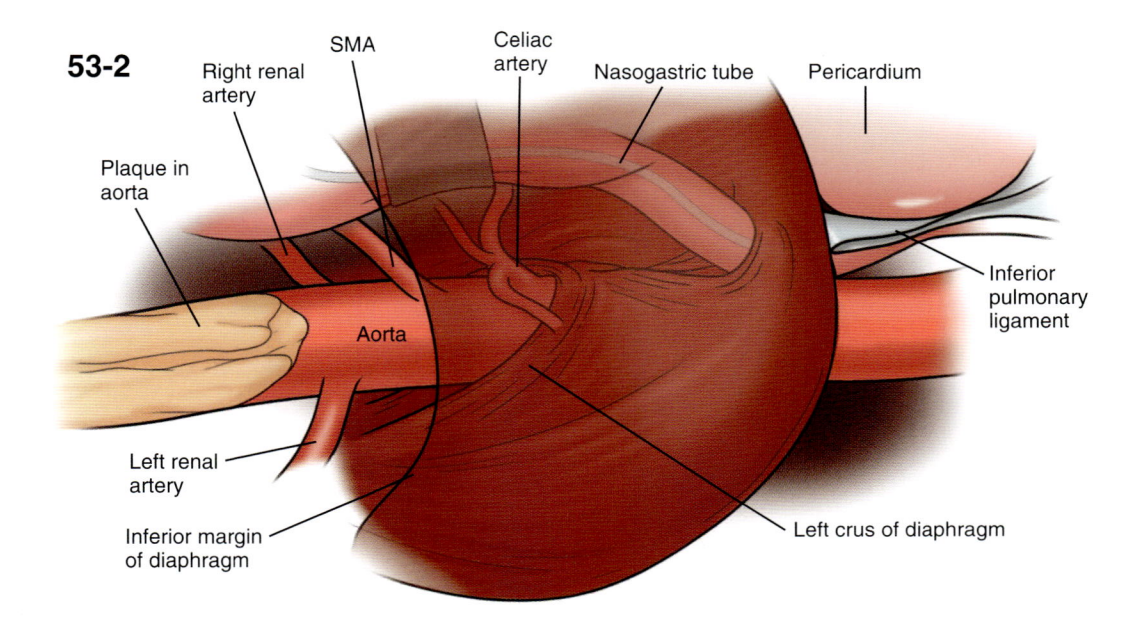

Figure 53-2 Exposure of perivisceral abdominal aorta.

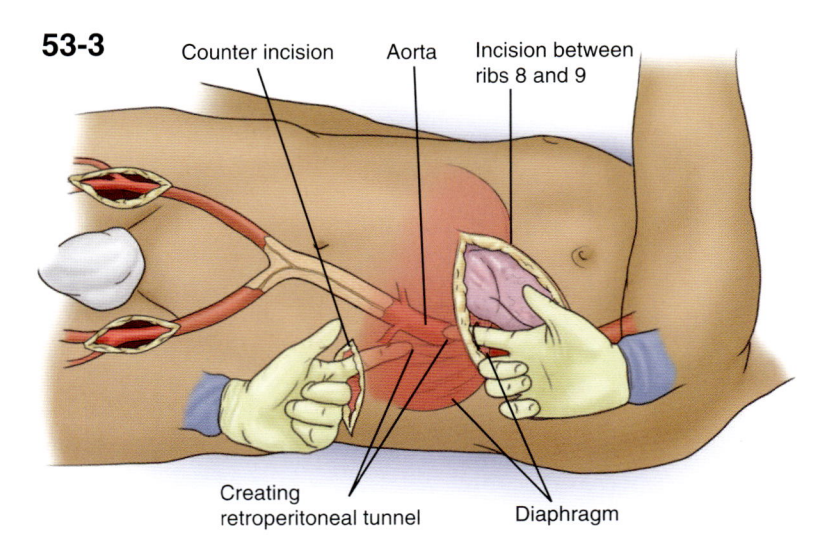

Figure 53-3 Retroperitoneal counter incision to facilitate tunnel between to chest and groins.

SURGICAL DETAILS `CONTINUED` In patients with anticipated extensive pelvic and intra-abdominal scarring and a plan for unilateral aortofemoral and suprapubic cross femoral bypass construction, a modified "thoracoabdominal" exposure can be used with no incision to the midline across the left rectus, and instead a vertical incision at the lateral edge of the left rectus muscle can be extended across the costal margin and the 8th interspace opened. Anterior and posterior abdominal fascial layers are divided lateral to the rectus, and I usually enter the lowest left hemithorax and divide the costal margin (see Chapter 40 for details). The retroperitoneal plane is then entered by separating overlying abdominal wall and underlying peritoneal lining beginning at the costal margin and proceeding inferiorly to the posterior rectus fascia. The next step is to expand this space with a sponge stick inferiorly down to the left psoas fascia and then dissect back superiorly sweeping the peritoneum (and abdominal contents) toward the right side of the abdomen and posteriorly along the psoas, lifting the left kidney in its abdomina/Gerota's fascia back toward the left hemidiaphragm. Separation of peritoneal lining off the diaphragm is aided by alternating pushing away the peritoneum and diaphragm muscle from each other with a sponge stick, electrocautery, or sharp dissection. Once the spleen is encountered, meticulous technique for mobilizing this aids with exposure. The entire left hemidiaphragm including the central tendon and left crus should be freed from the peritoneal membrane and tear in the diaphragm is not initially repaired and is repaired just before closing. At risk in this maneuver is the spleen, which can suffer a capsular tear and be a source of ongoing bleeding. An enlarged spleen, underlying hepatic disease, and prior abdominal operations with residual peri-splenic adhesions increase risk of splenic injury, and if a capsular tear occurs, I have a low threshold for performing splenectomy early in the operative sequence. A limited circumferentially oriented lateral opening of the left hemidiaphragm is done with open costal margin to aid aortic exposure. A fixed retractor system is set up (either Omni or Buckwalter (Symmetry Surgical, Antioch, TN) with an oval ring and deep blades applied superiorly at the costal margin, a countering shallow blade on the lower divided rib, and additional malleable or fixed blades retracting inferior structures. The left crus posterior to the left renal artery is divided (a key gateway) and extended superiorly to the supraceliac aorta. Division of a larger neurovascular trunk at the lower left crus is needed and small phrenic arteries off the aorta can be divided. Dissection exposure of least three-quarters of the supraceliac and paravisceral aortic circumference is needed. The proximal end-to-side anastomosis can be created off the supraceliac or even suprarenal aorta but celiac, SMA, and left renal branches require control or even temporary clamping, and large posterior lumbar arteries need temporary clip application to prevent back-bleeding through the aortotomy during anastomosis (**FIGURE 53-4**). The pararenal aorta can be used as well (after dividing the lumbar venous branch and mobilizing the left renal vein superiorly) if spared from more inferior aortic bifurcation and pelvic scarring from prior inflow operations.

Tunnels are created before bypass construction. The left ureter is protected within the infrarenal aortic region only if preperitoneal tunneling of the right aortofemoral graft limb is needed across the pelvis. This plane is created with digits from both of the surgeon's hands "connecting" from inferiorly under the right inguinal ligament, under the right rectus abdominis muscle and from superiorly in left retroperitoneal space under the rectus abdominis and over the inferiorly decompressed bladder (**FIGURE 53-4**).

An umbilical tape is passed through the tunnel to allow later safe aortic clamp delivery of the graft limb. The left aortofemoral graft limb is easily tunneled through the retroperitoneal space under the inguinal ligament to the left femoral vessel. `CONTINUES`

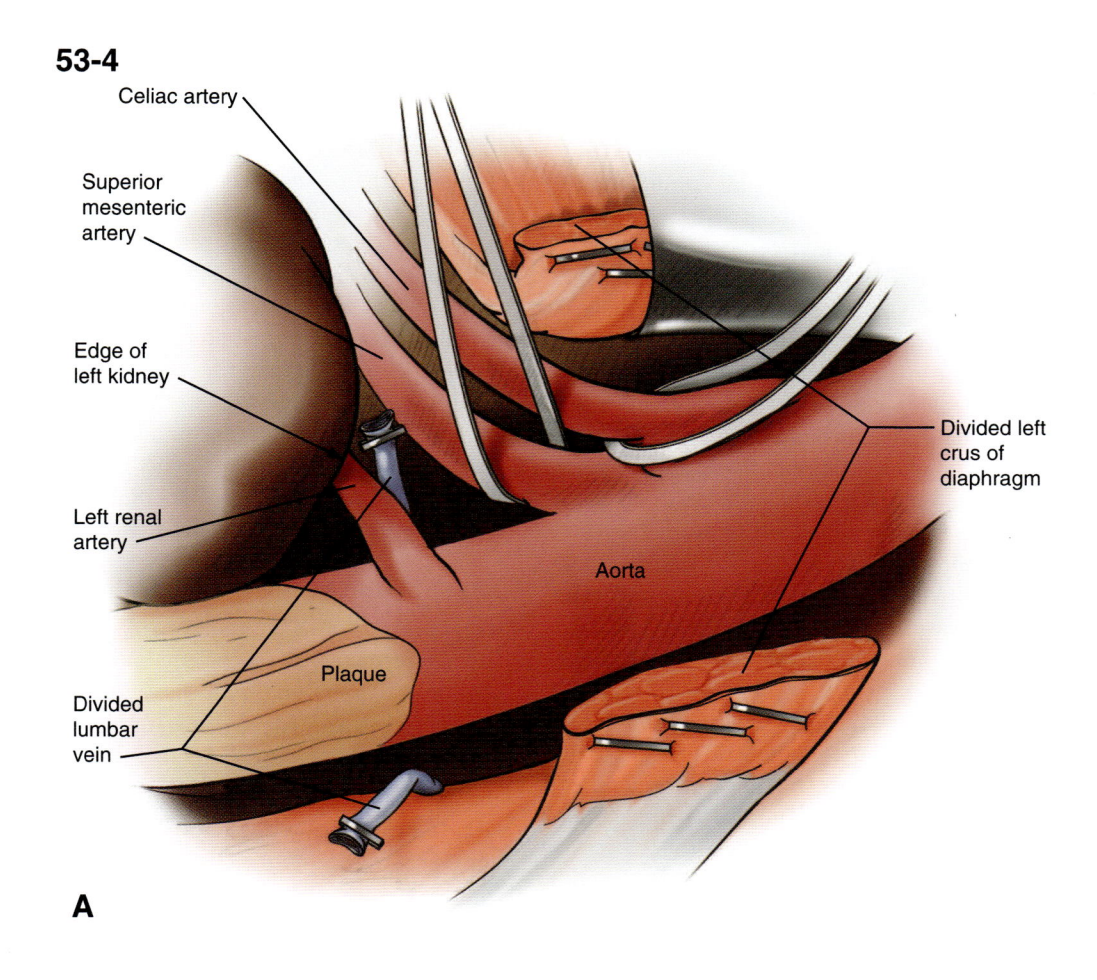

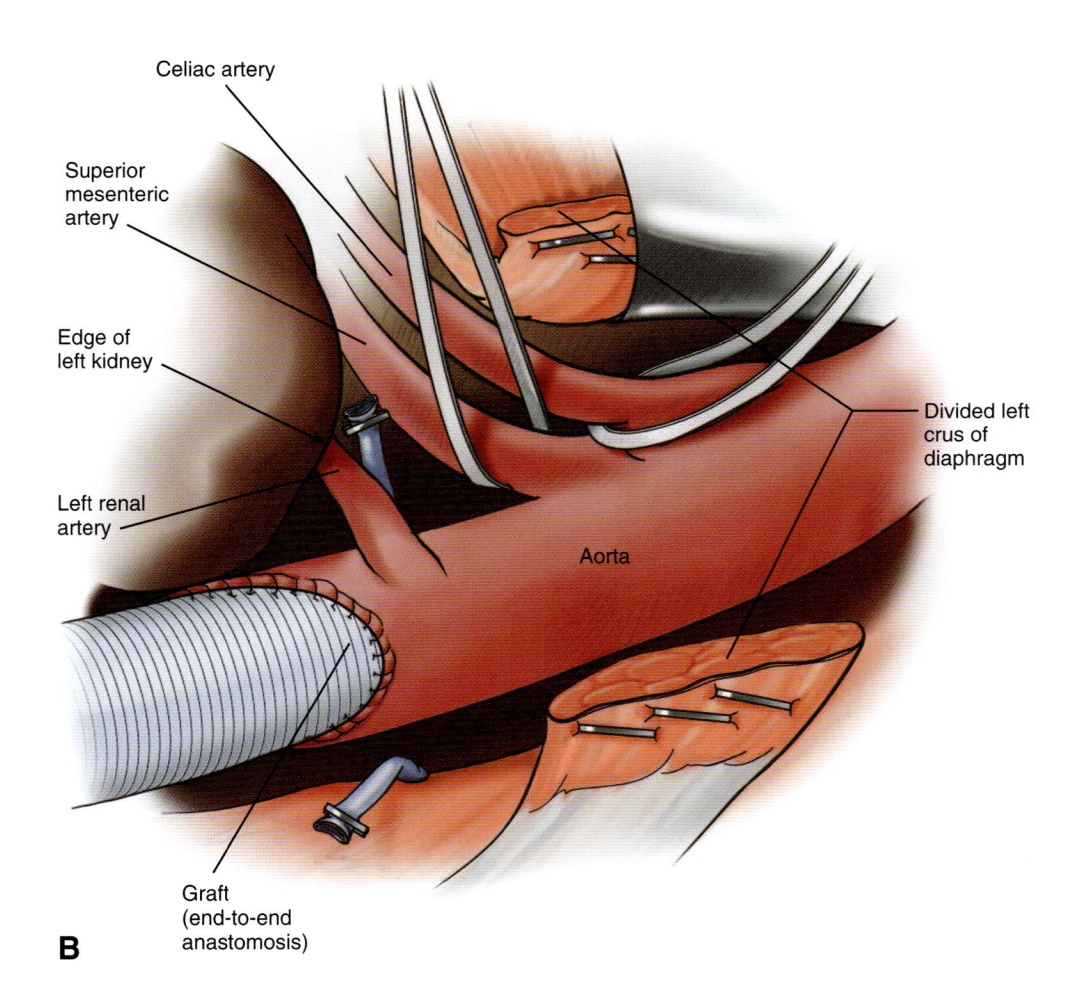

Figure 53-4 A. The crus of the diaphragm are the gateway to the retroperitoneal perivisceral aorta. B. End-to-end proximal anastomosis.

SURGICAL DETAILS <CONTINUED> Selection of the prosthetic graft conduit depends on the planned reconstruction. For a bifurcated TBF, I prefer a preconstructed PTFE 16 × 8 mm or 14 × 7 mm (for smaller diameter vessels) (WL Gore, Flagstaff, AZ) but these shorter length grafts, even preserving a long proximal body, may not be long enough for a preperitoneal tunneled right aortofemoral limb in taller individuals. Similar diameter Dacron bifurcated grafts are longer and can be used instead. For a unilateral aorto-left-femoral bypass then a ringed 8-mm PTFE can be used. After systemic heparinization, partial occluding Lambert-Kay or aortic Satinsky curved clamps can be applied to the para-visceral aorta. Curved long vascular clamps (with/without separate visceral branch clamping) may be applied completely across the aorta proximally and distally for smaller diameter aortas or partially calcified walls. A longitudinal arteriotomy 3 cm long is made and a spatulated end-to-side anastomosis is made with 4-0 polypropylene suture (RB-1 needle preferred) (FIGURE 53-5). For occluded aortas, it is easier to do end-to-end anastomosis.

Pledgeted repair sutures may be needed with more diseased aortic wall. Distended graft limbs are tunneled to femoral anastomotic sites. Significant laxity in the right preperitoneal aortofemoral limb is needed when all retracted peritoneal contents are allowed back into the left retroperitoneal space. Femoral anastomoses are made sequentially after appropriate adjunct reconstruction. Continuous-wave Doppler assessment of arterial flow in visceral branches, outflow iliofemoral vessels are done before and after heparin reversal with protamine.

After hemostasis is assured, the peritoneal cavity is explored to assure an intact splenic capsule, viable left colon, and the nasogastric tube repositioned if needed, and is then closed. A 32 F curved left thoracostomy tube is placed two intercostal spaces above the left retroperitoneal opening and positioned over the left hemidiaphragm. I try to partially close the left crus with a "figure-of-8" suture superiorly. The left hemidiaphragm is closed with a running polypropylene suture and brought through the lower intercostal space without trying to close the friable lateral-most portion of the diaphragm. This suture is then tied to an adjacent para-costal suture and results in a negligible lateral diaphragmatic defect. Interrupted absorbable sutures close the para-costal opening. Posterior and anterior abdominal fascial layers are closed separately with running looped absorbable suture to minimize bulging of the partially denervated (small intercostal nerves) flank muscles.

POSTOPERATIVE CARE Immediate postoperative extubation can be considered in lower-risk patients with low intraoperative blood loss (<800 mL) and no hemodynamic lability. Otherwise, extubation in the ICU can be done when hypothermia, residual metabolic acidosis (base deficit <5), hypoxemia, hypercarbia, hypotension, hypovolemia, and coagulopathy have been corrected. Occasionally, a coagulopathic patient in the operative room requires open abdominal packing, temporary vacuum-assisted negative pressure dressing use, and return to the operating room in 24 to 48 hours for abdominal wound closure. Patients are monitored in the ICU according to institutional care standards, and overall postop management does not differ from other open aortic procedures. When TBF is used after prior failed open inflow bypasses, I prefer indefinite clopidogrel 75 mg daily with or without aspirin 81 mg daily. ■

SUGGESTED READINGS

Back MR, Johnson BL, Shames ML, Bandyk DF. Evolving complexity of open aortofemoral reconstruction done for occlusive disease in the endovascular era. *Ann Vasc Surg.* 2003;17:8.

Brewster DC. Current controversies in the management of aortoiliac occlusive disease. *J Vasc Surg.* 1997 Feb;25(2):365-379.

Sampson RH, Showalter DP, Lepore MR Jr, Nair DG, Dorsay DA, Morales RE. Improved patency after axillofemoral bypass for aortoiliac occlusive disease. *J Vasc Surg.* 2018 Nov;68(5):1430-1437.

Scali ST, Schmit BM, Feezor RJ, Beck AW, Chang CK, Waterman AL, et al. Outcomes after redo aortobifemoral bypass for aortoiliac occlusive disease. *J Vasc Surg.* 2014 Aug; 60(2):346-355.

53-5

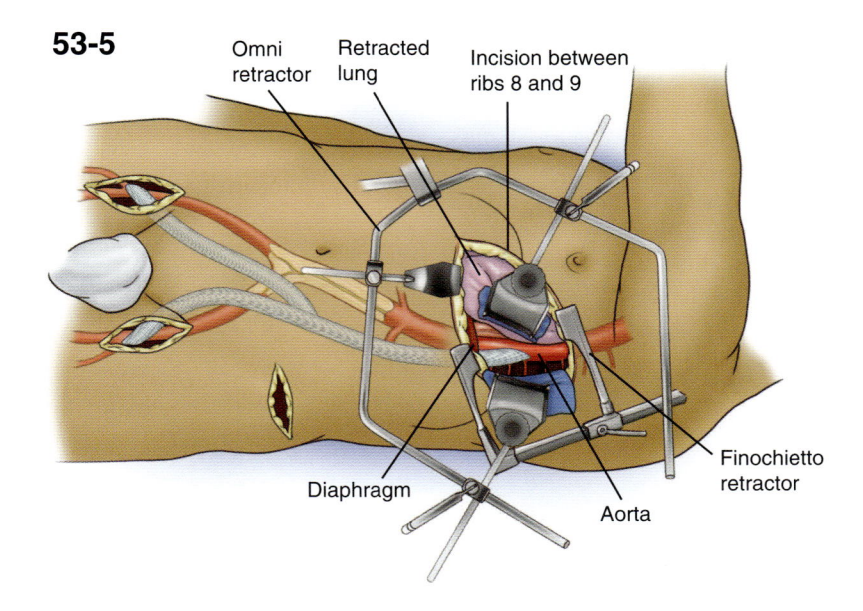

Omni retractor

Retracted lung

Incision between ribs 8 and 9

Diaphragm

Aorta

Finochietto retractor

Figure 53-5 Completed thoracobifemoral bypass.

Extra-Anatomic Bypass: Axillo-Bifemoral, Axillo-Unifemoral and Femoro-Femoral Bypasses

Russell H. Samson, MD, FACS, DFSVS

INDICATIONS Most extra-anatomic procedures are performed for limb-threatening ischemia. However, extra-anatomic grafts have also been used to combat prior aortic graft infection or occlusion, or for acute occlusions due to dissecting aneurysm. In most cases, extra-anatomic bypass is chosen because the patient is a high risk for an aortofemoral graft. Other reasons include hostile aorta making direct aortic surgery impractical, prior failed aortic revascularization, hostile abdomen, or morbid obesity.

NONINVASIVE AND CLINICAL PREOPERATIVE WORKUP All patients should undergo routine physiologic studies of their upper extremity arteries in addition to their lower extremity evaluation. Unexpectedly low arm blood pressures or differential between left and right arms will usually imply an inflow issue that needs to be corrected prior to axillofemoral bypass. Further, these studies will help determine the side most likely to provide the best inflow for such bypasses. If both axillary arteries are suitable donors, the right side is usually chosen since the left side is more predisposed to develop atherosclerosis. Prior to axillo-femoral bypass, CTA evaluation of the subclavian and axillary arteries is recommended in all patients irrespective of the physiologic upper extremity studies since unsuspected inflow pathology can result in failure to improve symptoms or, more importantly, graft occlusion. Duplex evaluation of the subclavian/axillary arteries is not required. If a hemodynamically significant lesion in a donor artery is suspected, then preoperative angioplasty and stenting may still allow that vessel to be utilized. CTA or aortic/runoff diagnostic arteriography should be performed to assess the infrainguinal arteries, if not already obtained during workup for possible aortic surgery or an endovascular intervention. Whenever possible, patients who are not on a statin should be started on this medication preoperatively. Preoperative antiplatelet agents are not prescribed. If time permits and medical consultation agrees, antiplatelet agents other than aspirin are stopped 7 days prior to the procedure. Because of underlying conditions that usually are found in these patients, most will have had a cardiac workup prior to surgery. However, preoperative cardiac clearance is not necessary in all patients.

SURGICAL TECHNIQUE

AXILLO-BIFEMORAL BYPASS AND AXILLO-UNIFEMORAL BYPASS: All procedures are performed under general anesthesia. If an arterial line is required during Axillo-femoral bypass, it should be placed in the contralateral arm. A rolled sheet is placed transversely under the shoulders and the donor arm abducted 90° and placed on an arm board (**FIGURE 54-1**). Keeping the arm abducted reduces the possibility that the graft can be avulsed off the anastomosis with postoperative elevation of the arm. This complication has been reported when surgeons position the arm adducted to the torso. Antiseptic chlorhexidine prep starts at the chin and ends in the mid-thigh bilaterally. An adhesive betadine-impregnated plastic drape is applied to the chest wall, abdomen, and thighs to isolate the graft from skin contact and resulting contamination. A cardiac surgery drape works well for these procedures. The axillary artery is exposed with an incision that is placed obliquely from an inch below the clavicular head to the mid-humeral head. Sometimes placement can be aided by palpating the axillary artery prior to making the incision. Electrocautery is utilized to dissect the subcutaneous tissue. The cephalic vein may be visualized and should be spared. The incision is deepened by splitting the fibers of the pectoralis major. Crossing veins and small muscular arteries will be encountered both medially and laterally and may need to be divided. Medially the medial pectoral nerve may be encountered and should be preserved. The axillary artery is divided into three parts by the pectoralis minor muscle with the first part proximal, the second posterior, and the third part distal (**FIGURE 54-2**). CONTINUES ▶

54-1

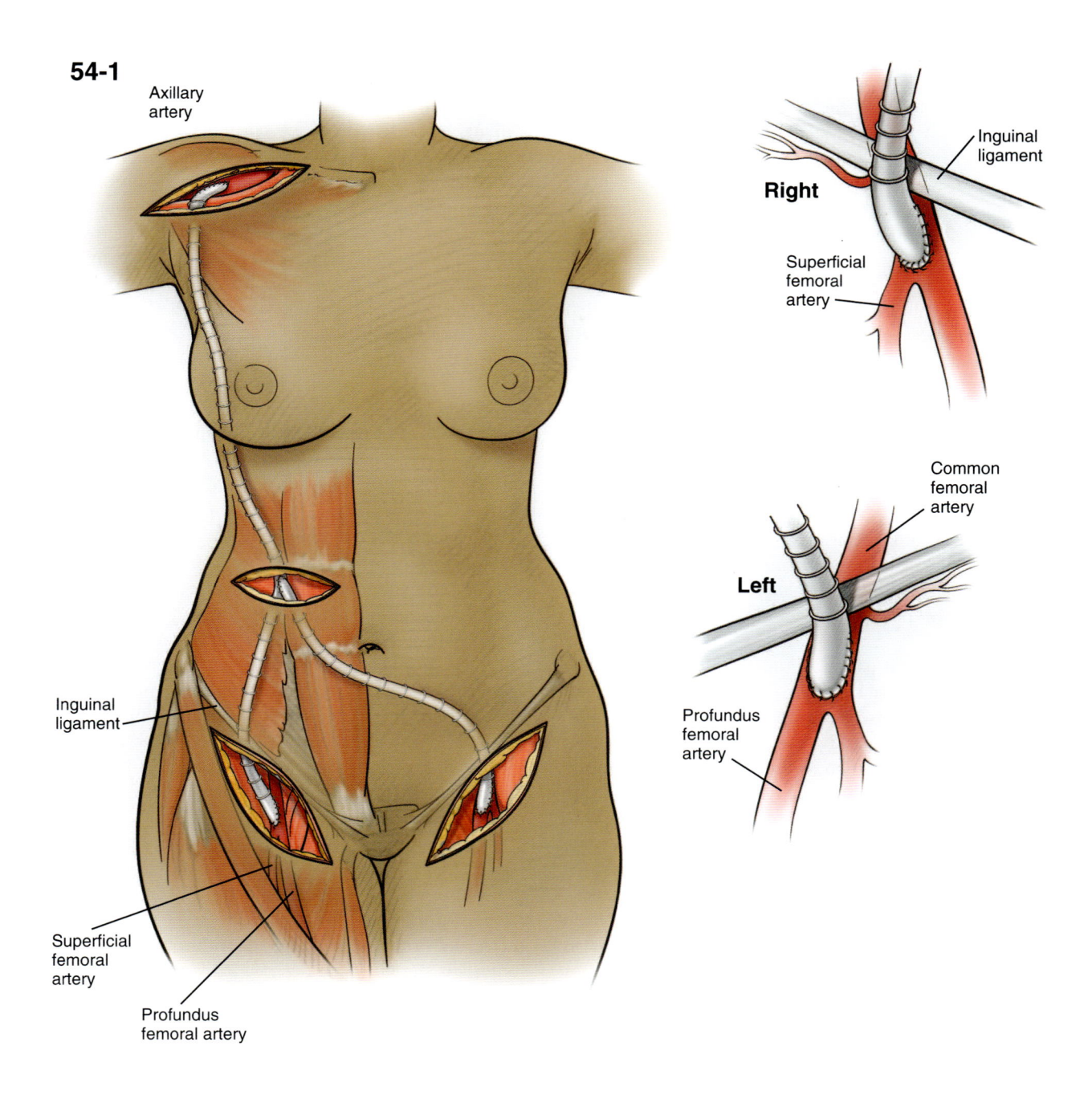

54-2

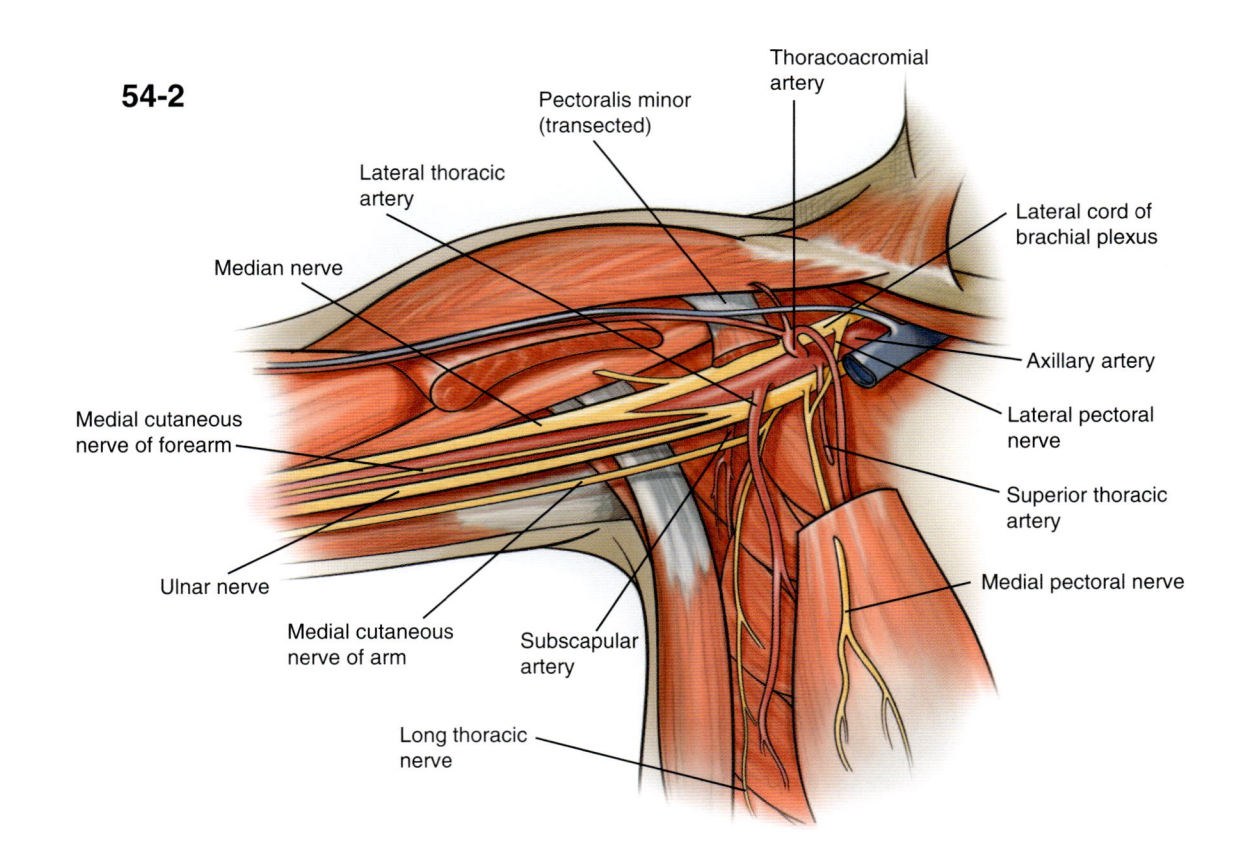

SURGICAL TECHNIQUE *AXILLO-BIFEMORAL BYPASS AND AXILLO-UNIFEMORAL BYPASS:* CONTINUED Although the proximal axillary artery can be exposed medial to the pectoralis minor muscle, satisfactory exposure usually will be aided by dividing this muscle, providing exposure to the second part of the axillary artery as well (FIGURE 54-3). Division causes no lasting disability. It is advisable to palpate the axillary artery to locate the most advantageous site for pectoralis minor division. The muscle is encircled by the surgeon's thumb and index finger, raised anteriorly, and divided using cautery. This will prevent inadvertent injury to the underlying brachial plexus and nerves.

The proximal anastomosis will usually be performed between the first and second parts of the axillary artery. In this area the axillary artery will be surrounded by the medial, lateral, and posterior cords of the brachial plexus but the anterior wall will be clearly visible. The axillary vein will partially cover the anterior portion of the first part of the axillary artery but will be more caudal in relation to the second part. The third part of the artery is significantly covered by neural structures, including the origin of the median and ulnar nerves and the medial cutaneous nerve of the forearm, thus making dissection inadvisable (FIGURE 54-2). Three branches of the axillary artery will be encountered during adequate dissection. Medially will be the thoracoacromial artery arising anteriorly and the superior thoracic artery from the inferior aspect, and laterally the long thoracic artery which usually arises from the lower border of the axillary artery. All can be sacrificed with impunity.

The femoral arteries are exposed using oblique groin incisions below the inguinal ligament. Although some surgeons prefer a vertical incision, an oblique incision heals better, and excellent exposure can be obtained by lengthening the incision laterally and lifting the inguinal ligament using retractors affixed to the table. The common, deep, and superficial femoral arteries should all be dissected to allow adequate inspection.

Polyexpandedtetrafluorethylene (ePTFE) (heparin-bonded or otherwise coated) as well as Dacron grafts have been utilized for these extra-anatomic grafts. The author's preference is an 8-mm ringed heparin-bonded ePTFE (Propaten) graft manufactured by Gore Medical (WL Gore & Associates, Flagstaff, AZ) Adding rings may prevent compression of the graft if the patient lies on their side, compressing an axillofemoral graft against the rib cage. Further, heparin bonding has been shown to improve patency rates of femoral-popliteal ePTFE bypass and may do the same for these grafts. Gore Medical also manufactures two lengths of a preconstructed axillo-bifemoral graft, thus obviating the need to perform an anastomosis to the crossover femoral. Furthermore, the configuration of the preconstructed graft results in an inverted "Y" shape after insertion (FIGURE 54-1), which may improve flow dynamics and long-term patency. Accordingly, if the surgeon prefers to construct an axillo-bifemoral bypass from two individual grafts, it is advisable that the anastomosis to the crossover be performed from a counter incision in the flank like what is required for the preconstructed graft (FIGURE 54-1) rather than arising distally in the ipsilateral groin region (FIGURE 54-4). It is possible that flow dynamics are not as linear as would occur using the flank take-off and may be related to the reported increased failure rates of the crossover portion of the bypass rather than the vertical limb.

An extra anatomical tunnel is created using an 8-mm tunneler starting under the pectoralis major. The author recommends the Scanlan (Scanlan International, Inc., Saint Paul, MN) plastic tunneler since its flexibility is useful. A long alligator clamp placed within the tunneler adds support during the tunneling. Tunneling from the groin toward the shoulder is not advised since there have been anecdotal occurrences where the tunneler has inadvertently penetrated the chest cavity using such an approach. The tunnel should be placed just posterior to the anterior axillary line so that the patient will be less likely to lie on the graft if they are a side sleeper. In most patients the tunneler will reach the ipsilateral groin if an axillo-unifemoral bypass is being performed. However, when an axillo-bifemoral bypass is constructed, a 2- to 3-cm counter incision is placed in the lower flank as high up on the flank as possible but still distal enough to allow the short limb of the axillo-bifemoral bypass graft to reach from the counter incision to the ipsilateral femoral artery. The tunneler is then pushed out through the counter incision. The **vertical limb of the axillo-bifemoral bypass graft is brought through** the tunneler from the counter incision into the axillary artery incision and positioned such that junction of the ipsilateral and contralateral limbs is visible in the counter incision. The femoral limbs of the graft are brought into the femoral incisions using an aneurysm clamp

passed subcutaneously from the groin incisions to the counter incision. Invariably, the long limb will reach the contralateral femoral artery. Rarely, extensions will be required to either limb but may be necessary in very tall patients or those with a very corpulent abdomen. In very obese patients, the surgeon should take into consideration that the abdominal bulge may not be as protuberant with the patient lying on the operating table and so extra length may be necessary so that stress is not put on the graft when the patient stands up postoperatively. Patients are then heparinized (the author uses 5000 units of heparin for all patients irrespective of weight, but weight-based doses can be given). Usually, all three anastomoses can be completed before further heparinization is necessary.

The axillary anastomosis is performed first. However, prior to performing the anastomosis, the graft will have to be trimmed and beveled. The surgeon needs to position it so that once anastomosed the graft will lie in a somewhat loose, lazy "C"-shaped turn such that if the patient elevates their arm directly above the head, there will be no tension on the anastomosis (FIGURE 54-3). The arteriotomy is placed anteriorly on the axillary artery. It is not advisable to place the anastomosis on the inferior or caudal aspect of the axillary artery as illustrated or described in older texts. These texts assume that the graft comes into the artery in the same plane, whereas it dives down from the anterior chest wall to the front of the artery. This old technique involves dividing inferior arising branches, placing clamps on the artery front to back and then rotating the clamps, and thus the artery, to bring this inferior aspect into view. Once the anastomosis is completed and the clamps released the artery rotates back into its original position. Therefore, only the anterior portion of the anastomosis may remain visible. However, the inferior position of the anastomosis can cause an unnatural sharp bend in the first part of the graft, which may lead to graft occlusion. Further, if the graft remains patent but then later occludes, redo surgery is more complicated since visualization of the entire anastomosis requires transection of the graft.

A 15-mm arteriotomy is used for the anastomosis with silastic loop control. An eye caliper is used to measure this distance, and the eye caliper is also used to measure how the graft is to be trimmed with a curved Metzenbaum scissors. Matching the two lengths creates a smooth anastomosis and prevents crinkling edges that can result in bleeding. The anastomosis is started at the heel, which is based laterally on the arteriotomy. Once completed, a hydrogel clamp is applied just distal to the anastomosis, taking care not to injure surrounding nerves. Silastic loops are released allowing flow into the distal arteries. Needle-hole bleeding can be limited by utilizing 4-0 thread on a C-1 needle. Topical thrombin or other hemostatic agents can be placed in the wound if necessary.

The ipsilateral femoral anastomosis is performed next but not fully completed. A hydrogel clamp is then placed on the contralateral limb in the counter incision and the graft is flushed by briefly releasing the axillary artery flow. The ipsilateral anastomosis is completed, and flow restored to that side. The graft is never flushed with saline since it may result in subsequent weeping of plasma through the graft pores. Similarly, flow into a completed proximal and distal anastomosis should not be allowed until vessel loops have been removed from the runoff arteries. Arterial flow into an occluded outflow can also result in subsequent serous fluid weeping and seroma formation.

The contralateral anastomosis is then completed in similar fashion, this time flushing by briefly releasing the clamp on the contralateral graft in the counter incision. Like for the ipsilateral anastomosis, it is generally advised that the anastomosis be performed across the common into the first few millimeters of the deep femoral artery even if the superficial femoral artery is patent since it is not unusual that the superficial femoral artery, which is patent currently, may become significantly diseased or occluded at a later stage. For both the ipsilateral and contralateral sides, it may be necessary to reconstruct a femoral bifurcation if the superficial femoral artery and deep femoral artery are patent but the common femoral is severely diseased. On occasion, endarterectomy may be required. If so, placing a bovine pericardial patch and then anastomosing the graft to the patch may prove beneficial. Protamine reversal is used in all patients. Topical thrombin or other topical agents may be utilized to decrease needle-hole bleeding if this is encountered.

All incisions are closed using a 3-0 absorbable suture for the subcutaneous tissue and 4-0 subcuticular suture. In the author's practice skin staples are also utilized. Pectoralis minor is not reattached, and pectoralis major should not require suture since it usually reapproximates after removal of the retractors. CONTINUES

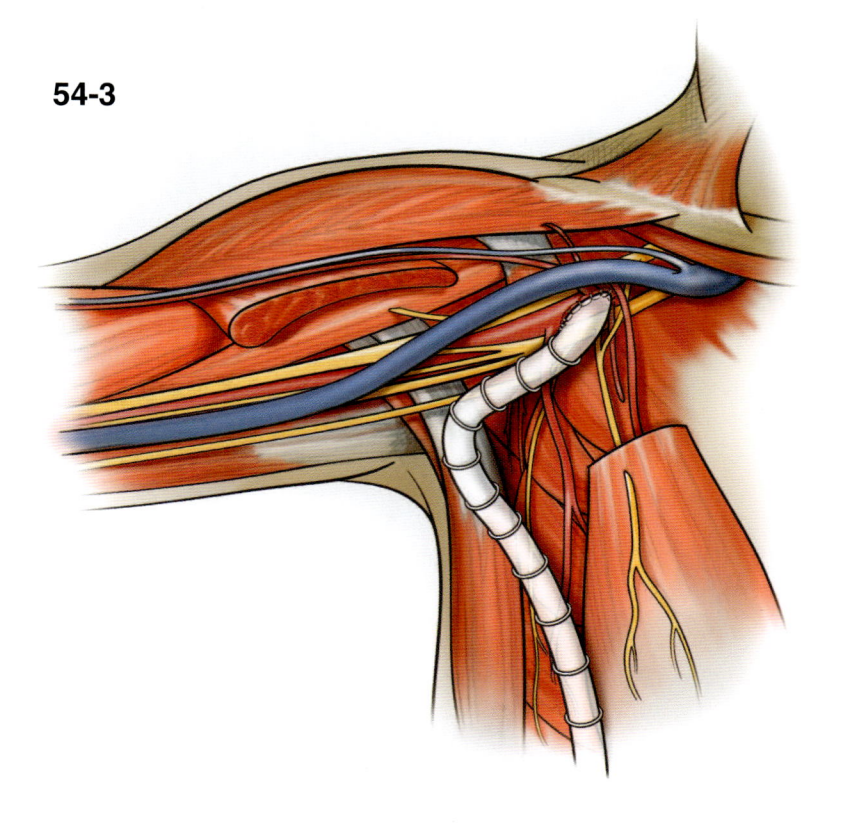

54-3

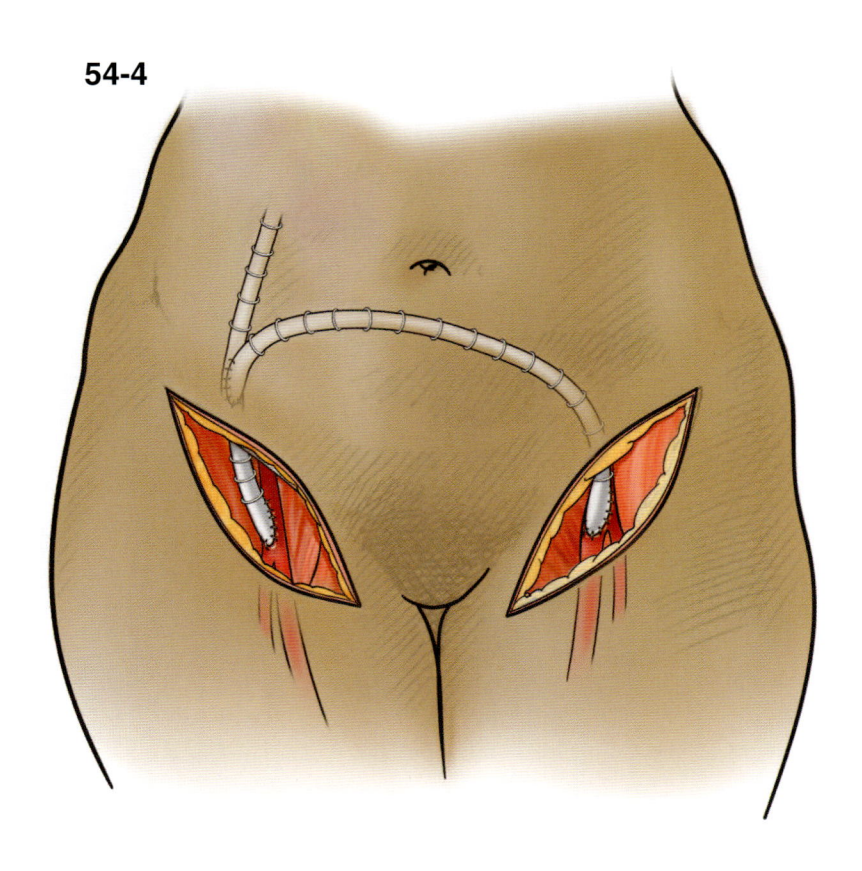

54-4

SURGICAL TECHNIQUE *FEMORO-FEMORAL BYPASS*: ◀ CONTINUED
General or spinal anesthesia can be utilized for these procedures. Skin prep, draping, and groin incisions are made as for axillo-bifemoral bypass. The ringed 8-mm ePTFE is delivered from side to side using a curved aneurysm clamp. The donor side is performed first. If the common femoral, origin of the superficial femoral, and deep femoral arteries are widely patent, the anastomosis should be placed as proximal on the common femoral as possible with the heel distal. This allows a slightly "S"-shaped graft configuration (FIGURE 54-5) rather than the upside down "C" like the crossover limb of a constructed axillo-femoral bypass (FIGURE 54-4). If not, the anastomosis can be placed more distally in the common, sometimes even with the toe being in the deep femoral artery.

The distal anastomosis should be constructed in a similar fashion to the contralateral limb of an axillo-bifemoral graft (see above).

FOLLOW-UP PROTOCOL Most patients do not require ICU care and can resume diet immediately. Routine postoperative management is prescribed. Prophylactic anticoagulants are not utilized unless required for indications unrelated to graft patency. Antiplatelet regimen usually involves aspirin and clopidogrel. Skin staples in the pectoral and counter incisions are removed at 1 week and groin staples usually on the tenth postop day.

Patients are encouraged to follow up every 6 months for a clinical evaluation, ankle-brachial indices, and color duplex evaluation of the graft as well as the inflow and outflow arteries. Color duplex and ankle-brachial indices are obtained outside of regular follow-up if there is any clinical indication of incipient graft failure. If this is confirmed, CTA and/or diagnostic arteriography should be added. The finding of a hemodynamically significant stenosis in the inflow or outflow is usually managed by an endovascular technique. This can usually be managed by a brachial artery approach or direct puncture of the graft where it lies over a rib or pubic bone. ∎

SUGGESTED READINGS

Ascer E, Veith FJ, Gupta SK, Scher LA, Samson RH, White-Flores SA, et al. Comparison of axillounifemoral and axillobifemoral bypass operations. *Surgery*. 1985;97:169-175.

Blaisdell FW, Hall AD. Axillary-femoral artery bypass for lower extremity ischemia. *Surgery*. 1963; 54:563-568.

Louw JH. Splenic-to-femoral and axillary-to-femoral bypass grafts in diffuse atherosclerotic occlusive disease. *Lancet*. 1963;1:1401-1402.

Samson RH, Showalter DP, Lepore MR Jr., Nair DG, Dorsay DA, Morales RE. Improved patency after axillofemoral bypass for aortoiliac occlusive disease. *J Vasc. Surg.* 2018;68(5):1430-1437.

54-5

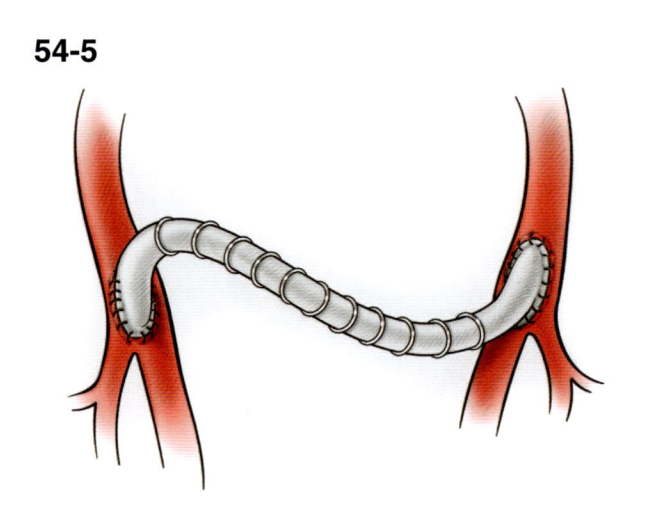

AORTA AND ILIAC INTERVENTIONS

Daniel Clair, MD • Daniel Mason, DO

INDICATIONS Endovascular intervention is currently a key component in the treatment of aortoiliac occlusive disease. Indications for endovascular intervention in these vessels include rest pain, tissue loss, and life-limiting claudication. While this type of severe claudication may commonly present as buttock and thigh pain, patients may develop calf pain and leg numbness. Severe aortoiliac atherosclerosis is associated with the classic triad of symptoms described by Henri Leriche as claudication of the buttocks and thighs, absent femoral pulses, and impotence.

The assessment of aortoiliac occlusive disease begins with a thorough history and physical followed by risk stratification, noninvasive studies, and imaging. History should include exercise or walking capacity, previous surgeries, vascular interventions, and comorbidities. The most common comorbidities include chronic tobacco use, hypertension, coronary artery disease, and chronic renal insufficiency. If the patient is under the age of 50 and presents with an aortic occlusion, a hypercoagulable state should be suspected. On physical exam, severe aortoiliac disease causes absent or diminished femoral and distal pulses; however, patients may have intact pulses in the femoral and pedal positions. More severe disease can often be associated with lower extremity ulcers and nonhealing wounds. Furthermore, risk stratification and comorbidity optimization is often needed for those with concomitant cardiac, pulmonary, and renal diseases.

While in the past digital subtraction angiography was considered the gold standard of imaging, this technique is now often performed intraoperatively as part of the revascularization procedure. Preoperative axial imaging studies are critical for surgical planning, and noninvasive vascular tests allow for functional assessment of the patient. Pulse volume recordings with toe pressure measurements and segmental pressures assess baseline disease severity. The baseline measurements provide a useful objective measure of success following revascularization, or a recurrence of a disease during follow-up appointments. Segmental pressures performed with a standardized walking test (often referred to as exercise ABIs or segmental pressures with stress testing) allow for an assessment of the degree of impairment patients experience. Axial imaging is best obtained with computed tomographic angiography of the abdomen, pelvis, and lower extremities and should allow visualization of contrast runoff into the distal vessels. When severe disease is present, this may require delayed imaging of the lower extremities to allow contrast to traverse collateral vessels into the distal vasculature. If the patient suffers from renal insufficiency, often associated with aortoiliac occlusion, arterial duplex ultrasonography can aid in preoperative axial vessel assessment. However, the quality of arterial duplex ultrasonography can be limited by obesity, bowel gas, and calcifications. Magnetic resonance angiography is an option and has the advantage of avoiding contrast and radiation. However, this imaging modality often overestimates stenosis and is associated with less detail in anatomic reconstruction. Axial imaging is important to assess the degree of stenosis in the aorta and iliac arteries as well as the common femoral arteries and femoral bifurcation. Additionally, it is important to have adequate assessment of the origins of the superficial femoral arteries and perhaps more importantly, the profunda femoris arteries.

POSITION The patient is placed in a supine position on a radiolucent operating table with the patient's head at the edge of the operating table. If an aortic or proximal common iliac artery occlusion is being treated, it can be helpful to have the left arm abducted and placed on an arm board. This allows for the option of antegrade access to the aortoiliac region if femoral retrograde recanalization of an occlusion proves difficult. The left side is preferred to avoid devices crossing the aortic arch vessel origins and increasing the risk for stroke. The right arm is usually tucked into the patient's side. It is helpful to have imaging monitor access in multiple planes to allow the operating surgeon to work comfortably from either side of the table and at either position (above or below) if left arm access is utilized.

OPERATIVE PREPARATION Prior to initiation of the case, surgical planning is discussed with the vascular team to ensure supplies are available. Computed tomography angiography of the aorta and bilateral lower extremities is performed to allow for preoperative planning. The caliber of the aorta, bilateral common femoral arteries, external iliac arteries, and common iliac arteries is determined to select for the appropriate size of sheaths, stents, and balloon catheters. Helpful preoperative information includes planned lengths and diameters of the aortic segment to be treated and the diseased iliac segments. Additionally, preoperative assessment should clarify if femoral endarterectomy is needed to improve artery outflow following treatment of the aortoiliac segment. Depending on the extent of disease, the interventionalist may plan for concurrent procedures of distal lower extremity angioplasty or surgical revascularization. Computed tomography angiography will allow identification of the location and severity of calcifications. Calcifications at the access site are a relative contraindication for closure devices due to increased risk of plaque rupture and may necessitate a cutdown to close the arteriotomy, or alternatively may provide an indication to use manual pressure to seal the access site in the groin.

Ideally, the vascular suite consists of a hybrid operating room, with a dedicated fixed C-arm for fluoroscopy, a motorized radiolucent operating table, and high-definition monitors allowing visualization in multiple planes from the operating table. For more complex endovascular procedures, the room should be prepared to accommodate conversion to an open procedure. Having the capability to convert procedures makes performance of hybrid procedures routine. The patient should be positioned in a manner that allows the C-arm to approach the patient from the head of the bed to allow for visualization of the entire aorta and iliac arteries. A side approach for imaging systems is needed in certain instances, such as imaging through the entire aortoiliac segment and the common femoral arteries in tall patients. This approach is necessary if concomitant distal revascularization is to be performed. **CONTINUES ▶**

For most percutaneous procedures, local anesthesia with sedation can be utilized. However, both patient and physician should understand that occasionally during complex interventions conversion to general anesthesia may be required. When extensive interventions are planned, two large-bore peripherally inserted venous access catheters should be utilized. Similarly for complex interventions, placement of an arterial line for continuous invasive pressure monitoring is helpful. The sphygmomanometer and arterial line should be placed on the right arm when considering using the left arm for access. Use of a Foley catheter for urinary drainage may also be necessary in these situations.

After the patient is sedated, the surgical field is prepped from umbilicus to distal thighs, including bilateral groins. The left arm is prepped from mid-forearm to the shoulder. A sterile drape is used to cover the perineal region. The entire field is prepped with 2% chlorhexidine via sterile applicator and allowed to dry for 3 minutes. The surgical sites are then draped in sterile fashion.

INCISION AND EXPOSURE   For percutaneous procedures, the common femoral arteries should be accessed in a retrograde direction with the use of micropuncture technique under ultrasound guidance. Ultrasound guidance has been proven to reduce access time, access attempts, and access site complications. Significant disease in the common femoral arteries or disease at the femoral artery bifurcation mandates an open or hybrid approach. This approach would entail femoral artery endarterectomy in addition to intervention in the aortoiliac segment. While reports have provided evidence that the common femoral artery may be treated with interventional therapy, in most situations this vessel is best treated with endarterectomy and patch angioplasty. To reduce infection risk, biologic-based patches should be utilized and if significant infection risk is present, autogenous tissue should be utilized. Maximizing the outflow with this hybrid approach ensures the best chance for long-term success. For those undergoing hybrid procedures, longitudinal incisions are made bilaterally to expose both femoral arteries and their bifurcations. Extensive exposure of the vessel allows the surgeon to perform an extended endarterectomy.

Exposure of the inguinal ligament with dissection of the lower edge of this ligament allows for mobilization of the ligament and surgical exposure of the distal external iliac artery. Proximal to the inguinal ligament there is often a crossing vein which can be easily injured. It is often best to electively divide this vessel between ligatures to avoid venous bleeding from a deep portion of the wound. The distal external iliac artery should be mobilized and isolated to allow for later clamp placement. Dissection is then carried distally on the artery to a point beyond the common femoral bifurcation. Branches along the common femoral artery will often include the superficial circumflex iliac artery, superficial epigastric artery, superficial external pudendal artery, and deep external pudendal artery. Preserving these vessels is important because they provide blood supply to the skin and soft tissue in the area of the incision. It is also helpful to position the initial skin incision slightly lateral to the artery itself, which can keep the dissection away from the saphenous vein and allows medial mobilization of inguinal lymph nodes, thus reducing the risk of postoperative lymphatic leak. Dissection of the superficial femoral artery should be carried at least 4 to 5 cm beyond the origin of this vessel, while dissection of the profunda femoris artery is often easily carried beyond the first branch point of this vessel. Frequently, a vein branch crosses slightly beyond the origin of the profunda and this vein should be carefully dissected and divided between ligatures. Isolating the branches of the profunda artery allows for easier performance of an eversion endarterectomy and allows excellent visualization of the origin of this vessel after the endarterectomy has been performed. Femoral artery endarterectomy and patch angioplasty procedures can be performed before or after the interventional portion of the procedure. When endarterectomies are performed before the procedure, the sheath can be delivered directly through the patch. However, when utilizing devices larger than 10 French, insertion following the endarterectomy can damage the reconstructed vessel, especially when the patient has extensive calcification in the femoral artery. Endarterectomy in the presence of severe calcification can lead to extensive thinning of the remaining femoral artery wall, and attempting to place large devices through these vessels can lead to significant disruption of the vessel wall. **CONTINUES** ▸

INCISION AND EXPOSURE `CONTINUED` After endovascular access is obtained, place a sheath and associated guidewire. If the occlusion or disease is easily crossed with access from below, advance the guidewire proximal to the diseased segment and insert a pigtail catheter. Using this catheter, obtain arteriograms of the area of the vasculature to be treated and identify the location of important vessels, including the superior mesenteric, renal, and collateral arteries. Additionally, the arteriogram will confirm guidewire placement in the aorta. If the occlusion cannot be traversed from below, access should be obtained from a vessel that allows for imaging above the area of disease. This can be performed from the left brachial or even left radial artery. Once again, access should be obtained under ultrasound guidance in retrograde fashion with the wire and catheter advanced into the descending thoracic aorta and ultimately into the abdominal portion of the aorta above the area of occlusion. Aortography should be performed to identify visceral and renal vessel origins and their relationship to the level of occlusion (FIGURE 55-1, FIGURE 55-2).

DETAILS OF PROCEDURE After access has been obtained, the patient should be systemically heparinized with 80 to 100 units/kg of heparin. The most commonly utilized wire for traversing an occlusion is a 0.035″ stiff, hydrophilic wire. Using this wire in conjunction with a hydrophilic crossing catheter, traverse the occlusion. This process may involve rotating the wire or catheter continuously and manipulating the wire through the lesion. Often the most challenging portion of the traversal is the access across the upper aspect or cap of the occlusion. This may involve adding support to the system to allow adequate forward pressure to engage the top of the lesion. It is often advantageous to "bury the system," or to advance sheath, catheter, and wire as a unit into the top of the occlusion. Next, begin wire rotation and advancement, moving the catheter forward in conjunction with the wire as feasible. After crossing the cap of the lesion and advancing distally in the occlusion, the wire may enter a subintimal plane and advancement of a wire loop may be used to complete lesion traversal. It is often easier to re-enter the true lumen distal to the iliac artery origin, as the atherosclerotic plaque in the iliac vessels becomes thinner and less calcified distally. Once the wire is thought to be through the lesion, one should aspirate through the catheter to confirm blood return for affirmation of the catheter position within a patent vessel. Once this has been completed, angiography should be performed to confirm the intraluminal position. After the catheter is confirmed to be in a patent vessel distally, the wire can be snared from the groin to allow through-and-through access and an easy method to advance devices. Alternatively, a rigid wire can be positioned from the proximal access. Once the through-and-through or rigid wire access is obtained, the channel can be dilated with a relatively small diameter balloon. Depending upon the native vessel size, either a 5-mm or 6-mm diameter balloon can be used to dilate the tract. The sheath from the groin can then be brought through this channel, and wire access from below into the patent vessel above can be achieved. Attention is then brought to creating a channel through the contralateral iliac system. For this stage of the procedure, it is helpful to use preoperative axial imaging in conjunction with intraoperative angiographic imaging to identify the location of the aortic bifurcation. A short-tipped angled catheter can then be advanced from the proximal access site into the channel. The catheter is positioned slightly above the bifurcation and angled toward the contralateral iliac system. If the catheter is advanced at this point without the wire, it will engage the occlusion, allowing for wire advancement through the contralateral iliac artery and traversal through the contralateral iliac system. The wire should be used in conjunction with the catheter, both of which may require rotation to allow advancement, similar to the procedure performed at the upper aspect of the vessel occlusion. Once again, confirmation of position within a patent vessel is performed, the wire is snared from below and a channel created with a relatively small diameter balloon. The sheath is then advanced through the channel and wire advanced from below into the patent system above. Often from each groin, a catheter is advanced over the through-and-through wire into the aorta above the occlusion, thus maintaining access through the lesion at all times. The wire is then withdrawn from above and a new wire positioned in the aorta from the groin catheter. This technique assures each wire is maintained in the same channel that has been created. Once the access through the occlusion has been achieved from each groin, treatment can be initiated (FIGURE 55-3). Treatment is performed utilizing measurements from axial images obtained preoperatively with calibrated angiography performed intraoperatively. It is important to remember that the aorta does not need to be dilated to the aortic wall. Instead, a channel needs to be created with adequate diameter to supply reasonable flow to the lower extremities allowing for normal activity (FIGURE 55-4). In most situations, 10- to 12-mm diameter channels in the aorta will provide adequate blood supply. While covered stents have proven to be more effective in the treatment of complex iliac lesions, the same has not been shown for aortic disease. For this reason, use of large diameter self-expanding stents is usually adequate to treat aortic occlusions with favorable outcomes. More recently, larger diameter venous stents with extensive wall coverage and stable deployment systems have been utilized. Covered stents (either balloon expandable or self-expanding) have been utilized when dilated to at least 10 or 12 mm. In most situations, re-creation of the aortic bifurcation provides excellent flow and can preserve the ability to gain access across the aortic bifurcation. When placing the aortic stent, it is best to deploy this stent from the most challenging groin access to recanalize. This assures the system has wire access maintained during the entire stenting portion of the procedure. After aortic stent placement, the wire from the contralateral femoral access site is then repositioned within the aortic stent. It has been helpful to position both femoral sheaths in the most proximal iliac artery to allow imaging of the bifurcation with contrast injection from the side not being used for stent deployment. Additionally, this allows the surgeon to easily mark the location of the aortic bifurcation while deploying the aortic stent. If a self-expanding stent has been used, the stent should be post-dilated with an appropriately sized balloon (usually either 10 or 12 mm in diameter) (FIGURE 55-5). After the aortic stent has been positioned proximally to the aortic bifurcation, covered iliac stents should be positioned. Because of the ability to achieve precise positioning, we have found balloon-expandable covered stents to be advantageous. It is appropriate to attempt to achieve the apposition of the upper aspect of these stents, but to avoid extensive "raising of the bifurcation." Once these stents have been expanded, the balloons should be advanced partially into the aortic stent and inflated to ensure adequate expansion of the upper aspect of these stents and the lower aspect of the aortic stent. `CONTINUES`

55-1

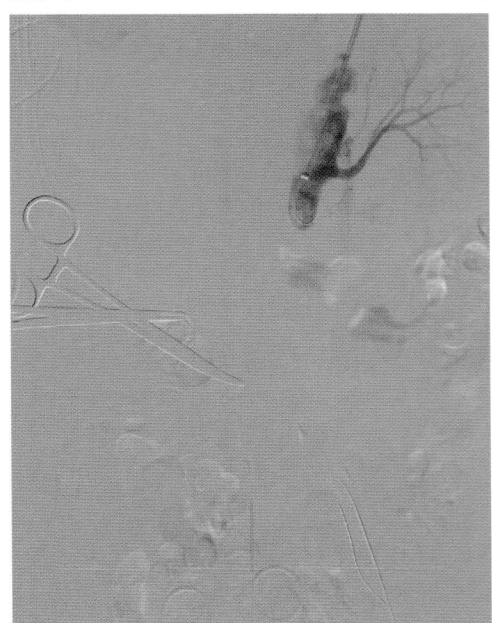

55-2

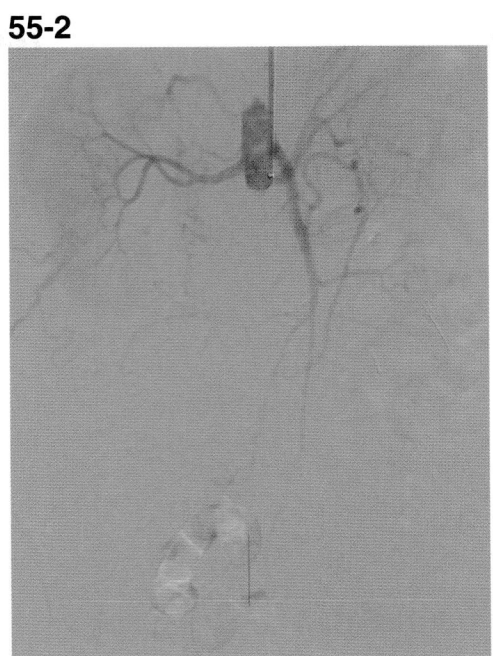

55-3

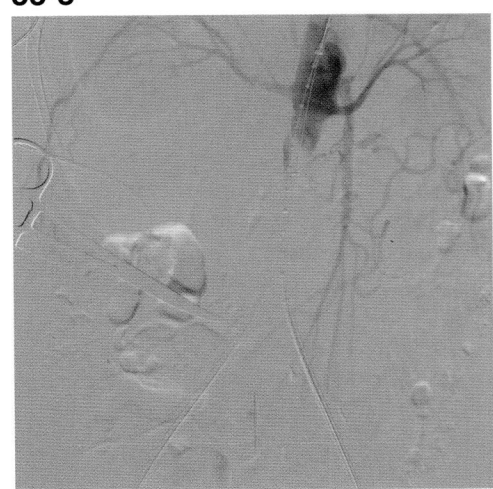

55-4

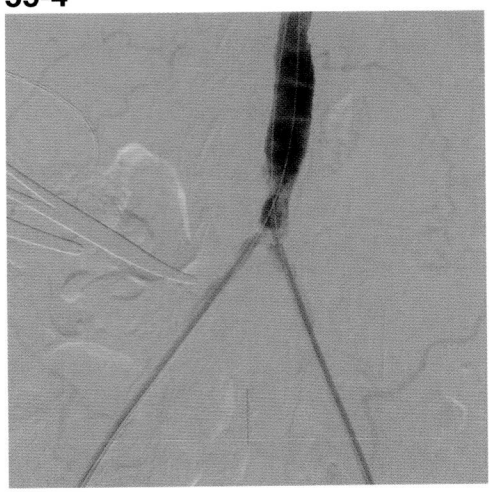

55-5

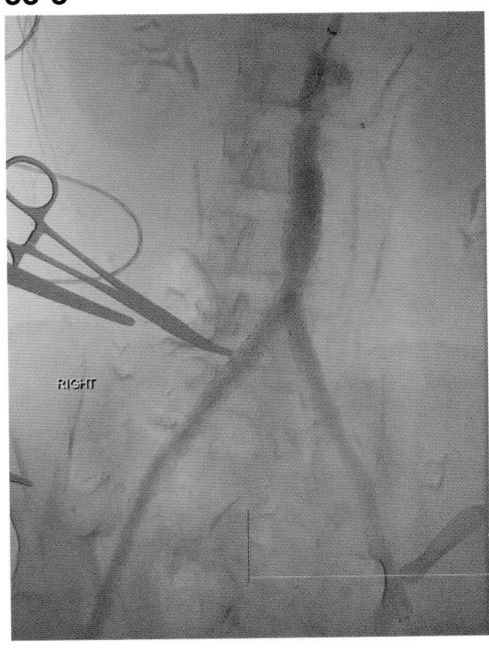

DETAILS OF PROCEDURE **CONTINUED** Simultaneous balloon inflation assures the stents will dilate similarly and balloon inflation can be taken through the entirety of the aortic stent to achieve a symmetric flow channel (**FIGURE 55-6**). The remainder of the procedure is identical to treating iliac artery disease. Stents should be extended to completely cover the area of disease. Preservation of internal iliac flow is preferred if feasible. The use of self-expanding stents in the external iliac arteries is preferred.

Special mention should be made regarding the situation in which an occlusion of the aorta abuts the renal arteries. This situation poses a particular risk for embolization of debris into the renal arteries. There are several options that have been used to address this situation. These options include lysis of proximal thrombus, placement of protective balloons, and stent deployment proximally with distal transition of the stent. The use of lytics is controversial, as many of these patients present with long-standing occlusion and lytic therapy is not as successful in this situation. Despite this concern, in many instances lytic therapy can resolve some of the proximal thrombotic burden and reduce the risk for proximal embolization into renal or visceral vessels. When performing lysis, it is important to have an adequate flow channel established, as some debris from the lysis is inevitable. If this debris flows into the renal arteries rather than down the aorta, it can lead to impairment of renal flow and renal dysfunction. A flow channel allows this debris to pass downstream where the continued effects of lysis dissolve the thrombus. A channel is created with inflation of 5- to 6-mm angioplasty balloons through the iliac systems. Ten- to 20-cm infusion catheters are then positioned through the occlusion, and lysis is continued overnight. Intervention can then be performed the following day, and in most instances the proximal thrombus has been removed and stenting has a much lower risk for renal embolization in this situation. An alternative strategy is to utilize the upper extremity access to place angioplasty balloons in the renal arteries during the time of aortic stent deployment. This technique is very effective in alleviating risk to the kidneys but requires a large enough arm access to allow dual balloon access (**FIGURE 55-7**). While protecting the renal arteries, this does not protect the superior mesenteric artery, and debris can be embolized proximally into this vessel, particularly during balloon inflation in the aortic stent. Finally, deploying a self-expanding aortic stent over the lower half of the renal arteries and then withdrawing the delivery system to cover the upper aspect of the debris is another protective strategy. This can keep the debris from entering the renal arteries, but this is not always completely protective. It is important to recognize renal and visceral embolization as potential complications and to assess for these complications after placement of the aortic stent. Completion angiographic evaluation should include images of these vessels (**FIGURE 55-8**).

Completion imaging should be performed before removing the femoral sheaths. Imaging at this stage of the procedure can be performed from the upper extremity access through a flush catheter or from one of the femoral sheaths. Visualization of the renal arteries should be included in the angiographic images. In some instances, selective catheterization of the renal arteries and the superior mesenteric arteries should be performed. Increasingly in performing these complex revascularizations, the use of post-procedure intraoperative axial imaging has become helpful. Use of intravascular ultrasound or on-table CT imaging allows visualization of the stented segment, the degree or adequacy of stent expansion, and assessment of stent irregularity. This imaging can reduce the need for early re-intervention and assure the primary reconstruction is optimized. Following completion of the angiographic and axial imaging, the sheaths can be removed. When hybrid procedures are being performed, the sheath access sites in the patch can be repaired directly. Alternatively, if the reconstruction has been performed prior to the endarterectomy, balloon control can be used proximally while the femoral endarterectomy is performed. If percutaneous reconstruction was performed, the use of closure devices reduces the need to hold compression on the vessel which has only recently been revascularized. When deploying closure devices, it is critical to assure the distal aspect of iliac stents are not damaged during closure device deployment. This may necessitate fluoroscopic imaging during device deployment.

COMPLICATIONS Complications of these interventions can occur at nearly every point in the procedure. It is critical to be aware of these complications and to understand how to potentially prevent them from occurring. Access site complications can occur at any site. Female gender and larger sheath size are associated with increased risk. Additionally, brachial artery access has a higher rate of complications than femoral artery access. The relative size difference in the artery increases its risk of occlusion and therefore hand ischemia. Additionally, the risk for pseudoaneurysm is higher with this approach as well. For larger sheath sizes in this location, especially those over 7 French, surgical closure of the access eliminates the risk of these complications. Endovascular repair also carries a risk of retroperitoneal hematoma formation. Formation is more likely when thrombolysis is performed. Hematoma formation can be reduced by minimizing the number of access sites, assuring accurate access below the inguinal ligament and adequate compression following sheath removal. Alternatively, closure devices have been shown to reduce bleeding at access sites and allow earlier mobilization of patients.

Pseudoaneurysms can also form following endovascular treatment and have differing treatments for differing severities. If a pseudoaneurysm is suspected, duplex ultrasound should be obtained. A pseudoaneurysm smaller than 2 cm may resolve spontaneously, but ultrasound-guided compression has also been used in these situations with good success. Most pseudoaneurysms are currently treated with direct ultrasound-guided thrombin injection into the neck of the pseudoaneurysm. While thrombin injection can be associated with increased risk of main artery occlusion, when properly administered this treatment is highly effective in the majority of situations and is extremely low risk. With this approach, pseudoaneurysms with neck diameters of greater than 5 mm carry a higher risk of complications, and surgical treatment should be considered primarily in this setting. Surgical intervention is also indicated when a pseudoaneurysm leads to neurologic impairment, overlying skin changes, skin necrosis, or extensive bleeding from ruptured pseudoaneurysm. Reduction of access site complications can be achieved by using ultrasound guidance for percutaneous access, which ensures direct access to the desired arterial location.

Another rare but potentially fatal complication is iliac artery rupture. This complication is common with severe calcification or small diameter vessels. Following dilation of previously occluded iliac arteries, imaging to assess for rupture should be performed. Ideally, the diagnosis is made prior to hemodynamic changes with immediate post-dilation angiography. When extravasation is noted, the balloon can be reinserted and inflated to relatively low pressure to occlude the area of rupture. This will allow the anesthesia team to administer volume and the surgical team to acquire necessary endovascular equipment to seal the rupture with a covered stent. Prior to deflating the balloon, the proceduralist should assure that the device is prepared for insertion, the sheath size is adequate for introduction, the team is prepared to rapidly insert sheath and position and deploy the device as needed, and the anesthesia team has needed support and adequate resuscitation has been given and available. At this stage of the procedure, if the sheath size is inadequate a larger diameter sheath must be available and prepared. It is often helpful for the surgeon to verbally describe the plan so all of the team members understand the planned order of events. When imaging does not reveal evidence of rupture, as may rarely occur, rupture should be suspected when significant blood pressure drop is seen via the arterial line with accompanying tachycardia. Rupture can be prevented by correctly assessing artery diameter and calcifications on preoperative computed tomographic angiography, and in situations where the vessel is felt to be at higher risk (heavy calcification, diminutive vessel diameter) proactive use of covered stent for treatment of this region allows for comfortable dilation of this segment. **CONTINUES**

55-6

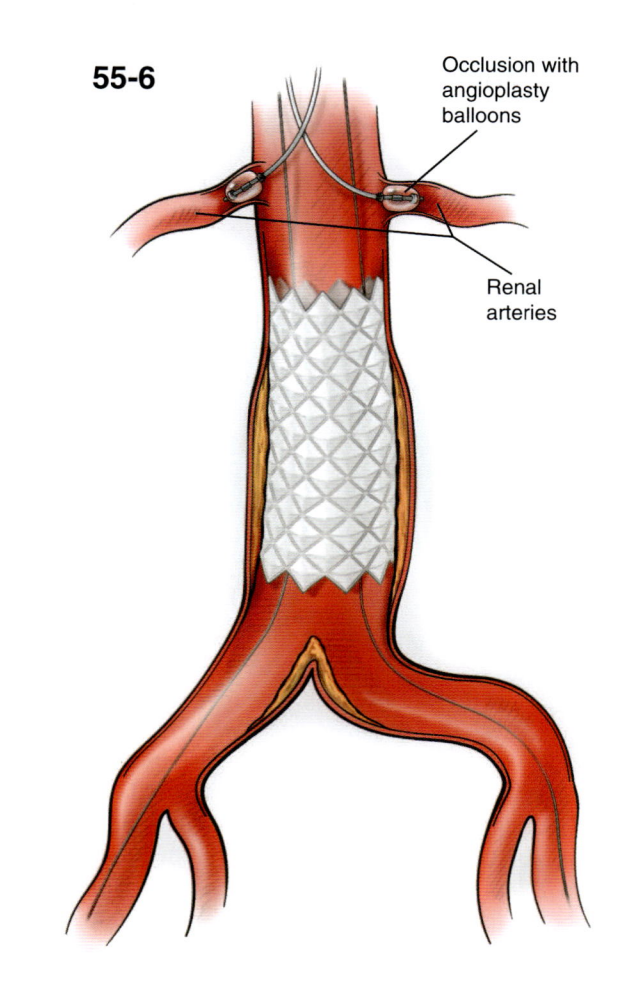

Occlusion with angioplasty balloons

Renal arteries

55-7

55-8

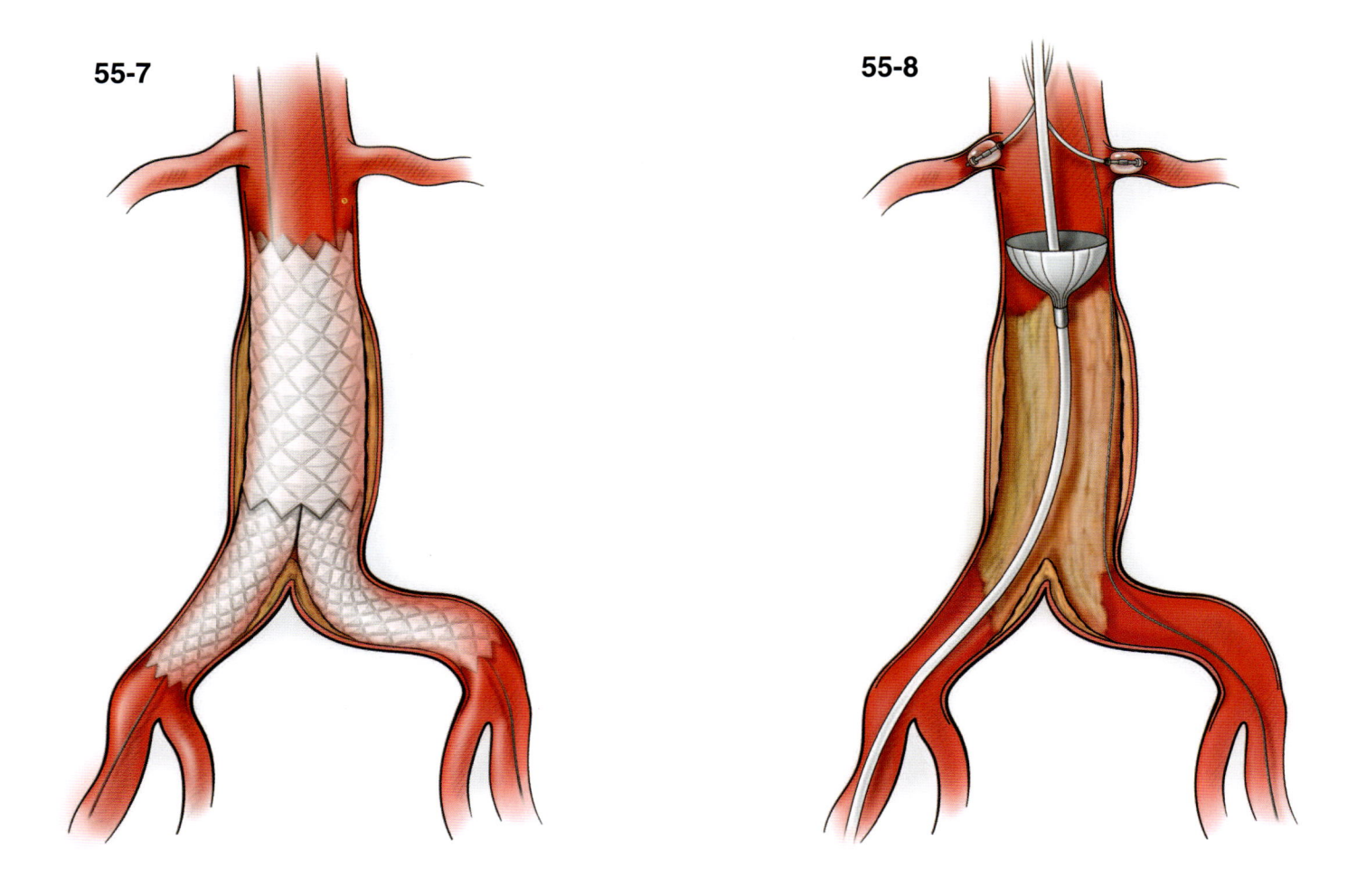

COMPLICATIONS `CONTINUED` Distal embolization can be a significant complication that can lead to devastating consequences. Manipulation of any piece of endovascular equipment in the vasculature can create detrimental emboli, and a number of techniques can be used to reduce the risk of this adverse consequence. Immediately following endovascular access, the patient should be therapeutically anticoagulated with heparin. Careful manipulation of any endovascular equipment, including wires, catheters, and balloons, can decrease the risk of emboli. One should ensure devices are advanced carefully within the lumen of the vessel and that methodical advancement is performed. Extended angioplasty times (>30 seconds) have been shown to reduce both embolization and flow-limiting dissection. Finally, stent placement after smaller caliber balloon dilation can allow the stent to be delivered precisely and to trap potential embolic debris and potentially reduce embolization. After completing a complex intervention, imaging of the entire lower limb vasculature should be performed to assure no embolic debris has complicated the procedure and blocked the distal vasculature. If embolic debris is identified, it should be pursued with aspiration or other means of embolus retrieval.

During any interventional procedure that involves the use of contrast material, acute renal injury can be encountered. Given the relatively common association of aortoiliac disease, diabetes mellitus, and renal insufficiency, one should be cognizant of the patient's underlying level of renal dysfunction. In the perioperative setting, acute renal failure can be a result of contrast toxicity or renal embolism. The risk can be decreased by minimizing contrast and provision of adequate intravenous fluids before and after surgery. If the creatinine is above 1.5 mg/dL, sodium bicarbonate infusion may aid in preventing this complication. Standard contrast mixtures can be further diluted and still allow adequate resolution for intervention, particularly in the lower extremities. Additionally, the use of CO_2 angiography can nearly eliminate the need for contrast angiography. If acute renal failure does occur, treatment is supportive with diligent attention to ensuring adequate volume status as well as close monitoring of electrolyte status and urine output.

CLOSURE The authors prefer the use of a suture mediated closure device for sealing vessel access. However, in situations of extensive scarring or vessel wall calcification, alternative closure devices may be utilized. These devices have been proven to reduce hematoma and pseudoaneurysm formation, but leave a foreign body and thus by their nature have an inherent infection risk. Thus when using closure devices, careful attention to sterile technique is imperative. It is helpful to assess the pulse in the vessel distal to the access site following the procedure to assure the closure device has not led to vessel occlusion, which can rarely occur. If the pulse is inadequate or there is concern regarding the flow through the access point, ultrasound can be utilized to assess the flow through the area of interest.

Closure of the femoral artery exposure in hybrid operations is an important part of assuring an excellent outcome. Closure is best performed in layers utilizing monofilament absorbable suture material (Monocryl or polydioxanone [PDS] sutures). Braided sutures have the potential to increase infection risk and should be avoided. The femoral sheath is reapproximated initially, sealing the femoral vessels and patch of the endarterectomy site from the upper layers of the closure. Two additional subcutaneous layers of resorbable, monofilament tissue approximation follow the sheath closure and the skin is approximated with subcuticular suture. Finally, skin adhesive is applied superficially to seal the wound completely. While vacuum-assisted closure devices have had some proven benefit to reduce infection rates in high-risk patients, these devices are not routinely utilized.

POSTOPERATIVE CARE The primary goal of postoperative care is to monitor for the main contributors of postoperative mortality, which include cardiac, pulmonary, and renal dysfunction. As many aortoiliac occlusion patients are advanced in age, it is critical to initiate early mobilization and physical therapy. Aggressive, early mobilization can reduce length of stay and increase discharge to home after these procedures. After the procedure, the patient is admitted to the hospital, keeping the patient supine for no more than 2 to 4 hours. If the brachial artery was accessed percutaneously, without surgical incision closure, the arm is kept extended with the use of a stiff arm board for 4 hours. An Ace wrap can be used to help reduce swelling and to keep latent compression on the access site. Initially following the intervention, neurovascular checks should be performed every hour with instructions to include motor and sensory evaluations along with assessment of distal pulses or auscultation of pedal Doppler signals. Generally, the patient can have their home medications restarted. One should confirm the patient is on a statin and dual antiplatelet therapy for the next 4 to 6 weeks. If the patient had presented with a hypercoagulable state, or another indication for anticoagulation for other causes, anticoagulation medication should be restarted the next day. In most instances, patients with complex percutaneous reconstructions can be discharged after 1 night in the hospital. For those patients undergoing hybrid revascularization, hospitalization for 1 or 2 nights may prove necessary. If the patient previously suffered from significant limitations of their activity related to their vascular insufficiency, a brief stay in a rehab center may be required to help improve the patient's activity level.

Patients are scheduled for a postoperative follow-up appointment in 4 weeks. For those patients who have undergone complex endovascular reconstruction of their aorto-iliac segment, CT angiography allows visualization of the reconstruction. This imaging study should be combined with noninvasive testing of the adequacy of the revascularization with segmental pressure assessment including documenting the ABI readings. If one has already obtained adequate axial imaging during the procedure or early afterward, then duplex imaging of the iliac vessels can provide a baseline from which to follow the patient and should be combined with segmental pressure assessments and pulse volume recordings. If there are no issues or complications, visits are performed every 6 months for the first year and then annually thereafter. At each appointment, a thorough history should be obtained to assess for symptoms, and a physical exam should be performed which should include a full pulse, motor, sensation, and skin exams. Skin exams should involve investigation for abnormal skin changes or foot wounds as well as site checks for vascular access devices. Evidence of re-stenosis may include new onset of related symptoms, a duplex showing >50% diameter reduction, doubling of peak velocities, or a drop in ABI greater than 0.15. ■

SUGGESTED READINGS

Cameron JL. Aortoiliac occlusive disease. In: *Current Surgical Therapy.* Philadelphia, PA: Elsevier; 2020:968-976.

Clair DG, Beach JM. Strategies for managing aortoiliac occlusions: access, treatment and outcomes. *Expert Review of Cardiovascular Therapy.* 2015;13(5):551-563. doi:10.1586/14779072.2015.1036741

Kashyap VS, Pavkov ML, Bena JF, et al. The management of severe aortoiliac occlusive disease: Endovascular therapy rivals open reconstruction. *Journal of Vascular Surgery.* 2008;48(6). doi:10.1016/j.jvs.2008.07.004

Mwipatayi BP, Sharma S, Daneshmand A, et al. Durability of the balloon-expandable covered versus bare-metal stents in the Covered versus Balloon Expandable Stent Trial (COBEST) for the treatment of aortoiliac occlusive disease. *Journal of Vascular Surgery.* 2016;64(1). doi:10.1016/j.jvs.2016.02.064

Ray JJ, Eidelson SA, Karcutskie CA, et al. Hybrid revascularization combining iliofemoral endarterectomy and iliac stent grafting for TransAtlantic Inter-Society Consensus C and D aortoiliac occlusive disease. *Annals of Vascular Surgery.* 2018;50:73-79. doi:10.1016/j.avsg.2017.11.061

Schneider PA. The infrarenal aorta, aortic bifurcation, and iliac arteries: advice about balloon angioplasty and stent placement. In: *Endovascular Skills: Guidewire and Catheter Skills for Endovascular Surgery.* Boca Raton, London, New York: CRC Press; 2020:313-327.

Taeymans K, Groot Jebbink E, Holewijn S, et al. Three-year outcome of the covered endovascular reconstruction of the aortic bifurcation technique for aortoiliac occlusive disease. *Journal of Vascular Surgery.* 2018;67(5):1438-1447. doi:10.1016/j.jvs.2017.09.015

Obturator Bypass

C. Yvonne Chung, MD • Matthew R. Smeds, MD

INDICATION An obturator bypass is an extra-anatomic bypass that provides in-line flow from an inflow vessel in the pelvis to an outflow vessel in the upper leg via the obturator foramen of the pelvis. Customary inflow sources include the common or external iliac artery or a limb of an existing prosthetic bypass, and the usual outflow vessels may include the deep or superficial femoral arteries or the popliteal artery. The primary use of this procedure is to exclude placing a prosthetic bypass graft through an infected femoral triangle, particularly when no autogenous conduit is available, or a "hostile" groin due to prior procedures, radiation, or malignancy. Modern series with significant numbers of cases are lacking; however, mid-term patencies have been reported as high as 88% at 2 years, with a significant number of reinterventions in these often complex and sick patients.

PREOPERATIVE PREPARATION A thorough history and physical exam with particular attention to previous vascular interventions is important in preoperative planning. Prior abdominal surgeries, gynecologic surgeries, and hernia repairs that may impede exposure of the obturator canal are also pertinent to note. CT imaging helps in evaluating the extent of infection, if the procedure is being performed for this indication, while providing anatomic details of the external iliac and obturator arteries as well as patency of above-knee popliteal artery as a potential bypass target. Vein mapping by duplex ultrasound identifies availability of autogenous conduit if appropriate to use.

ANESTHESIA General anesthesia with endotracheal intubation is routine. An arterial line provides continuous hemodynamics monitoring as well as convenient sampling for blood gases and activated clotting time after heparin administration. A Foley catheter should be placed for bladder decompression to aid in surgical exposure and minimize risk of bladder injury. Large-bore peripheral intravenous catheters can provide sufficient access for medication and fluid administration without the need for central venous access.

POSITION AND OPERATIVE PREPARATION The patient is positioned supine with a slight Trendelenburg position to aid in retraction of bowel from the lower abdomen. In the case of groin infection, the infected area is first excluded from the bypass surgical field with sterile surgical prep and covered with Ioban. Surgical prep is then fully performed again over the groin Ioban to include the abdomen up to the xiphoid process, groin, and ipsilateral leg circumferentially to the toes. Ioban is placed again over the abdomen, groin, and thigh to minimize skin contaminants to the surgical field and bypass conduit.

INCISION AND EXPOSURE An oblique incision along a dermatome line extending from 3 cm medial to the anterior superior iliac spine to 2 cm above the pubic symphysis is created. Fascial layers of the external oblique, internal oblique, and transversalis abdominis are divided along the direction of their fibers until the peritoneum is exposed and kept intact (**FIGURE 56-1**). A self-retaining retractor set with adjustable retractor blades is used for exposure.

DETAILS OF PROCEDURE The peritoneum and intraperitoneal content are swept medially with sponge sticks to expose the psoas muscle. Inferior epigastric vessels along the deep surface of the rectus abdominus muscle are identified and preserved to maintain all collaterals if possible. The ureter crosses the psoas and external iliac artery and should be identified and protected. Using a self-retaining retractor set, deep retractor blades are positioned superiorly and medially for retraction of the peritoneal contents. The lateral femoral cutaneous nerve travels along the lateral pelvic wall, and injury to the nerve from retraction should be avoided. With the retroperitoneum exposed, the common, external, and internal iliac arteries are identified, dissected, and encircled with silastic vessel loops. The common and external iliac arteries lay along the medial border of the psoas muscle (**FIGURE 56-2**), the latter of which exits the pelvis posterior to the inguinal ligament. Injury to the iliac vein, which lays posterior to the artery, should be carefully avoided as it can lead to significant blood loss. **CONTINUES ▶**

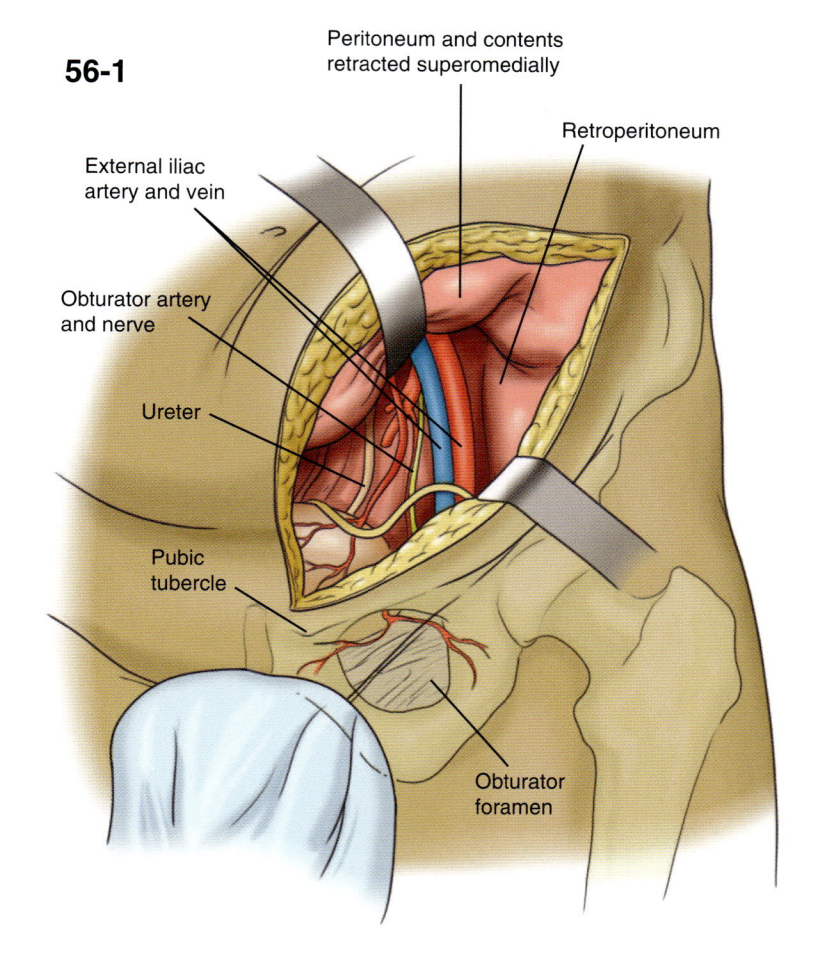

Figure 56-1 Retroperitoneal incision.

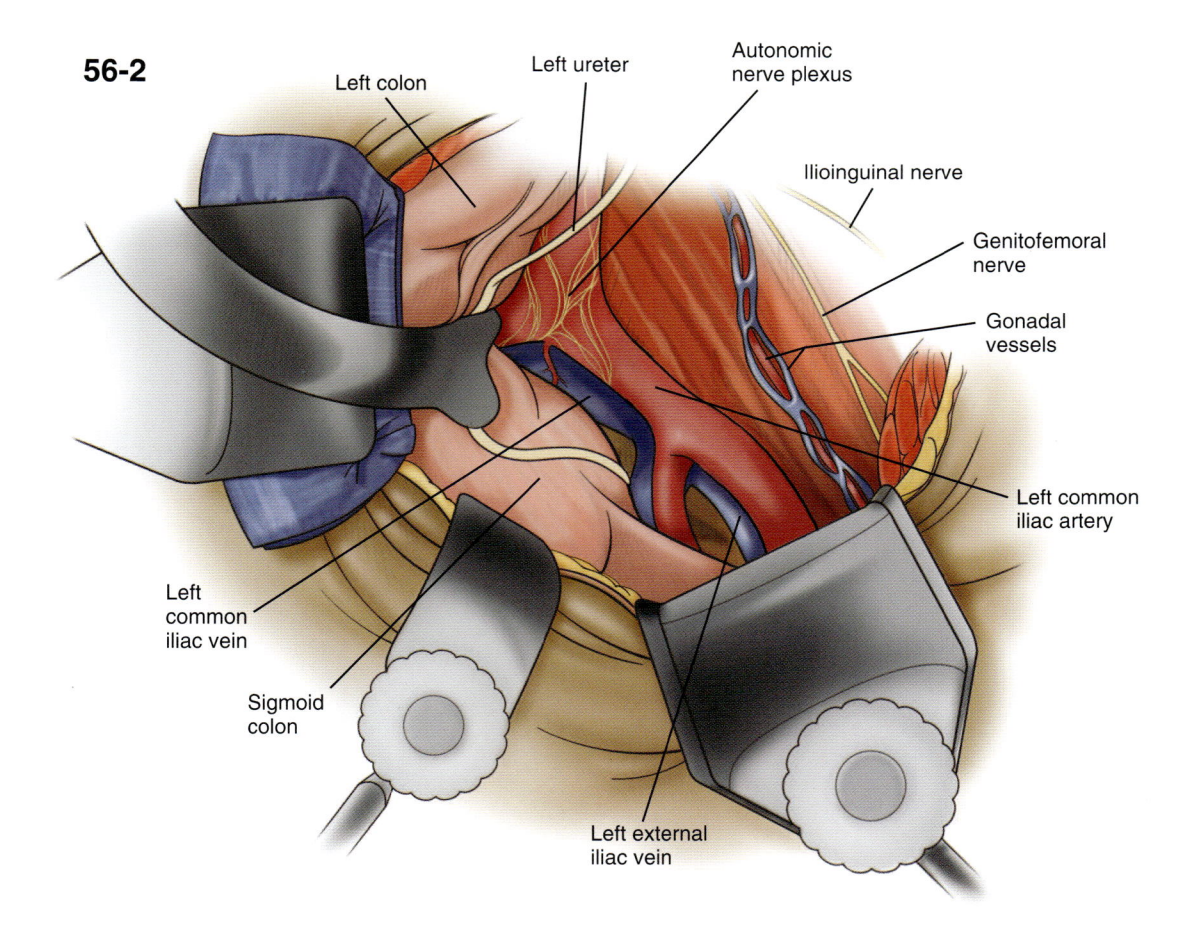

Figure 56-2 Exposure of external iliac artery and obturator foramen with colon mobilized.

DETAILS OF PROCEDURE `CONTINUED` Once inflow vessels are controlled, exposure of the distal bypass target is performed with the abdominal retractors relaxed to allow hip flexion and external rotation. A medial mid-thigh incision is created below the adductor longus tendon. The subcutaneous tissue is divided down to the sartorius. The sartorius is retracted posteriorly and the adductor magnus anteriorly to identify the neurovascular bundle at the adductor hiatus. The distal superficial femoral artery or above-knee popliteal artery is dissected and isolated with silastic vessel loops (FIGURE 56-3). Returning to the abdomen, the retractors are re-expanded while protecting the bladder anteromedially and the rectum posteromedially. The obturator foramen is identified by tracing downward along the pubic ramus and is approached medial to the external iliac vein and posterior to the superior pubic ramus. The obturator artery, a branch of the anterior division of the internal iliac artery, and the obturator nerve pass through this foramen (FIGURE 56-4). `CONTINUES`

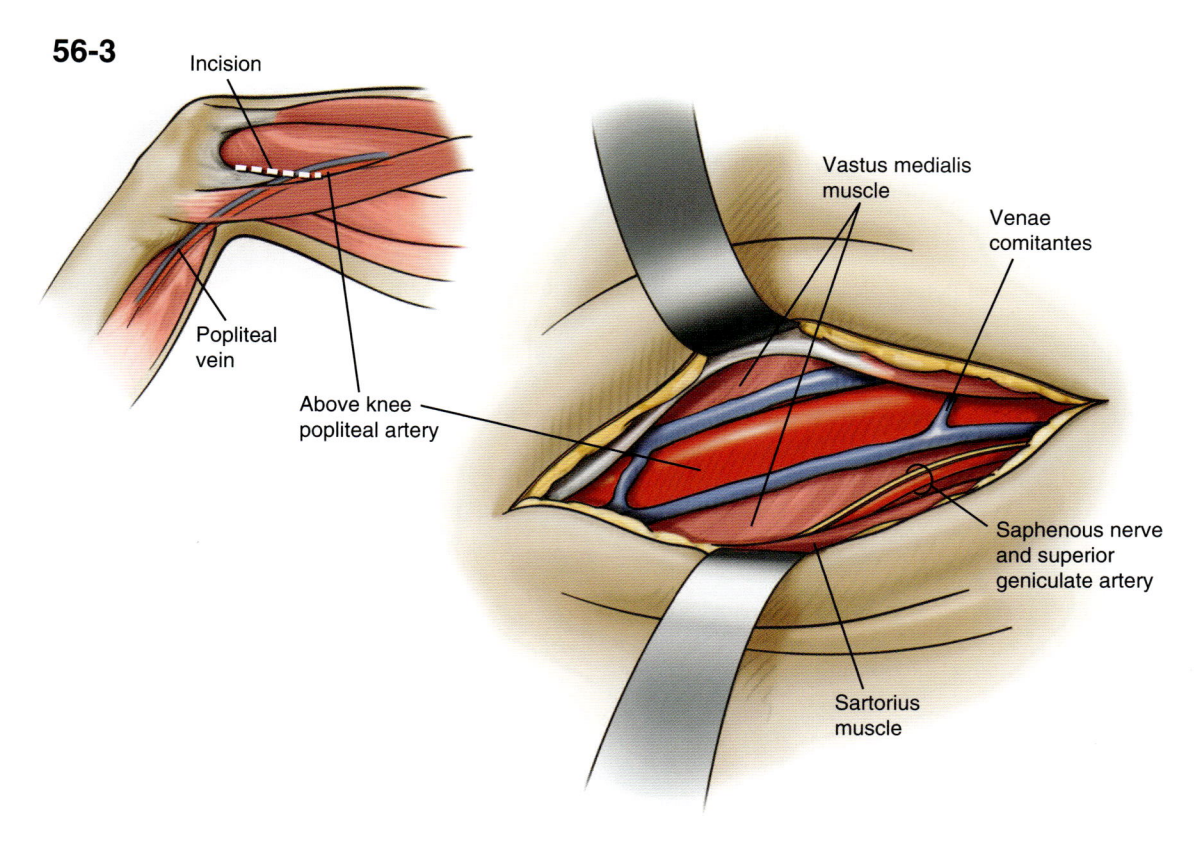

Figure 56-3 Above knee popliteal artery exposure.

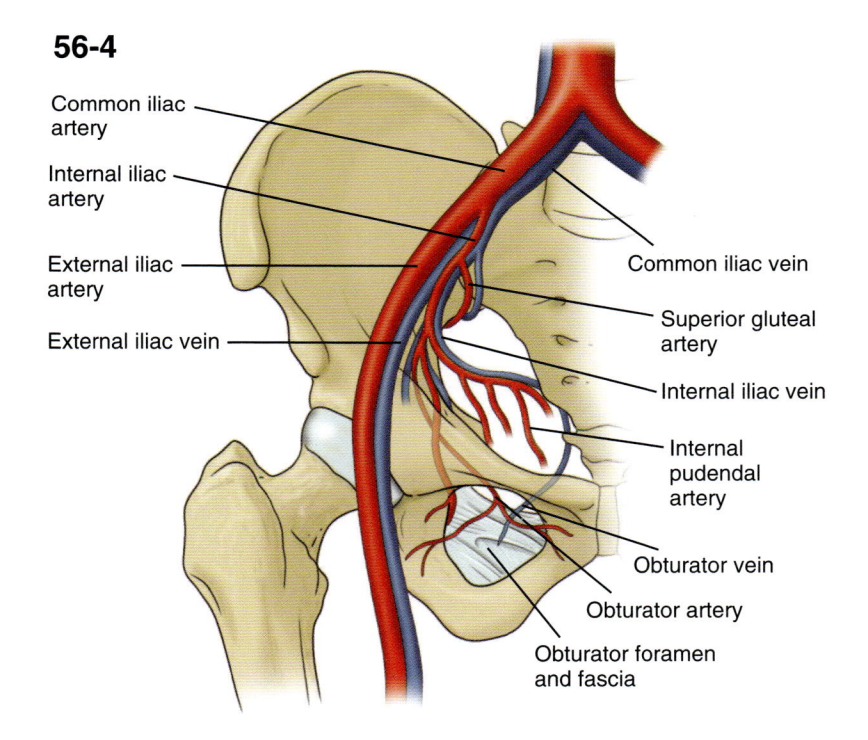

Figure 56-4 Dissection of obturator foramen and fascial band.

DETAILS OF PROCEDURE `CONTINUED` In males, the spermatic cord crosses the obturator neurovascular bundle and should be preserved, while in females, the crossing round ligament can be divided. The obturator neurovascular bundle passes through the lateral portion of the foramen, therefore the graft should be tunneled through the anteromedial part of obturator membrane. The foramen membrane may be tough and require sharp incision or electrocautery followed by blunt dilation. The tunnel may be developed bluntly using a curved aortic clamp. In the thigh, the tunnel courses between the adductor magnus posteriorly and adductors brevis and longus anteriorly (FIGURE 56-5).

Tunneling from the top down with a slightly curved sheathed tunneler can help avoid trauma to rectum, bladder, and vagina. An 8-mm externally reinforced PTFE graft is passed through this tunnel from the donor artery in the pelvis to the target artery in the leg (FIGURE 56-6). In rare instances, the inflow may be taken from the contralateral iliac artery. In these cases, the graft is tunneled through the space of Retzius between the bladder and pubic symphysis.

Systemic heparin is administered with goal ACT of at least 250 seconds and maintained while the arterial anastomoses are created. Proximal and distal clamps are placed and a longitudinal arteriotomy is made in the common or external iliac artery. The inflow anastomosis is created between this arteriotomy and the graft using 5-0 or 6-0 Prolene or PTFE suture in a running manner. Once the anastomosis is hemostatic, flow is restored to the native artery while the graft is clamped. The distal anastomosis is created in a similar fashion once the graft is trimmed to length. After completion of the anastomoses, the quality of pulsation and flow is interrogated with palpation and handheld Doppler at the outflow artery. After the bypass is completed, the external iliac artery distal to the inflow anastomosis may be ligated if necessary.

CLOSURE Meticulous hemostasis is achieved in both wounds. Protamine sulfate is given for heparin reversal. The abdominal fascia is reapproximated in anatomic layers with running 0 or 1 monofilament suture. The distal incision fascia and subcutaneous layers of both incisions are closed with absorbable sutures. Skin is closed with subcuticular Monocryl, and skin glue is applied to both incisions. Once both incisions are cleaned and dried, Ioban drape is reapplied over both to avoid potential contamination from the infected groin, if applicable.

Groin debridement is then performed if appropriate. Excision of infected arterial segment may be necessary, though the superficial and deep femoral arteries should be kept in continuity, if possible, as the profunda will be perfused retrograde from the distal anastomosis.

POSTOPERATIVE CARE Postoperative care is provided in a monitored setting where assessment of lower extremity perfusion is performed frequently, and any concerning change is addressed immediately. Without violation of the peritoneum, intestinal ileus is generally avoided, and the patient's diet may be advanced as tolerated. Appropriate antibiotic coverage for groin infection, if necessary, is continued through the perioperative period. ■

SUGGESTED READINGS

Bath J, Rahimi M, Long B, Avgerinos E, Giglia J. Clinical outcomes of obturator canal bypass. *J Vasc Surg.* 2017 Jul;66(1):160-166.

Guida PM, Moore SW. Obturator bypass technique. *Surg Gynecol Obstet.* 1969 Jun;128(6):1307-1316.

Reddy DJ, Shin LH. Obturator bypass: technical considerations. *Semin Vasc Surg.* 2000 Mar;13(1):49-52.

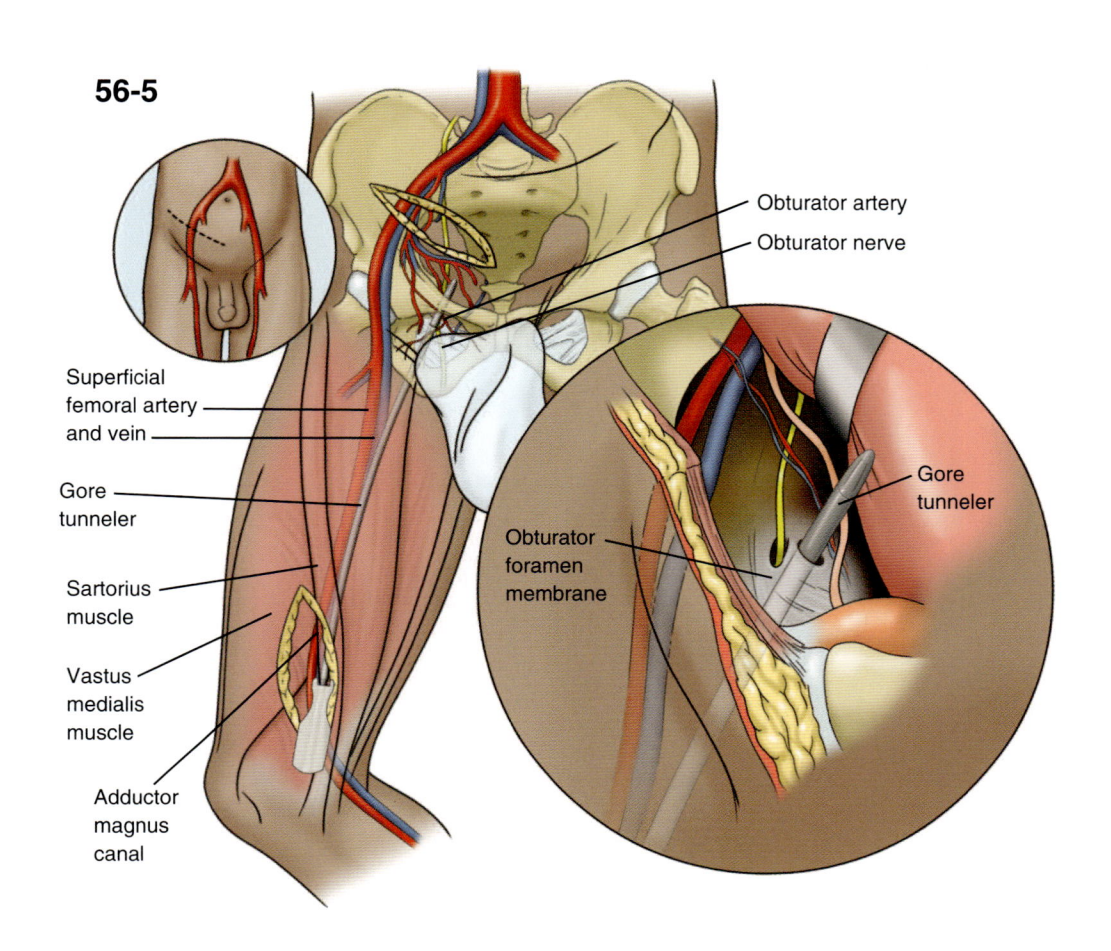

Figure 56-5 Creating tunnel and avoiding the groin.

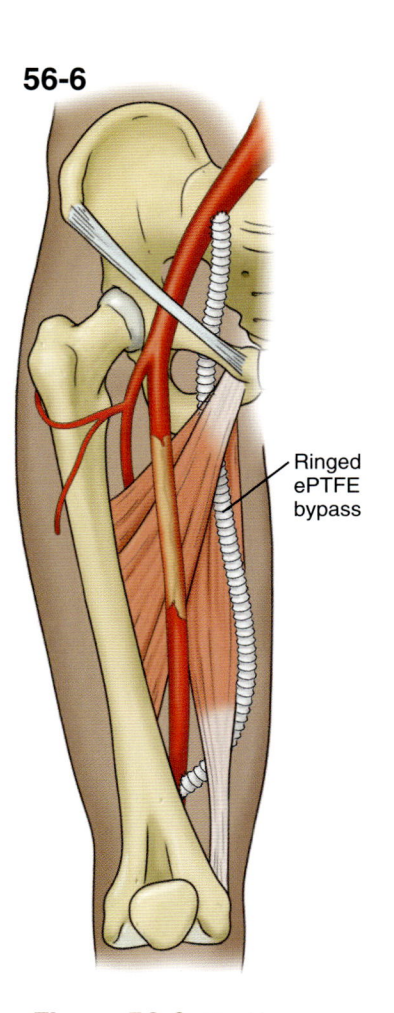

Figure 56-6 Final bypass.

Section XII

LOWER EXTREMITY OCCLUSIVE DISEASE AND ANEURYSMS OPEN

Femoral Endarterectomy and Profundaplasty +/– Iliac Stenting (Hybrid)

Brian Grant, MD • Hosam El Sayed, MD • Jean M. Panneton, MD

INDICATIONS Common femoral artery (CFA) atherosclerotic disease represents a key area of treatment in the management of patients with advanced peripheral arterial disease and chronic limb-threatening ischemia. CFA atherosclerotic disease can present as isolated calcific and bulky disease, or as a subset of multilevel atherosclerotic disease involving the iliac arteries and distal aorta.

Despite advances in endovascular technology, open intervention remains the gold standard for CFA atherosclerotic disease. Endovascular techniques in this location are generally associated with increased technical failure and poor long-term patency when compared with open surgical repair. Additionally, the profunda femoris artery (PFA) is a critical vessel for perfusion of the thigh musculature and collateral distal flow in the setting of a significantly diseased superficial femoral artery (SFA). It is at increased risk for occlusion, thrombosis, or embolization with endovascular intervention. In conjunction, atherosclerotic disease in the iliac arteries can severely impede arterial inflow and is responsible for debilitating symptoms. Hybrid reconstructions such as femoral endarterectomy and profundaplasty with retrograde iliac stenting allow for avoidance of more morbid procedures and are increasingly being used for multilevel reconstructions.

A thorough history and physical is performed with emphasis on the arterial status of the lower extremities. The patient is optimized with cardiovascular risk factor modification, smoking cessation, and initiation of antiplatelet agents. All these measures help with secondary prevention of cardiovascular morbidity. Statin therapy is extremely important for its plaque stabilization and cardioprotective effects.

Preoperative imaging to assess both vascular anatomy and physiology aids in operative planning. Preoperative ankle-brachial index (ABI) with segmental and toe pressures is mandatory to establish baseline perfusion and to allow for post-intervention comparison. Additionally, lower extremity segmental arterial pressures can identify a component of inflow (iliac) or outflow (femoral-popliteal) disease. Anatomical studies including computed tomography angiography (CTA), magnetic resonance angiography (MRA), and digital subtraction angiography (DSA) are utilized for diagnosis and to aid in preoperative planning of clamp sites.

ANESTHESIA General anesthesia is commonly employed, and local/regional anesthesia is preferred in patients with significant cardiopulmonary comorbidities. However, recent studies have not demonstrated decreased perioperative cardiac complications with local/regional anesthesia. Large-bore intravenous access and invasive hemodynamic monitoring via arterial line are recommended.

POSITION AND OPERATIVE PREPARATION A hybrid room or an operating room with x-ray compatibility is necessary. The patient is placed in supine position, and the lower abdomen, bilateral groins, and the ipsilateral leg are circumferentially prepped and draped in standard fashion. Standard prophylactic antibiotics are administered.

INCISION AND EXPOSURE The CFA is palpated at the mid-inguinal point, midway between the pubic symphysis and the anterior superior iliac spine below the inguinal ligament. The artery is generally easily palpable due to the calcified arterial wall. The type of incision is guided by surgeon preference, but a longitudinal incision is preferred as it has the advantage of being extended for more proximal and distal exposure as needed. Sharp dissection is performed through the subcutaneous tissues and deep fascia, keeping medial to the sartorius muscle to expose the femoral sheath. Dissection is carried out in a vertical soft tissue plane overlying the artery, avoiding the creation of dissection flaps with resultant devascularization and potential dead space. If lymphatics are encountered, they should be securely ligated with suture or surgical clips to reduce the risk of seroma or lymphocele formation. The femoral sheath is entered using sharp dissection. The CFA is dissected from inguinal ligament proximally onto the proximal SFA distally (**FIGURE 57-1A**). Cephalad retraction of the inguinal ligament aids in exposure of the distal external iliac artery. Anatomic variants branching off the CFA are also dissected circumferentially. Care should be taken to avoid injury to the inferior epigastric and deep circumflex iliac arteries at the junction between the common femoral and external iliac arteries at the inguinal ligament level. The profunda femoris usually originates posterior-laterally from the CFA at the level where the vessel changes caliber, and where the CFA continues as the SFA. A key gateway to exposure of the PFA includes mobilization of the SFA and retracting it medially (**FIGURE 57-1B**). The overlying lateral femoral circumflex vein usually requires ligation and division to allow for exposure of the proximal profunda femoris. Occasionally, you will need to go further distal and ligate the crossing profunda femoral vein.

The extent of exposure of femoral vessels depends on the location of the disease and the length of vessel needed to ensure safe clamp placement and avoidance of clamp injury. The inguinal ligament may be partially divided if more proximal exposure of the external iliac artery is necessary, but should be reapproximated at the end of the operation to avoid hernia formation.

DETAILS OF PROCEDURE

FEMORAL ENDARTERECTOMY AND PROFUNDAPLASTY: The patient is systemically heparinized with 100 units/kg of unfractionated heparin, with additional dosing if required to achieve an activated clotting time (ACT) greater than 250 seconds. Clamps or vessel loops are applied to the distal external iliac artery, SFA, and PFA arteries. Clamp orientation is important with reference to residual plaque, and care is taken to avoid crushing the clamp. In general, clamps are placed in the AP position rather than medial lateral. Other smaller branches are controlled with traction using silastic loops. Occasionally, due to heavy and extensive calcification within the external iliac artery, the use of balloon occlusion can be employed with a 5- to 8-mm Fogarty type balloon with stop cocks attached. A longitudinal arteriotomy is performed on the anterior surface of the CFA and extended beyond the length of the plaque. The length of the arteriotomy is determined by the underlying length of plaque. In general, the clamps should be placed approximately 2 cm above and below the proposed arteriotomy site. The arteriotomy may extend distally over either the ostium of the profunda femoris (most commonly) or SFA, depending on which vessel is more diseased and requiring more intervention (**FIGURE 57-2**). One can also extend the incision along both and use a larger pantaloon patch.

The arteriotomy should not involve the crotch of the bifurcation. In cases where the SFA is patent, the arteriotomy extends into it beyond any significant plaque. In cases where the SFA is occluded, the arteriotomy is extended into the profunda. A freer elevator is utilized to create a cleavage plane within the media of the femoral artery (**FIGURE 57-3A**).

Attention to the depth of the cleavage plane is prudent to avoid excessive thinning and weakening of the remaining arterial wall. A very deep endarterectomy plane may lead to destruction of the vessel and the need for complete vessel replacement with an interposition graft. A smooth feathering of the plaque is created in both the proximal and distal endpoint by gradually decreasing the depth of the cleavage plane. Care should be taken during this process distally, where the direction of pulling on the plaque should be from distal to proximal against the direction of flow to allow for creation of a smooth feathering and distal endpoint. Occasionally, this is facilitated by transecting the edge of the plaque to obtain a distal endpoint. Intimal tacking at the distal endpoints can be performed with 7-0 Prolene suture. This prevents dissection propagation distally once flow is restored (**FIGURE 57-3B**). **CONTINUES ▶**

57-1

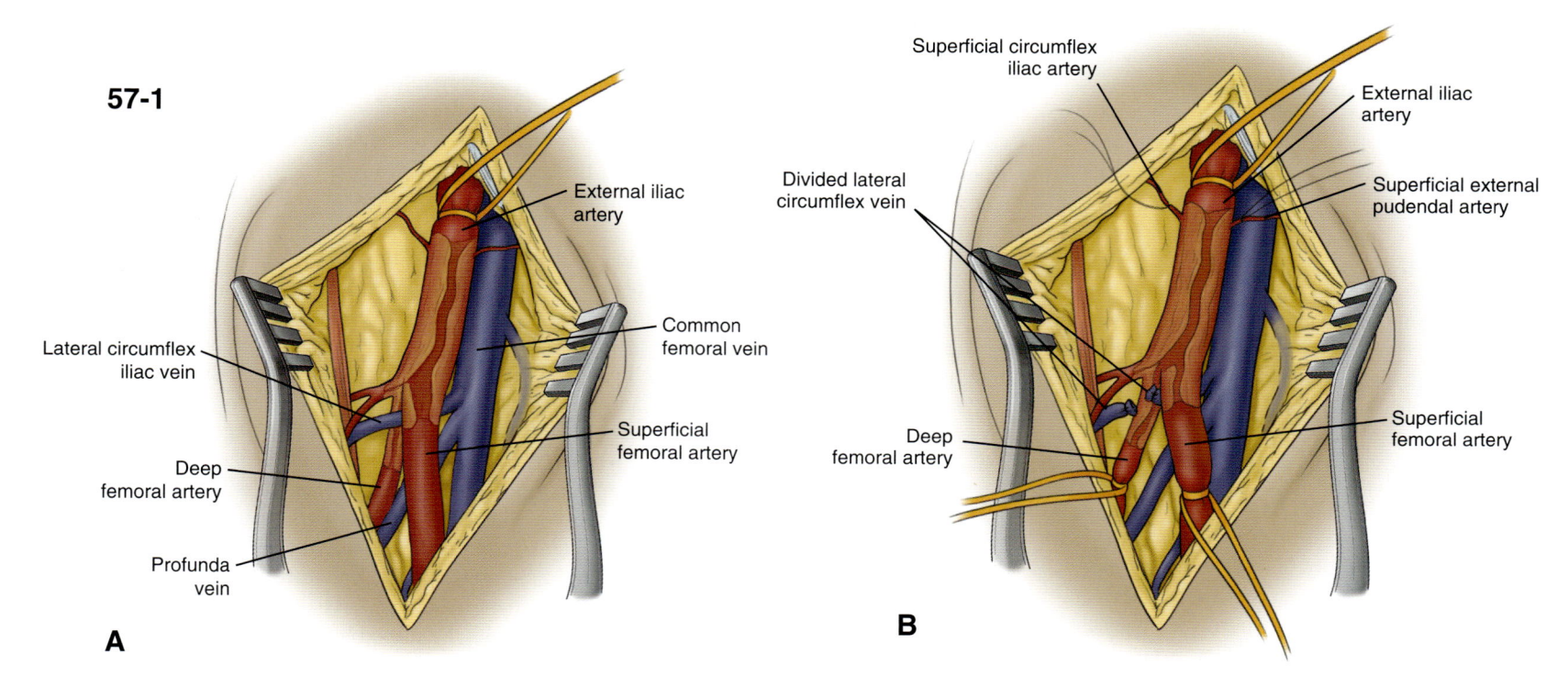

Figure 57-1 A. Femoral arteries dissection and exposure. B. Medial retraction of the SFA to expose the profunda femoris artery (PFA).

57-2

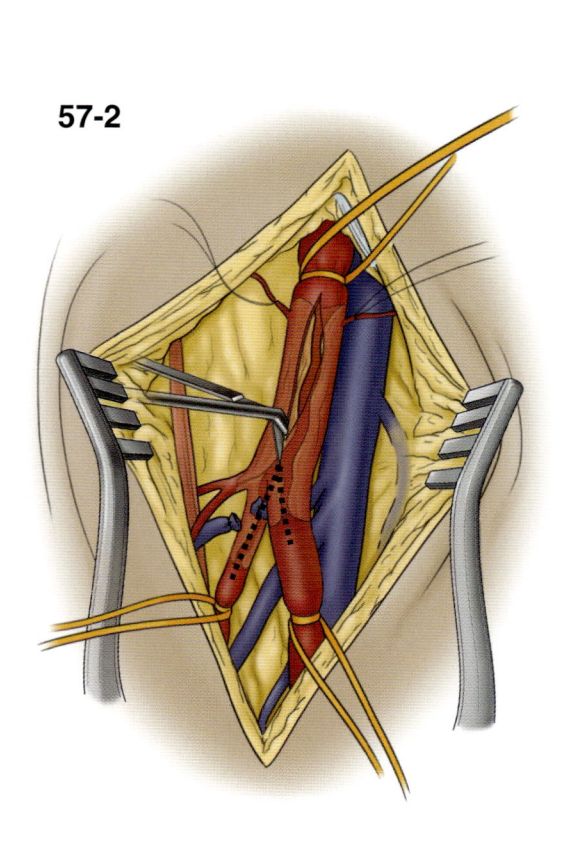

Figure 57-2 Femoral artery arteriotomy extended over both the SFA and PFA.

57-3

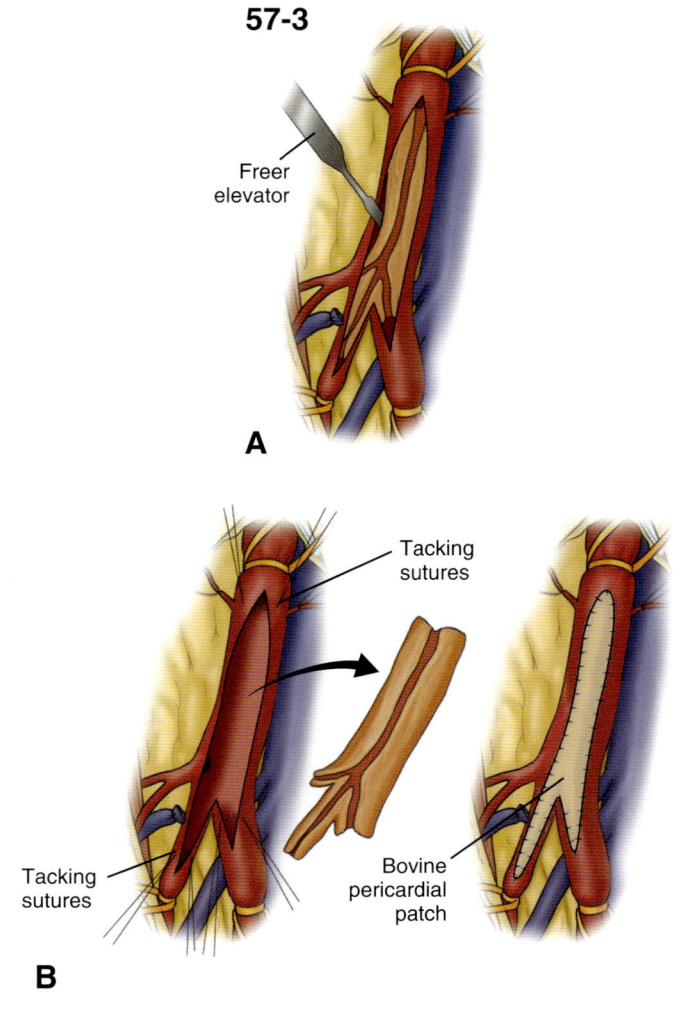

Figure 57-3 A. Development of endarterectomy plane. B. Plaque removed with intima tacked down to avoid dissection and bovine patch anastomosis.

DETAILS OF PROCEDURE *FEMORAL ENDARTERECTOMY AND PROFUNDAPLASTY:* `CONTINUED` Some patients only have focal orificial profunda disease, in which case an eversion-type endarterectomy can be performed. The cleavage plane should be reviewed and the residual arterial wall inspected for residual plaque or shreds (fronds) of the external elastic membrane or circular muscle fibers. This identification process is facilitated by heparinized saline irrigation.

Patch angioplasty is performed with either autologous vein, biologic, or prosthetic patches. Most commonly, a bovine pericardial patch is used. However, if there is concern for an infected field, the ipsilateral or contralateral great saphenous vein is best. The patch is then trimmed to size and secured to the edges of the arteriotomy with 5-0 or 6-0 Prolene sutures (FIGURE 57-4).

Patch closure can be performed with a single straight patch or a single Y-shaped pantaloon patch. Alternatively, syndactylization can be used by suturing together the arteriotomies of the profunda femoris and SFA to create a single common channel, which is then closed with a single patch. The clamps are released sequentially to allow for back-bleeding, reclamped, and then the anastomosis completed. Suture line hemostasis is achieved with repair 5-0 or 6-0 Prolene suture.

ILIAC ARTERY STENTING: In conjunction with femoral endarterectomy, adjunctive iliac artery stenting may be performed to treat additional proximal atherosclerotic disease affecting inflow. Iliac artery stenting can be divided into four phases: vessel access, crossing of the lesion, vessel preparation, and stenting. A key variation in the technique is at the access phase. In general, wire access into the iliac arterial system can be obtained either before or after femoral endarterectomy. It is within this phase of the operation that significant morbidity and technical difficulty can be encountered.

We prefer to obtain wire access into an intact CFA prior to performing endarterectomy, to limit our chances of creating a dissection. Accessing the intact femoral artery has a higher chance of staying in the true lumen while crossing the iliac lesion into the distal aorta. Using a 21G Micropuncture needle, we access a less heavily calcified segment of CFA under direct visualization. A micro-wire followed by a 4 French sheath is placed. A 0.035″ hydrophilic wire is advanced into the external iliac artery, and then advanced into the aorta (FIGURE 57-5).

Note should be made of any resistance to ensure a dissection plane is not created. A directional catheter is used to navigate through the iliac arterial system in either luminal or subintimal fashion. In cases of iliac artery occlusion, where subintimal crossing is performed, we aim to re-enter in the proximal common iliac artery. Re-entry into the distal aorta may be necessary and may mandate contralateral common iliac artery stenting—termed kissing stents. In cases of difficult re-entry, re-entry catheters can be utilized. This is done to prevent the ipsilateral stent from occluding the contralateral common iliac artery (see below). Once the lesion is crossed, an initial diagnostic angiogram via the catheter in the infrarenal aorta is performed to ensure true lumen location (see Chapter 55 for details). Occasionally, the guidewire cannot be passed retrograde, and percutaneous approach from the contralateral femoral artery or the brachial artery can be considered. In these cases, wire flossing is commonly used. This allows for a shorter working length and more control when performing retrograde stenting.

Once the iliac artery is crossed, the femoral endarterectomy is performed. The proximal clamp is placed with wire in place and the endarterectomy performed as above. Prior to completion of the patch, two techniques can be used to exteriorize the wire. First, the patch can be punctured with a Micropuncture or 18G needle, and the wire brought through the patch. The second option is leaving a few stitches loose to allow for sheath placement between the patch and native vessel. A disadvantage of the latter is the potential requirement of arterial clamping due to poor apposition and seal. Routing the wire through the patch allows for maintenance of continuous flow to the extremity by avoiding clamps. If the patch is punctured, the wire should be brought through the needle, the anastomosis completed, clamps removed, and flow restored. The puncture site should be distal on the patch to ensure adequate length of purchase for sheath placement. A U-stitch with 5-0 Prolene may be placed either pre- or post-puncture to allow for hemostasis after stenting. The size of sheath required will depend on the stent size but in general, a 7 French sheath is placed.

Selection of Balloon and Stent Dimensions Typical balloon and stent sizes used to treat iliac lesions range from 6 to 12 mm. Appropriate sizing may be assisted by angiographic measurements with calibrated catheters or intravascular ultrasound. Balloon and stent oversizing by 5 to 10% is recommended except for heavily calcified lesions that may rupture. Near occlusive iliac lesions may require pre-dilation. Balloon inflation should be gradual to avoid trauma to adjacent normal caliber vessel. Increased attention should be given to any change in hemodynamic status which may indicate arterial rupture during iliac artery angioplasty. Technical success is judged by residual stenosis of less than 30% and a systolic pressure gradient of less than 10 mmHg. `CONTINUES`

57-4

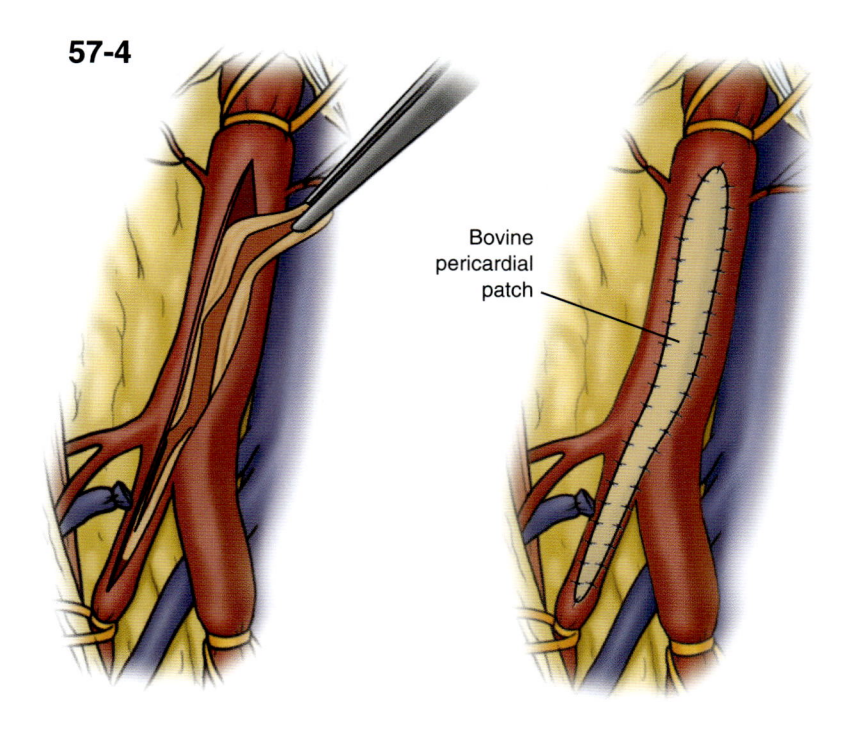

Figure 57-4 Different types of profundaplasty. Extension of patch angioplasty onto PFA.

57-5

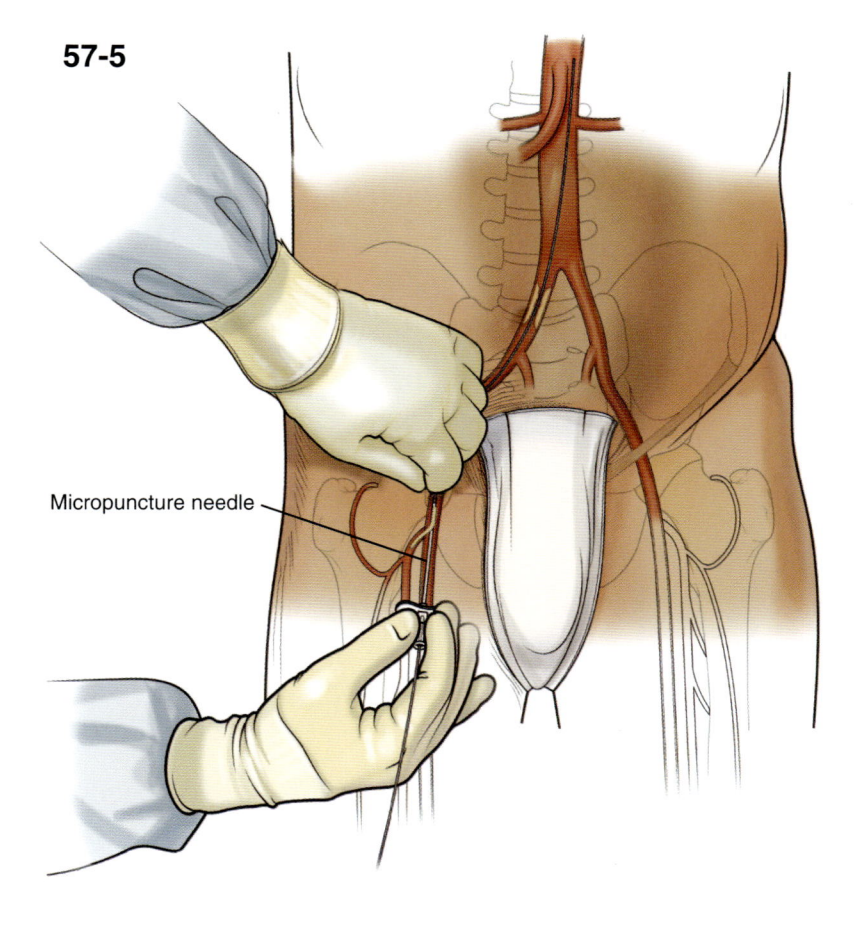

Figure 57-5 Initial steps of wire access for Iliac artery stenting. Initial wire access through the bovine patch.

DETAILS OF PROCEDURE *ILIAC ARTERY STENTING: Selection of Balloon and Stent Dimensions* **CONTINUED** A variety of stents can be used to treat aortoiliac lesions. Recent studies, such as the VBX FLEX study, demonstrated the durability of covered stents to treat stenoses in the iliac arteries. It is our preference to use balloon expandable covered stents in the common iliac arteries and self-expanding covered stents in the more tortuous external iliac arteries. In addition to improved patency, the presence of a covered stent allows more aggressive dilation of calcified vessels, as they will minimize extravasation (**FIGURE 57-6A**). Contralateral access may be required for common iliac stenting at the bifurcation in a "kissing" fashion using balloon expandable stents (**FIGURE 57-6B**).

Once in the appropriate position, the stent is deployed according to manufacturer instructions and pre-balloon angioplasty if size expansion is required or residual stenosis is observed. Completion angiogram is performed to ensure appropriate stent placement and the absence of dissection or perforation. An additional antegrade intervention may be done to treat distal arterial stenosis. In this scenario, the sheath can be "flipped" without losing access, or removed totally and reinserted in the antegrade direction. Wire, catheter, and subsequently the sheath are removed. The arteriotomy is closed with a preexisting U-stitch.

Endarterectomy vs. Stenting First There are advantages to the order in which stenting is performed prior to or after endarterectomy. The operator must be cognizant of the risk of retrograde dissection of the proximal endarterectomy flap with wire passage. If the endarterectomy is performed first and there is a small residual plaque, it is helpful to tack down the flap with interrupted Prolene sutures to avoid the wire dissecting. Any abnormal wire behavior should be noted and investigated. Obtaining wire access prior to endarterectomy obviates this risk. Additionally, performing the endovascular intervention after the endarterectomy ensures there is no stagnant blood flow in the newly placed stent while the arteries are clamped. In comparison, placing stents into the distal iliac arteries before common femoral endarterectomy often precludes the ability to use a clamp for proximal control of inflow into the CFA because of concern over crushing the stent. In this scenario, proximal control is achieved with balloon inflation.

CLOSURE Intraoperative Doppler assessment in the SFA and profunda femoris distal to the endarterectomized segments should be performed. Consideration should be given for protamine administration to reverse anticoagulation. Wound exploration for hemostasis and lymphatic leaks is conducted. Multilayered wound closure should be performed with anatomical reapproximation of the femoral sheath, and deep and superficial fascia.

For re-explored groin dissections, consideration should be given to adjunctive dressings that will aid in preserving a clean and dry surgical field. The use of incisional negative pressure wound therapy, for example Prevena Incision Management System (KCI, San Antonio, TX), can aid in this process. Distal pulses should be evaluated prior to reversal of anesthesia.

POSTOPERATIVE CARE/FOLLOW UP Depending on intraoperative course and preexisting comorbidities, many patients will be admitted to a step-down or intermediate care unit for continued recovery. Antiplatelet therapy should be continued due to the newly deployed stent. Noninvasive assessment of hemodynamics via ABIs and duplex ultrasound of the lower extremities should be performed at the 1-month follow-up visit. The patient should then be followed every 6 months for 2 years and then annually. ■

SUGGESTED READINGS

Dosluoglu HH, Lall P, Cherr GS, Harris LM, Dryjski ML. Role of simple and complex hybrid revascularization procedures for symptomatic lower extremity occlusive disease. *J Vasc Surg.* 2010 Jun;51(6):1425-1435. e1. doi: 10.1016/j.jvs.2010.01.092. PMID: 20488323.

Kashyap VS, Pavkov ML, Bena JF, et al. The management of severe aortoiliac occlusive disease: endovascular therapy rivals open reconstruction. *J Vasc Surg.* 2008 Dec;48(6):1451-1457, 1457.e1-3. doi: 10.1016/j.jvs.2008.07.004. Epub 2008 Sep 19. PMID: 18804943.

Mwipatayi BP, Thomas S, Wong J, Temple SEL, Vijayan V, Jackson M, Burrows SA; Covered Versus Balloon Expandable Stent Trial (COBEST) Co-investigators. A comparison of covered vs bare expandable stents for the treatment of aortoiliac occlusive disease. *J Vasc Surg.* 2011;54:1561-1570.

Panneton JM, Bismuth J, Gray BH, Holden A. Three-year follow-up of patients with iliac occlusive disease treated with the Viabahn balloon-expandable endoprosthesis. *J Endovasc Ther.* 2020 Oct;27(5):728-736. doi: 10.1177/1526602820920569. Epub 2020 Apr 24. PMID: 32329658.

Piazza M, Ricotta JJ 2nd, Bower TC, Kalra M, et al. Iliac artery stenting combined with open femoral endarterectomy is as effective as open surgical reconstruction for severe iliac and common femoral occlusive disease. *J Vasc Surg.* 2011 Aug;54(2):402-411. doi: 10.1016/j.jvs.2011.01.027. Epub 2011 Apr 30. PMID: 21531527.

Sidawy AN, Perler BA. *Rutherford's Vascular Surgery and Endovascular Therapy.* 9th ed. Elsevier; 2019.

Stanley J, Veith F, Wakefield T. *Current Therapy in Vascular and Endovascular Surgery.* 5th ed. Elsevier; 2014.

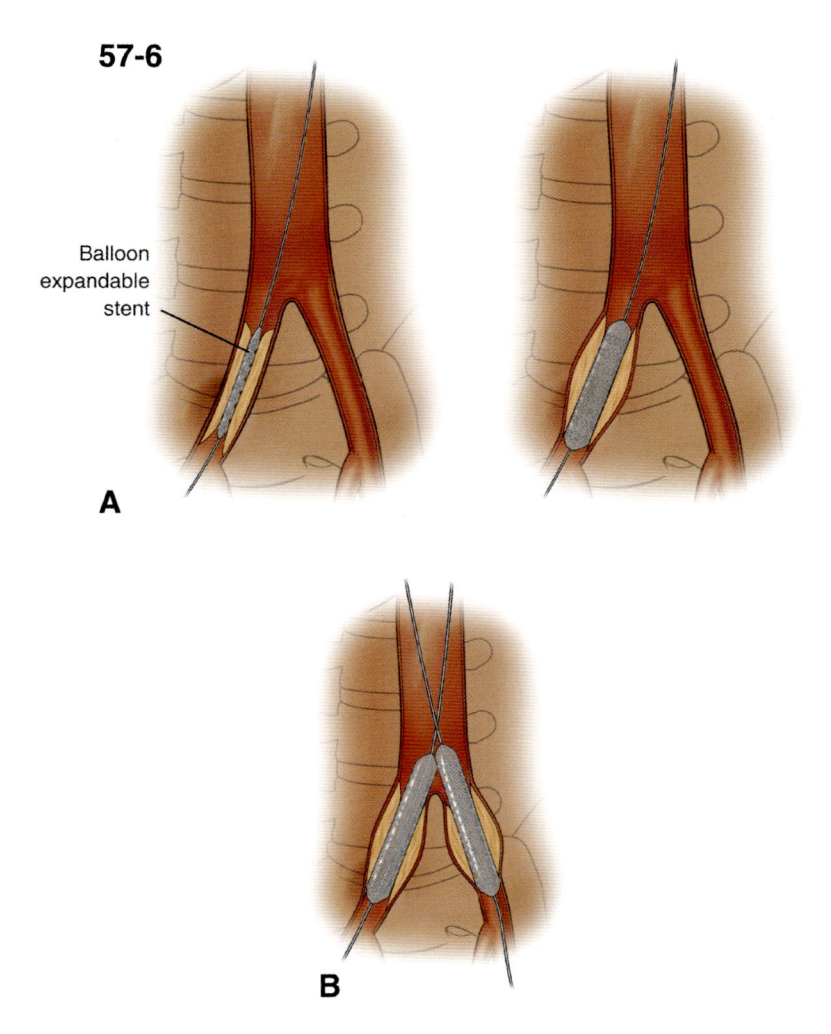

Figure 57-6 A. Retrograde iliac artery stenting. B. Bilateral retrograde iliac artery stenting with kissing stents.

Exposure of the Femoral and Popliteal Vessels for Above Knee and Below Knee Bypasses

April J. Boyd, MD, PhD

INDICATIONS Femoral popliteal bypass procedures are performed for lifestyle-limiting claudication, ischemic rest pain, tissue loss, popliteal aneurysm repairs, trauma, stent thrombosis, and in some circumstances for acute on chronic arterial occlusion.

POSITION AND OPERATIVE PREPARATION In most cases, the patient is supine, and their entire leg is prepped from the toes distally and up to the umbilicus. We advise prepping in both legs in the unusual event that the vein is inadvertently not of adequate quality, so the other side is immediately available without having to re-prep and risk contamination. Signals in each foot should be documented and marked.

INCISIONS, EXPOSURE, AND DETAILS OF THE PROCEDURE

BYPASS CONDUIT: The greater saphenous vein is the conduit of choice for most bypass procedures. Please refer to Chapter 4 for details of vein harvest. However, when this is not available, the cephalic and basilic arm veins will suffice if they are appropriate size. It is generally agreed that greater than 3.0 mm constitutes a good vein, 2.5 to 3.0 mm is a marginal vein, and under 2.5 mm is an inadequate vein. The vein harvest may be done through a long continuous incision, separate skip incisions, or harvested endoscopically. The vein is marked distended to avoid twisting during tunneling, and the proximal and distal ends are noted. If adequate vein is not available, ringed ePTFE with heparin coating (Propaten; WL Gore Inc, Flagstaff, AZ) is the best prosthetic conduit (usually 6 mm diameter).

APPROACH TO THE COMMON FEMORAL ARTERY

Infra-Inguinal Approach The common femoral artery and its branches are best approached through a vertical skin incision placed directly over the femoral pulse. In cases where the pulse is reduced or nonpalpable, this artery is best appreciated slightly medially along a line from the pubic tubercle to the anterior superior iliac spine. Nonpulsatile, calcified arteries can be felt by moving the fingers back and forth along this line, as one will feel the vessel "roll" under the fingers. In very obese patients, marking the location with ultrasound just prior to incision can be helpful. In addition, superiorly retracting the pannus with surgical tape (outside the sterile surgical field) can be helpful in a very obese patient. It is crucial to ensure that dissection is directly onto the common femoral artery, as this decreases the likelihood of wound complications, such as skin necrosis.

Following a vertical incision, a self-retaining retractor is placed, with care not to injure surrounding structures. Visualization of the common femoral vein or saphenous vein indicates too medial an approach, whereas twitching of the leg muscles or direct visualization of the femoral nerve indicates too lateral an approach. Clusters of lymph nodes are best mobilized to the medial side of the incision to prevent subsequent lymphatic leakage and lymphocele formation. Any lymphatic vessels encountered crossing the vessels of interest should also be clipped or ligated for the same reason. The femoral sheath is then incised to reveal the common femoral artery. Atherosclerotic inflammation can make dissection in the plane between the common femoral artery and vein difficult, risking bleeding should the vein be inadvertently injured.

If severe atherosclerotic disease is encountered in the common femoral artery and there is concern about controlling inflow, or an endarterectomy is considered in conjunction with the bypass, then dissection can be directed superiorly under the inguinal ligament to a disease-free region of the external iliac artery. The superficial epigastric artery (medial) and superficial circumflex iliac artery (lateral) branches are identified and encircled with vessel loops. Inferior retraction on these branches aids in exposure of the external iliac artery, which is dissected free beneath the inguinal ligament and encircled with a vessel loop (FIGURE 58-1A). Care should be taken not to injure the circumflex iliac vein as it passes over the surface of the external iliac artery just beneath the inguinal ligament. If required, this crossing vein can be ligated for more proximal exposure of the external iliac artery.

The common femoral artery is then dissected inferiorly to point where there is a notable change in vessel caliber, typically 3 to 5 cm below the inguinal ligament, which indicates the bifurcation into the superficial and deep (profunda femoris) branches of the common femoral artery. The superficial femoral artery (SFA) generally continues in the same plane. The SFA is the gateway to the profunda femoris artery (PFA), and retracting it medially facilitates exposure; the PFA normally travels in a posterior lateral direction (FIGURE 58-1B). If a caliber change is not appreciated within 5 cm of the inguinal ligament, then one should be aware of normal anatomic variants with the PFA branching-off high under the inguinal ligament, posteromedial, or distally off the SFA. The medial and lateral circumflex artery branches of the PFA can also arise from the common femoral artery in approximately 20 to 25% of cases. To avoid unnecessary bleeding, it is a good rule to check for posterior common femoral artery branches before performing an arteriotomy.

Invariably the PFA has crossing veins, most notably the lateral femoral circumflex vein. These branches are divided for more distal exposure of the artery. More distal exposure of the PFA will also involve dissection between the adductor longus muscle (medially) and vastus medialis muscle (laterally), whereas exposure of the very distal PFA involves dissection between the adductor longus (anteriorly) and gracilis muscle (posteromedially). Exposure of the most distal PFA may avoid complications of a recurrent dissection of the femoral vessels or provide outflow for shorter-distance bypass conduits when vein is in short supply. The proximal anastomosis can come off of the common femoral artery, the SFA, or the PFA (FIGURE 58-2).

Transverse Suprainguinal Approach The common femoral artery can also be approached through a suprainguinal transverse incision two fingerbreadths superior to the inguinal ligament. This approach limits the exposure of the superficial and profunda femoris arteries and is therefore not ideal for endarterectomy procedures. It can be used if the skin in the inguinal crease is inflamed or macerated. The subcutaneous tissues and Scarpa's fascia are divided until the inguinal ligament is identified. The inguinal ligament then retracted superiorly. The femoral sheath is opened longitudinally, exposing the common femoral artery.

MEDIAL EXPOSURE OF THE POPLITEAL ARTERY

Supra-Geniculate Above-Knee Popliteal Artery Exposure With the patient in the supine position, the knee is flexed to approximately 30° with a roll under the mid-thigh. However, others prefer for exposure for the above-knee (AK) popliteal artery a roll placed just below the knee, and for the below-knee (BK) popliteal artery exposure, a roll placed just above the knee. The leg is then rotated laterally and an approximately 10 cm longitudinal incision is made between the edges of the vastus medialis muscle (anterior) and the sartorius muscle (posterior-medially). The incision runs inferiorly from the medial femoral condyle to a point overlying the adductor magnus tendon. If the saphenous vein incision does not run too posterior, then that incision can be used, but one should be cautious against creating skin flaps. Also, caution is necessary to not injure the saphenous vein, which lies posterior-medially in the subcutaneous tissues, or the saphenous nerve as it runs parallel to the saphenous vein. The incision is then deepened through the subcutaneous tissue and fascia aided by a self-retaining retractor, and the sartorius muscle is retracted posteriorly and vastus medialis anterior. The popliteal fossa is entered when the deep fascia is incised just above the sartorius muscle. The AK popliteal artery lies in a popliteal fat pad. If a patient does not have occlusive disease, the popliteal pulse can be palpated against the posterior aspect of the femur. However, in general this incision is done for an occluded SFA, and therefore auscultation with a Doppler can aid in isolating the artery. The popliteal artery is isolated anterior-medial to the popliteal vein (FIGURE 58-3); if it is necessary to move more distally, it can be found distally between the two heads of the gastrocnemius muscle and beneath the popliteus muscle. Several collateral geniculate branches of the popliteal vein may require ligation and division to improve isolation of the popliteal artery with this approach. **CONTINUES** ▶

58-1

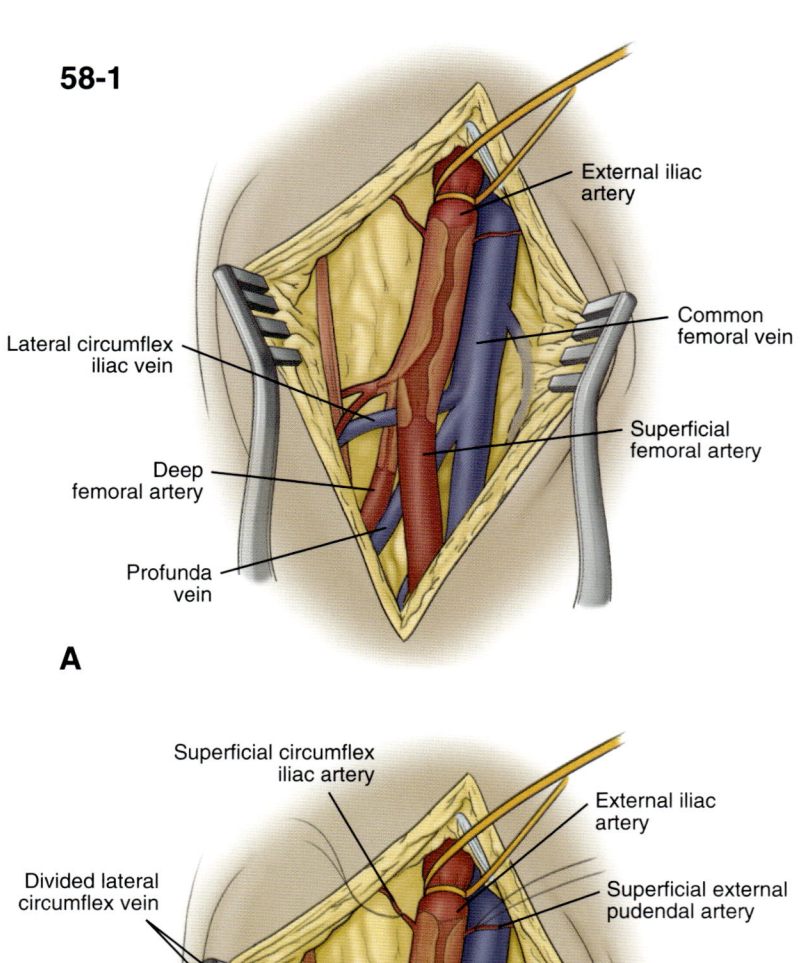

Lateral circumflex iliac vein

Deep femoral artery

Profunda vein

External iliac artery

Common femoral vein

Superficial femoral artery

A

58-2

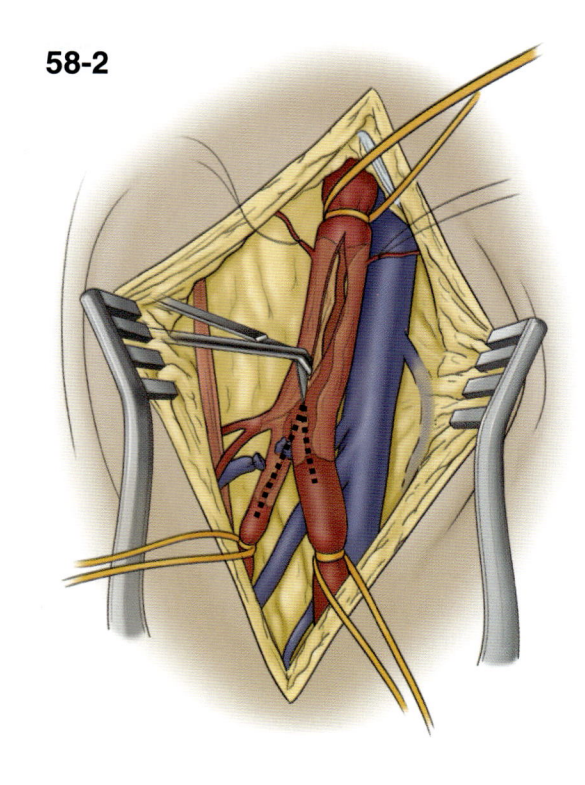

Superficial circumflex iliac artery

External iliac artery

Divided lateral circumflex vein

Superficial external pudendal artery

Deep femoral artery

Superficial femoral artery

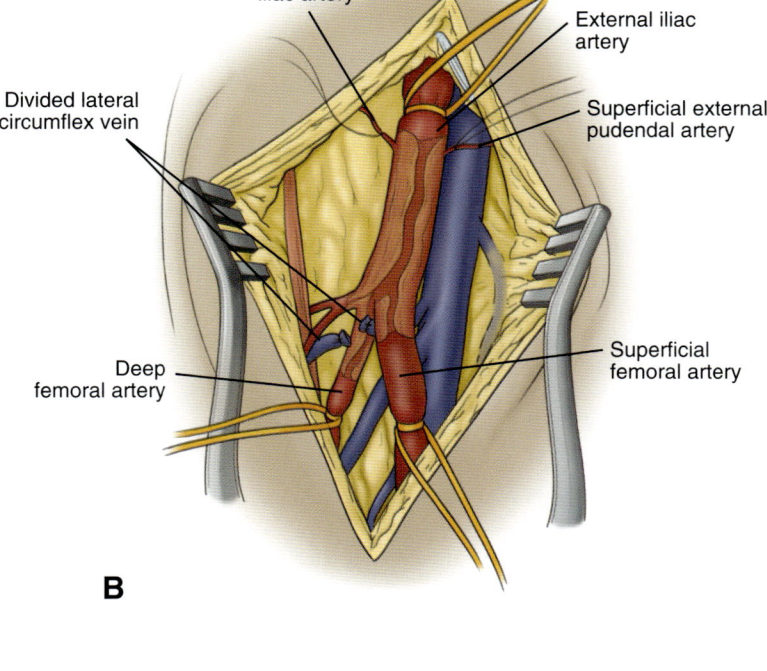

B

58-3

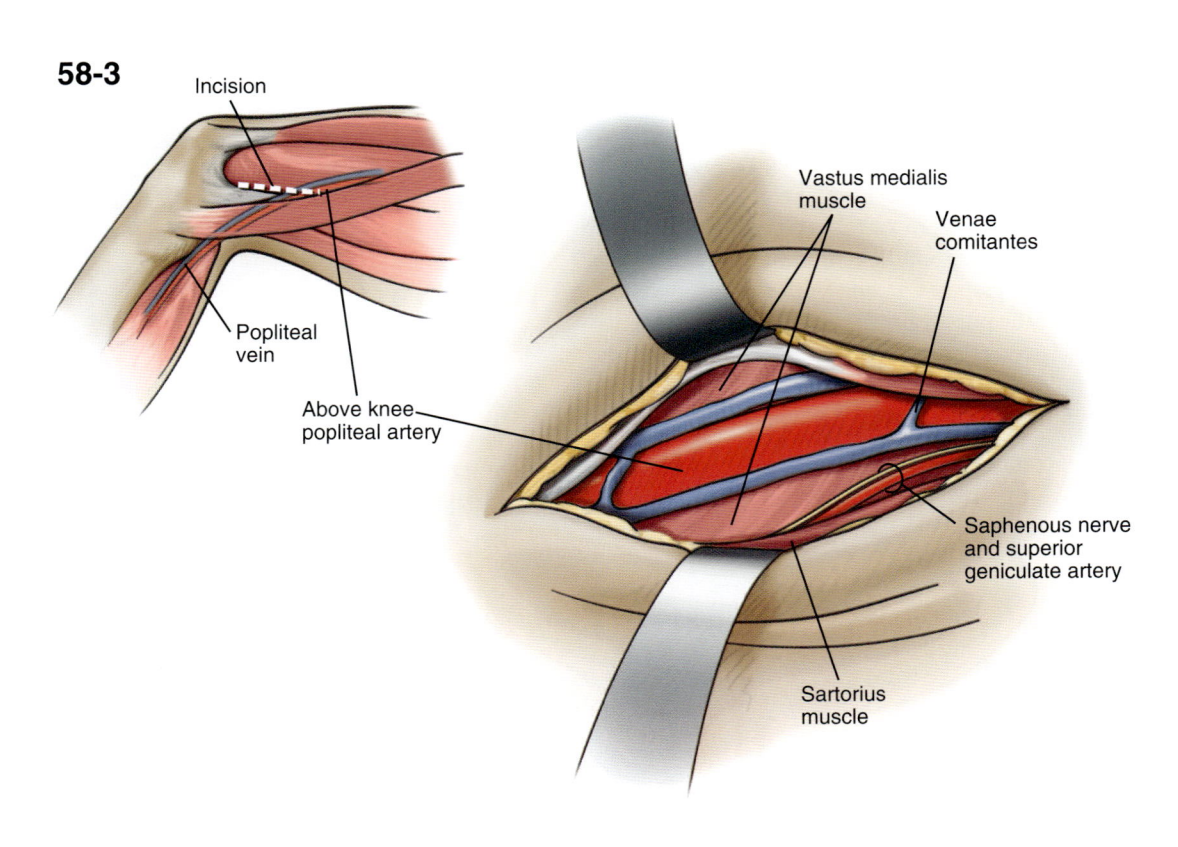

Incision

Popliteal vein

Above knee popliteal artery

Vastus medialis muscle

Venae comitantes

Saphenous nerve and superior geniculate artery

Sartorius muscle

INCISIONS, EXPOSURE, AND DETAILS OF THE PROCEDURE *MEDIAL EXPOSURE OF THE POPLITEAL ARTERY Infrageniculate (BK) Exposure* ◄CONTINUED This is a common approach to the BK popliteal artery and/or proximal tibial vessels. With the patient in the supine position, the knee is flexed 30 degrees and rotated laterally with a roll placed above the knee. An incision is made 1 to 2 cm inferior to the border of the tibia just anterior to the saphenous vein. The incision is deepened through the subcutaneous tissue with the use of a self-retaining retractor to the crural fascia, which is then incised proximal to the semitendinosus tendon (FIGURE 58-4). The gracilis, sartorius, semitendinosus, and semimembranosus muscle tendons can be divided to provide better exposure, but in general should be reattached anterior to prevent knee instability. The medial head of the gastrocnemius muscle, which is the gateway to the BK popliteal artery, can then be retracted posteriorly to expose the neurovascular bundle. It is not necessary to mobilize the soleus (the gateway to the proximal tibial vessels) unless access to the tibioperoneal trunk or anterior tibial artery is required. The tibial nerve, which lies posterior-medial to the artery, is identified and protected as popliteal vein is retracted posteriorly to expose the popliteal artery which is anterior-lateral to the vein. Division of crossing popliteal vein branches may be necessary improve exposure of the artery.

Tunneling and Anastomosis For reversed-vein bypass grafts originating from the femoral artery and planned medial approached popliteal artery, the bypass can be tunneled in several ways. An anatomic tunnel for the AK popliteal artery is done underneath the adductor canal and sartorius (FIGURE 58-5A), paying attention that the proximal graft stays underneath and not through the sartorius muscle.

For the BK popliteal artery, the anatomic tunnel is created by starting between both heads of the gastrocnemius muscle (FIGURE 58-5A). A counter-incision similar to exposure of the AK popliteal artery can be helpful. The advantage of an anatomic tunnel is that it gives protection for the bypass from superficial wound breakdown. One can also do a subcutaneous tunnel that runs in the subcutaneous tissue in the course of the vein harvest, and then traverse across the suprageniculate or infrageniculate popliteal fossa. For vein bypasses, it is recommended that the proximal anastomosis is performed before tunneling, and then the bypass tunneled while distended with blood.

Posterior Approach to the Popliteal Artery This approach is useful for popliteal aneurysms and popliteal entrapment syndrome. See Chapter 64 for details of the exposure.

LATERAL EXPOSURE OF THE POPLITEAL ARTERY

Suprageniculate (AK) Exposure The lateral approach to the suprageniculate AK popliteal artery is rarely used but is an important alternate route to this artery when medial exposure is complicated by infection or when a lateral bypass route is preferred. With the patient in the supine position, the knee flexed at 30 degrees and rotated medially with a roll behind the mid-thigh, a 10- to 12-cm longitudinal skin incision in made between the vastus lateralis and biceps femoris muscles. Subcutaneous tissues are then dissected, and the iliotibial band is incised. On deepening the incision, the tendon of the biceps femoris muscle is noted inserting into the superior aspect of the fibular head. A self-retaining retractor is placed, and the popliteal fossa is entered. The neurovascular bundle (common peroneal nerve, popliteal artery, and vein) can be palpated in the popliteal fad pad. The nerve is retracted inferiorly, and the popliteal vein and its branches are dissected from the artery, and it is encircled with vessel loops and mobilized close to the surface.

Lateral Infrageniculate (BK) Exposure Like the lateral suprageniculate approach, the lateral infrageniculate approach is even more rarely used because of the need to remove the proximal portion of the fibula. This approach may be necessary if there is infection, an open wound, or scarring from multiple prior medial approaches to the popliteal artery. With the patient in the supine position, a longitudinal incision is made from the fibular head distally over the proximal third of the fibula. The common peroneal nerve which encircles the fibula just below its head should be noted and protected. The biceps femoris tendon and the ligamentous attachments of the upper fourth of the fibular head are divided by blunt and sharp dissection, staying as close to the bone as possible. The deep and superficial branches of the peroneal nerve are dissected free and retracted anteriorly. Two holes are drilled into the bone at the site of planned transection, while a retractor is placed deep to the fibula to protect the vessels and nerves. The fibula is then transected with a rib cutter. With the bone removed, the popliteal artery is found anterior to the popliteal vein and tibial nerve. The popliteal artery is isolated and encircled with vessel loops. With more distal dissection, isolation of the proximal tibial vessels is also possible without muscle division.

For bypass grafts originating from the femoral artery to the laterally approached suprageniculate and infrageniculate popliteal artery, a tunnel is created in the subcutaneous tissue and the vein conduit is distended and marked before being tunneled, to prevent twisting or kinking of the conduit (see Chapter 61). The course of the bypass follows a curvilinear path in the subcutaneous tissue along the anterior thigh toward the mid-lateral femoral condyle and then into the popliteal fossa. Whether the infrageniculate popliteal artery is approached medially or laterally in bypass procedures, sufficient length of bypass conduit to allow the flexed knee to fully straighten without tension is required.

CREATING ANASTOMOSIS For a detailed review please see Chapters 2, 4, and 5. Patients are heparinized with 80 to 100 units/kg of heparin, and the activated clotting time (ACT) is kept above 250 seconds. While atraumatic vascular clamps (or balloon catheters in cases of severe calcification) are necessary for the femoral anastomosis, an atraumatic tourniquet is preferred for vessel control when performing the distal anastomosis. Herein, the leg is elevated and an Esmark bandage is used to drain the leg of venous blood. The tourniquet is inflated to between 250 and 300 mmHg (FIGURE 58-6). In the setting of severe calcium where the vessels can not be compressed, 2F Fogarty catheters can be used extraluminally for control.

Prior to deflating the tourniquet, and atraumatic clamp or pull dog is used to occlude the conduit, and the vessels are forward- and back-flushed. The anastomosis is completed and the torniquet deflated and then let down just before the final completion of the distal anastomosis.

CLOSURE Prior to closure, an on-table angiogram or duplex ultrasound are used to insinuate the bypass anastomosis, and distal pedal signals confirmed with a Doppler. Protamine sulfate is used to reverse heparinization. The wounds are then closed in several layers, paying close attention not to make it so tight as to compress the graft. Closure is done in multiple layers with absorbable sutures in the subcutaneous tissue and mattress nylon sutures or skin staples on the skin.

POSTOPERATIVE CARE The patient's blood pressure should be meticulously controlled and kept between 100 and 140 mmHg. Antiplatelet agents and statin therapy are proven to augment long-term patency and limb salvage, as well and Warfarin and direct thrombin inhibitors. ■

SUGGESTED READINGS

Massoud TF, Fletcher EW. Anatomical variants of the profunda femoris artery: an angiographic study. *Surg Radiol Anat.* 1997;19(2):99-103. doi: 10.1007/BF01628133. PMID: 9210243.

Veith FJ, Ascher E, Cayne NS. Unusual surgical exposures to avoid scarred or infected standard access routes to the common femoral, deep femoral, and popliteal arteries. *J Vasc Surg.* 2016 Oct;64(4):1160-1168. doi: 10.1016/j.jvs.2016.03.472. Epub 2016 Aug 25. PMID: 27566930.

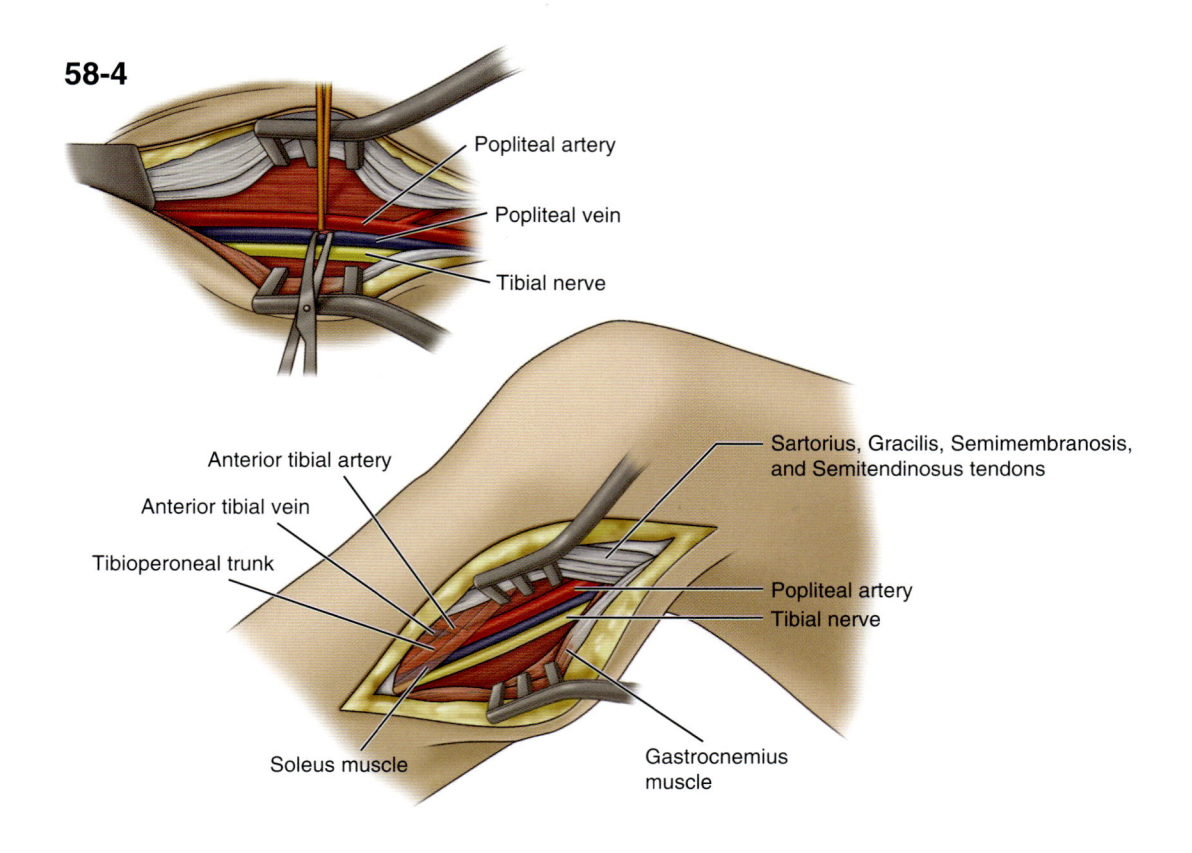

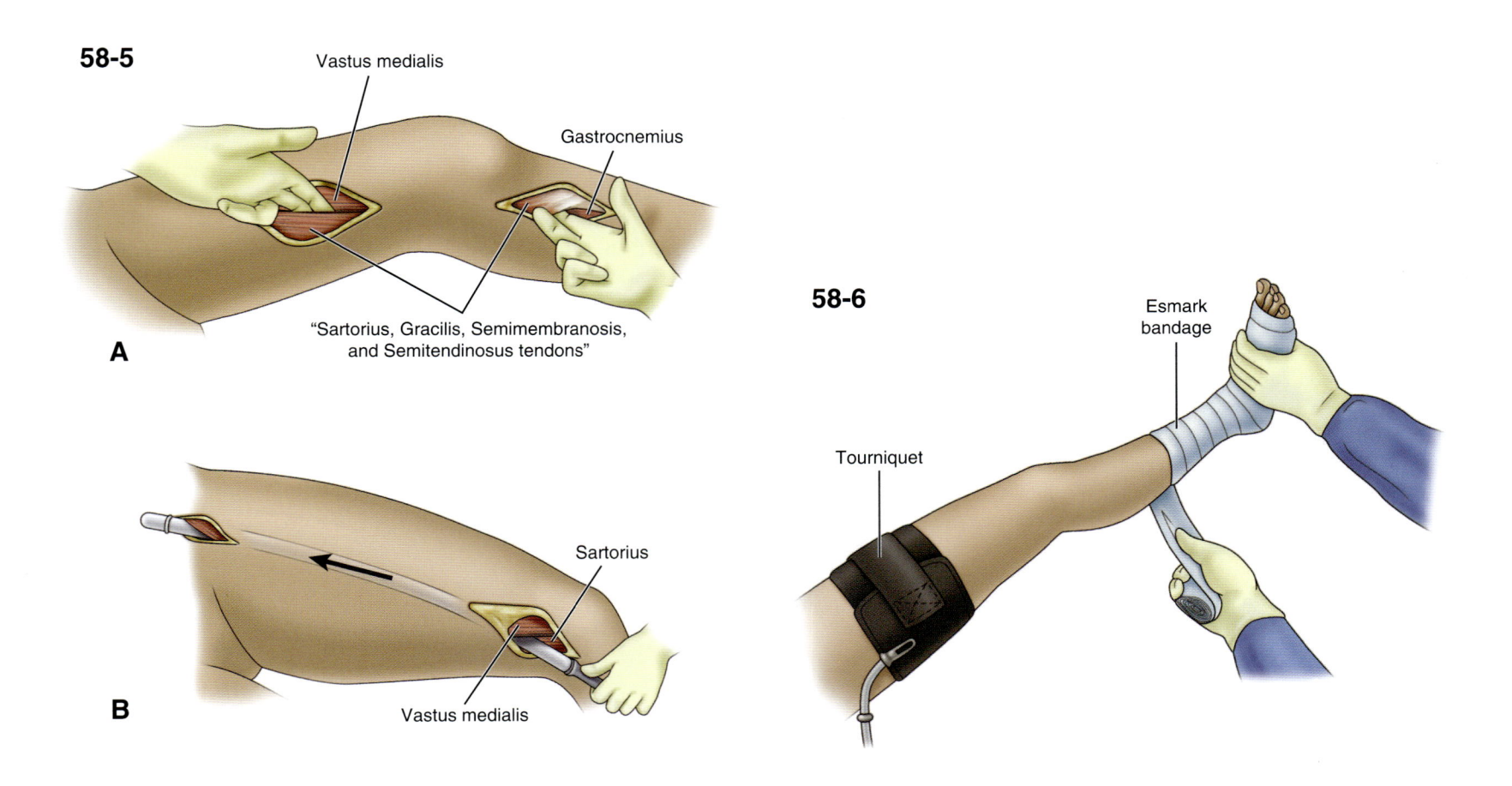

FEMORAL-TIBIAL IN SITU BYPASS

John Landau, MD, MSc • Luc Dubois, MD, MSc

INDICATIONS Despite the ever-growing sophistication of endovascular therapies for chronic limb ischemia, the femoral-tibial insitu bypass remains the gold standard for lower limb revascularization, particularly in patients with challenging anatomy and limited tibial run-off. Primarily indicated for the treatment of limb-threatening ischemia, this approach boasts excellent durability when measured against other procedures. By minimizing the handling and dissection of the saphenous vein and having a better size match with the inflow and outflow sites, in situ bypass is often advantageous when compared to the reversed vein configuration and can be done without having to expose the entire saphenous vein, thus minimizing wound morbidity.

Surgical planning is individualized to the patient's anatomy and is based on preoperative imaging. CT angiogram in the arterial phase is typically utilized to assess the patient's arterial and venous anatomy. In certain cases, a catheter-based angiogram may be necessary to delineate appropriate distal arterial targets, particularly in patients with calcified tibial vessels (diabetics, renal failure) where the calcification may obscure patency assessment and complicate outflow target selection. A duplex ultrasound can confirm the saphenous vein's suitability. Anatomic requirements for the procedure are centered around a suitable saphenous vein which is at least 3 mm in diameter and also is nonsclerotic and nondiseased. Suitable inflow site for the proximal anastomosis should be available at the level of the common femoral artery or proximal superficial or profunda femoris arteries. In some cases, it may be necessary to perform an endarterectomy and patch angioplasty of the common femoral artery in order to provide a suitable proximal anastomotic site. The distal anastomosis should be constructed at the outflow vessel that provides the best direct inline flow to the foot.

PREOPERATIVE PREPARATION Patients should have appropriate imaging studies available as discussed above. In addition, appropriate medical therapy including an antiplatelet and a statin are important both in minimizing cardiovascular complications and in maximizing graft patency. It is of tremendous value for the surgeon to perform or repeat the ultrasound of the saphenous vein at the time of the procedure. This allows the surgeon to mark out the position of the vein and its major branches (**FIGURE 59-1**) in order to limit the extent of the incision required to expose the vein. It also allows the surgeon to note any sclerotic areas of the saphenous vein or the presence of a duplicated system that may alter the surgical plan.

ANESTHESIA These procedures can be performed under either spinal/regional or general anesthesia. If spinal/regional is chosen, then the surgeon must ensure the procedure does not take longer than the regional anesthesia time; which may be a consideration if an extended profundoplasty or extensive femoral endarterectomy and patching is paired with the in situ bypass. It is generally not possible to conduct in situ bypass using local anesthesia alone given the extent of the dissection and incisions. Some literature has suggested reduced mortality with a spinal or regional approach when compared to general anesthesia.

POSITIONING The patient is positioned supine with the operative leg gently flexed at the knee and externally rotated at the hip to allow access to both the lower leg and the groin. Any hair is removed using clippers immediately before sterilizing the skin. Skin prep is carried out on the entire leg circumferentially from the umbilicus to the ankle using an alcohol-based chlorhexidine solution. We utilize a clear sterile bag to isolate the foot from the surgical field so that foot reperfusion can be monitored during the procedure.

DETAILS OF THE PROCEDURE

INCISION AND EXPOSURE: To minimize operative time, a two-surgeon team is advantageous as both can work simultaneously when exposing the vein and arterial segments. One team begins in the groin with an oblique incision which is carried down along the course of the saphenous vein. It is easier to isolate the saphenous vein and its branches first before arterial exposure using a self-retaining retractor and judicious dissection with scissors. Branches of the saphenofemoral junction are isolated and suture ligated on the saphenous vein side with 3-0 or 5-0 silk suture depending on branch size. The saphenofemoral junction should be skeletonized in order to facilitate harvest of the saphenous vein flush with the femoral vein. Once the vein is prepared in the groin, the common femoral, superficial femoral, and profunda femoris are isolated and vessel looped (**FIGURE 59-2**).

A second team working in the lower leg begins by simultaneously exposing the saphenous vein through a longitudinal incision. This incision is typically placed one finger-breadth below the edge of the tibia, but can be modified based on the location of the vein as dictated by the ultrasound. The portion of the vein below the knee is dissected free and again the branches are suture ligated using 5-0 or 3-0 silk. Once the vein is dissected and mobilized, the arterial target can be exposed. If the intended target is the popliteal, posterior tibial, or peroneal arteries, these can be exposed through the same lower leg incision. If the anterior tibial artery is being used as the outflow site, a separate longitudinal incision will be required along the lateral aspect of the lower leg, between the muscle bellies of the tibialis anterior and extensor digitorum longus.

VEIN PREPARATION AND PROXIMAL ANASTOMOSIS: Once the vein and arterial targets are exposed and controlled, the patient receives systemic heparinization and the saphenofemoral junction is clamped with a Cooley or Satinsky clamp. The vein is transected using a 15-blade scalpel flush with the saphenofemoral junction (**FIGURE 59-3**). It is possible to take a small portion of the anterior wall of the femoral vein with the saphenous vein in order to improve the size of the venous "hood" available for the proximal anastomosis, although care must be taken not to narrow the femoral vein during this step. The resultant venotomy is closed using a two-layer 5-0 Prolene running Blaylock suture. It is imperative to then remove the first set of valves from the saphenous vein at this stage using direct visualization and Potts scissors. If this first set of valves is missed, it will be difficult to access using a valvulotome without damaging the proximal anastomosis. The vein is then set aside, being careful to note the orientation to prevent twisting of the proximal portion of the vein. The arteries of the groin are then clamped and any adjunctive endarterectomy or profundoplasty is carried out at this stage. The proximal anastomosis is then constructed in an end-side fashion using running 6-0 Prolene (**FIGURE 59-4**) with endothelial apposition (**FIGURE 59-5**). It is important not to stretch the vein too tightly during this stage in an effort to reach more proximally, as this may affect flow dynamics and can result in poor distensibility of the vein. Once the proximal anastomosis is completed, the proximal portion of the vein is unclamped. Distally the vein is ligated and transected, ensuring there is adequate length to reach the intended target vessel. The vein is then serially dilated using heparinized saline with care taken not to overdistend the vein, and any missed branches are oversewn with 7-0 Prolene.

CONTINUES ▶

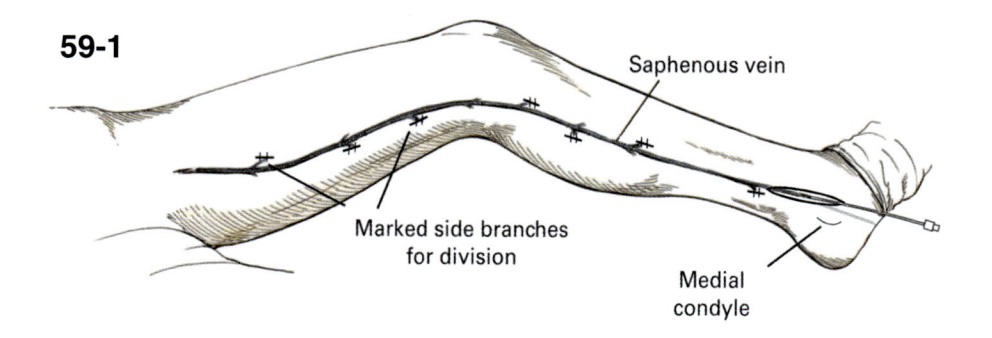

59-1

Saphenous vein

Marked side branches
for division

Medial
condyle

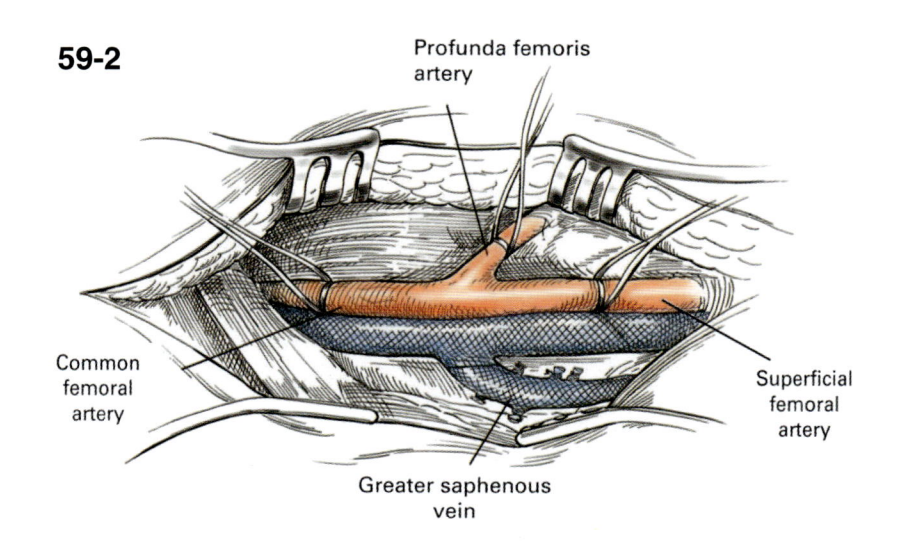

59-2

Profunda femoris
artery

Common
femoral
artery

Superficial
femoral
artery

Greater saphenous
vein

59-3

Saphenous
vein cuff

Femoral
vein

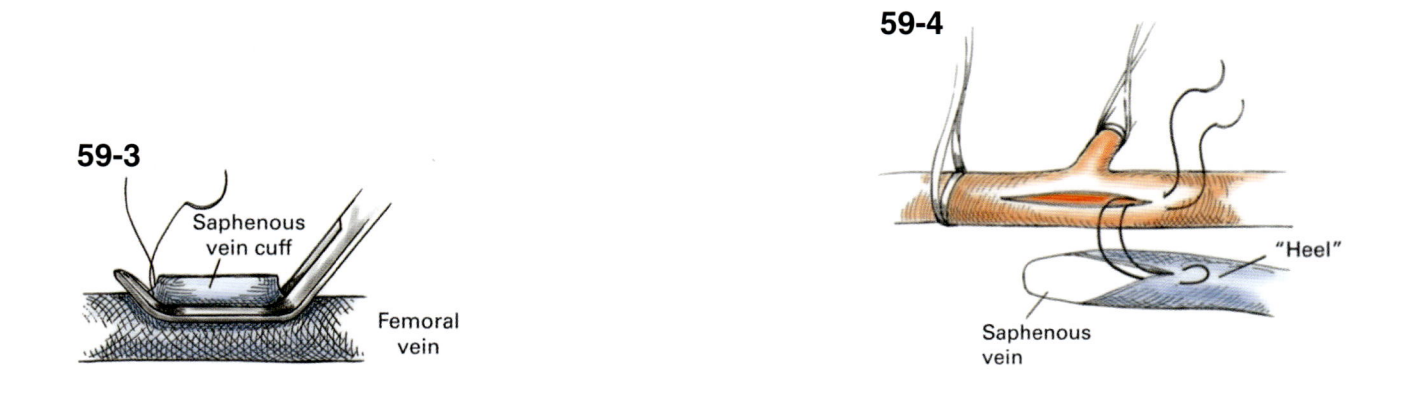

59-4

"Heel"

Saphenous
vein

59-5

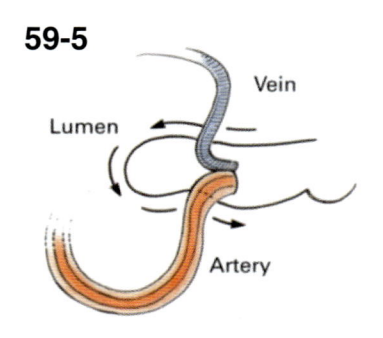

Vein

Lumen

Artery

DETAILS OF THE PROCEDURE *VALVE LYSIS AND LIGATION OF BRANCHES*: **CONTINUED** Valve lysis is then carried out using a valvulotome once pulsatile flow is established in the proximal portion of the vein. Different types are available; we typically use either the LeMaitre valvulotome (FIGURE 59-6) or the Mills valvulotome. The benefit of the LeMaitre valvulotome is that one does not have to expose the entire vein, while to use the Mills, the vein must be completely exposed and the Mills introduced via side branches. It is recommended to use at least two passes of the valvulotome to ensure that all valves have been lysed, which should result in robust, pulsatile flow through the vein (FIGURE 59-7). Absence of pulsatile flow at this stage may suggest hemodynamically significant arteriovenous fistulas through patent side branches of the saphenous vein. A bulldog clamp is then placed on the end of the vein. The preoperatively marked incisions in the thigh are then incised and the branches exposed and ligated along the course of the saphenous vein. We typically try to avoid making long incision flaps, particularly across the knee joint. A hand-held continuous wave Doppler probe is used in between skip incisions with distal vein compression to find any missed branches; once the Doppler indicates only obstructed flow along the entire vein, it is ready for distal anastomosis.

DISTAL ANASTOMOSIS AND COMPLETION STUDIES: If the intended target is the anterior tibial artery, we typically tunnel the vein from medial to lateral through the interosseous membrane. After exposing the interosseous membrane from both a medial and lateral approach, we incise the membrane so that it will admit at least two fingertips to prevent compression. If the saphenous vein is very superficial below the knee we will often tunnel the distal portion of the vein lateral to the medial head of the gastrocnemius muscle by incising the fascia overlying the sartorius muscle above the knee and passing the vein deep through this subsartorial tunnel behind the knee. If a tunnel is required, care must be taken not to twist or kink the vein.

The intended target vessel is then proximally and distally clamped and opened with a scalpel longitudinally, and the vein is transected and spatulated (FIGURE 59-8) making sure to check the necessary length with the leg straightened. In order to optimize flow dynamics at the anastomosis, relatively long anastomosis should be constructed measuring at least 15 mm in length. Once the anastomosis is completed, flow should be documented using pulse exam and at minimum hand-held continuous wave Doppler with a biphasic unobstructive signal in both the vein and the outflow vessel beyond the anastomosis. If any doubt exists about the quality of the flow or the reperfusion of the foot, an angiogram can be performed. We find it best to insert a Micropuncture kit at the proximal anastomosis, as this can also be used as an access point should anything require an endovascular "touch-up."

CLOSURE Once an adequate technical result is confirmed, all incisions are closed using absorbable suture for the deeper layers and skin staples or running subcuticular monofilament suture. Occlusive dressings are applied and a "window" is left in the dressing (often using a clear Tegaderm) to allow monitoring of the graft signal in the early postoperative period using Doppler.

POSTOPERATIVE CARE Technical defects causing immediate graft failure typically occur in the first 24 to 48 hours postoperatively, and the graft signal and foot perfusion need to be carefully monitored during this time. Patients should be continued on an antiplatelet agent and a statin postoperatively, and consideration should be given to the addition of IV heparin in those patients at higher risk of graft thrombosis (small vein, diseased outflow, history of thrombophilia). A postoperative duplex ultrasound should be obtained when able to do so, typically within the first 4 to 6 weeks after surgery, to detect any early stenoses or retained valves which may be addressed to preserve patency of the bypass. A well-constructed in situ bypass in patients with appropriate anatomy will typically have an excellent 5-year patency in excess of 70 to 80%. ∎

SUGGESTED READINGS

El-Sayed HF: Bypass surgery for lower extremity limb salvage: vein bypass. *Methodist Debakey Cardiovasc J.* 2012 Oct-Dec;8(4):37-42.

Hoballah J, Bunch C, Sharp W. Femoral to posterior tibial/peroneal artery in situ bypass. In: Lumley J, Hoballah J, eds. *Vascular Surgery.* Springer Surgery Atlas Series. Springer, Berlin, Heidelberg; 2009.

Levine AW, Bandyk DF, Bonier PH, Towne JB. Lessons learned in adopting the in situ saphenous vein bypass. *J Vasc Surg.* 1985;2(1):145-153.

Mills JL. Infrainguinal disease: surgical treatment. In: Sidawy AN, Perler BA, eds. *Rutherford's Vascular Surgery and Endovascular Therapy.* 9th ed., 2019;1438-1462.

Watelet J, Soury P, Menard JF, et al. Femoropopliteal bypass: in situ or reversed vein grafts? Ten-year results of a randomized controlled trial. *Ann Vasc Surg.* 1997;11:510-519.

59-6

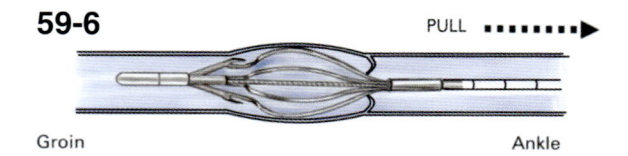

PULL ▪▪▪▪▪▪▪▶

Groin

Ankle

59-7

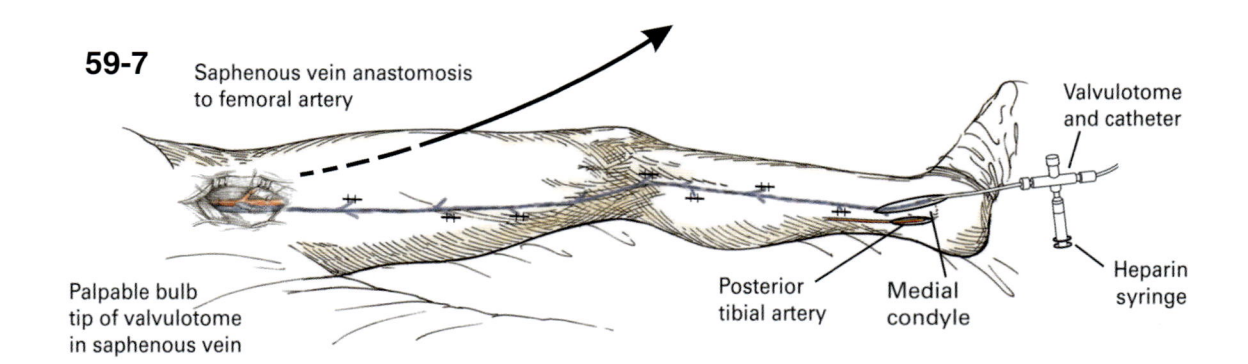

Saphenous vein anastomosis
to femoral artery

Valvulotome
and catheter

Heparin
syringe

Posterior
tibial artery

Medial
condyle

Palpable bulb
tip of valvulotome
in saphenous vein

59-8

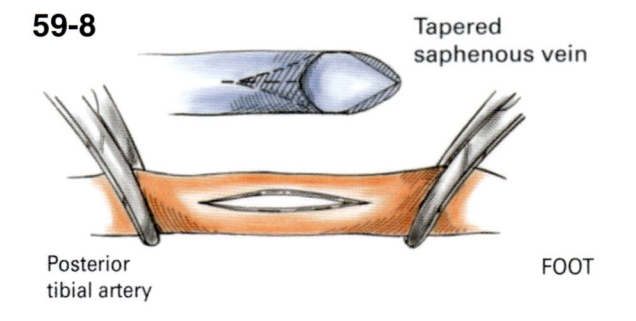

Tapered
saphenous vein

Posterior
tibial artery

FOOT

EXPOSURE OF TIBIAL VESSELS

Randolph Guzman, MD

INDICATIONS Exposure of the tibial vessels in the legs is an essential basic skill for vascular surgeons. It is important to review the anatomy and principles of exposure of these vessels. These vessels can be the distal target outflow vessels for bypasses typically originating from the femoral (common, superficial, or profunda) or popliteal arteries. Tibial artery bypasses typically are performed for ischemic rest pain or tissue loss.

Although these target vessel exposures are typically used for bypassing atherosclerotic disease for critical limb ischemia, they can uncommonly also be used for the treatment of traumatic distal arterial injuries as well as embolic, aneurysmal, or even as a proximal inflow source for more distal bypasses. Proper knowledge, appreciation, and review of the anatomy and principles of tibial artery exposure are essential in enhancing the comfort level of surgeons to maintain open surgical options in appropriately selected patients.

Adequate imaging is critically important in determining the target vessel. Although computed tomography angiograms (CTA) are in common use, this modality may have significant limitations with respect to visualization of distal vessels, particularly in the presence of calcification, as well as individual patient variability, protocol technique, and contrast timing. If there is any concern about adequate visualization, conventional angiography remains the gold standard and should be performed preoperatively or intraoperatively to ensure that the optimal target vessel is selected preoperatively.

INCISION AND OPERATIVE PREPARATION Patients are usually in the supine position. The incisions depend on the target vessel and are described in detail.

DETAILS OF THE PROCEDURE

ANATOMY OF THE TIBIAL VESSELS: The gateway to understanding the exposure of the tibial vessels is appreciating the anatomy of the compartments of the leg and the course of the three tibial arteries in these compartments. Of the four leg compartments (anterior, lateral, superficial posterior, deep posterior), only two of the compartments contain the three tibial arteries supplying the leg. The anterior compartment contains the anterior tibial artery while the deep posterior contains the posterior tibial and peroneal arteries. The anterior tibial artery is the first branch off the popliteal artery and arises just below the popliteus muscle (FIGURE 60-1). From the popliteal fossa posteriorly, the anterior tibial artery enters the anterior compartment as it traverses the interosseous membrane in between the two proximal heads of the tibialis posterior muscle. Although less commonly performed, on occasion using the lateral approach is not feasible due to wounds or tunneling concerns; medialization of the proximal anterior tibial artery with distal incision at least 5 cm in length through the interosseous membrane is a technically demanding option. For the lateral extra-anatomic approach, the proximal anterior tibial artery emerges laterally and transitions to the anterior compartment, so the exposure is now done through lateral skin incisions. The artery emerges lateral to the tendon of the extensor hallucis muscle at the level of the ankle and distally. The gateway for proximal exposure for the anterior tibial artery is understanding its relationship with the tibialis anterior muscle Most proximally, the anterior tibial artery is situated deep and lateral to the tibialis anterior muscle lying on the interosseous membrane. As it courses more distally, it then becomes more superficial to lie near the lateral surface of the tibia as it eventually runs more medially at the ankle to become the dorsalis pedis artery. On the skin surface, this translates to a line originating proximally just anterior-medial to the fibular head to a point distally midway between the tibia and fibula. The skin incisions for exposure of the anterior tibial artery reflect the approximations of the course of the anterior tibial artery. Proximally, the incision starts about two fingerbreadths posterolateral to the tibia, followed by incision of the underlying deep fascia. The fascial incision can be extended proximally and distally to facilitate exposure of the muscle without extending the skin incision. **CONTINUES**

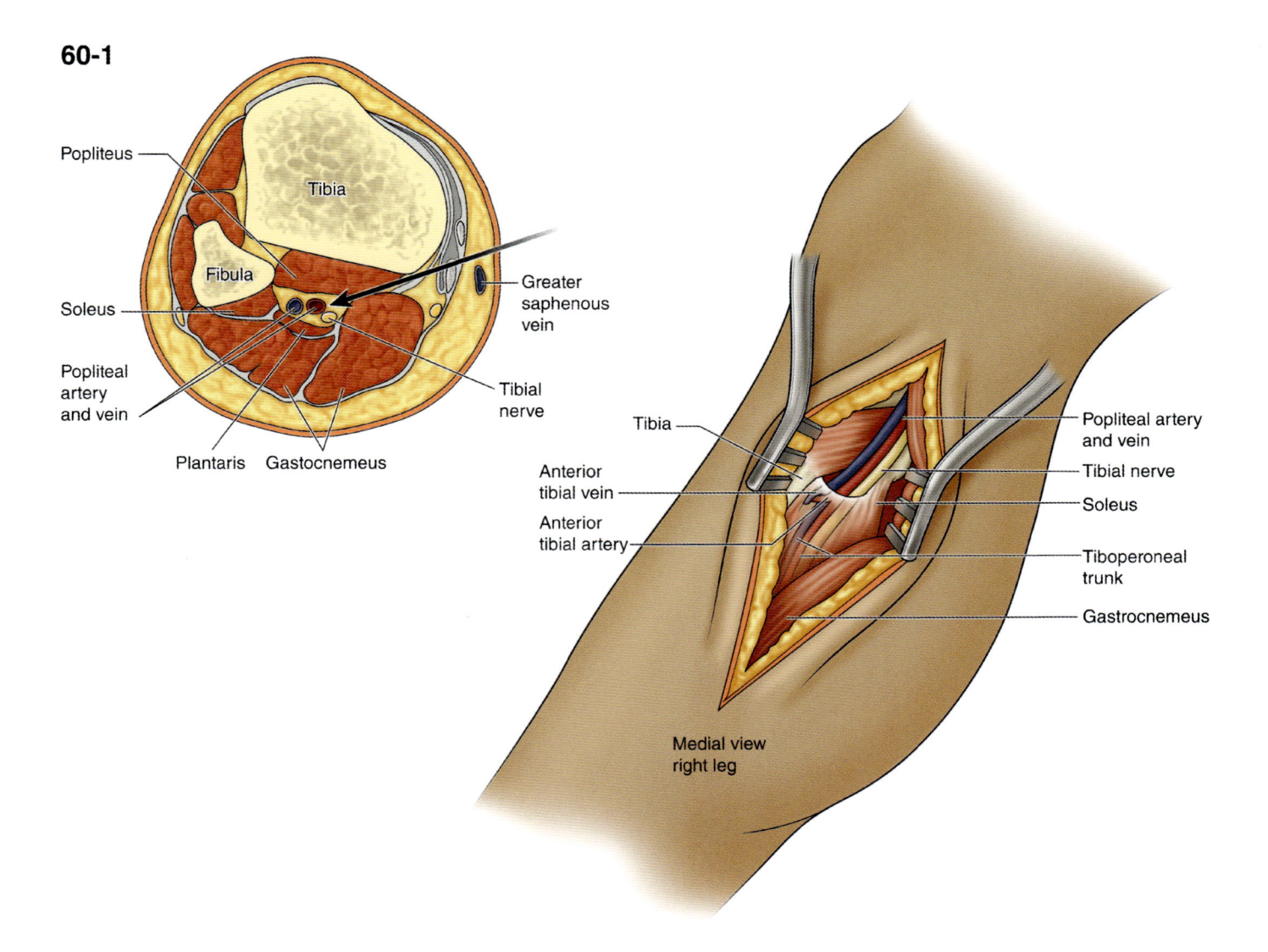

60-1

Figure 60-1 The four compartments o the leg and the course of the three tibial arteries are shown. Medial exposure of anterior tibial artery showing anterior tibial vein.

DETAILS OF THE PROCEDURE *ANATOMY OF THE TIBIAL VESSELS:*
CONTINUED The plane between the tibialis anterior and extensor digitorum longus muscles is developed and splayed open with self-retaining
retractors (FIGURE 60-2). The anterior tibial artery is then found lying
on the interosseous membrane surrounded by its accompanying veins
bilaterally. The skin incisions for the mid and distal anterior tibial artery
are similar, made one to two fingerbreadths lateral to the tibia. It is worth
mentioning in terms of exposure that the tibialis anterior muscle becomes
more tendinous distally, making exposure easier and more superficial.
Another point for exposure distally is that the anterior tibial artery is also
enveloped more distally by the muscle of the extensor hallucis muscle. Most
surgeons prefer to tunnel the bypass laterally in the subcutaneous tissue
(i.e., extra anatomic). A thigh counter-incision done halfway can be helpful.
If one cannot tunnel the graft laterally, an approximate 4-cm incision of
the interosseous membrane from the lateral side, at the graft, can then be
brought through this. Caution should be taken to not kink or twist the
graft when tunneling, and herein marking the vein is mandatory. In this
scenario, tunneling the bypass medial to lateral is done after proximal
tunneling of the graft, which is done like a BK popliteal bypass except for
the last step. CONTINUES

60-2

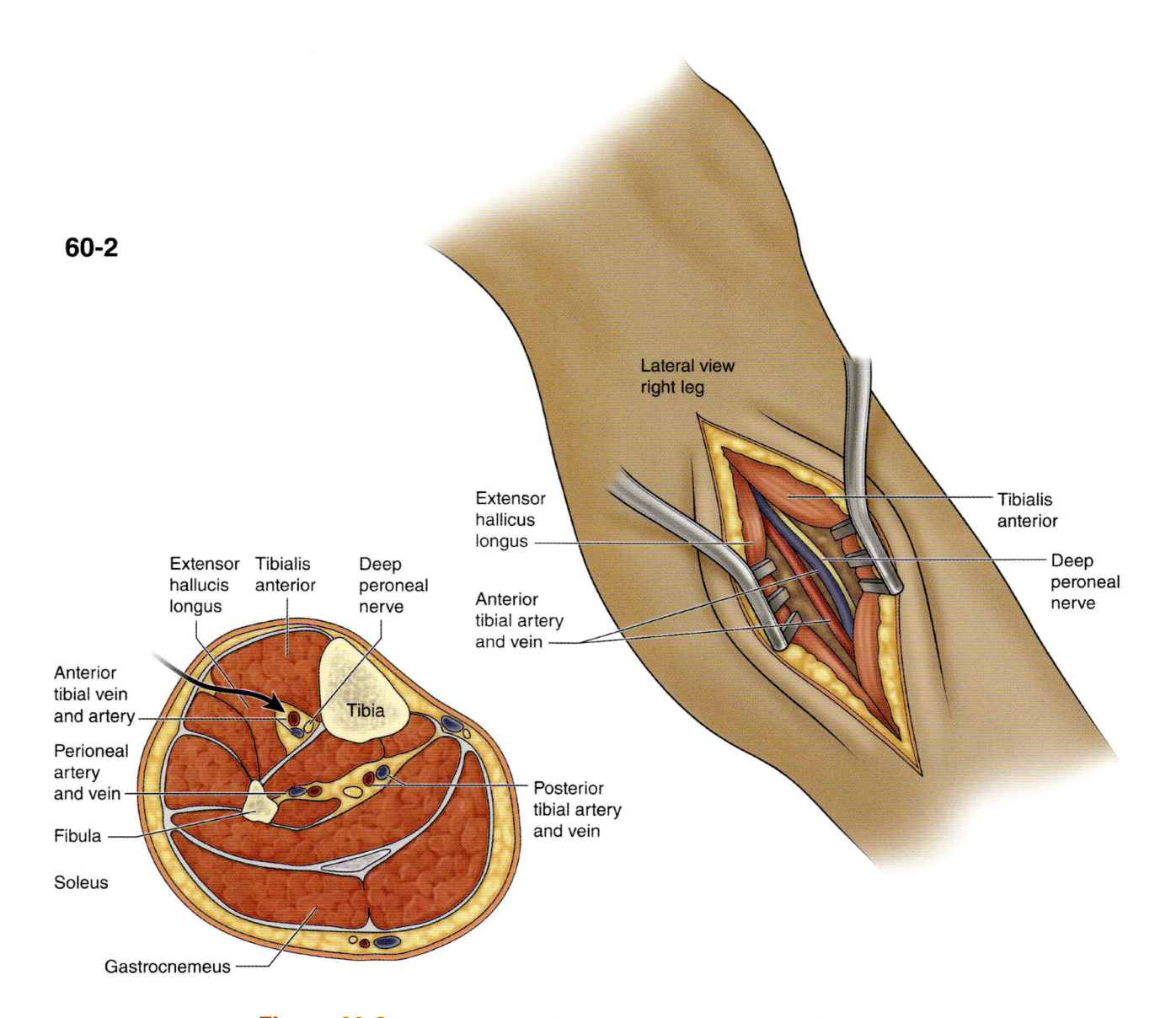

Figure 60-2 Lateral incision showing tibia, muscles, vessel, and nerves.

DETAILS OF THE PROCEDURE *TIBIAL PERONEAL TRUNK, PROXIMAL POSTERIOR TIBIAL ARTERY, AND PROXIMAL PERONEAL ARTERY:* **◄ CONTINUED** The next segment of artery for exposure past the anterior tibial artery is the tibioperoneal trunk and posterior tibial artery. Exposure of the tibioperoneal trunk is easily done by following the popliteal artery exposure distally. The popliteal artery continues distally as the tibioperoneal trunk and is exposed by incising the tendinous arc of the overlying soleus muscle. This tendinous arc of the soleus muscle is the gateway to the tibioperoneal trunk artery (**FIGURE 60-3**). The simplest way to do this is to locate the firm tendinous portion of the soleus muscle as you dissect anterior to the distal popliteal artery past the origin of the anterior tibial artery. Once this tendinous arc is identified, the musculotendinous portion is released along the tibia with cautery or by sharp dissection. Be careful when using cautery as the tibial nerve lies just deep to this. This can be aided with the use of a right-angle clamp or the tip of index finger which is placed underneath this tendinous arch. This can be done for an extended length, exposing the tibioperoneal trunk as far distally as required, which allows one to see the origins of the posterior tibial and peroneal arteries. Another gateway during this exposure is the anterior tibial vein crossed at the takeoff of the anterior tibial artery, and ligating this opens the tibial peroneal trunk. There may be additional small veins that are encountered distally during the dissection that may need to be clipped or tied for hemostasis. Sometimes it is easier to expose the tibioperoneal trunk from the posterior aspect, depending on the configuration of accompanying veins that may hinder exposure from the anterior aspect. The origins of the posterior tibial artery and peroneal artery are then easily found by continuing the dissection distally. **CONTINUES ►**

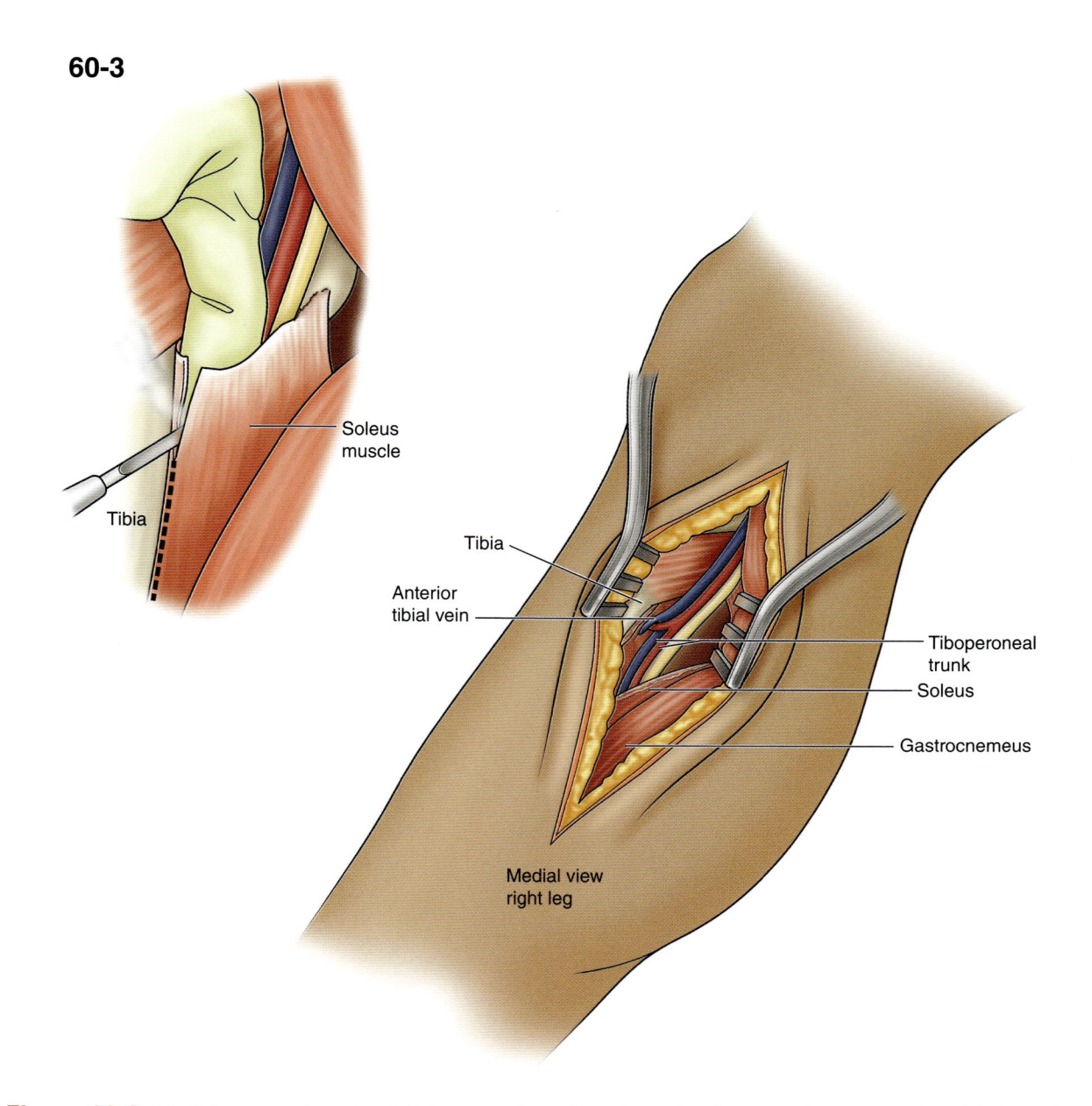

60-3

Soleus muscle

Tibia

Tibia

Anterior tibial vein

Tiboperoneal trunk

Soleus

Gastrocnemeus

Medial view right leg

Figure 60-3 Medial approach to the tibial peroneal trunk, and proximal peroneal and posterior tibial arteries.

DETAILS OF THE PROCEDURE *TIBIAL PERONEAL TRUNK, PROXIMAL POSTERIOR TIBIAL ARTERY, AND PROXIMAL PERONEAL ARTERY:* CONTINUED For the posterior tibial artery exposure, if the posterior tibial artery requires separate exposure distal and separate to the popliteal artery, the incision is dictated by the course of usable saphenous vein. The vein is mobilized for length in the usual fashion. If the vein is not used the entire length, then the incision can be made two fingerbreadths medial to the tibia. The gateway for exposure of the proximal posterior tibial is identical to exposing the tibial peroneal trunk as described but extending and deepening the exposure and entering the deep posterior compartment. As above, following incision of the deep fascia, this medial portion of the gastrocnemius muscle is retracted posteriorly. Taking down the proximal soleus muscle with division of the soleus muscle fibers more deeply will then expose the underlying posterior tibial artery lying within the deep compartment fascia. Anatomically, the posterior tibial artery courses deep from near the popliteal fossa to emerge more medially and superficially toward the ankle. The exposure for the distal posterior tibial artery is easier and more straightforward than the proximal and is found between the flexor digitorum longus muscle and flexor hallucis muscles (FIGURE 60-4). The saphenous vein stays anterior to the medial malleolus, and a separate incision is required to expose the most distal part of the posterior tibial artery. This incision is found in line in the groove of the ankle at the posterior aspect of the medial malleolus where the posterior tibial pulse is typically palpated.

The incisions for exposure of the peroneal artery are like the exposure for the posterior tibial artery and the tibial nerve. Once the posterior tibial artery is found, the tibial nerve is easily located more laterally; this is the gateway to the peroneal artery, which is found laterally (FIGURE 60-5). Feeling for the fibula is a simple maneuver to assure you are headed in the correct direction, as the peroneal artery lies medial to it. Anatomically, the peroneal artery courses from the midline and courses more laterally distally resting near the medial aspect of the fibula at the ankle. Exposure of this distal portion of the peroneal is somewhat more difficult as it is enveloped by the flexor hallucis muscle more distally. This is typically the most difficult exposure of all the tibial vessels. The mid and distal peroneal arteries shift away from the posterior tibial nerve and become enveloped by the flexor hallucis muscle. Persistence as well as meticulous dissection is required to expose the peroneal artery, as accompanying veins can be particularly fragile and one may need to use a tourniquet to decompress the veins, which allows for easier exposure. In cases that are difficult to access from the medial approach, or with infected field, one may approach the peroneal artery from a lateral incision. This requires resection of approximately 10 cm of the fibula. It also allows for deep compartment decompression.

CONTINUES

60-4

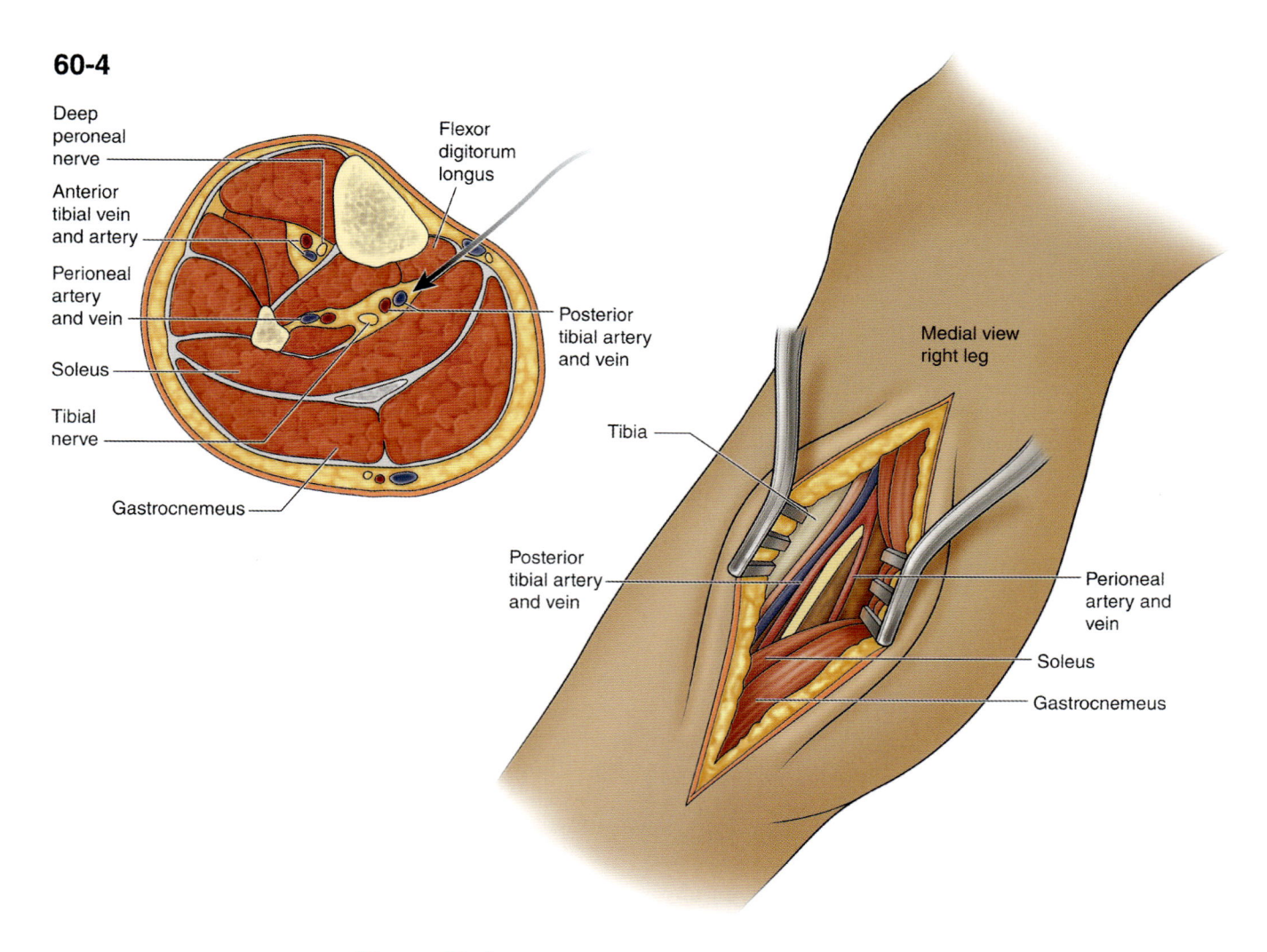

Figure 60-4 Exposure of the distal posterior tibial artery.

60-5

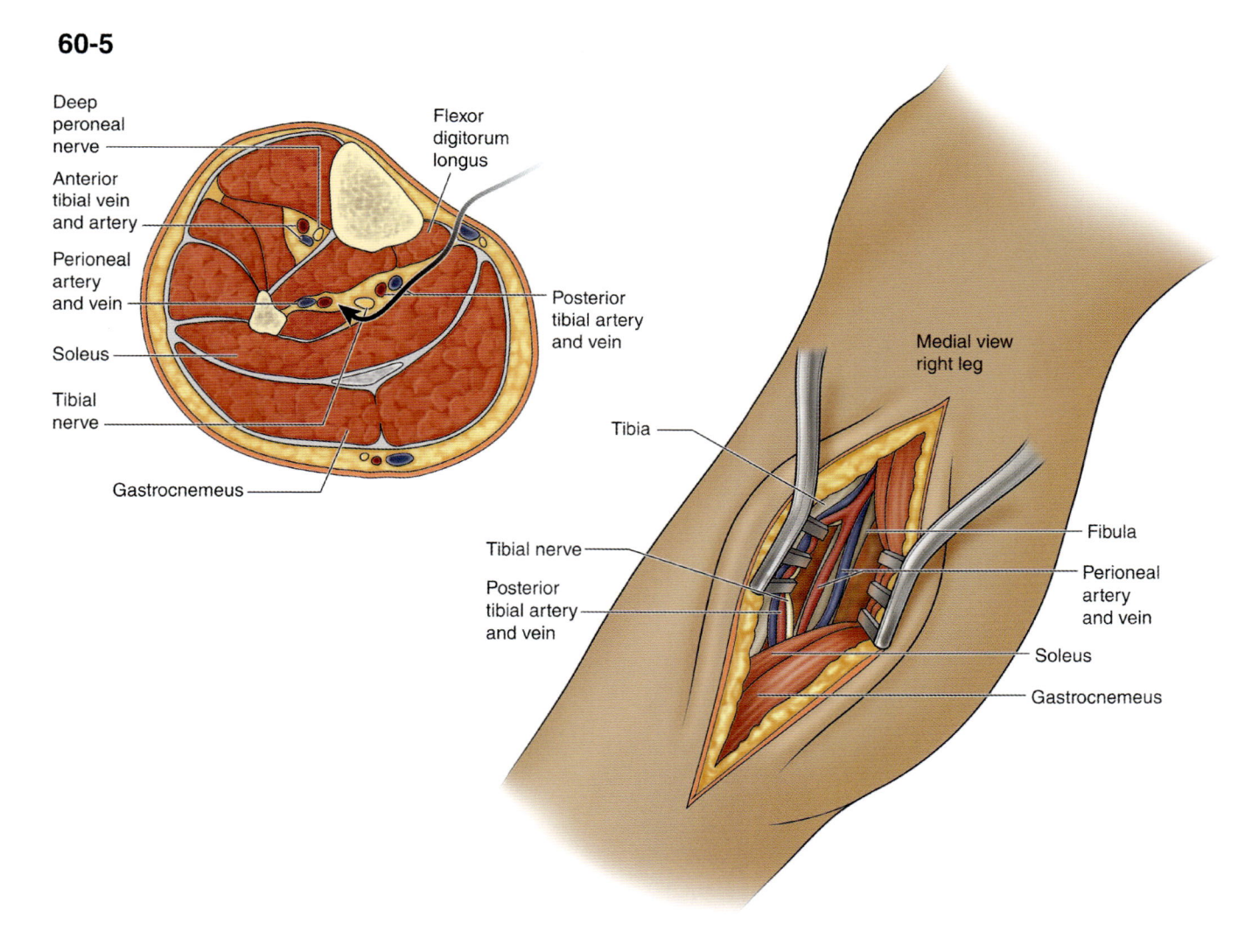

Figure 60-5 The medial exposure of the peroneal and posterior tibial artery is shown with corresponding incisions.

DETAILS OF THE PROCEDURE *TIBIAL PERONEAL TRUNK, PROXIMAL POSTERIOR TIBIAL ARTERY, AND PROXIMAL PERONEAL ARTERY:* `CONTINUED` A Gigli saw is ideal for this. One should caution against getting too deep with the Gigli saw, as the peroneal artery lies immediate deep to the fibula (FIGURE 60-6).

POSITIONING The patient is placed in a supine position. The leg is prepped and draped in routine fashion. Similar to the positioning for a popliteal exposure, the thigh is propped up with a bundle of two to three towels, with the leg slightly flexed for exposure of the posterior tibial and peroneal vessels. For exposure of the anterior tibial artery, the same position can be used for the proximal and mid-anterior tibial artery and is helped by rotating the table away from the surgeon. Alternatively, the leg can be left flat for the proximal exposure of the anterior tibial artery. For more distal exposure of the anterior tibial artery, the leg tends to rotate laterally, making the exposure less ergonomic. Rotating the bed away from the surgeon again may help in this this situation but I often will just wrap the forefoot with a green towel, rotate the foot medially, and fix it to the contralateral side of the bed with non-piercing towel clips. This serves to rotate the distal leg medially and keep it in a fixed position. It is extremely valuable to obtain an on-table angiogram of the target vessel prior to performing the distal anastomosis; this assures you are beyond all distal disease. The technique is done by simply inserting a 23G butterfly needle into the exposed artery and injecting straight contrast through a 5-cc syringe followed by flushing with 0.9% saline. After performing the proximal anastomosis, the graft is tunneled anatomically as described in Chapter 58.

The arterial bypasses are done as previously described. We prefer not to use clamps or vessel loops on the tibial vessels, and a tourniquet inflated to 250 to 300 mmHg usually decompresses the veins and allows for adequate visualization of the lumen to perform an anastomosis (see Chapter 60). In addition, it is highly recommended to not expose the entire artery circumferentially, only the anterior surface. This prevents unwarranted venous bleeding and reduces distal spasm. If the vessels are too calcified to compress with a tourniquet, 2F Fogarty embolectomy catheters inflated with air are useful alternatives. An atraumatic bulldog clamp is used on the vein graft just prior to deflating the tourniquet, which allows the vessels to be forward- and back-flushed.

ADJUNCTIVE MANEUVERS FOR PROSTHETIC GRAFTS: If there is no adequate autogenous vein available, one can use either a 6-mm ringed heparin bonded Propaten prosthetic graft (WL Gore Inc, Flagstaff, AZ) or a cadaver saphenous vein. In these circumstances, it has been demonstrated that an adjunctive measure can improve patency. These maneuvers include distal anastomotic measures (FIGURE 60-7) such as a Taylor patch, a Linton patch, a St. Mary's hood, or a distal arterial-venous fistula.

CLOSURE Prior to closure, an on-table angiogram is mandatory to check for defects in the bypass anastomosis, and distal pedal signals should be confirmed with a Doppler. Protamine sulfate is used to partially reverse heparinization. The wounds are then closed in several layers, paying close attention not to make it too tight, which would compress the graft. Closure is done in multiple layers with absorbable sutures in the subcutaneous tissue and mattress nylon sutures or skin staples on the skin.

POSTOPERATIVE CARE The patient's blood pressure should be meticulously controlled and kept between 100 and 140 mmHg. Antiplatelet agents and statin therapy are proven to augment long-term patency and limb salvage, as well as Warfarin and direct thrombin inhibitors. ■

SUGGESTED READINGS

Agur A, Dalley A. *Grants's Atlas of Anatomy*. Wolters Kluwer; 2020.

Chaikof E, Cambria R. *Atlas of Vascular Surgery and Endovascular Therapy: Anatomy and Technique*. Elsevier Health Sciences; 2014.

Huber TS, Back MR, Flynn TC, Harward TR, Culp WC, Carlton LM, Seeger JM. Intraoperative prebypass arteriography for infrageniculate revascularization. *Am J Surg*. 1997 Aug;174(2):205-209. doi: 10.1016/s0002-9610(97)00083-4.

McVay CB. Surgical Anatomy. Volume 1. *Anson & McVay Surgical Anatomy*. Saunders; 1984.

Pansky B, Gest R. *Lippincott's Concise Illustrated Anatomy: Back, Upper Limb and Lower Limb*. Lippincott; 2011.

Wind G, Valentine RJ. *Anatomic Exposures in Vascular Surgery*. 3rd ed. Lippincott Williams & Wilkins; 2013.

60-6

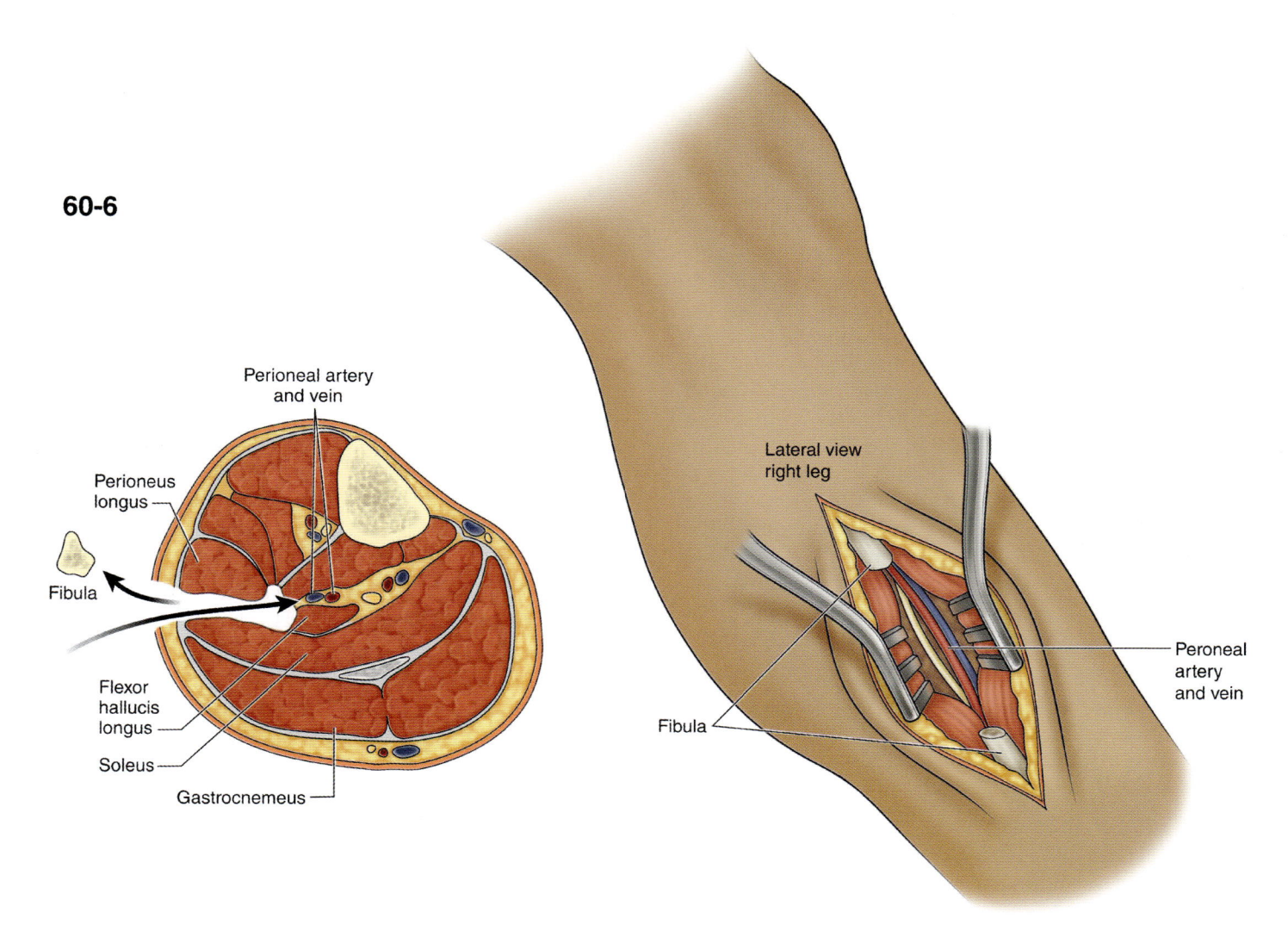

Figure 60-6 Lateral exposure of the peroneal artery is shown.

60-7

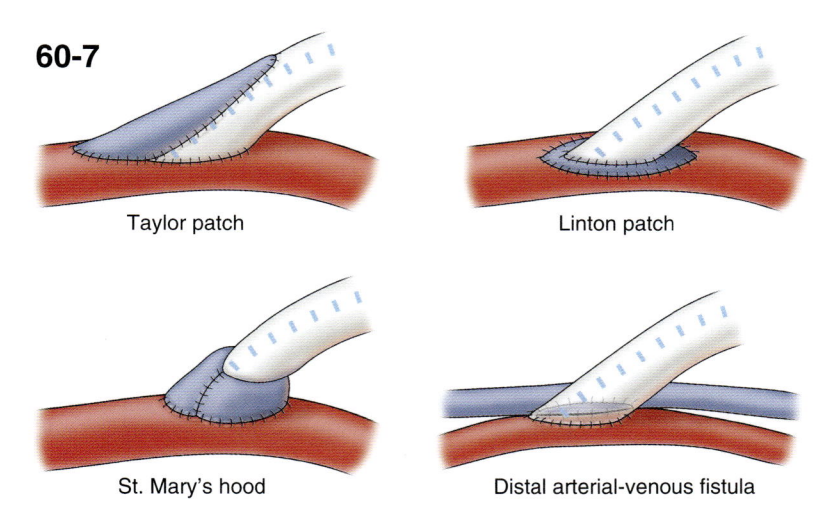

Taylor patch

Linton patch

St. Mary's hood

Distal arterial-venous fistula

Figure 60-7 Adjunctive mneuvers to improve outflow vessel patency.

FEMORAL-TIBIAL BYPASS USING REVERSED SAPHENOUS VEIN OR ARM VEINS

Derek J. Roberts, MD, PhD, FRCSC • Sudhir K. Nagpal, MD, FRCSC, FACS

INDICATIONS The indications for femoral-tibial bypass are most frequently chronic limb-threatening ischemia (CLTI), which includes ischemic rest pain, tissue loss, and/or gangrene. Autologous greater saphenous vein (GSV) is the preferred conduit for these bypasses given their improved patency and limb salvage rates when compared to prosthetic or composite grafts. We generally use the best available conduit for femoral-tibial bypass and do not save vein(s) for future potential operations. Our preference is to use ipsilateral and then contralateral GSV (if that leg has an ankle-brachial index [ABI] of at least 0.60 to assure there is enough blood flow to heal the incision), followed by spliced saphenous veins, continuous or spliced arm veins, and then cryopreserved vein or heparin-bonded, expanded polytetrafluoroethylene with an interposed Miller vein cuff of another adjunctive maneuver (see Chapter 60).

Indications for use of a reversed as opposed to in-situ GSV orientation include: (1) patients at high-risk for wound complications (because the graft can be tunneled anatomically); (2) when the proximal anastomosis must be constructed cephalad to the saphenofemoral junction; and (3) patients with a fragile, somewhat small-caliber GSV, which may be prone to injury during valve lysis. However, most commonly, decisions regarding use of a reversed instead of in-situ bypass graft is based on surgeon preference and experience. Advantages of the reversed orientation include the ability to tunnel the graft anatomically and avoid performing valve lysis, which can damage the vein. Disadvantages include: (1) the need for greater surgical manipulation of the vein; (2) size mismatch between the arteries and vein at the anastomoses; (3) the potential adverse hemodynamic effect of intact valves; and (4) the fact that intact valves complicate graft thrombectomy.

PREOPERATIVE ASSESSMENT

PHYSICAL EXAMINATION: In addition to the peripheral vascular physical examination, the lower limbs are assessed for prior surgery, chronic venous disease, infections, and tissue loss or gangrene. When arm vein harvest may be required, we examine the cephalic and basilic veins from wrist to shoulder with a proximal tourniquet inflated.

RISK FACTORS AND CARDIAC TESTING: Patients should have their vascular risk factors treated and undergo cardiac testing as per current clinical practice guideline recommendations.

VASCULAR IMAGING: Bilateral lower extremity noninvasive physiologic testing for ankle brachial index and pressure measurements is required. We recommend a preoperative computed tomography angiogram of the abdomen and pelvis with runoff to the feet. This is used to determine if iliac endovascular intervention is required, and to select inflow and outflow targets. It is imperative to obtain digital subtraction arteriography (DSA) in patients with calcified tibial arteries and where the tibial artery target is unclear. Using well-established protocols, duplex ultrasound is the time-honored instrument for measurement of the size of the greater saphenous vein, and if inadequate, bilateral arm vein mapping should be obtained. A vein diameter ≥3 mm is optimal, because a smaller diameter is a powerful independent predictor of failure of bypass patency.

INFLOW SELECTION: The common femoral, superficial femoral, profunda femoris, or popliteal artery may be used for inflow. The inflow pulse should be strong and not distal to an upstream significant stenosis. Common femoral endarterectomy with patch angioplasty is not an uncommon concomitant procedure during femoral-tibial bypass, and occasionally the proximal vein anastomosis can function as the patch angioplasty. Significant stenoses of the iliac or superficial femoral arteries proximal to intended inflow sites may be treated with angioplasty and stenting preoperatively or during the case. If there are any questions as to the adequacy of the inflow, pressure measurements of the inflow vessel with provocative nitroglycerin or papaverine can help determine if a proximal lesion is hemodynamically significant. In patients with significant groin scarring from previous femoral cutdowns, the proximal anastomosis may be performed onto the profunda femoris artery to avoid redo-exposure.

OUTFLOW SELECTION: The least calcified tibial artery that provides in-line flow to the foot is chosen for outflow. When sufficient high-quality vein graft exists and both tibial arteries provide in-line flow, then angiosome-directed revascularization is considered. When tibial artery targets are not available, the peroneal artery is used and affords similar patency results.

POSITIONING The patient is placed in supine position on a radiolucent operating table with both arms abducted (or one arm tucked to facilitate C-arm entry if concomitant endovascular iliac intervention is planned). When arm vein harvest is planned, we place the prepared arm on a wide arm board.

PREPARATION AND DRAPING The entire ipsilateral lower limb is shaved and the GSV mapped using ultrasonography to avoid creating skin flaps and to identify branches (**FIGURE 61-1A**).

When the ipsilateral GSV is absent or there is concern about its quality, the contralateral lower limb or upper limb with the largest diameter or highest quality arm veins are also shaved and their veins mapped. In obese patients, we tape the pannus cephalad to assist with groin exposure. Limbs considered for vein harvest are circumferentially painted with chlorhexidine or betadine (open wounds). The foot and/or hand are then placed in a transparent bag. A rest made of bundled sterile towels or surgical gowns is placed under the thigh to allow the calf muscles to dangle and aid in exposure.

DETAILS OF PROCEDURE

VEIN GRAFT HARVEST

GSV The longitudinal femoral artery incision is extended in an oblique fashion posterior-medially over the greater saphenous vein. Oblique incision can be made over the common femoral artery pulse proximally and angled medially distally toward the marked GSV (see Chapter 5 for details). The GSV is identified and all branches up to the saphenofemoral junction are ligated and divided. The anterior accessory saphenous vein branch is preserved and used for patch angioplasty if an iliofemoral endarterectomy or extended profundaplasty is planned. Skip incisions can help reduce tissue flaps and tissue ischemia over the GSV (**FIGURE 61-1B**).

The last incision is longer and is used to also expose the posterior tibial or peroneal artery or create the tunnel to the anterior tibial artery. We commonly use four skip incisions for proximal tibial bypasses and five for more distal bypasses. When dissecting the GSV around the knee, extra caution must be taken to prevent inadvertent injury, as the vein is superficial and tends to increasingly branch at this location, and it is not a good place for skip incisions.

Arm Veins The cephalic, basilic, and median cubital veins may be used for bypass conduits. Use of the forearm cephalic vein may be limited by phlebitis or intraluminal webs caused by repeated cannulation. In the arm, the cephalic vein is often thin walled, while the basilic vein has a larger diameter. The basilic-cephalic loop graft is a U-shaped graft with the vertex of the U formed by the median cubital veins. This graft is harvested by making skip incisions directly over the vein-mapped cephalic and basilic veins in the arm and median cubital veins in the antecubital fossa. (**FIGURE 61-2**).

When the larger diameter basilic vein is used as the proximal, non-reversed portion of the loop graft, a Mills or other valvulotome may be introduced through a median cubital vein side branch and used to lyse its valves instead of those of the thin-walled cephalic vein; the vertex of the loop graft is then straightened, after which the thin-walled cephalic vein is maintained in the reversed position as it has a better size match to the tibial arteries.

If the forearm cephalic vein is adequate, it is dissected in continuity from the wrist to the deltopectoral groove to maximize the harvested length of vein. The basilic vein can then be spliced in the reversed fashion to increase length for a tibial bypass as needed. This formation negates valve lysis in a fragile vein. **CONTINUES ▶**

61-1

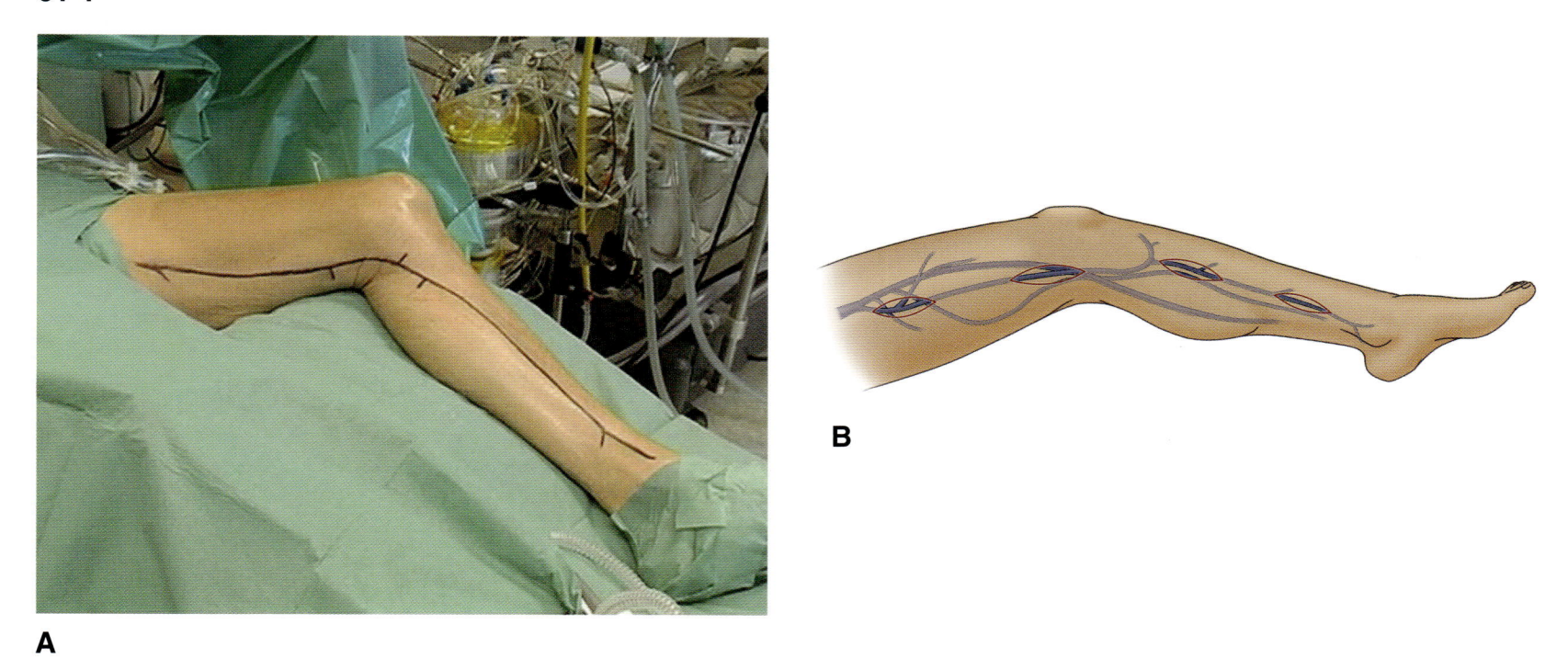

A

B

Figure 61-1 Intraoperatively mapped GSV (A) and skip incisions over mapped GSV to harvest the vein for reversed bypass (B).

61-2

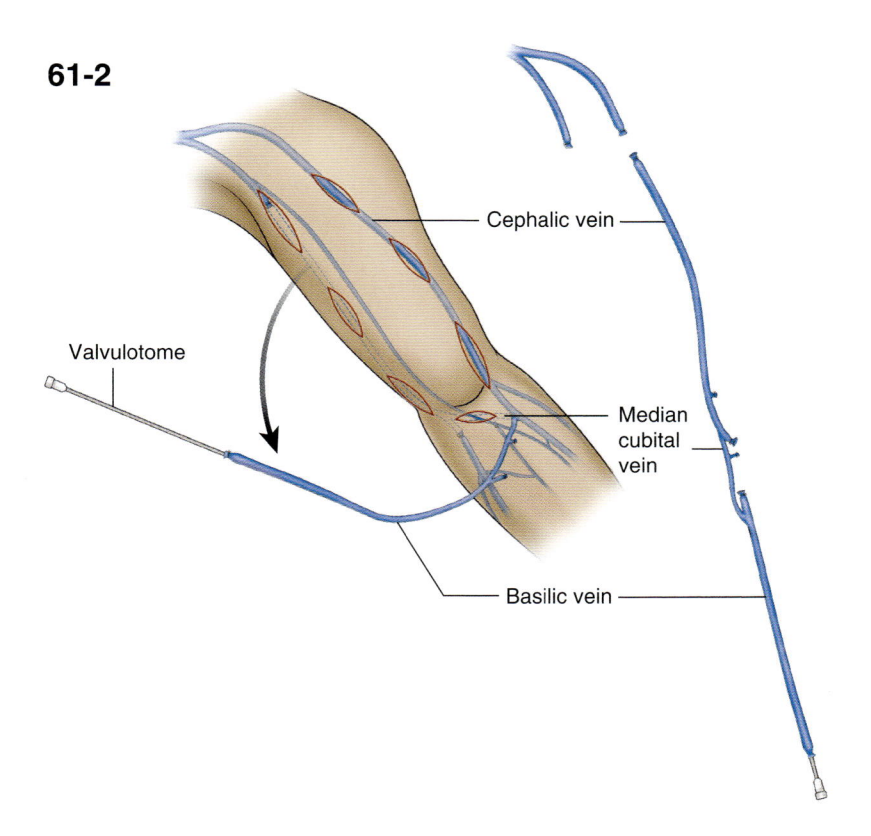

Figure 61-2 Arm vein harvest with skip incisions over the vein-mapped cephalic, median cubital, and basilic veins to create a basilic-cephalic loop graft.

DETAILS OF PROCEDURE *TECHNIQUE:* `CONTINUED` When harvesting vein grafts, the ventral, usually branch-free, surface of the vein is first unroofed in the periadventitial plane (see Chapter 5 for details of vein harvesting). A vessel loop is then placed around the vein to facilitate atraumatic vein traction and identification of branches. To avoid impingement on the lumen of the vein, branches are ligated 2 mm away from the wall and divided between 3-0 or 2-0 silk ties and metal clips. With the assistance of a narrow, deep Richardson retractor, we then develop a plane anterior to the vein under the skin bridge at the distal end of the incision. Using an index finger, this plane is carefully propagated caudally under the skin. With the vein located deep to the finger, the skin is incised and intervening adipose tissue is squeezed and then incised with electrocautery to unroof the vein. This process of creating skip incisions is followed down the leg or along the arm until sufficient vein is harvested. Before the vein is removed, the caudal aspect is marked and two medium-sized clips or a silk tie are placed on the residual stump. The vein is transected above the clips and pulled through the skip incisions. A Darrah clamp or Lauer are placed on the proximal aspect of the GSV, or arm vein, and the proximal vein is sutured ligated with 2-0 silk or 6-0 Prolene (two layers). If in doubt about a branch or deep tissue, it is better to have a normal uninjured vein, and skip incisions should be abandoned for a continuous incision.

VEIN GRAFT PREPARATION: The vein graft is placed into a basin containing heparinized saline until the surgeon is ready to inspect its integrity. The distal end of the graft is then cannulated with an olive-tipped or 18-gauge intravenous cannula connected to a 20-cc syringe containing heparinized saline. Injection of heparinized saline into the vein gently distends it (high pressures should be avoided) and identifies non-ligated branches and iatrogenic vein wall injuries. If areas of the vein are sclerotic or have a small diameter (<2.5 mm), consideration should be given to splicing better quality and larger diameter segments of harvested vein together.

PROXIMAL ANASTOMOSIS: The proximal anastomosis is performed most often end-to-side to the inflow artery using double-armed 6-0 polypropylene suture in a parachuted fashion. The inflow artery is opened with a 15-blade and the arteriotomy is extended with Potts scissors. If a concomitant iliofemoral endarterectomy or extended profundaplasty is required, the endarterectomized artery can be patched with a longitudinally opened accessory saphenous vein branch, bovine pericardial patch, or endarterectomized occluded superficial femoral artery. If the distal reversed vein has a small caliber, a side-branch can be split open in conjunction with the vein and incorporated into the anastomosis to increase its diameter (see Chapter 59).

VEIN SPLICING: If vein splicing is required, the ends of the reversed veins to be spliced are obliquely beveled to create a diamond shape. The heel and toe of the anastomosis are tacked together with two 7-0 Prolene sutures and then run toward each other to reduce the purse-stringing effect that can occur during vein-to-vein anastomoses (**FIGURE 61-3**). It can be helpful to use an 8F pediatric feeding tube when sewing the anastomosis to prevent back-walling the anastomosis.

TUNNELING: The bypass may be tunneled subcutaneously, anatomically, or subcutaneously and anatomically. Before the vein graft is tunneled, the inflow is unclamped and two medium-sized clips are placed on the end of the reversed vein graft. The anterior aspect of the vein graft is marked while it is "live" to prevent subsequent kinking. It is best to tunnel the graft distended and marked to prevent twisting. To tunnel subcutaneously, either the vein bypass is tunneled though the bed of the recently harvested GSV or a 65-cm GORE tunneler is used to tunnel the graft subcutaneously (superficial to the crural fascia) through another plane. The method of tunneling anatomically is explained in Chapters 60 and 62 (**FIGURE 61-4**). Finally, the tunnel to the anterior tibial artery can be performed anatomically through the interosseous membrane or extra-anatomically through a lateral subcutaneous tunnel created from the groin.

DISTAL ANASTOMOSIS: As the tibial arteries are small in diameter, frequently calcified, and prone to vasospasm, we only unroof their ventral surface enough to permit performance of the distal anastomosis and do not dissect them circumferentially. The venous blood from the leg is then exsanguinated with an Esmarch bandage wrapped circumferentially and tightly around the leg starting at the foot and working up to the thigh (**FIGURE 61-5**). A mid-thigh tourniquet is then inflated to 250 to 300 mmHg for proximal control. The tibial artery is opened with an 11-blade and the arteriotomy is extended with micro-Potts scissors. The length of bypass graft required is subsequently measured with the knee fully extended. The heel and toe are marked before the bypass is cut. An end-to-side anastomosis is then performed with a double-armed 7-0 polypropylene suture in a parachuted fashion (see Chapter 4 for anastomosis creation). A continuous-wave Doppler examination is used to confirm an acceptable Doppler signal in the tibial artery before and after the anastomosis.

COMPLETION STUDIES: The bypass graft is punctured near the hood of the proximal anastomosis with a 2qG butterfly needle, an 8-gauge angiocatheter or Micropuncture 4-French sheath and connected to arterial line extension tubing. Hand-injection DSAs are then performed. If there is evidence of vasospasm on the angiogram, 50 to 100 μg of nitroglycerin (diluted in saline to 10 μg/mL) or 30 mg of papaverine is slowly injected into the vein, and then a subsequent DSA is done to confirm resolution.

CLOSURE The subcutaneous tissues of the groin wound, thigh, and leg are reapproximated in two layers with absorbable sutures. We do not recommend reapproximating the crural fascia of the leg, as this and postoperative edema can compress the graft. When we are concerned about subcutaneous tissue quality, we close the skin with interrupted, vertical mattress 3-0 nylon sutures. Otherwise, the skin is reapproximated with staples or 4-0 absorbable subcuticular sutures.

POSTOPERATIVE CARE

POSTOPERATIVE CARE: A Bair hugger covered by warm blankets is applied over the lower limbs in the recovery room to promote artery dilation. Dressings are removed on the second postoperative day. Leg elevation and gentle compression garments (if the graft is not tunneled superficially) are used to treat post-bypass edema.

FOLLOW-UP: Clinical examination, ABIs, and duplex ultrasound are performed early after bypass; at 3, 6, and 12 months for the first year, and at least biannually thereafter. More frequent surveillance is performed when uncorrected abnormalities are identified on duplex ultrasound or when vein grafts other than GSV are used. ■

61-3

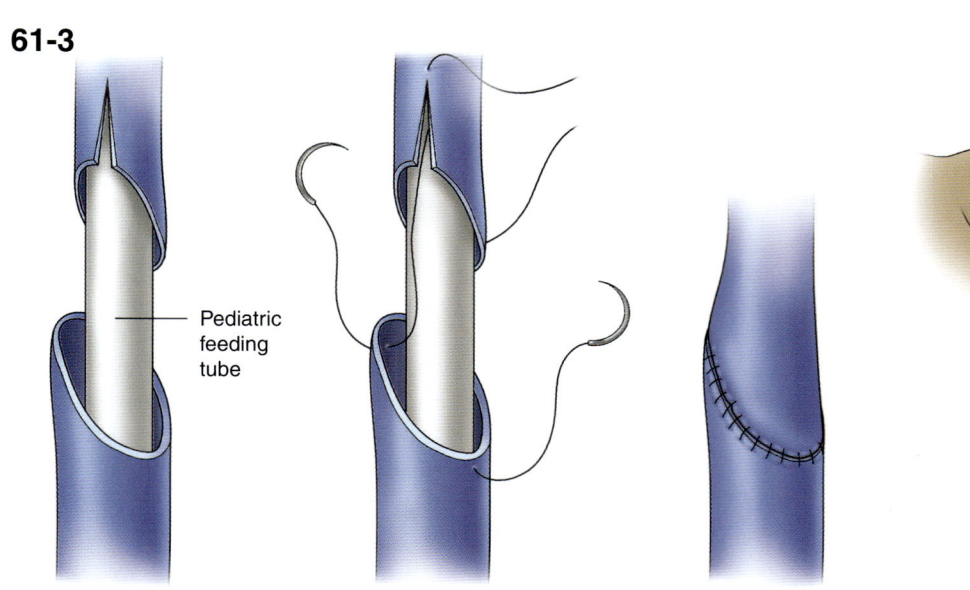

Figure 61-3 Spliced vein graft, making sure both grafts have the same valve orientation.

61-4

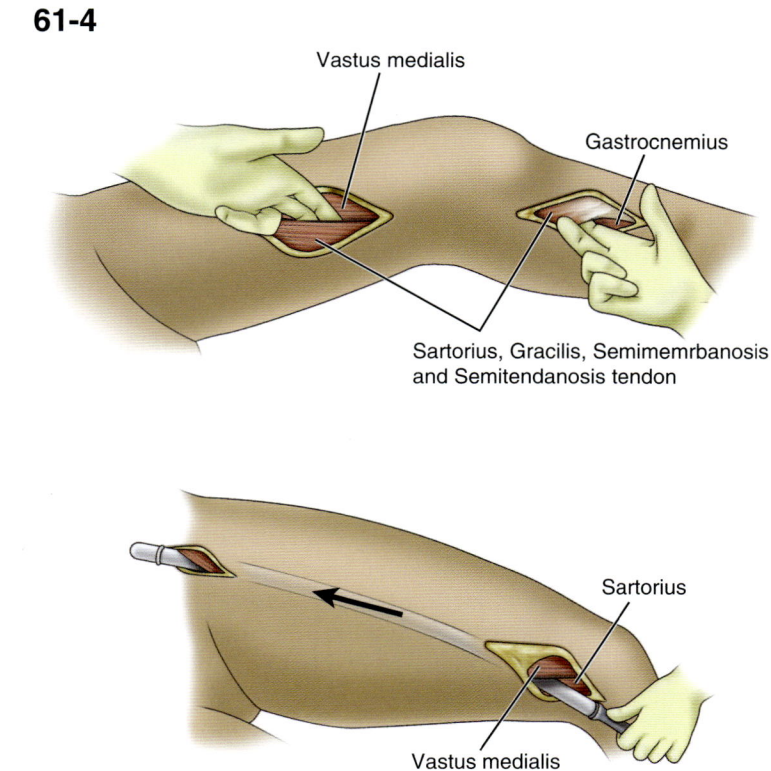

Figure 61-4 Creation of tunnels.

61-5

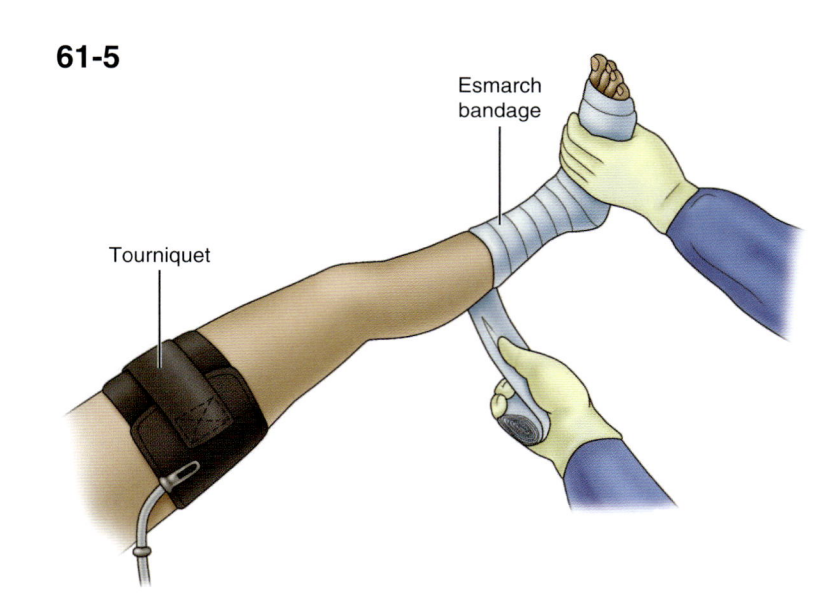

Figure 61-5 Tourniquet placement after esmark exsanguination of venous blood.

PEDAL BYPASS

Clara Gomez-Sanchez, MD • Michael S. Conte, MD

INDICATIONS Some of the most challenging cases in lower extremity arterial occlusive disease are those in patients with extensive tibial and inframalleolar disease. Diabetes is associated with more distal distribution of atherosclerosis in the leg, and the combination of diabetic foot wounds and ischemia can be particularly devastating. While patients with proximal disease may be more likely to complain of claudication pain in large muscle groups, the effects of isolated infrageniculate disease may be underrecognized until the point of chronic limb threatening ischemia (CLTI) with tissue loss or ischemic rest pain. A fundamental tenet of revascularization in CLTI, particularly with tissue loss, is to restore in-line flow to the ankle and foot. There are multiple series that demonstrate excellent rates of limb salvage with pedal revascularization.[1-3] Based on these data, bypass to the dorsalis pedis or plantar arteries is indicated in selected patients with CLTI and severe tibial disease who do not have a more proximal artery available with in-line flow to the foot.

PREOPERATIVE PLANNING A comprehensive evaluation of the patient should include a complete history and physical exam, with particular attention to cardiovascular and pulmonary risk factors as well as ambulatory and functional status. The surgeon should document a complete pulse exam and carefully examine the extremity for wounds and signs of infection. Noninvasive studies including measurement of ankle and toe pressures are fundamental in establishing the degree of ischemia. The Society for Vascular Surgery threatened limb classification system based on wound, ischemia, and foot infection (WIFI) grading stratifies patients into those at highest risk of limb loss and greatest potential benefit for revascularization.[4]

Successful bypass surgery depends on meticulous selection of the inflow position, conduit, and outflow target. While all three factors are important, conduit quality is preeminent in distal bypass surgery. The inflow vessel should be a healthy segment of artery with no hemodynamically significant proximal disease. In patients with isolated infrapopliteal disease, distal origin grafts arising from the superficial femoral or popliteal artery have equivalent patency rates to those originating from the common femoral artery.[5] Patients with severe multilevel disease may need additional procedures to address inflow prior to pedal bypass. It is acceptable to perform iliac stenting, common femoral endarterectomy, or even endovascular treatment of mild to moderate superficial femoral artery (SFA) disease to allow optimization of inflow to a distal graft origin. However, we caution against selecting a graft inflow position distal to an intervention for long-segment SFA disease or chronic total occlusions, and the popliteal pulse should be easily palpable if a below-knee proximal anastomosis is selected.

Selection of the proximal graft origin must take into account not only the health of the inflow artery, but also the length of good quality conduit available. Studies have demonstrated superiority of autologous vein as the conduit for tibial and pedal bypass, with the ipsilateral greater saphenous vein (GSV) as the ideal choice.[3,6-9] Some patients have limited length of adequate caliber GSV (3 mm or larger), so use of an acceptable distal inflow site may shorten the graft length required. When GSV is not available, the upper extremities should be evaluated for conduit; spliced arm veins offer fair alternatives when the lower extremity veins are inadequate. Intraoperative evaluation of the vein when distended under direct vision may identify areas of decreased caliber or fibrotic segments that were not noticed on preoperative ultrasound. If a spliced vein graft is required, it is preferably constructed with no more than three segments. If the patient does not have adequate length of autologous vein available, they may not be a reasonable candidate for a pedal bypass.

For popliteal-to-pedal bypass, one may choose between using the proximal (translocated) or distal GSV for conduit. Vein grafts may be reversed or non-reversed with valve lysis. We generally favor using the proximal GSV, as it is larger in caliber and keeps the harvest incisions away from the more ischemic distal extremity. Proximal GSV presents a significant size mismatch with the pedal vessels; thus, we often employ it in a non-reversed orientation with valvulotomy. However, if the distal GSV is used for conduit, it is generally larger at the ankle and readily used in a reversed fashion. It can also be left in situ. The harvest incision for the saphenous vein in the lower leg should be made carefully with the future graft tunnel in mind. Any wound breakdown overlying the graft position could threaten the revascularization.

Cross-sectional imaging is useful for the evaluation of inflow disease, but offers insufficient resolution of the small vessels of the lower leg and foot for selection of a pedal bypass target. We recommend digital subtraction angiography in all candidates for infrapopliteal bypass. An adequate angiogram requires both anterior-posterior and lateral projections of the foot, and the runoff should extend to the toes. The inframalleolar targets of interest are the dorsalis pedis and tarsal arteries or the terminal branches from the posterior tibial artery, the common, medial, or lateral plantar arteries. It is important to recognize that anatomic variants, especially of the dorsalis pedis and its branches, are not rare and that tarsal branches can be mistaken for the dorsalis pedis if only a single foot view is obtained. These vessels are small and often calcified, so precise selection of the best location for anastomosis is critical to success of the bypass. The vessel diameter at the selected location should be at least 2 mm but ideally closer to 2.5 mm.

PATIENT POSITIONING AND EQUIPMENT The patient is positioned supine with both groins prepped into the field, as well as the affected limb circumferentially and any additional sites as needed for conduit harvest. A padded surgical bump may assist with positioning when dissecting out the distal superficial femoral or popliteal arteries, as well as supporting the leg in external rotation for dissection of the plantar arteries on the foot. A sterile tourniquet should be available on the field for the distal anastomosis and may also be used for the proximal anastomosis depending on the position selected. In the case of highly calcified vessels, it may not be feasible to employ the tourniquet, and atraumatic vascular clamps should be available. Slim taper point needles (e.g., Ethicon VISI-BLACK needles) may be helpful when suturing heavily calcified vessels.

SURGICAL EXPOSURE Previous chapters detail the surgical approach to the common and superficial femoral arteries, the popliteal artery, and saphenous vein harvest (Chapter 5, 59, 60). If any inflow procedures such as a femoral endarterectomy are indicated, these should be completed first. Duplex ultrasound using a high resolution (e.g., 15 MHz) transducer can be helpful to localize the pedal and plantar arteries and areas of calcification prior to incision and exposure.

DORSALIS PEDIS AND TARSAL ARTERIES: The dorsalis pedis artery is identified by intraoperative ultrasound slightly lateral to the extensor hallucis longus tendon prior to incision. A longitudinal incision 3 cm in length is made over the artery in the proximal foot and through the thin layer of subcutaneous tissue. The inferior aspect of the extensor retinaculum is incised as needed. The artery is quite superficial in this position and cessation of flow during anastomosis is best achieved with a sterile tourniquet, so the dissection can typically be quite limited if the identified segment appears minimally diseased (**FIGURE 62-1**).

In the case that the dorsalis pedis itself is inadequate, the terminal branches may be employed as recipient vessels instead and/or the bypass graft hooded over the branch points. For exposure of the lateral tarsal branch, the proximal dorsalis pedis is exposed just distal to the edge of the inferior extensor retinaculum. The dissection is continued until the branch point of the lateral tarsal artery, which can be identified coursing toward the head of the fifth metatarsal. More distal exposure of the lateral tarsal branch may be achieved by laterally retracting the extensor digitorum longus tendons, but may additionally require division of the first and second tendon as well as transection of the extensor hallucis brevis muscle.

Once the distal target is exposed on the dorsum of the foot, our preference for graft tunneling is subcutaneous, crossing anteriorly over the tibia in the distal leg such that the graft approaches the dorsalis pedis in a straight, caudally directed fashion (**FIGURE 62-2**). One potential disadvantage of using the distal greater saphenous vein is proximity between the harvest incision and the tunneled graft at the ankle. If the skin closure over graft or at the distal anastomosis is under tension (e.g., due to edema), it may be prudent to perform a relaxing incision to prevent breakdown and graft exposure. An alternative option is to tunnel the graft anatomically through the interosseous membrane and within the anterior compartment, which may be necessary if the length of vein is marginal, when skin quality is poor, or when nearby wounds pose a threat. **CONTINUES ▶**

62-1

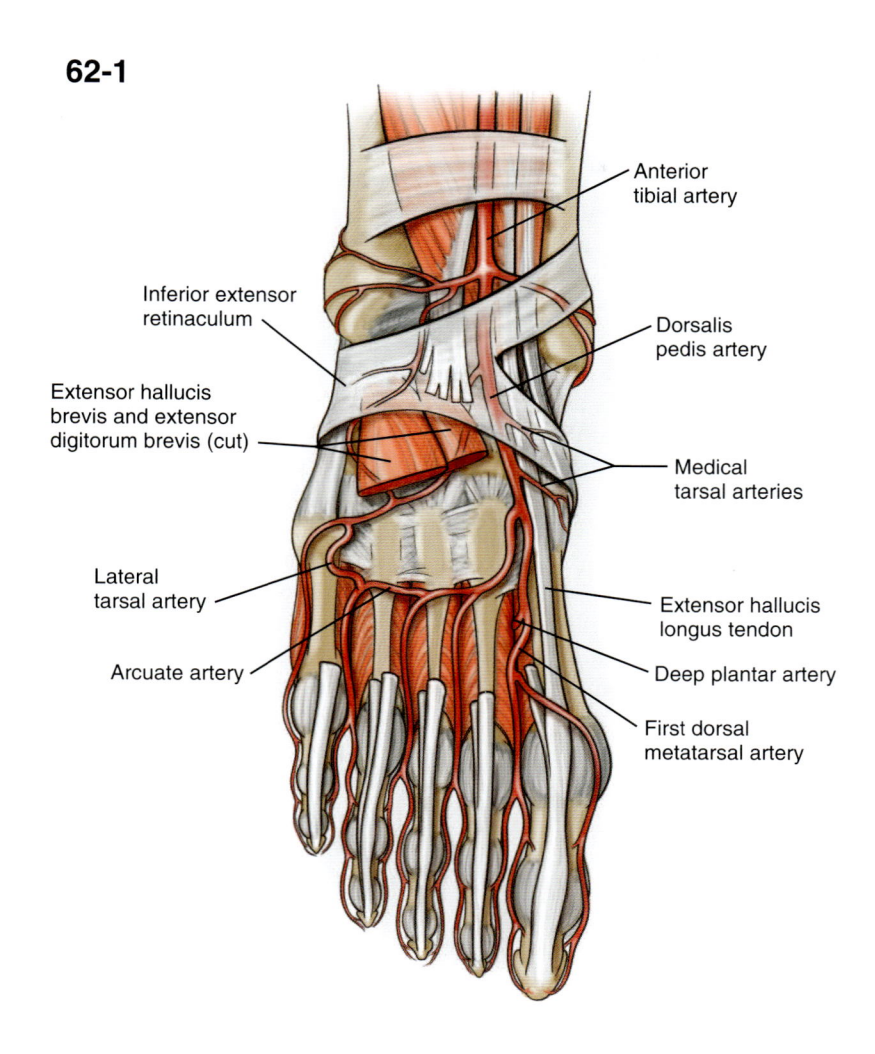

Anterior
tibial artery

Inferior extensor
retinaculum

Dorsalis
pedis artery

Extensor hallucis
brevis and extensor
digitorum brevis (cut)

Medical
tarsal arteries

Lateral
tarsal artery

Extensor hallucis
longus tendon

Arcuate artery

Deep plantar artery

First dorsal
metatarsal artery

62-2

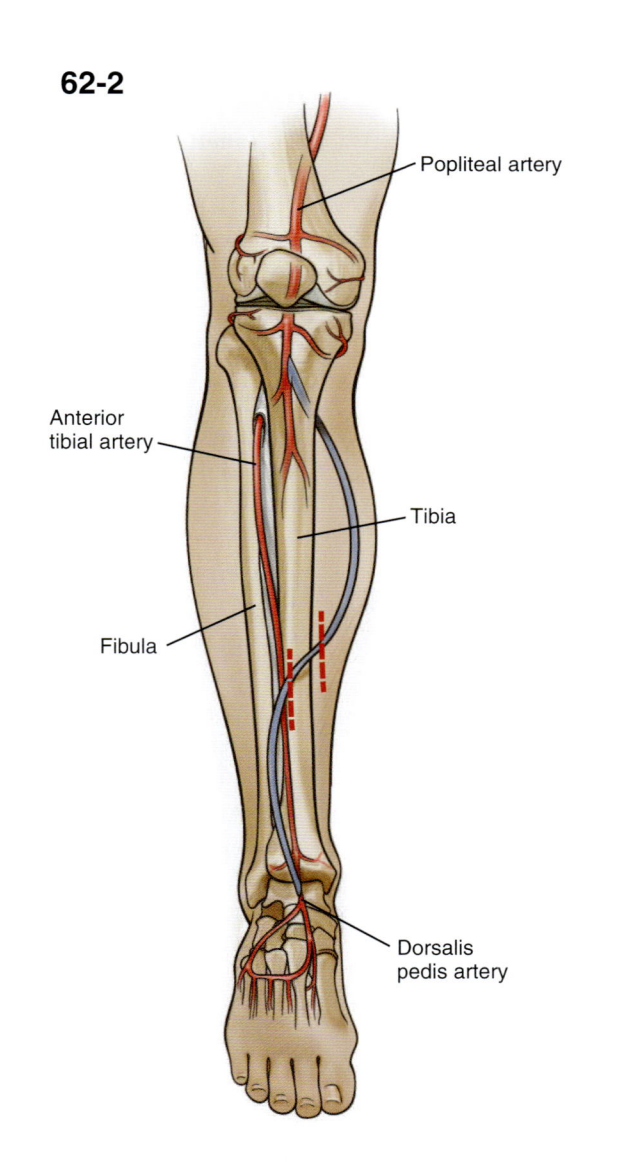

Popliteal artery

Anterior
tibial artery

Tibia

Fibula

Dorsalis
pedis artery

SURGICAL EXPOSURE *PLANTAR ARTERIES:* CONTINUED The posterior tibial artery terminates in the common plantar artery, which passes under the flexor retinaculum and bifurcates into the lateral and medial plantar arteries. These tend to be deeper in the foot under thick plantar fascial tissue. The leg is externally rotated and exposure starts with an incision in the medial foot just inferior to the malleolus to identify the transition of the posterior tibial into the common plantar artery as it passes under the flexor retinaculum. This allows for identification of the origins of the plantar arteries at their branch point. The lateral plantar is typically more inferior, while the medial is superior and often the smaller of the two. Preoperative angiography is essential for deciding which of the branches to hood the graft onto and can be augmented by palpation and duplex ultrasound intraoperatively. The medial plantar aponeurosis is incised and the abductor hallucis muscle must be transected to expose the plantar bifurcation and main branches as they travel onto the plantar surface (FIGURE 62-3).

Tunneling for plantar bypass is typically subcutaneous on the medial aspect of the leg and travels anatomically behind the medial malleolus to provide protection to the graft during flexion and extension of the ankle (FIGURE 62-4). The graft should be measured with the foot in full dorsiflexion to ensure adequate length without tension during ambulation and will have some redundancy when the foot is at rest or plantarflexed.

ANASTOMOSIS After creating the tunnel, the patient should be systemically heparinized prior to clamp control or exsanguination of the leg with an Esmarch bandage and inflation of a tourniquet. The proximal anastomosis with the popliteal artery is described in detail elsewhere. Briefly, we recommend an end-to-side anastomosis in a running fashion with the hood of the bypass extending approximately 2 cm, usually employing a 5-0 or 6-0 polypropylene suture. Proximal control is released to allow the graft to distend in order to mark the top side of the conduit and guide it carefully through the tunnel without twisting. The length of graft should be measured while distended and marked prior to inflating the tourniquet for distal vascular control.

A longitudinal arteriotomy is created with a micro-scalpel on the pedal artery and extended with fine Potts scissors for a length of at least 6 mm. Gentle interrogation with lacrimal probes (1–2 mm) confirms that the selected portion of the vessel has a patent outflow tract. The vein graft is measured and trimmed at the distal extent of the anastomosis and then spatulated to match the length of the arteriotomy. We recommend using a parachuting technique with 6-0 or 7-0 polypropylene suture with fine needle size (e.g., Ethicon BV-1) to allow meticulous visualization of the sutures in the heel and toe of the graft. The anastomosis is then sutured in a continuous running fashion from each side. The tourniquet is released to flush and de-air the graft when the anastomosis is nearly completed. We recommend completion imaging with both a duplex ultrasound and a completion angiogram to evaluate technical success and runoff into the foot.

Some patients have extremely calcified arteries, which can make the anastomosis technically challenging. We strongly recommend against trying to perform a formal endarterectomy in these small, fragile vessels. However, medial calcification can often be gently fractured with a DeBakey forceps and any loose fractured pieces of intimal plaque gently teased out of the lumen. The vessel should be thoroughly flushed with heparinized saline to clear any debris and back- and forward-bleeding checked prior to completing the anastomosis.

WOUND CLOSURE AND DRESSINGS Interrupted subcutaneous sutures (e.g., 3-0 Vicryl) are placed to begin closure over the graft and the distal anastomosis. We recommend closing the skin with interrupted nylon mattress sutures for careful approximation of the skin edges without causing undue tension. The graft pulse and distal signals should be checked after the skin closure to confirm the graft has not been compressed by the closure. After sterile dressings are applied, a gentle ACE wrap can be used with windows cut into the fabric for regular pulse exams. Especially with bypass to the plantar vessels, a posterior splint or boot may be helpful to maintain the foot in a neutral position. The splint should be placed by the surgeon to be absolutely sure that no pressure is placed on the bypass graft or the immediate outflow.

POSTOPERATIVE CARE Wounds at the ankle and foot are at particularly high risk of complication without aggressive management of lower extremity edema. Bedrest is generally ordered for the first 24 hours, with strict elevation above the level of the heart at all times when in bed. Even once off bedrest, patients should be strictly counseled to maintain elevation at all times except when actively ambulating for short periods. When sitting, the leg should not be left in a completely dependent position for prolonged periods of time. Intravenous fluids should be used judiciously to maintain perfusion while actively monitoring elements such as urine output, daily weights, and labs to avoid fluid overload. This is particularly important in patients with a history of heart failure and chronic renal disease, who may require diuresis to assist with mobilizing perioperative fluids. Sutures are left in place for 3 weeks postoperatively. Antibiotics are tailored to treatment of any ongoing foot infections and are unnecessary in the absence of concurrent infection. All patients are maintained on antiplatelet therapy, generally with aspirin 81 mg daily; low dose anticoagulation with rivaroxaban 2.5 mg twice daily may be beneficial in patients who do not otherwise have indications for anticoagulation or dual antiplatelet therapy.[10,11] ∎

REFERENCES

1. Pomposelli FB, Kansal N, Hamdan AD, Belfield A, Sheahan M, Campbell DR. A decade of experience with dorsalis pedis artery bypass: Analysis of outcome in more than 1000 cases. *J Vasc Surg*. 2003;37(2):307-315.

2. Ascer E, Veith F, Gupta S. Bypasses to plantar arteries and other tibial branches: An extended approach to limb salvage. *J Vasc Surg*. 1988;8 (4):434-441.

3. Hughes K, Domenig CM, Hamdan AD, et al. Bypass to plantar and tarsal arteries: An acceptable approach to limb salvage. *J Vasc Surg*. 2004;40(6):1149-1157.

4. Mills JL, Conte MS, Armstrong DG, et al. The Society for Vascular Surgery Lower Extremity Threatened Limb Classification System: Risk stratification based on Wound, Ischemia, and foot Infection (WIfI). *J Vasc Surg*. 2014;59(1):220-234.e2.

5. Reed AB, Conte MS, Belkin M, Mannick JA, Whittemore AD, Donaldson MC. Usefulness of autogenous bypass grafts originating distal to the groin. *J Vasc Surg*. 2002;35(1):48-55.

6. Nierlich P, Enzmann FK, Metzger, et al. Alternative venous conduits for below knee bypass in the absence of ipsilateral great saphenous vein. *Eur J Vasc Endovasc Surg*. 2020;60:403-409.

7. Schanzer A, Hevelone N, Owens CD, et al. Technical factors affecting autogenous vein graft failure: observations from a large multicenter trial. *J Vasc Surg*. 2007;46(6):1180-1190.

8. McGinigle KL, Pascarella L, Shortell CK, et al. Spliced arm vein grafts are a durable conduit for lower extremity bypass. *Ann Vasc Surg*. 2015;29(4):716-721.

9. Almasri J, Adusumalli J, Asi N, et al. A systematic review and meta-analysis of revascularization outcomes of infrainguinal chronic limb-threatening ischemia. *J Vasc Surg*. 2018;68(2):624-633.

10. Bonaca MP, Bauersachs RM, Anand SS, et al. Rivaroxaban in peripheral artery disease after revascularization. *N Engl J Med*. 2020;382(21):1994-2004.

11. Anand SS, Eikelboom JW, Connolly SJ, et al. Rivaroxaban with or without aspirin in patients with stable peripheral or carotid artery disease: An international, randomised, double-blind placebo-controlled trial. *Lancet*. 2018;391(10117):219-229.

62-3

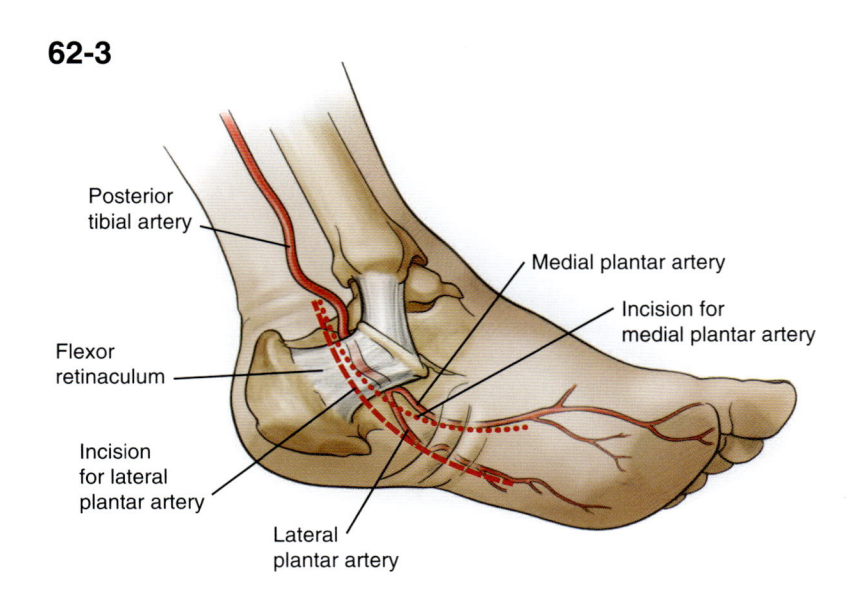

62-4

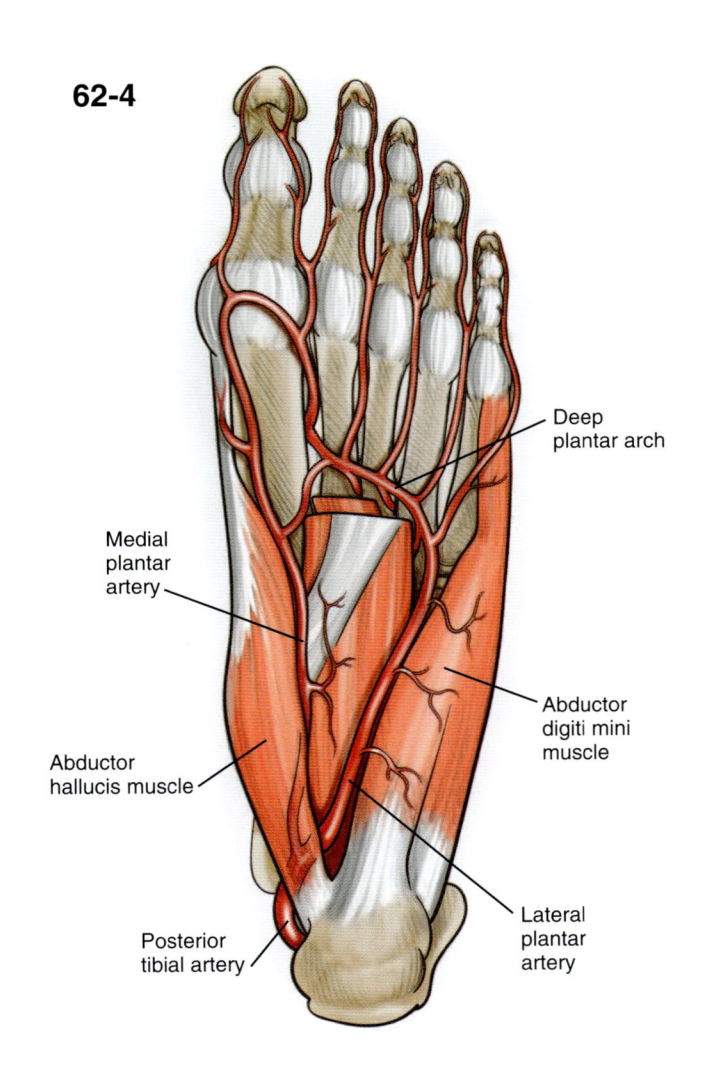

OPEN EXPOSURE FOR FEMORAL AND POPLITEAL ANEURYSM REPAIR

Asha Behdinan, MD • Kathryn L. Howe, MD, PhD

PART I: FEMORAL ARTERY ANEURYSMS

INTRODUCTION Lower extremity aneurysms have the second highest incidence of aneurysmal disease, following the infrarenal aorta and iliac arteries. They are, however, often associated with aortic aneurysms and aneurysms in the contralateral limb. The presence of a femoral aneurysm confers a 50 to 90% risk of concomitant aortic aneurysm. Femoral aneurysms typically arise in the common femoral artery (CFA), and are categorized as either true aneurysms or pseudoaneurysms.

CFA diameter ranges from 0.8 to 1.0 cm, with a true aneurysm being defined as a uniform dilatation of the artery greater than or equal to 1.5 times its normal size. True aneurysms involve all three layers of the vessel wall, while pseudoaneurysms do not. Instead, pseudoaneurysms are saccular projections arising from a defect in the vessel wall containing flow from the native artery into the adjacent tissue.

True femoral aneurysms may be asymptomatic in up to 40% of patients, but can present with pain, compressive symptoms (including leg edema, neuropathic pain, weakness, skin changes, and palpable pulsatile mass), or lower extremity ischemia secondary to distal embolization. These patients rarely present with isolated ruptures of their femoral aneurysms.

To confirm diagnosis, the first-line imaging modality is duplex ultrasonography; however, CT angiography (CTA) or magnetic resonance angiography (MRA) can be used to delineate anatomic features and plan for surgical repair.

Symptomatic patients (described above) must be treated in order to prevent or limit the effects of neurogenic compression, thrombosis, and embolization. For those with asymptomatic femoral artery aneurysms, they are often treated nonoperatively until reaching a size threshold of 2.5 cm, or signs of distal ischemia appear.

Treatment options for femoral artery true and pseudoaneurysms can be categorized into open, endovascular, or hybrid approaches. This chapter focuses on the role of open surgical intervention for this pathology. This treatment modality consists of either aneurysm exclusion with an interposition graft (using either autologous or prosthetic conduits), direct repair, or patch angioplasty.

PREOPERATIVE PLANNING Patients presenting with isolated lower extremity artery aneurysms require imaging (duplex or cross-sectional) to identify aneurysmal disease at other arterial sites, including the aorta, iliac arteries, popliteal arteries, and contralateral femoral artery. CTA and MRA can be useful to identify anatomic variations, look for evidence of distal embolization and occlusive disease, or determine arterial measurements necessary for endovascular therapy. However, duplex ultrasound is the preferred imaging modality for femoral pseudoaneurysm assessment.

Patients must also be assessed for systemic infection, as the presence of a mycotic aneurysm could preclude use of endovascular treatment options.

In patients with pseudoaneurysms, use of anticoagulation, pregnancy, and aneurysm neck dimensions are important to help guide treatment. Those who require systemic anticoagulation, have ongoing infection, allergy to antithrombotic agents, and have wide aneurysm necks are typically not amenable to ultrasound-guided thrombin injections, and require open repair.

POSITIONING The patient is placed in a supine position with both legs and the lower abdomen prepped and draped in sterile manner. The arms can either be tucked or left extended at 80 degrees based on surgeon preference.

PROCEDURE
- Incision
  - The common femoral artery is identified via palpation of the femoral pulse, or landmarks (midway between anterior superior iliac spine and pubic symphysis).
  - A longitudinal/curvilinear skin incision over the common femoral artery is made.
- Exposure (FIGURE 63-1)
  - The underlying subcutaneous tissue is incised using electrocautery until the aneurysm is encountered.

- Dissection is then extended cephalad until the inguinal ligament is identified.
- The proximal common femoral artery is then identified at the level of the inguinal ligament, which is exposed circumferentially and controlled using a silastic vessel loop.
- The distal end of the dissection is then carried out to identify the superficial femoral artery (SFA) and profunda artery, which are both exposed circumferentially and controlled with silastic vessel loops.
- Systemic heparin (100 units/kg) is administered, circulating for 3 to 5 minutes.
- The distal external iliac artery/proximal CFA, SFA, and profunda are clamped.
- *Pearl: Ensure ligation of the* vein of pain *(deep circumflex iliac vein) if obtaining high proximal control.*
- *True aneurysm*: The aneurysm sac is opened longitudinally with a number 11 blade, and arteriotomy is extended using Potts scissors. The aneurysm is then transected in a transverse fashion to prepare for repair.
- *Pseudoaneurysm*: The aneurysm sac is opened either longitudinally or transversely with a number 11 blade and extended with Potts scissors until the arterial wall defect is identified.
- Anastomosis/Repair
  - *True aneurysm*: An end-to-end interposition graft using 8-mm PTFE/Dacron or autologous saphenous vein is placed with a running 5-0 or 6-0 polypropylene suture.
  - *Pseudoaneurysm*: The arterial wall defect is identified and repaired primarily or repaired with bovine pericardial patch or autologous vein patch angioplasty with a 5-0 or 6-0 polypropylene suture.
- Closure
  - The subcutaneous tissues are closed in two to three layers using 3-0 Vicryl sutures and the skin closed with staples or running subcuticular suture.

POSTOPERATIVE CARE AND COMPLICATIONS Postoperatively, the patient is placed on best medical therapy for risk factor modification. Distal flow is confirmed using either duplex ultrasonography or arteriography. Clinical follow-up exams are typically conducted at 1-month, 3-month, and 6-month intervals with repeat imaging to ensure patency of the repair.

Complications associated with the procedure include distal embolization, wound infection, lymphatic leak/drainage, thrombosis or occlusion of graft, blood loss, and femoral nerve injury.

PART II: POPLITEAL ARTERY ANEURYSMS

INTRODUCTION Popliteal artery aneurysms (PAA) have the highest incidence of peripheral artery aneurysms, accounting for over 70%. Over half the patients have an aneurysm in the contralateral popliteal artery, and 30 to 50% have a concomitant abdominal aortic aneurysm. The majority are true aneurysms, arising most commonly from degenerative or atherosclerotic disease. Arterial wall stress from repetitive joint use has also been studied as a factor for loss of mechanical integrity leading to aneurysm formation.

Patients typically present with lower extremity ischemia secondary to thrombosis or distal embolization, with symptoms ranging from mild claudication to acute limb ischemia (ALI). When patients present with ALI, they have a high likelihood of limb loss due to chronically occluded tibial vessels from previous thromboembolic events, making revascularization challenging. Patients may also present with compressive symptoms from a large popliteal mass, including limb edema, venous thromboembolism, and neuropathic pain. Exceedingly rarely, patients present with rupture of the aneurysm. Asymptomatic popliteal artery aneurysms can also be discovered incidentally on workup for other aneurysmal disease. *Pearl: The most common cause of a mass behind the knee is a Baker cyst, not PAA.*

The typical diameter of the popliteal artery is 0.7 to 1.1 cm, with most clinicians identifying a size threshold for repair of asymptomatic popliteal aneurysm as 2 cm in diameter. It is also accepted that all symptomatic PAAs are repaired given the high incidence of ischemic complications and limb loss.

63-1

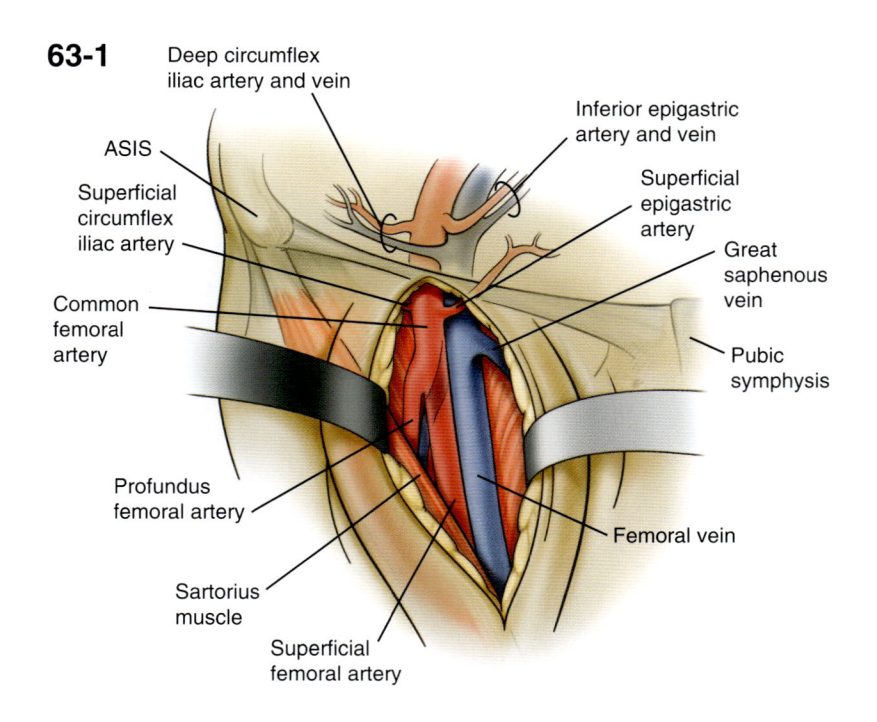

PREOPERATIVE PLANNING Duplex ultrasonography is the first-line imaging modality used for diagnosis and size estimation of PAAs. CTA/MRA can also be used for further evaluation of arterial anatomy, thrombus burden, and outflow vessels for operative planning. Angiography remains the gold standard for determining the patency of distal limb perfusion. For patients requiring arterial bypass, duplex ultrasonography can also be used for vein mapping to identify an autologous conduit.

Prior to intervention, the patient must be on appropriate risk factor modification, including an antiplatelet agent and cholesterol-lowering medication. Surgical options include open, endovascular, and hybrid procedures. This chapter focuses on open treatment modalities; however, endovascular and hybrid techniques can be used to recanalize outflow through thrombolytic therapy in preparation for open surgical repair. Currently, arterial bypass with ligation or interposition grafting remains the gold standard for treatment of such aneurysms.

POSITIONING

MEDIAL APPROACH: A medial approach is indicated in patients with small, fusiform aneurysms that do not require decompression as part of repair. Advantages include familiarity of this approach for vascular surgeons and avoiding the popliteal fossa.

The patient is placed in a supine position with both legs and the lower abdomen prepped and draped in sterile manner. The arms can either be tucked or left extended at 80 degrees based on surgeon preference.

POSTERIOR APPROACH: A posterior approach is indicated in patients with large aneurysms exhibiting symptoms of compression within the popliteal fossa, or with distorted anatomy from mass effect.

The patient is placed in the prone position with the affected limb fully prepped and draped in sterile manner. For patients undergoing greater saphenous vein harvest, the procedure begins with the patient supine, and later transferred to the prone position.

PROCEDURE (PER APPROACH)

MEDIAL APPROACH (FIGURE 63-2)

- Exposure of below-knee popliteal artery
  - A 10- to 12-cm longitudinal skin incision is created 1 to 2 cm posteromedial to the tibia.
  - Underlying subcutaneous tissues are incised using electrocautery to the level of the fascia, which is then also incised in a similar fashion.
  - The heads of the gastrocnemius muscle are retracted using a self-retainer, allowing for entrance into the popliteal space.
  - The tendons of the semimembranosus and semitendinosus muscles are split as required, exposing the popliteal vessels. The popliteal artery is mobilized for a length of 2 cm and controlled using silastic vessel loops.
- Exposure of above-knee popliteal artery
  - The above-knee popliteal artery is exposed through the medial incision used for GSV harvest along the border of the sartorius muscle above the knee.
  - Subcutaneous tissues are incised using electrocautery, to the level of the adductor tendon on the anterior border and sartorius muscle posteriorly, which are retracted.
  - The underlying fascia is incised, and the popliteal artery and distal SFA are exposed, mobilized, and controlled using silastic vessel loops.
- Anastomosis/Repair
  - Systemic heparin (100 units/kg) is administered, circulating for 3 to 5 minutes.
  - The GSV is transected, and the stump is suture-ligated.
  - The SFA is clamped. A longitudinal arteriotomy is made in the SFA using a number 11 blade and extended with Potts scissors for 1 cm.
  - Harvested GSV is either reversed or non-reversed (requires valvulotomy) and the end for proximal anastomosis is spatulated.
  - Proximal anastomosis is performed using running 5-0/6-0 polypropylene suture.
  - Valvulotomy is performed if the GSV is non-reversed and strong pulsatile flow confirmed.
  - The vein graft is checked for hemostasis and passed through an anatomic, subcutaneous, or subfascial tunnel to the distal popliteal artery.

- The popliteal artery is then suture-ligated proximal and distal to the aneurysm using 2-0/3-0 polypropylene sutures.
- *Pearl: The aneurysm sac should be ligated as close to the aneurysm as possible to promote thrombosis and decrease likelihood of expansion from collateral vessels.*
- Distal control of the popliteal artery is obtained using clamps/silastic vessel loops. The vein graft is transected to the appropriate length and an anastomosis is created in either an end-to end or end- to-side fashion between the distal popliteal artery, and vein graft is performed using 5-0/6-0 polypropylene sutures.
- Hemostasis at all surgical sites is confirmed.
- Closure
  - Subcutaneous tissue and skin of the proximal incision are closed in multiple layers.
  - The fascia overlying the sartorius muscle and in the popliteal space is closed with 3-0 Vicryl sutures.

POSTERIOR APPROACH (FIGURE 63-3)

- Incision
  - An S-shaped incision is made at the medial side of the distal thigh extending laterally across the crease of the calf, ending lateral to the proximal small saphenous vein, which is ligated.
  - *Pearl: If the small saphenous vein is of adequate caliber, the incision can be extended, and the vein harvested.*
- Exposure
  - *Pearl: Dissection should occur on the anterior surface of the aneurysm to avoid damage to the tibial and peroneal nerves lateral to the sac. The tibial nerve lies superficially, and the peroneal nerve heads laterally to the biceps femoris tendon.*
  - The proximal popliteal artery is identified and exposed as described above.
  - Dissection is continued along the surface of the aneurysm sac, the overlying fascia incised longitudinally, and the sural nerve is retracted. The distal popliteal artery is identified deep to the popliteal vein and controlled with silastic vessel loops.
  - Systemic heparin is administered, and proximal/distal control is obtained.
  - The aneurysm sac is opened and decompressed, and backbleeding vessels are suture-ligated from within the aneurysm sac.
  - Using harvested GSV/SSV or prosthetic conduit, a spatulated interposition bypass graft is used to reconstruct the popliteal artery in an end-to-end fashion using 6-0 polypropylene sutures.
  - *Pearl: End-to-side bypass with proximal ligation may be performed in cases where there is a large size discrepancy between the popliteal artery and conduit.*
  - The clamps are removed, and hemostasis is confirmed.
- Closure
  - Subcutaneous tissue is closed in the same manner as described above.
  - A drain may be left in situ for ongoing decompression.
  - *Pearl: These are difficult wounds to heal. Monitor closely for dehiscence.*

POSTOPERATIVE CARE AND COMPLICATIONS Postoperative care, complications, and follow-up are similar to that of femoral artery aneurysms as discussed above. Key principles include early mobilization, antiplatelet therapy, and annual surveillance after obtaining a postoperative baseline duplex. ■

SUGGESTED READINGS

Kassem M, Gonzalez L. *Popliteal Artery Aneurysm*. [online] Ncbi.nlm.nih.gov. 2021.

Leake AE, Segal MA, Chaer RA, Eslami MH, Al-Khoury G, Makaroun MS, Avgerinos ED. Meta-analysis of open and endovascular repair of popliteal artery aneurysms. *J Vasc Surg.* 2017 Jan;65(1):246-256.e2. doi: 10.1016/j.jvs.2016.09.029. PMID: 28010863.

Jacobowitz G, Cayne NS. In: *Rutherford's Vascular Surgery and Endovascular Therapy*. 9th ed. Chapter 83: Lower Extremity Aneurysms. Elsevier (Philadelphia, PA), 2019. pp. 1078-1094.

Saleem T, D'Cruz J, Baril D. *Femoral Aneurysm Repair*. [online] Ncbi.nlm.nih.gov. 2021.

63-2

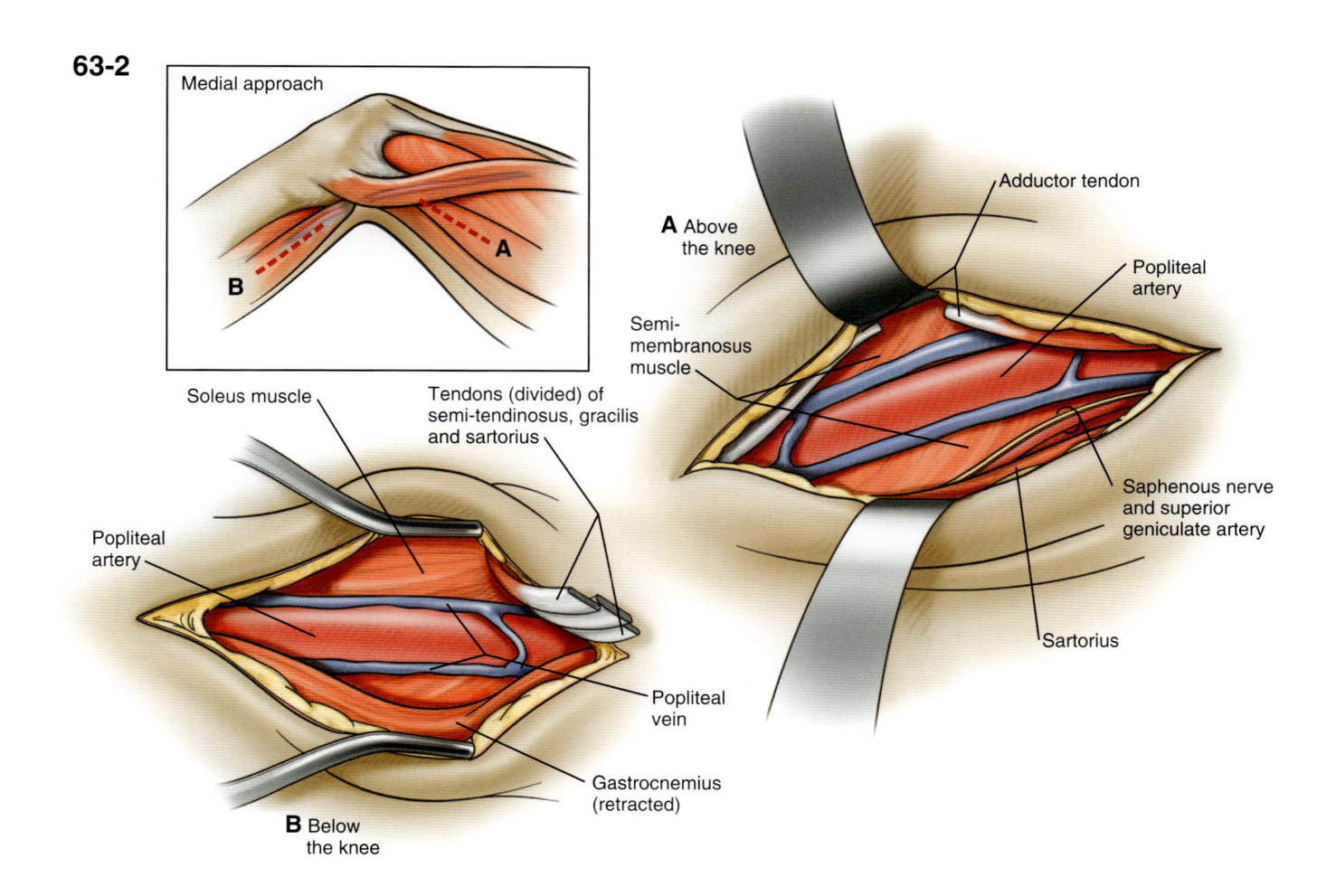

Medial approach

A Above the knee

Adductor tendon

Popliteal artery

Semi-membranosus muscle

Saphenous nerve and superior geniculate artery

Sartorius

Soleus muscle

Tendons (divided) of semi-tendinosus, gracilis and sartorius

Popliteal artery

Popliteal vein

Gastrocnemius (retracted)

B Below the knee

63-3

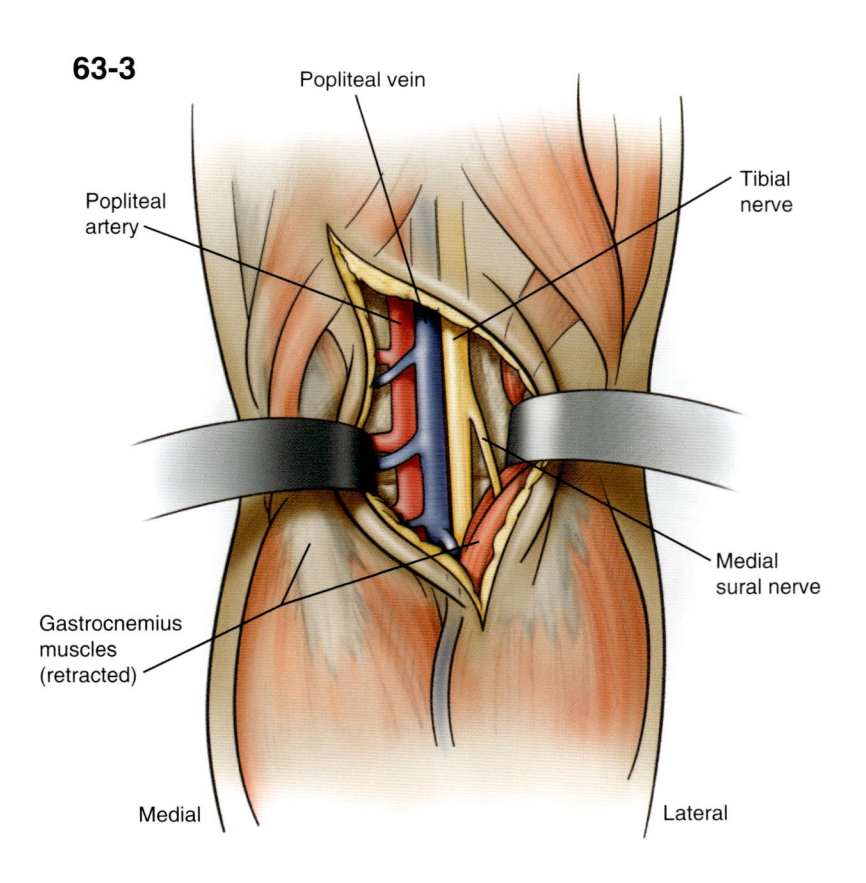

Popliteal vein

Popliteal artery

Tibial nerve

Medial sural nerve

Gastrocnemius muscles (retracted)

Medial

Lateral

Popliteal Entrapment Release

Patrick Vaccaro, MD

INDICATIONS Popliteal artery entrapment syndrome (PAES) is caused by abnormal anatomic variants of the gastrocnemius or popliteus muscle resulting in compression of the popliteal artery behind the knee with physical activity resulting in symptoms of claudication. Afflicted patients are typically young and physically active. While patients typically have normal distal pulses at rest on exam, passive dorsiflexion and active plantar flexion will result in diminished pulses. Initial diagnostic evaluation typically begins with noninvasive testing, including exercise ABIs which may demonstrate a decrease post exercise due to compression of the popliteal artery by the gastrocnemius. Arterial duplex imaging can also be utilized to visualize the artery in real time during calf muscle contraction and relaxation. MRA is particularly useful in delineating the abnormal anatomy in relation to the popliteal artery and can be useful for operative planning. Diagnostic angiography with neutral and provocative maneuvers for PAES is considered the gold standard for diagnosis with high documented sensitivity and specificity (FIGURE 64-1). Angiography is also useful for delineating arterial anatomy and runoff in cases of advanced disease with popliteal artery stenosis, occlusion, or embolization. Given its invasive nature, angiography is typically reserved for patients with a high index of suspicion for PAES. Appropriate and complete preoperative testing may also foreshadow the need for interposition grafting of the popliteal artery so that plans for saphenous vein procurement may be made ahead of time. There are six types of PAES (FIGURE 64-2) describing various anatomic variants resulting from specific embryologic phenomenon.

Type I results in a medially deviated popliteal artery with a normally positioned gastrocnemius. Type II is similar in that the popliteal artery is also medially deviated but this is secondary to an abnormal femoral insertion of the muscle. Type III entrapment results from embryologic remnants of the gastrocnemius remaining posterior to or surrounding a normally positioned artery. Type IV is secondary to the popliteal artery remaining in its embryologic position deep to the popliteus muscle or fibrous bands resulting in compression. Type V is when there are both venous and arterial involvements secondary to any of the above-described anatomic abnormalities. Type VI, also known as functional PAES, is when there are typical features of PAES but no anatomic abnormality to explain the symptoms. It is important to recognize and understand the various types of PAES to guide appropriate management intraoperatively. Typically, the treatment for PAES will involve myotomy, artery, and vein circumferential dissection and correction of the involved anatomic abnormality. In more advanced cases, where there has been arterial degeneration, vascular reconstruction may be necessary. In general, the principles of surgical treatment for PAES include release of arterial entrapment, restoration of normal anatomy, and restoration of arterial flow.

POSITION Although the operative site may occasionally be approached through a medial knee incision, in most cases the approach is posterior through the popliteal fossa. To facilitate this approach the patient is placed in the prone position with appropriate support and padding for the body, head, and neck.

OPERATIVE PREPARATION After routine skin preparation, the operative field is draped in the usual sterile fashion with circumferential exposure of the operative leg from the level of the upper thigh. This allows the surgeon the ability to flex and extend the leg during the actual exposure of the deep popliteal space.

64-1

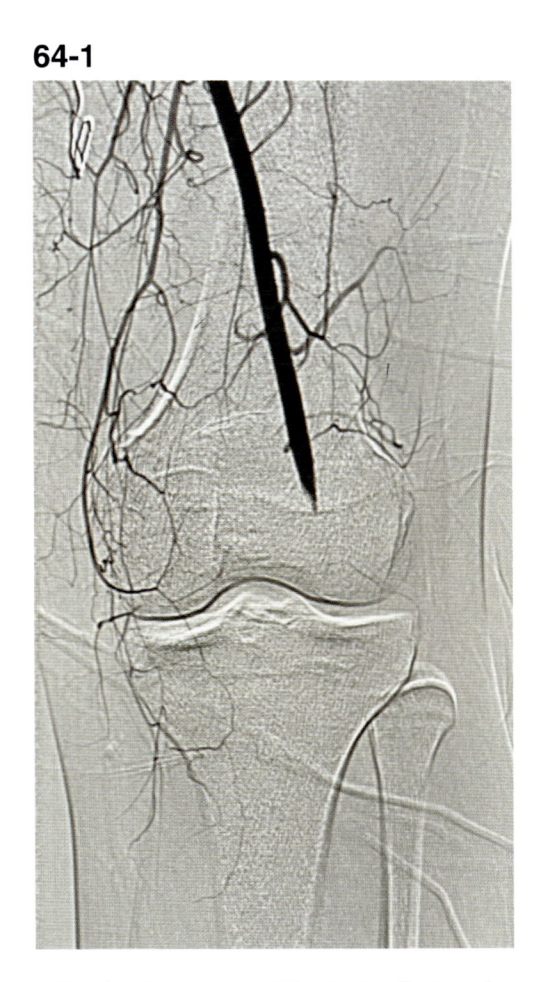

Figure 64-1 Angiogram of patient with popliteal entrapment with plantar flexion demonstrating occlusion of the popliteal artery.

64-2

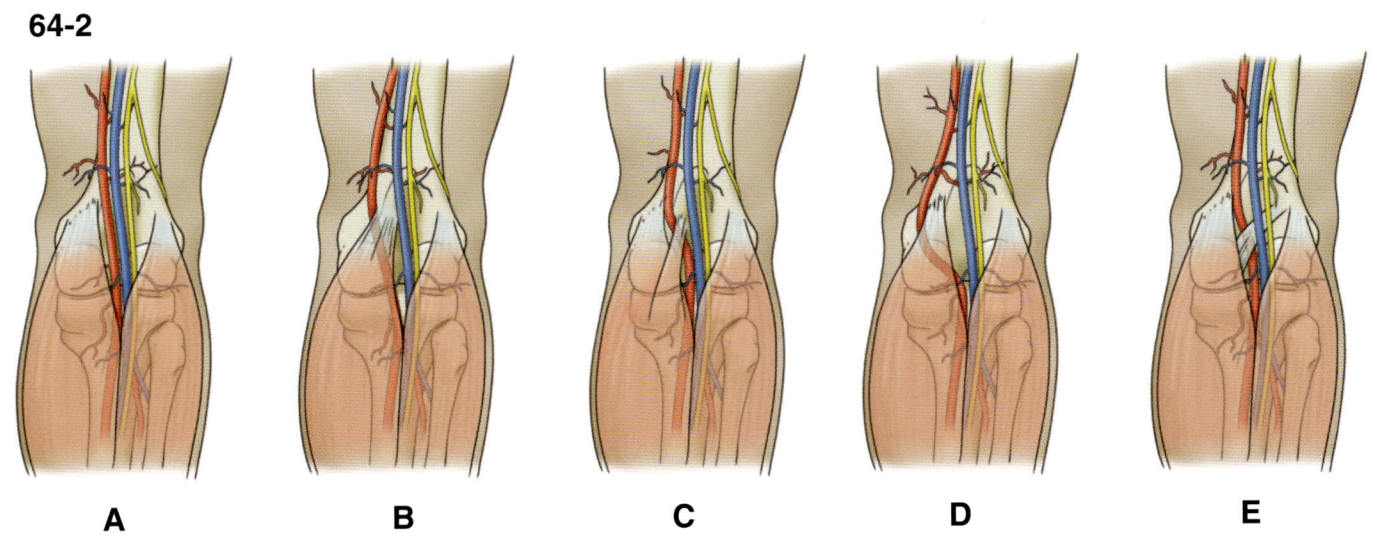

A   B   C   D   E

Figure 64-2 Depiction of various types of popliteal entrapment.

INCISION AND EXPOSURE   A generous S-shaped incision is made medially and cephalad to the posterior popliteal skin crease adjacent to the tendinous structures (FIGURE 64-3). It is then gently curved onto the actual skin crease and carried laterally for 4 to 5 centimeters and then curved inferiorly medial to the fibula. The incision is deepened to the superficial fascia and then using a combination of blunt and sharp dissection, the subcutaneous tissue is swept off the superficial fascia, developing superior and inferior skin flaps. These flaps are rolled back as far as possible and secured to the adjacent skin with fine silk suture. Tacking these flaps back avoids the need for retractors at the skin level. Bleeding points are controlled with cautery. At this point the fascia is carefully entered several millimeters medial to the midline and opened throughout the length of the incision, between the heads of the gastrocnemius muscles inferiorly and between semimembranosus and biceps femoris muscle superiorly with scissors. Before cutting, the fascia is carefully elevated off the underlying structures. As the inferior half of the fascia is opened, care is taken to avoid injury to the short saphenous vein and the sural nerve. These are important landmarks and the gateway to the popliteal vein and tibial nerve, respectively. Injury to the sural nerve can lead to long-term superficial pain, especially on the lateral side of the foot. The muscles are then gently separated with Weitlaner retractors, making sure not to encroach upon the tibial nerve laterally (FIGURE 64-4). The retractors are readjusted as the dissections are deepened. The dissection should remain as close to the artery as possible to avoid inadvertent injury to surrounding structures.

Through this approach, the popliteal artery is deep and medial to the popliteal vein. No matter the entrapment type, the popliteal artery is exposed in the superior aspect of the incision and circled with a vessel loop.

Keeping one's dissection in proximity to the popliteal artery is the gateway to making sure the cause of the condition is appropriately treated. Care is taken to separate the artery from the vein by gentle sharp and blunt dissection. Branches of the vein cross the artery and may be adherent to the arterial wall, causing minor compression on occasion, and should be divided between fine silk ligatures. In this fashion, the artery may be circumferentially mobilized several centimeters inferiorly between the heads of the gastrocnemius muscles. During the course of this dissection, the six variants of popliteal entrapment are handled as they are encountered and will be discussed below under Details of Procedure. The technic for reversed saphenous vein interposition grafting, when necessary, will also be discussed.

DETAILS OF PROCEDURE   On the basis of preoperative testing, the surgeon will have a suspicion for the type of entrapment they may encounter. Similarly, the degree of disease within the popliteal artery will be known ahead of time so that plans may be made for procurement of saphenous vein for interposition grafting. In Type I entrapment, the popliteal artery will deviate medially to a normally inserted medial head of the gastrocnemius muscle. In Type II entrapment, the medial deviation of the popliteal artery is due to an abnormal insertion site of the medial head of the gastrocnemius which may be to the medial femoral condyle or the intercondylar area. In both cases, by keeping dissection on the popliteal artery as previously discussed, the abnormality is easily recognized. In both cases the muscle causing the arterial deviation is cut with cautery at its insertion and mobilized inferiorly, allowing the artery to return to an unobstructed course. Care is taken to make sure there is no kinking of the artery due to elongation secondary to its abnormal course, and it is palpated to make sure there is no unrecognized intrinsic arterial disease. If necessary, a small section of the muscle may be excised to reduce the risk of abnormal reattachment of the muscle reproducing symptoms. Small intermuscular bleeding points are frequently encountered after transection and controlled with cautery. **CONTINUES ▸**

64-3

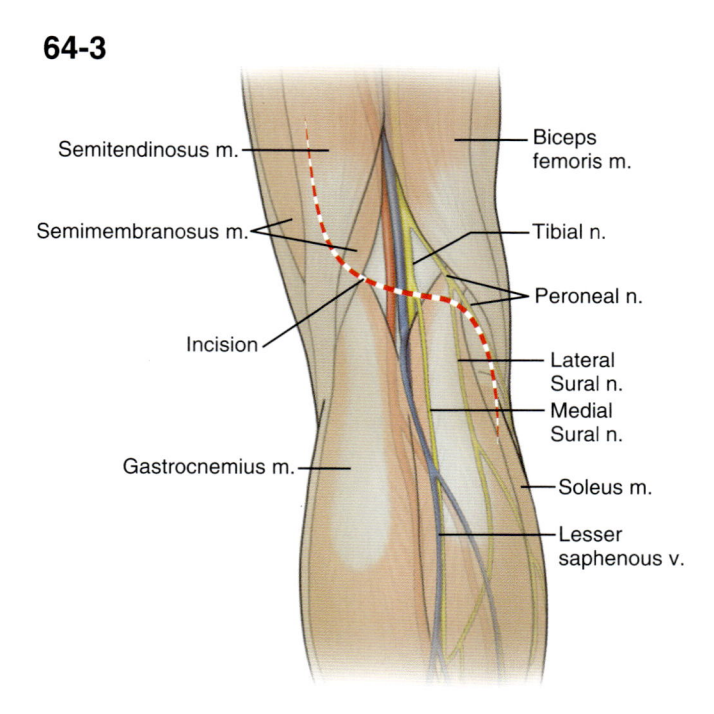

Figure 64-3 Incision and exposure of popliteal fossa.

64-4

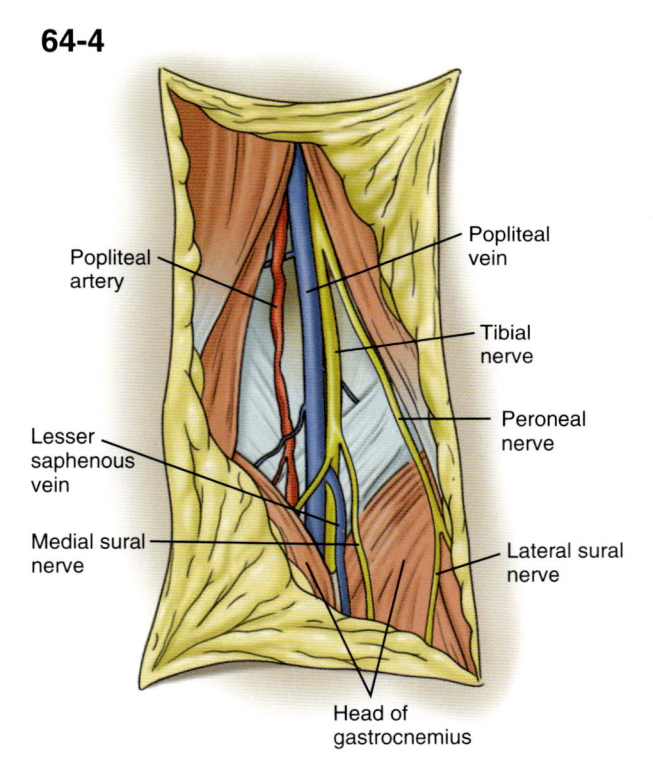

Figure 64-4 Tethered popliteal artery.

DETAILS OF PROCEDURE `CONTINUED` Type III entrapment is usually caused by an accessory muscle slip arising from the medial head of the gastrocnemius muscle crossing posteriorly and laterally to a normally placed popliteal artery (FIGURE 64-5). The muscle slip generally inserts in the intercondylar space. Dissection should remain on this muscle slip in the quest to identify its insertion point. In this case the muscle slip is carefully divided at its insertion to the femur and resected back to its origin from the gastrocnemius. Again, the artery is palpated for any undetected abnormality following adequate mobilization.

As opposed to Types I, II, and III, which are due to abnormal muscle variants of the medial head of the gastrocnemius, Type IV entrapment occurs more distally on the popliteal artery and is due to compression by the popliteus muscle. Dissection may be more difficult as the area between the heads of the gastrocnemius is entered due to an increase in small crossing veins and nerves. These small veins should be ligated and divided between fine silk sutures. The reaction between the artery and overlying muscle may be more intense in this type, and injury to the artery is carefully avoided as this muscle is widely resected and the compression relieved. Occasionally the artery may be adherent to the underlying bone and must mobilized. Occasionally, interposition grafting of the popliteal artery with saphenous vein may be necessary due to the degree of intrinsic scarring of the artery.

Type V entrapment may be caused by any of the previously mentioned muscle anomalies and differs only in that the popliteal vein is also entrapped. Due to the delicate nature of the venous wall, additional attention to detail is required to avoid needless venous injury during the dissection.

Type VI entrapment appears to be due to hypertrophy or lateral displacement of the medial head of the gastrocnemius, and its treatment requires circumferential mobilization of the most proximal extent. Placement of a Penrose drain around the medial head allows the operator to apply traction, facilitating transection of the muscle insertion with cautery at its most proximal position. Excision of 1 to 2 cm of the muscle reduces the chance of reattachment in a position to reproduce the symptoms.

Occasionally the popliteal artery may need to be replaced or bypassed due to the presence of intrinsic disease usually secondary to repeated trauma to the artery from the compressing muscle. The greater or small saphenous vein may be used, depending on adequate size determined preoperatively by duplex scan. If one is planning a posterior approach and the small saphenous vein is too small in caliber, the greater saphenous vein may first need to be removed with the patient in the supine position if the greater saphenous vein is also too small at the ankle. The groin wound is then closed, and the patient is flipped into the prone position and the leg prepped and draped again. The diseased segment of artery is excised, and an end-to-end interposition graft is performed. The technique for the performance of the vascular anastomoses is described elsewhere in this book.

CLOSURE Meticulous hemostasis must be obtained prior to closure to avoid a hematoma and the development of excess scarring. If heparin had been used for the performance of a bypass graft, it must be reversed with protamine sulfate. The subcutaneous tissue is closed with interrupted 2-0 or 3-0 absorbable suture and the skin is closed in a subcuticular fashion with a 4-0 absorbable suture. Paper tapes may be used to reinforce the closure, and it is covered with a dry, sterile dressing. A closed suction drain may be used at the surgeon's discretion.

POSTOPERATIVE CARE The patient is kept non-weight bearing with crutches for 5 to 7 days and advanced according to the surgeon's preferred protocol. ■

SUGGESTED READINGS

Altintas U, Helgstrand U, Hansen M, Stentzer K, Schroeder T, Eiberg J. Popliteal artery entrapment syndrome: ultrasound imaging, intraoperative findings, and clinical outcome. *Vasc and Endovasc Surg.* 2013;47(7):513-518.

Gokkus K, Sagtas E, Bakalim T, Taskaya E, Aydin AT. Popliteal entrapment syndrome. A systematic review of the literature and case presentation. *Muscles Ligaments Tendons J.* 2014;4(2):141-148.

Kim SY, Min SK, Ahn S, Min SI, Ha J, Kim SJ. Long-term outcomes after revascularization for advanced popliteal artery entrapment syndrome with segmental arterial occlusion. *J Vasc Surg.* 2012;55:90-97.

Turnipseed WD. Functional popliteal artery entrapment syndrome: a poorly understood and often missed diagnosis that is frequently mistreated. *J Vasc Surg.* 2009;49:1189-1195.

Turnipseed WD. Popliteal entrapment in runners. *Clin Sports Med.* 2012;31:321-328.

64-5

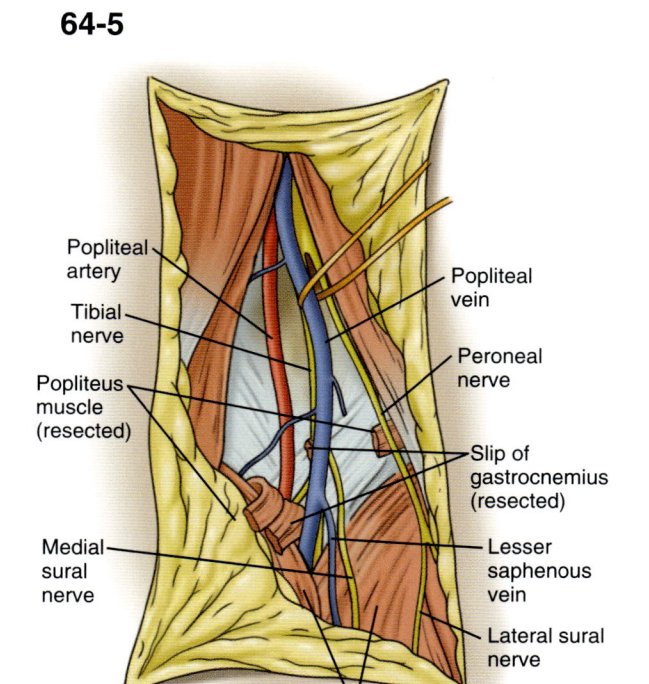

Figure 64-5 Popliteal artery dissected free with muscle removed.

LOWER EXTREMITY SFA, TIBIAL OCCLUSIVE DISEASE AND ANEURYSM ENDOVASCULAR

SUPERFICIAL FEMORAL ARTERY ENDOVASCULAR INTERVENTION

Sean A. Kennedy, MD • Sebastian Mafeld, MBBS

SUMMARY The gateway to success in endovascular femoropopliteal intervention does not lie in a particular tool or technical tip. Rather, it relies on a decision-making framework that demonstrates a thorough understanding of the patient, target lesion characteristics, and risk factors for restenosis. Endovascular treatment of the superficial femoral artery (SFA) and popliteal remains a rapidly evolving field. Consequentially, we hope to highlight the core principles underlying successful treatment that will apply not only today, but for the foreseeable future.

Appropriate patient selection for SFA/popliteal intervention is critical. Our practice pattern is conservative such that claudicants are typically not treated by endovascular means. An important question for surgeons performing endovascular procedures is how best to treat lesions in the distal femoral-popliteal segment. Endovascular practitioners are faced with a large range of devices, including plain balloons, drug-eluting balloons, cutting balloons, drug-eluting stents, bare metal stents, and atherectomy/lithotripsy devices yet with limited data. As such, there is no singular "perfect" endovascular treatment approach to the SFA/popliteal segment, and a variety of options are valid.

THE FEMOROPOPLITEAL SEGMENT: UNDERSTANDING THE ENVIRONMENT

MOVEMENT: The SFA passes through the adductor canal transitioning to the popliteal artery (PA) after exiting the adductor hiatus (AH). During hip and knee flexion, the SFA and popliteal arteries undergo deformations that include shortening, increased tortuosity, compression, and rotation in the axial plane. Such forces affect the whole femoropopliteal segment, most markedly the adductor canal, and accelerate atherosclerotic degeneration of this region (FIGURE 65-1). When stenting the adductor canal SFA/popliteal artery, each stent increases the rigidity of that segment, resulting in compensatory exaggerated motion in unstented adjacent arterial segments. Stents placed in these regions should be highly flexible, with high radial strength. Ideally, when stenting a segment it is better to use a single longer stent to cover the desired region instead of overlapping stents, as overlap further compounds the risk of stent kinking and failure.

With knee flexion, the forces on the popliteal artery also need to be considered. A common misconception is that the hinge-point of the popliteal artery is at the joint line itself. However, studies have demonstrated the hinge-point is in fact in the distal P1 or proximal P2 segment. Therefore, some groups have even advocated dynamic angiography with knee flexion to guide feasibility of stenting in a given patient.

CALCIFICATION: Calcification is an "enemy" of the endovascular practitioner as it can prevent effective angioplasty and stent expansion. Calcification is also a barrier to drug elution from coated balloons and stents. Even vessel location is of relevance with respect to atherosclerotic calcification, and proven therapies in one location may not translate to another. For example, compared to coronary arteries, SFA atherosclerosis has been shown to typically contain greater relative calcium and less lipid requiring added considerations for drug elution. Sirolimus- and everolimus-based stents, which have shown great benefit in coronary interventions, have not been shown to be of equal benefit in femoropopliteal disease. Furthermore, femoropopliteal atherosclerotic calcifications have been shown to frequently demonstrate bone-like osteoid metaplasia proliferation. Such rigid calcifications not only complicate endovascular and surgical interventions but the underlying cellular processes which lead to their development may represent potential areas for novel targeted therapies.

RISK FACTORS FOR RESTENOSIS: At the conclusion of endovascular intervention, a result must not only be satisfactory from an angiographic standpoint but durable and long-lasting. On this basis, consideration of risk factors for restenosis is critical to ensuring long-term patency. This includes patient-level, lesion-level, and therapy-related risk factors such as male gender, increasing age, hypercholesterolemia, critical limb-threatening ischemia (CLTI), prior interventions, smaller vessel diameter, longer target lesions with greater atherosclerotic load, presence of total occlusion, and increasing stented length.

GATEWAYS TO SUCCESS IN ENDOVASCULAR FEMOROPOPLITEAL INTERVENTION

Successful endovascular intervention can be distilled into three key principles:

1. Safe Access: Selecting your approach to a fem-pop lesion is critical to success. If a lesion is approximately 5 cm or more beyond the ostium of the SFA, an antegrade approach is favored. This allows closer proximity to the lesion with enhanced control and "pushability" of wires and catheters. The common femoral artery has traditionally been the access site of choice. However, evidence is emerging to support the safety and efficacy of direct SFA puncture. This can be useful if body habitus is unfavorable. A closure device is typically required to seal a SFA puncture, as there is no effective structure to compress against for hemostasis. Alternatively, an "up-and-over" approach (FIGURE 65-2) can be considered if there is proximal SFA disease preventing antegrade approach. Available cross-sectional imaging should be carefully reviewed pre-intervention, as iliac tortuosity and the presence of abdominal aortic endografts can render an "up-and-over" approach extremely difficult. In hostile groins, a brachial or even radial approach can be considered.

2. Safe Navigation: Based on preprocedural imaging and initial angiography, selecting key tools is essential to safely navigate the fem-pop segment. Every institution will have varying equipment, but basic tools such as a Bentson wire, Glidewire, and angled catheter (e.g., Kumpe) are the workhorses of fem-pop intervention. Adjunctive equipment, such as support catheters, chronic total occlusion (CTO) re-entry devices, and smaller 0.018 and 0.014 systems, are useful bailout strategies. An approach to navigation is provided in the section below regarding the most common lesion types encountered.

3. Safe Closure: No procedure is complete until successful hemostasis has been achieved. A perfect angiographic result can be compromised by failed hemostasis. Manual compression is the traditional gold standard and still has its place in a world of abundant closure devices. Ten to 15 minutes of compression for a 6Fr access is typically sufficient for hemostasis. Closure devices are useful hemostatic adjuncts. They have the advantage of earlier ambulation but predispose to unique complications themselves, including vessel occlusion. Of note, antegrade and SFA closure device use is typically "off-label," although accepted in practice. Ultrasound guidance during deployment of closure devices with an intravascular component is a useful adjunct to prevent mal-deployment due to arterial plaque.

65-1

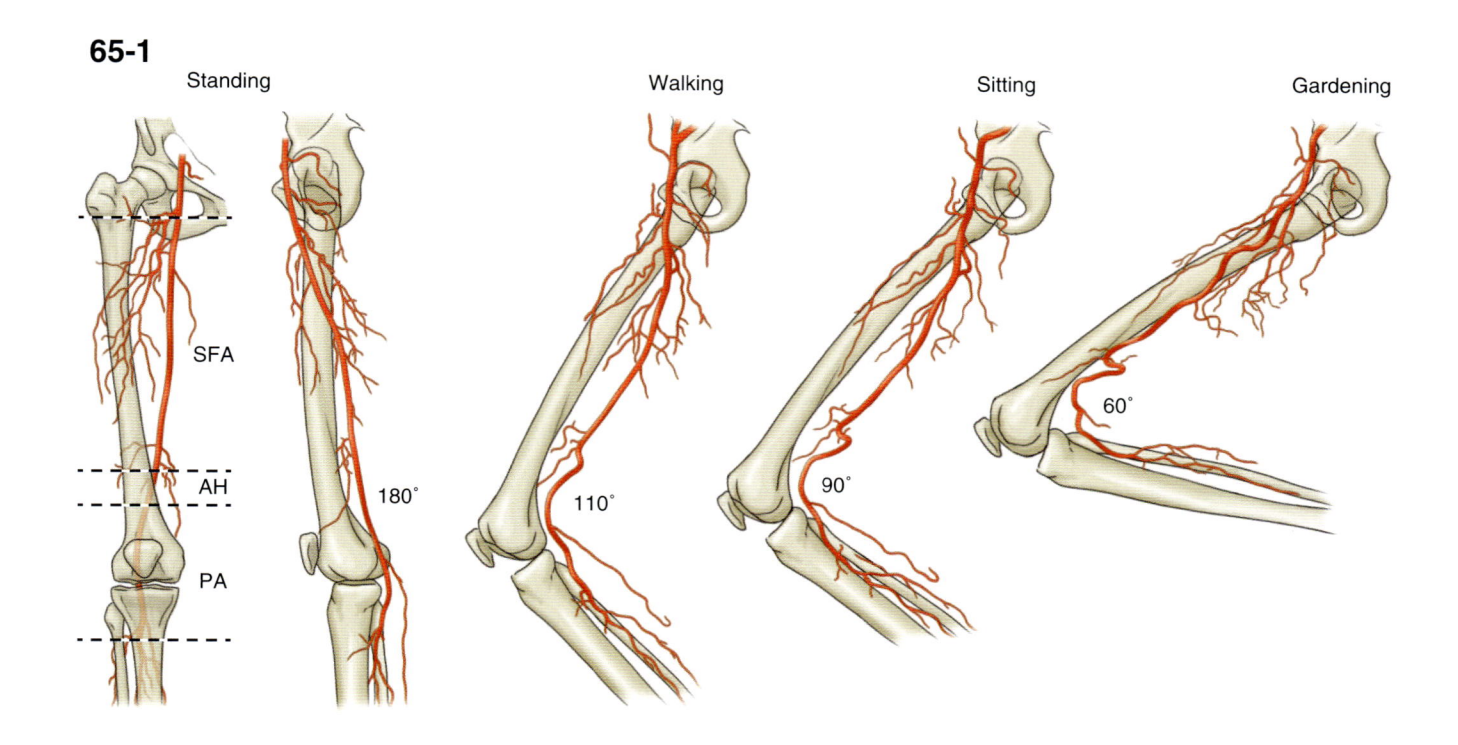

Standing   Walking   Sitting   Gardening

SFA

AH

PA

180°   110°   90°   60°

65-2

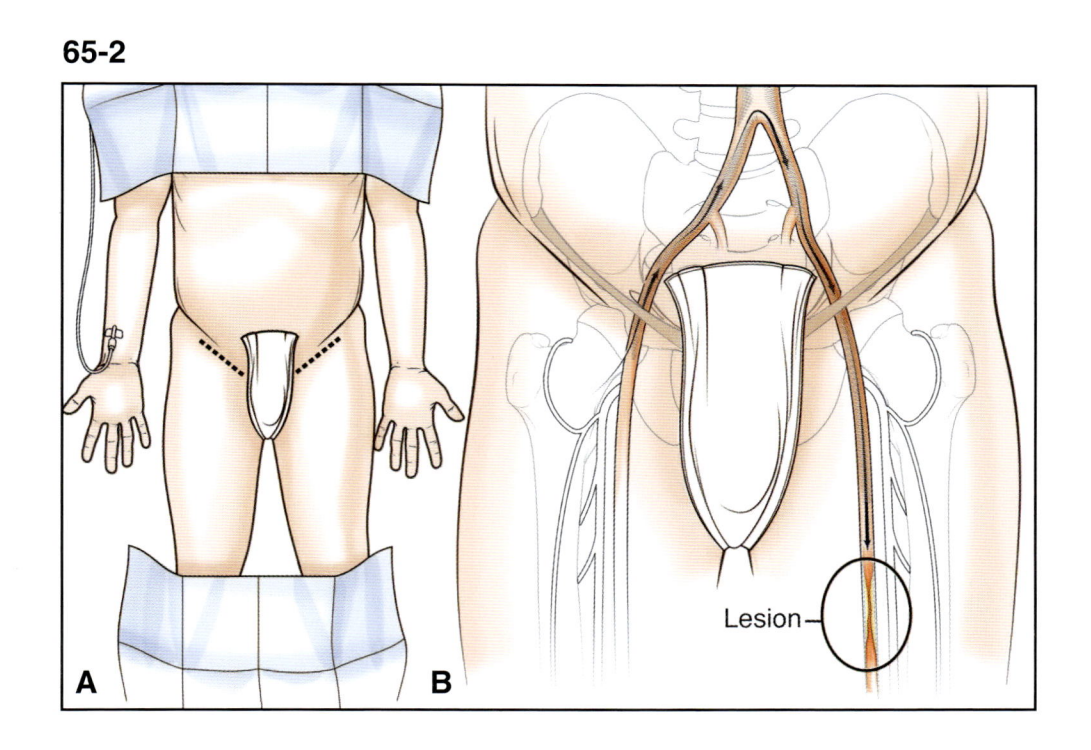

A   B

Lesion

KEY CONCEPTS TO FEMOROPOPLITEAL INTERVENTIONS

LEAVE NOTHING BEHIND: Conservative use of stents in the fem-pop segment is advised. Wherever possible, angioplasty-only approaches should be considered. Given the substantial movement-related physical stress faced by stents in this region, each stent left behind carries its own risk of stent-related complications, including fracture and in-stent restenosis.

VESSEL PREPARATION: Optimizing the vessel prior to both drug-coated technology deployment as well as certain stents is critical to success. Adequate disruption of calcium and predilatation of the vessel wall in a target lesion with a combination of plain angioplasty and adjunctive technologies where indicated, such as cutting balloons, atherectomy, and lithotripsy, has been shown to improve drug-elution efficacy in the vessel wall. Additionally, such preparation, particularly in calcified lesions, is critical to effective deployment of certain self-expanding stents like the SUPERA (Abbott, Santa Clara, CA). Inadequate vessel preparation in a heavily calcified SFA can lead to inadequate packing of SUPERA stent, most notably at the adductor hiatus (FIGURE 65-3). The stent in the affected section will have minimal radial force and be prone to restenosis and occlusion. This is prevented by excellent vessel preparation which allows tight packing of a SUPERA stent (FIGURE 65-4).

PAVE AND CRACK: Often, vessel calcification cannot be overcome with persistent stenosis despite repeated angioplasty. Some authors have advocated the concept of "pave and crack," whereby a flexible covered stent graft such as the VIABAHN (W.L. Gore & Associates, Inc., Flagstaff, AZ) is deployed into the calcified segment followed by aggressive angioplasty to disrupt the calcification, after which an additional stent such as a SUPERA may be placed to support the VIABAHN. The downside of using a covered stent-graft is potential loss of collaterals as well as reducing future ability to collateralize. There is emerging evidence that the SUPERA stent may be able to function as a multiflow modulator. On this basis, at the author's institution, in select circumstances where calcification cannot be overcome, focal overdilatation of the vessel to disrupt the calcification has been used, knowingly rupturing the artery. Rather than "paving" with a covered stent-graft beforehand, instead we use a SUPERA stent alone, thereby avoiding the need for stent-grafting.

SPECIFIC FEMOROPOPLITEAL TARGET LESION CONSIDERATIONS

The following scenarios represent the most common faced in fem-pop intervention. Each requires unique considerations, and approaches will vary depending on local practice patterns and health economic factors. Operators should have an algorithm for approaching each situation. Our typical practice is delineated below.

SHORT FOCAL STENOSIS: Plain balloon angioplasty. Our typical practice for SFA/popliteal angioplasty is to perform prolonged inflation of 2 to 3 minutes with appropriate heparinization. Prior studies have shown this to result in reduced residual stenosis and fewer flow-limited dissections. If there is an acceptable angiographic result, a drug-eluting balloon is considered if the aforementioned risk factors for restenosis are present. Stenting is reserved for persistent flow limitation or residual (>50%) stenosis. While the authors do not advocate a particular stent type, it is important to be aware that not all stents are created equal. If a residual stenosis is present, it is important to ensure the angioplasty balloon is appropriately sized to the vessel before proceeding directly to stenting. If there is marked focal calcification, atherectomy can be considered for debulking.

LONG SEGMENT STENOSIS: Plain balloon angioplasty for 2 to 3 minutes. If there is an acceptable angiographic result, a drug-eluting balloon or drug-eluting stent is considered if the aforementioned risk factors for restenosis are present. If the long segment stenosis is heavily calcified, we pursue aggressive plain angioplasty at high pressures sometimes to the point of vessel rupture in order to truly disrupt the calcified plaque. Depending on operator comfort, some may desire to "pave" the SFA beforehand with a covered stent-graft or prepare to deploy a SUPERA stent immediately after vessel "cracking." "Breaking" the calcium or "paving and cracking" a pathway is critical. This form of vessel preparation along with appropriate SUPERA stent deployment is a key to success in heavily calcified lesions. CONTINUES ▶

65-3

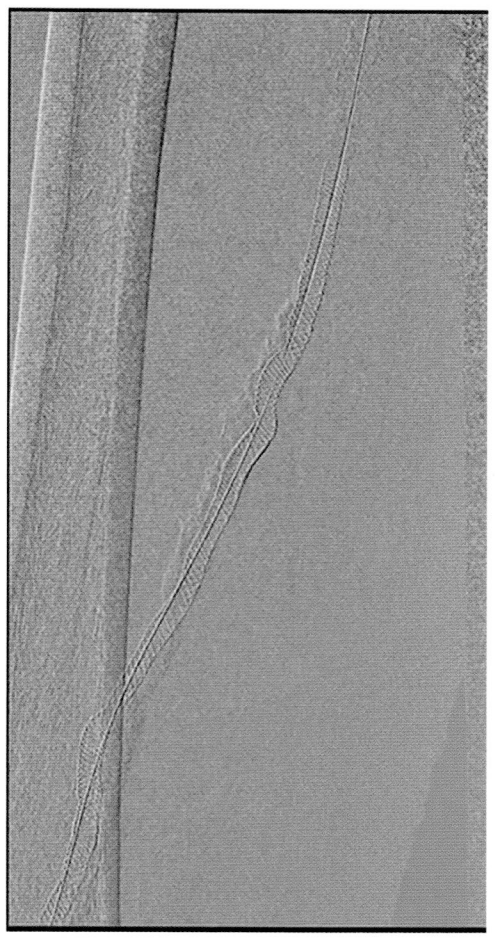

65-4

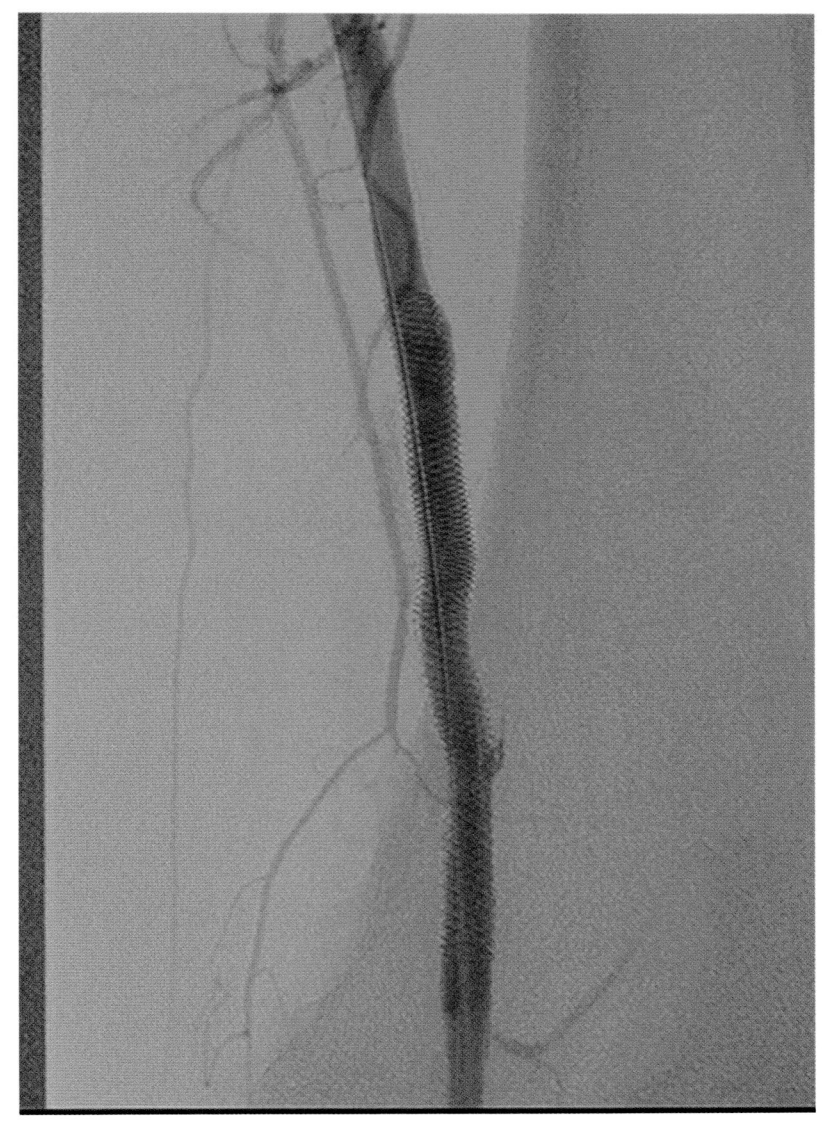

SPECIFIC FEMOROPOPLITEAL TARGET LESION CONSIDERATIONS

CHRONIC TOTAL OCCLUSIONS: `CONTINUED` Initially, we attempt to cross a chronic total occlusion via an antegrade approach. First, we start with 0.035 systems using an angled catheter such as a Kumpe or CXI Support Catheter (Cook Medical, Bloomington, IN) to provide support and directionality together with a Bentson wire. Adequate magnification or digital zoom of the lesion cap is helpful to guide initial entry. We interrogate the lesion with the wire backed by the catheter (FIGURE 65-5A). If this fails, we perform the same strategy with an 035 Glidewire. Another solution for particularly challenging lesions is to make gradual forward progress with serial 3- or 4-mm balloon angioplasty with wire advancement while the balloon is inflated. If we persistently fail to cross the lesion via these techniques, the same strategies can be employed in a subintimal approach with a Glidewire (FIGURE 65-5B). Here it is critical to re-enter the luminal segment of vessel as soon as possible. Gentle contrast injections should be done via a catheter when suspected luminal access is achieved. Strategies for re-entry should the wire alone fail include re-entry devices and balloon inflation to attempt to create a re-entry fenestration. In our experience, a common operator error in approaching CTOs is the failure to switch to retrograde approaches sooner in patients with CLTI. It is useful to set a predetermined time limit for antegrade attempts. This mental strategy helps with procedural decision-making in avoiding prolonged futile antegrade attempts. Care must be taken in the context of single vessel runoff so as not to potentially cause vessel injury that would preclude surgical bypass options. When a suitable retrograde target vessel is identified, we access the vessel with a Micropuncture needle under ultrasound and/or fluoroscopic guidance. A 014 or 18 wire is then used to attempt to cross the lesion in a retrograde manner. Crossing catheters and balloons can be used without a sheath to help in crossing these lesions. Once this is achieved, the wire can either be manipulated into an antegrade sheath/catheter or snared antegrade. With through-and-through access, excellent wire support and trackability is achieved, allowing the passage of balloons.

RESTENOSIS/OCCLUSION: For recurrent lesions in stent or in native vessel, we tend to use drug-coated balloons and stents. In-stent occlusion can be one of the most challenging circumstances to treat. While the cause may be related to neointimal hyperplasia, other causes such as stent fracture are commonly missed and should be considered. Careful assessment of dedicated magnified exposures of stents should be obtained in these circumstances to exclude subtle stent fracture. In such cases, relining with a covered stent may be needed to achieve a durable result. Atherectomy devices can also be considered for in-stent restenosis.

TIPS AND TRICKS

- Ipsilateral oblique angiography "opens" the CFA bifurcation, allowing improved identification of proximal SFA disease (FIGURE 65-6A and B).
- Review all available imaging prior to intervention. For example, in patients with duplex studies only, check if any previous cross-sectional studies are available. Even non-dedicated, non-vascular studies of the CT abdomen/pelvis can provide useful information for access planning, and may image more of the SFA than expected.
- Be mindful of the elongating the SUPERA stent. In the proximal SFA, if the stent elongates it may end too high.
- Do not commit yourself to a large sheath prior to performing angiography. Even with modern duplex ultrasound, CTA, and MRA technique, angiographic images are the true gold standard. We typically use a 4Fr micropuncture sheath to perform initial diagnostic angiography.
- Beware of the occlusion that can be crossed with ease; this may be fresh thrombus. Always ask the patient if their symptoms have changed acutely. If symptoms have changed dramatically in the days/weeks prior to intervention, reconsider your treatment approach, as other measures such as thrombolysis may be needed.
- Endovascular intervention is not benign. In patients with single-vessel runoff, aggressive endovascular intervention may entail a less favorable risk-benefit ratio compared to surgical bypass.
- Know when to stop. Treat the patient, not the images. Seeking angiographic perfection can lead an operator to overtreat and predispose to complications.
- Always ensure an adequate duration of dual antiplatelet medication is prescribed following the use of drug-eluting technology. ∎

SUGGESTED READINGS

Chan YC, Cheng SW, Cheung, GC, 2015. Predictors of restenosis in the use of helical interwoven nitinol stents to treat femoropopliteal occlusive disease. *J Vasc Surg.* 62;1201–1209. https://doi.org/10.1016/j.jvs.2015.05.030

Cui C, Huang X, Liu X, Li W, Lu X, Lu M, Jiang M, Yin M, 2017. Endovascular treatment of atherosclerotic popliteal artery disease based on dynamic angiography findings. *J Vasc Surg.* 65;82–90. https://doi.org/10.1016/j.jvs.2016.05.087

Dake MD, Fanelli F, Lottes AE, O'Leary EE, Reichert H, Jiang X, Fu W, Iida O, Zen K, Schermerhorn, M, Zeller T, Ansel GM, 2021. Prediction model for freedom from TLR from a multi-study analysis of long-term results with the Zilver PTX Drug-Eluting Peripheral Stent. *Cardiovasc Intervent Radiol.* 44;196–206. https://doi.org/10.1007/s00270-020-02648-6

Davaine J-M, Quillard T, Chatelais M, Guilbaud F, Brion R, Guyomarch B, Brennan MÁ, Heymann D, Heymann M-F, Gouëffic Y, 2016. Bone like arterial calcification in femoral atherosclerotic lesions: prevalence and role of osteoprotegerin and pericytes. *Eur J Vasc Endovasc Surg.* 51;259–267. https://doi.org/10.1016/j.ejvs.2015.10.004

Duda SH, Bosiers M, Lammer J, Scheinert D, Zeller T, Tielbeek A, Anderson J, Wiesinger B, Tepe G, Lansky A, Mudde C, Tielemans H, Bérégi JP, 2005. Sirolimus-eluting versus bare nitinol stent for obstructive superficial femoral artery disease: the SIROCCO II trial. *J Vasc Interv Radiol.* 16;331–338. https://doi.org/10.1097/01.RVI.0000151260.74519.CA

http://fyra.io, n.d. August 2015 Issue [WWW Document]. *Endovascular Today.* URL https://evtoday.com/issues/2015-aug (accessed 2.28.21a).

http://fyra.io, n.d. Biomechanical Forces in the Femoropopliteal Arterial Segment [WWW Document]. *Endovascular Today.* URL https://evtoday.com/articles/2005-june/EVT0605_F3_Smouse.html (accessed 2.28.21b).

http://fyra.io, n.d. SFA Disease: Deciding What to Leave Behind [WWW Document]. *Endovascular Today.* URL https://evtoday.com/articles/2019-jan/sfa-disease-deciding-what-to-leave-behind (accessed 2.28.21c).

Kennedy SA, Rajan DK, Bassett P, Tan KT, Jaberi A, Mafeld, S, 2021. Complication rates associated with antegrade use of vascular closure devices: a systematic review and pooled analysis. *J Vasc Surg.* 73;722–730.e1. https://doi.org/10.1016/j.jvs.2020.08.133

Litsky J, Chanda A, Stilp E, Lansky A, Mena C, 2014. Critical evaluation of stents in the peripheral arterial disease of the superficial femoral artery – focus on the paclitaxel eluting stent. *Med Devices (Auckl).* 7;149–156. https://doi.org/10.2147/MDER.S45472

MacTaggart J, Poulson W, Seas A, Deegan P, Lomneth C, Desyatova A, Maleckis K, Kamenskiy A, 2019. Stent design affects femoropopliteal artery deformation. *Ann Surg.* 270;180–187. https://doi.org/10.1097/SLA.0000000000002747

Maleckis K, Deegan P, Poulson W, Sievers C, Desyatova A, MacTaggart J, Kamenskiy A, 2017. Comparison of femoropopliteal artery stents under axial and radial compression, axial tension, bending, and torsion deformations. *J Mech Behav Biomed Mater.* 75;160–168. https://doi.org/10.1016/j.jmbbm.2017.07.017

Ormiston W, Dyer-Hartnett S, Fernando R, Holden A, 2020. An update on vessel preparation in lower limb arterial intervention. *CVIR Endovascular.* 3;86. https://doi.org/10.1186/s42155-020-00175-6

Poulson W, Kamenskiy A, Seas A, Deegan P, Lomneth C, MacTaggart J, 2018. Limb flexion-induced axial compression and bending in human femoropopliteal artery segments. *J Vasc Surg.* 67;607–613. https://doi.org/10.1016/j.jvs.2017.01.071

Rocha-Singh KJ, Zeller T, Jaff MR, 2014. Peripheral arterial calcification: prevalence, mechanism, detection, and clinical implications. *Catheter Cardiovasc Interv.* 83;E212–E220. https://doi.org/10.1002/ccd.25387

Zorger N, Manke C, Lenhart M, Finkenzeller T, Djavidani B, Feuerbach S, Link J, 2002. Peripheral arterial balloon angioplasty: effect of short versus long balloon inflation times on the morphologic results. *J Vasc Interv Radiol.* 13;355–359. https://doi.org/10.1016/S1051-0443(07)61736-9

65-5

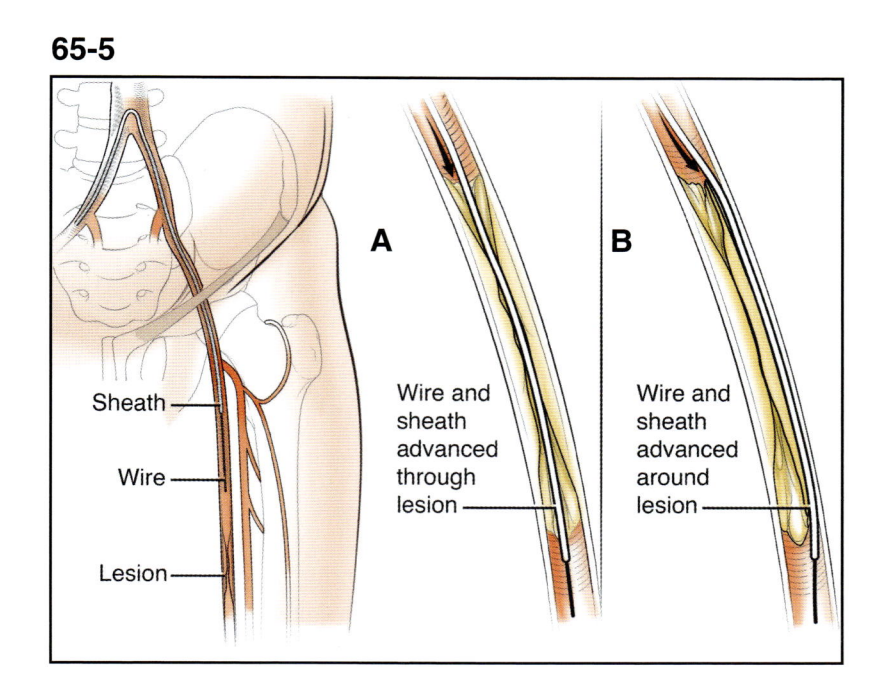

Sheath

Wire

Lesion

A Wire and sheath advanced through lesion

B Wire and sheath advanced around lesion

65-6

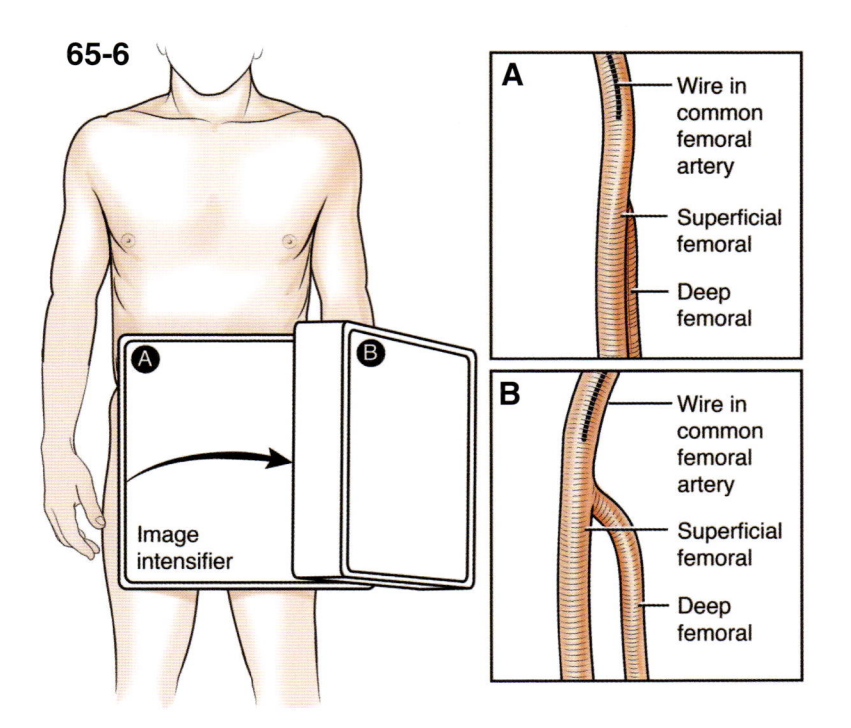

Image intensifier

A Wire in common femoral artery

Superficial femoral

Deep femoral

B Wire in common femoral artery

Superficial femoral

Deep femoral

TIBIAL ENDOVASCULAR INTERVENTION

Rebecca B. Hasley, MD, MPH • Jeffrey J. Siracuse, MD

INDICATIONS Endovascular interventions are commonly the first-line treatment for lower extremity vascular insufficiency. Infraopopliteal interventions are more common when treating chronic limb-threatening ischemia (CLTI). The specific indications for tibial and/or peroneal angiography/angioplasty are multiple and stem from symptoms related to acute and CLTI, including rest pain and tissue loss.

Prior to angiography, patients should be evaluated with history and physical, including complete pulse examination, motor and neurologic examinations, and characterization of any lower extremity wounds. Adjunct noninvasive studies, including ankle-brachial index, pulse volume recordings, toe pressures, and transcutaneous oxygen pressures can further characterize severity of limb ischemia and healing potential. Additionally, computed tomography angiography (CTA) or magnetic resonance angiography (MRA) with or without contrast can be used as adjuncts to localize disease burden and for preintervention planning.

POSITION The patient is placed in a supine position on fluoroscopy table; arms are tucked.

OPERATIVE PREPARATION After routine skin preparation, the operative field is draped to expose the ipsilateral and contralateral femoral access sites. Arm, popliteal, or pedal access sites may be prepped as well in select patients.

INCISION AND EXPOSURE After positioning and operative preparation have been be completed, proceed with local anesthesia and ultrasound-guided access of the common femoral artery (CFA). Ideal entry into the CFA is at the level of the femoral head. Alternate access sites include superficial femoral, popliteal, tibial, brachial, and radial arteries. We prefer contralateral CFA access as our default approach. Once the desired site has been chosen, access can be obtained using an 18- or 21-gauge needle. A 21-gauge needle will allow for use of a 0.018-inch guidewire, whereas an 18-gauge needle will allow for use of a 0.035-inch guide wire and may be useful if there is significant calcification or scarring in the access area. An omniflush is often used for an aortogram and to facilitate getting over the aortic bification. Once ipsilateral femoral access is achieved, the omniflush may be exchanged for an end hole catheter for dedicated extremity images.

For distal popliteal access, flexion of the knee as well as external rotation at the hip can facilitate successful access from a supine position (**FIGURE 66-1**). For ipsilateral pedal access, fluropscopic- or ultrasound-guided micropuncture access of the dorsalis pedis, peronal, or posterior tibial artery can be achieved distally (**FIGURE 66-2**).

DETAILS OF PROCEDURE Selection of endovascular intervention should be based on lesion location, length, presence of single or multiple stenoses, and presence of occlusions. The endovascular treatment options include percutaneous transluminal angioplasty (PTA), PTA with stenting, or atherectomy. PTA involves balloon angioplasty of stenotic lesions. The placement of stents may be either bare-metal or drug-eluting. Lastly, atherectomy is unique in that this technique removes plaques rather than covering or crushing them. Directional atherectomies are imaging-guided procedures that can selectively remove plaque from specific locations within the artery. Rotational atherectomies involve circumferential plaque removal.

Based on the initial angiography, one can decide which endovascular intervention would be most suited to the lesions. For some lesions, retrograde recanalization may be necessary for unfavorable tibioperoneal trunk anatomy, including long segments of disease or calcification, or small vessel diameter. Lastly, subintimal recanalization is an option for patients with total occlusions. A re-entry device may be used to facilitate entry into the true lumen. In these cases, subintimal angioplasty is achieved through purposeful exit of the lumen into the subintimal plane and then re-entry into the lumen distal to the total occlusion. Having crossed the occlusion, in the subintimal plane, we then proceed with balloon angioplasty with or without stent placement. With difficult-to-cross lesions, a bidirectional approach is often needed (**FIGURE 66-3**).

CLOSURE Arteriotomy closure may be achieved through manual pressure or the use of a closure device. If using manual compression, one should be careful to not completely occlude distal flow. As a general guideline, one should hold pressure for 3 minutes for every French size used. Additionally, we do not recommend manual pressure be used exclusively for sheaths larger than 8F.

Closure devices may also be used. Devices including plugs, suture-based devices, and compression assistants have demonstrated success but have not demonstrated superiority to the use of manual compression. One should also note the increased likelihood of distal ischemia as a complication with the utilization of these devices.

POSTOPERATIVE CARE Post-procedural care after tibioperoneal angioplasty includes bedrest, pulse checks, and may also include anticoagulation or antiplatelet therapy. Post-procedural complications can be related to access site, intervention, or systemic.

Access site complications include hematoma, thrombosis, arteriovenous fistulation, and pseudoaneurysm. Patients presenting with access site bleeding or hematoma can generally be managed with conservative treatment, including compression, physical exam monitoring, resuscitation, and anticoagulation reversal if needed. Access of the CFA above the inguinal ligament associated with post-procedure hemodynamic instability should raise concern for retroperitoneal hemorrhage and should be managed aggressively. If a pseudoaneurysm is suspected, then duplex ultrasound should be obtained, and management should be dependent on said findings.

Post-procedural complications related to angioplasty may include vessel rupture, dissection, embolization, acute arterial occlusion, and restenosis. Vessel rupture and dissection should be managed with reintervention and placement of covered stent. Embolization and acute arterial occlusion may be managed through percutaneous versus surgical thrombectomy. Restenosis may be managed initially through angiography and angioplasty.

Finally, complications related to contrast-induced nephropathy may occur post-procedurally. These complications may be averted through pre-procedure hydration, minimizing contrast used within the procedure, or alternatively, using carbon dioxide contrast. ■

66-1

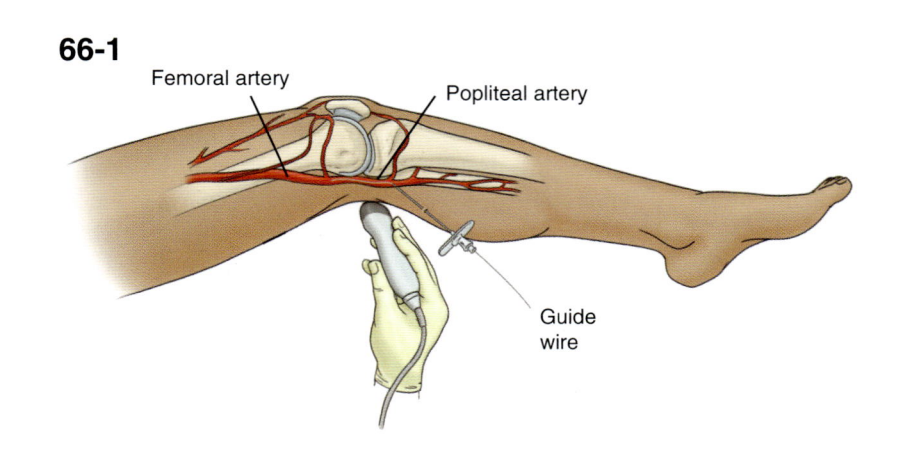

66-2

66-3

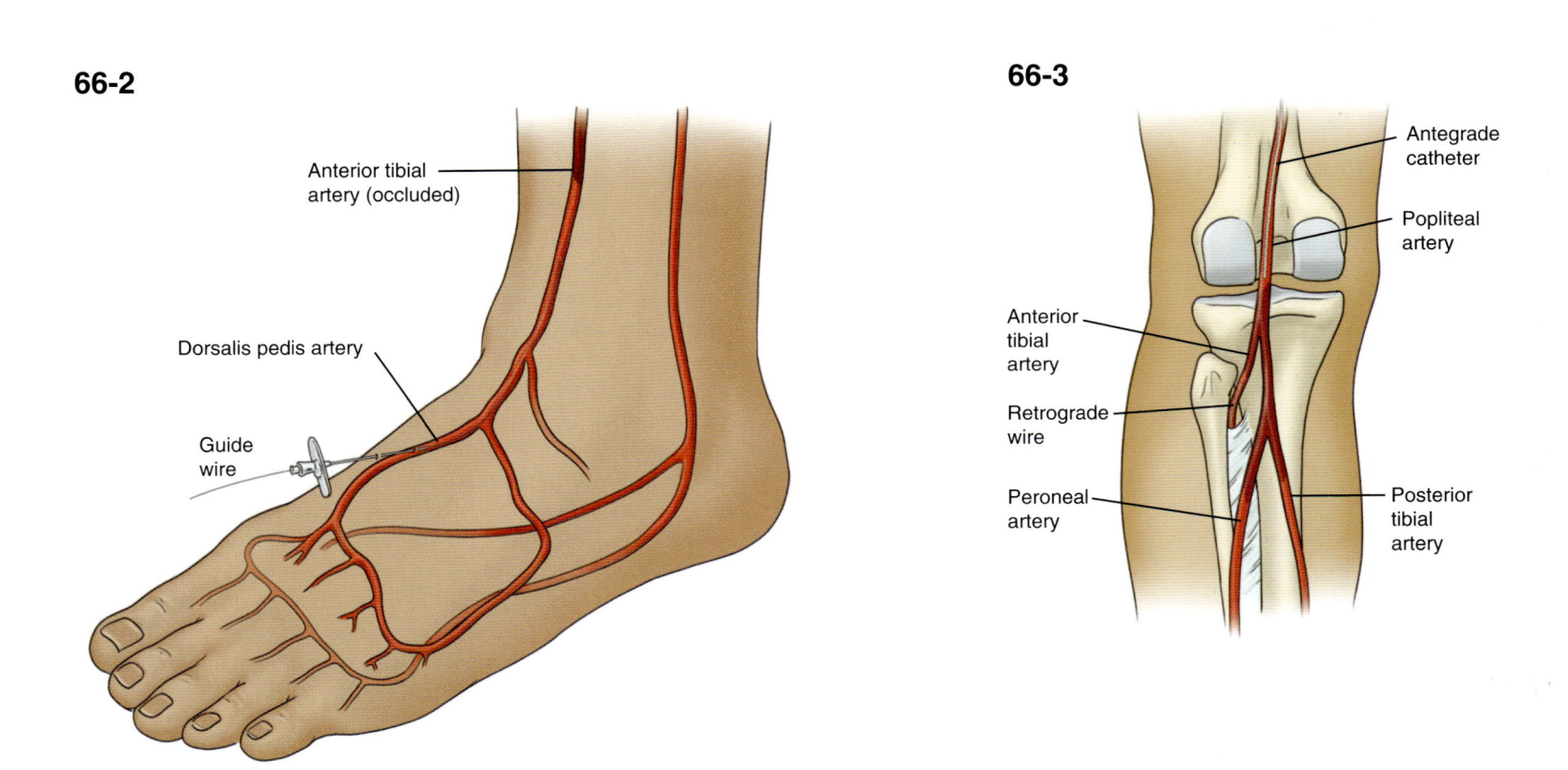

LOWER EXTREMITY ATHERECTOMY AND SUBINTIMAL RECANALIZATION

Venita Chandra, MD, FACS • Michael Paisley, MD

During lower extremity angiography and treatment of occlusive disease it is common to encounter dense, bulky calcific disease and long chronic total occlusions (CTO). This type of disease distribution is becoming increasingly common (with the increase in diabetes, and end-stage renal disease) and makes traditional revascularization options more difficult. Long-calcified CTOs are often difficult if not impossible to cross, and when crossed are often in a subintimal plane, thus requiring re-entry. Bulky calcified or dense fibrocalcific disease can make traditional percutaneous old balloon angioplasty (POBA) or other tools such as drug-coated peripheral balloons (DCB) and stenting less effective, and thus vessel preparation with atherectomy can be considered. The use of a variety of tips and tricks can help with management of these long complex lesions. This chapter will discuss some of these techniques, in particular subintimal recanalization and vessel prep with atherectomy.

INDICATIONS Preoperative lower extremity duplex ultrasound (DUS) with ankle brachial index (ABI) will offer baseline measurements of perfusion, areas of stenosis, and occlusion and can be compared to post-intervention studies on follow-up. Preoperative CT angiography is not mandatory and can add cost to the preoperative workup; however, if there is concern for suprainguinal inflow disease, unclear access options, or extent of calcific changes, obtaining cross-sectional imaging can provide information for planning inflow interventions and device selection, and more accurately characterize the extent of occlusions compared to ultrasound.

In long CTOs, particularly heavily calcified vessels, passage through the true lumen may be impossible, and creation of a subintimal plane is often the only mechanism of successful crossing. There are several techniques for re-entry utilizing common devices as well as specialized devices developed specifically for true lumen re-entry, which are often required if subintimal recanalization is performed.

The use of atherectomy has gained popularity as a tool to maximize lumen gain. There is a growing body of literature with varied outcomes, and several different technologies/approaches including orbital, directional, rotational, and photoablation (laser). Different technologies work better in different scenarios; however, in general patients with dense, bulky, or eccentric disease may benefit from the use of atherectomy, and the decision to utilize the technique is surgeon and patient dependent.

POSITION The patient is placed in the supine position with the arms padded and tucked to allow appropriate positioning of the imaging systems. Orientation of the patient relative to the imaging system will vary depending on the imaging system, planned access sites, and anatomic distribution of disease. Access options include retrograde contralateral femoral, ipsilateral antegrade femoral, and retrograde pedal sites. Radial access is also increasingly being used, but has a limited role in longer CTOs due to the decrease in pushability. Radial access is also of limited use in patients with more distant infrapopliteal disease extension. Planning and preparation for all access options is ideal and can provide an efficient transition between access sites; however, stationing a sheath as close to the lesion is optimal.

OPERATIVE PREPARATION The patient is prepared in a sterile fashion with skin preparation and draping of the operative field. The area prepped and included should encompass the bilateral groins and lower abdomen. Decision to prepare the entire lower extremity will be determined by need for possible pedal access, concomitant wound care or other interventions, and possible hybrid approach. Any infected or open wound should be prepped and isolated to avoid contamination of the other operative fields. In general, it is best to prepare any possible access site at the beginning of the case, to minimize the challenges encountered if deciding to utilize a different access site.

INCISION AND EXPOSURE Ultrasound-guided access is generally recommended, as it allows for the safest approach, using the micropuncture technique. Radiographic confirmation of appropriate access is ensured with angiography. Complete angiography of inflow, the lesion, and outflow should be performed before proceeding with the intervention. Particularly in long CTOs where subintimal recanalization may be used, it is important to understand where the true lumen reconstitutes to minimize extension of the subintimal dissection plane in normal reconstituted vessel.

DETAILS OF PROCEDURE After obtaining diagnostic angiography and deeming intervention is indicated, the sheath of choice is placed appropriately to provide a platform for intervention; again, the distal tip of the sheath should optimally be placed as close to the lesion as possible. Systemic heparin is universally given unless contraindicated and other systemic anticoagulation is given. During the diagnostic angiography, the level of reconstitution of the vessel beyond the occlusion should be noted and marked to provide a target for recanalization. The red arrows marking peroneal artery origin and reconstitution and blue arrows marking posterior tibial artery occlusion and reconstitution are displayed in FIGURE 67-1. After diagnostic angiography is performed with characterization of the lesions of interest and decision to intervene, the surgeon must then gain true lumen access proximal and distal to the lesion. Utilization of smaller platform 0.018- and 0.014-inch wire catheter systems can aid in crossing tight stenoses; however, long occlusions may need more supportive wire systems such as .035 system.

In CTOs, successful crossing of the lesions can either be true luminal or subintimal. Crossing stenotic lesions is often possible in a true luminal fashion without creation of a subintimal plane. These lesions can be nearly occlusive, and utilization of a 0.018- or 0.014-inch platform and wires with hydrophilic tips can allow for true luminal passage of near-occlusive lesions. Steps prior to attempting to cross the stenosis that can aid in success include placing the sheath as close to the lesion as possible to provide more stability, utilizing coaxial crossing catheters, and thoughtful escalation of wires. Wires most well suited to attempt a true lumen passage are generally hydrophilic coated with a softer tip but enough stiffness beyond the tip to provide pushability. Examples include Hydro ST (Cook Medical, Bloomington, IN), Glidewire Advantage (Terumo Medical, Somerset, NJ), and Command ST (Abbott Vascular, Santa Clara, CA). While attempts to stay within the true lumen should always be made, attempts at crossing long-calcified CTOs are often challenging and can require wire escalation to stiffer CTO wires, and also often result in subintimal plane being formed.

Initial access into the cap of occlusion and entry into the subintimal plane is achieved by selection of the origin of the occluded artery and placement of the tip of the catheter at the proximal occlusion with subsequent advancement of a wire. Sometimes a stiffer wire is required at this point to initiate the plane. After the wire is advanced several millimeters into the subintimal plane, advancement of the catheter can be attempted to aid in support of the wire as the subintimal plane is traversed toward the reconstituted artery. Often, when beginning the subintimal recanalization, a loop in the distal end of the wire is created, and it is important to maintain a small loop during this process as one advances the wire and catheter (FIGURE 67-2). Care should be taken to avoid creation of very large loops, however, as it is helpful to keep the subintimal plane smaller to assist in re-entry. Utilizing roadmap features or marking the location of the reconstituted vessel are recommended, as care should always be taken to avoid extension of the distal dissection far beyond the reconstitution of true lumen. Subintimal planes also carry a higher risk of perforation. Signs of perforation include a very large wire loop or the wire traveling far outside the expected path of the marked artery, and can be confirmed with angiography.

As mentioned previously, re-entry into true lumen is a key component to the success of subintimal recanalization. Sometimes after crossing the lesion in the subintimal plane the surgeon crosses into the true lumen and notes the wire easily traveling in the distal vessel at the level of reconstitution; however, any looping of the wire tip, resistance to passage of the wire, or the wire traveling outside of the expected course of the vessel should be noted and redirection of the wire attempted with catheter reinforcement. When the wire appears to be in a dissection plane beyond the level of reconstitution of the vessel and the true lumen cannot be gained, further techniques often need to be employed.

There are a number of tips and tricks to assist with re-entry. The use of stiffer CTO wires, wires with bent tips (such as that Medtronic Enteer wire or the Abbott Proceed wire), or the use of angled catheters can help drive a wire across into the true lumen. If changing your wire/catheter combinations is unsuccessful, you can then consider either the use of a re-entry device, the CART technique, or an alternative access.

67-2

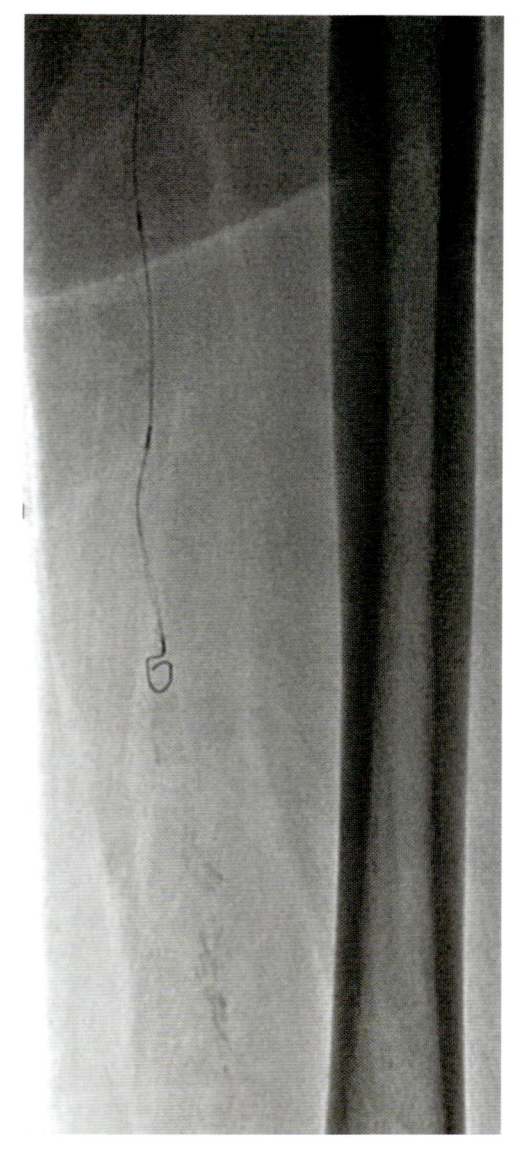

67-1

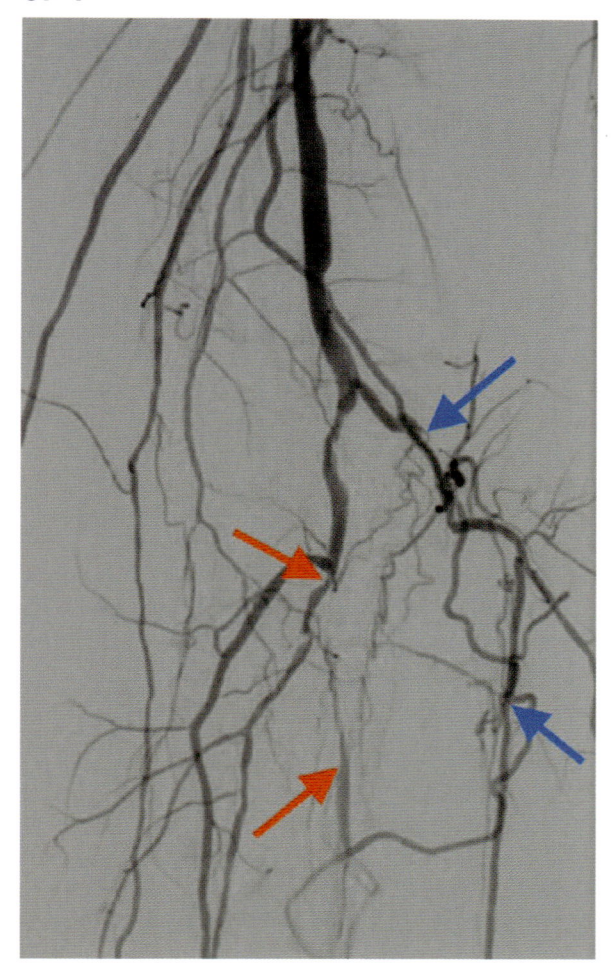

DETaILS OF PROCEDURE ◀CONTINUED▶ Following successful crossing of the lesions, one must then decide about treatment. The decision to perform atherectomy is made based on the characteristics of the lesion to be treated and surgeon preference for debulking of significant calcific disease. Atherectomy can be a useful adjunct to help with plaque modification and luminal gain; however, these benefits need to be balanced with the increased time and cost they may add to the case. There is no definition of what level of calcification qualifies as an indication for atherectomy, and it should be used as an adjunctive tool to "prepare" the vessel or modify the plaque for angioplasty with the goal of increasing luminal gain with balloon or stent angioplasty. Different types of atherectomy devices are available for use and are classified as directional, rotational, orbital, and laser. When deciding to use atherectomy, consideration should be given to the use of a distal embolic protection device such as SpiderFX (Medtronic, Minneapolis MN). Although the clinical significance of the use of distal embolic protection is not well known, it is generally used when treating thrombotic lesions, total occlusions, and when distal runoff involves only a single vessel. Some devices have instructions for use that allow treatment of a lesion with a subintimal segment, in stent restenosis or infrageniculate lesions. Careful attention must be paid to the recommended indications and limitations of each device based on the individual devices instructions for use (TABLE 67-1).

Directional atherectomy devices have internally housed blades that oppose the area of plaque to be treated via an opening on the side of the device (FIGURE 67-3, panel 1). Antegrade advancement of the device while opened and activated actuates the atherectomy blades to remove plaque along the segment of interest (FIGURE 67-3, panel 2). It is then withdrawn after closing the device to pack the atherectomized material into the tip of the device (FIGURE 67-3, panel 3), repositioned with rotation of the device to change the apposition of the arterial wall, and the vessel is retreated. The HawkOne, SilverHawk, and TurboHawk (Medtronic, Minneapolis, MN), and Pantheris (Avinger Vascular, Redwood City, CA) have specifications for eccentric calcium and CTOs with a subintimal segment and are passed via 6- to 8-French sheaths depending on the device size selected.

Rotational atherectomy devices generally employ a diamond-tipped burr that when actuated spins concentrically and ablates plaque in a monodirectional fashion. These devices are delivered via 5- to 7-French sheaths and have specifications for infrageniculate lesions with the Boston Scientific Rotoblator. Other devices include the Boston JetStream, which can treat thrombotic lesions in addition to eccentric calcium and in stent restenosis.

Orbital atherectomy utilizes an eccentrically mounted diamond-coated crown that uses centrifugal force to "orbit" around edge of the vessel lumen when actuated in the area of disease and abrades calcium from the vessel wall. The DiamondBack 360 (Cardiovascular Systems, Inc.) is the only orbital device with a peripheral intervention specification at this time, and can be used below the knee and in eccentric plaque. It is delivered via 4- to 6-French sheaths depending on the burr size. Selection of burr size and the device's rotational speed will be determined by the desired lumen of the vessel being treated. Generally, a larger crown and faster speeds of rotation

will achieve a larger luminal diameter, and this must be tailored the vessel being treated.

Laser atherectomy devices utilize ultraviolet light via fiberoptics at the tip of the device to ablate or vaporize plaques. Phillips Medical has two devices: the TurboElite with indications for eccentric plaque, CTOs, and thrombotic lesions, and the TurboPower that has a specification for in stent restenosis.

Careful device selection, taking in to account the patient's disease location, characteristics, and limitations of the device is crucial to a favorable outcome and familiarizing oneself with a device before utilization in a procedure is paramount. While each device has its own considerations, in general slow passage of the device with careful evaluation of the lesions treated and evaluation of post-treatment outflow are key technical aspects of atherectomy's utilization.

Post-atherectomy balloon or stent angioplasty is then employed in a standard fashion; examining distal outflow to rule out distal embolization is particularly important after atherectomy. After all interventions are completed, routine completion angiography is performed.

CLOSURE Closure of the access is directed by the site of access and characteristics of the vessel. Small diameter calcified vessels may not accept a closure device. Pressure can be held with reversal of heparinization.

POSTOPERATIVE CARE Immediate postoperative care includes appropriate cares mandated by the type of access with duration of bedrest, access site, and bilateral limb assessments. The patient should be assessed in the postoperative care unit frequently with neurovascular exams and access site assessments. Patients who undergo interventions should be started on an antiplatelet regimen if not already on one; generally clopidogrel 150-mg loading dose followed by 75 mg daily for 6 weeks, then 81 mg aspirin daily. General management of comorbid conditions, any wounds, statin therapy, regular physical activity, and smoking cessation should be standard in the management of peripheral arterial disease patients and there is no exception in these interventions.

Postoperative follow-up includes DUS with ABI within 4 to 6 weeks of intervention. Generally, 6-month follow-up with DUS and ABIs followed by annual follow-up with DUS and ABIs is recommended. If the patient has a clinical worsening in symptoms, nonhealing of wounds, or progressive tissue loss, imaging should be repeated earlier to assess for restenosis. ■

SUGGESTED READINGS

Finn M, Ingrassia J, Parikh S. Plaque modification in endovascular procedures in patients with infrainguinal disease. *Intervent Cardiol Clin.* 2020;9:125-137.

Korosoglou G, Giusca S, Andrassy M, et al. The role of atherectomy in peripheral artery disease: current evidence and future perspectives. *Vasc Endovasc Rev.* 2019;2(1):12-18.

Schneider P. Complex lower extremity revascularization. In: *Endovascular Skills: Guidewire and Catheter Skills in Endovascular Surgery.* 4th ed. Boca Raton, FL CRC Press; 2019.

TABLE 67-1 ATHERECTOMY TYPES AND LESIONS TO CONSIDER FOR TREATMENT

Atherectomy Type	Highly Calcified	Thrombotic Lesion	Subintimal	In-Stent Stenosis
Directional	Yes	No	Yes	No
Rotational	Yes/No	Yes/No	Yes/No	Yes/No
Orbital	Yes	No	No	No
Laser	Yes	Yes	Yes	Yes

67-3

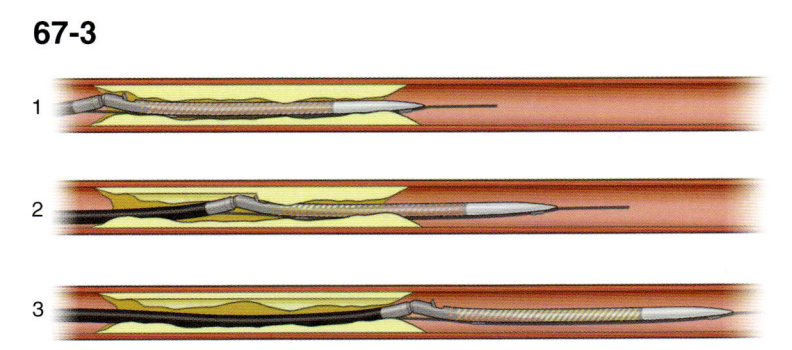

PEDAL INTERVENTIONS

Giuseppe Papia, MD, MSc

INDICATIONS The healing of very distal wounds in the foot for limb salvage and amputation prevention are the main indications for pedal vascular interventions. These advanced interventions are performed to achieve continuous inline vascular flow to target ulcers and nonhealing wounds. As such, it is key to note that all proximal inflow vessels must be treated first prior to attempting pedal reconstruction; otherwise the pedal intervention itself is likely not to achieve limb salvage. Often pedal interventions can be staged in separate settings, treating tibial vessels first rather than being performed all at once. The treatment of proximal tibial lesions alone can often achieve wound healing. However, ongoing ischemia despite tibial revascularization and failure of wound healing indicates the tibial intervention is not enough to perfuse the target lesion on the foot, and the next step is to revascularize the vessels of the foot. The pedal artery anatomy lateral view (**FIGURE 68-1A**) and anterior view (**FIGURE 68-1B**) are displayed.

An angiosome-directed approach is used when possible to target the specific tissue arteries to achieve perfusion of the target tissue zone. The greater the number of tibial vessels that are opened, thus increasing perfusion to more angiosomes (**FIGURE 68-2**), the higher the chance of achieving limb salvage. This speaks to the importance of perfusing bordering angiosomal tissue in addition to the target angiosomal tissue. Thus, if one is unsuccessful in perfusing the target angiosomal vessel, opening vessels of bordering angiosomes can also be significant to heal wounds and save limbs. Finally, it is important to note that there can be a wide variability in angiosomes between patients, especially in patients with diabetes and with dialysis-dependent renal failure. This latter group in particular is very challenging, as they may have severe distal disease and may not have a complete pedal arch. A pedal-plantar loop technique to revascularize the wound bed may be key to achieving wound healing and amputation prevention.

TOOLS Imaging is critical to identifying patient anatomy, target lesions, and subsequent approach for pedal interventions. Imaging of the foot anatomy with high resolution equipment is key to performing these procedures and minimizing radiation exposure and contrast dose. Pedal interventions can be very challenging with a simple conventional C-arm. Patients are placed in a supine position and imaging of the foot is performed both with foot in a lateral position and the image intensifier in the opposite oblique, and from an antero-posterior view.

Sheaths: Long 5French or 6French sheaths (90–110 cm if using a retrograde approach up and over the aortic bifurcation) to be placed in the distal popliteal artery for support of your system, for infusion of medication, and for contrast injections.

Wires: A complement of long (300 cm) 0.014 support wires with steerable tips and CTO wires with various weighted tips are recommended. These will allow for adequate length for attacking lesions either from an antegrade or retrograde approach as well as enough length for catheter and balloon exchanges.

Catheters: A complement of 0.014 support catheters 120 to 150 cm in length to aid the crossing of lesions and direct injection of vessels for optimal imaging. These can be angled or straight, as the operator prefers.

Angioplasty balloons: Long low profile over-the-wire (OTW) angioplasty balloons 1.5 to 3 mm in diameter to allow treatment of pedal and tibial lesions while minimizing the number of balloon inflations. A shaft length of 130 to 150 cm is recommended to ensure lesions can be reached over a long system. We recommend OTW balloon system for best support and crossing for pedal interventions.

Medications: Heparin to be given at a dose of 100 U/kg for anticoagulation. Nitroglycerin (20- to 100-μg doses) to treat vasospasm and for microvascular recruitment.

APPROACH Patients are placed in a supine position. An antegrade approach or a retrograde approach for sheath placement in the common femoral artery can be used with local anesthetic at the puncture site. With the sheath parked in the popliteal artery, one can obtain good images with contrast injected at low doses close to the site of treatment. Hand injections of 5 to 10 cc of 50% dilute contrast are used to define the anatomy and identify target lesions. This position is also ideal for infusion of medications such as nitroglycerine. Further catheter-directed imaging in specific tibial arteries can also be performed and will give the best resolution. Pedal interventions can be subdivided into three general approaches depending on target and anatomy: a direct antegrade approach, an indirect retrograde approach via the pedal-plantar loop, and a transcollateral approach.

DIRECT ANTEGRADE APPROACH: Once the anatomy is defined, the goal is to achieve in-line continuous blood flow to the target lesion. The patency of pedal procedures is quite poor, and ultimately the more vessel perfusion one can establish to the foot the higher the likelihood of limb salvage. We would approach the target angiosome vessel first in a conventional antegrade fashion with a steerable wire and support catheter rapidly spinning the wire attempting to cross the lesion and to remain intraluminal, avoiding subintimal dissections as much as possible. Remaining intraluminal avoids the challenge of re-entry when going subintimal in these small arteries. Support catheters 0.014 can be used to cross lesions and allow for direct-contrast injections to confirm the lesion has been crossed and flow is directed toward the wound. A long low-profile (2 mm) angioplasty balloon provides excellent wire support for crossing lesions and avoids an exchange over very long systems when treating the lesion. Angiograms can be performed through these balloon lumina. One trick, as it is a small 0.014 lumen, is to use an 8-mL coronary control syringe with 50% dilute contrast, which can make these injections much easier. We advocate for long inflations for 2 to 3 minutes at profile with balloons that cover the entire target lesion.

If one is unable to cross with this conventional support wire system, one would move next to a dedicated CTO wire to drill through the CTO. A gentle angle is placed at the wire tip and constant drilling with a torque device is performed while avoiding a loop in the wire. As progress is made through the occlusion with the wire, which can be small gains at a time, one should gently continue to advance and support the wire tip with the catheter or balloon slowly moving through the CTO. CTO wires come in increasing weighted tip loads, and the strength can be advanced from lower tip load to higher as progress is stalled, noting however that the higher the tip load, the greater the chance of perforation. When the wire tip becomes too distorted, be sure to change to a fresh CTO wire and continue drilling. Finally, if progress cannot be made with a CTO wire then one could revert to a conventional wire with loop and perform a subintimal technique to attempt to establish flow. The challenge of subintimal dissections is to not injure healthy distal vessels or compromise possible surgical targets. For calcific lesions at the proximal dorsalis pedis or distal posterior tibial artery, dorsiflexing and plantarflexing the foot can sometimes help to straighten and change the orientation of the arteries and help to cross lesions at these sites.

INDIRECT RETROGRADE APPROACH VIA THE PEDAL-PLANTAR LOOP: When the target angiosome vessel cannot be crossed, preventing in-line continuous flow directly, an attempt can be made to cross it retrograde via the pedal arch by entering the foot from the opposite tibial vessel and thus approaching the occlusion from the other side. The steps and approach to crossing the occlusion from this retrograde approach is the same as described above. The added advantage here is the ability to open and angioplasty the pedal-plantar loop, which may be occluded and may add to perfusion of the vascular bed. **CONTINUES ▶**

68-1

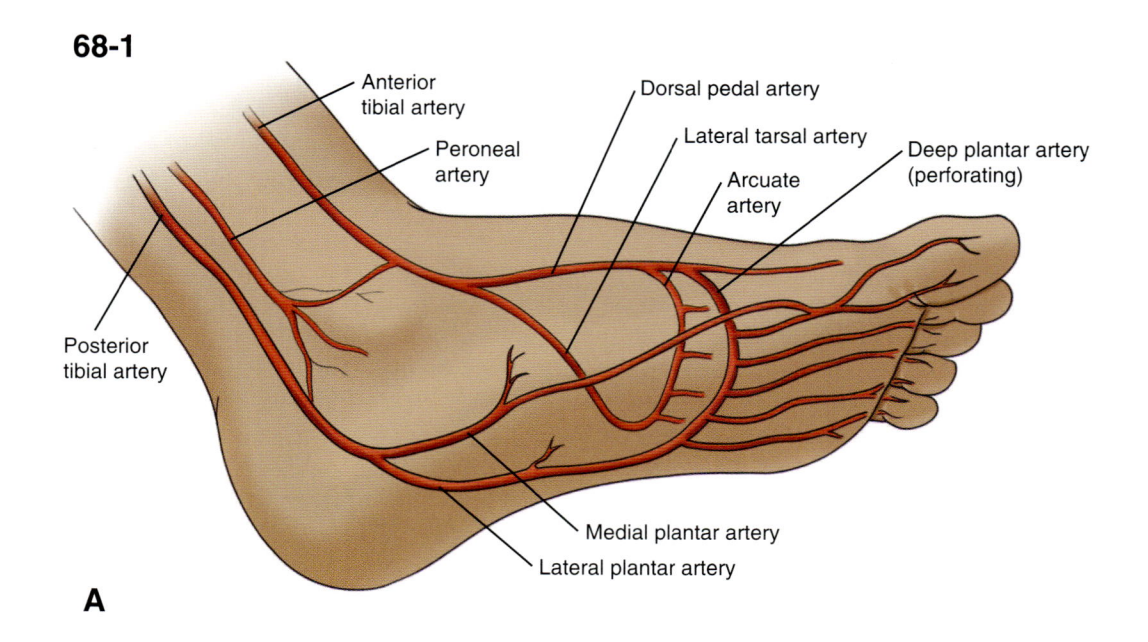

Anterior
tibial artery

Peroneal
artery

Dorsal pedal artery

Lateral tarsal artery

Arcuate
artery

Deep plantar artery
(perforating)

Posterior
tibial artery

Medial plantar artery

Lateral plantar artery

A

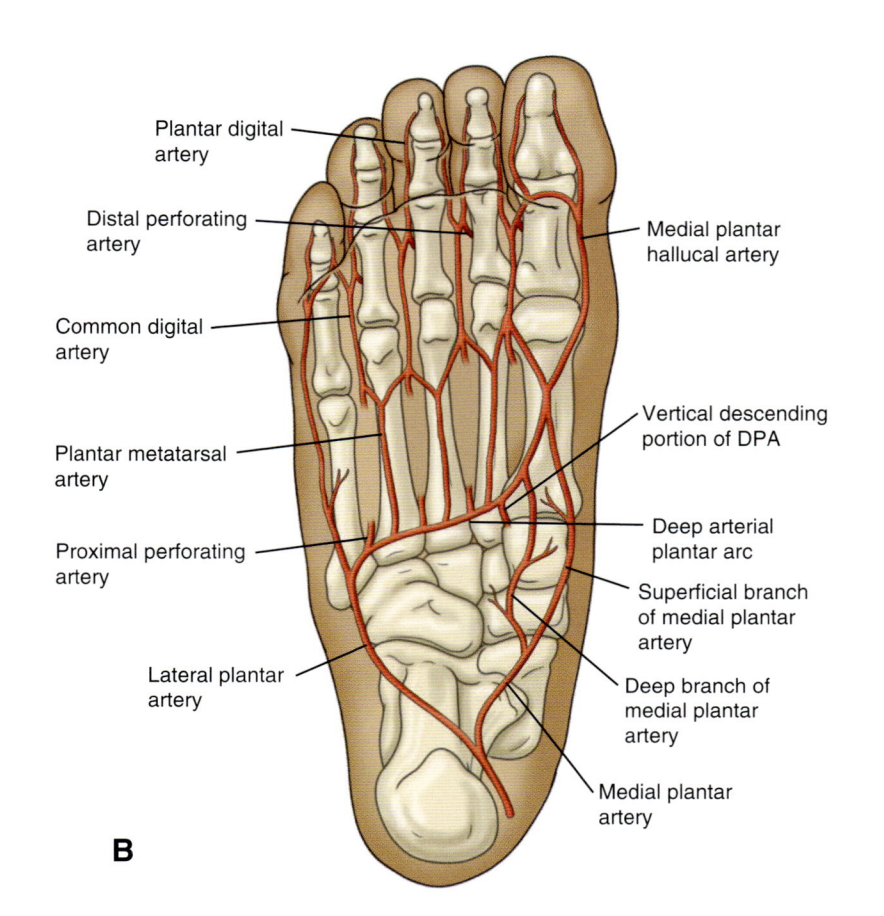

Plantar digital
artery

Distal perforating
artery

Common digital
artery

Plantar metatarsal
artery

Proximal perforating
artery

Lateral plantar
artery

Medial plantar
hallucal artery

Vertical descending
portion of DPA

Deep arterial
plantar arc

Superficial branch
of medial plantar
artery

Deep branch of
medial plantar
artery

Medial plantar
artery

B

68-2

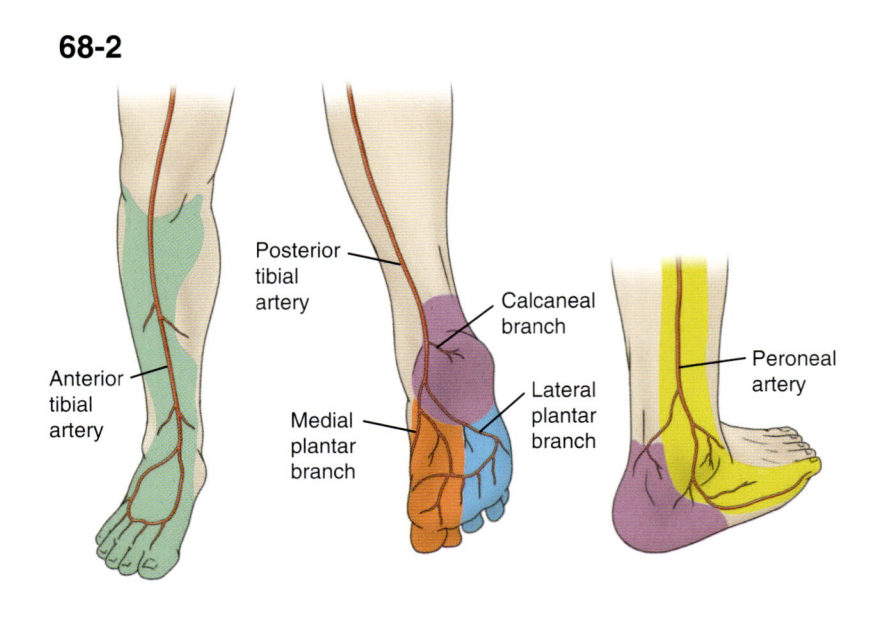

Posterior
tibial
artery

Calcaneal
branch

Anterior
tibial
artery

Medial
plantar
branch

Lateral
plantar
branch

Peroneal
artery

APPROACH `CONTINUED` Patients with diabetes and renal failure have variable and challenging pedal arterial anatomy, and angiosomes can be isolated. Angiosomes should only serve as a guide in the patient in terms of determining target vessels. Pedal flow can be compartmentalized with little to no crossover between anterior and posterior pedal circulation. Thus, crossing and opening the pedal-plantar loop in these patients allows the plantar circulation to perfuse the dorsal circulation and vice versa, thus maximizing perfusion of wounds. The pedal-plantar loop technique of revascularization allows contralateral flow to perfuse the ulcers and can be key in pedal interventions for limb salvage if one cannot establish direct blood flow with good ulcer perfusion via the main target tibial artery, the caveat being that if one establishes direct in-line flow successfully there is no need to risk damaging vessels by further attempting to open the pedal arch. The operator has to balance successful perfusion with not doing too much and risking that success. However, when the foot has diffuse disease with poor distal distribution of flow, the so-called desert foot, the pedal-plantar loop technique can be vital to wound healing and saving the limb. A combination of approaches depending on the anatomy are used to open flow from the dorsalis pedis to the lateral plantar artery. An 0.014″ wire around the pedal arch to recannulize the arch vessels and the dorsalis pedis can achieve in-line flow to a pedal wound (FIGURE 68-3A). Long low-profile balloons are inflated around the loop for 2 to 3 minutes (FIGURE 68-3B). Nitroglycerine is given to account for any spasm, but to also open the microvasculature.

TRANSCOLLATERAL APPROACH: Sometimes the severity of the disease in the tibial and pedal vessels does not allow for recannulation via a more conventional antegrade or retrograde approach. Vessels are far too calcified and diseased to open, or the occlusions are so long-standing that the vessels are atretic and nonexistent. At this point a final approach that can be considered is to take advantage of well-established collaterals to approach pedal arteries in order to open and increase blood flow to ischemic tissue. It is unconventional to approach these procedures via non-named collateral vessels; however, limb salvage can be achieved by taking advantage of them. Often important collateral branches can exist from the distal peroneal arteries which can be well established in these patients and therefore used to traverse into the pedal arteries and open and augment flow to wounds. Angioplasty of these distal perforators can help achieve increased in-line flow and to an open pedal vessel. Finally, in extreme cases retrograde punctures of digital arteries to access the deep pedal arch of the foot have also been described for limb salvage. ∎

SUGGESTED READINGS

Ferraresi R, Palena LM, Mauri G, Manzi M. Tips and tricks for a correct "endo approach". *J Cardiovasc Surg.* 2013;54:685-711.

Hizing E, Schreve M, et al. Below the ankle angioplasty in patients with critical limb ischemia: a systematic review and meta-analysis. *J Vasc Interv Radiol.* 2019;1-8.

Lee AC, Khuddus MA. Pedal arch revascularization. *EndovascToday.* May 2014.

Manzi M, Palena LM. Treating calf and pedal vessel disease: the extremes of intervention. *Semin Intervent Radiol.* 2014;31:313-319.

Nakama R, Watanabe N, et al. Clinical outcomes of pedal artery angioplasty for patients with ischemic wounds. *JACC.* 2017;10(1).

Palena LM, Manzi M. Extreme below-the-knee interventions: retrograde transmetatarsal or transplant arch access for foot salvage in challenging cases of critical limb ischemia. *J Endovasc Ther.* 2012;19:805-811.

68-3

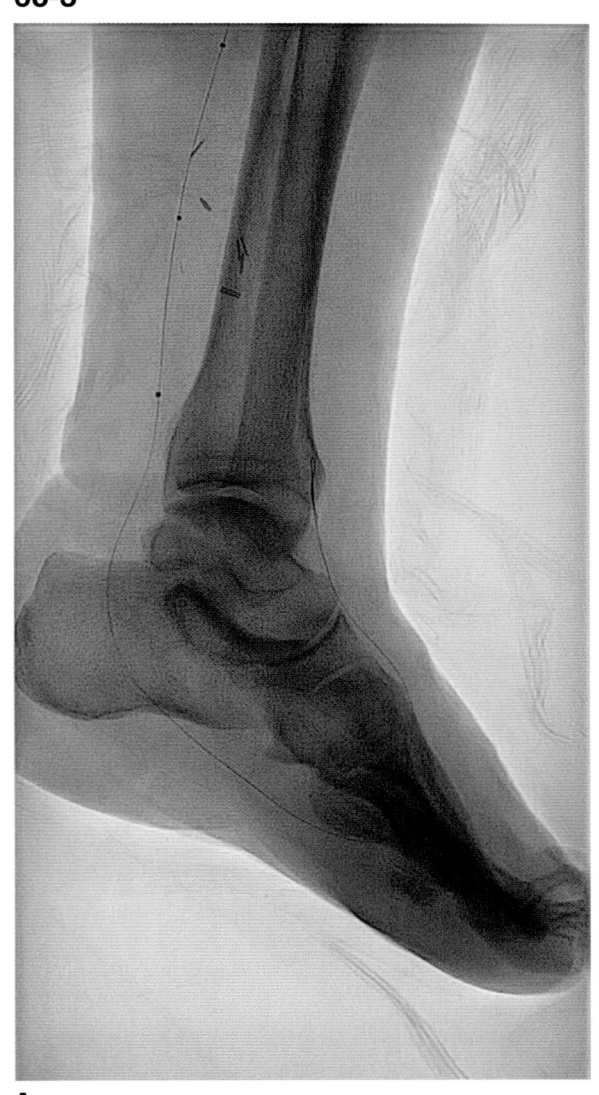

A

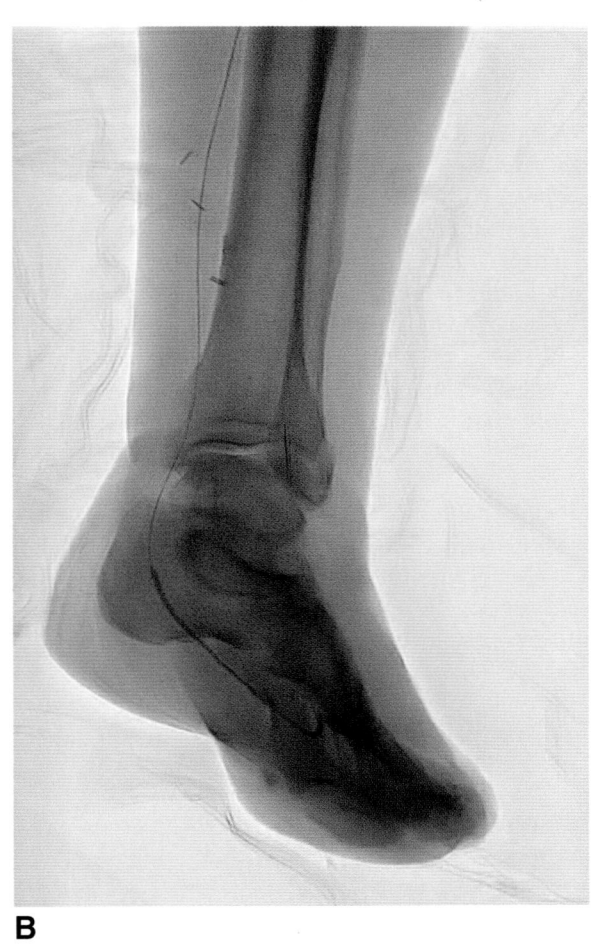

B

ARTERIAL THROMBOLYSIS

Afsha Aurshina, MD • **Anil Hingorani, MD**

INDICATIONS Catheter-directed intra-arterial thrombolysis (CDT) is a standard treatment for patients with acute and subacute limb ischemia of lower extremity arteries and bypass grafts. Due to its potential benefits of being safer and more effective than systemic thrombolysis, its use in current practice has substantially increased.(1, 2) Clinical and technical success have been observed, especially in acute cases with fresh thrombus or emboli. CDT is thus the first-line treatment of choice for acute limb ischemia (ALI) patients with symptoms of <14 days duration. The PEARL (PEripheral Use of Angiojet Rheolytic Thrombectomy with variety of catheter Lengths) registry further justifies the addition of pharmacomechanical thrombectomy (PMT) to CDT.(3)

Patients with viable limbs (Category I ischemia), do not require immediate invasive thrombolysis. These patients are usually admitted and started on anticoagulation while clinical workup is continued. CDT can then be scheduled and performed several hours after presentation. For marginally threatened limb (Category IIa), CDT is indicated urgently. For immediately threatened limb (Category IIb), surgical revascularization is preferred, to establish immediate perfusion and salvage the limb.(4) However, in patients with high cardiovascular risks from comorbidities, thrombolysis may be preferred. A standard technique or choice of thrombolytic agent has not been defined and is usually based on the discretion of the operating surgeon, based on limb viability, thrombus characteristics, and risk of hemorrhage.

PREOPERATIVE PREPARATION A diagnosis of ALI is usually determined after thorough clinical examination and duplex ultrasound (DUS) imaging.(5) The DUS imaging, in addition to location and extent, contributes data describing thrombus as fresh or chronic. The location and extent of thrombus is to be independently reviewed by the operating surgeon. For patients with Category I ischemia or when diagnosis of ALI is suspected, computed tomography angiography can further help define the extent of stenosis or occlusion if the duplex exam is not conclusive. Patients with severe limb ischemia are immediately initiated on systemic anticoagulation using weight-based intravenous infusion of unfractionated heparin (UFH) at 18 units/kg/hour after the initial bolus in the emergency room (80 units/kg).

ANESTHESIA Local anesthesia with moderate conscious sedation is the most commonly employed technique for CDT. An anesthesiologist is usually necessary for monitoring of hemodynamic status throughout the procedure. The specific anesthetic agents given to the patient are left to the discretion of the anesthesiologist. Ultrasound-guided periadventitial administration of local anesthetic is performed by the operating surgeon to provide sufficient pain control during the procedure. Careful ultrasound-guided access is paramount to avoid femoral hematoma formation during thrombolysis.

POSITION AND OPERATIVE PREPARATION The patient should be placed in a supine position on a table compatible with fluoroscopy, preferably in a dedicated angiography suite. The neck, elbow, and knees should be adequately supported and arms secured at patient's side to prevent injury. Urinary catheterization is routinely performed, after initiation of sedation, to closely monitor fluid and hemodynamic status during thrombolysis.

INCISION AND EXPOSURE After routine skin preparation, proper exposure, and administration of local anesthesia, intravascular access is obtained using an ultrasound-guided micropuncture system, to minimize bleeding, into a compressible segment of the affected artery. Prior meta-analysis of randomized data have demonstrated the utility of using ultrasound guidance for the puncture in terms of reducing complications.(6) In addition, puncture of the least calcified portion of the vessel may facilitate successful hemostasis with the vascular closure device upon completion.

The most commonly used access site for lower extremity thrombolysis is the common femoral artery (CFA). A crossover catherization from contralateral CFA is preferred for accurate puncture into the CFA. This is easier to achieve from a retrograde approach. Puncture into the brachial artery, ipsilateral CFA, popliteal artery, or direct graft puncture are alternatively used based on location of occlusive lesion. A small skin incision, if necessary, should be approximated to the size of sheath to minimize bleeding. Avoid puncture of the posterior wall of the CFA to decease risk of groin and retroperitoneal hematoma. A 4 to 5 Fr Micropuncture access set can be employed to decrease risk of inadvertent puncture.

DETAILS OF PROCEDURE Once access is obtained, angiographic confirmation can be performed. This additionally gives an assessment for suitability of puncture closure device placement. A complete diagnostic angiography of the affected limb can then be performed to accurately identify the location and extent of thrombus, with delayed imaging to visualize the tibial runoff vessels. In cases of embolic occlusion, consider bilateral lower extremity angiography to identify any asymptomatic lesions.

The micropuncture cannula is then upsized to a 6 Fr sheath to accommodate the 5 Fr thrombolysis catheters and all potentially necessary devices for adjunctive balloon angioplasty or mechanical thrombectomy. After placement of sheath, another weight-based bolus dose of UFH (80 units/kg) is to be administered.

A stiff, hydrophilic guidewire is typically utilized to probe the occlusive lesion and cross it. The ease of transversing the occlusion helps determine of the consistency of the thrombus, (guidewire traversal test) (**FIGURE 69-1**). Embolic occlusions are typically easy to cross because of the lack of a thick platelet-rich fibrin plug. Very rarely, if the occlusion cannot be traversed, an end-hole catheter can be placed at the proximal end of the occlusion to initiate thrombolysis. It takes a few hours of thrombolysis for the proximal fibrin plug to soften and return to the operating room to continue thrombolysis.

Using the Fast Track thrombolysis protocol, suction thrombectomy can initially be performed to debulk the thrombus using the Angiojet or the Penumbra systems. This is followed by pharmacomechanical thrombectomy (PMT). The dose of the tPA used for the power pulse depends on the volume of the thrombus. We vary the dose from 4 to 10 mg of tPA. In about 80% of cases, we are able to use the Fast Track protocol in a single session for eliminating the thrombus and revascularizing the limb (**FIGURE 69-2**). Once tPA is delivered, it is allowed to dwell for additional 10 to 20 minutes. In occasional cases, the thrombus can be macerated using a non-drug–eluting balloon followed by repeat suction thrombectomy for further debulking and removal of remnants of thrombus. In some cases, the Fast Track protocol does not completely clear the thrombus given the extent of thrombus, and thrombolysis is continued for 6 to 24 hours. This is an essential step to remove resilient thrombus and confirm areas of arterial stenosis. **CONTINUES** ▶

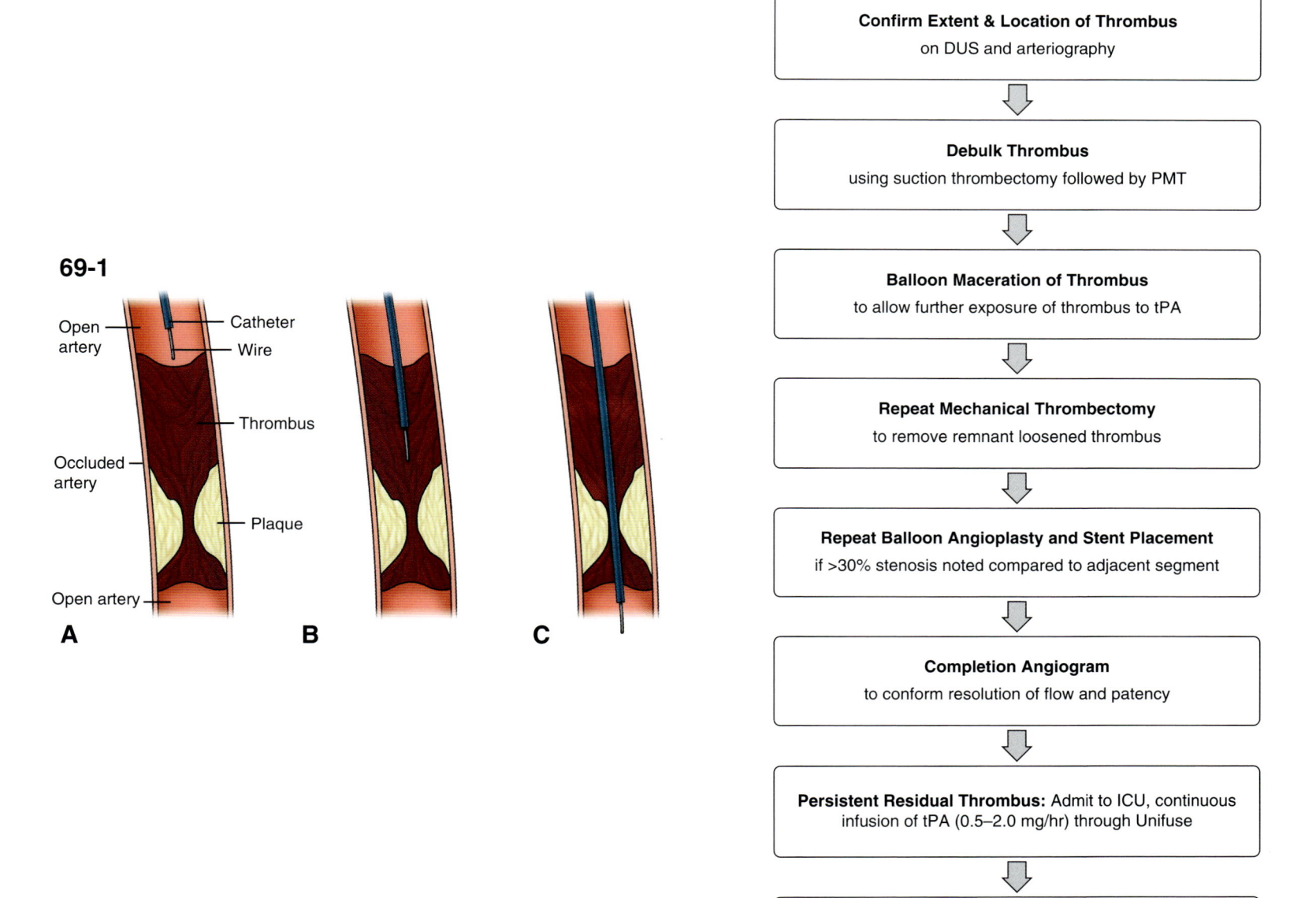

69-1

Open artery — Catheter

Wire

Thrombus

Occluded artery

Plaque

Open artery

A   B   C

69-2

Diagnosis of Ali
by physical examination and DUS

Medical Rx
Immediate systemic anticoagulation with UFH (80 U/kg)
and drip

Confirm Extent & Location of Thrombus
on DUS and arteriography

Debulk Thrombus
using suction thrombectomy followed by PMT

Balloon Maceration of Thrombus
to allow further exposure of thrombus to tPA

Repeat Mechanical Thrombectomy
to remove remnant loosened thrombus

Repeat Balloon Angioplasty and Stent Placement
if >30% stenosis noted compared to adjacent segment

Completion Angiogram
to conform resolution of flow and patency

Persistent Residual Thrombus: Admit to ICU, continuous
infusion of tPA (0.5–2.0 mg/hr) through Unifuse

Post-Operative care:
3–6 months of Factor Xa inhibitor with Follow-up within 1 week,
then q3 months for 1 year and then q6 months thereafter

Figure 69-2 The FastTrack Thrombolysis Protocol for management of
ALI.

DETAILS OF PROCEDURE CONTINUED In these cases, lysis is continued using Alteplase (0.5–2 mg/hour) with a multi-hole infusion catheter, while the patient is closely monitored in the surgical intensive care unit for hemorrhage or hemodynamic instability. The use of a multi-side hole infusion catheter (i.e., Unifuse, Cragg-McNamara) (**FIGURE 69-3A**) allows even distribution along the length of the thrombus and decreases the need for catheter repositioning. The infusion area should be embedded in the thrombus (**FIGURE 69-3B**). Concomitant heparin infusion of 500 units/ hour (subtherapeutic) is administered via the sheath to prevent sheath thrombosis. Parameters including complete blood count, fibrinogen level, and activated partial thromboplastin time are to be monitored. Repeat angiography often reveals a culprit lesion that led to the thrombosis. In those cases, balloon angioplasty and stenting or other endovascular interventions are considered.

CLOSURE Meticulous hemostasis should be obtained to prevent formation of hematoma. An arterial closure device can be deployed after completion angiogram, to decrease duration of post-procedure immobility and need for manual compression.

POSTOPERATIVE CARE Immediately after the procedure, patients with total or near-total resolution of residual thrombus are transferred to a standard surgical floor and observed for hemodynamic stability, pain control, access site hemostasis, and distal perfusion. Patients are discharged home once oral anticoagulation is initiated. During the interim period, patients are anticoagulated with intravenous UFH.

Postoperative medical management involves oral anticoagulation. Usually, an oral Factor Xa inhibitor is prescribed for 6 months. The duration of anticoagulation is dependent on the underlying cause of the thrombosis. If the underlying cause of the thrombosis is corrected, than 3 to 6 months of anticoagulation is used. If patients are already on antithrombotic regimen, the same anticoagulant is usually continued. After 3 to 6 months, if anticoagulation is to be discontinued it is recommended to maintain antiplatelet therapy for life.

FOLLOW-UP All patients undergoing thrombolysis should be seen in the vascular clinic within 1 week of procedure, followed by every 3 months postoperatively for the first year and every 6 months thereafter with a physical examination and DUS. ∎

REFERENCES

1. The STILE Investigators. Results of a prospective randomized trial evaluating surgery versus thrombolysis for ischemia of the lower extremity. The STILE trial. *Ann Surg.* 1994;220(3):251-66; discussion 66-68.

2. Ouriel K, Veith FJ, Sasahara AA. Thrombolysis or peripheral arterial surgery: Phase I results. TOPAS Investigators. *J Vasc Surg.* 1996;23(1):64-73; discussion 4-5.

3. Leung DA, Blitz LR, Nelson T, Amin A, Soukas PA, Nanjundappa A, et al. Rheolytic pharmacomechanical thrombectomy for the management of acute limb ischemia: results from the PEARL Registry. *J Endovasc Ther.* 2015;22(4):546-557.

4. Rutherford RB, Baker JD, Ernst C, Johnston KW, Porter JM, Ahn S, et al. Recommended standards for reports dealing with lower extremity ischemia: revised version. *J Vasc Surg.* 1997;26(3):517-538.

5. Katzen BT. Clinical diagnosis and prognosis of acute limb ischemia. *Rev Cardiovasc Med.* 2002;3 Suppl 2:S2-6.

6. Sobolev M, Slovut DP, Lee Chang A, Shiloh AL, Eisen LA. Ultrasound-guided catheterization of the femoral artery: a systematic review and meta-analysis of randomized controlled trials. *J Invasive Cardiol.* 2015;27(7):318-323.

7. Ascher E, Chait J, Pavalonis A, Marks N, Hingorani A, Kibrik P. Fast-track thrombolysis protocol: a single-session approach for acute iliofemoral deep venous thrombosis. *J Vasc Surg Venous Lymphat Disord.* 2019;7(6):773-780.

8. Gagne PJ, Gasparis A, Black S, Thorpe P, Passman M, Vedantham S, et al. Analysis of threshold stenosis by multiplanar venogram and intravascular ultrasound examination for predicting clinical improvement after iliofemoral vein stenting in the VIDIO trial. *J Vasc Surg Venous Lymphat Disord.* 2018;6(1):48-56 e1.

69-3

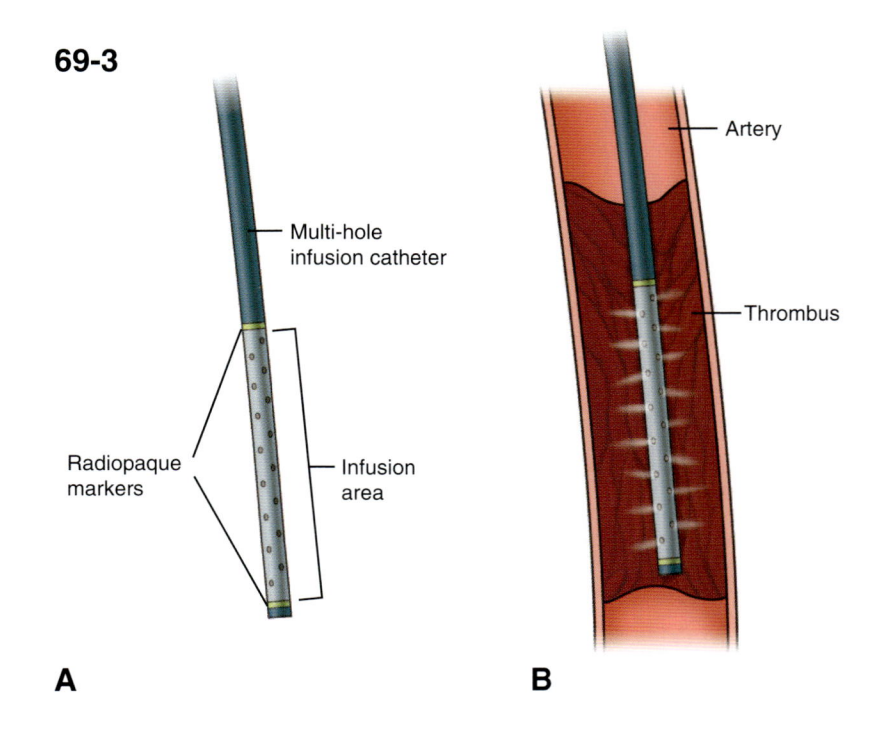

Multi-hole infusion catheter

Radiopaque markers

Infusion area

A

Artery

Thrombus

B

ENDOVASCULAR POPLITEAL ANEURYSM REPAIR

Armin Farazdaghi, MD • **Randall R. De Martino, MD, MS**

INDICATIONS Popliteal artery aneurysms, though uncommon in the general population, account for the predominant portion of peripheral artery aneurysms. Risk factors include male sex, advanced age, and aneurysms in other locations. They are most often associated with atherosclerotic degeneration. Treatment of popliteal artery aneurysms is indicated in symptomatic patients, or in asymptomatic patients after aneurysm size surpasses 2 cm. Symptomatic patients most often present with thrombotic or embolic events, with a wide range of acuity including limb-threatening ischemia, chronic limb ischemia, and more uncommonly, rupture. In patients who are acutely symptomatic, initial treatment with catheter-directed thrombolytic therapy may restore the vessel lumen patency and outflow branches that are prone to embolic occlusion. This will permit open or endovascular treatment to follow. Additional factors that necessitate the need for repair include diseased tibial runoff that would risk limb survival with further embolization from the intraluminal thrombus associated with the aneurysm.

Endovascular repair has become more commonplace, as treatment is associated with decreased morbidity and comparable durability. Patients selected for endovascular repair are preferably those with normal runoff and focal aneurysmal extent allowing for treatment with the fewest stent grafts possible. This will also be relevant in patients with notable size discrepancies between the proximal and distal landing zone, which will require more pieces and has been associated with lower patency. In contrast, patients with single vessel runoff would be best served with open bypass with autologous venous conduit. Patients with nickel allergies should also be offered open repair due to the nitinol component of the Viabahn stent graft.

PREOPERATIVE PREPARATION Preoperative preparation should include optimization of the patient's cardiovascular risk factors. Imaging to assess for abdominal aortic aneurysms and contralateral popliteal aneurysm should be performed due to the high rates of concomitant disease, as well as CT angiogram of the pelvis and bilateral lower extremities with anatomical assessment of access options, vessel tortuosity, size, and runoff. Additionally, vessel size of the proximal and distal landing zone will dictate the feasibility of endovascular repair with Viabahn stent, size ranging from 5 to 13 mm.

ANESTHESIA Anesthesia with moderate conscious sedation should be used, with local anesthetic used at the access site. General anesthesia is not typically necessary.

POSITION AND OPERATIVE PREPARATION The patient is positioned supine. For totally percutaneous cases, bilateral groins are prepped. If open vessel access is needed, the field should include this region as well.

INCISION AND EXPOSURE In straightforward cases, our preference is for percutaneous access in a retrograde fashion with ProGlide suture–mediated closure, given the facility of this technique for other large sheath endovascular procedures. However, for patients with tortious iliac artery systems, surgical bifurcated grafts, or aortic endografts, ipsilateral access is preferred. This can easily be done via open exposure of the ipsilateral superficial artery (SFA). Percutaneous access is established with ultrasound and fluoroscopic guidance, ensuring that a healthy femoral artery segment over the femoral head is selected. For open access, the ipsilateral SFA should be evaluated for a segment free from significant atherosclerotic disease and calcification. Local anesthetic is injected and a longitudinal incision is made at the level of proximal SFA deemed optimal for access, often just below the inguinal crease.

DETAIL OF PROCEDURE Once the location for percutaneous access is identified, it is instilled with local anesthetic. The CFA is then cannulated in retrograde fashion with a 21-gauge Micropuncture needle under ultrasound guidance, and 0.018 wire advanced under fluoroscopic guidance and upsized to a 5 Fr sheath using a Seldinger technique. For sheath sizes >9 Fr, two ProGlide Perclose sutures are used in an 11 and 1 o'clock position for later closure. Smaller access can use a single suture. The patient is then given systemic heparin, 100 units/kg, with a goal ACT greater than 250 seconds. The contralateral SFA is then selected after up-and-over access

of the aortic bifurcation, and the appropriately sized sheath (7–12 Fr) is advanced into the contralateral extremity. Arteriogram is then performed to better visualize the lesion and to better assess for stent graft length measurements and distal runoff vessels. Arteriogram of a symptomatic 2.7-cm popliteal artery aneurysm with mural thrombus that presented following recent distal embolization is displayed in (**FIGURE 70-1**). If there are significant discrepancies or concern for stent sizing, we recommend confirmation with intravascular ultrasound (IVUS). It is critical to ensure proper size, as excess will result in graft infolding that can lead to thrombosis. Undersized grafts will not properly exclude the aneurysm and will be prone to migrate.

Glidewire and Kumpe catheter are used to cross the popliteal aneurysm. The glidewire is then exchanged over the catheter for a stiffer wire, such as an Amplatz. The stent graft should be approximately 10 to 20% oversized to ensure adequate seal at the proximal and distal landing zones. The distal landing zone should ensure the ostia of the anterior tibial or TP trunk are not covered. The Viabahn stent graft device should be prepared and deployed in accordance with the device IFU. Post-deployment transluminal balloon angioplasty is performed in accordance with the IFU recommendation based on device size to ensure it is fully expanded without infolding. Repeat intravascular ultrasound can be utilized to ensure adequate apposition and full expansion of the stent graft. If there is a size discrepancy between the proximal and distal landing zones, the smaller piece should be deployed first. Typically, the smaller piece is needed distally. The larger piece should overlap into the smaller piece with at least 5 cm of overlap to ensure adequate seal and reduce the risk of Type III endoleak.

Completion angiography is performed to exclude the presence of Type I or III endoleak, with the knee in both the flexed and extended position. Arteriogram following deployment of 8 mm × 10 cm Gore Viabahn stent with excellent seal without coverage of the anterior tibial or TP trunk is displayed in (**FIGURE 70-2**). Finally, the CFA access is closed by tightening the sutures placed at the beginning of the case.

POSTOPERATIVE CARE/FOLLOW-UP Postoperative care for all patients should entail establishing a baseline utilizing duplex ultrasound noninvasive studies, including ABI, segmental pressures, and Doppler of the operative extremity. The aforementioned baseline imaging should be obtained at 1 month, followed by repeat studies for surveillance at 3 months, 6 months, 12 months, and yearly thereafter. Duplex surveillance ultrasound at 24 months demonstrates a widely patent endovascular repair (**FIGURE 70-3**).

Patients should remain on dual antiplatelet therapy postoperatively for at least 1 month if the repair results are excellent with patent multivessel runoff. Continuing patients on mono versus dual antiplatelet therapy will need to be carefully considered in subsequent follow-up visits and are dependent on the number of stents, length of repair, and runoff. ■

SUGGESTED READINGS

Antonello, M, Frigatti P, Battocchio P, et al. Open repair versus endovascular treatment for asymptomatic popliteal artery aneurysm: results of a prospective randomized study. *J Vasc Surg.* 2005;42,(2):185-193.

Curi MA, Geraghty PJ, Merino OA, et al. Mid-term outcomes of endovascular popliteal artery aneurysm repair. *J Vasc Surg.* 2007;45(3):505-510.

Ghotbi R, Sotiriou A, Schönhofer S, Zikos D, Schips K, Westermeier W. Stent-graft placement in popliteal artery aneurysms: midterm results. *Vasc Dis Manage.* 2007;4(4):123-127.

Golchehr B, Zeebregts CJ, Reijnen MMPJ, Tielliu IFJ. Long-term outcome of endovascular popliteal artery aneurysm repair. *J Vasc Surg .* 2018;67(6):1797-1804.

Huang Y, Gloviczki P, Oderich GS, et al. Outcomes of endovascular and contemporary open surgical repairs of popliteal artery aneurysm. *J Vasc Surg.* 2014: 60(3):631-638.

Tielliu IFJ, Verhoeven ELG, Zeebregts CJ, Prins PR, Bos WTGJ, van den Dungen JJAM. Endovascular treatment of popliteal artery aneurysms: is the technique a valid alternative to open surgery? *J Cardiovasc Surg.* 2007;48(3):275-279.

Wain RA, Hines G. A contemporary review of popliteal artery aneurysms. *Cardiol Rev.*2007;15(2):102-107.

70-1

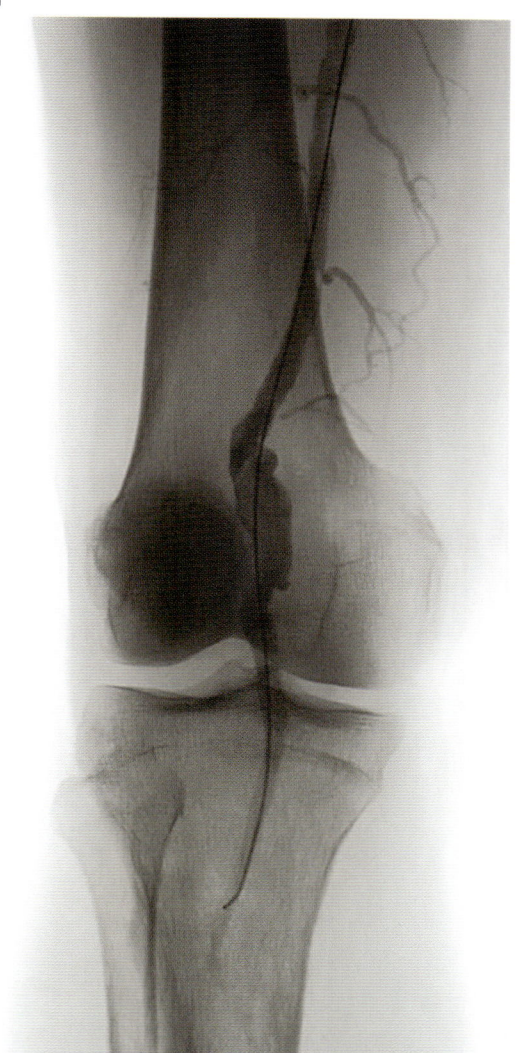

70-2

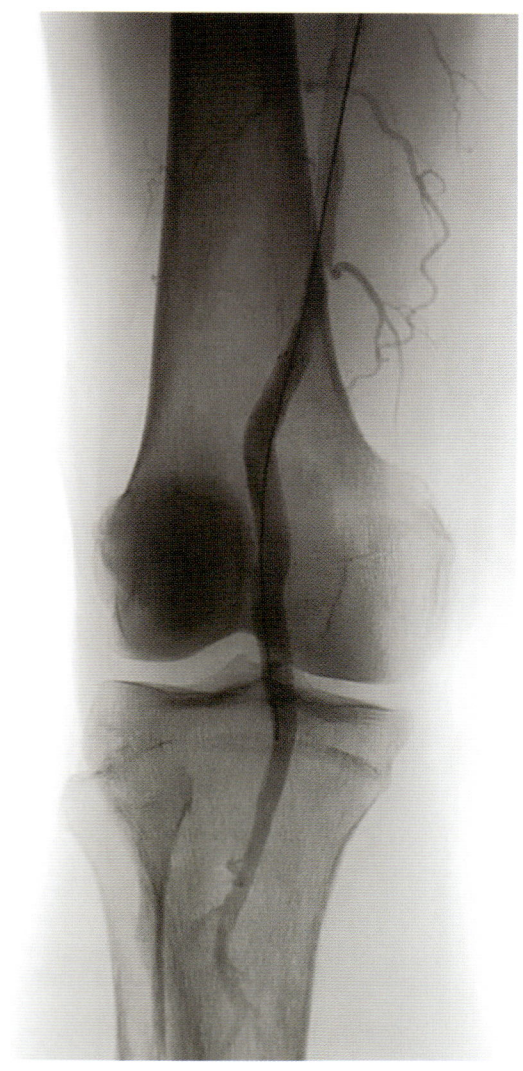

70-3

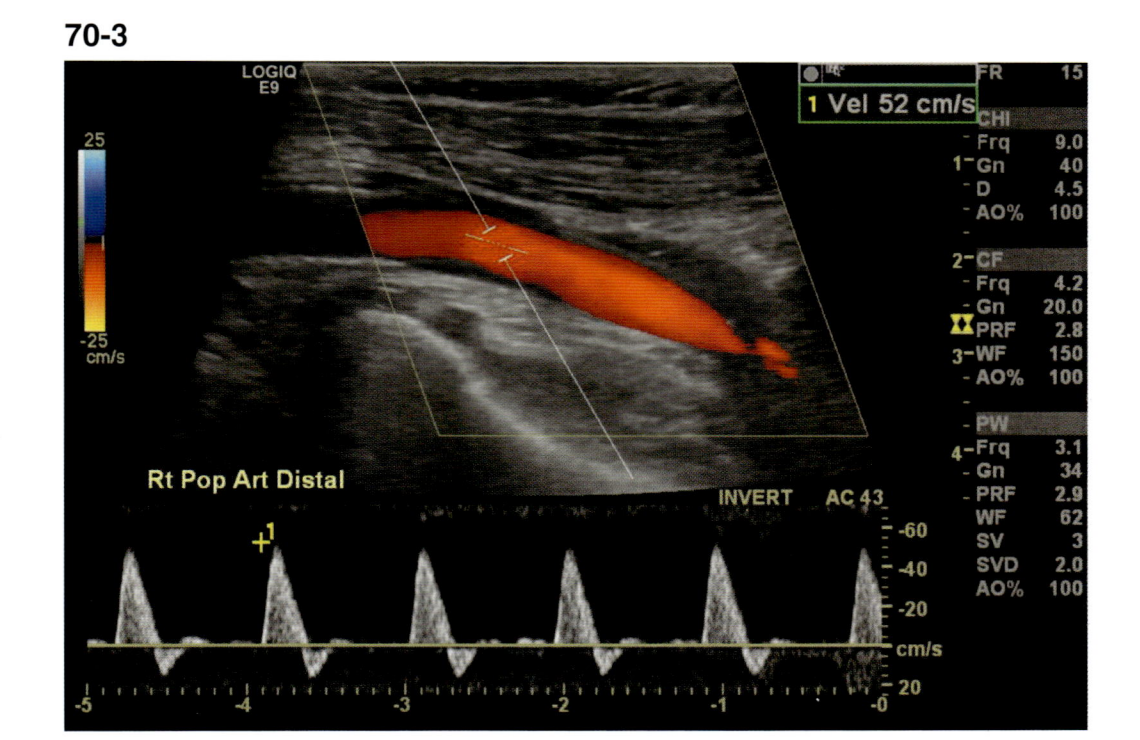

Section XIV
VEINS AND INFERIOR VENA CAVA

Inferior Vena Cava Filter Placement and Retrieval: Endovascular

Anand Brahmandam, MBBS • Cassius Iyad Ochoa Chaar, MD, MS

INFERIOR VENA CAVA FILTER PLACEMENT

INDICATIONS Venous thromboembolism (VTE), comprising deep vein thrombosis (DVT) and pulmonary embolism (PE), is a major public health problem and contributes to significant morbidity and mortality. The cornerstone for the treatment of VTE is anticoagulation. However, vena cava interruption is indicated to prevent PE in patients with contraindication to anticoagulation or failure of anticoagulation. The Prevention du Risque d'Embolie Pulmonaire par Interruption Cave (PREPIC) trials showed that permanent IVC filter placement in addition to anticoagulation led to a 4% PE risk reduction in PE at 12 days.[1] At 8-year follow-up in the PREPIC trial, there was a 9% PE risk reduction and a 10% increase in risk of recurrent DVT, with no difference in survival.[2] On the other hand, the PREPIC-2 trial showed that placement of retrievable IVC filters in high-risk patients with PE in addition to anticoagulation did not affect outcomes.[3] The most recent standards of practice are based on a multi-society consensus documents which recommend against the routine placement of IVC filters for prophylaxis or relative indications.[4-6] Very selectively, IVC filter placement can be considered in trauma patients, during the perioperative period for patients at high risk for VTE, or for patients undergoing advanced therapies for PE.

PREPROCEDURAL PLANNING The gateway to successful IVC filter deployment is adequate preprocedural planning. A thorough preoperative medical record review with a specific focus on anatomic factors pertinent to filter deployment, such as location of DVT and extent of DVT-sectional imaging could be very helpful to identify the presence of anatomic variants, such as duplicated IVC, mega cava (IVC diameter >30 mm), IVC atresia, or a left-sided IVC. The majority of commercially available IVC filters can be inserted via jugular or femoral access.[7] It is important to confirm that the appropriate kit is utilized for the chosen access site. The right common femoral vein or the right internal jugular vein are preferred for venous access. This is due to the relatively straight alignment of these veins with respect to the long axis of the IVC. In patients with lower extremity DVT, ensure that the common femoral vein selected for access is devoid of thrombus. Consideration of IVC anatomy is pertinent for decisions relating to the type of filter and intended filter position. Retrievable IVC filter placement is contraindicated in patients with IVC diameter >30 mm. The Gianturco-Roehm Bird's Nest filter (Cook Medical, Bloomington, IN) is a permanent filter approved for use in IVC diameter of 30 to 40 mm. In addition, IVC filter placement is contraindicated in the presence of IVC atresia or IVC thrombus. Deployment of IVC filters in a suprarenal configuration through a jugular approach can be considered in these scenarios or in pregnant women with a contraindication to anticoagulation. Preprocedural prophylactic medication for patients with a contrast allergy must be administered. In patients with chronic kidney disease or contrast allergy, carbon dioxide venography can be considered. In addition to preoperative imaging, ultrasound examination of the chosen access vein is recommended to confirm patency and lack of DVT in the procedure room prior to access.

POSITION AND OPERATIVE PREPARATION The patient is placed supine on a radiolucent operating table, with both arms abducted to facilitate tucking. If filter placement is planned through a jugular venous access, a right-sided approach is recommended, and this is facilitated by turning the head toward the left side. Routine skin preparation and sterile draping of the neck access site or bilateral groins is suggested. In most patients, IVC filter placement can be performed with local anesthesia and moderate sedation.

ACCESS AND VENOGRAPHY Ultrasound-guided venous access of the common femoral or internal jugular vein is obtained with a 21-gauge Micropuncture needle, corresponding 0.018″ wire and Micropuncture sheath to avoid iatrogenic injury (FIGURE 71-1, femoral approach). A 6 Fr sheath is then placed in the common femoral vein, following which ascending venography of the iliac veins and IVC is performed through the sheath or via a marker pigtail catheter (FIGURE 71-2). This is done to ensure that the iliac veins and the IVC are free of thrombus, and to assess for any anatomic variation. The level of the drainage of the lowest renal vein is determined and the diameter of the IVC is measured 1 to 2 cm below it. The diameter of the IVC should be less than 28 to 30 mm depending on the type of filter used and its instructions for use (IFU). The size of the IVC changes significantly with hydration status, and measurements of the diameter should be done during the procedure and documented regardless of prior measurements based on other types of imaging.

FILTER DEPLOYMENT The delivery sheaths for commercially available IVC filters range between 7 and 12 Fr, and the delivery sheaths containing the IVC filter have radio-opaque markers to aid the operator with optimal positioning. These delivery sheaths are designed such that the IVC filters are deployed by unsheathing using a "pin-and-pull" technique. Under fluoroscopic guidance, the 6 Fr sheath is exchanged over a 0.035″ wire for the corresponding IVC filter delivery system. Existing radio-opaque markers, bony landmarks (FIGURE 71-3), and a fluoroscopic roadmap can be used to aid the operator with optimal positioning and angle. The IVC filter is then unsheathed by the "pin-and-pull" technique. We typically deploy the IVC filter with the tip just below the lowest renal vein (FIGURE 71-4). It is important to note that after successful deployment of the filter, the delivery catheter must be retracted under fluoroscopic guidance to ensure complete detachment of the filter. A completion venogram, performed through the delivery sheath, is essential to document optimal positioning of the filter in relation to the renal veins.

CLOSURE After satisfactory deployment of the IVC filter, the delivery sheath is removed, and manual pressure is held for 15 minutes to facilitate hemostasis at the access site.

POSTOPERATIVE CARE For deployment through a femoral access, post-procedural bedrest is recommended, where the patient remains supine and flat for at least 3 hours. For filter deployment through a jugular access, post-procedural bedrest for 3 hours is recommended. During this time, the patient should be monitored for bleeding or hematoma formation.

INFERIOR VENA CAVA FILTER RETRIEVAL

INDICATIONS Since the introduction of retrievable IVC filters in 2003, these devices have gained popularity resulting in increased utilization. However, due to rise in filter-related complications, the Food and Drug Administration (FDA) alerted physicians in 2010 to consider IVC filter retrieval when protection from PE is no longer warranted. Based on a decision-analysis model, an ideal IVC filter retrieval window was determined to be between 29 and 54 days after placement.[8] The current standard of practice is to consider IVC filter retrieval once patients can safely resume anticoagulation or the risk for PE decreases. Several studies have demonstrated that increased dwell times result in a higher rate of failure to retrieve and are associated with a higher rate of procedural complications.[9-11] Based on this, it is important to note that the ideal timing for IVC filter retrieval and the decision to retrieve an IVC filter is multifactorial and should be individualized, guided by a risk-benefit profile that incorporates filter dwell time, patient symptoms, and the risk of bleeding or recurrent VTE.

PREPROCEDURAL PLANNING A thorough medical evaluation of the patient, including coagulation profiles, renal function, ambulatory status, and hypercoagulability workup, is required prior to consideration of IVC filter retrieval. Often a multidisciplinary risk-benefit assessment is warranted in patients with VTE and risk factors for recurrent bleeding. The most recent standards of practice do not recommend any routine cross-sectional imaging prior to removal unless clinically indicated. When IVC filters have a dwell time greater than 1 year, we obtain contrast-enhanced cross-sectional imaging in the form of a computed tomography (CT) scan of the abdomen and pelvis to assess for tilt, position of the apex or hook of the filter, extent of strut penetration, and importantly, the presence of thrombus. The presence of thrombus in the IVC filter warrants deferral of retrieval to a later date, after thrombus resolution within the filter and the IVC. Based on the CT scan, the hook of the filter may not be accessible by standard retrieval techniques and that would be crucial in planning the approach and the type of advanced endovascular techniques warranted. Anticoagulants should be held for a brief period prior to filter retrieval, especially if the retrieval procedure is expected to be challenging and advanced endovascular techniques are anticipated. Like IVC filter placement, prophylactic premedication for patients with a contrast allergy must be appropriately administered, and selective use of carbon dioxide angiography in patients with chronic kidney disease can decrease the use of nephrotoxic contrast. **CONTINUES ▶**

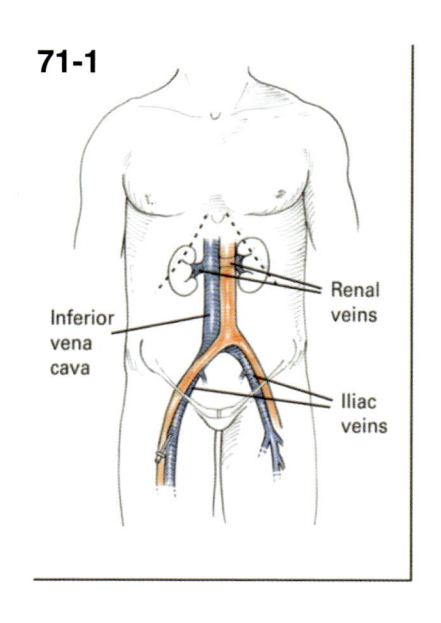

71-1

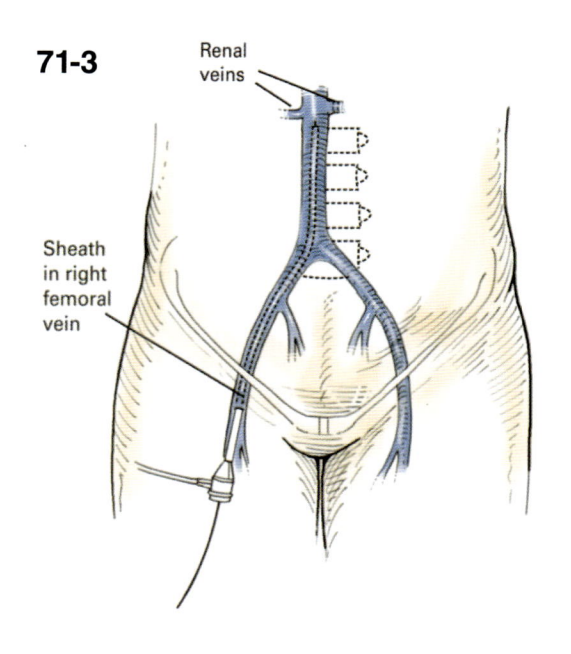

71-3

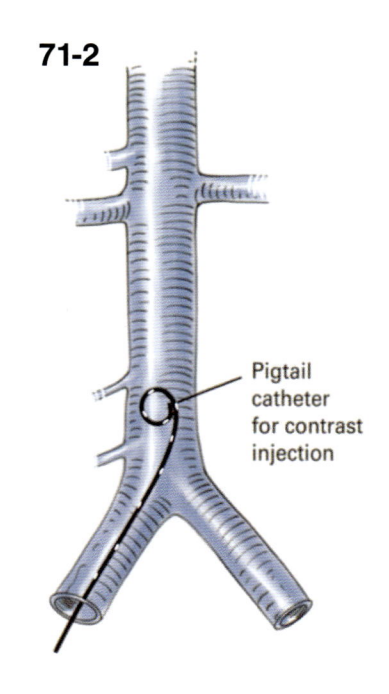

71-2

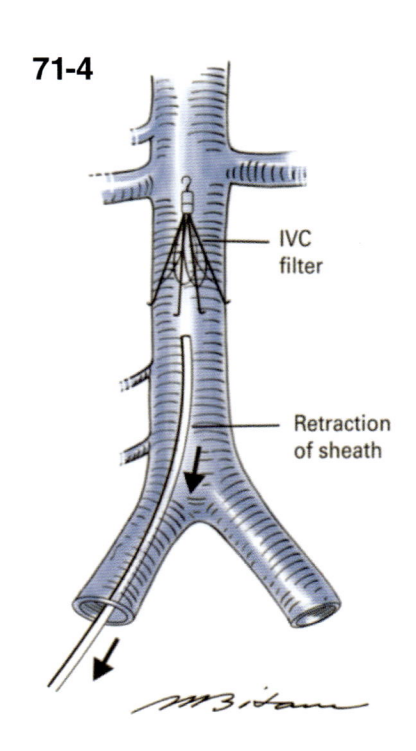

71-4

POSITION AND OPERATIVE PREPARATION Since the majority of the IVC filter retrievals are performed through a jugular venous access, the patient is placed supine on a radiolucent operating table with both arms abducted and tucked, followed by routine skin preparation of the neck. For IVC filters with prolonged dwell times, bilateral groins should be prepped and sterilely draped. A second femoral access is sometimes used for challenging IVC filter retrievals. While IVC filter retrieval can be safely performed in most patients with local anesthesia and moderate sedation, use of general anesthesia is preferred for patients with prolonged filter dwell times or increased filter tilt.

ACCESS AND VENOGRAPHY Ultrasound-guided venous access of the right internal jugular vein is obtained using a 21-gauge micropuncture needle, the corresponding 0.018″ wire and Micropuncture sheath to avoid iatrogenic injury. A 6 Fr sheath is then introduced into the jugular vein, following which a soft angled 0.035″ Glidewire (Terumo, Somerset, NJ) is navigated into the IVC under fluoroscopic visualization. Next, a Glide catheter (Terumo, Somerset, NJ) is introduced over the wire and a venogram of the IVC is performed to ensure the absence of thrombus within the filter or the IVC.

TECHNIQUES OF IVC FILTER RETRIEVAL

STANDARD RETRIEVAL: The decision to retrieve the filter is made after initial venography is performed. The gateway to successful IVC filter retrieval involves two key components. The first step involves securing the filter and aligning its long axis with the retrieval system. The second step involves collapsing the filter into the retrieval system and freeing the struts from the IVC wall. Standard IVC filter retrieval is performed by capturing the filter hook with a snare (FIGURE 71-5A), followed by collapsing the entire filter in toto into the retrieval sheath (FIGURE 71-5B). Currently, there are various kits commercially available for IVC filter retrieval, such as the Günther-Tulip retrieval set (Cook Medical, Bloomington, IN), the Recovery Cone system (Bard Peripheral Vascular, Tempe, AZ), or the ALN Optional filter extraction kit (ALN Implants, Chirurgicaux, France). IVC filter retrieval with these commercially available kits involves capture of the filter hook with a single-loop snare (Günther-Tulip retrieval set) or a cone (Recovery Cone system). In addition to an access needle and guidewire, the Günther-Tulip retrieval set comprises a 11 Fr 60-cm sheath and a 6.3 Fr snare. The Recovery Cone system consists of a 10 Fr 75-cm sheath, Y-adapter and the recovery cone. After jugular venous access is obtained as detailed previously, the 6 Fr sheath is exchanged over an Amplatz wire (Boston Scientific, Boston, MA) for a 10 or 11 Fr sheath under fluoroscopic visualization, based on the preferred commercially available kit. It is imperative that the introduction of the larger sheath through the heart is done over a stiff wire with continuous fluoroscopic visualization to avoid any iatrogenic injuries, which can be devastating. The sheath is then positioned in the suprarenal IVC and the snare or recovery cone are opened above the IVC filter. The hook of the filter is then engaged by the retrieval snare or recovery cone system. Once satisfactory hook-capture is achieved, the entire filter is retrieved in toto by advancing the introducer sheath until the recovery cone or retrieval snare and the entire filter are within the sheath. Completion venography can then be performed through the introducer sheath to assess for extravasation or thrombus formation. **CONTINUES▶**

71-5

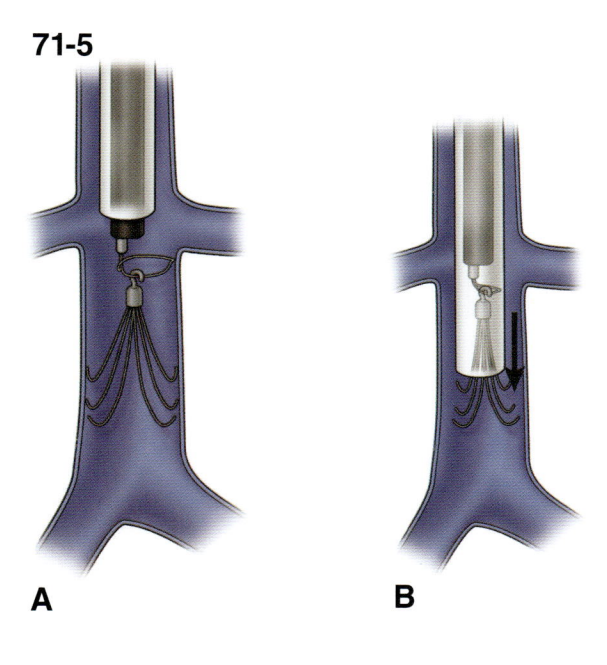

A   B

TECHNIQUES OF IVC FILTER RETRIEVAL *ADVANCED RETRIEVAL:*

CONTINUED Certain anatomic factors such as filter tilt, hook apposition to the IVC wall, scarring and fibrosis around the filter hook or struts, or a prolonged dwell time can make filter retrieval challenging. In these scenarios, advanced retrieval techniques are usually required for successful IVC filter retrieval. Numerous techniques have been described, but we preferentially use the wire-loop retrieval technique.[12,13] A 16 Fr stiff sheath at least 40 cm in length (Cook Medical, Bloomington, IN) is positioned in the suprarenal IVC and offers a rigid support system for disengaging the filter hook or struts. An Omni flush catheter (AngioDynamics, Latham, NY) is then introduced beyond the filter and formed such that the apex of the filter is hooked by this catheter. A soft 0.035″ Glidewire (Terumo, Somerset, NJ) is then introduced through the Omni flush catheter into the suprarenal IVC, which is then snared with the EN Snare device (Merit Medical, South Jordan, UT), introduced through the 16 Fr sheath in a "buddy-catheter" fashion. (**FIGURE 71-6A**). This wire-loop is then recaptured into the 16 Fr sheath and exteriorized. The 16 Fr sheath is then advanced over this wire-loop, under fluoroscopic visualization, to engage the filter hook and collapse the filter struts (**FIGURE 71-6B**). We administer low-dose systematic heparin (3000–5000 units) to prevent thrombus formation in or around the sheath, as those cases can sometimes have a longer duration than expected. Engaging the hook of the filter sometimes requires multiple attempts with repositioning of the direction of the sheath compared to the long axis of the filter and the wire loop. That repositioning can be achieved by gently changing the direction of the sheath at the level of the neck outside the body, and that would shift the angle of the tip of the sheath in the IVC for a few degrees which is usually sufficient to align the tip of the sheath with the hook of the IVC filter. Multiple fluoroscopic projections and the use of radiographic magnification is often necessary to confirm hook engagement by the sheath as demonstrated in the technical video.[14] It is important to note that continued traction on the wire-loop in combination with forward tension and a gentle rotational torque on the 16 Fr sheath is often required to separate the struts from the wall of the IVC and collapse the filter. Moreover, in cases with hook or strut fibrosis, a significant amount of force is often applied by the operator on this entire system. After successful filter retrieval, a completion venogram is performed through the sheath to rule out extravasation or thrombus formation in the IVC. Of note, it is important to routinely flush the introducer sheath every 15 minutes to prevent thrombus formation within the sheath.

CLOSURE

After successful retrieval of the IVC filter and completion venography, the sheath is removed. Access site hemostasis is achieved with manual pressure for at least 30 minutes, given the large caliber of the sheath. A figure-of-eight or horizontal mattress stitch using nonabsorbable 2-0 or 3-0 sutures can be used as a supplement to manual pressure.

POSTOPERATIVE CARE

Similar to IVC filter placement, post-procedural bed rest is recommended for a period of 3 to 4 hours after filter retrieval. During this time, the patient should be monitored for bleeding or an access site hematoma. Patients can most often be discharged home on the same day, and anticoagulant agents can be resumed after 24 hours from IVC filter retrieval. ■

REFERENCES

1. Decousus H, Leizorovicz A, Parent F, et al. A clinical trial of vena caval filters in the prevention of pulmonary embolism in patients with proximal deep-vein thrombosis. Prevention du Risque d'Embolie Pulmonaire par Interruption Cave Study Group. *N Engl J Med.* 1998;338:409-415.
2. Group PS. Eight-year follow-up of patients with permanent vena cava filters in the prevention of pulmonary embolism: the PREPIC (Prevention du Risque d'Embolie Pulmonaire par Interruption Cave) randomized study. *Circulation.* 2005;112:416-422.
3. Mismetti P, Laporte S, Pellerin O, et al; Group PS. Effect of a retrievable inferior vena cava filter plus anticoagulation vs anticoagulation alone on risk of recurrent pulmonary embolism: a randomized clinical trial. *JAMA.* 2015;313:1627-1635.
4. Kaufman JA, Barnes GD, Chaer RA, et al. Society of Interventional Radiology Clinical Practice Guideline for Inferior Vena Cava Filters in the treatment of patients with venous thromboembolic disease. Developed in collaboration with the American College of Cardiology, American College of Chest Physicians, American College of Surgeons Committee on Trauma, American Heart Association, Society for Vascular Surgery, and Society for Vascular Medicine. *J Vasc Interv Radiol.* 2020;31:1529-1544.
5. Kearon C, Akl EA, Ornelas J, et al. Antithrombotic therapy for VTE disease: CHEST Guideline and Expert Panel Report. *Chest.* 2016;149:315-352.
6. Jaff MR, McMurtry MS, Archer SL; American Heart Association Council on Cardiopulmonary CCP, Resuscitation, American Heart Association Council on Peripheral Vascular D, American Heart Association Council on Arteriosclerosis T and Vascular B, et al. Management of massive and submassive pulmonary embolism, iliofemoral deep vein thrombosis, and chronic thromboembolic pulmonary hypertension: a scientific statement from the American Heart Association. *Circulation.* 2011;123:1788-1830.
7. Rectenwald JE. Vena cava interruption. In: Chaar, CIO, ed. *Current Management of Venous Diseases.* Cham: Springer International; 2018:419-432.
8. Morales JP, Li X, Irony TZ, Ibrahim NG, Moynahan M, Cavanaugh KJ Jr. Decision analysis of retrievable inferior vena cava filters in patients without pulmonary embolism. *J Vasc Surg Venous Lymphat Disord.* 2013;1:376-384.
9. Avgerinos ED, Bath J, Stevens J, et al. Technical and patient-related characteristics associated with challenging retrieval of inferior vena cava filters. *Eur J Vasc Endovasc Surg.* 2013;46:353-359.
10. Al-Hakim R, Kee ST, Olinger K, Lee EW, Moriarty JM, McWilliams JP. Inferior vena cava filter retrieval: effectiveness and complications of routine and advanced techniques. *J Vasc Interv Radiol.* 2014;25:933-939; quiz 940.
11. Brahmandam A, Skrip L, Mojibian H, et al. Costs and complications of endovascular inferior vena cava filter retrieval. *J Vasc Surg Venous Lymphat Disord.* 2019;7:653-659 e1.
12. Brahmandam A, Aurshina A, Ochoa Chaar CI. Retrieval of inferior vena cava filters. In: Chaar CIO, ed. *Current Management of Venous Diseases.* Cham: Springer International; 2018: 433-450.
13. Iliescu B, Haskal ZJ. Advanced techniques for removal of retrievable inferior vena cava filters. *Cardiovasc Intervent Radiol.* 2012;35:741-750.
14. Ochoa Chaar CI, Kostiuk V, Gholitabar N. The wire loop technique for IVC filter removal. *J Vasc Surg Cases Innov Tech.* 2021;7(3):369-370. Published 2021 May 20. doi:10.1016/j.jvscit.2021.04.017.

71-6

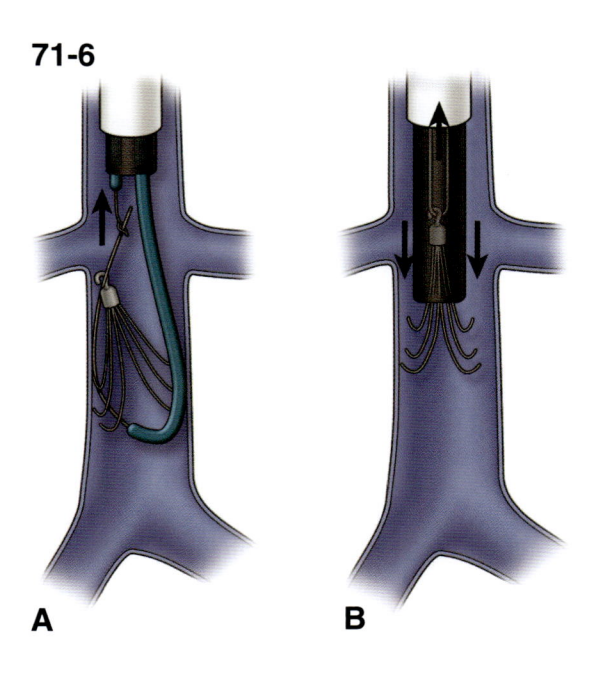

A   **B**

INFERIOR VENA CAVA FILTER REMOVAL: OPEN

Steven Abramowitz, MD • Edward Woo, MD

INDICATIONS Standard and advanced endovascular techniques are highly successful at removing long-dwelling filters regardless of filter design. However, not all filters can be successfully removed by endovascular means. Inferior vena cava (IVC) filters with significant tilt due to either technical error at the time of placement or subsequent migration can see either apical ingrowth into the caval wall or perforation through the cava itself, thus rendering endovascular retrieval dangerous or technically challenging. Failed endovascular retrieval can also cause structural or conformational change to the filter, precluding future endovascular retrieval attempts. Furthermore, the design of some irretrievable IVC filters may lead to extensive caval wall adhesion or caval erosion contraindicating endovascular removal.

Retained IVC filters can lead to a myriad of potential complications for patients. The most common complication, IVC thrombosis, can be of greater concern in the setting of a malpositioned filter. Even in filters that are appropriately located within the cava, tine penetration of the IVC is often seen on cross-sectional imaging. While tine perforation is often asymptomatic, pericaval tines can be problematic and associated with infection, visceral injury, aortic perforation, ureteral erosion, hemorrhage, and vertebral penetration. Structurally compromised filters can lead to distal embolization resulting in myocardial perforation, pulmonary artery puncture, pulmonary hemorrhage, and pulmonary artery thrombosis. Patients with symptomatic IVC filter–related complications, high-risk pericaval structure involvement, significant loss of filter integrity, or at significant risk for IVC thrombosis due to a retained filter can benefit from open surgical filter removal when endovascular techniques have failed or are contraindicated.

PREOPERATIVE PREPARATION In preparation for open IVC filter retrieval, cross-sectional imaging plays a key role in preoperative planning. Identification of the filter type, anatomic location, structural integrity, and pericaval involvement of the IVC filter being removed will dictate the safest operative approach for open retrieval. Both computed tomographic (CT) scanning and magnetic resonance imaging (MRI) can be used to assess the type of filter, the anatomic location of the filter, and any filter-associated IVC thrombus. However, preoperative CT scanning may be superior in identifying pericaval structural involvement due to tine penetration into the surrounding structures. Endoscopy or colonoscopy is typically not required even if viscus involvement is suspected. Inferior vena cavography can also be helpful in perioperative planning.

The type of IVC filter being retrieved and associated complications necessitating open retrieval determine both operative exposure and retrieval technique. In patients without viscus involvement, visualization of intraperitoneal structures may not be necessary, and a retroperitoneal approach may be employed. A midline or chevron incision also affords adequate exposure. When the duodenum or pancreas is involved, general surgery assistance is requested. If the filter extends beyond the renocaval confluence, a transabdominal approach is preferred. For patients with retrievable IVC filters or non-retrievable IVC filters where significant tilt, wall adherence, or apex penetration through the cava wall precludes standard, loop-snare, or endobronchial retrieval by endovascular means, endovenectomy may not be required for filter removal. Filters with significant fracture, extensive wall apposition, or caval erosion/damage will require venotomy and possible cava repair with a patch angioplasty or even interposition graft. A review of prior endovascular retrieval attempts in conjunction with cross-sectional imaging will clarify the need for either a retroperitoneal or transabdominal approach with or without venotomy and caval reconstruction.

POSITION AND OPERATIVE PREPARATION General anesthesia is recommended, as complete paralysis is required. Routine placement of large-bore or central venous access as well as an arterial line are recommended due to the potential for blood loss. The use of intraoperative blood salvage is advised when caval reconstruction is being performed unless there is concern for extensive viscus injury leading to bacterial contamination. For transabdominal approach, the patient should be placed standardly supine on the operating room table with arms outstretched, prepped widely. If a retroperitoneal approach is being employed, a bump should be placed under the right flank to elevate the patient.

INCISION AND EXPOSURE

RETROPERITONEAL APPROACH: A transverse incision should be made two fingerbreadths above the umbilicus extending from the lateral margin of the right rectus to the palpated bony prominence of the eleventh rib (**FIGURE 72-1**). The external oblique aponeurosis and underlying muscle fibers are divided, and dissection between the fibers of the underlying internal oblique is performed while flaps of the muscle body may be raised to allow for retraction. The transversus abdominus muscle and transversalis fascia are then opened laterally to expose the interface between the fascia and the peritoneum. The peritoneum is then mobilized posteromedial, creating a plane to reveal first the psoas muscle and then the IVC. Care is taken to identify the ureter and preserve its attachment to the peritoneum for safe retraction.

TRANSABDOMINAL APPROACH: A vertical midline incision is made, and the peritoneum is entered in the standard fashion. Care should be taken to explore the abdominal cavity when viscus involvement is suspected. Upon encountering any penetrating filter tines, the tines should be cut with wire cutters as flush to the cava as exposure will allow. The lateral attachments of the ascending colon are dissected free, and medial reflection of the colon and mesentery is performed. Duodenal mobilization with medial reflection by sharp dissection of the second and third portions of the duodenum will reveal the underlying vena cava (**FIGURE 72-2**).

When filter tine perforation has caused a significant enterotomy, primary repair of the bowel with seromuscular sutures should be performed. It is acceptable to use wire cutters to separate the filter from the duodenum and/or pancreas if minimal involvement, leaving healed-in small tines in place, as this is no different than metal staples for a bowel anastomosis. One routinely should plan on being able to control the IVC superior to the renal veins even if an IVC clamp is used. If suprarenal cava control is required, dissection of bilateral renal cava confluence is performed.

DETAILS OF PROCEDURE With either a retroperitoneal or transperitoneal exposure, once the IVC is visualized, the location of the IVC filter is determined (**FIGURE 72-3**). The anterior and lateral surface of the IVC required for filter removal and vascular control is cleared of areolar tissue. If the struts penetrate the aorta, proximal and distal control should also be obtained. Care is taken to avoid any personal injury from protruding tines. Silastic vessel loops or vascular tape is then used to circumferentially control the vena cava proximal and distal to the identified IVC filter. Avoid avulsion of any posterior lumbar veins. Visualized lumbar veins may be controlled or clipped to limit back-bleeding during cava venotomy, or oversewn from the inside. **CONTINUES** ▶

72-1

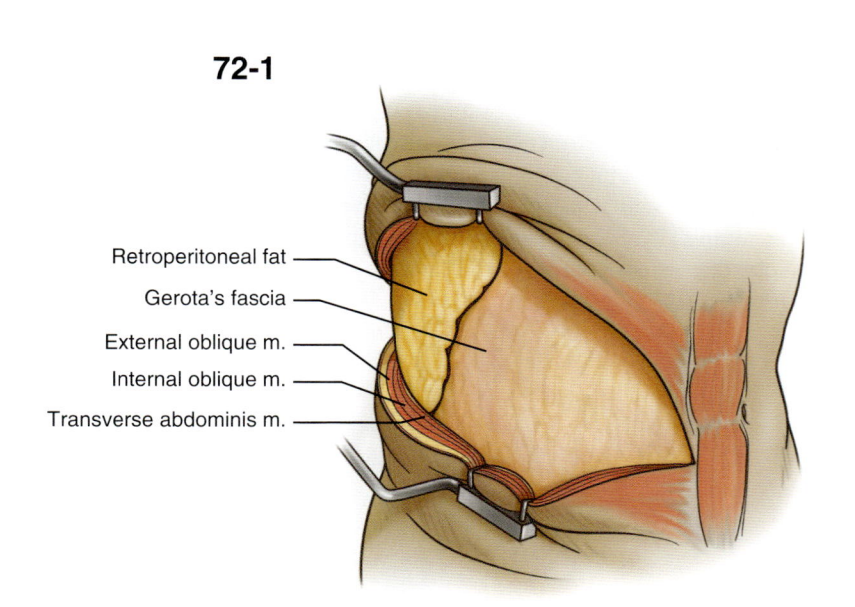

Retroperitoneal fat
Gerota's fascia
External oblique m.
Internal oblique m.
Transverse abdominis m.

72-2

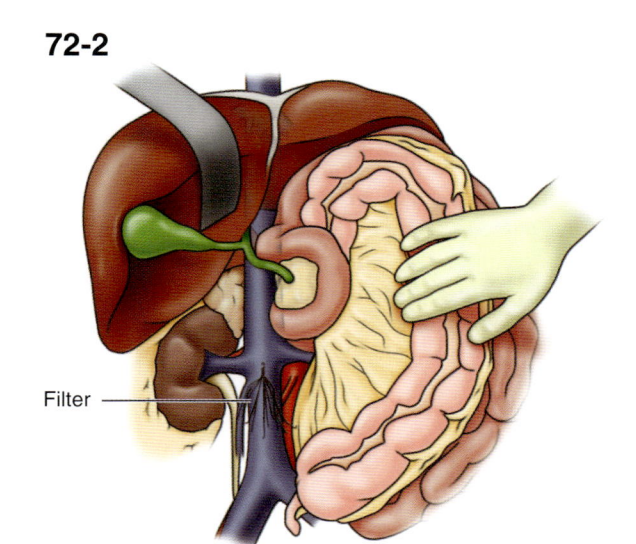

Filter

72-3

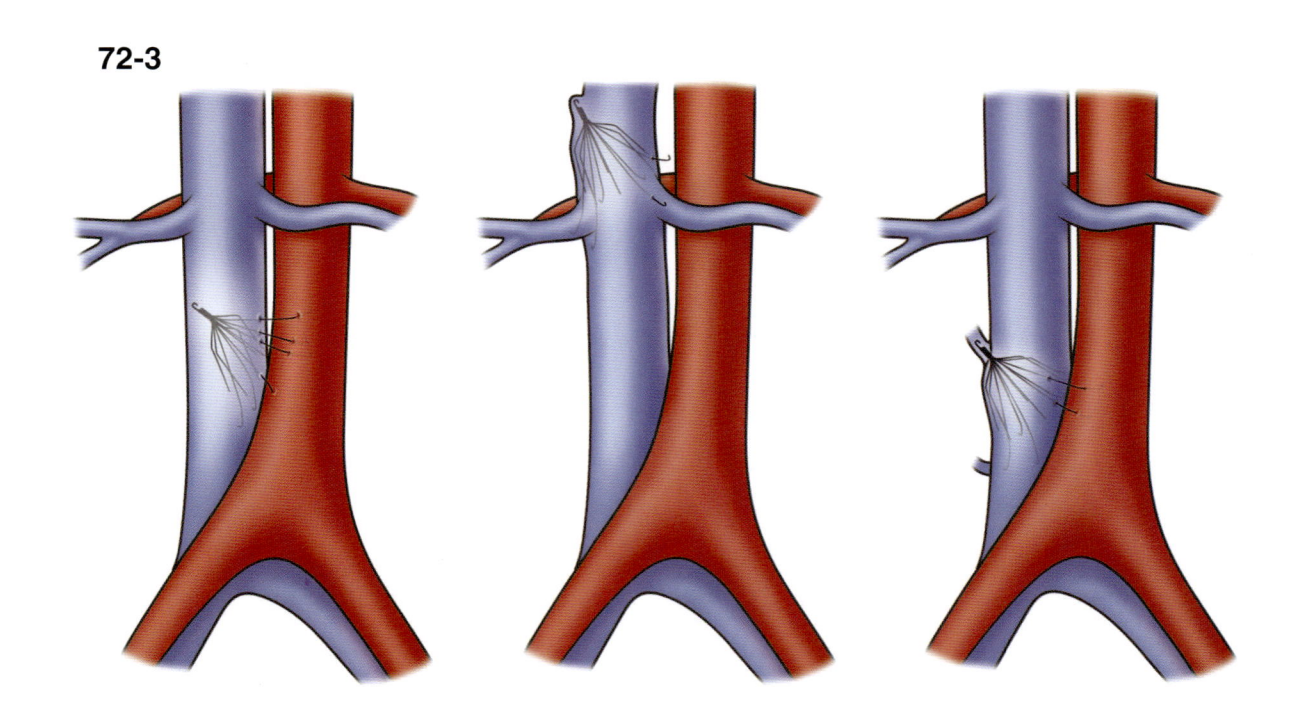

DETAILS OF PROCEDURE *VENOTOMY-SPARING TECHNIQUE*: **CONTINUED** A venotomy-sparing technique may be used to remove an unfractured IVC filter. This technique is best employed in cases where excessive tilt has caused the apex of conical filters to embed into or protrude through the lateral or anterior caval wall. The patient is heparinized, and vascular clamps are placed after careful dissection of the IVC proximal and distal to the filter location. Protruding tines are cut to allow for easier removal of the IVC filter. Two options exist: the first is to clamp the IVC above and below the filter. The apex of the filter is then identified exterior to the vena cava wall or palpated at its point of wall adherence. A prolene suture is then used to perform a purse-string suture surrounding the filter apex. An incision is then made over or around the apex.

The filter apex or hook is then grabbed with a hemostat, the filter pulled out, and then the purse string is tied down (**FIGURE 72-4A**). A second similar technique uses a sheath to recapture the filter. Herein, once the apex is visualized, after the venotomy a suture or .014″ nitinol wire is passed behind the apex of the IVC filter. If a retrieval hook is present in the filter design, the suture or wire may be passed under the hook. The looped material is then passed through a 14 to 16F short sheath. The sheath is then advanced to recapture the filter in a manner similar to that of a standard endovascular snare technique, and the sheathed filter is then withdrawn. The purse-string suture is then tied, while the sheath is removed

(**FIGURE 72-4B**). Any remaining IVC defects are oversewn using prolene suture. Flow is restored to the IVC, heparin reversed with protamine sulfate, and hemostasis is obtained.

RETRIEVAL WITH VENOTOMY AND CAVAL REPAIR: In situations where there is significant caval erosion, the filter apex lies posteriorly, or the IVC filter design precludes resheathing the filter in the method described above, a venotomy can be performed to remove the IVC filter. In this instance, the patient is again anticoagulated, and clamps are placed on the vena cava proximal and distal to the location of the IVC filter. The renal veins can be clamped as needed. A longitudinal venotomy is then performed directly overlying the filter after visualized protruding tines are cut flush with the cava wall (**FIGURE 72-5A**). A large side-biting Satinsky or Lambert K clamp may be needed to control posterior lumbar vein bleeding if there is significant venous bleeding that cannot be controlled. The IVC filter is then manually extracted under direct visualization. Endovenectomy of synechiae or webbing is required in addition to removing filter remnants to restore intraluminal patency. Once the filter is removed, assessment of the remaining IVC is performed, and any denuded segments are resected. Denuded or perforated areas of the cava are repaired primarily with pledgeted suture. **CONTINUES**

72-4

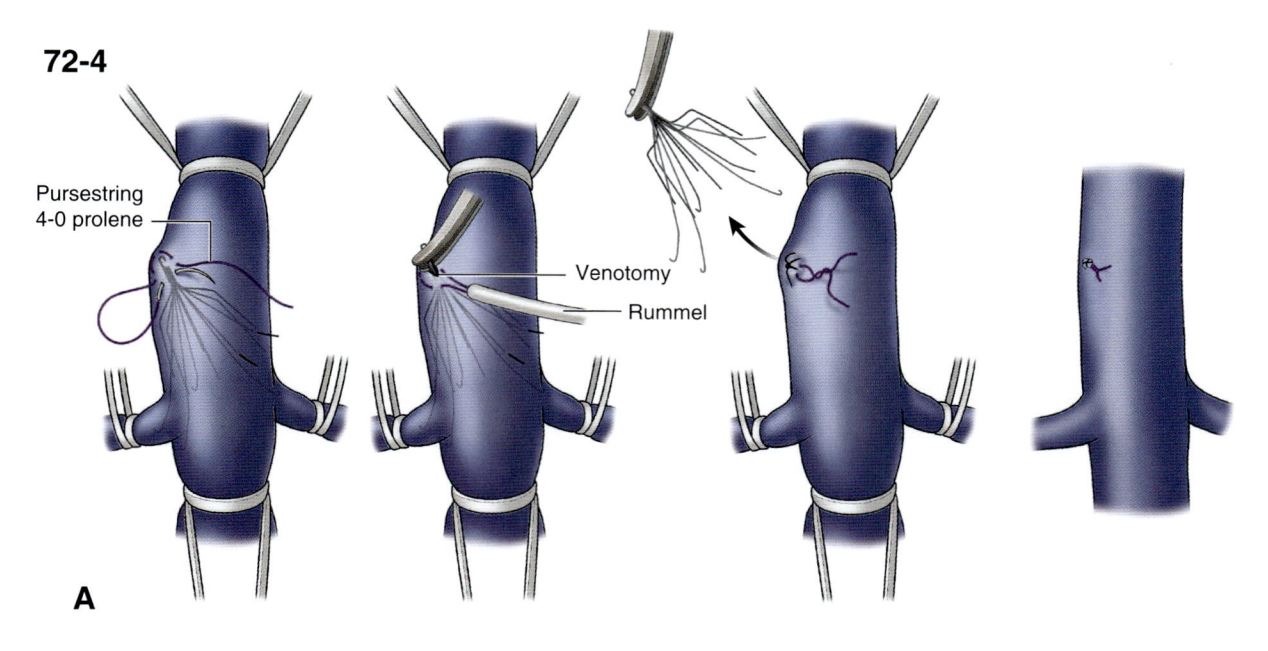

Pursestring
4-0 prolene

Venotomy

Rummel

A

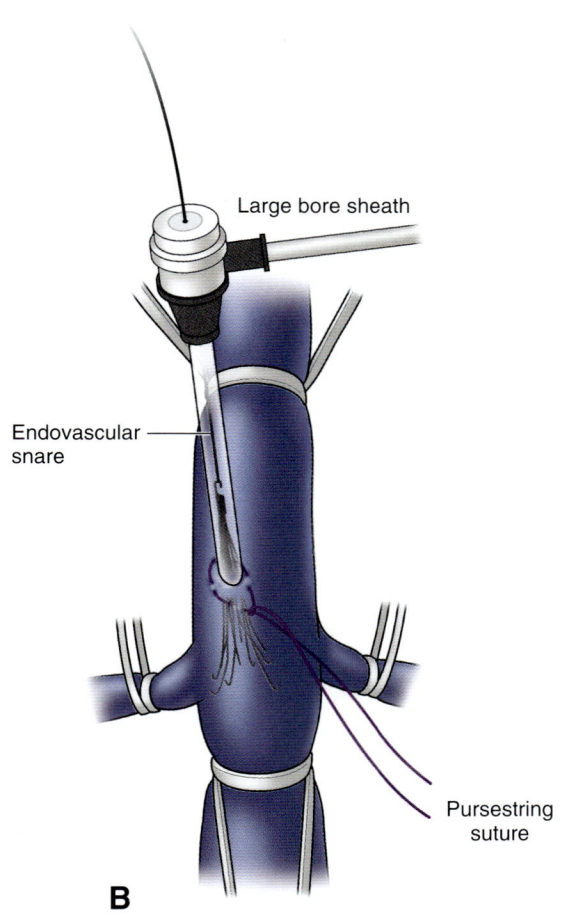

Large bore sheath

Endovascular
snare

Pursestring
suture

B

DETAILS OF PROCEDURE *RETRIEVAL WITH VENOTOMY AND CAVAL REPAIR*: ◀**CONTINUED**▶ Primary repair of the venotomy can be safely performed if there is no luminal compromise. Frequently there is concern for luminal narrowing due to cava wall resection, and in that scenario a large bovine pericardial patch or prosthetic patch can be used to prevent cava stenosis (**FIGURE 72-5B**). In very rare circumstances, the IVC may be circumferentially involved or damaged beyond operative repair. In this instance, the lumbar veins are oversewn from within the venotomy site, and a short interposition bypass with ringed ePTFE can then be performed upon resection of the involved cava segment (see Chapter 76). Upon completion of whichever repair is performed, flow is restored, heparin reversed, and hemostasis is then obtained.

CLOSURE   A Valsalva maneuver may be used to assess hemostasis. Retractors should be removed and the peritoneum allowed to fall back into place. A drain is not required. The surgical field should be copiously irrigated, given the likelihood for viscus involvement and enterotomy repair. The bowel should be inspected for any missed enterotomies and then returned to its normal anatomic location. Retroperitoneal or abdominal closures are done in the standard fashion.

POSTOPERATIVE CARE   In addition to standard postoperative care for those patients undergoing retroperitoneal or transabominal surgery, care must be taken to ensure adequate venous thromboembolic event prophylaxis in this patient population. Many patients undergoing open IVC filter retrieval are on long-term anticoagulation for underlying hypercoagulable disorders or recurrent venous thromboembolic events. Endothelial injury as a result of venotomy or venotomy-sparing filter removal in conjunction with limited mobility after open surgical intervention predisposes this patient population to an elevated risk of caval thrombosis, iliofemoral deep vein thrombosis (DVT), and pulmonary embolism (PE). Early resumption of anticoagulation is recommended, and periprocedural anticoagulation in those patients not previously on anticoagulation therapy is preferred. Pneumatic compression is also recommended for all patients to mimic the calf-pump muscle and improve venous return.

A high degree of suspicion should be maintained for DVT and PE in these patients post-procedurally. Operators should have a low threshold to work up a PE by CT scan. The same is true for obtaining a duplex to work up potential DVT. If either a PE or a DVT is confirmed, indirect CT venography of the abdomen and pelvis should be performed to assess the IVC. Should the patient experience new bilateral lower extremity edema, indirect CT venography of the IVC is recommended regardless of the presence of DVT on duplex. ■

SUGGESTED READINGS

Charlton-Ouw K, Afag S, Leake S, et al. Indications and outcomes of open inferior vena cava filter removal. *Ann Vasc Surg.* 2018;46(2):205c-205e.

Connolly P, Balachandran V, Trost D, Bush D. Open Surgical inferior vena cava filter retrieval for cava perforation and a novel technique for minimal cavotomy filter extraction. *J Vasc Surg.* 2012;56:256-259.

Go, M, Keller-Biehl, L, Starr, J. penetration of the inferior vena cava and adjacent organs after filter placement is associated with retrievable filter type and length of time in place. *J Vasc Surg Venous Lymphat Disord.* 2014 Apr;2(2):174-178.

Lee J, So Y, Choi Y, Park S, Heo E, Kim D. Clinical course and predictive factors for complication of inferior vena cava filters. *Thomb Res.* 2014;133:538-543.

Malek J, Kwolek C, Conrad M. Presentation and treatment outcomes of patients with symptomatic inferior vena cava filters. *Ann Vasc Surg.* 2013;27:84-88.

Manzur M, Ochoa C, Ham S, et al. Surgical management of perforated inferior vena cava filters. *Ann Vasc Surg.* 2017 Jul;42:25-31.

Rana M, Gloviczki P, Kalra M, Bjarmason H, Huang Y, Fleming MJ. Open surgical removal of retained and dislodge inferior vena cava filters. *Vasc Surg.* 2015;3(2):201-206.

72-5

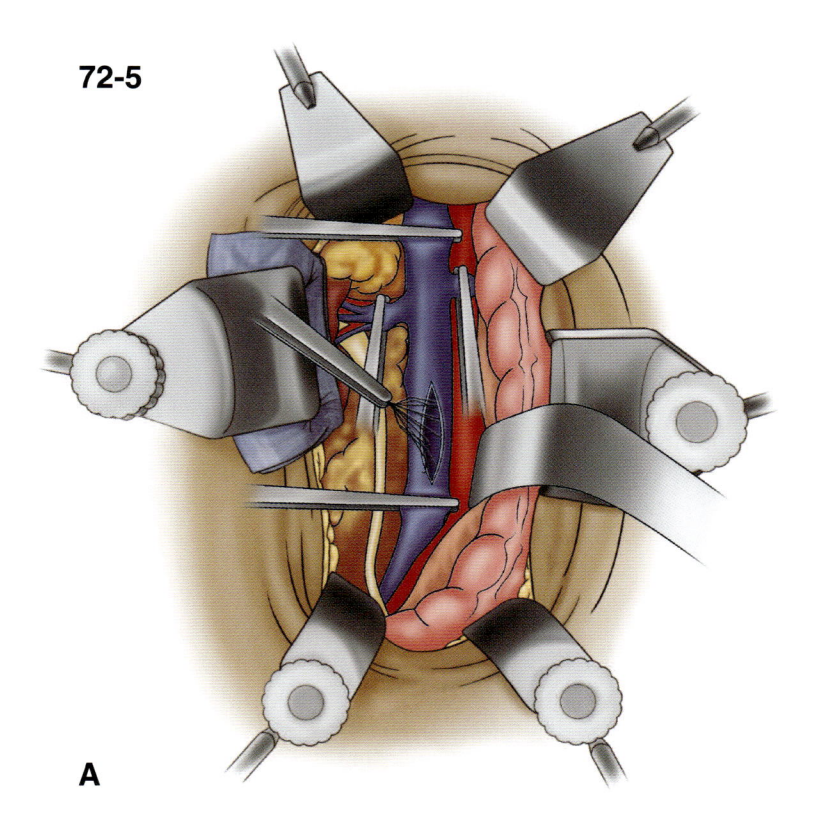

A

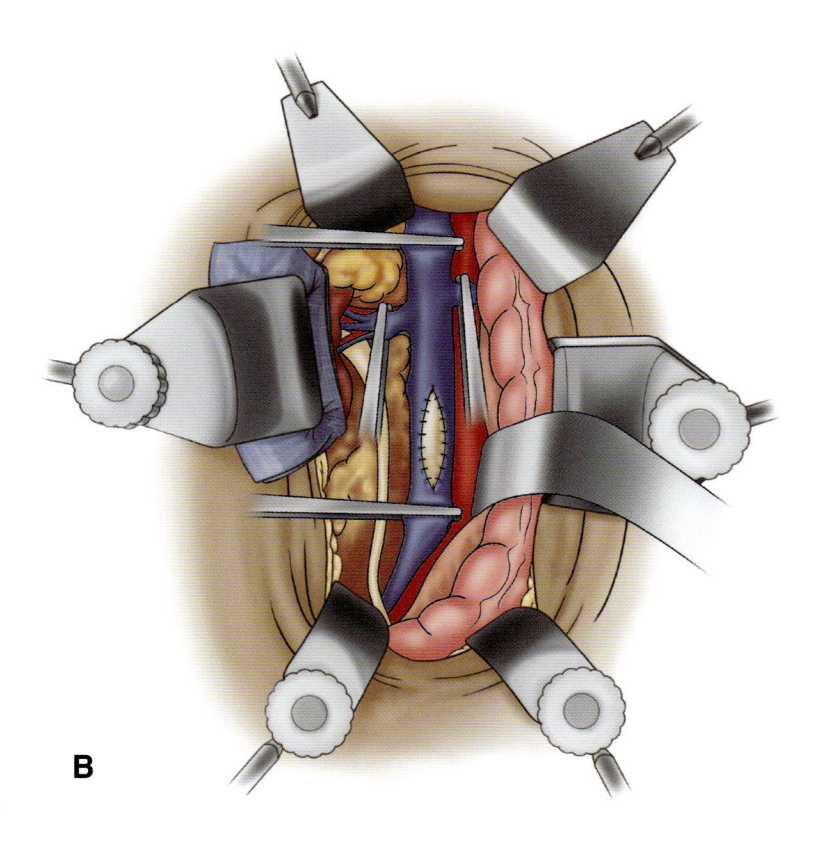

B

CHAPTER 73

MICROPHLEBECTOMY

Sherry D. Scovell, MD

INDICATIONS The main indications for microphlebectomy are visible and palpable varicose veins of the lower extremity with or without associated venous-related symptoms, such as heaviness, aching, and fatigue. In symptomatic patients, visible varicose veins are often associated with underlying superficial venous hypertension, such as an incompetent great saphenous vein, small saphenous vein, or anterior accessory of the great saphenous vein. If superficial venous insufficiency is diagnosed, it must be treated prior to or concomitant with the removal of the associated tributary varicose veins or the patient will likely experience continued symptoms and may develop recurrent varicose veins. It is prudent to obtain a venous insufficiency ultrasound to evaluate the deep and superficial venous systems for evidence of insufficiency. If there is no evidence of superficial venous insufficiency, microphlebectomy is performed as a stand-alone procedure.

PREOPERATIVE PREPARATION Prior to performing microphlebectomy, a complete history with documentation of previous vein procedures and personal and family history of venous insufficiency, deep and superficial vein thrombosis, and hypercoagulable state should be noted. The Caprini score may be used as a risk assessment tool for venous thromboembolism in high-risk patients.

On the day of the procedure, high-quality photographs documenting the location and extent of the varicose veins should be taken. When the patient is in a standing position, varicose veins are engorged secondary to venous hypertension. However, during the procedure venous pressure will decrease, as the patient will be in Trendelenburg position. As a result, the varicosities will be challenging to visualize, and it is imperative that they be mapped with the patient in a standing position prior to the procedure. The veins may be mapped via visual inspection and/or palpation. For increased clarity of vein mapping or when removing smaller diameter veins, transillumination is a useful adjunct. Surgical marking pens should be employed for mapping. There are multiple methods of marking that may be used to indicate the exact location of the varices to be removed. It is our preference to trace the outline of the vein and place a dot over the area where the vein is most prominent. Permanent markers should be avoided as they can lead to inadvertent tattooing of the skin. Once the patient is placed in supine position, it may be helpful to recheck the exact location of the varicose veins with transillumination in patients with redundant or lax skin, as the vein location may shift with changes in patient position.

When marking the veins, it is important to note and discuss with the patient the proximity of nerves to the varicose veins and the theoretic risk of injury to these nerves. Tributary varicose veins in the distribution of the great saphenous along the medial aspect of the mid to distal calf may be in close proximity to the saphenous nerve. The saphenous nerve is prone to injury during microphlebectomy of a superficial segment of distal calf great saphenous vein or tributary varicose veins in this region. Small saphenous vein tributary varicosities may be in close proximity to the sural nerve in the lower posterior calf below the inferior border of the gastrocnemius muscle. Care should be taken when performing microphlebectomy on varicose veins overlying the Achilles tendon for this reason.

Of utmost importance, the common peroneal nerve originates as a branch of the sciatic nerve just cephalad to the popliteal fossa. It then courses laterally in the popliteal fossa and deep to the biceps femoris muscle and its tendon until it becomes extremely superficial over the lateral head and neck of the fibula, where is it prone to injury during microphlebectomy. Microphlebectomy incisions in the region of the lateral head and neck of the fibula should be avoided due to potential injury of the common peroneal nerve or one of its branches. Lateral superficial varicosities, which cross over the head and neck of the fibula, may be removed by making incisions several centimeters cephalad to and several centimeters caudal to this area. The residual varix, which lies over the head and neck of the fibula, should decompress.

ANESTHESIA Although there are some centers in which microphlebectomy is still performed in the operating room, this procedure is most often performed in an office or ambulatory setting with the use of tumescent anesthesia, which is a dilute local anesthetic solution comprised of lidocaine with epinephrine and the addition of sodium bicarbonate. Originally described for liposuction procedures by Klein in 1987, it was modified for use in venous procedures by Cohn and colleagues in 1995. A typical mixture includes 500 mL of a 0.9% sodium chloride solution, 30 mL of 1% lidocaine with 1:100,000 epinephrine, and 5 mL of 8.4% sodium bicarbonate, although the concentrations may vary slightly by physician preference. It is instilled into the perivascular space either manually via a syringe or, more commonly, through the use of a peristaltic roller pump for more efficient delivery. Hydrodissection of the veins from the surrounding subcutaneous tissue and assistance in exsanguination of the vein are added advantages of tumescent anesthesia. The addition of epinephrine aids in local vasoconstriction to decrease bleeding during the procedure and prolongs the local action of lidocaine by slowing its systemic absorption, thus decreasing its toxicity. The sodium bicarbonate serves as a buffer to decrease pain during administration of the acidic lidocaine solution. Use of oral anxiolytic medications is a helpful adjunctive measure, especially in patients with heightened anxiety, although it does not provide any analgesia.

POSITION The positioning of the patient will depend upon whether an ablation procedure will be performed simultaneously and the location of the varicose veins to be removed. If microphlebectomy is being performed as a stand-alone procedure, the patient should be positioned to allow full access to the varicose veins to be removed. When treating varicose veins on the medial aspect of the thigh and calf, the leg is typically flexed and externally rotated. When treating varicose veins on the posterior thigh and calf, the prone position is most advantageous. Multiple positions, including supine, prone, and lateral, may be necessary to access all of the target veins to be removed. When the patient is awake, they are able to participate in turning to allow adequate exposure to the areas being treated.

When removing the varicose veins, especially if they are large in diameter, it is beneficial to place the patient in Trendelenburg position to decrease venous engorgement and thus overall bleeding and post-procedure bruising. The patient is kept in this position until the compression stocking is applied at the end of the procedure.

DETAILS OF PROCEDURE The technique described is a modification of the original Muller technique from 1966, which emphasized the use of local anesthesia, small 2-mm incisions, absence of vein ligatures and skin sutures, post-procedure compression, and immediate ambulation.

After the patient is properly positioned on the table, the leg is prepped and draped in the normal sterile manner. The patient is placed in Trendelenburg position, which aids in assuring a bloodless surgical field. One percent lidocaine plain is used to anesthetize the skin prior to instilling the tumescent anesthesia into the subdermal tissue manually using a 21-gauge or 27-gauge, 7 cm long spinal needle and either a 30 or 60 mL syringe or a peristaltic roller pump for more efficient delivery. The classic peau d'orange effect on the overlying skin will be evident after instillation. To minimize patient discomfort, consecutive injections should be administered in an area that is already well anesthetized. Micro incisions are created using the pre-procedure mapping as a guide. As one of the goals of this procedure is to keep the incisions between 1 and 3 mm and cosmetically appealing, the incisions may be made using the tip of the #11 surgical scalpel (**FIGURE 73-1**), a 15-degree ophthalmologic blade, or an 18-gauge standard or filter needle. These small incisions should be fashioned along Langer's lines in an attempt to aid healing and minimize scarring.

Once the puncture is created, a hook or fine-tipped clamp is inserted into the incision, taking care to avoid trauma to the surrounding skin or tissue, and used to exteriorize the vein segment, which is elevated as a vein loop (**FIGURE 73-2**). If needed, a spatula may be used to carefully dissect the vein from the surrounding tissue, although this is also accomplished through instillation of tumescent anesthesia. For microphlebectomy, the varicosities to be removed are in the subcutaneous tissue; therefore the hook should not need to be inserted more than several millimeters in depth. There are multiple options available for hooks and spatulas, all of which have slightly different characteristics, including the Mueller-style hook, Ramlet phlebectomy hook, Oesch-style hook, and the Varady hook, to name just a few. Fine-tipped clamps, such as the Jacobson micro mosquito forceps, are ideal for exteriorization as well (**FIGURE 73-3**). As this step is performed blindly, it is important to use the markings as a guide. The vein should be easily extracted from the incision, and one should avoid removing surrounding periadventitial tissue, which may include small cutaneous nerves with the vein. If the periadventitial tissue is retrieved with the vein, it should be separated from the vein and preserved. **CONTINUES ▶**

73-1

Stab
phlebectomy

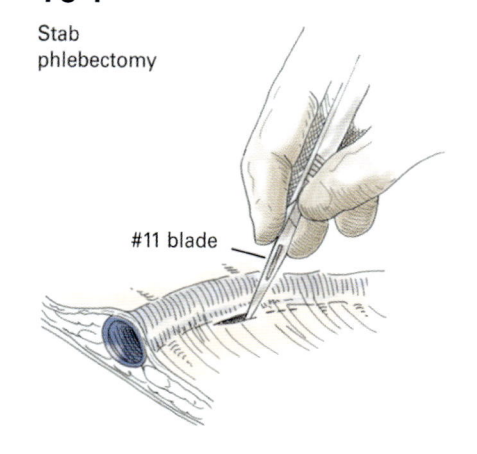

#11 blade

73-2

Vein hook

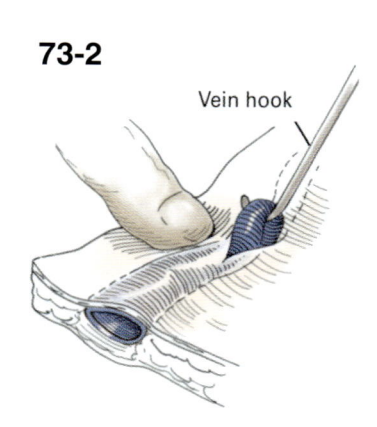

73-3

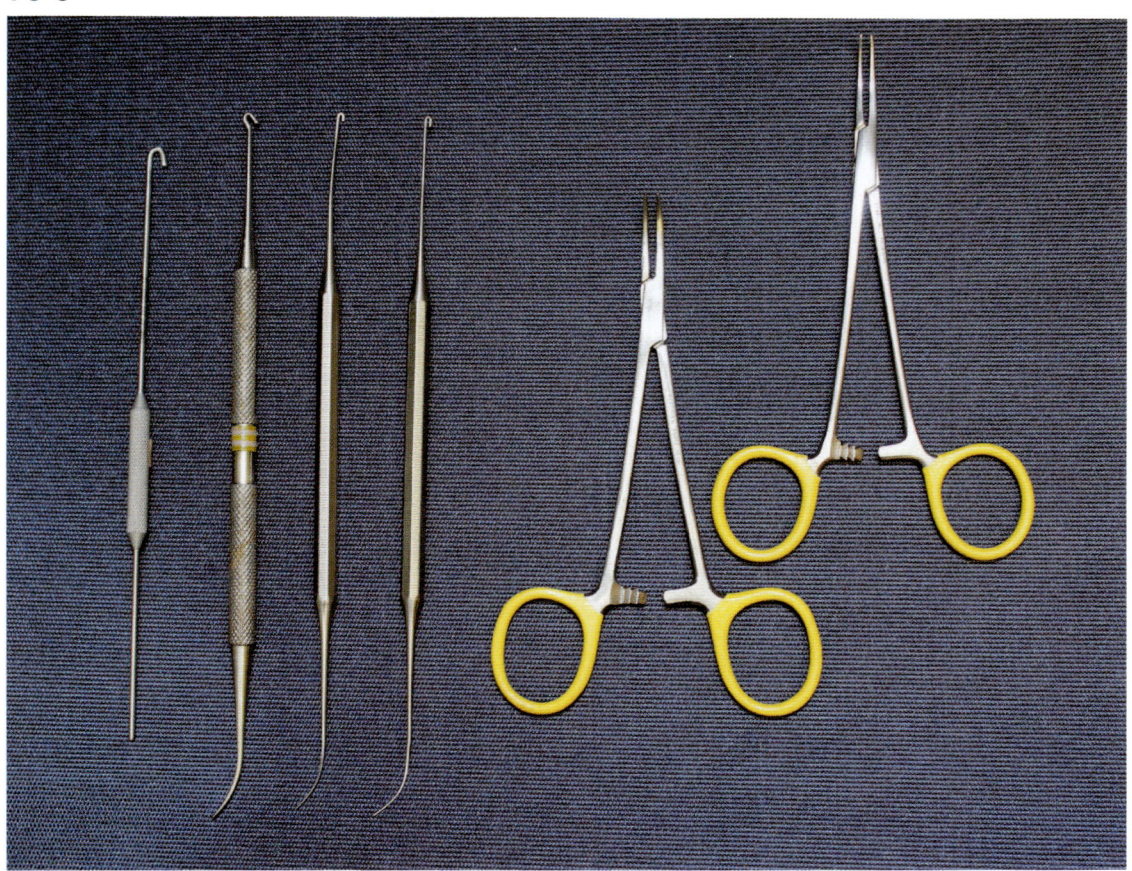

DETAILS OF PROCEDURE CONTINUED Once a loop of varix is exteriorized, Jacobson micro mosquito forceps and Halstead mosquito clamps are used for extraction of the varix. The two segments of the loop are identified and clamped separately. The vein is divided at this time to facilitate removal of the maximum length of vein (**FIGURE 73-4**). Using a back-and-forth, windshield-wiper movement with aid of the spatula if necessary, the proximal segment of vein is slowly removed. It is helpful to use two mosquito clamps together in this step. One mosquito clamp stabilizes the vein and prevents it from retracting back into the incision, while the other clamp is used to grasp the vein just above the skin and gently pull in a back-and-forth manner. When tension is placed on the varix, it will eventually tear. The same technique is repeated for the distal vein segment.

There are several ways to determine where the next incision should be fashioned. The length of the vein segment removed can be used to gauge where the next incision should be placed. When tension is put on the vein, the adjacent skin will often dimple or exhibit a divot where it is tethered by the surrounding connective tissue, which can also be used to estimate the location of the next incision in conjunction with the vein mapping. It is prudent to attempt to remove as much vein as possible between incisions. If large segments of vein are retained between incisions, they often become inflamed and thrombose, which can cause post-procedure discomfort and phlebitis.

Occasionally, the patient may experience pain or burning when retrieving a vein segment. Often this sensation will occur if a cutaneous nerve is in proximity. Dissecting the vein free from the surrounding tissue prior to extraction will often prevent this from occurring. As mentioned previously, care should be taken when removing vein segments in close proximity to the saphenous, sural, and common peroneal nerves.

CLOSURE The vein segments are typically not suture-ligated but thrombose secondary to post-procedure compression. The small incisions are easily able to be approximated with quarter-inch Steri-Strips without the need for sutures, and covered with Tegaderm dressings to contain any blood-tinged tumescent anesthesia, which may leak out of the incisions and onto the compression stockings. ABD pads are placed over the incisions for additional compression to assist with hemostasis when the patient stands, and a medical grade, thigh-high compression stocking is donned over the pads. Alternatively, a compression wrap may be utilized. Immediate ambulation is encouraged, as is leg elevation when seated.

POSTOPERATIVE CARE The patient should continuously wear compression stockings for at least 24 hours post procedure. Ambulation is encouraged, with leg elevation when seated. Nonsteroidal anti-inflammatory medication will decrease inflammation and thus discomfort. Narcotics are typically not required. Supplementation with ice over the compression stocking is also helpful to decrease inflammation. The compression stocking and dressings may be removed 24 hours after the procedure, and the patient may shower. Patients should avoid bathing and swimming for at least 1 week. Aerobic exercise should be avoided for at least 1 week, but activities of daily living may be resumed after 24 to 48 hours. ■

SUGGESTED READINGS

Almeida JI, Raines JK. Principles of ambulatory phlebectomy. In: Bergan JJ, ed. *The Vein Book*. Burlington, MA: Elsevier Academic Press; 2007:247-255.

Bahl V, Hu HM, Henke PK, et al. A validation study of a retrospective venous thromboembolism risk scoring method. *Ann Surg.* 2010;251:344-350.

El-Skeikha JE, Nandhra S, Carradice D, et al. Clinical outcomes and quality of life 5 years after a randomized trial of concomitant or sequential phlebectomy following endovenous laser ablation for varicose veins. *Br J Surg.* 2014;101:1093-1097.

Geersen DF, Shortell CEK. Phlebectomy techniques for varicose veins. *Surg Clin N Am.* 2018;98:401-414.

Giannas J, Bayat A, Watson SJ. Common peroneal nerve injury during varicose vein operations. *Eur J Vasc Endovasc Surg.* 2006;31(4):443-445.

Kerver ALA, van der Ham AC, Theeuwes HP, et al. The surgical anatomy of the small saphenous vein and adjacent nerves in relation to endovenous thermal ablation. *J Vasc Surg.* 2012;56:181-188.

Klein JA, Jeske DR. Estimated maximal safe dosages of tumescent lidocaine. *Anesth Analg.* 2016;122:1350-1359.

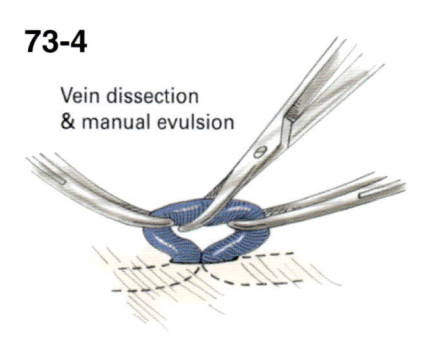

73-4

Vein dissection
& manual evulsion

SAPHENOUS VEIN ABLATION

David Szalay, MD

INDICATIONS Saphenous vein incompetence is a common clinical entity that can lead to the development of varicose veins, pain, edema, and secondary skin changes. More severe consequences of saphenous incompetence and varicose veins include superficial thrombophlebitis, varicosity bleeding, and venous ulcers. The traditional treatment for saphenous incompetence has been surgical ligation and stripping, but in the past two decades practice has moved increasingly toward endovenous ablation or closure of incompetent saphenous veins. Endovenous ablation avoids significant anesthesia, reduces periprocedural pain, facilitates early recovery, and minimizes both wound complications and risk of saphenous or sural nerve injury. With appropriate patient selection and technique, the long-term success of saphenous ablation is comparable or superior to surgery.

A number of endovenous techniques that have shown to be successful in the treatment of saphenous incompetence. These techniques can be generally categorized as thermal/heat-induced ablation using laser (Endovenous Laser Ablation [EVLA]) or radiofrequency (Radiofrequency Ablation [RFA]), which require tumescent anesthetic, or non-thermal/non-tumescent techniques such as Cyanoacrylate Embolization (CE) or MechanicoChemical Ablation (MOCA). We describe EVLA below.

PREPROCEDURE ASSESSMENT AND PATIENT SELECTION A focused history should determine contributing factors, symptoms, and complications related to venous disease. The patient is examined in both the standing and supine position to document the size and location of any varicosities, secondary skin changes of venous disease, and the possible presence of associated peripheral arterial disease. A full venous duplex of the lower extremities is performed—ideally with the patient standing—to assess deep venous patency and competence, reflux at the saphenofemoral and saphenopopliteal junctions, and the presence of complete or segmental reflux along the great, small, or accessory saphenous veins. Size, patency, tortuosity, and duplications of the saphenous veins are noted as well as the presence of any contributing or significant incompetent perforating veins. We recommend that pretreatment photographs also be taken to facilitate postprocedural comparison.

POSITION The patient position is determined by the vein(s) targeted for ablation. The great saphenous and anterior (anterolateral) accessory saphenous veins are treated with the patient supine, while the small saphenous veins are treated with the patient prone. The procedure table should allow for variable height and have the capability to place the patient in the Trendelenburg position.

PROCEDURAL PREPARATION AND ACCESS Skin preparation is applied circumferentially, and draping is positioned to allow full limb access. To facilitate duplex guidance, an ultrasound probe is then draped in a sterile sleeve.

Endovenous access of the targeted vein(s) is the first key procedural step and is common to all ablation techniques. Appropriate selection of the access site(s) is an essential step which will improve both immediate procedural and long-term procedural success. Access plans should first be determined during preprocedural consultation and confirmed again on ultrasound immediately prior to the procedure. Whenever possible, the vein should be accessed at or below the lowest point of reflux, or below the lowest perforating vein that communicates with the saphenous segment, to reduce the risk of persistent or recurrent sources of reflux. Tortuosity, scarring, or near-occlusion of the vein above the access site may impede the subsequent passage of wires, sheaths, and catheters. In these cases the use of multiple access site(s)—above and below non-traversable segments— may be required to facilitate complete closure of the targeted vein. When more than one vein (or vein segment) is to be treated, it is generally best to access what is determined to be the most difficult vein first (size, location, tortuosity, etc.), as local or generalized vasospasm may make the

subsequent venipunctures more challenging. Vein segments that lie below the superficial/"saphenous" fascia and above the muscle fascia are generally easier to access, as they are easier to image, are mostly straight, and tend not to "roll" given their fixed position. When access must be obtained through a more superficial segment or tributary, the target should be healthy, non-tortuous, and allow for easy passage of the wire and sheath into the the subfascial segment.

Once the access site(s) is/are selected, venipuncture is performed under ultrasound guidance with either transverse (FIGURE 74-1) or longitudinal visualization. Transverse orientation of the ultrasound probe allows confirmation that the needle is centered on the vein, while longitudinal orientation can show a longer segment of the vein and better visualize the wire passing into the lumen of the vein. Local anesthetic is applied to the skin and subcutaneous tissue only, as instillation around the vein may induce vasospasm. Needle entry into the vein lumen is confirmed via tactile feedback as a "pop" is felt as the lumen is entered, visually as a "flash" of blood into the access needle is observed, and sonographically on ultrasound guidance. If there is difficulty passing the wire, a very subtle pullback/push-in or rotation of the needle may be required as the bevel is up against the vein wall.

CATHETER PLACEMENT All ablation techniques require successful placement of the treating fiber to the most proximal extent of target vein segment.

When a long sheath is required, wire access should first be obtained across the targeted vein segment into the deep system (through the saphenofemoral junction). The long laser sheath with cm markers is used. An estimate of distance from insertion point to saphenofemoral junction is performed using external landmarks (FIGURE 74-2). The sheath is then tracked over the wire (FIGURE 74-3), and sheath positioning relative to the target saphenofemoral junction is confirmed using ultrasound. Of note, there are also now laser fibers that can be passed along the length of the target vein without the need for a full-length sheath.

Various maneuvers can be employed to facilitate passage of wires, sheaths, and/or catheters through difficult segments, including gentle external pressure (manually or with the ultrasound probe), repositioning the leg with minor rotation, extension or flexion, and the concurrent flushing of the access sheath with saline to help dilate the vein. It is good practice to have extra wires of varying size and characteristics as well as sheaths available to problem-solve in the exceptional case and to supplement what is provided in the procedural kit. Recall that additional or alternative access sites are always an option if a vein segment is ultimately impossible to negotiate.

TUMESCENCE Tumescent anesthesia is required for ablation techniques that use thermal energy to close the vein. Tumescent anesthesia for these procedures involves instilling a circumferential layer of fluid along the entire length of the treated vein. This fluid layer, which is typically dilute lidocaine (0.1 or 0.2%) without epinephrine serves as a "heat sink" which minimizes transfer of heat to surrounding tissues. The associated external pressure also decreases lumen diameter and improves device apposition to the vein wall. Ultrasound imaging is again key to ensure complete and adequate coverage of the vein. The tumescence is delivered through a 22-gauge needle via hand-filled syringes or by means of a pressurized tumescent pump. When delivered into the interfascial plane where possible, the tumescent will typically track quite nicely and encompass the vein with a classic ultrasound appearance often referred to as "Cleopatra's eye." Superficial segments must have adequate tumescence to ensure separation of the vein from overlying skin.

While uncommon given the dilute local anesthetic used, if there is concern about the total amount of local given one can either further dilute the solution or simply use plain normal saline/lactated Ringer's solution.

CONTINUES ▶

74-1

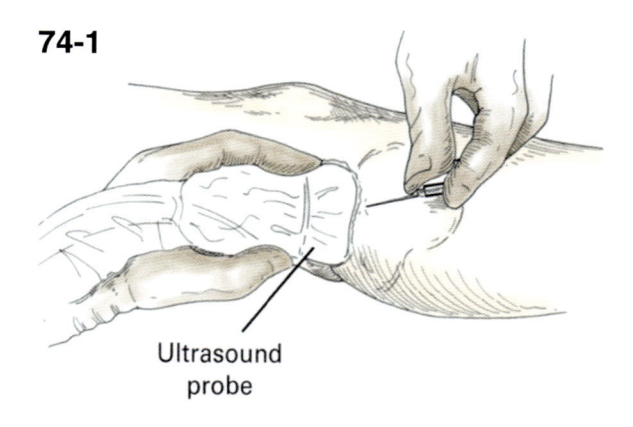

Ultrasound
probe

Figure 74-1 (Reproduced with permission from Ellison E, Zollinger, Jr. RM, Pawlik TM, Vaccaro PS, Bitans M, Baker AS. eds. *Zollinger's Atlas of Surgical Operations*, 11e. New York: McGraw-Hill Education; 2022.)

74-2

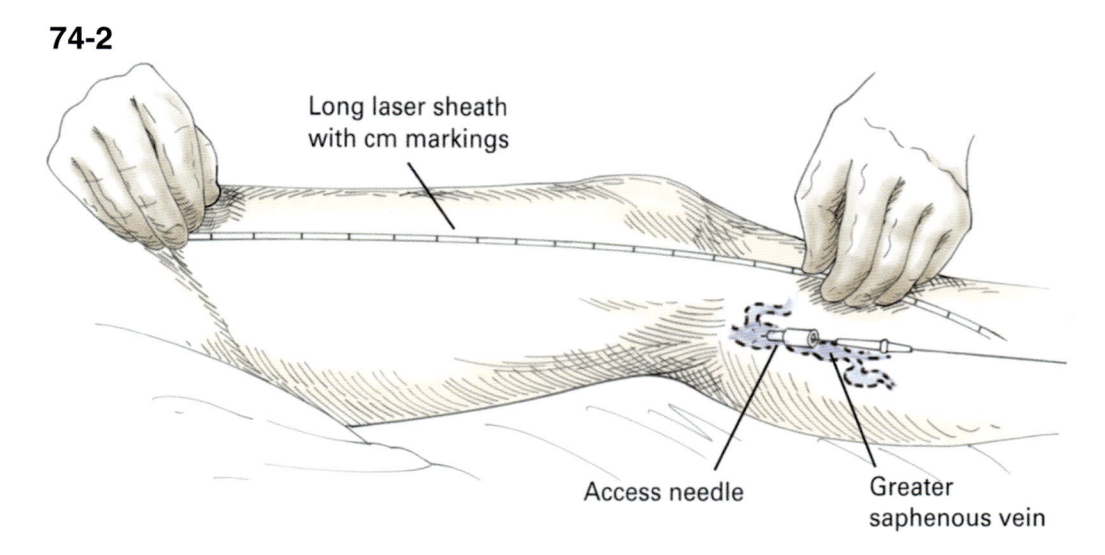

Long laser sheath
with cm markings

Access needle

Greater
saphenous vein

Figure 74-2 (Reproduced with permission from Ellison E, Zollinger, Jr. RM, Pawlik TM, Vaccaro PS, Bitans M, Baker AS. eds. *Zollinger's Atlas of Surgical Operations,* 11e. New York: McGraw-Hill Education; 2022.)

74-3

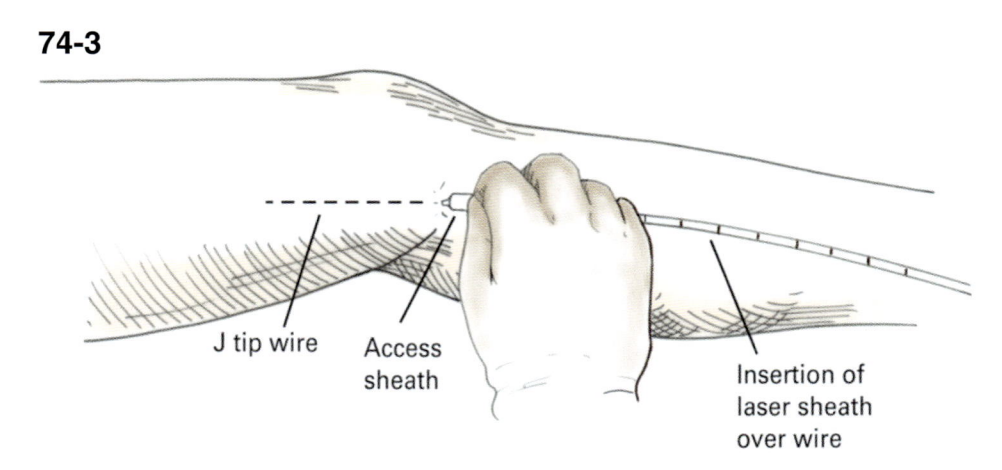

J tip wire   Access
sheath

Insertion of
laser sheath
over wire

Figure 74-3 (Reproduced with permission from Ellison E, Zollinger, Jr. RM, Pawlik TM, Vaccaro PS, Bitans M, Baker AS. eds. *Zollinger's Atlas of Surgical Operations,* 11e. New York: McGraw-Hill Education; 2022.)

ABLATION OR CLOSURE The final procedural step is closure or ablation of the vein. All techniques follow the overlying principle of closing the targeted vein from the most proximal extent and progressively pulling back the treatment catheter. During this step, Trendelenburg positioning may help empty or reduce volume in the targeted vein and its tributaries. Specific considerations for each technique are outlined below.

THERMAL TECHNIQUES

LASER ABLATION It is our practice to start the laser ablation at least 15 to 20 mm (and no closer) from the junction with the deep system. The laser fiber is pulled back from groin to skin entrance along with the sheath (FIGURE 74-4). The suggested "pullback rate" for the first 10 cm is generally slower than the remaining length (maximum of 2 mm/sec) and the total energy delivered in KJoules is captured on the laser console. The amount of energy delivered per vein area can be calculated, but in practicality we advise as slow and steady pullback as the patient tolerates. Transmission of heat into superficial tributaries may cause transient local discomfort, which is addressed by adding more anesthetic and "pulsing" the laser in shorter bursts through the area.

RADIOFREQUENCY ABLATION RFA catheters are configured to deliver 20-second thermal cycles over a 7-cm length. The most proximal segment is treated with two cycles, with the subsequent lower segments treated with at least one cycle. Markings on the catheters/sheaths help guide position and pullback time.

CYANOACRYLATE EMBOLIZATION This technique delivers a proprietary cyanoacrylate adhesive along the length of the vein. Glue catheter position should begin at least 5 cm from the targeted deep system junction. The ultrasound probe is essential to both confirm the position of the catheter tip and apply consistent external pressure, compressing the vein to promote adhesion and limit proximal propagation of the adhesive. The compression time is a minimum of 3 minutes near the junction and then for at least 30 seconds as the catheter is pulled back in 3-cm lengths. Additional adhesive volume can be used at one's discretion for dilated vein segments or at the junction with large tributaries. Near completion, care should be taken to avoid depositing glue into the subcutaneous tissue as this can cause local irritation and seromas. This can be ensured by pulling the glue catheter back into the outer sheath before removal.

MECHANICOCHEMICAL ABLATION MOCA Uses the concurrent process of mechanical disruption of the endothelium and delivery of a sclerosing agent to close the vein during the catheter pullback process. With wire rotation activated and simultaneous sclerosant infusion, a pullback rate of 1 to 2 mm/sec is recommended. If the catheter sticks to the vein wall, some local anesthetic together with a gentle "tug" may be required to free the tip.

For all procedures it is essential to adhere to the principles and guidance as outlined in their respective IFU(s). On completion and catheter/sheath removal, a few minutes of external pressure is typically sufficient for hemostasis followed by the application of Steri-Strips and/or a small bandage at the access site(s).

POSTPROCEDURAL CARE We place all patients in Class II compression (30–40 mmHg) post ablation irrespective of technique. External compression of the veins and tributaries may improve outcomes and seems to reduce postprocedural discomfort. The duration of compression is variable between practices, but we advise our patients to wear compression continuously for 48 hours and then subsequently off at bedtime only for an additional 5 days. Patients are encouraged to ambulate immediately following treatment and at least two to three times per day in the 2 weeks following intervention. We advise the use of low-dose, over-the-counter NSAIDs to mitigate inflammation and discomfort if there is no contraindication to their use. Plain acetaminophen can also be used if required. Most patients can resume regular daily activities immediately but may want to avoid strenuous or repetitive lower extremity work or exercise for about a week.

An in-office ultrasound is performed at about 7 to 10 days to confirm closure and ensure no deep venous clot. We then see the patient again at 8 weeks to determine procedural success and assess the need for additional or adjuvant treatments. ∎

74-4

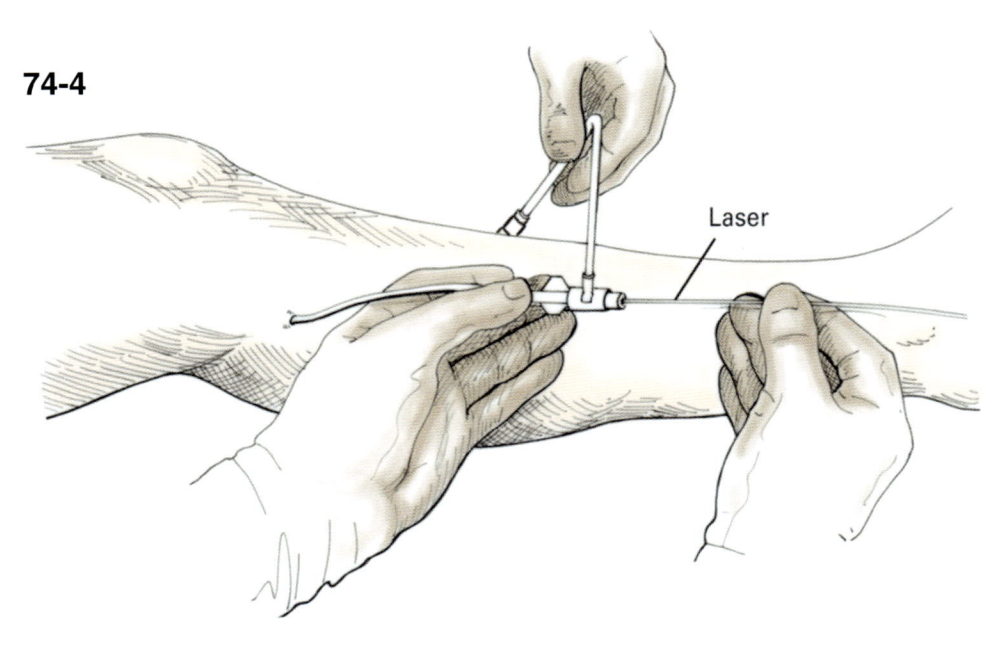

Laser

Figure 74-4 (Reproduced with permission from Ellison E, Zollinger, Jr. RM, Pawlik TM, Vaccaro PS, Bitans M, Baker AS. eds. *Zollinger's Atlas of Surgical Operations,* 11e. New York: McGraw-Hill Education; 2022.)

High Ligation and Stripping

Harold Davis Waller, MD • Julianne Stoughton, MD

INDICATIONS Currently in the United States, the role of vein stripping (VS) or high ligation and stripping (HLS) has been limited due to the emergence and availability of both thermal and non-thermal vein ablation methods.[1] The indications for HLS have changed, but this remains an important tool for the surgeon in some unique situations where ablation is not available or advisable. Treatment with HLS or endovenous ablation (EVA) is considered when ambulatory venous hypertension exists due to refluxing truncal veins, and when signs or symptoms of chronic venous insufficiency are present and nonresponsive to conservative measures. The obliteration of refluxing veins (by HLS or EVA) helps to reduce the ambulatory venous hypertension which, if left untreated, can lead to eventual skin changes and ulceration. Treatment also helps to diminish the risk of thrombosis of superficial veins and reduces patient symptoms. These symptoms of refluxing superficial veins are related to dilation by hydrostatic pressure and have been described by patients as heaviness, aching, swelling, throbbing, and itching ("HASTI" symptoms).[2] Ultimately, later stages of venous insufficiency may result in the development of enlarged varicosities, leg edema, skin changes, and ulceration.[3]

Since the advent of thermal and non-thermal EVA, the primary indications for HLS currently include veins that are close to the skin (subdermal), truncal veins with enlarged or complex deep vein junctions which may require ligation, and veins with markedly enlarged vein diameters. The success rate of EVA diminishes with exceptionally enlarged vessel sizes, and VS can be an excellent choice to avoid recanalization or failure of ablation in those patients.[4] When done with the modern techniques, including ultrasound guidance, tumescent local anesthesia, and inversion stripping, this method can be well tolerated with minimal recovery and acceptable risk. Our current method for HLS is a modification of perforate-invaginate stripping method using a flexible Codman stripper without the acorn tips. Dissection is minimized by localizing the saphenofemoral junction (SFJ) and distal venotomy targets using intraoperative duplex ultrasound. The perivenous trauma of vein avulsion is minimized by inverting and invaginating the vein during removal. Postoperative pain and bleeding are minimized by ultrasound-guided infiltration of the saphenous sheath with tumescent anesthesia with epinephrine.

CONTRAINDICATIONS The most recent varicose vein guidelines document recommends EVA over HLS, but this is grade 1B level of evidence and does not consider the minimally invasive methods of stripping described below.[5] There are several situations where stripping and ligation are not advisable. HLS can be problematic when patients are on full-dose anticoagulation. If needed, patients can undergo HLS when on prophylactic dosing of anticoagulants, but there can be a significant risk of bleeding when patients are fully anticoagulated. Additionally, HLS should be avoided when incisions are planned in areas of unhealthy skin (such as areas of lipodermatosclerosis and severe thinning with hyperpigmentation). Tortuous veins which are not amenable to stripper catheter or wire advancement are not able to be stripped. Finally, HLS of previously thrombosed and recanalized veins with significant periadventitial scarring is not ideal due to excessive bleeding risk and technical difficulty due to the chronically fibrotic veins.

OPERATIVE PREPARATION Therapeutic doses of anticoagulation are held for at least 3 days preoperatively and the INR is corrected to less than 1.5 if necessary before any incision is made in order to reduce the risk of postoperative hematoma and bleeding. Prophylactic doses of anticoagulation can be continued if needed for higher-risk patients. For example, ½ mg/kg/day enoxaparin, 10 mg rivaroxaban, and so on. Only patients requiring prophylactic antibiotics for patient-specific indications (such as recent joint replacement or cardiac valvular disease) are given the antibiotics parenterally prior to incision.

Duplex ultrasound focused on areas of reflux in the superficial, perforating, and deep systems is obtained preoperatively. The refluxing saphenous vein segments can be marked to determine the path of reflux and to help determine incision sites and aid in the administration of tumescent local anesthesia. Before the operation, the patient should stand to encourage venous distension, and visualized varicosities are marked percutaneously if simultaneous ambulatory phlebectomy is planned.

Depending on surgeon and anesthesia preferences, the operation can be performed under general, regional, or local anesthesia. Our preference is for monitored anesthesia care (MAC) with the addition of local tumescent anesthesia.

POSITION After preoperative percutaneous marking in the standing position, the patient is placed in the supine position on the operating table. Since the advent of endovenous ablation, stripping has not often been chosen as a treatment option in the small saphenous vein system. Prior to incision, the table is subsequently adjusted to a head down (Trendelenburg) position to minimize venous distension and to lower the risk of bleeding.

After routine circumferential leg skin preparation, the operative field is draped to expose the anterior superior iliac spine superiorly and laterally, the groin crease medially, and the foot is covered to allow full access to the entire leg and groin.

INCISION AND EXPOSURE We use intraoperative duplex ultrasound to evaluate the SFJ and to specifically pinpoint the junctional tributaries, as they can be highly variable and difficult to locate with a smaller groin incision. We then use the ultrasound to choose the sites for our proximal and distal incisions. Finally, we assess the course of the saphenous vein, noting any areas of varicosity, tortuosity, and large perforators or tributaries along the length. Intraoperative duplex ultrasound can reduce tissue trauma by limiting exploratory subcutaneous dissection.

DETAILS OF PROCEDURE A small oblique incision is made on our marked proximal incision site and dissection is carried through the subcutaneous tissue in a vertical axis to limit injuries to underlying structures, namely lymphatics. After identification of the great saphenous vein (GSV), dissection proceeds cephalad to expose the SFJ (**FIGURE 75-1**). Care should be taken to ensure that the exposed vessels represent the SFJ as veering off course during dissection can result in unintended injury to the femoral vein or artery. Once the SFJ is clearly identified, the GSV is encircled with a vessel loop and tributaries in the immediate vicinity are ligated and divided. Our attention now turns to the pre-marked distal incision site.

A very small vertical incision is made over the pre-marked distal incision site and dissection is carried through the subcutaneous tissue to identify the distal GSV, which is encircled with a vessel loop. Using tension to draw the vein up, the vein is ligated approximately 1 cm distally to the planned venotomy site. Again, applying proximal tension with the vessel loop to expose the vein and prevent bleeding, a transverse venotomy is made in the vein through which the head of the flexible stripper is inserted (**FIGURE 75-2**). **CONTINUES** ▶

75-1

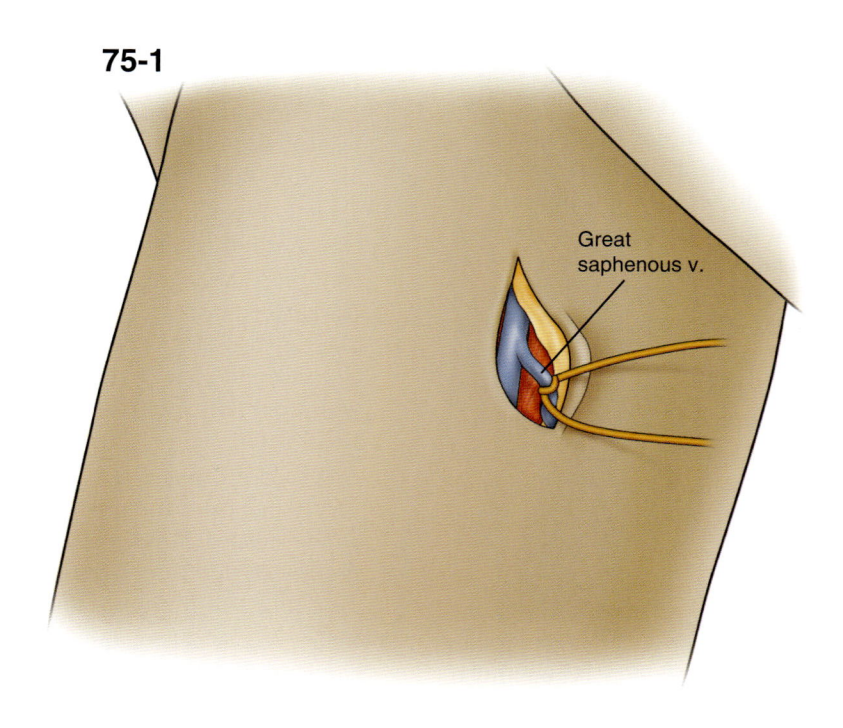

Great
saphenous v.

75-2

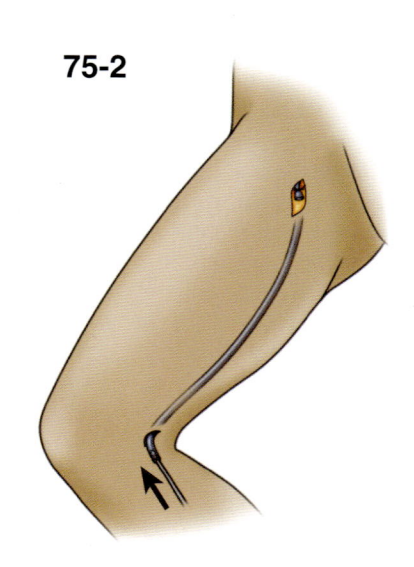

DETAILS OF PROCEDURE CONTINUED The stripper can be palpated and followed by ultrasound along the pre-marked course of the GSV as it is advanced within the vein toward the groin. It should travel with minimal resistance. We turn our attention back to the proximal incision to observe the stripper head distending the GSV at the SFJ. A transverse venotomy is made over the stripper head and the stripper is pulled through. At this time, the proximal GSV is suture ligated and divided near to the femoral vein. Note that ligation too proximal to the femoral vein can result in its narrowing, whereas ligation too distal can result in a longer stump which may thrombose and subsequently embolize. With the stripper head protruding from the proximal end of the now divided GSV, a suture is used to secure its divided end to the head of the stripper, leaving a long tail of suture which will be used as countertraction. Prior to stripping the vein, tumescent anesthesia is injected into the saphenous sheath along the course of the vein. If there are any tributary veins along the length of the GSV, they can be anesthetized with additional tumescent for adequate hemostasis and analgesia.

An assistant then pulls the stripper at the knee in the direction of the patient's feet while the surgeon assures inversion of the vein, allowing the vein to be pulled inside-out. This allows for minimal trauma to any perivenous tissue attachments and is usually done with minimal resistance. As the stripper head is pulled through the distal venotomy, the vein invaginates (**FIGURE 75-3**). Further tension is applied as the full length of the now-invaginated GSV is delivered through the distal venotomy. The distal vein is subsequently divided proximal to the previously placed suture tie and is removed from the field intact and inside-out with suture along its length.

If the vein is torn during invaginated stripping, the suture can be pulled back up to the groin to retrieve the stripper catheter. If necessary, the small acorn tip can be attached and used to complete stripping of the remaining GSV remnants.

CLOSURE The groin incision is closed in layers with absorbable suture. The scarpa's fascia layer is closed with interrupted 4-0 Vicryl, and the skin is closed in a running subcuticular fashion with 5-0 Monocryl or similar absorbable suture. The distal incision may require closure with a single subcuticular suture or, in some cases, may be closed by approximation with a Steri-Strip.

POSTOPERATIVE CARE After skin closure on the OR table, the incisions are padded with gauze to control any leakage of blood and/or tumescent fluid. A 20- to 30-mmHg thigh-high compression stocking is applied to the limb and an additional Ace wrap is applied for light compression. Ice packs are applied to the medial thigh for pain control and to reduce postoperative swelling and bruising. The patient is encouraged to stand in the postoperative area and to remain ambulatory in the immediate postoperative period. The Ace wrap should be removed on the evening of postoperative day 0. The patient's pain should be well controlled with either NSAIDs, Tylenol, or an alternating regimen of the two medications. Ice packs are also an excellent adjunct for pain control and swelling reduction. The compression stocking should be worn during the day for 2 weeks postoperatively. There are no significant activity restrictions, but heavy weight lifting is discouraged in the first 1 to 2 weeks postoperatively. Patients are encouraged to call their surgeon with any concerns including significant bruising and bleeding. A postoperative checkup is usually scheduled for 1 month post-procedure. Patients are then seen again 6 months post procedure. ■

REFERENCES

1. Carruthers TN, Farber A, Rybin D, Doros G, Eslami MH. Interventions on the superficial venous system for chronic venous insufficiency by surgeons in the modern era: an analysis of ACS-NSQIP. *Vasc Endovascular Surg.* 2014 Oct-Nov;48(7-8):482-490.

2. Bendix SD, Peterson EL, Kabbani LS, Weaver MR, Lin JC. Effect of endovenous ablation assessment stratified by great saphenous vein size, gender, clinical severity, and patient-reported outcomes. *J Vasc Surg Venous Lymphat Disord.* 2021 Jan;9(1):128-136.

3. Lurie F, Passman M, Meisner M, et al. The 2020 update of the CEAP classification system and reporting standards. *J Vasc Surg Venous Lymphat Disord.* 2020 May;8(3):342-352.

4. Harlander-Locke M, Jimenez JC, Lawrence PF, Derubertis BG, Rigberg DA, Gelabert HA. Endovenous ablation with concomitant phlebectomy is a safe and effective method of treatment for symptomatic patients with axial reflux and large incompetent tributaries. *J Vasc Surg.* 2013 Jul;58(1):166-172.

5. Gloviczki P, Comerota AJ, Dalsing MC et al. Society for Vascular Surgery; American Venous Forum. The care of patients with varicose veins and associated chronic venous diseases: clinical practice guidelines of the Society for Vascular Surgery and the American Venous Forum. *J Vasc Surg.* 2011 May;53(5 Suppl):2S-48S.

6. Keller WL. A new method of extirpating the internal saphenous and similar veins in varicose conditions: a preliminary report. *NY Med J.* 1905;82:385.

7. Mayo CH. Treatment of varicose veins. *Surg Gynecol Obstet.* 1906;2:385.

8. Babcock WW. A new operation for extirpation of varicose veins of the leg. *NY Med J.* 1907;86:153-156.

9. Myers TT. Results and technique of stripping operation for varicose veins. *JAMA.* 1957;163(2):87-92

10. Fullarton GM, Calvert MH. Intraluminal long saphenous vein stripping: a technique minimizing perivenous tissue trauma. *Br J Surg.* 1987 Apr;74(4):255.

11. Goren G, Yellin AE. Minimally invasive surgery for primary varicose veins: limited invaginated axial stripping and tributary (hook) stab avulsion. *Ann Vasc Surg.* 1995 Jul;9(4):401-414.

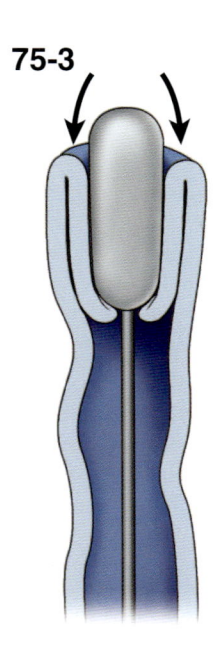

75-3

CHAPTER 76

INFERIOR VENA CAVA TUMOR RESECTION

Graham Roche-Nagle, MD

INDICATIONS Primary and secondary tumors of the vena cava are rare and often malignant. They either originate in the vein wall, invade the walls secondarily, or grow within the vena cava as tumor thrombus causing obstruction. They can also cause extrinsic compression of the inferior vena cava (IVC) lumen. The most frequent primary tumor of the IVC and superior vena cava (SVC) is leiomyosarcoma, which are malignant tumors of smooth muscle cells that can originate in any location but occur most often in the uterus, retroperitoneum, or intraabdominal region. Leiomyosarcoma of IVC was first described by Dzsinich et al. in 1992. Renal cell carcinomas are the most frequent secondary tumors involving the IVC and are more frequent in occurrence than leiomyosarcomas.

Leiomyosarcomas of vascular origin are particularly rare tumors, occurring mainly in the IVC. The International Registry of Inferior Vena Cava Leiomyosarcomas revealed that these tumors involve the IVC in 60% of patients and most tumors occur in the lower (44.2%) or middle (50.8%) region of the IVC, while only a small number of tumors occur in the upper third or suprahepatic region (4.2%). There are no definitive symptoms, but typical symptoms include leg swelling, dyspnea, and a general feeling of being unwell accompanied by weight loss and abdominal and/or back pain.

These tumors are polypoid or nodular, are firmly fixed to the vessel wall, and demonstrate less intratumor hemorrhage or necrosis than other sarcomas. The most frequent growth pattern is intraluminal; however, the tumor can invade across the vein wall into nearby organs in advanced situations. Such biologic behavior makes it difficult to differentiate a primary venous leiomyosarcoma from other IVC tumors. Frequently, cases with malignancies invading or obstructing the vena cava have distant metastases to the lung, liver, kidney, bone, and pleura at the point of the diagnosis, or they are too frail to undergo an operation. There are few successful treatment options available, and resection often is the only prospect for cure or palliation of symptoms. Partial resection of the caval wall, with either primary or patch closure, is more often chosen over graft replacement if adequate margins can be obtained, since it is less risky and simpler to perform. Reconstruction of IVC depends of tumor location and its extension, and depending on the oncologic staging, in some circumstances only resection and no reconstruction is required if the vena cava is occluded and venous collaterality is well established.

Adequate imaging is most important in preoperative planning. Resectability is determined by invasion of adjacent structures and not the extent of the IVC involvement. Often a right nephrectomy, and sometimes enterotomy are needed, depending on invasion of other organs. A computed tomography scan with intravenous contrast of arterial and delayed venous views provides the necessary information. In selected patients, a magnetic resonance venogram can help determine resectability. The technical challenges in this operation relate to the mobilization of the tumor from the retroperitoneal surface and the control of suprahepatic IVC.

POSITION The patient is placed in a supine position.

OPERATIVE PREPARATION After routine skin preparation, the operative field is draped to expose the abdomen.

INCISION AND EXPOSURE Several incisions are adequate depending on the extent of operation, including midline, a right subcostal incision with midline extension, or traditional chevron. On occasion, for tumors invading the retrohepatic and renal veins, a combined midline incision with median sternotomy is necessary for supradiagphragmatic control of the IVC. After retractor placement and initial evaluation for the presence of intraabdominal metastatic disease, right medial visceral rotation is performed by identifying the white line of Toldt and dividing it lateral to the ascending colon from the base of the cecum and continued up to the hepatic flexure (see Chapter 74), The mesentery of the right colon and small bowel is dissected off the retroperitoneum to its root. The duodenum is Kocherized by incising its lateral peritoneal attachments and is then mobilized until the head of the pancreas is exposed to the uncinate process and its posterior aspect visualized (see Chapter 74). The cecum and small bowel are swept out of the pelvis and toward the patient's left upper quadrant. A complete right medial visceral rotation exposes the IVC from the inferior border of the liver (suprarenal portion) to its bifurcation (**FIGURE 76-1**).

DETAILS OF PROCEDURE The caudal extent of the IVC tumor is ascertained by intraoperative ultrasound (IVUS) if available. The anterior medial surface of the aorta is dissected at this level, and all the lymphatic tissues covering the aorta are lifted and turned toward the IVC. An aortocaval window is then entered and the plane between the IVC and the retroperitoneal surface comes into view and dissection continued until the right side of the IVC is reached. By skeletonizing the anterior–medial surface of the aorta in a cranial direction, the right renal artery and left renal vein are reached and exposed. Ligating adjacent lumbar veins allows the back wall of the vena cava to be visualized. When the perirenal segment is involved, individual control of the right and left renal vein is essential. The left renal vein may be occluded, and there is no need for left renal artery control if the left gonadal and/or adrenal veins are patent and not part of the resection. Control of the right renal artery during right renal vein occlusion is recommended due to minimal collateral venous drainage for the right kidney, which can lead to organ congestion. If an expeditious repair is anticipated, this may not be necessary. Alternatively, intermittent release of the right renal vein control can be done if the increase in blood loss is acceptable.

If exposure of the suprahepatic IVC and hepatic vein confluence is required, liver mobilization begins with dissection of the ligamentum teres which is divided. The falciform ligament is divided with cautery and the left lateral section of liver is taken down from the diaphragm and the right liver is mobilized from the diaphragm after the division of the coronary and triangular ligaments until the anterior surface of the suprahepatic IVC is exposed (**FIGURE 76-2A**). The junction between the origin of the middle hepatic vein (MHV) and the IVC is defined by sharp dissection. The right lobe of the liver is gently rotated to the left to visualize the retrohepatic vena cava (**FIGURE 76-2B**). Both the right and left diaphragmatic veins draining into the IVC can be divided in order to lengthen the free segment of suprahepatic IVC so that a vascular clamp can be placed. **CONTINUES** ▶

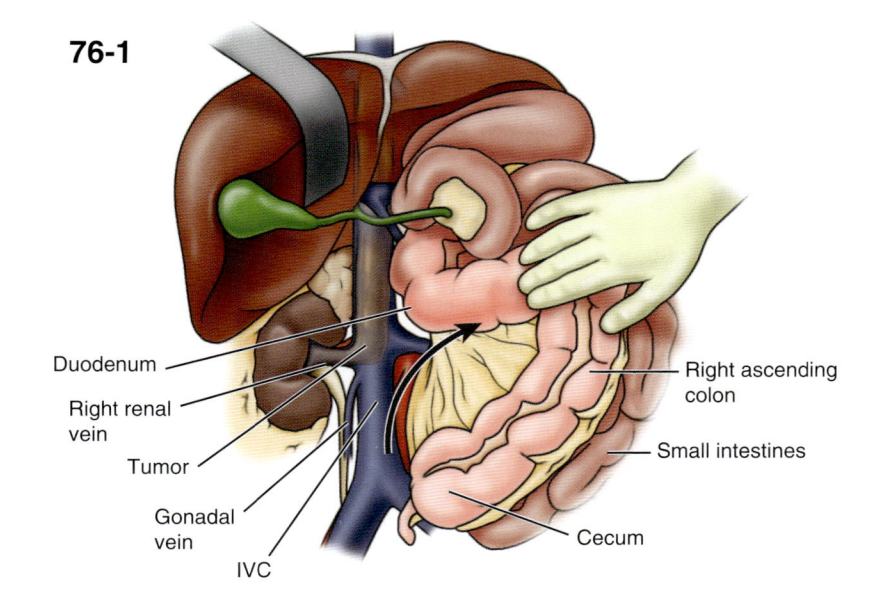

76-1

Duodenum

Right renal vein

Tumor

Gonadal vein

IVC

Right ascending colon

Small intestines

Cecum

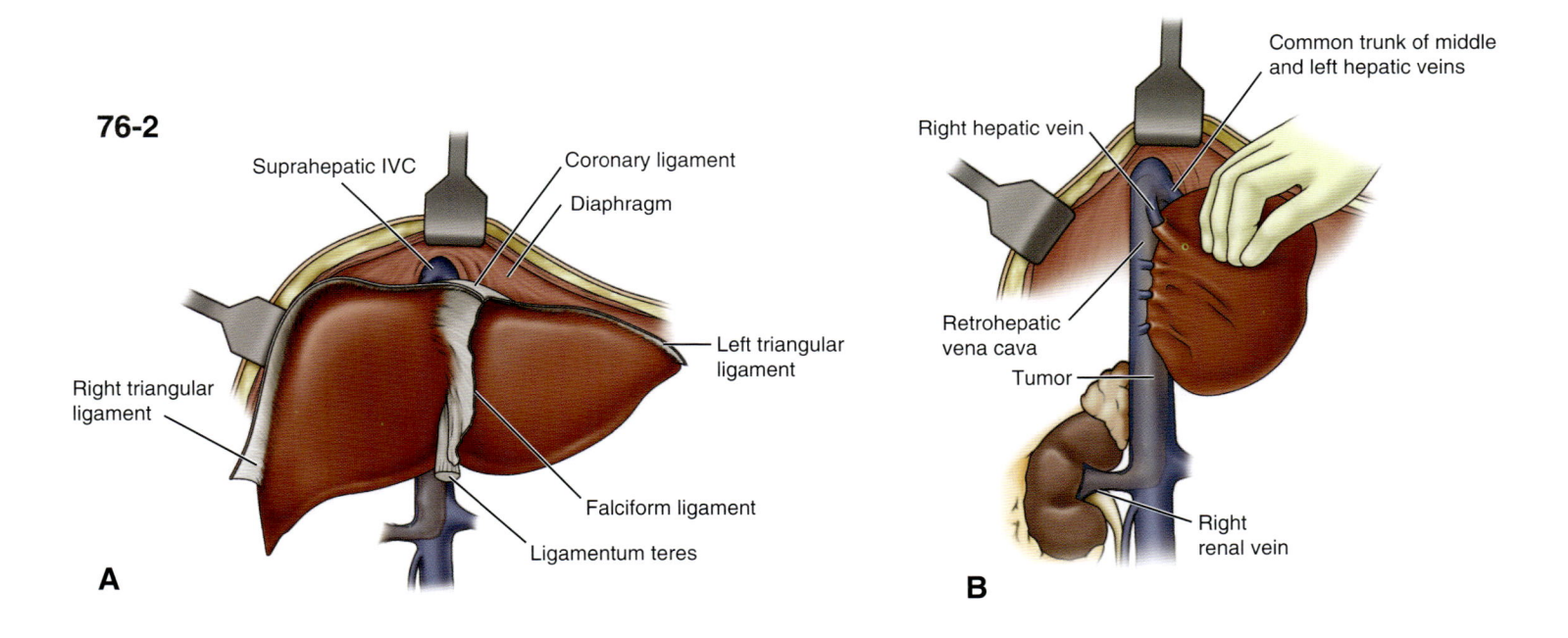

76-2

A

Suprahepatic IVC

Coronary ligament

Diaphragm

Left triangular ligament

Right triangular ligament

Falciform ligament

Ligamentum teres

B

Common trunk of middle and left hepatic veins

Right hepatic vein

Retrohepatic vena cava

Tumor

Right renal vein

DETAILS OF PROCEDURE `CONTINUED` Once appropriate exposure has been obtained, heparin is now given intravenously by the anesthesiologist at the surgeon's discretion. After vascular control is achieved, a cavotomy is performed and the tumor extracted. If required, the tumor can be milked back into the cavotomy site and a vascular clamp applied (FIGURE 76-3). Heparinized saline is used to irrigate the field, allowing free removal of clot. The reconstruction of IVC will depend on tumor location and its extension. If partial resection of the caval wall has been performed, it can be repaired with either primary or patch closure. Primary repair can be performed if <50% narrowing of the IVC lumen will result. Otherwise, patch repair is recommended. In the absence of potential intraoperative contamination, a bovine pericardium patch or polytetrafluoroethylene (PTFE) patch can be used. For circumferential replacement, ringed reinforced PTFE graft is our choice. The graft size chosen is usually smaller than the IVC (typically 16 mm). The rings will help prevent compression by adjacent structures and graft collapse during inspiration. If there is potential contamination, autogenous material is preferred. Autologous graft for circumferential replacement includes a paneled vein graft or superficial femoral vein. Alternatively, a cryopreserved vein graft can be used. The renal veins are reimplanted directly onto to the graft or a short interposition graft as feasible (FIGURE 76-4A). Prosthetic grafts need to be isolated from the visceral organs, and wrapping them with a large bovine pericardial patch offers tissue coverage (FIGURE 76-4B).

Primary resection without caval reconstruction is performed if there has been chronic caval tumor thrombosis with minimal leg symptoms and adequate collaterals. Aggressive volume rescuscitation is very important for allowing patients to tolerate IVC clamping. During unclamping, the patient is placed in Trendelenburg, a Valsalva maneuver is induced, and the graft is filled with heparinized saline to avoid air embolism. Upon completion, a Doppler or duplex ultrasound study is performed to verify an unobstructed blood flow. Compression stockings are used throughout the procedure and postoperatively until the patient is ambulatory.

CLOSURE Meticulous hemostasis must be obtained to prevent retropertoneal hematoma. If heparinization has been used, protamine sulfate may be given to reverse anticoagulation. When prosthetic reconstructions are performed, the graft is covered with surrounding tissue or an omental flap, or both, to avoid contact with adjacent organs. If not available, then a large bovine patch is placed to cover the prosthetic. Routine fascial closure is performed with subsequent skin closure.

POSTOPERATIVE CARE Compression stockings are used postoperatively until the patient is ambulatory. We advocate for the use of routine systemic anticoagulation for 3 months after IVC reconstruction to prevent VTE and graft thrombosis events. Some authors recommend patients having IVC reconstruction receiving only antiplatelet therapy with aspirin. Bleeding into the wound may occur from excessive anticoagulation, improper hemostasis, seeping from the suture line, or postoperative hypertension. The patient should remain under physiologic monitoring for the postoperative period. Postoperative hypotension must be avoided by adequate blood and fluid replacement. Early postoperative screening for DVT should be considered, especially in cases with large tumor burden or when graft reconstruction is performed. ■

SUGGESTED READINGS

Bower TC. Primary and secondary tumors of the inferior vena cava. In: Gloviczki P, Yao JST, eds. *Handbook of Venous Disorders*. London: Hodder Arnold; 2009:529-550.

Gaignard E, Bergeat D, Robin F, Corbière L, Rayar M, Meunier B. Inferior vena cava leiomyosarcoma: what method of reconstruction for which type of resection? *World J Surg*. 2020;44:3537–3544.

Hicks CW, Glebova NO, Piazza KM, Orion K, Pierorazio PM, Lum YW, Abularrage CJ, Black JH 3rd. Risk of venous thromboembolic events following inferior vena cava resection and reconstruction. *J Vasc Surg*. 2016 Apr;63(4):1004-1010.

Mingoli A, Cavallaro A, Sapienza P, Di Marzo L, Feldhaus RJ, Cavallari N. International registry of inferior vena cava leiomyosarcoma: analysis of a world series on 218 patients. *Anticancer Res*. 1996;16:3201-3205.

Serrano C, George S. Leiomyosarcoma. *Hematol Oncol Clin North Am*. 2013 Oct;27(5):957-974.

Wachtel H, Gupta M, Bartlett EK, Jackson BM, Kelz RR, Karakousis GC, Fraker DL, Roses RE. Outcomes after resection of leiomyosarcomas of the inferior vena cava: a pooled data analysis of 377 cases. *Surg Oncol*. 2015 Mar;24(1):21-27

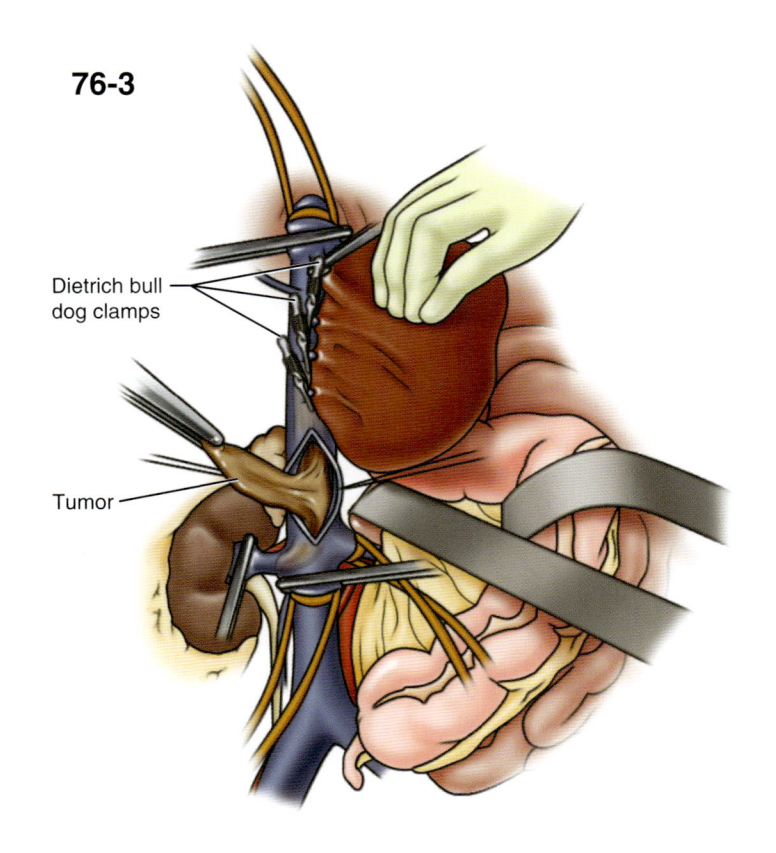

76-3

Dietrich bull dog clamps

Tumor

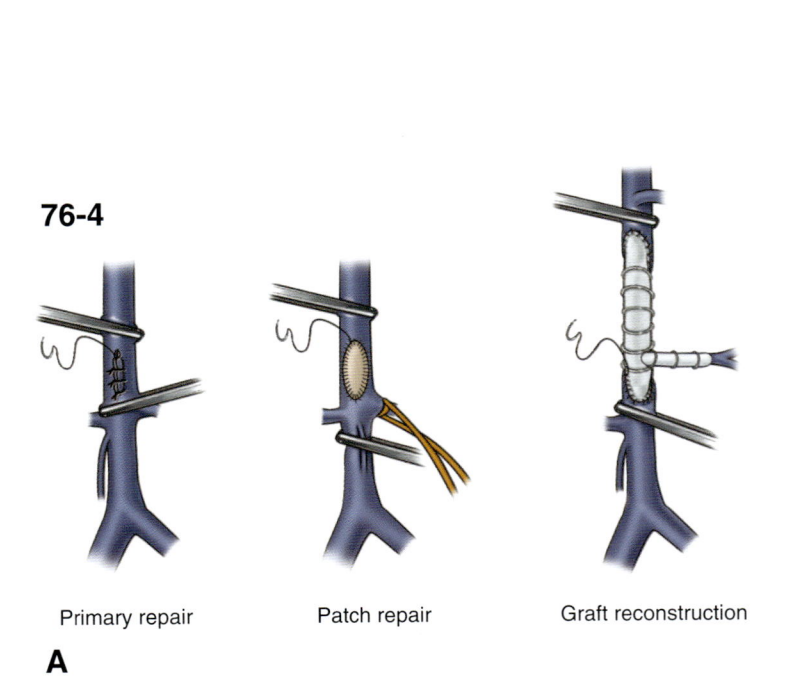

76-4

Primary repair

Patch repair

Graft reconstruction

A

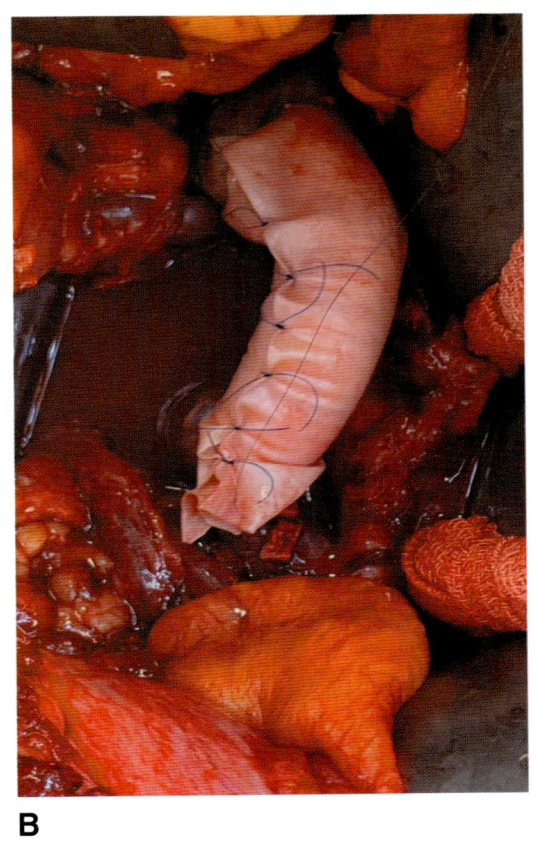

B

ANTERIOR SPINE EXPOSURE

Victor Davila, MD • **Samuel R. Money, MD**

INDICATIONS Orthopedic spine and neurosurgical teams are the primary drivers of offering an intervention for symptomatic spinal anatomy. From the perspective of the exposure team (vascular surgery) the primary evaluation for operative suitability relies on the likelihood of safely obtaining exposure to the spine. There are alternatives to anterior lumbar interbody fusion (ALIF), such as a posterior approach or a lateral approach, which can be performed solely by the spine team. Therefore, if the exposure team does not believe that the operation can be accomplished safely, an alternative should be considered.

POSITION The patient is placed in the supine position with the arms placed on arm boards to the side. A radiolucent operating table is needed because of fluoroscopy use to ensure the desired spinal level(s) are localized. Fluoroscopy is also used to aid in determination of the center of the vertebral body or disk space. The surgeon should position table-mounted bars at the level of the axilla on the left or right side of the patient to allow for self-retaining retractor affixation. A small roll or bump is placed at the level of the iliac crest to ensure normal slope and spine curvature. This also aids in minimizing steep angles for interbody prosthesis insertion during the spinal portion of the procedure. The authors also routinely place a pulse oximeter on the left hallux and check a baseline oxygen saturation and waveform after positioning. This serves as an early warning system if the iliac artery is compressed or damaged during the operation. The abdomen from the xyphoid to the pubis and laterally to the mid axillary line is included in the sterile field.

OPERATIVE PREPARATION Patients undergo a multidisciplinary consultation with the neurosurgery/orthopedic spine team and the spine exposure team (vascular surgery). The neurosurgery/orthopedic spine team discusses the indication for and expected goals of the operation. Consultation with vascular surgery consists of a full evaluation of previous abdominal surgeries, arterial anatomy for occlusive disease, and venous anatomy for aberrant structures. Herein, a CT angiogram is very helpful. Special attention should be paid to prior hernia repairs with mesh located in the preperitoneal space. Laparoscopic inguinal hernia repairs generally obliterate the space used to access the retroperitoneum and provide exposure to the spine. Open inguinal hernia repairs do not generally make this exposure more difficult. Previous laparoscopic procedures are generally not contraindications to proceeding with the exposure of the anterior spine, as port sites do not cause dense and widespread scar tissue formation. Previous ostomy creation or reversal can make maintaining dissection in the retroperitoneal space difficult.

The physical examination continues with an evaluation of the lower extremities for signs of peripheral arterial disease and venous occlusion. Significant lower extremity swelling should be noted and causes of venous occlusion (DVT, tumor, etc.) should be investigated.

Risks include damage to abdominal structures (solid organ injury, ureteral injury, vascular injury, nerve injury), wound complications, seroma formation requiring drainage, and retrograde ejaculation. All males considering having children or additional children should consider sperm storage preoperatively. Cross-sectional imaging should be reviewed, which can indicate aortic or iliac aneurysms, degree of calcification, and large branches in the area of dissection. For patients with scoliosis, cross-sectional imaging can also help establish the relative positions of structures that may not reside in their normal anatomical locations.

Type and screen and adequate intravenous access for potentially aggressive resuscitation should be obtained prior to starting the operation.

INCISION AND EXPOSURE/DETAILS OF PROCEDURE An infraumbilical incision approximately 8 to 10 cm in length is made along the midline 2 cm below the umbilicus, but some prefer to make a left paramedian incision. If higher levels are in need of exposure, the incision can be extended in a curvilinear fashion to the left side of the umbilicus, or even a hockey stick transplant incision. The incision is carried down to the linea alba and the fascia is cleared of subcutaneous tissue 3 to 4 cm to the left of the linea alba in a manner similar to performing an open component separation for abdominal wall reconstruction. Two to three cm lateral and parallel to the linea alba, the fascia is incised over the left rectus muscle. The rectus is swept laterally and the preperitoneal space is entered. In the event that more medial exposure is needed, it is also helpful to expose the medial edge of the rectus abdominus (**FIGURE 77-1**). A large handheld retractor is used to retract the rectus muscle and abdominal sidewall laterally while the retroperitoneal plane is developed. A sweeping motion with the hand or a sponge stick aiming at the ipsilateral femoral head is useful to proceed with the dissection. The epigastric vessels are usually encountered at this point and can be sacrificed with bipolar electrocautery or suture ligation. Once the psoas muscle is identified, a self-retaining retractor is utilized to maintain the exposure. The author's preference is a Thompson retractor with four swivel renal vein retractors and two non-swivel retractors (**FIGURE 77-2**). If more cephalad exposure is needed, the lateral attachments of the semilunar line can be freed with blunt dissection or electrocautery and retracted toward the head. After the psoas muscle is identified, the iliac artery and vein are usually well visualized or can be palpated. The ureter must be identified next and swept medially and placed under the renal vein retractors, and the common and external iliac arteries are dissected free (**FIGURE 77-3**). The dissection is then carried over to the medial aspect of the left iliac vein. A key gateway to this procedure for both L4-L5 and L5-S1 procedures is early identification and division of the ascending iliolumbar vein. Tearing this vein ends in significant hemorrhage with difficult to control bleeding, as the vein will retract into the spinal canal. The ascending iliolumbar vein can drain into either the common iliac vein or external iliac vein, and there can be multiple veins. They should be ligated and clipped on the vein and either ligated or double clipped distally, followed by transection with an 11 blade. **CONTINUES ▶**

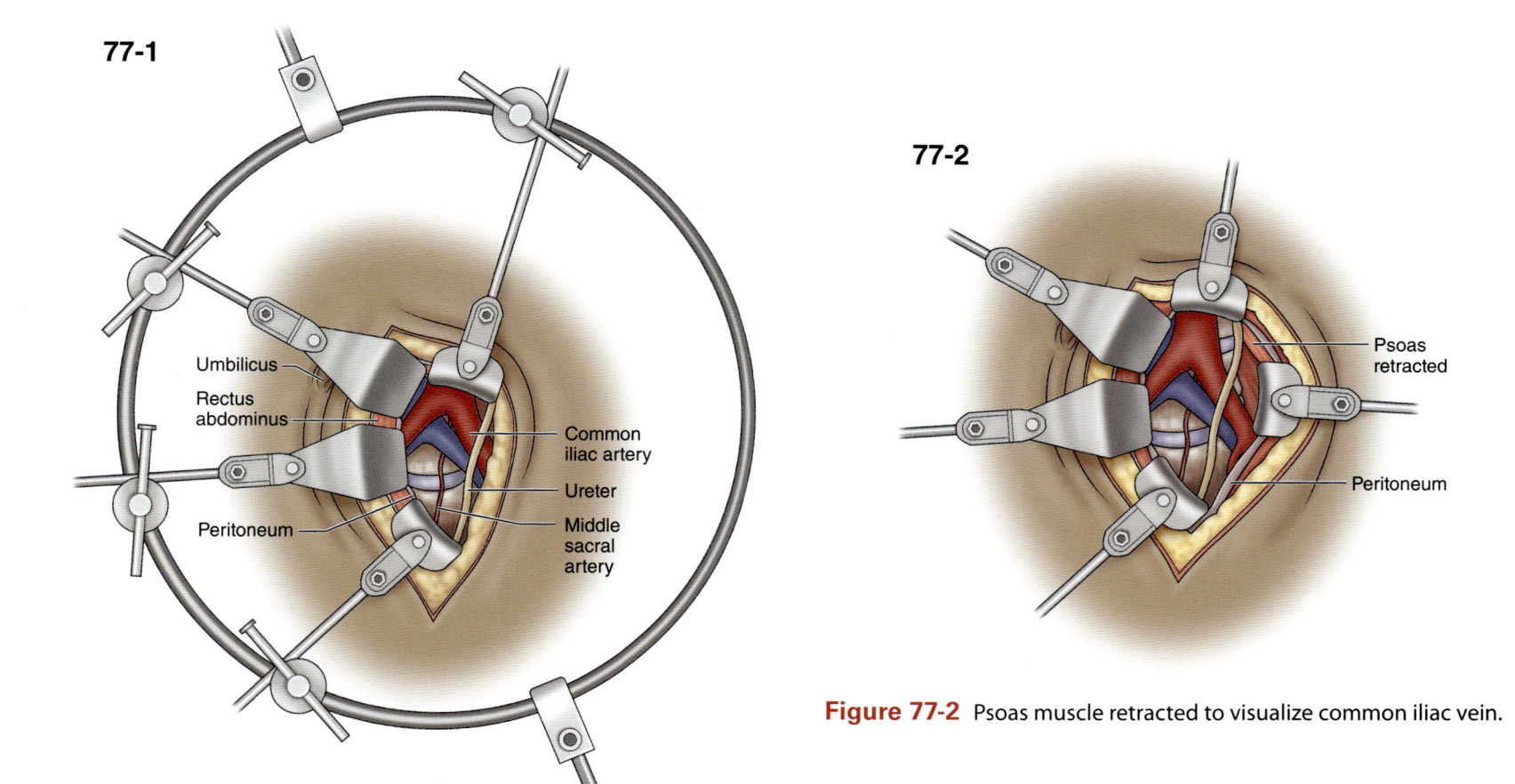

Figure 77-1 Retracted retroperitoneal and psoas muscle.

Figure 77-2 Psoas muscle retracted to visualize common iliac vein.

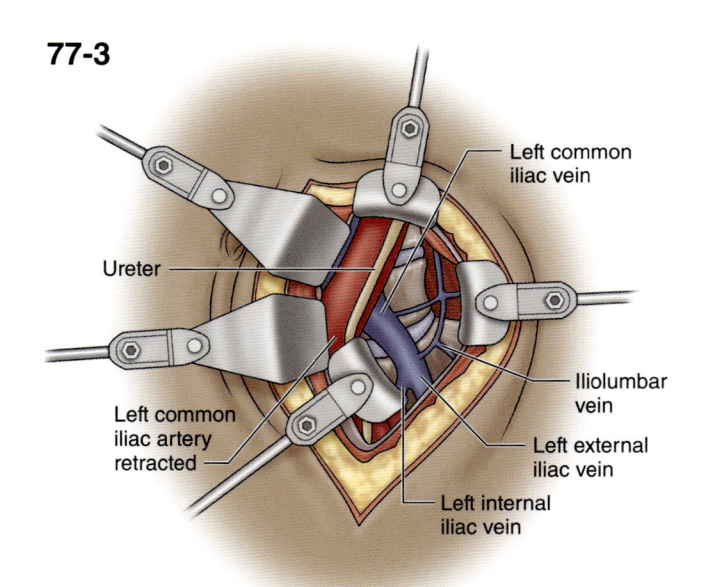

Figure 77-3 Ureter retracted and left common iliac artery mobilized and retracted, with exposure of common iliac vein and iliolumbar vein.

INCISION AND EXPOSURE/DETAILS OF PROCEDURE CONTINUED For exposure of the L4-S1 disk space, depending on the course of the overlying iliac artery and vein, more often the left common and external iliac arteries and left external iliac vein are retracted medially and to the right side to facilitate exposure (**FIGURE 77-4A**). When placing the retractors, one should avoid aggressive or extreme force, which could end up causing a vascular injury. Occasionally, the common iliac arteries can be splayed apart with lateral retraction providing access (see below). More cephalad, the aorta can be mobilized to the right of the spinal column as necessary. The middle sacral artery and vein are ligated or coagulated with a bipolar electrocautery and transected, and the ends mobilized cephalad and caudad to expose the L4-L5 disk space.

For L5-S1 exposure, it is easiest for the spine surgeon to access this area between the aortic bifurcation (**FIGURE 77-4B**). The left external and common iliac artery are mobilized and now retracted laterally. Attention must be paid to the pulse oximeter on the left hallux when significant retraction of the artery occurs. Any dampening of the arterial waveform or decrease in the pulse oximetry should prompt relaxation and repositioning of the retractors.

The renal vein retractors can be slotted on either side of the vertebral body to allow for full visualization of the disk space. As the retractors are placed, the drop-off between L5 and S1 is easily palpated. The middle sacral artery and vein are ligated or coagulated with a bipolar electrocautery and transected, and the ends mobilized cephalad and caudad to expose the L5-S1 disk space.

Avoid excessive retraction at the superior portion of the incision as it risks injury to the aortic bifurcation and left common iliac vein. Also, placing an inferior hand held renal vein retractor in the midline helps facilitate insertion of the prosthetic disc by the spine team. Discussion with the spine team regarding which anatomic level will be addressed first in multilevel cases should occur to provide appropriate exposure of the disk spaces in the correct order. The authors would like to note that the renal vein retractors themselves are excellent dissection tools and can bluntly dissect and maintain retraction in one motion. Appropriate x-rays are taken to confirm the disc space prior to turning the case over to the spine team.

Bleeding can occur at any time during the exposure and therefore the requisite vascular surgical clamps, sutures, and hemostatic control devices should be ready in the event they are needed. Appropriate suture (5-0 Prolene) for vascular repair or ligation (3-0 silk) is usually sufficient. A laparoscopic knot pusher is very useful for tying down in this sometimes-confined space and should be readily available, in addition to long-armed bipolar coagulation forceps.

CLOSURE After the interbody prosthesis has been inserted, the surgical bed is inspected for hemostasis (**FIGURE 77-5**). Vigorous irrigation of the wound bed should be avoided if bone morphogenetic protein was used in the interbody, as this can lead to its dispersal in the surgical bed instead of remaining at the level of the fusion. Hemostasis should be achieved and can be aided by hemostatic products on top of the fusion at each level. Long-acting local anesthesia can be administered to the surgical bed with attention paid to the transverse abdominis plane (TAP) to anesthetize the nerves supplying the anterior abdominal wall. The retractor system blades are removed from the field and the peritoneum is allowed to return to its normal resting position. If more than one vertebral level was exposed or there was extensive retroperitoneal dissection achieving exposure of one level, some consider a drain important, which can be placed through the left lower quadrant of the abdomen with the drain in the lateral retroperitoneal space. Fluid collections rarely encompass or are in close association with the vertebral body and are usually in the lateral or anterolateral portions of the dissection plane. The fascia is approximated with permanent suture. The subcutaneous tissue and skin are reapproximated.

POSTOPERATIVE CARE Patients are monitored for return of bowel function, and diet is advanced per surgeon judgement. With a single-level exposure, most patients can tolerate a diet on post operative day 1. Patients undergoing multiple level exposures, prolonged operating time, and extensive dissection (secondary to challenging anatomy or previous surgery) may be better served with introduction of regular diet after objective evidence of return of bowel function (bowel sounds or passing of flatus). The lower extremities should be evaluated for signs and symptoms of deep vein thrombosis. Occasionally, patients will report a sense of left lower quadrant fullness. If symptomatic, cross-sectional imaging can identify fluid collections, which can be addressed with percutaneous drain placement. Aspiration alone usually results in fluid reaccumulating and need for repeat percutaneous intervention. Fluid drained percutaneously should be evaluated to ensure that it is not related to a structural injury such as the ureter (fluid creatinine) or a cerebrospinal fluid leak (beta-2 transferrin). ■

SUGGESTED READINGS

Gumbs AA, Shah RV, Yue JJ, Sumpio B. The open anterior paramedian retroperitoneal approach for spine procedures. *Arch Surg*. 2005 Apr; 140(4):339-343.

Manunga J, Alcala C, Smith J, et al. Technical approach, outcomes, and exposure-related complications in patients undergoing anterior lumbar interbody fusion. *J Vasc Surg* 2021;73:992-998.

77-4

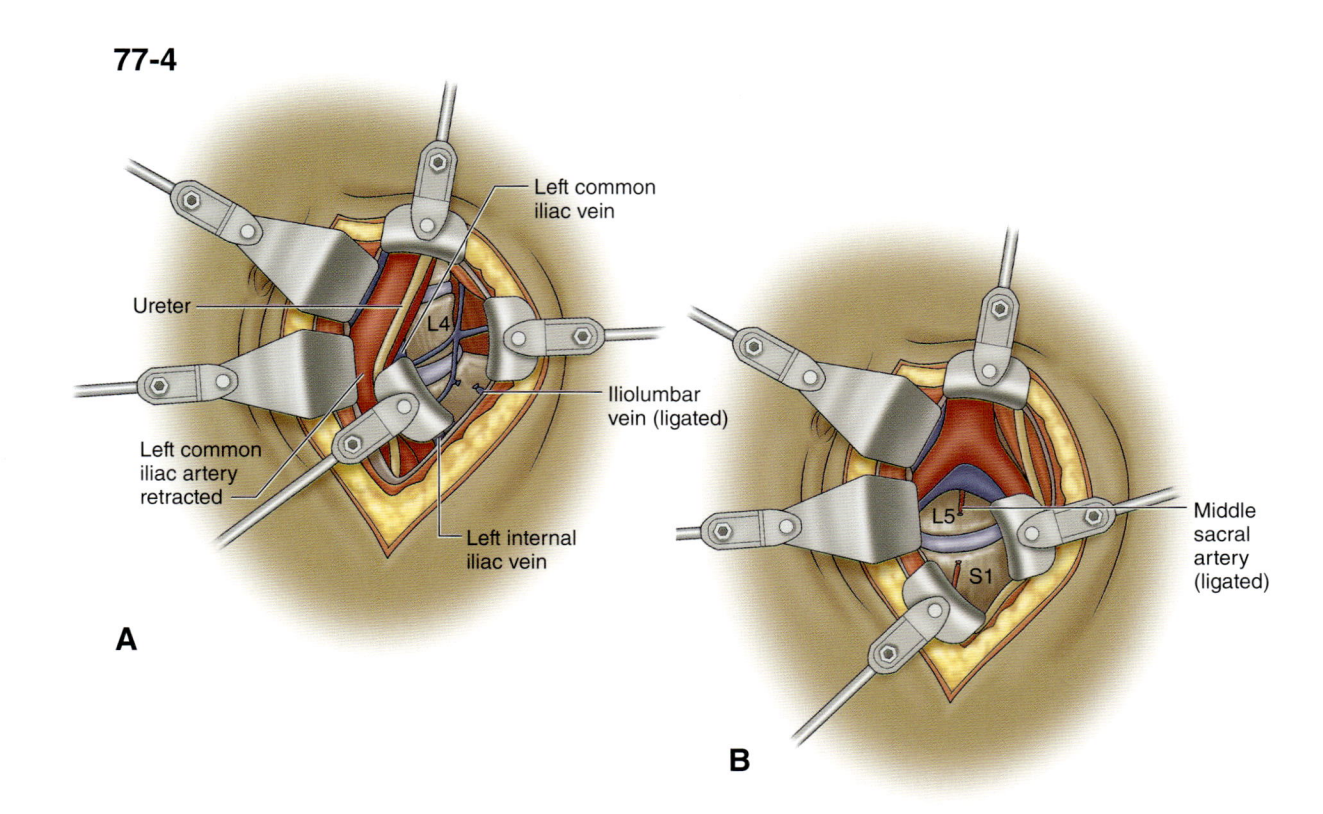

Left common iliac vein

Ureter

L4

Iliolumbar vein (ligated)

Left common iliac artery retracted

Left internal iliac vein

A

L5

S1

Middle sacral artery (ligated)

B

Figure 77-4 A. L4-L5 exposed laterally, common iliac vein retracted medially with iliolumbar vein ligated. B. L5-S1 exposed medially with middle sacral artery coagulated or ligated.

77-5

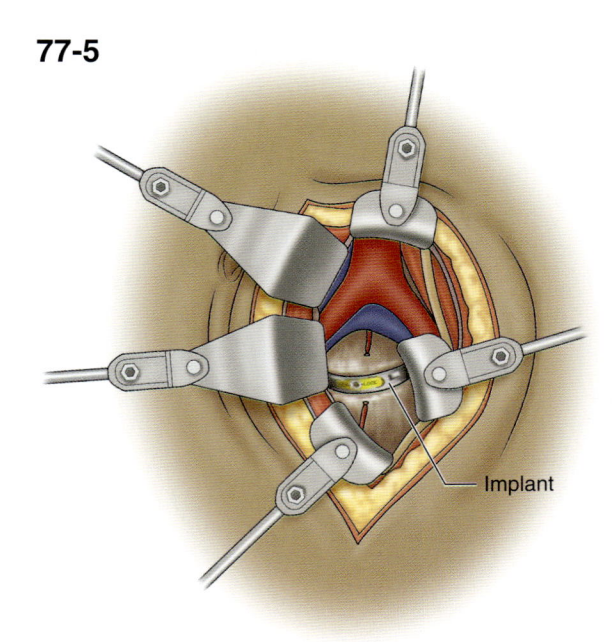

Implant

Figure 77-5 Disc implanted.

INDEX